Textbook of Operative Dentistry

FOURTH EDITION

Other CBS Books by the Same Author

✦ **Pre-Clinical Conservative Dentistry**, second edition
✦ **Fundamentals of Dental Radiology**, fourth edition
✦ **Community Dentistry**

Textbook of Operative Dentistry

FOURTH EDITION

Vimal K Sikri
MDS, DOOP (PU), DEME (AIU), FICD

Professor and Head
Department of Conservative Dentistry and Endodontics

and

Principal
Punjab Government Dental College and Hospital
Amritsar, Punjab
India

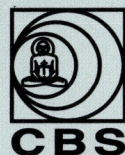

CBS Publishers & Distributors Pvt Ltd

New Delhi • Bengaluru • Chennai • Kochi • Kolkata • Mumbai • Pune
Hyderabad • Nagpur • Patna • Vijayawada

Disclaimer

Science and technology are constantly changing fields. New research and experience broaden the scope of information and knowledge. The author has tried his best in giving information available to him while preparing the material for this book. Although, all efforts have been made to ensure optimum accuracy of the material, yet it is quite possible some errors might have been left uncorrected. The publisher, the printer and the author will not be held responsible for any inadvertent errors, omissions or inaccuracies.

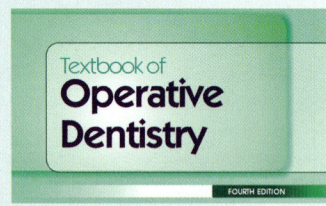

ISBN: 978-81-239-2887-6

Copyright © Author and Publisher

Fourth Edition: 2016
First Edition: 2002
  Reprint: 2003, 2004, 2005, 2006
Second Edition: 2008
  Reprint: 2009, 2010, 2012
Third Edition: 2014

All rights reserved. No part of this book may be reproduced or transmitted in any form or by any means, electronic or mechanical, including photocopying, recording, or any information storage and retrieval system without permission, in writing, from the author and the publisher.

Published by Satish Kumar Jain and produced by Varun Jain for
CBS Publishers & Distributors Pvt Ltd
4819/XI Prahlad Street, 24 Ansari Road, Daryaganj, New Delhi 110 002, India.
Ph: 23289259, 23266861, 23266867   Website: www.cbspd.com
Fax: 011-23243014   e-mail: delhi@cbspd.com; cbspubs@airtelmail.in
Corporate Office: 204 FIE, Industrial Area, Patparganj, Delhi 110 092
Ph: 4934 4934   Fax: 4934 4935   e-mail: publishing@cbspd.com; publicity@cbspd.com

Branches

- **Bengaluru:** Seema House 2975, 17th Cross, K.R. Road, Banasankari 2nd Stage, Bengaluru 560 070, Karnataka
  Ph: +91-80-26771678/79   Fax: +91-80-26771680   e-mail: bangalore@cbspd.com
- **Chennai:** 7, Subbaraya Street, Shenoy Nagar, Chennai 600 030, Tamil Nadu
  Ph: +91-44-26680620, 26681266   Fax: +91-44-42032115   e-mail: chennai@cbspd.com
- **Kochi:** Ashana House, No. 39/1904, AM Thomas Road, Valanjambalam, Ernakulam 682 018, Kochi, Kerala
  Ph: +91-484-4059061-62-64-65   Fax: +91-484-4059065   e-mail: kochi@cbspd.com
- **Kolkata:** 6/B, Ground Floor, Rameswar Shaw Road, Kolkata-700 014, West Bengal
  Ph: +91-33-22891126, 22891127, 22891128   e-mail: kolkata@cbspd.com
- **Mumbai:** 83-C, Dr E Moses Road, Worli, Mumbai-400018, Maharashtra
  Ph: +91-22-24902340/41   Fax: +91-22-24902342   e-mail: mumbai@cbspd.com
- **Pune:** Bhuruk Prestige, Sr. No. 52/12/2+1+3/2 Narhe, Haveli (Near Katraj-Dehu Road Bypass), Pune 411 041, Maharashtra
  Ph: +91-20-64704058, 64704059, 32392277   Fax: +91-20-24300160   e-mail: pune@cbspd.com

Representatives

- **Hyderabad** 0-9885175004   • **Nagpur** 0-9021734563
- **Patna**   0-9334159340   • **Vijayawada** 0-9000660880

Printed at: HT Media Ltd., Noida

to
My Father
(1927–1996)

*Who taught me the first lesson of life
and gave me the light of learning*

Preface to the Fourth Edition

Once a student asked, Sir, how to learn more? I answered, please stay with the question for a longer period. What I wanted to emphasize was to keep impinging the plethora of questions around you; slowly and slowly you will find answers and that is all about learning. Another way of learning is to 'teach' and by teaching you will 'learn'. Learning is only the kindling of the flame. We do 'know' so much in life but rarely 'understand'. Learning, a timeless pleasure and a valuable treasure, is all about understanding.

I, being my self-critic, keep evaluating my books regularly. The flaws observed in the third edition have been corrected and the fourth edition in your hands is new and updated version of the subject of *Operative Dentistry*. The language is kept lucid along with self-explanatory photographs and diagrams. Almost all chapters are updated; adding new text, simplifying the language and modifying the diagrams. I hope the present edition is in 'must-read' category for the students pursuing *Operative Dentistry* as a career.

I am grateful to my colleagues Dr Renu Sroa, Professor, and Dr Baljit Sidhu, Assistant Professor, for their constant help and motivation. I am also thankful to my ex-students, Dr Priyanka Setia and Dr Ibadat Preet and my students, Dr Meghna Mittal, Dr Shaveta Seth, Dr Tejinderpal Singh, Dr Komalgeet Kaur, Dr Jasbir Kaur and Dr Neha Mengi for checking and rechecking the manuscript.

I acknowledge the understanding and patience of my gracious wife, Dr Poonam; my sons, Dr Ankit, Dr Arpit, and my sweet bitiya, Dr Annupriya.

I request all the students and teachers to go through the present edition and suggest areas of improvement.

Vimal K Sikri

Preface to the First Edition

Controversies, undoubtedly, are the positive signs of scientific progress. Until and unless there is difference of opinion in any treatment modality, further research will not be possible. All those clinicians who openly admit controversies help the scientific world to grow and flourish.

The book in your hands is the outcome of inherent controversies in operative dentistry as seen and observed by me during my teaching assignments in the Government Dental College, Amritsar, for more than two decades. With more than a dozen books already available on operative dentistry, what is the need for writing another book, I asked myself? Dentistry like other sciences is dynamic and requires an original approach from a writer for a major thrust in research. He who stirs the minds of others and inclines them more and more to experimentation contributes his real worth to this noble profession. I admit in all humility that I have tried a bit in this direction. On account of gradual evolution in every field of operative dentistry coupled with tremendous research in the dental materials, Operative Dentistry is being presented in a new light. Outdated subjects have been ignored and a couple of subjects which are the need of the day have been included.

Operative dentistry is the mother of all branches of dentistry. Many specialties of dentistry have sprung from it. Notwithstanding, operative dentistry has acquired new dimensions and a new significance with the evolution of ceramics and composites. The chapters on "Composites" and "Ceramics" are given a new look in this book. Various clinical cases and laboratory techniques have been quoted to substantiate the point. The chapter on "Color and its Application" is added since it is the need of today's aesthetic world.

Keeping in view the depth and importance of the subjects, the topics on "Bonding", "Finishing and Polishing", "Microleakage" and "Cervical Lesions" are presented as separate chapters. The basics in the subject have not been compromised. They are given an elaborate treatment in this book.

In order to make this book as comprehensive as possible, several eminent academicians were invited to support and write a few pages from their experience. Dr Beena Rani Goel of Bagalkot is among a few clinicians who undertakes "Direct Filling Gold" restorations. Her experience and expertise have been included. Dr S Balagopal of Chennai, a dynamic teacher, has also contributed his clinical cases on "Glass Ionomer Cements". Dr Subba Rao of Chennai (Matrices), Dr Nageshwar Rao of Dhanwad (Cast Restorations) have contributed a lot to this book. The contribution of two ladies, Dr Poonam Sikri and Dr Sarang Sharma is unique. Their contribution is inbuilt in the text and their inspiration, writing and editing have been instrumental in a big way for the publication of this book.

I have reasons to believe that this book will serve the much expected purpose of inspiring students, teachers, clinicians and others, interested in the vital study of "operative dentistry".

I shall be highly indebted to the reader, if he has any useful suggestions for improving the quality of the book in the next edition.

Vimal K Sikri

Contributors

1. **Dr Beena Rani Goel**
   Ex-Professor and Head
   PMNM Dental College and Hospital
   Bagalkot 587101
   Ph.: 0831-470140

2. **Dr R Nageshwar Rao**
   Ex-Chairman
   SDM College of Dental Sciences and Hospital
   Sattur, Dharwad 580009
   Ph.: 0836-468231

3. **Dr CV Subba Rao**
   Ex-Professor and Head
   TN Govt. Dental College
   Chennai
   Ph.: 044-8261827

4. **Dr D Majumdar**
   Ex-Principal
   Dr R. Ahmed Dental College, Kolkata
   Ph.: 09331035537

5. **Dr S Balagopal**
   Vice Principal
   Tagore Dental College
   Rathinamangalam
   Chennai 600048
   Ph.: 09444039411

6. **Dr Poonam Sikri**
   Principal
   Desh Bhagat Dental College
   Muktsar, Punjab
   Ph.: 09876070555

7. **Dr Sarang Sharma**
   Associate Professor
   ESIC Hospital, Rohini, New Delhi
   Ph.: 09811966639

8. **Dr Poonam Bogra**
   Professor and Head
   DAV Dental College
   Yamunanagar, Haryana
   Ph.: 0416023112

9. **Dr Subha Anirudhan**
   Reader
   Sri Ramakrishna Dental College and Hospital
   SNR College Road, Nava India
   Coimbatore, Tamil Nadu 641006
   Ph.: 9786078340

10. **Dr Renu B Sroa**
    Professor
    Govt Dental College and Hospital
    Amritsar 143001, Punjab
    Ph.: 0972893115

11. **Dr Rajat Dang**
    Reader
    MM Institute of Dental Sciences
    Mullana, Ambala, Haryana
    Ph.: 09996487253

12. **Dr Garima Malhotra**
    Sr. Lecturer, ITS Dental College
    Greater Noida, UP
    Ph.: 09211177907

13. **Dr Roopa Nadig**
    Director, PG Studies
    Dayananda Sagar College of Dental Sciences
    Shavige Malleshwara Hills, Kumaraswamy Layout
    Bangalore 560078
    Ph.: 09845011424

14. **Dr CL Satish Babu**
    Professor and Head
    V. S. Dental College, K.R.Road
    Bangalore 560004
    Ph.: 09448458424

15. **Dr Jagat Bhushan**
    Professor and Head
    HS Judge Dental College, PU Campus
    Chandigarh
    Ph.: 09855442735

16. **Dr Ibadatpreet Kaur**
    Postdoctoral research scholar
    Baba Farid University of Health Sciences
    Faridkot, Punjab
    Ph.: 09501114426

17. **Dr HL Usha**
    Principal
    VS Dental College, KR Road
    Bangalore
    Ph.: 09880518186

18. **Dr KK Wadhwani**
    Dean
    KG Medical University
    Lucknow
    Ph.: 09415001259

Contents

Preface to the Fourth Edition vii
Preface to the First Edition ix
Contributors xi

1. Introduction to Operative Dentistry 1–6

Evolution of operative dentistry 1
Beginning of dental science 2
Dentistry in 20th century 4
Future of operative dentistry 4
Chronology of major events in
 operative dentistry 4

2. Nomenclature 7–22

Systems having similar notation in each
 segment 7
System having different notation in each
 segment 8
FDI system 9
Nomenclature related to various surface
 of tooth 10
Terminology related to caries 10
Affected and infected dentin 12
Nomenclature related to cavity preparation 13
Various walls in a cavity preparation 14
Various angles in a cavity preparation 17
Bevel 17
Angles in occlusal cavity (class I) 17
Angles in proximoocclusal cavity in
 posterior teeth (class II) 18
Angles in proximal cavity (class III) 18
Angles in proximoincisal cavity in anterior
 teeth (class IV) 18
Angles in buccal and lingual cavity (class V) 18
Angles in mesioocclusodistal cavity 19
Classification of different cavities 19
Dr GV Black classification 19
Modification of Black classification 19
Dr GJ Mount classification 21
Dr Vimal Sikri classification 22

3. Occlusion 23–51

Ideal vs normal occlusion 24
Functional occlusion 24
Nonfunctional occlusion 25
Physiologic and nonphysiologic occlusion 25
Centric relation 25
Centric occlusion and MIP 26
Potential contact areas of posterior surface 27
Relationship between centric occlusion and
 centric relation 27
Guidance of occlusion 28
Occlusal designs and schemes 30
Occlusion and restorative dentistry 31
Articular analysis 32
Types of articulators 33
Facebow records 34
Articulation of casts 35
Interocclusal records 35
Occlusal records for restoring a single
 posterior tooth 36
Occlusal records for restoring all posterior
 teeth in a single arch 36
Reasons for restoring the normal anatomical
 form of an individual tooth 37
Considerations in restoring individual teeth 37
Occlusal adjustments prior to restoration 38
Procedure for occlusal examination 39
Elimination of premature contacts 39
Protrusion and posterior contacts 41
T-scan system 41
Occlusal considerations during tooth
 preparation 41
Role of contact areas 44
Role of marginal ridge 45
Reasons for modifying occlusal table 44
Relationship between toothwear and
 restorative materials 45
Transferable records 46
Nontransferable records 48
Final checking of the casting for occlusion 48
Full mouth rehabilitation 50

4. Periodontal Restorative Interface 52–62

Dentogingival unit 52
Preservation of periodontium 53
Contour 53
Height of epithelial attachment 54
Proximal contact areas 54
Methods of testing a contact area 55
Embrasures 55
Occlusal surface 55
Margins 57
Surface finish and texture 57
Trauma from occlusion 57
Etiology 57
Effects of occlusal disharmony 59

Diagnostic signs of traumatic occlusion	59
Aims of occlusal equilibration	61
Diagnosis of premature contacts	61
Occlusal adjustment by grinding	62

5. Dental Caries 63–79

Definitions	63
Classification of caries	63
Etiology of dental caries	65
Acidogenic theory	65
Proteolytic theory	66
Proteolysis chelation theory	66
Bioelectric phenomenon	67
Levine's theory	69
Bandlish theory	69
Systemic theory	70
Contributory factors in dental caries	71
The host factors	71
Microflora	72
Substrate or diet	73
Time	73
The histopathology and chemical events in caries process	73
Caries of enamel	74
Caries of dentin	75
Caries of cementum	75
Arrested caries	75
Secondary caries	76
Epidemiology	77
Microbiology	77
Histopathology	78
Differentiating secondary caries with residual caries	79

6. Diagnosis and Treatment Planning 80–107

Definition	80
History of patient	80
Clinical examination	81
Caries risk assessment	84
Caries activity tests	86
Caries diagnosis	90
ICDAS	91
Nyvad's system	92
CART	93
Conventional radiography	94
Xeroradiography	95
Digital enhancement	96
Computer image analysis	96
Subtraction radiography	97
CBCT	97
Electronic caries monitor	99
Optical caries monitor	99
Fibre optic transillumination	99
Digital imaging fiberoptic transillumination	100
Ultraviolet illumination	100
Transillumination with near infrared light	100
Laser auto fluorescence	100
Quantitative laser fluorescence	100
DIAGNOdent caries detector	101
Infra-red fluorescence	102
Endoscope/videoscope	102
Dye penetration method	102
Carbon dioxide laser	103
Terahertz imaging	104
Multi-photon imaging	104
Optical coherence tomography	104
Infrared thermography	104
LED technology (Midwest caries ID)	105
ACIS (CarieScan)	105
Frequency domain infrared photothermal radiometry and modulated luminescence	105

7. Instruments, Instrumentation and Sterilization 108–151

Hand cutting instruments	108
Metal used in the manufacture of hand instruments	108
Design characteristics of hand cutting instruments	109
Instrument nomenclature	110
Instrument formula	110
Direct and lateral cutting instruments	110
Classification	111
Chisels	112
Excavators	112
Modified forms of chisels	112
Miscellaneous	114
Instrument grasp	114
Sharpening of hand instruments	115
Rotary cutting instruments	115
Dental handpieces	116
Speed ranges and uses	117
Common features of rotary instruments	117
Dental burs	118
Classification	118
Bur shapes	118
Bur sizes	119
Design of dental burs	120
Factors influencing the cutting effectiveness and efficiency of bur	121
Abrasive instruments	123
Factors influencing the abrasive efficiency and effectiveness	124
Disposable diamond abrasives	124
Different methods of cutting	125
Operating positions	127
Sterilization of instruments	129
Terminology	129
Categorization of dental instruments and other commonly used items	130
Presoaking and cleaning	130

Packaging	131
Methods of sterilization	132
Control of sterilization	142
Cleaning and disinfection of handpieces	142
Cleaning, disinfection and sterilization of burs	143
Infection control	143
Methods for infection control	145
Future developments	150

8. Matrices, Retainers and Wedges 152–162

Slow separation	153
Rapid or immediate separation	153
Matrices	154
Classification of matrices	154
Matrices for class II, MOD and complex restorations	154
Matrices for class III direct tooth-colored restorations	156
Matrices for class IV preparations for direct tooth-colored restorations	157
Matrices for class V preparations for direct tooth-colored restorations	158
Matrix retainers	158
Wedges	160

9. Isolation of the Operating Field 163–176

Isolation from moisture	163
Direct methods	163
Rubber dam	163
Cotton rolls and cotton holders	169
Gauze pieces	170
Absorbent pads	170
Evacuation systems	170
Gingival retraction cord	171
Indirect methods	173
Isolation from soft tissues	173
Retraction of cheeks, lips, and tongue	173
Retraction of gingiva	174
Physicomechanical means	174
Chemical means	174
Electrosurgical means	175
Surgical means	176

10. Principles of Cavity Preparation 177–195

Outline form	177
Modification of outline form	179
Enameloplasty	180
Cusp capping	180
Resistance and retention forms	181
Convenience form	185
Removal of remaining carious dentin	185
Pulp protection	186
Cavity varnish	186
Finishing the enamel walls and margins	186
Toilet of cavity	188
Forces exerted during occlusion/mastication and their resolution	190
Mechanical functions of marginal ridges	192
Application of stresses and their distribution in individual restorations	194

11. Interim Restorations 196–210

Rationale	196
Various interim restorative materials	196
Gutta-percha	197
Dental cements	197
Zinc oxide eugenol cements	197
Modified zinc oxide eugenol cement	198
Cavit	202
Zinc phosphate cement	203
Modified zinc phosphate cements	206
Zinc silicophosphate cements	206
Polycarboxylate cements	206
Calcium hydroxide	208
Prefabricated crowns	209
Indirect acrylic restorations	209

12. Silver Amalgam 211–243

Advantages	211
Disadvantages	211
Composition of alloy	211
Effect of constituent metals on the properties of amalgam	212
Manufacturing of alloy	213
Alloy mercury reaction	213
Cavity preparation	214
Class I	214
Class II	217
Class III	221
Class IV	223
Class V	223
Class VI	224
Conservative cavity preparation	224
Minimal intervention dentistry	226
Repair of defective restorations	226
Manipulation of silver amalgam	227
Failures of dental amalgam	230
Gallium alloys	234
Bonded amalgam restorations	235
Fluoridated amalgam	238
Amalgam restorations and oral environment	239
Mercury and its management	240

13. Cast Restorations 244–283

Definition	245
Indications	245

Contraindications	246
Advantages/disadvantages	247
Basic concepts of cavity design	247
Principles of cavity preparation	248
Types of margins in cast restoration	252
Bevels	253
Types and design features of facial and lingual flares	254
Variations in proximal marginal design	254
Cusp capping/onlay	255
Pin-retained cast restorations	256
Tucker's technique	256
Fabrication of cast restorations	258
Impression technique	258
Construction of the die and working model	261
Preparing the wax pattern	266
Removing the pattern	268
Investment of pattern	273
Casting machines	274
Casting techniques	277
Thermal expansion technique	277
Hygroscopic expansion technique	277
Casting defects	280

14. Complex Restorations 284–313

Classification of coronal tooth destruction	284
Extra retentive devices	285
Indications	286
Advantages/disadvantages	287
Classification of pins	287
Direct pins	287
Cemented pins	287
Friction locked pins	289
Threaded pins	289
Pins materials	292
Principles of pin placement	292
Pinhole preparation	295
Pin bending and pin trimming	296
Pin removal	296
Class II pin retained restorations	297
Class III and Class IV pin retained restorations	297
Class V pin retained amalgam	299
Pin amalgam foundation	299
Pins, stresses and tooth	300
Pins, stresses and restorative material	301
Factors affecting retention of pins in tooth structure	302
Factors affecting retention of pins in restorative material	303
Complications during pin placement procedure	304
Failures of pin retained restorations	307
Effect of pins on pulp	307
Pin retained cast restorations	308
Restoration of a single tooth with cast restoration utilizing pins	309

15. Direct Filling Gold 314–334

Properties of pure gold	314
Types of direct filling gold	315
Annealing/degassing	317
Condensation/compaction of direct filling gold	319
Biological properties of pure gold	322
Indications	323
Contraindications	323
Cavity preparation and restoration	324
Class I cavity	324
Class V cavity	326
Class III cavity	329
Class II cavity	332
Summarizing the advantages and disadvantages of DFG restorations	333

16. Bonding in Dentistry 335–362

Definitions	335
Types	335
Factors affecting adhesion	336
Tooth as a substrate for bonding	337
Conditioning enamel and etching	337
Bonding to dentin	340
Priming	342
Dentin bonding agents	343
Mechanism of dentin bonding	343
Evolution of dentin bonding agents	345
Role of water in the bonding process	351
Bonding in other clinical situations	356
Additives for dentin-enamel adhesion	357
Success/failures of adhesive	358
Water treeing phenomenon	359
Nanoleakage and water treeing	360
Functional implications of water treeing	360

17. Composites 363–403

Composition	363
Evolution of composites	365
Properties of composites	365
Advances in composites	365
Curing of composites	370
Configuration factor	373
Cavity preparation for composites	374
General consideration for composites restorations	374
Placement of composites	379
Establishing proximal contacts	387
Failures in composite restorations	388
Composite laminates and veneers	390
Illusion	391

Composite inlays	393
Classification of composite inlays	393
Cavity preparation	394
Repairing composite restorations and porcelains fused to metal restorations with composite resins	398

18. Glass-Ionomer Cement 404–422

Composition	404
Dispensing	405
Classification	405
Setting reaction	406
Physical and mechanical properties	407
Modified glass ionomer cements	409
Metal modified glass-ionomer cement	409
Resin modified glass-ionomer cement	410
Compomers	410
Giomers	411
Antibacterial GIC	412
Fluoride recharge material	412
Clinical placement of glass-ionomer	413
Clinical applications	417
Reaction of pulp to glass-ionomer cement	422

19. Minimal Invasive Dentistry 423–432

Early diagnosis of caries	423
Assessment of individual caries risk	424
Radiographic assessment of caries depth and progress	424
Decreasing risk of further demineralization and arresting existing lesions	424
Remineralization of existing lesions	425
Restoring cavitated lesions using minimal tooth preparation	426
Atraumatic restorative treatment (ART)	426
Repair rather than replacement of defective restorations	430

20. Dental Ceramics 433–475

Terminology	433
Classification	434
Composition	434
Coloring and opacifying dental porcelain	437
Additives in dental porcelain	438
Properties of porcelain	438
Strengthening dental porcelain	439
Condensation of dental porcelain	440
Firing procedure	441
All ceramic systems	442
Aluminous porcelain (Hi Ceram)	443
Leucite reinforced porcelain (Optec HSP)	445
Duceram LFC	445
Injection moulded glass ceramic/leucite reinforced hot pressed glass ceramic (Optec OPC)	446
Infiltrable ceramic/high alumina ceramic (In ceram)	446
Castable glass ceramic (DICOR)	447
Castable apatite ceramic (Cera Pearl)	449
Machinable ceramic	449
Polycrystalline ceramics	450
Porcelain inlays	451
Cavity preparation	451
Fabrication of porcelain inlays	454
Inlays fired on a platinum foil	454
Porcelain inlays fired on refractory dies	459
Inlays made by lost wax technique	460
Castable glass ceramic (DICOR)	460
Castable apatite ceramic (Cera Pearl)	462
Pressed glass ceramic (IPS Empress)	463
Machined ceramic inlays	463
Copy milling technique	463
CAD-CAM generated porcelain inlays	464
Porcelain laminates/veneers	466
CAD-CAM/CAD-CIM	471

21. Finishing and Polishing 476–494

Microabrasion and macroabrasion	477
Burnishing	477
Objectives of finishing and polishing	478
Health hazards during finishing and polishing	479
Finishing and polishing instruments	479
Abrasive materials	481
Finishing and polishing of amalgam restorations	481
Finishing and polishing of composite restorations	483
Finishing and polishing of glass-ionomer restorations	488
Finishing and polishing of direct gold restorations	489
Finishing and polishing of cast gold restorations	489
Finishing of non-precious alloy restorations	491
Finishing and polishing of porcelain restorations	492

22. Microleakage 495–513

Clinical implications of microleakage	495
Restorative materials and microleakage	496
Role of smear layer in microleakage	497
Factors controlling the bacterial penetration at tooth restoration gaps	498
Microleakage around amalgam restorations	498

Microleakage around glass-ionomer restorations	500
Microleakage around composite restorations	500
Microleakage around direct gold restorations	505
Microleakage around cast restorations	505
Microleakage around porcelain restorations	506
Methods to detect microleakage	507
Nanoleakage	511

23. Pulpal Reactions 514–529

Pulp-dentin organ	515
Physiology of pulp-dentin organ	515
Composition of dentin and pulp	515
Factors influencing pulpal response to dental restorative material	516
Intensity of pulpal response	517
Stages of pulpal inflammation	518
Test for evaluation of biocompatibility	520
Restorative materials and pulpal reactions	521
Pulpal reaction to tooth preparation	524
Pulpal reaction to caries	525
Pulpal reaction to trauma	527
Pulpal reaction to vital bleaching	528

24. Tooth Substance Loss 530–555

Attrition	530
Cervical lesions	532
Carious cervical lesions	532
Non-carious cervical lesions	532
Abrasion	533
Erosion	534
Abfraction	541
Biomechanics of class V cavity	544
Measurement of tooth substance loss	544
Treatment of tooth substance loss	545
Treatment of carious cervical lesion	545
Treatment of non-carious cervical lesion	546
Treatment of attrition	552

25. Geriatric Restorations 556–569

Medical history	556
Psychological considerations	557
Age changes in dental tissues	557
General effects of aging	557
Mechanism of aging	557
Age changes in enamel	558
Age changes in dentin	558
Age changes in pulp	559
Age changes in cementum	560
Age changes in bone	561
Age changes in periodontium	561
Clinical implications	561
Aging and cumulative effects of diseases	563
Treatment planning for elderly	564
Restorative management of common oral diseases in elderly	565
Considerations for prescribing medicines to the elderly	568

26. Dentin Hypersensitivity 570–579

Definition	570
Incidence and prevalence	570
Etiology and predisposing factors	570
Exposure of dentin as a result of loss of cementum	571
Exposure of dentin as a result of loss of enamel	572
Factors affecting measurement of hypersensitivity	572
Methods used to measure tooth hypersensitivity	572
Diagnosis	573
Management of hypersensitivity	573
Treatment modalities for dentinal hypersensitivity	574
Prevention	577
Newer techniques	577

27. Management of Deep Carious Lesions 580–589

Response of pulpo-dentinal complex in different stages of lesion progression	580
Arrested caries	580
Histopathology of dentinal caries	581
Effective depth (RD) and pulpal response	582
Prognosis of deep carious lesions	582
Repairability of pulpo-dentinal complex	582
Caries indicator dyes	583
Treatment modalities of deep carious lesions	583

28. Esthetic Dentistry 590–601

Esthetic principles	590
Analysis of esthetic smile	593
Examining the dentofacial composition	595
Treatment planning in esthetic dentistry	596
Cosmetic contouring	596
Diastema closure	597
Diastema closure with direct bonding composite application	597
Guidelines for anterior adhesive anterior restoration	598
Layering techniques	598

Contents

Direct composite pre-fabricated veneers
  (Componeers)   599
Lumineers   599
Lasers in esthetic dentistry   599
Ethics and esthetic dentistry   600

29. Color and its Application   602–619

Source of light   602
Optical characteristics   602
Color   604
Structure and function of eye   605
Perception of color   605
Metamerism   606
Fluorescence   607
Opalescence   607
Basic color schemes   607
Color harmonies   607
Additive color theory   608
Subtractive color theory   608
Color systems   608
Dimensions of color   609
Optics of natural teeth   612
Dental shade guides   613
Shade-taking devices   614
Guidelines for clinical shade selection   615
Procedure for shade matching in porcelain
  restorations   616

30. Tooth Discoloration and Bleaching   620–637

Tooth discoloration and staining   620
Classification of tooth discoloration   620
Bleaching of teeth   621
Vital tooth bleaching   621
Bleaching agents for vital bleaching   622
In-office bleaching   622
Preparation of patient for bleaching   622
Dentist prescribed bleaching   624
Non-vital bleaching   627
Side effects of non-vital bleaching   629
Laser assisted tooth whitening   631
Over the counter products   632
Additional materials used during
  bleaching procedure   633
Safety issues in bleaching   634
Advancements in bleaching   636

31. Laser in Operative Dentistry   638–647

Principle of laser   638
Laser device   638
Laser delivery system   639
Laser emission modes   639
Mechanism of action   639
Laser-tissue interaction   639
Types of lasers   640
CO_2 laser   641
Nd:YAG laser   641
Argon laser   641
Er:YAG laser   641
Uses of lasers in conservative dentistry   642
Excimer laser   645
Laser hazards   646

Appendix   649
Index   651

Introduction to Operative Dentistry

Operative dentistry, the mother of all branches of dentistry, deals with restoration of teeth that are defective because of trauma, disease or any other abnormality to achieve functions and esthetics. Operative dentistry includes restorative dentistry, preventive dentistry and esthetic dentistry. The ultimate aim is to prevent the destruction of teeth followed by restoring the damaged tooth to its function.

DEFINITIONS

Operative dentistry is defined as the branch of dentistry which deals with the diagnosis, prognosis, treatment and prevention of defects of teeth, restoring them to their form, function and esthetics; thereby, maintaining the stomatognathic system.

Mosby's medical dictionary defines operative dentistry as 'the phase of dentistry concerned with restoration of teeth that are defective through disease, trauma or abnormal development to a state of normal function, health and esthetics, including preventive, diagnostic, biologic, mechanical and therapeutic techniques as well as material and instruments science on application.'

Mosby's dental dictionary defines operative dentistry as 'the branch of dentistry that deals with the esthetic and functional restoration of the hard tissues of individual teeth.'

EVOLUTION OF OPERATIVE DENTISTRY

Since literature was meager in ancient days, the genesis of dental practice could not be ascertained. Early efforts were made in dentistry by the Europeans and the Arabians and they were interested mainly in gold work prosthesis. Gold is considered to be one of the oldest materials used in dentistry.

As early as 2700 BC, Etruscans and Phoenicians were practicing gold crowns. The practice continued up to 500-700 BC. Hippocrates (460-370 BC), the father of medicine, was born in 460 BC in Cos (Greece). Many of his writings have references of teeth, their formation, eruption and other maladies. In his book 'On Affection' he observes; in case of toothache, if the tooth is decayed and loose, it must be extracted. If it is neither decayed nor loose, but still painful, it is necessary to dessicate it by cauterizing. Splinting of loose mandibular anterior teeth by gold wires has been shown in Fig. 1.1 (an ancient photograph). Restorative aspect was not practiced during that period. Celsus (25 BC–50 AD) was perhaps the first to recommend filling of large cavities with paper, lead and other substances somewhere around 1st century AD. Dental amalgam was first used by a Chinese, Su Kung, in 650 AD. The use of gold leaf to fill cavities was perhaps the most significant development of medieval and early modern period from standpoint of restorative dentistry. It is known with certainty that gold leaves were used extensively at the time of Columbus.

Oral hygiene measures were adopted by various religious sects. Both Hindus and Muslims made it mandatory to follow the oral hygiene measures meticulously.

Sushruta was perhaps the first dental anatomist in the world who had described the anatomy of jaw bones with great accuracy. He also described that the

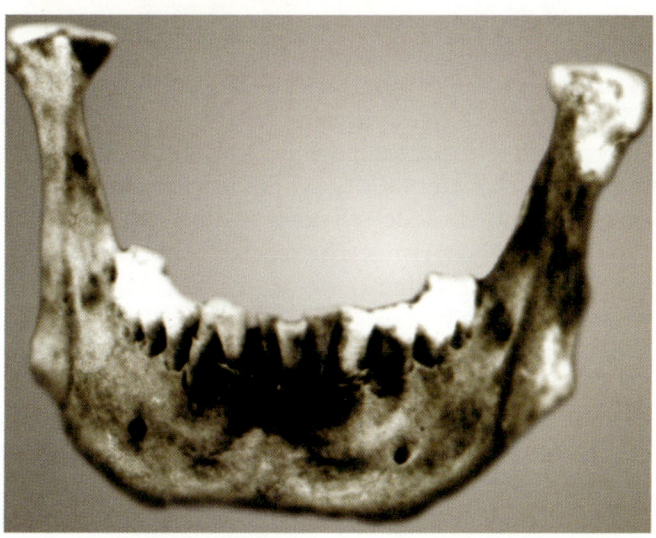

Fig. 1.1: Splinting of mandibular anterior teeth with gold wires

lower third molar could press the inferior dental nerve. The chief contribution to dentistry (from the beginning of Christian era to about 1500 AD) seems to be a shift from prosthesis to restoration of carious teeth. According to Arabian author Rhazes (841–926), carious teeth were filled with ground mastic, alum and honey during that period.

A description of removal of carious matter from teeth before filling with gold leaf was given by Giovanni da Vigo (1460–1525) in his article 'Practica Copiosa in arte chirugica' (1514).

Andreas Vesalius (1514–1564) in his book on anatomy 'De humani Corporis fabrica' published in 1543, categorically said that teeth were not bones. However his opinion that teeth grow throughout life was later discarded.

Ambroise Pare (1517-1590) is credited with having prepared artificial tooth from bone and ivory. Later Jacques Guillemeau (1550–1613) who was a pupil of Pare, prepared a paste by fusing together certain waxes, gums, ground mastic, powdered pearl and white coralle. He used this paste as a filling material.

Beginning of Dental Science (1600–1840)

It was during this period that the foundation for considering dentistry as a science was laid down. Prior to that, dentistry was merely an art practiced by barbers, surgeons or artisans.

In the beginning of 17th century wax models used in connection with prosthetic work were first mentioned by Mathaeus Gottfried Purmann. Charles Allen (1687) gave first written material on dentistry 'Operator for the Teeth'. By the beginning of 19th century, dentistry was no longer in hands of barbers/artisans but was practiced by professionally minded dentists/surgeons.

Pierre Fauchard (1678–1761), popularly known as father of dentistry (Fig. 1.2), described the materials and practices of his time in his book 'Traite des dents' (Treatise on the Tooth). He was among few scholars who described the causes of tooth decay and their prevention. He suggested humoral imbalance as the main cause for dental decay. Earlier the explanation of caries and toothache was attributed to the tooth worm. At that time, the restorative materials mentioned were lead, tin and gold, though his preference was for tin.

He brought a new dignity and decorum to the dentist's office by insisting that the patient be seated in an arm chair which is steady and firm, suitable and comfortable, the back of which should be of horse hair or with a soft pillow raised more or less according to the stature of the patient and particularly to that of the dentist.

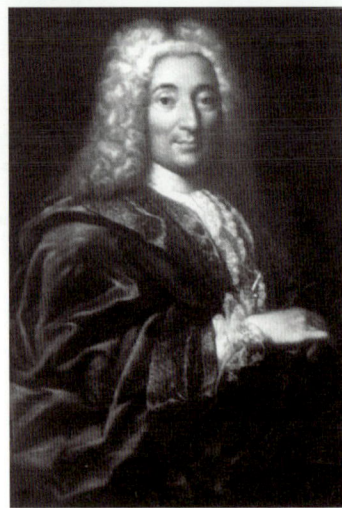

Fig. 1.2: Pierre Fauchard (1678-1761)

Robert Bunon (1702–1748), a well known dentist of that era, challenged the belief that maxillary canines should never be extracted because this would damage the eyes. He also refuted the notion that the pregnant women should not be given dental treatment.

John Hunter (1728–1793) published a book, 'The Natural History of Human Teeth' in 1771, which dealt mostly with dental anatomy, anatomy of jaws and muscles of mastication. He was the pioneer in coining the terms *incisors, canines* and *premolars*. He also gave the idea that the teeth do not grow throughout life.

Low fusing metal alloy was introduced by Jean Darcet in 1770. Bowdet (1775) made the first reference to use gold base to support ivory teeth with gold pins. A baked porcelain complete denture was made in a single block by French dentist Dubois de Chemant in 1788. Josiah Flagg (1790) invented first dental chair with adjustable headrest and extended armrest for holding instruments (Fig.1.3). Since then, there is

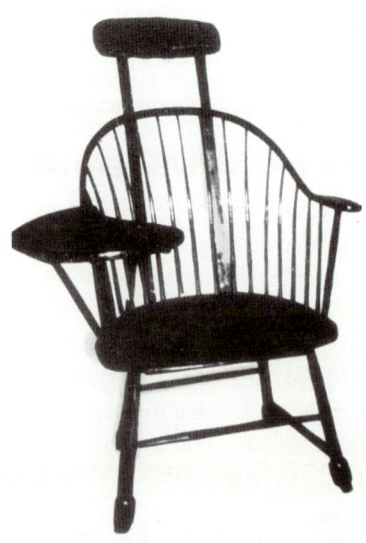

Fig. 1.3: First dental chair

Introduction to Operative Dentistry

continuous improvement in the design of dental chair to provide better comforts both to the patient and the operator (Figs 1.4 and 1.5).

R.C. Skinner contributed maximum in the dental literature. His book 'A Treatise on the Human Teeth' practically a sixteen page pamphlet was published in 1801. The book mainly dealt with dental diseases and their prevention.

The combination of silver and mercury to form 'silver paste' was announced by M. Taveau of Paris in 1826. This was the beginning of dental amalgam which is recognized as one of the outstanding developments in the field of dentistry.

Chapin Harris (1806–1860) published his book 'The Dental Art: A Practical Treatise on Dental Surgery' regarding various aspects of dentistry. He was also instrumental in starting the first scientific journal 'American Journal of Dental Sciences' on 1st June, 1839. He was so attached with the journal that for the first ten years, he bore all the expenditure himself.

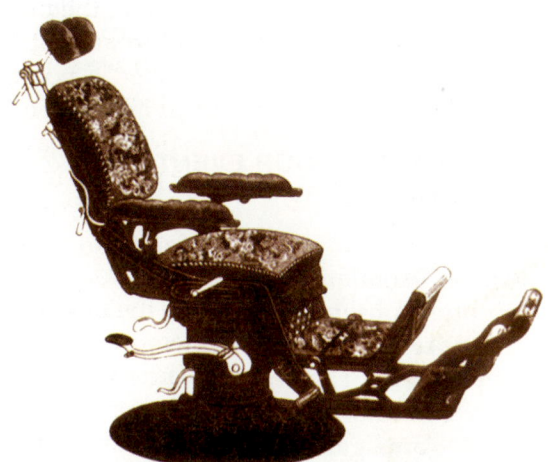

Fig. 1.4: Improved dental chair

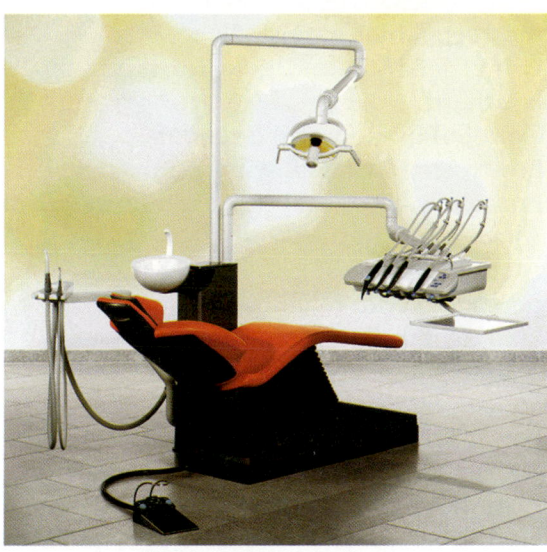

Fig. 1.5: Modern dental chair

Period of Improvement in Dentistry (1840–1900)

On 6 March 1840, first dental college 'Baltimore College of Dental Surgery' came into existence with only five admissions.

In 1840, American Society of Dental Surgeons was established and a couple of years later they banned the use of silver amalgam. In 1845, Amalgam pledge was taken by the members of society. Later in 1855, Dr. Townsend of Philadelphia proposed a combination of four parts of silver and five parts of tin. This was unbalanced alloy having poor edge strength but this was used until about 1863. Dental profession remained hesitant about the use of amalgam until G.V. Black (1885) in his article 'Physical characteristics of filling materials', suggested a formula for amalgam so that it neither expanded nor contracted and also hardness was sufficient. His contributions for operative dentistry are unmatched. His writings might be more than hundred years old but are followed even today. *Greene Vardiman Black* is rightly remembered as the father of operative dentistry (Fig. 1.6).

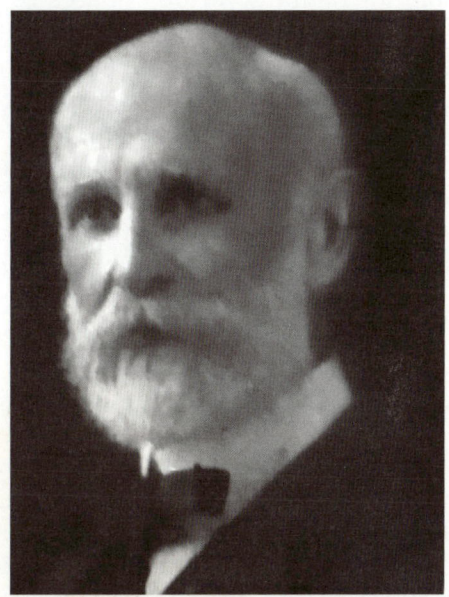

Fig. 1.6: Greene Vardiman Black (1836–1915)

Gutta-percha, an exudate of trees of Sapodilla family, was discovered in India in 1842. Gutta-percha along with zinc-oxide eugenol was used for purpose of temporary fillings as advocated by Hill in 1848.

Zinc-oxide eugenol cement was introduced in 1858. These were very easy to handle and manipulate even in the presence of moisture, well tolerated by pulp and provided good marginal seal; but lacked strength, had prolonged setting time and low resistance to abrasion.

In 1871, a translucent cement (silicate cement) was introduced by Fletcher in England. Dr. Pierce introduced zinc phosphate cement in 1879.

Gas and gasoline furnaces were introduced by Charler (1889) for high fusing porcelain inlays and electric furnace was introduced by Lewitt Ellsworth Custer (1894).

Dentistry in 20th Century

With the beginning of 20th century, the quality of restorative material were refined and improved.

William H. Taggart (1855-1933) introduced casting method for inlay in 1907. Lane suggested the idea of casting by using investment containing high percentage of silica to Plaster of Paris at 650°C to compensate for casting shrinkage. Schen (1932) developed a technique employing hygroscopic expansion of investment to compensate for shrinkage of casting. Sonder (1942) recognized that thermal expansion of investment was greatly inhibited by rigid metal casting ring and advocated lining the ring with soft asbestos.

Gaylor in 1935 provided first modern description of chemistry of amalgam reaction. She was also responsible for naming various phases as gamma, gamma 1, gamma 2. Innes and Youdelis (1963) presented improved alloy containing high copper content (12%) in form of silver-copper eutectic spheres. This new alloy was named admixed alloy. Further, Asgar (1974) developed single composition high copper alloy.

Self-curing acrylic resins for anterior restorations was developed in Germany in 1937 by Walter Wright.

In an effort to improve the physical properties of unfilled acrylic resins, Bowen of National Bureau of Standards developed a polymeric restorative material reinforced with silica particles commercially known as composite.

Polycarboxylate cement was introduced by Dennis Smith in 1968. This cement was only dental cement with true adhesive qualities.

Glass-ionomer cement was invented by Wilson and Kent (1971), with the need to improve upon the properties of silicates and polycarboxylate cements, so as to give adherence to tooth and a better seal. Improvements in all these materials continued with the advent of antibacterial composites, Giomers, etc.

FUTURE OF OPERATIVE DENTISTRY

The future of operative dentistry seems to be bright. The explosive developments of new technology will continue. The armamentarium for prevention and diagnosis will flourish. A chair-side litmus paper test will be a valuable tool to analyze the status of the pulp. Nanotechnology, i.e. fabrication of very small size machines is being tried in medical field. Medical nanorobots have been proposed for pharmaceutical research, clinical diagnosis, rewriting DNA sequences in cells repairing brain damage, etc. This technology will be utilized in dentistry too. Nanodentistry may evolve through several stages of technical developments, initially using genetic engineering, tissue regeneration and later involving growth of new tooth in vitro. One day the complete replacement of dentition should become feasible with installation of biologically autologous tooth replacement. Nanodentistry can also result in renaturation procedure which means replacement of old amalgam fillings with biological materials.

In addition to all these, the durability and appearance of teeth can also be increased by replacing the upper enamel with covalent bonded artificial materials like sapphire and diamond which have more strength and hardness. Other changes, which can be predicted in dentistry, are the development of caries vaccinations, lasers replacing high speed handpieces, three-dimensional radiographs and last but not the least the computer helping to enhance both delivery and predictability of dental procedures. The future dentists, in all probability, will see convenient and better dentistry.

CHRONOLOGY OF MAJOR EVENTS IN OPERATIVE DENTISTRY

1400: Use of gold in leaf form for filling teeth by Joannes Arculanus.
1538: Important observations on development of teeth by Andreas Versalius.
1560: Preparation of artificial teeth from bone and ivory by Ambroise Pare.
1650: Copper amalgam by Stocker.
1684: Use of wax in taking impressions of the teeth by Matthaeus Gottfried Purmann.
1687: First written material on dentistry "Operator for the Teeth" by Charles Allen.
1728: Use of lead, tin and gold for filling by Pierre Fauchard.
1767: Gold foil by Robert Woffendale.
1770: Low fusing metal alloy by Jean Darcet.
1774: Porcelain as dental restorative material by Alexis Duchateau.
1789: A French dentist De Chemant patented 1st porcelain tooth material.
1790: First dental chair by Josiah Flagg.
1806: 26 different shades of porcelain by Guiseppangelo Fonzi.
1808: Fonzi Italian dentist invented terrometallic porcelain tooth that was held in place by platinum pin or frame.
1812: Non-cohesive gold for filling by Marcus Bull.
1818: Father of amalgam – Dr. Louis Regnart.

Introduction to Operative Dentistry

1819: Bell's Putty (a kind of silver amalgam) by Charles Bell.
1826: "Silver paste" (a mixture of silver and mercury) introduced by M. Taeveau.
1838: Hand drill with adjustable head by John Lewis.
1838: Condensation of gold foil by E. Meritt.
1839: American Journal of Dentistry was published.
1840: First dental college of the world, i.e. Baltimore Dental College.
1840: First national dental organisation, i.e. The American Society of Dental Surgeons.
1845: Dental drill by William Rogers.
1848: Gutta percha temporary stopping by Hill.
1855: Cohesive annealed gold foil by Robert Arthur.
1857: Impression compound by Stent.
1858: Flexible engine cable by Charles Merry.
1861: Zsigmondy/Palmer Notation.
1862: Angled handpiece by Charles Merry.
1864: Rubber Dam by Sanford C. Barnum.
1868: Textbook of operative dentistry by Dr. Jonathan Taft.
1871: Dental engine by Morrison.
1871: Steel matrix for proximal cavities by Louis Jack.
1872: Carborundum disc by Robert Arthur.
1873: Silicate cement by Fletcher.
1873: Gold shell crowns by J.B. Beers.
1873: Zinc oxide and clove oil by Chisolm.
1875: Separators by Jarvis.
1879: Zinc phosphate cement by Dr. Pierce.
1885: "Physical character of filling material" book published by Dr. G.V. Black
1889: W.D. Miller – Chemicoparasitic Theory
1890: "Descriptive anatomy of human teeth" book published by G.V. Black.
1897: 1st diamond dental bur by William and Schroeder.
1903: Dr. Charles Land patented 1st ceramic crown.
1907: Practical method of casting of gold inlay by W.H. Taggart.
1910: High silica investment material by Von Horn.
1915: Pin retention by Burgess.
1925: Agar-agar compound by Poller.
1930: Calcium hydroxide paste by Hermann.
1935: Chemistry of reaction of amalgam and phases.
1937: Reversible hydrocolloids by Sears.
1937: Acrylic resins by Walter Wright.
1941: Silver wires (which were later called silver cones or silver points) by Jasper.
1944: Gottelib – Proteolytic theory.
1951: Rubber base impression materials.
1951: Ultrahigh speed air rotor handpieces.
1953: Fluid turbine type handpieces by Nelson and Nelson.
1955: Phenomenon of acid etching by Buonocore.
1955: Schatz and Martin-Proteolysis chelation theory.
1958: Cemented pins by Dr. Miles Markley.
1959: 1:1 ratio of mercury: alloy by Dr. Wilmer Eames.
1960: Composite by R.L. Bowen.
1960: Friction lock pins by Dr. Philip Goldstein.
1963: High copper alloy (Admixed type) by Innes and Youdelis.
1963: Vita Zahnfabrik introduced 1st commercial porcelain.
1965: Mclean and Hughes introduced aluminous porcelain.
1966: Self- threading pins by Going.
1967: Eggers lura proposed sucrose chelation theory.
1968: Polycarboxylate cement by Smith.
1971: Glass Ionomer Cement by Wilson and Kent.
1971: Dental notation by FDI, i.e. Federation Dentaire Internationale.
1972: 1st Machinable mica glass ceramic Macor M. was patented by Corning Glass Works Co.
1973: Duret et al first used CAD-CAM.
1974: Single composition high copper alloy by Asgar.
1976: Base metal alloys by Bauer and Eden.
1980: Amalgapin by Shavell.
1980: L.K. Bandlish introduced Bandlish theory of dental caries.
1982: Nakabayashi introduced concept of bonding.
1983: Simmons introduced miracle mix.
1984: Adair and Grossman developed castable glass ceramic (DICOR).
1984: Microabrasion concept is introduced by McClosky.
1985: Hobo S. and Iwata T. developed castable apatite ceramic (Cerapearl).
1985: Mclean and Gasser developed glass cermet.
1989: Wholwend et al developed injection moulded glass ceramic.
1989: 1st resin modified glass-ionomer (Vitrebond) was developed by 3M.
1991: Kerby et al developed stainless steel glass-ionomer cement.
1992: Arita A. et al developed SiC added GIC.
1993: Dentsply launched Dyract, 1st compomer.
1994: Imazato et al developed antibacterial composite containing MDPB.
1995: High viscosity glass-ionomer cements was introduced.
1996: Flowable resin was introduced.
1997: Heraeus Kulzer introduced packable composites.
1998: Ceramay introduced leucite reinforced porcelain.
1998: Mount introduced newer classification of carious/lesions.

1999: Sikri suggested modified classification of caries/cavities.
1999: Deb et al developed SrO added GIC.
2000: Fast setting GIC was introduced by 3M ESPE (Ketac Cem)
2002: Shofu introduced Giomers.
2003: Lohbauer et al developed fiber reinforced GIC.
2003: Mazzaoui et al developed CPP-ACP added GIC.
2004: Tjandrawinata et al developed glass-ionomer containing spherical silica.
2005: Pamir et al developed Titanium tetrafluoride added GIC.
2005: Hurrell-Gillingham et al developed Fe_2O_3 containing GIC.
2005: Boyd et al developed zinc based GIC.
2005: Bertolini et al developed Niobium Silicate GIC.
2005: Gu et al developed Yttria, ZrO_2 stabilized GIC.
2006: Gu et al developed hydroxyapatite and hydroxyapatite/ZrO_2 in GIC.
2006: Prentice et al developed boric acid containing GIC.
2007: 3M ESPE introduced siloranes containing composite.
2009: Tan S.X. et al developed antibacterial titanium oxide silver Core-Shell composite.
2010: Poly quaternary ammonium salts containing antibacterial GIC.
2010: Kerr introduced Vertise flow, self adhering flowable composite.
2010: Dentsply introduced smart dentin replacement technology.
2010: Sevinc B.A. and Hanley L. introduced antibacterial dental composite containing ZnO nanoparticles.
2010: 'Biodentine' was introduced by Septodont having applications similar to that of MTA
2011: Kerr introduced 'sonic fill' composite filling system, whereby ultrasonic energy allows composite to be evenly distributed in cavities up to 5.0 mm.
2012: Coltene Whaledent introduced 'componeers' as direct ready made composite veneers having a thickness of 0.3 mm, requiring no tooth preparation for application.

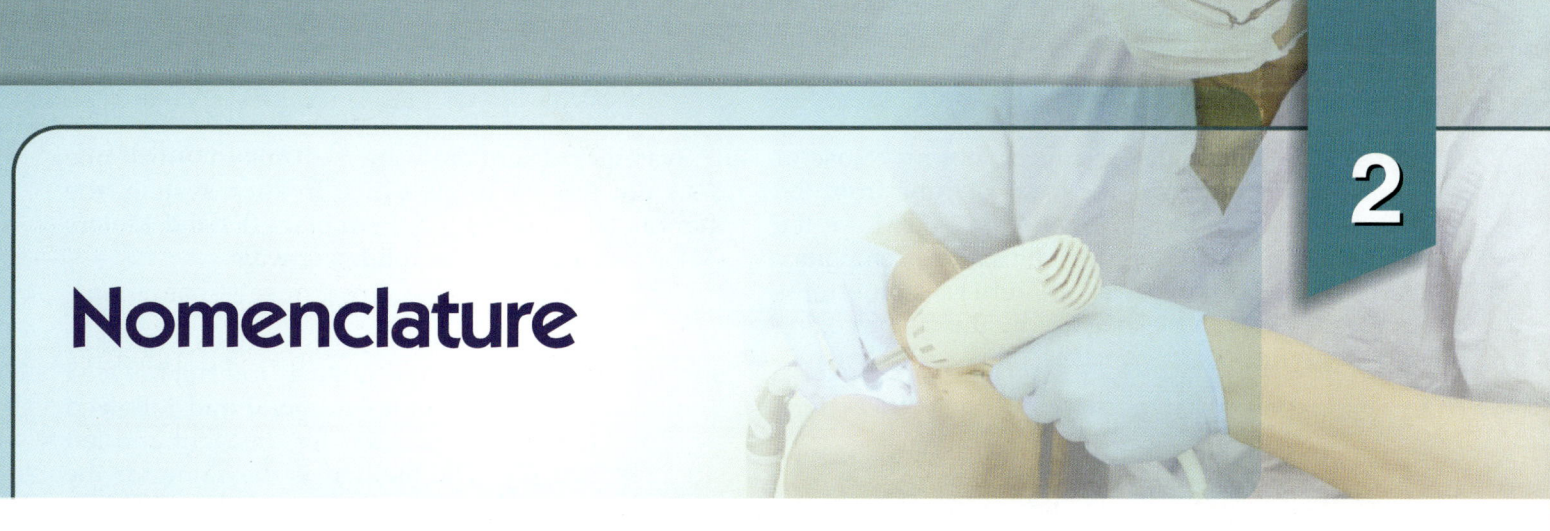

Nomenclature

For understanding the concepts of operative dentistry, it is essential that the clinician be thoroughly familiar with the technical terms used during the treatment. These terms also help in recording the patient's signs and symptoms, which can be useful during subsequent visits of the patient. Let us first be familiar with the notation systems, i.e. the systems used for denoting teeth in the arch.

The majority of the tooth notation systems fall into two categories:
A. Those having a similar notation for the teeth in each segment and
B. Those having a different notation for the teeth in each segment

Tooth notation systems were originally developed for designating permanent teeth, later supplementary systems for the temporary dentition were established, often by adding to the symbols used in the basic systems.

In the description of various systems that follows, the method used for denoting temporary teeth is given second to the method used for denoting permanent teeth.

A. SYSTEMS HAVING A SIMILAR NOTATION IN EACH SEGMENT

System 1: The oldest known method in this group still in use is probably 'Zsigmondy system' (Zsigmondy, 1861). The central incisor of each segment is given the number '1' and the numbers then run in a distal direction. The segments are shown as the patients' upper right, upper left, lower right and lower left segments respectively.

The Zsigmondy system is frequently employed both in Europe and America. It is also common in Australia and Japan. In English speaking countries it, is generally known as *Palmer's Notation* (Palmer, 1891).

Zsigmondy's System Permanent teeth															
R	8	7	6	5	4	3	2	1	1	2	3	4	5	6	7	8	L
	8	7	6	5	4	3	2	1	1	2	3	4	5	6	7	8	

The temporary teeth are indicated merely by altering the Arabic numerals to Roman ones. Sometimes temporary teeth are designated with the letters a – e or with capital letter A – E instead of Roman numerals I-V or letter D (deciduous) placed after the number of the tooth or a small 'd' is placed before the number of the tooth. The temporary teeth may also be indicated by the addition of the letter 'm' after the number of the tooth.

Different variants for temporary teeth										
R	V	IV	III	II	I	I	II	III	IV	V	L
R	e	d	c	b	a	a	b	c	d	e	L
	e	d	c	b	a	a	b	c	d	e	
R	E	D	C	B	A	A	B	C	D	E	L
	E	D	C	B	A	A	B	C	D	E	
R	5D	4D	3D	2D	1D	1D	2D	3D	4D	5D	L
	5D	4D	3D	2D	1D	1D	2D	3D	4D	5D	
R	d5	d4	d3	d2	d1	d1	d2	d3	d4	d5	L
	d5	d4	d3	d2	d1	d1	d2	d3	d4	d5	
R	5m	4m	3m	2m	1m	1m	2m	3m	4m	5m	L
	5m	4m	3m	2m	1m	1m	2m	3m	4m	5m	

System 2: There is another system which employs both the angle signs and the numerals 1 to 8 for enumerating the permanent teeth and A to E for enumerating the temporary teeth. It is exactly opposite to the above mentioned Zsigmondy's system. In this system, notation begins with number 1 for the third molar and with the letter A for the second temporary molar. It ends with 8 and E for the permanent and deciduous central incisors, respectively.

R	1	2	3	4	5	6	7	8	8	7	6	5	4	3	2	1	L
	1	2	3	4	5	6	7	8	8	7	6	5	4	3	2	1	
R	A	B	C	D	E	E	D	C	B	A	L
	A	B	C	D	E	E	D	C	B	A	

System 3: Other angle systems do not make use of numerals, but designate the teeth (starting from the central incisor) as: $I_1, I_2, C, P_1, P_2, M_1, M_2$ and M_3, i.e. the initial letters of their respective Latin names. Temporary teeth are shown with small letters, sometimes supplemented with the letter d (deciduous) preceding the letter symbol.

Permanent teeth
$R \dfrac{M_3\ M_2\ M_1\ P_2\ P_1\ C\ I_2\ I_1\ \vert\ I_1\ I_2\ C\ P_1\ P_2\ M_1\ M_2\ M_3}{M_3\ M_2\ M_1\ P_2\ P_1\ C\ I_2\ I_1\ \vert\ I_1\ I_2\ C\ P_1\ P_2\ M_1\ M_2\ M_3} L$

Temporary teeth
$R \dfrac{dm_2\ dm_1\ dc\ di_2\ di_1\ \vert\ di_1\ di_2\ dc\ dm_1\ dm_2}{dm_2\ dm_1\ dc\ di_2\ di_1\ \vert\ di_1\ di_2\ dc\ dm_1\ dm_2} L$

The system 3 is employed mainly in Holland.

System 4: This 4 is another older system which was invented by Dane, Haderup (1887, 1891). According to this system, the teeth are numbered in each segment starting with number 1 for the central incisor. The teeth are then numbered from 1 to 8 in a distal direction. The tooth numbers in the upper jaw are combined with a plus sign, those in the lower jaw with a minus sign. These signs are placed to the right of the numeral if the tooth is situated on the right side of the jaw and to the left of the numeral if the tooth is situated on the left side of the jaw. Temporary teeth were originally shown by the addition of the letter L placed before the numeral. After a few years, this was altered to another form, whereby 0, also placed before the numeral, substituted the letter L. In central Europe, the temporary teeth are indicated by Roman numerals (without the addition of 0) in conjunction with + and − signs.

Haderup's system
$R \dfrac{8+\ 7+\ 6+\ 5+\ 4+\ 3+\ 2+\ 1+\ \vert\ +1\ +2\ +3\ +4\ +5\ +6\ +7\ +8}{8-\ 7-\ 6-\ 5-\ 4-\ 3-\ 2-\ 1-\ \vert\ -1\ -2\ -3\ -4\ -5\ -6\ -7\ -8} L$

Different variants for temporary teeth
$R \dfrac{05+\ 04+\ 03+\ 02+\ 01+\ \vert\ +01\ +02\ +03\ +04\ +05}{05-\ 04-\ 03-\ 02-\ 01-\ \vert\ -01\ -02\ -03\ -04\ -05} L$
$R \dfrac{V+\ IV+\ III+\ II+\ I+\ \vert\ +I\ +II\ +III\ +IV\ +V}{V-\ IV-\ III-\ II-\ I-\ \vert\ -I\ -II\ -III\ -IV\ -V} L$

Haderup's system is practically the only one used in Sweden, Denmark, Norway, Finland and Iceland. Along with other systems, it is also used in Germany, Italy, Switzerland, Yugoslavia, Poland and Czechoslovakia.

System 5: There are some systems in which one does not use the angle signs. In such system, the Incisors (I), Canines (C), Premolars (P) and Molars (M) are indicated in the following way:

$I_1, I_2, C, P_1, P_2, M_1, M_2$ and M_3

The upper jaw is indicated by the letter s (superior) and the lower jaw by the letter i (inferior) placed immediately after the index numeral and followed by d or s (dexter and sinister) for the right and left side, respectively. The method is the same for the temporary teeth, the difference being that small letters are used to represent the teeth, i.e. i1, i2, c, m1, m2. The system is used in Holland and some other countries.

System 6: This system is very similar to System 5 having the same letter and index numeration for the teeth but here the segment is identified by the position of the index in relation to the alphabetical letter of the tooth. For the upper right segment, the index is placed higher than and to the left of the alphabetical symbol of the tooth; for the upper left segment, higher and to the right of it. For the lower right segment, the index is placed lower and to the left of the alphabetical symbol of the tooth; for the left segment, lower and to the right of it. This system is employed in South Africa.

$$R \dfrac{{}^3M\ {}^2M\ {}^1M\ {}^2P\ {}^1P\ {}^1C\ {}^2I\ {}^1I\ \vert\ I^1\ I^2\ C^1\ P^1\ P^2\ M^1\ M^2\ M^3}{{}_3M\ {}_2M\ {}_1M\ {}_2P\ {}_1P\ {}_1C\ {}_2I\ {}_1I\ \vert\ I_1\ I_2\ C_1\ P_1\ P_2\ M_1\ M_2\ M_3} L$$

System 7: This system manages without the use of angle signs. In this system, the teeth are numbered 1–8 from the central incisor to the last molar. The teeth of the upper jaw are indicated by a capital D (droite) or G (gaucha) for the right or left side respectively and is placed immediately prior to the number of the tooth. The teeth of the lower jaw are indicated by a small d or g.

Temporary teeth are indicated by substituting Roman numerals for the Arabic ones. This system is used to a limited extent in France, while a variant occurs in Romania.

$$R \dfrac{D8\ D7\ D6\ D5\ D4\ D3\ D2\ D1\ \vert\ G1\ G2\ G3\ G4\ G5\ G6\ G7\ G8}{d8\ d7\ d6\ d5\ d4\ d3\ d2\ d1\ \vert\ g1\ g2\ g3\ g4\ g5\ g6\ g7\ g8} L$$

B. SYSTEMS WITH DIFFERENT NOTATION IN EACH SEGMENT

Several systems which employ different notations for the teeth in different segments are in use. The most common of these systems are the 'Army system', 'Navy system', 'Universal system' and the 'Bosworth system'. These are as follows:

Nomenclature

System 8:

The Army System
R $\dfrac{8\ 7\ 6\ 5\ 4\ 3\ 2\ 1\ \vert\ 1\ 2\ 3\ 4\ 5\ 6\ 7\ 8}{16\ 15\ 14\ 13\ 12\ 11\ 10\ 9\ \vert\ 9\ 10\ 11\ 12\ 13\ 14\ 15\ 16}$ L

System 9:

The Navy System
R $\dfrac{1\ 2\ 3\ 4\ 5\ 6\ 7\ 8\ \vdots\ 9\ 10\ 11\ 12\ 13\ 14\ 15\ 16}{17\ 18\ 19\ 20\ 21\ 22\ 23\ 24\ \vdots\ 25\ 26\ 27\ 28\ 29\ 30\ 31\ 32}$ L

System 10:

The Universal System
R $\dfrac{1\ 2\ 3\ 4\ 5\ 6\ 7\ 8\ \vdots\ 9\ 10\ 11\ 12\ 13\ 14\ 15\ 16}{32\ 31\ 30\ 29\ 28\ 27\ 26\ 25\ \vdots\ 24\ 23\ 22\ 21\ 20\ 19\ 18\ 17}$ L

System 11:

The Bosworth System
R $\dfrac{8\ 7\ 6\ 5\ 4\ 3\ 2\ 1\ \vert\ 1\ 2\ 3\ 4\ 5\ 6\ 7\ 8}{H\ G\ F\ E\ D\ C\ B\ A\ \vert\ A\ B\ C\ D\ E\ F\ G\ H}$ L

On the basis of these four systems, the designation for the temporary teeth can be made for each system on two different principles (1) retain the designation of the first five teeth in each segment and indicate that they are temporary teeth by making some addition to the symbol of the tooth (2) retain the method for designating the teeth, but substitute for the numbers of the permanent teeth. Substitutions can be in the form of alphabetical letters or different numerals. The temporary teeth will in this case, have quite different symbols from the permanent teeth.

The first alternative may be illustrated with adaptations of the Navy system in which the second temporary molar on the right side of the upper jaw retains the number '4' and the second temporary molar on the left-hand side of the lower jaw retains the number '29'. The first variant indicates that deciduous teeth are indicated by putting a ring round the number of tooth (4,29). In a second variant, this is shown by the addition of '1/2' to the number of permanent tooth ($4^{1/2}$, $29^{1/2}$). The Universal system may be adapted in a similar way. In this case, the temporary teeth are indicated by placing the letter 'T' (temporary) in front of the number of the corresponding temporary tooth. Another adaptation of this system is to write the number of the tooth after the letter D (D4, D29).

Examples of the second alternative, i.e. those in which the method of designating the teeth is retained but different symbols are used are modification of the Navy System, in which the temporary teeth of the upper jaw are number from I–X, beginning with the second temporary molar on the right side, and those in the lower jaw from XI–XX. Another system is to use the letters A-J for the temporary teeth of the upper jaw and the letters K-T for the lower jaw.

Variants of the Navy System for Temporary Teeth
R $\dfrac{\text{I}\ \ \text{II}\ \ \text{III}\ \ \text{IV}\ \ \text{V}\ \vert\ \text{VI}\ \ \text{VII}\ \ \text{VIII}\ \ \text{IX}\ \ \text{X}}{\text{XI}\ \ \text{XII}\ \ \text{XIII}\ \ \text{XIV}\ \ \text{XV}\ \vert\ \text{XVI}\ \ \text{XVII}\ \ \text{XVIII}\ \ \text{XIX}\ \ \text{XX}}$ L
R $\dfrac{A\ \ B\ \ C\ \ D\ \ E\ \vert\ F\ \ G\ \ H\ \ I\ \ J}{K\ \ L\ \ M\ \ N\ \ O\ \vert\ P\ \ Q\ \ R\ \ S\ \ T}$ L

This second variant is also to be found adapted to the Army system and the Universal system, where they are respectively:

Army System
R $\dfrac{E\ \ D\ \ C\ \ B\ \ A\ \vert\ A\ \ B\ \ C\ \ D\ \ E}{J\ \ I\ \ H\ \ G\ \ F\ \vert\ F\ \ G\ \ H\ \ I\ \ J}$ L

Universal System
R $\dfrac{A\ \ B\ \ C\ \ D\ \ E\ \vert\ F\ \ G\ \ H\ \ I\ \ J}{T\ \ S\ \ R\ \ Q\ \ P\ \vert\ O\ \ N\ \ M\ \ L\ \ K}$ L

With the Bosworth system, the temporary teeth are indicated in the following way:

R $\dfrac{D5\ \ D4\ \ D3\ \ D2\ \ D1\ \vert\ D1\ \ D2\ \ D3\ \ D4\ \ D5}{DE\ \ DD\ \ DC\ \ DB\ \ DA\ \vert\ DA\ \ DB\ \ DC\ \ DD\ \ DE}$ L

The Universal system has also a variant employing the letter 'D' for temporary or deciduous teeth as follows:

R $\dfrac{D1\ \ D2\ \ D3\ \ D4\ \ D5\ \vert\ D6\ \ D7\ \ D8\ \ D9\ \ D10}{D20\ D19\ D18\ D17\ D16\ \vert\ D15\ D14\ D13\ D12\ D11}$ L

Sometimes the letter is placed after the numerals.

System 12: Finally, there is a system that is the exact mirror image of the Navy system, that is, both the upper and the lower jaw are numbered from left to right.

R $\dfrac{16\ 15\ 14\ 13\ 12\ 11\ 10\ 9\ \vert\ 8\ 7\ 6\ 5\ 4\ 3\ 2\ 1}{32\ 31\ 30\ 29\ 28\ 27\ 26\ 25\ \vert\ 24\ 23\ 22\ 21\ 20\ 19\ 18\ 17}$ L

FDI SYSTEM

The Federation Dentaire Internationale (FDI)/Two digit system is accepted all around the world but not very much in USA. This tooth notation system was developed by Dr. J. Viohl and accepted by the Federation Dentaire Internationale in a meeting in 1971. It is considered as one system, which makes visual sense, cognitive sense and computer sense. It fulfils the following basic requirements:

FDI System

Permanent Teeth

```
              Maxillary
  18 17 16 15 14 13 12 11 : 21 22 23 24 25 26 27 28
R ..................................................L
  48 47 46 45 44 43 42 41 : 31 32 33 34 35 36 37 38
             Mandibular
```

Primary Teeth

```
              Maxillary
     55 54 53 52 51 : 61 62 63 64 65
R ..........................................L
     85 84 83 83 81 : 71 72 73 74 75
             Mandibular
```

- Simple to teach and understand
- Readily communicable in print and telephone
- Easy to speak in conversation and dictation
- Easy to enter into a computer
- Easily adaptable to standard charts used in general practice

The FDI two digit system identifies each of the 32 permanent teeth with a two digit number, the first digit indicating the quadrant (1 to 4, starting from upper right quadrant clockwise to lower right quadrant) and the second digit indicating the tooth type (1 to 8, starting from central incisor to the third molar). The 20 primary teeth are represented in a similar fashion: Quadrant as 5 to 8 and tooth type as 1 to 5.

Nomenclature Related to Various Surfaces of the Tooth

Different surfaces of the tooth are named according to their adjoining anatomic structures. These are given in Table 2.1.

Caries involving any of these surfaces is denoted by that particular surface name used as a prefix before the word 'caries', e.g. Caries on the mesial surface of the tooth is referred to as mesial caries. Caries involving two surfaces say mesial and occlusal is referred to as mesio-occlusal (MO) caries. Caries involving three surfaces say mesial, occlusal and distal is referred to as mesio-occluso-distal (MOD) caries.

Anatomical tooth crown and clinical tooth crown: Portion of the tooth that is covered with enamel is referred to as the anatomical tooth crown. Portion of the tooth that is exposed in the oral cavity is referred to as the clinical tooth crown.

Anatomic tooth root and clinical tooth root: Portion of the tooth that is covered with cementum is referred to as the anatomical tooth root. Portion of the tooth that is not visible in the oral cavity is referred to as the clinical tooth root.

TERMINOLOGY RELATED TO CARIES

What is Dental Caries?

Dental caries is an infectious and microbiological disease that results in localized dissolution and destruction of the calcified tissues of the tooth.

According to the location, caries can be:

a. Primary caries
   - Pit and fissure caries
   - Smooth surface caries
   - Root surface caries
   - Residual caries
b. Secondary/recurrent caries
   - Adjacent to restoration margins
   - Beneath the restoration

According to the amount of tooth involvement caries can be:

c. Incipient caries
d. Advanced/cavitated caries

According to the rate of progression caries can be:

e. Acute caries
f. Chronic caries

a. Primary Caries

The original carious lesion in the tooth is referred to as the primary caries. Depending upon its location on the tooth, the pattern of caries progression varies and also influences the cavity preparation. Caries can be located in the pits and fissures, on smooth surfaces and root surfaces (Figs 2.1A and B).

Pit and Fissure Caries

Caries beginning in the pits and fissures of teeth is referred to as pit and fissure caries. Pits and fissures are those areas of the teeth where there is imperfect coalescence of developmental enamel lobes. Because of incomplete fusion of enamel, these areas are

Table 2.1: Different surfaces of the tooth

Facial surfaces	Labial surface	Facing towards the lip
	Buccal surface	Facing towards the cheeks
Lingual surface		Facing towards the tongue
Palatal surface		Facing towards the palate
Mesial surface		Facing towards the midline
Distal surface		Facing away from the midline
Incisal surface		Functioning edges of the incisors and canines
Occlusal surface		Functioning/masticating surfaces of the premolars and molars
Cervical portion		Portion of the tooth related to the cervical line or necks of teeth
Gingival portion		Portion of the tooth close to the gingiva

Nomenclature

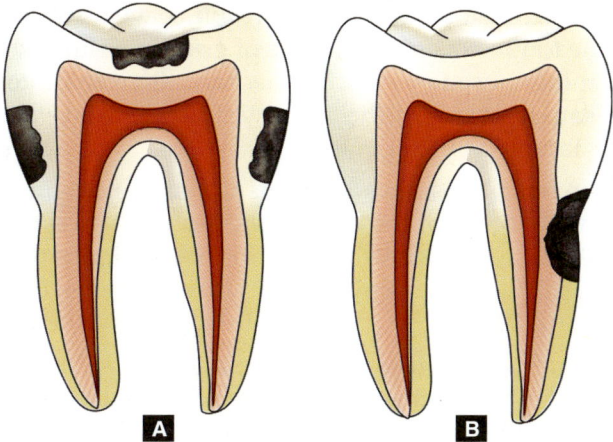

Figs 2.1A and B: Caries on different surfaces of teeth; **(A)** in pits and fissures and on smooth surfaces and; **(B)** on roots surface

susceptible to food impaction and hence caries. On the contrary, grooves and fossae are areas where there is perfect coalescence of developmental enamel lobes, which makes them less susceptible to caries. These areas usually do not lodge food and are easily cleaned by the normal cleansing procedures. Pit and fissure caries usually begins as a small point penetration at the bottom of the pit and fissure. From here, it fans along the enamel rods to the dentino-enamel junction. On reaching the dentino-enamel junction, caries spreads laterally at the junction and then penetrates towards the pulp through the dentinal tubules. Diagrammatic representation of pit and fissure caries can be seen as two cones, base to base, with the apex of the enamel cone at the point of entry in enamel and the apex of the dentin cone towards the pulp (Fig. 5.11). Because of its pin point origin, pit and fissure caries may not be clinically visible in its early stages until the caries has spread largely, undermining the enamel in which case the lesion is seen as a bluish discoloration of the tooth or as a cavitation after the overlying unsupported enamel has been lost under the forces of mastication.

These caries are prevalent in the following areas:
- Pits and fissures on the occlusal surfaces of premolars and molars and occlusal 2/3rd of buccal and lingual surfaces of molars
- Pits on the lingual surfaces of upper incisors
- Any other surface where the pit is abnormally present

Smooth Surface Caries

Smooth surface caries does not begin in the pits and fissures but on relatively smooth surfaces of the tooth that have been covered with plaque for quite some time. Unlike pit and fissure caries, smooth surface caries initially involves a larger area of enamel on its outer surface. Caries then spreads along the enamel rods to the dentino-enamel junction. At the junction, it spreads laterally and then towards the pulp through the dentinal tubules. Diagrammatic representation of smooth surface caries can be seen as two cones, the apex of each cone pointing towards the pulp. The apex of the enamel cone contacts the base of the dentin cone (Fig. 5.10).

These caries are prevalent in the following areas:
- Cavities on the proximal surfaces of incisors, canines, premolars and molars.
- Cavities in the gingival third of the facial and lingual surfaces of all the teeth.

Root Surface Caries

Root surface caries is also at times referred to as senile caries and begins on the roots of teeth that have been exposed to the oral environment and covered with plaque for quite some time. The progression of this type of caries is rapid and hence should be detected and checked in time. Because of the increasing number of elderly who are retaining teeth, the prevalence of root caries is also increasing for the last few years.

Residual Caries

Caries that remains after the cavity preparation has been complete is referred to as residual caries, which may have been left behind either intentionally by the operator or by accident. Residual caries at the dentino enamel junction or enamel walls is not acceptable. Only affected dentin can be left behind.

b. Secondary Caries

Secondary caries is also at times referred to as recurrent caries and begins around or beneath the restoration (Fig. 5.14). Its occurrence is suggestive of an improper seal between the tooth and restoration where microleakage may occur predisposing to the development of caries.

c. Incipient Caries

Incipient caries is at times also referred to as initial caries or reversible caries. It is just the beginning of the caries activity and the lesion is evident as a white opaque area on the surface of the enamel. Surfaces inflicted by incipient caries are fairly hard and only minor surface roughening may be present. Unlike hypoplastic white areas which are visible irrespective of whether the tooth surface is dry or wet, incipient caries becomes visible only when the tooth surface is dried. At this stage, the lesion is in a reversible state, i.e. can be remineralized provided oral hygiene measures are followed and the plaque removed and controlled. A remineralized lesion may continue to be white or turn brownish black because of external staining. Such dark areas, referred to as arrested caries, are hard to touch and appear even when the tooth surface is dry or wet.

d. Advanced/Cavitated Caries

Caries that has progressed to the dentino-enamel junction and is no longer reversible is called *advanced caries*. When the overlying enamel breaks down, the lesion is known as cavitated caries. At this stage, the lesion cannot be remineralized and requires cavity preparation and restoration for treatment.

e. Acute Caries

Caries of a rapid onset and spread is referred to as acute caries, e.g. nursing bottle caries or rampant caries. Lesions are light yellow in color, soft and highly infectious.

f. Chronic Caries

Caries of a slower onset and spread is referred to as chronic caries. Lesions may be present in only few locations in the mouth. They are hard and dark brown to black in color. Their dark color is because of enough time for external staining to occur.

AFFECTED AND INFECTED DENTIN

Carious dentin can be grossly divided into two zones (1) infected dentin or the outer zone and (2) affected dentin or the inner zone (Fusayama, 1979). Infected dentin is characterized by irreversibly denatured collagen, which is infiltrated with bacteria and is not remineralizable. Affected dentin is characterized by reversibly denatured collagen, which is not infiltrated with bacteria and is remineralizable. Infected dentin should be removed while affected dentin can be left behind during cavity preparation. It is believed that affected dentin either remineralizes or becomes sterile once the cavity is thoroughly restored.

Clinically, it may be difficult to precisely distinguish between the two zones of dentin caries but still a guide that helps in distinguishing between them is as follows: (1) Infected dentin is darker than the affected dentin (2) Infected dentin is softer to touch than the affected dentin. However, this guide may provide to be of little use in acute caries where the discoloration is very slight and not readily distinguishable. A more accurate guide to distinguish between the two is the application of 1.0% solution of acid red in propylene glycol. This dye stains only the irreversibly denatured collagen, i.e. infected dentin.

OTHER DEFECTS IN THE TOOTH STRUCTURE

Attrition: It is defined as the loss of tooth structure occurring as a result of frictional contact between opposing teeth (Fig. 2.2).

Abrasion: Lesions formed as a result of wearing away of the tooth substance because of grinding, rubbing or scraping caused by external mechanical means, like in repeated contact of the teeth with foreign objects or substances (Fig. 2.2).

Abfraction: These are wedge shaped defects in the cervical region of the tooth believed to be a result of tensile stress concentrated in this area consequent to occlusal forces in some remote area (*see* Figs 23.9A, 24.2 and 24.3).

Erosion: Lesions formed as a result of dissolution of tooth structure subsequent to chemical attack of either endogenous or exogenous origin, or combined chemico-mechanical attack. Depending upon the source of chemicals usually acids, erosion may be intrinsic or extrinsic (Fig. 2.3).

Fracture: Any break in the continuity of the tooth surface is referred to as a fracture (Fig. 2.4).

Enamel hypoplasia: Defective formation of the enamel that may occur because of injury to the ameloblasts is called enamel hypoplasia. Hypoplasia may be seen as a deformed tooth or pits and grooves on the tooth surface. It is seen as opaque white to light brown area with smooth hard surface (Fig. 2.5).

Hypocalcification: Defective mineralization of the tooth is referred to as hypocalcification. It is seen as an opaque white area that is soft to an explorer touch (Fig. 2.6).

Amelogenesis imperfecta: This is a heredity condition in which enamel is defective. It may be either hypoplastic or hypocalcified or both. The teeth may appear normal or extremely unsightly.

Dentinogenesis imperfecta: This is a heredity condition in which only dentin is defective but enamel is normal. Enamel is loosely attached to the underlying dentin and is lost early in the life.

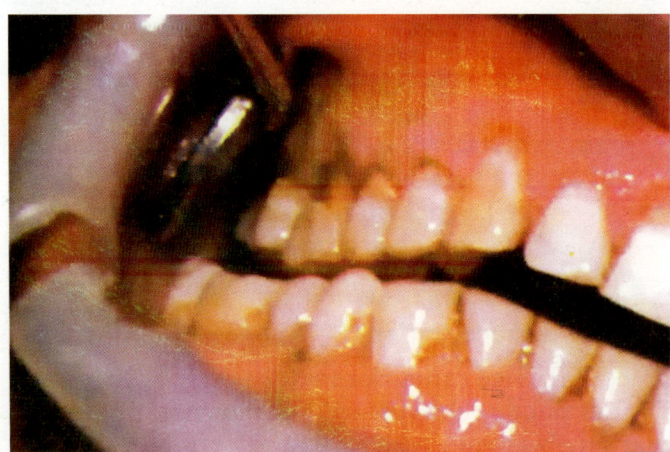

Fig. 2.2: Attrition in anterior teeth and abrasion in maxillary posterior teeth

Nomenclature

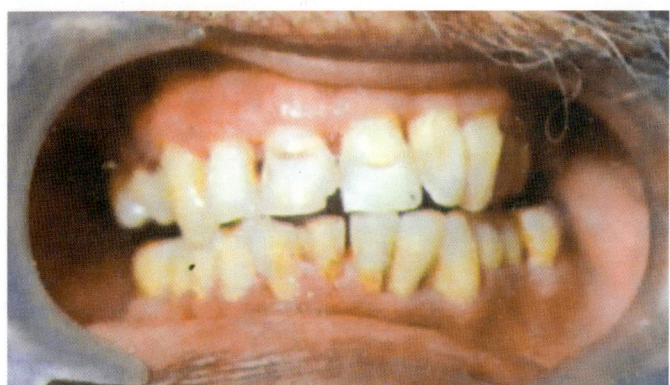

Fig. 2.3: Erosion lesions in maxillary anterior teeth

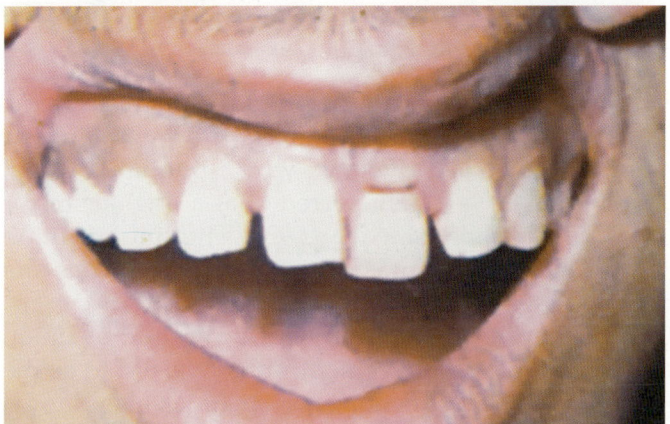

Fig. 2.4: Fracture in maxillary central incisor

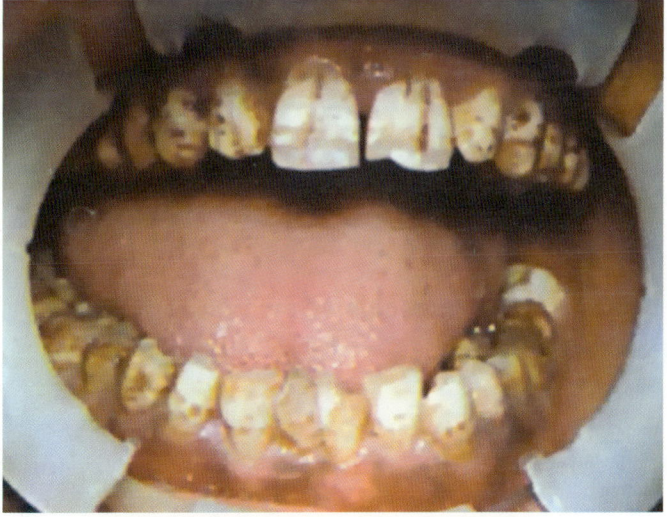

Fig. 2.5: Generalised enamel hypoplasia

NOMENCLATURE RELATED TO CAVITY PREPARATION

Cavity: A cavity refers to a defect in enamel or in both enamel and dentin, subsequent to the destruction caused by dental caries.

Cavity preparation: Cavity preparation is the alteration of defective, diseased or injured tooth structure by dental surgical procedures and subsequently shaping

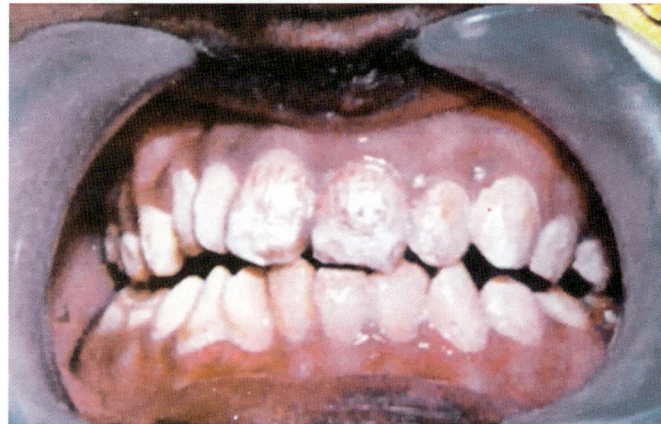

Fig. 2.6: Enamel hypocalcification

the remaining enamel and dentin to receive a restorative material such that the tooth is returned to its normal form, function, health and esthetics (where needed).

Intracoronal cavity preparation: Cavity that is prepared in the interior of the tooth is referred to as the intracoronal cavity preparation.

Extracoronal cavity preparation: Cavity preparation that involves the external surfaces of the tooth and has walls that results from removal of most or all of the enamel is referred to as the extracoronal cavity preparation, e.g. a crown preparation.

Simple Cavities

Cavities involving only one surface of the tooth are called simple cavities (Fig. 2.7), e.g. Mesial (M), Distal (D), Facial (F), Lingual (L), Occlusal (O) and Incisal (I) cavities.

Compound Cavities

Cavities involving two adjoining surfaces of the tooth are called compound cavities (Fig. 2.8). For example:
- (MO) – Mesioocclusal cavity
- (MB) – Mesiobuccal cavity
- (ML) – Mesiolingual cavity
- (DO) – Distoocclusal cavity
- (DB) – Distobuccal cavity
- (DL) – Distolingual cavity

Complex Cavities

Cavities involving more than two adjoining surfaces of the tooth are called *complex cavities* (Fig. 2.9), for example:
- Mesioocclusodistal cavity (MOD cavity)
- Mesioincisodistal cavity (MID cavity)
- Facioocclusolingual cavity (FOL cavity)

Pit and Fissure Cavities

Cavities involving the pits and fissures of anterior and posterior teeth are referred to as pit and fissure cavities.

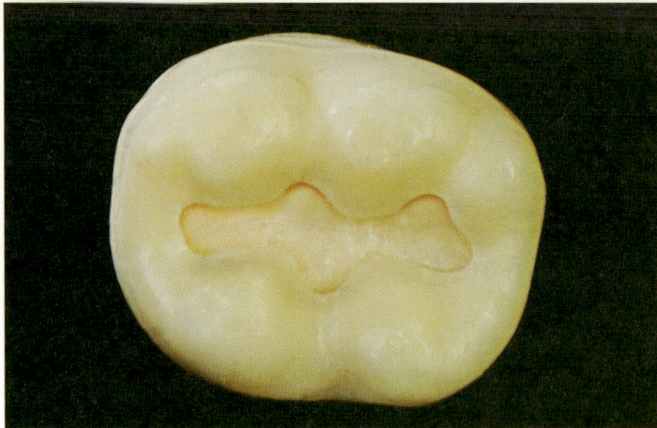

Fig. 2.7: Simple cavity

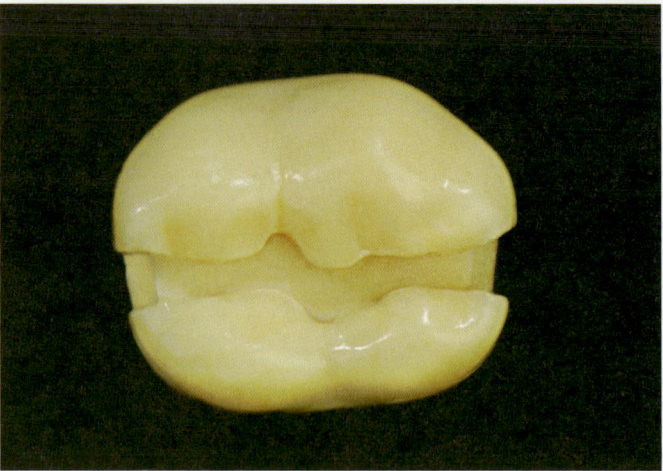

Fig. 2.9: Complex cavity

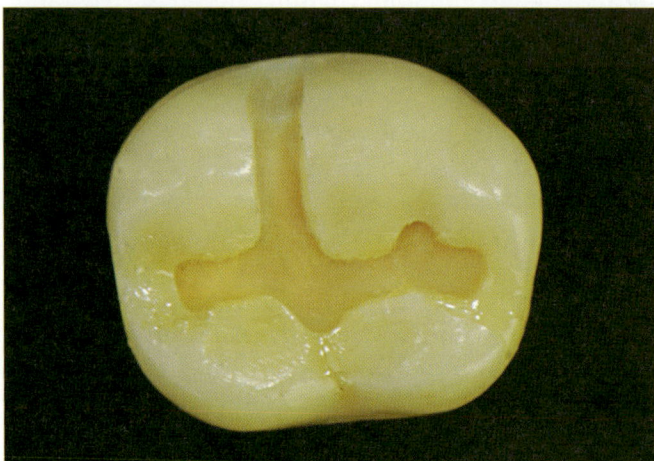

Figs 2.8: Compound cavity

Step: An auxiliary extension of the main cavity on to an adjoining surface is referred to as a step. For example, in a class III cavity with a lingual dovetail, the lingual dovetail is referred to as a lingual step.

Dentino-enamel junction (DEJ): The line of union between enamel and dentin is referred to as the dentino-enamel junction.

Cemento-enamel junction (CEJ): The line of union between enamel and cementum is referred to as the cemento-enamel junction. It is at times also known as the cervical line.

Different walls of the cavity are named according to the surfaces towards which they face (Table 2.2).

Walls in an Occlusal Cavity (Class I) (Fig. 2.10)

- Facial wall
- Lingual wall
- Mesial wall
- Distal wall
- Pulpal wall

Walls in a Proximoocclusal Cavity (Class II) (Fig. 2.11)

Occlusal portion

- Facial wall
- Lingual wall
- Mesial or distal wall (any one of these, depending on which surface the cavity is present)
- Pulpal wall

Proximal portion

- Facio proximal wall
- Linguo proximal wall
- Gingival wall
- Axial wall

Walls in a Proximal Cavity (Class III) (Fig 2.12)

- Facial wall
- Lingual wall

Smooth Surface Cavities

Cavities involving the prepared smooth surfaces of the teeth are referred to as smooth surface cavities.

Various Walls in a Cavity Preparation

Wall: Any surface of the cavity is referred to as a wall.

Internal wall: Surface of a prepared cavity that does not extend to the exterior of the tooth is referred to as an internal wall.

External wall: Surface of a prepared cavity that extends on to the exterior of the tooth is referred to as an external wall.

Enamel wall: That portion of the cavity wall which is composed of enamel is called an enamel wall.

Dentin wall: That portion of the cavity wall which is composed of dentin is called a dentin wall.

Floor/seat of the cavity: Any cavity wall that is flat and perpendicular to the forces directed occlusogingivally is referred to as a floor/seat of the cavity, e.g. pulpal and gingival walls. Flat floors provide stabilization/resistance form to the cavity.

Nomenclature

Table 2.2: Different walls in a cavity preparation		
Facial walls	Labial wall	Wall facing towards the lips
	Buccal wall	Wall facing towards the cheeks
Lingual/Palatal walls		Walls facing towards the tongue and palate, respectively
Incisal/Occlusal walls		Walls facing towards the incisal and occlusal portions of the tooth, respectively
Mesial/distal walls		Walls facing towards the mesial and distal aspects of the tooth, respectively
Axial wall		Wall nearest the pulp and parallel to the long axis of the tooth in cavities present on the axial surfaces
Pulpal wall		Wall nearest the pulp and perpendicular to the long axis of the tooth in cavities present on the occlusal surface or incisal edges of the teeth
Gingival wall		Wall facing the gingiva
Subpulpal wall		When the pulp chamber is accessed and the roof of the pulp chamber removed, the floor of the pulp chamber left behind is referred to as the subpulpal wall

- Gingival wall
- Axial wall

Walls in a Proximo Incisal Cavity (Class IV)

Incisal step
- Facial wall
- Lingual wall
- Mesial or distal wall (any one of these depending on which surface the cavity is present)
- Pulpal wall

Proximal portion
- Facioproximal wall
- Linguoproximal wall
- Gingival wall
- Axial wall

Walls in Facial and Lingual Cavities (Class V)
(Fig. 2.13)
- Mesial wall
- Distal wall
- Occlusal/incisal wall
- Gingival wall
- Axial wall

Walls in a Mesioocclusodistal Cavity

Mesial proximal box
- Facioproximal wall
- Linguoproximal wall
- Gingival wall
- Axial wall

Distal proximal box
- Facioproximal wall
- Linguoproximal wall
- Gingival wall
- Axial wall

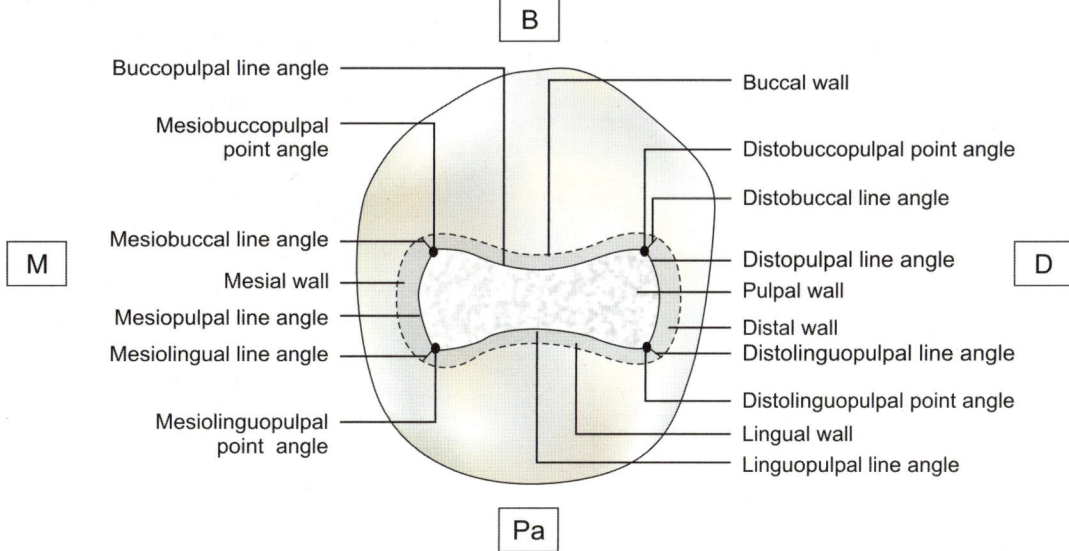

Fig. 2.10: Walls and angles in an occlusal Class I cavity (maxillary first premolar)

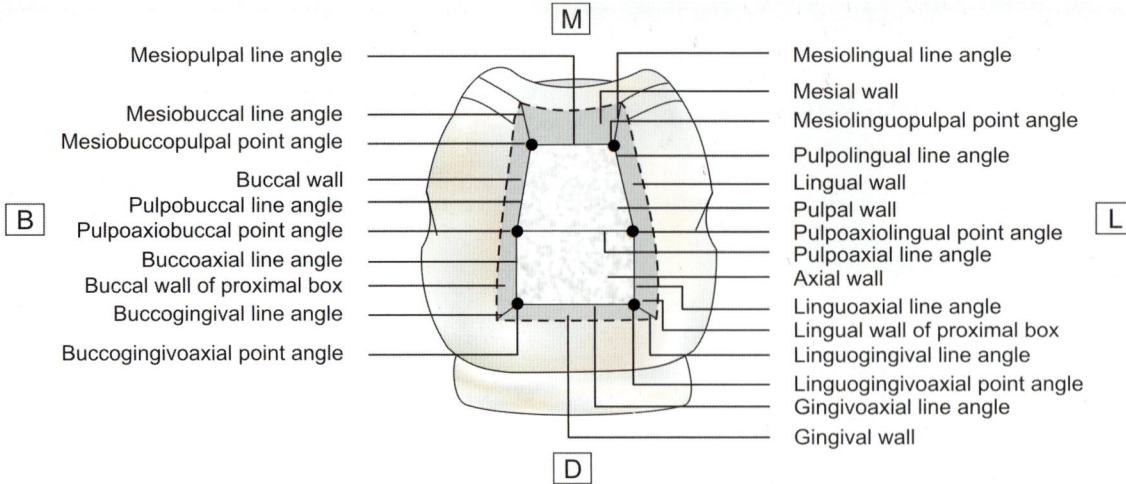

Fig. 2.11: Walls and angles in a Class II cavity (mandibular first molar)

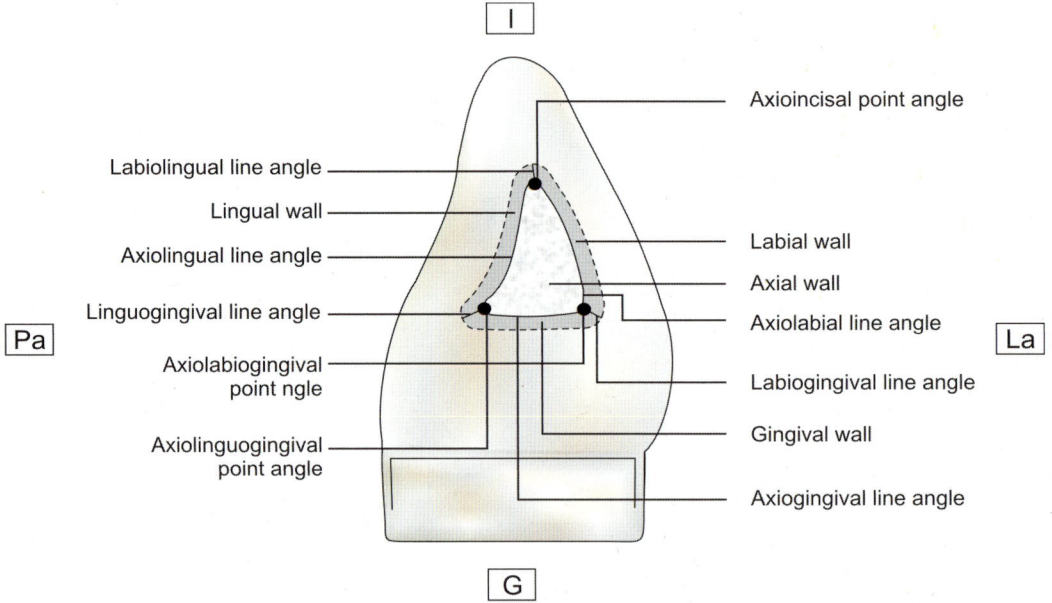

Fig. 2.12: Walls and angles in a Class III cavity (maxillary canine)

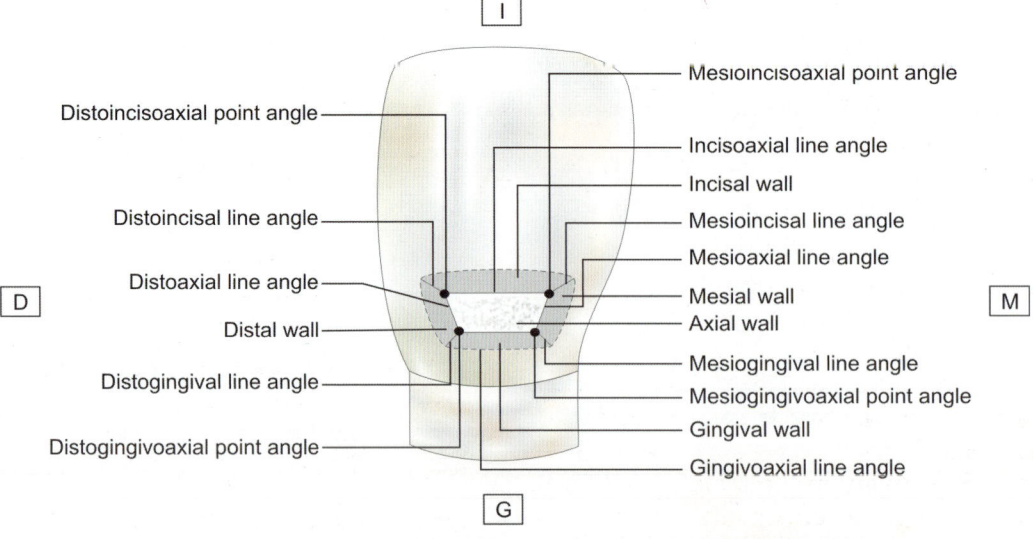

Fig. 2.13: Walls and angles in a Class V cavity (maxillary central incisor)

Occlusal portion
- Facial wall
- Lingual wall
- Pulpal wall

Various Angles in a Cavity Preparation

Angle: Junction of two or more surfaces of a prepared cavity is marked by an angle.

Line angle: The angle formed at the junction of two adjoining walls in a cavity preparation is referred to as a line angle. For example, angle formed between a mesial wall and a pulpal wall is called a mesiopulpal line angle.

Point angle: The angle formed at the junction of three adjoining walls in a cavity preparation is referred to as a point angle. For example, angle formed at the junction of mesial, buccal and pulpal walls is called a mesio-bucco-pulpal point angle.

Axial line angle: Any line angle parallel to the long axis of the tooth is called an axial line angle.

Pulpal line angle: Any line angle horizontal to the long axis of the tooth is called a pulpal line angle.

Cavosurface angle: Angle formed at the junction of the cavity wall and the unprepared tooth surface is referred to as the cavosurface angle. The junction between the cavity wall and the unprepared tooth surface is actually referred to as the cavosurface margin.

Bevel

Bevel, in dictionary terminology, is defined as any angle other than 90°, between the planes or surfaces. Earlier, bevel was placed only on cavosurface margins and defined as the rounding off of cavosurface margins at an angle.

Now with the bevels being given at various other surfaces of prepared teeth, it is defined as 'any abrupt incline between the two surfaces of prepared tooth or between the cavity wall and the cavosurface margins in the prepared cavity'.

Bevels are basically given to reduce the marginal errors (space between restoration and tooth surface).

Different types of bevels are:
a. *Partial bevel:* It involves part of the enamel wall (Fig. 2.14A). Such type of preparation is indicated in direct filling gold restorations. A few authors advise giving partial bevel in composite restorations to have more surface area.
b. *Short bevel:* It involves the entire enamel wall (Fig. 2.14B). This type of bevel is best suited in cast gold restorations.
c. *Inverted bevel:* It is given on the labial shoulder of metal ceramic crowns to effectively improve the esthetics at the margins (Fig. 2.14C).
d. *Reverse bevel:* A reverse bevel is placed at the dentinal portion of the cervical wall towards the axiogingival line angle (Fig. 2.14D). The hydrostatic pressure during cementing a cast restoration can produce a rotational displacement of the casting with flat gingival walls. This effect is resisted by the reverse bevel resulting in even seating of the cast restoration.

How to Combine Terms?

When one word is to be formulated by combining the names of two or more surfaces/walls, the 'al' ending of the prefix word is changed to an 'o', e.g. if mesial and occlusal is to be combined, the word so formulated is mesioocclusal and similarly if mesial, distal and occlusal have to be combined, the word so formulated is mesiodistoocclusal.

Angles in an Occlusal Cavity (Class I) (Fig. 2.10)

Line Angles
- Mesiofacial
- Mesiolingual
- Distofacial
- Distolingual
- Faciopulpal
- Linguopulpal
- Mesiopulpal
- Distopulpal

Point Angles
- Mesiofaciopulpal
- Distofaciopulpal

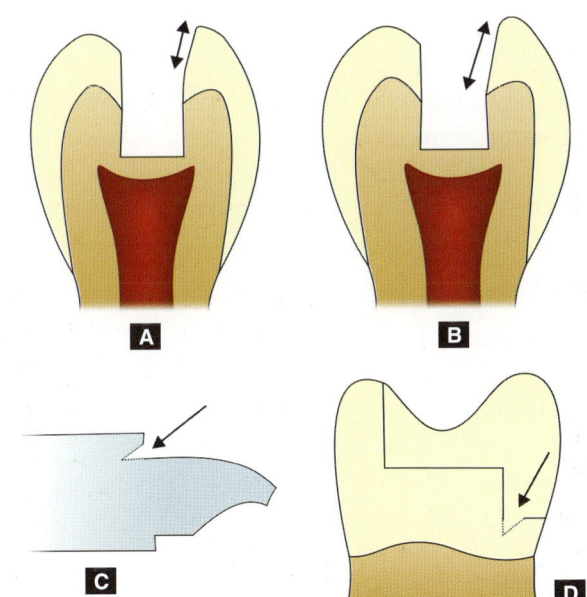

Figs 2.14A to D: Bevels: **(A)** Partial bevel; **(B)** Short bevel; **(C)** Inverted bevel and **(D)** Reverse bevel

- Mesiolinguopulpal
- Distolinguopulpal

Angles in a Proximoocclusal Cavity in Posterior Teeth (Class II) (Fig. 2.11)

Occlusal Portion

Line Angles

- Faciodistal or faciomesial
- Linguodistal or linguomesial
- Faciopulpal
- Linguopulpal
- Mesiopulpal/distopulpal
- Axiopulpal (this line angle is common to both the occlusal and proximal portions of the cavity preparation)

Point Angles

- Distofaciopulpal or Mesiofaciopulpal
- Distolinguopulpal or Mesiolinguopulpal
- Facioaxiopulpal ⎤ These point angles are
- Linguoaxiopulpal ⎦ common to both the occlusal and proximal portions of the cavity preparation

Proximal Portion

Line Angles

- Faciogingival
- Linguogingival
- Facioaxial
- Linguoaxial
- Axiogingival

Point Angles

- Faciogingivoaxial
- Linguogingivoaxial

Angles in a Proximal Cavity in Anterior Teeth (Fig. 2.12)

Line Angles

- Faciogingival
- Linguogingival
- Facioaxial
- Linguoaxial
- Axiogingival
- Faciolingual (incisal)

Point Angles

- Facioaxiogingival
- Linguoaxiogingival
- Faciolinguoaxial (axio incisal)

Angles in a Proximoincisal Cavity in Anterior Teeth (Class IV)

Incisal Step

Line Angles

- Faciomesial or faciodistal
- Linguomesial or linguodistal
- Faciopulpal
- Linguopulpal
- Mesiopulpal or distopulpal
- Axiopulpal (This line angle is common to both the occlusal and proximal portion of the cavity preparation).

Point Angles

- Faciomesiopulpal or faciodistopulpal
- Linguomesiopulpal or linguodistopulpal
- Facioaxiopulpal ⎤ These point angles are
- Linguoaxiopulpal ⎦ common to both the occlusal and proximal portions of the cavity

Proximal Portion

Line Angles

- Facioaxial
- Linguoaxial
- Faciogingival
- Linguogingival
- Axiogingival

Point Angles

- Faciogingivoaxial
- Linguogingivoaxial

Angles in Buccal and lingual Cavities (Class V) (Fig. 2.13)

Line Angles

- Mesioocclusal/Mesioincisal
- Distoocclusal/Distoincisal
- Mesiogingival
- Distogingival
- Occlusoaxial/Incisoaxial
- Gingivoaxial
- Mesioaxial
- Distoaxial

Point Angles

- Mesioocclusoaxial/Mesioincisoaxial
- Distoocclusoaxial/Distoincisoaxial
- Mesiogingivoaxial
- Distogingivoaxial

Nomenclature

Angles in Mesioocclusodistal Cavity

Mesial Proximal Box

Line Angles

- Facioaxial
- Linguoaxial
- Faciogingival
- Linguogingival
- Axiogingival
- Axiopulpal (This line angle is common to the occlusal and proximal portion of the cavity preparation)

Point Angles

- Facioaxiogingival
- Linguoaxiogingival
- Facioaxiopulpal ⎤ These point angles are
- Linguoaxiopulpal ⎦ common to both the occlusal and proximal portions of the cavity preparation

Distal Proximal Box

Line angles

- Facioaxial
- Linguoaxial
- Faciogingival
- Linguogingival
- Axiogingival
- Axiopulpal (This line angle is common to both the occlusal and proximal portions of the cavity preparation)

Point angles

- Facioaxiogingival
- Linguoaxiogingival
- Facioaxiopulpal ⎤ These point angles are
- Linguoaxiopulpal ⎦ common to both the occlusal and proximal portions of the cavity preparation

Occlusal Portion

Line angles

- Faciopulpal
- Linguopulpal

Other Commonly used Terms

Extension for prevention: It is the extension of the cavity preparation into areas that are caries susceptible. This principle was conceived by *Marshall Ebb* and later adopted by *G.V. Black*. But nowadays, clinicians are overdoing with this principle and more conservative preparations are becoming popular because of the caries immunity provided by preventive measures like fluoride therapy, improved hygiene and diet, enameloplasty, pit and fissure sealants, etc.

Enameloplasty: It is a conservative procedure in which narrow pits and fissures in the enamel can be ground off with a flame shaped bur to a smooth saucer shaped surface that is easily cleaned.

Prophylactic odontotomy: It is again a conservative procedure in which the developmental pits and fissures are minimally cut and restored with amalgam.

Pit and fissure sealant application: It is a procedure in which resin sealant is applied on to the deep pits and fissures without cutting any tooth structure. It is a non-invasive procedure.

Preventive resin restoration: It is a procedure in which a small bur is used to explore suspicious pits and fissures which are subsequently restored with composite and resin sealant.

Classification of Different Cavities

Dr. G.V. Black gave the first classification of cavities more than a hundred years ago (Table 2.3). It is still being widely used and universally accepted. Though Black originally divided the lesions in five categories; *Simon* later added the sixth (Fig. 2.15).

Modification of Black's Classification

Black's parameters for classification were controlled by a number of factors. These factors are still being followed with slight modifications to it. Black suggested:

Table 2.3: Classification of cavities as given by Dr. G.V. Black; Simon later added class VI cavity	
Class I cavities	Cavities beginning in the structural defects like pits and fissures that occur on the occlusal surfaces of premolars and molars, the occlusal two thirds of the buccal and lingual surfaces of the molars, the lingual surfaces of incisors and any other aberrant locations.
Class II cavities	Cavities in the proximal surfaces of premolars and molars
Class III cavities	Cavities in the proximal surfaces of incisors and canines, but not involving the incisal angle
Class IV cavities	Cavities in the proximal surfaces of incisors and canines but also involving the incisal angle
Class V cavities	Cavities in the gingival third of facial and lingual surfaces of all the teeth
Simon later added a sixth category as follows:	
Class VI cavities	Cavities on the incisal edges and cusp tips of all the teeth (Fig. 2.15)

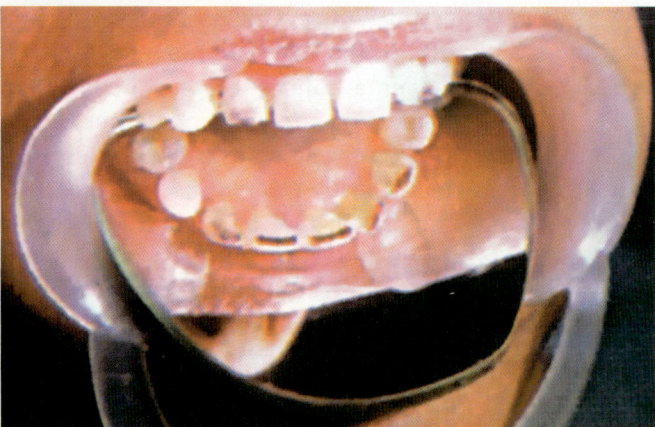

Fig. 2.15: Caries involving incisal edges of maxillary teeth

- Removal of tooth structure to gain access and to improve visibility.
- Removal of all traces of affected dentin from the floor of the cavity.
- Provision of mechanical retentive designs.
- Concept of extension for prevention.
- Keeping cavosurface margins at 'self cleansing' areas.

With the advent of newer adhesive restorative materials, fluorides, etc. the clinicians started following different cavity designs. The concepts given by Black became controversial and debatable. Tunnel preparations and slot preparations were introduced to avoid undue cutting of marginal ridge. However, all these procedures were discarded with time; either because of excessive marginal leakage at the cervical margins or weakening of the marginal ridge. The removal of caries was also not properly accomplished with these procedures.

The knowledge of the presence of two layers of carious dentin, one being infected and the other being affected; and also the phenomenon of remineralization of the affected dentin by fluorides and fluoride releasing restorative materials led to the belief that the affected part of dentin could be left as such.

The mechanical retention design in cavities has been questioned. 'Acid etching followed by bonding provides sufficient retention', was the initial thinking of researchers. The concept was soon challenged and various studies observed that only etching and bonding didn't provide sufficient retention. Therefore, though adhesive restorative dentistry has markedly improved the marginal adaptability of restorative materials to cavity walls but these are not ideal substitutes for retention form of cavity as given by Black.

The concept of 'extension for prevention' and keeping the proximal cavosurface margins in 'self cleansing' areas has also been questioned. Inspite of this, the validity of these principles in operative dentistry still exists.

Though Black's classification of cavities/carious lesions is simple, easily followed and universally accepted, certain areas of teeth where caries may occur have been overlooked. Also the spectrum of individual class is a little longer. For example:

i. Carious lesions at line angles of different teeth are not included (Figs 2.16A and B).
ii. Carious lesions on the labial surfaces of anterior teeth other than in cervical third are not included (Figs 2.17A and B).
iii. Carious lesions on the lingual surfaces of anterior teeth other than in the cervical third and pits are not included (Fig. 2.18).
iv. Proximal lesions, whether at one side or two sides are taken in one class. MOD cavities are always controversial in Black's classification. Few authors have designated MOD as class VI without any unanimity for its acceptance.

Mount (1998) has also classified carious lesions/cavities according to site and size as given in Table 2.4. He expresses a carious lesion by site and size.

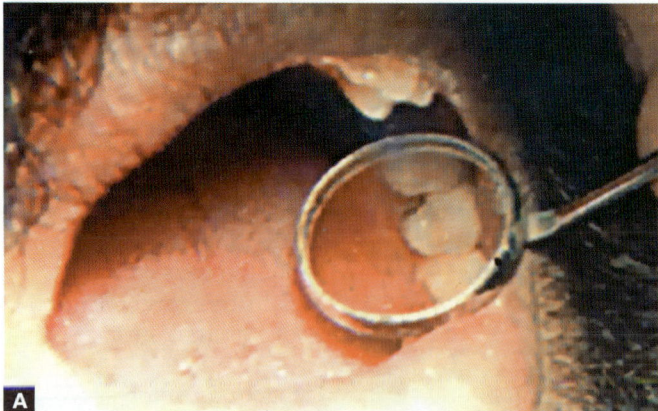 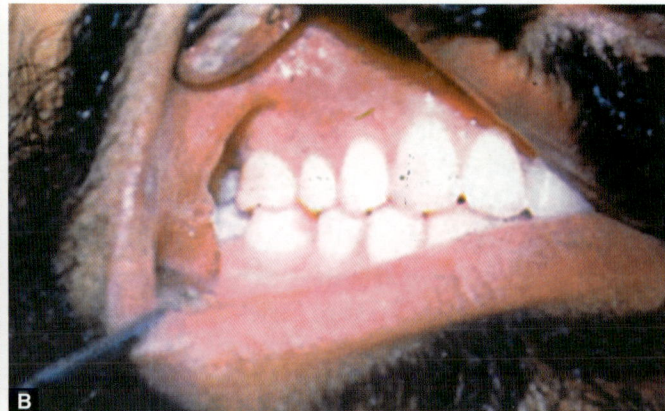

Figs 2.16A and B: (A) Caries involving distopalatal line angle of maxillary left first premolar; (B) Caries involving mesiobuccal line angle of mandibular right first molar

Nomenclature

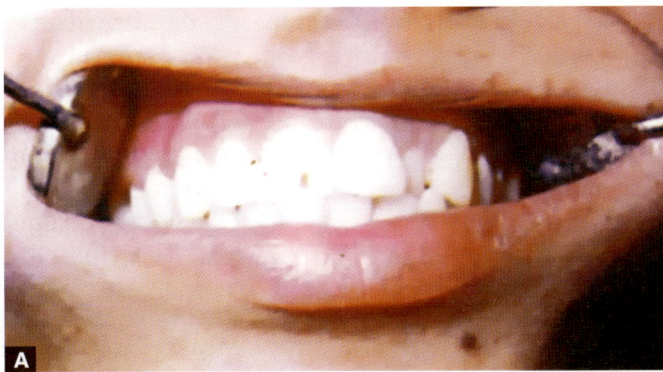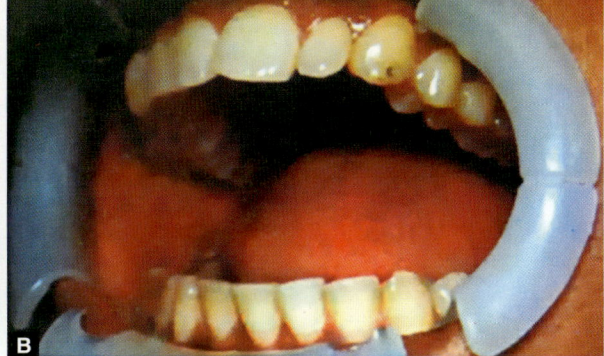

Figs 2.17A and B: (A) Carious lesion on the labial surface of maxillary right central incisor other than in cervical third; **(B)** Carious lesion on the labial surface of maxillary left canine other than in cervical third

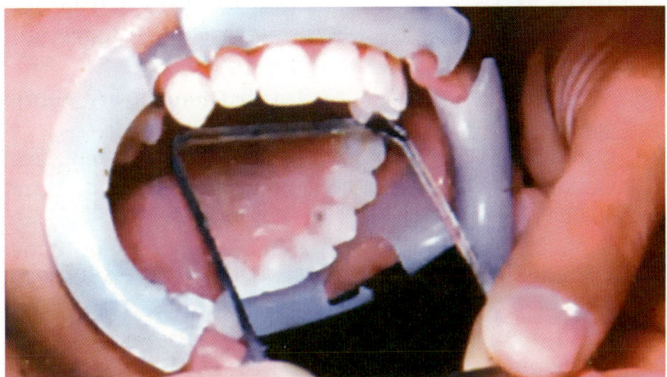

Fig. 2.18: Caries at the cingulum area

Table 2.4: Classification of carious lesions/cavities as given by Mount (1998)

	Site				
		Minimal	Moderate	Enlarged	Extensive
Size		1	2	3	4
Pit/fissure	1	1.1	1.2	1.3	1.4
Contact areas	2	2.1	2.2	2.3	2.4
Cervical	3	3.1	3.2	3.3	3.4

The explanation of sizes is:

1. Minimal involvement of dentin. Treatment by remineralization alone.
2. Moderate involvement of dentin. Treatment by cavity preparation. Remaining enamel is sound, well supported by dentin and not likely to fail under normal occlusal load. That is, the remaining tooth structure is sufficiently strong to support the restoration.
3. The cavity is enlarged beyond moderate size. The remaining tooth structure is weakened to the extent that cusps and incisal edges are split, or are likely to fail if left exposed to occlusal or incisal load. The cavity needs to be further enlarged so that the restoration be designed to provide support and protection to the remaining tooth structure.
4. Extensive caries with bulk loss of tooth structure has already occurred.

The proposed classification by Mount provides options for treatment planning, keeping in mind treatment by adhesive restorative materials. Though this concept is not entirely unfair, but there is always a subjectivity in deciding the size of the lesion. It may become difficult for an undergraduate to differentiate between different sizes; one half deciding it as size 3 and the other half as size 4 for the same lesion. Secondly, treatment planning varies with operator to operator. Thirdly, the carious sites mentioned earlier which are missing in Black's classification are also missing in this classification. Contact caries (site 2) whether on one side or two sides is taken as one, which is always misleading. And also clubbing root caries with crown caries creates confusion amongst readers.

Keeping in view the simplicity and acceptability of Black's classification, it should not be totally changed; however, little modifications will cover the areas left by Black. I propose a new modified classification, which is tabulated in Table 2.5.

The Class IV cavity of Black is not included in this classification, since with the advent of newer materials and techniques incisal edge involvement can be tackled safely. The proposed classification does not include root caries. I am of the firm belief that root caries should be dealt separately and in no way be clubbed with the crown caries. Class II Div. II clearly shows the involvement of both mesial and distal surfaces of posterior teeth and hence no confusion with the classification for MOD cavities. The changes are only in the Class IV and Class V cavities proposed by Black. Class V proposed by Black is class IV Div. I in the proposed classification and Class IV Div. II are the lesions at the cervical line angles. Class V in this proposed classification is added afresh and includes the lesions, which were not included in Black's classification.

Table 2.5: Classification of cavities as proposed by Dr. V.K. Sikri (1999)

Class	Div.	Description
Class I	Div. I	Cavities involving pits and fissures of occlusal surfaces
	Div. II	Cavities involving buccal and lingual pits of posterior and anterior teeth
Class II	Div. I	Cavities involving one proximal surface of posterior teeth
	Div. II	Cavities involving both proximal surfaces of posterior teeth
Class III	Div. I	Cavities involving one proximal surface of anterior teeth
	Div. II	Cavities involving both proximal surfaces of anterior teeth
Class IV	Div. I	Cavities on cervical one third of labial and lingual surfaces of all the teeth
	Div. II	Cavities on labial and lingual line angles of all the teeth
Class V	Div. I	Cavities on labial surfaces of anterior teeth other than cervical one third
	Div. II	Cavities on lingual surfaces of anterior teeth other than pits and cervical one third
Class VI	Div. I	Cavities on incisal edges
	Div. II	Cavities on occlusal cusp tips

The proposed classification is simple, includes all the surfaces which can be carious and the spectrum of each class is limited. Finally, the record keeping would be easier and the operator's subjectivity has also been taken care of. I believe, the proposed classification would be accepted for future use.

BIBLIOGRAPHY

1. Alhouri, N., Watts, D.C., McCord, J.F. and Smith, P.W.: Mathematical analysis of tooth and restoration contour using image analysis. Dent. Mater.: 20, 839, 2004.
2. Black, G.V. and Black, A.D.: A work on operative dentistry. Sixth eden. pp. 203, Medico Dental Publishing Co., London, 1924.
3. Blinkhorn, A.S., Choi, C.L.K. and Paget, H.E.: An investigation into the use of the FDI tooth notation system by dental schools in the U.K. Eur. J. Dent. Educ.: 2, 39, 1998.
4. Fusayama, T.: Two layers of carious dentin: diagnosis and treatment. Oper. Dent.: 4, 63, 1979.
5. Mount, G.J.: A new cavity classification. Aust. Dent. J.: 43, 153, 1998.
6. Osborne, J.W., Howell, M.L.: Marshall h. Webb and extention for prevention: A litreture review. Quint. Int, 30, 399, 1999.
7. Papa, J., Cain, C. and Messer, N.H.: Efficiency of tunnel restoration in the removal of caries. Quint. Int.: 24, 715, 1993.
8. Sigurjons, H.: Extension for prevention: Historical development and current status of G.V. Black's concept. Oper. Dent.: 8, 57, 1983.
9. Sikri, V.: Is it necessary to change Black's classification? J.C.D.: Vol. 2., No.1, 35, 1999.
10. Simon, W.J.: Clinical Operative Dentistry. W.B. Saunders Company, Philedelphia, 1956.
11. Van Noort, J.M.: Controversial aspects of composite resin. B.D.J.: 155, 380, Dec. 10, 1983.

Occlusion

The need for restorative dentistry has been steadily increasing with the improvement in the socioeconomic status and the awareness to preserve the natural teeth among the population. The basic objective of restorative dentistry is to develop the form, function and esthetics of the teeth to be in harmony with the stomatognathic system. We can achieve these objectives by understanding the nature of occlusion and functions of stomatognathic system.

The term *occlusion* is defined as *the static relationship between incising or masticating surfaces of maxillary and mandibular teeth or tooth analogues.*

Occlusion is also defined as 'the relationship between the occlusal surfaces of the maxillary and mandibular teeth when they are in contact'.

Different specialities of dentistry have different concepts of occlusion.

a. The prosthodontists follow the concept of *balanced occlusion*. They believe that the functional stability and effectiveness of complete dentures is maintained when there are simultaneous bilateral tooth contacts in lateral and protrusive excursions.
b. The orthodontists follow the concept of *morphologic occlusion*. According to them, the mesiobuccal cusp of maxillary first molar shall fall into the mesiobuccal groove of the mandibular first molar. Only when this relationship exists will the dentition be strong and stable and not produce any trauma to the periodontium. Based on this maxillomandibular relationship various types of occlusion have been classified.

- *Class I occlusion (neutro-occlusion or orthognathic)*: The mesiobuccal cusp of the maxillary first molar falls into the buccal groove of mandibular first molar (Fig. 3.1) and one or more teeth are crowded, malposed, rotated, in crossbite or in open bite, etc.
- *Class II occlusion (disto-occlusion or retrognathic)*: The mesiobuccal cusp of the maxillary first molar falls into the the embrasure between the mandibular second premolar and mandibular

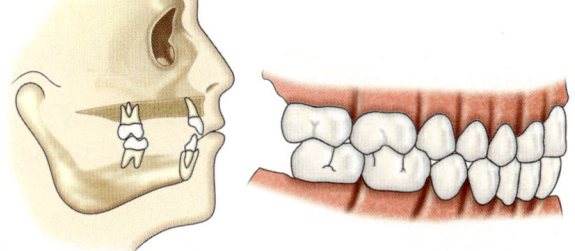

Fig. 3.1: Class I occlusion or normal occlusion

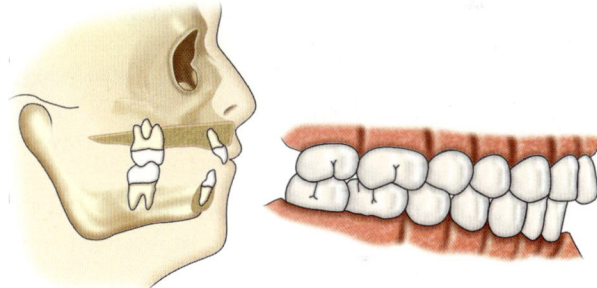

Fig. 3.2: Class II occlusion or disto-occlusion

first molar (Fig. 3.2), i.e. the mandible has moved distally than in class I occlusion.
- *Class III occlusion (mesio-occlusion or prognathism)*: The mesiobuccal cusp of the maxillary first molar falls into the embrasure between the mandibular first molar and mandibular second molar, i.e. the mandible has moved mesially than in class I occlusion (Fig. 3.3).

c. The third concept is the *functional/physiologic occlusion*, which is followed by operative dentists and periodontists. A functional occlusion is one which can function efficiently without pain and remains in a state of health regardless of the relationship between the maxillary and mandibular teeth, i.e. the relationship may be a class I, class II or class III molar relationship, or any other occlusal scheme but in case it is functioning efficiently without any pathological manifestations, the occlusion is physiologic.

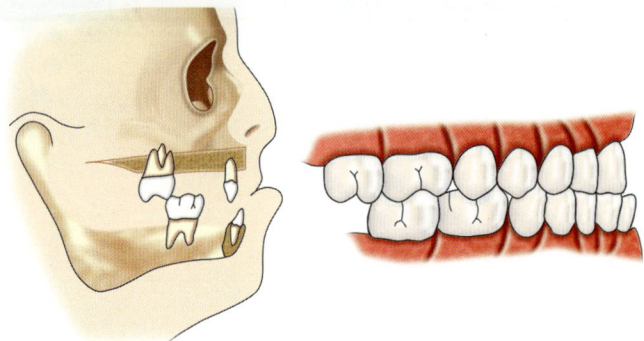

Fig. 3.3: Class III occlusion or mesio-occlusion

The characteristic features of functional occlusion are:
- Centric occlusion should produce stable maxillo-mandibular relationship at correct vertical dimension of occlusion. There should be an acceptable interocclusal distance between the vertical dimension of rest and vertical dimension of occlusion.
- Bilateral simultaneous contact between the supporting cusps and respective fossae or marginal ridges to ensure even and axial distribution of occlusal forces. Also, when in centric occlusion the condyles should be symmetrically related in their fossae.
- Initial contact in centric relation should preferably be bilateral and the subsequent 'slide in centric' should be in an anterior direction and 1.0 mm or less in extent.
- There should be harmony between the cuspal inclines during working and nonworking movements of the condyles.
- No premature contact should be present in any mandibular movements.
- On lateral excursion, either canine guidance or group function should be present on working side, with no contacts on nonworking side.
- On protrusion, there should be posterior disocclusion (no posterior contact).
- The masticatory forces should be distributed over as many teeth as possible in the intercuspal position (ICP).
- Bilateral contacts should be present between the posterior teeth in the retruded cuspal position (RCP).
- Structural harmony between occlusion and the temporomandibular joints helps in achieving neuromuscular harmony.

IDEAL VS NORMAL OCCLUSION

An ideal occlusion may be defined as *the most dynamic position, arrangement and relationship of one tooth with another tooth, of one arch with another arch and of both the arches with the base of the skull so as to perform the optimal functions of mastication, phonetics and esthetics maintaining the integrity and longevity of the individual tooth and the stomatognathic system.*

An ideal occlusion is difficult to achieve in any individual. A variety of occlusal patterns are present in different individuals and hence it is very difficult to define an ideal occlusal pattern. In operative dentistry, clinicians should prefer achieving a functional occlusion.

There is no unanimity in using the term *ideal occlusion*. Two different individuals can have different occlusions but if the occlusion is physiologic, it is normal for that particular person. The arrangement of the natural teeth, deviant though it may be, is still normal for that individual, as long as the function is satisfactory without pain or discomfort and without damage to supporting structures. No change is hence indicated even if the occlusion does not fit in the pattern of theoretical ideal occlusion. Such an occlusion is termed *normal*.

FUNCTIONAL OCCLUSION

The term *functional occlusion* is defined as *the contacts of maxillary and mandibular teeth during mastication and deglutition.*

Functional occlusion occurs in the segment of arch towards which the mandible moves and is divided into two—*lateral functional* and *protrusive functional occlusion*.

a. *Lateral functional occlusion* is predominantly guided by canines but involves sharing of contact by other posterior teeth in the functional working segment. There are two potential ranges of lateral functional contact on multicusped posterior teeth.
   i. The facial range of lateral functional occlusion involves mandibular facial cusps moving from their area of centric contact facially and slightly distally across the lingual inclines of maxillary facial cusps. Ideally, the lower cusp tips will pass through the embrasure spaces or grooves and the actual functional contact will occur on the distal inclines or ridges of these cusps. These facial range contacts may include all the cusps in the segment.
   ii. The lingual range of lateral functional contacts involves the tracking of maxillary palatal cusp tips from their areas of centric contact up the facial inclines of mandibular lingual cusps lingually. The lingual range of lateral functional contacts in natural dentition is undesirable. They are usually eliminated by occlusal adjustment or avoided when restorations are fabricated.
b. *Protrusive functional occlusion* occurs when the mandible moves forward, i.e. all mandibular anterior teeth will contact along the palatal inclines of maxillary anterior teeth. Frequently, protrusive contact will also involve the mesial incline of mandibular first premolar in contact with the palatal

surface of maxillary canines. The remainder of posterior teeth should be discluded by the guiding influence of anterior teeth during protrusive excursion.

NONFUNCTIONAL OCCLUSION

Nonfunctional occlusion or balancing contacts are undesirable in the natural dentition. However, in certain cases, a balanced nonfunctional occlusion may be necessary to provide adequate tooth guidance for mandibular excursion. Like functional occlusion, nonfunctional occlusion is also divided into two–*lateral nonfunctional* and *protrusive nonfunctional* occlusion.

a. *Lateral nonfunctional occlusion:* The contact occurs on the opposing inclines between the two zones of centric contact. When the mandible moves towards the lateral functioning side, the mandibular facial cusps on the nonfunctioning side move obliquely, lingually and mesially towards the maxillary palatal cusps along their facial inclines. Zone of potential nonfunctional lateral contacts hence can occur on lingual inclines of mandibular facial cusps and facial inclines of maxillary palatal cusps.

b. *Protrusive nonfunctional occlusion:* The contact may occur on either or both the right and left posterior segments. Two potential ranges can be seen:
   i. The facial range of protrusive nonfunctional occlusion occurs when the mesial cusp ridges of mandibular facial cusps contact the distal slopes of triangular ridges of maxillary facial cusps. These contacts are nonfunctional since they occur in the posterior segment during anterior movements of mandible and thus may interfere with protrusive functional contact of anterior teeth.
   ii. The lingual range of protrusive nonfunctional contacts occurs when distal cusp ridges of maxillary palatal cusps contact the mesial slope of triangular ridges of mandibular lingual cusps. The direction of the movement of the mandibular buccal cusps, during working (W), nonworking (NW), and protrusive (P) mandibular movements are shown in Figs 3.4 and 3.5, respectively.

PHYSIOLOGIC AND NONPHYSIOLOGIC OCCLUSION

Physiologic occlusion is defined as occlusion in harmony with the functions of masticatory system.

Nonphysiologic occlusion is defined as the occlusion which leads to or associated with traumatic lesions or disturbances in supporting structures of teeth, muscles and temporomandibular joint.

Occlusion should be examined before planning the restorative procedures to identify the signs and symptoms of nonphysiologic occlusion to correct them, if necessary.

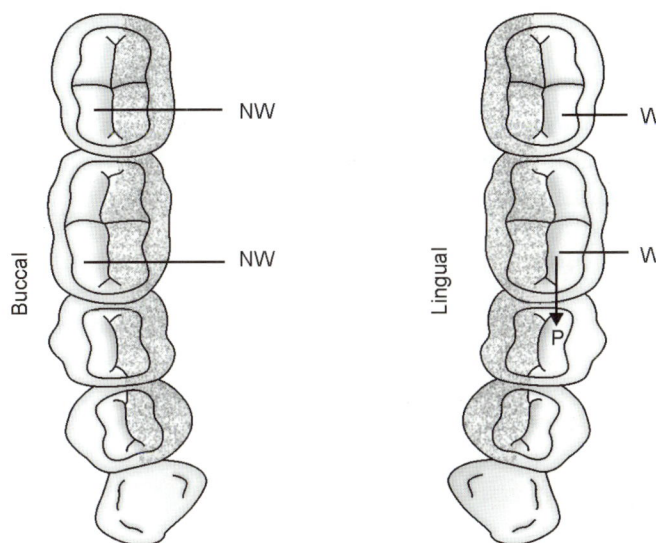

Fig. 3.4: The direction of movement of the mandibular buccal cusps (in arch) during working (W), nonworking (NW) and protrusive (P) mandibular movements

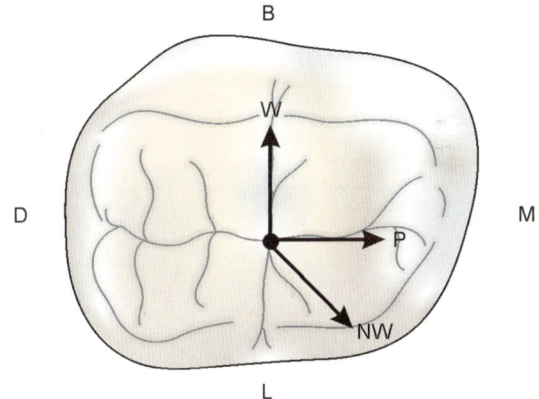

Fig. 3.5: The direction of movement of mandibular buccal cusps during working (W), non-working (NW) and protrusive (P) movements

CENTRIC RELATION

The definition of centric relation has undergone sea changes since the time it was first defined, despite the fact that the centric relation remains the same. Currently, the centric relation is defined as *"maxillomandibular relationship in which the condyles articulate with the thinnest avascular portion of their respective discs with the complex in an anterior superior position against the slopes of the articular eminences. This position is independent of tooth contact and clinically discernible when the mandible is directed superiorly and anteriorly. It is restricted to a purely rotatory movement about a transverse horizontal axis.*

The normal relationship of mandibular condyle to glenoid fossa and related structures is shown in Fig. 3.6. There are two schools of thought about the preciseness of centric relation. One school of thought believes it to be a precise location, whereas the other school of thought believes in some freedom from this position. The freedom in the antero-posterior direction is referred to as "long centric", while the freedom in the medio-lateral position is referred to as "wide centric" (Fig. 3.7).

In centric relation the mandible is in its terminal position and will rotate along a horizontal axis which is referred to as the *terminal hinge axis*. The condyles rotate around terminal hinge axis and the lower incisors also arc about 20–25 mm. This arc of movement is termed the *terminal arc of closure*. And the teeth make an initial contact during this closure called the *retruded contact position*.

CENTRIC OCCLUSION AND MAXIMAL INTERCUSPAL POSITION (MIP)

Centric occlusion is the position of maximum intercuspation of teeth which is in harmony with the neuromascular mechanism.

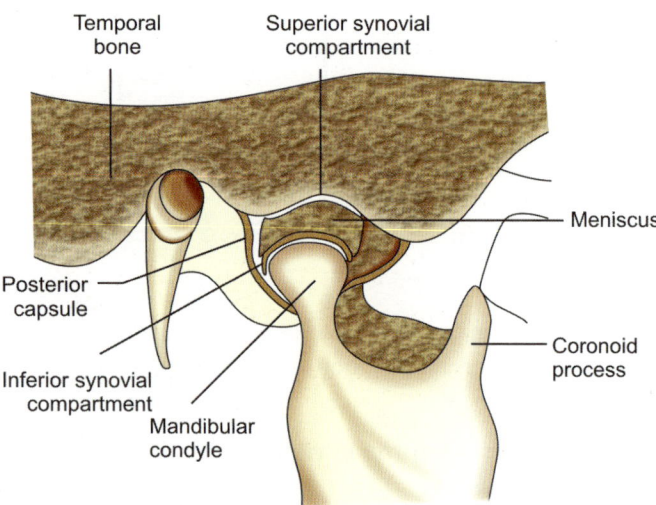

Fig. 3.6: Anatomy of temporomandibular joint (Schematic representation)

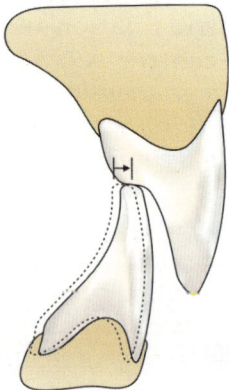

Fig. 3.7: Centric relation and the possible movement

Centric occlusion is defined as the occlusion of opposing teeth when the mandible is in centric relation. This may or may not coincide with the maximal intercuspal position.

Maximal Intercuspal Position is defined as the complete intercuspation of opposing teeth independent of condylar position, sometimes referred to as the best fit of the teeth regardless of the condylar position – also called maximal intercuspation.

Centric occlusion should always coincide with most retruded position of mandible while rehabilitating edentulous patients with complete dentures. However, only in a very small percentage of individuals with natural dentition, the centric occlusion will coincide with the centric relation. This is the principle of point centric concept.

However in most of the individuals with natural dentition, the centric occlusion is about 1 mm anterior to true centric relation. This is sliding centric or wandering centric. It is also called *long centric relation*. Normally in centric occlusion or maximal intercuspal position, the palatal cusps of maxillary molars contact the central fossae or the marginal ridges of mandibular molars, while the buccal cusps of mandibular molars contact the central fossae in marginal ridges of maxillary molars. These cusps are known as *supporting cusps*. The buccal cusps of maxillary and the lingual cusps of mandibular teeth that do not contact the opposing fossae and marginal ridges are called *nonsupporting cusps*. They are also called guiding cusps

In centric occlusion or maximal intercuspal position, the maxillary teeth overlap the mandibular teeth. The horizontal overlap of maxillary incisors to mandiular incisors is called *overjet* and the vertical overlap of maxillary incisors is known as *overbite*. The horizontal overlap of the posterior teeth is called *buccal overjet* and will help in preventing the cheek or tongue bite. The normal occlusal anatomy of maxillary first molar and mandibular first molar is depicted in Figs 3.8 and 3.9, respectively.

The cusps of posterior teeth are divided into four inclines. Each incline is named by the direction it faces. In mandibular molars, the inclines will be: mesiobuccal incline, distobuccal incline, mesiolingual incline and distolingual incline. For convenience, the inclines are further divided into two: outer incline and the inner incline. The inner inclines are surfaces between the cusp tip and the central fossa. Outer inclines are the surfaces that face outward towards the cheeks or tongue starting from the cusp tip.

Contacts that occur on cuspal inclines are called *poded contacts*. Stable centric contacts may contact two, three or four opposing inclines and hence are termed

Occlusion

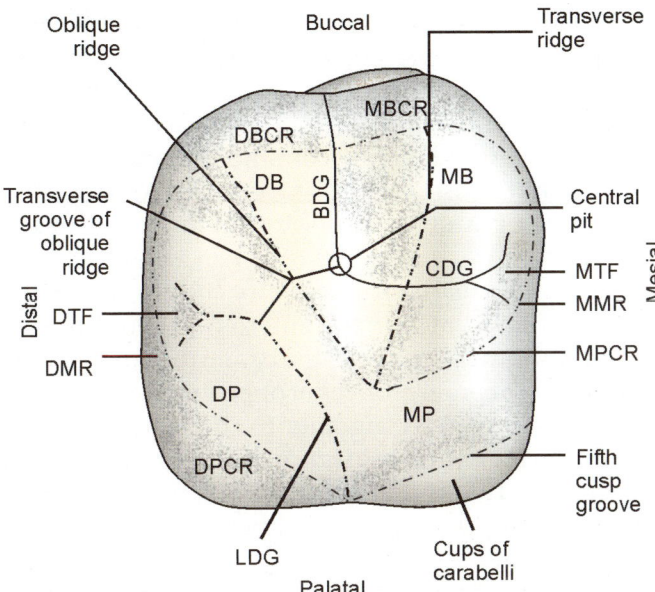

Fig. 3.8: Occlusal anatomy of maxillary 1st molar : MB-Mesiobuccal cusp, DB-Distobuccal cusp, DP-Distopalatal cusp, MP-Mesiopalatal cusp, BDG-Buccal developement groove, LDG-Lingual developmental groove, CDG-Central developmental groove, MTF-Mesial triangular fossa, DTF-Distal triangular fossa, MBCR-Mesiobuccal cusp ridge, DBCR-Distobuccal cusp ridge, DPCR-Distopalatal cusp ridge, MPCR-Mesiopalatal cusp ridge

bipoded contacts, tripoded contacts and *quadrapoded contacts*, respectively.

The maximal intercuspal position (MIP) does not coincide with the centric relation or retruded contact position in about 90% of the individuals while only in 10% of the individuals the maximal intercuspal position (MIP) coincides with centric relation or retruded cuspal position.

Potential Contact Areas of the Occlusal Surface

In an ideal arrangement of teeth, the facial to lingual zones of potential contact of maxillary posterior teeth are (Fig. 3.10):

Zone 1: Lingual inclines of facial cusps—lateral functional contact (facial range)
Zone 2: Central groove area—centric contact (facial range)
Zone 3: Facial inclines of palatal cusps—lateral nonfunctional contact
Zone 4: Lingual cusp tips-centric contact (lingual range)
Zone 5: Lingual inclines of palatal cusps—lateral functional contact (lingual range)

In an ideal arrangement of teeth, the facial to lingual zones of potential contact of mandibular posterior teeth are (Fig. 3.10):

Zone 1: Facial incline of facial cusp—lateral functional contact (facial range)
Zone 2: Facial cusp tips—centric contact (facial range)
Zone 3: Lingual inclines of facial cusps—lateral nonfunctional contact
Zone 4: Central groove area—centric contact (lingual range)
Zone 5: Facial inclines of lingual cusps–lateral functional contact (lingual range)

The cusp tips and lingual inclines of lingual cusps of mandibular posterior teeth normally have no contact potential. Similarly, the cusp tip and buccal inclines of buccal cusps of maxillary teeth normally have no contact potential.

Relationship Between Centric Relation and Centric Occlusion

Centric occlusion is also termed Intercuspal contact position (ICP). During closure of mandible in centric relation, the mandible slides forward to a position where the maxillary and mandibular teeth intercuspate maximum in centric occlusion.

Mostly there is an anterior and upward slide of the mandible from centric relation to centric occlusion. This slide, which occurs on the inclines of the premolars

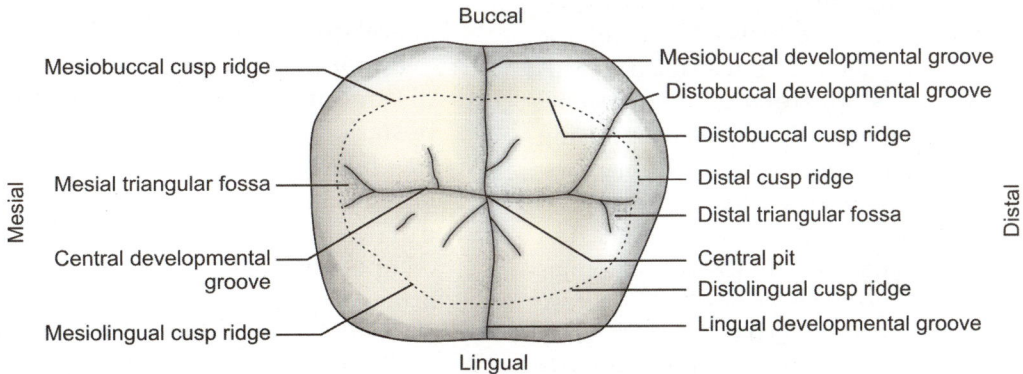

Fig. 3.9: Occlusal anatomy of mandibular first molar

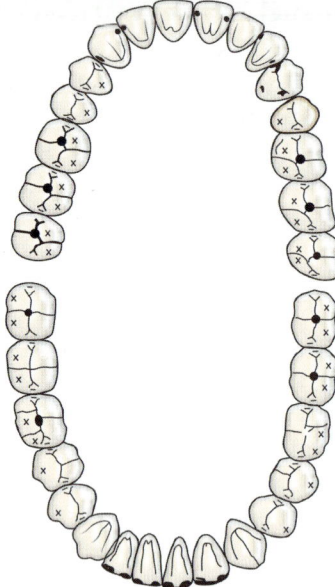

Fig. 3.10: Contact areas of mandibular and maxillary teeth in centric (x) contacts the (•) on the opposing teeth

and molars that come in contact during motion, seldom increases one millimeter. This slide and the actual contact varies from individual to individual. As the mandible slides from its initial point of premature contact in centric relation to centric occlusion, the condyles move downward and forward against the articular eminence. Rarely, the initial tooth contact in centric relation is that of maximum intercuspal relation of teeth. In such cases, where centric occlusion coincides with centric relation there is no slide of the mandible. Only if the patient and the musculature is relaxed, the clinician can guide the mandible into centric relation.

GUIDANCE OF OCCLUSION

Guidance is the influential effect of the temporomandibular joint and dental occlusion on the direction of mandibular movements. The following features help understanding the guidance of occlusion:

i. *Supporting cusps/Centric holding cusps/Stamp cusps* are the palatal cusps of maxillary molars and bicuspids and the buccal cusps of mandibular molars and bicuspids. The incisal edges of the mandibular anterior teeth are also used in this designation. Centric stops are the areas of contact that the supporting cusp makes with opposing teeth, e.g. Mesiopalatal cusp of maxillary first molar (supporting cusp) makes contact with central fossa (centric stop) of mandibular first molar. Supporting cusp-central fossa contact has been compared to mortar and pestle. Therefore the supporting cusp cuts, crushes and grinds fibrous food against the ridges forming the concavity of the fossa.

During restorative procedures, it is important that supporting cusps are not contacting the opposing teeth in a manner, which will result in lateral deflection of teeth. Rather the restorations should provide contact on smooth concave fossae so that masticatory stresses are directed approximately parallel to the long axis of the tooth.

ii. *Nonsupporting cusps/Noncentric holding cusps/Shear cusps* are located in the antero-posterior plane in facial and lingual embrasures or in the developmental grooves of opposing teeth creating an alternate arrangement when the teeth are in normal interdigitation. These cusps have sharper ridges that shear food as they pass close to the supporting cusp ridges during chewing momentum.

The supporting cusps have the following features compared to nonsupporting cusps:
- Supporting cusps contact the opposing teeth in intercuspal position. They support vertical dimension of face.
- These are nearer to the faciolingual centre of tooth than nonsupporting cusps.
- Their outer incline has a potential for contact.
- These have broader, much rounder cusp ridges than nonsupporting cusps.

iii. *Guiding inclines* are the bucco-occlusal inclines (lingual inclines of buccal cusps) of maxillary posterior teeth, lingual inclines of maxillary anterior teeth and the linguo-occlusal inclines (buccal inclines of lingual cusps) of mandibular posterior teeth.

The guiding inclines are the planes that determine the path of supporting cusps during normal and protrusive excursions.

iv. *Incisal guidance* is a direct product of vertical and horizontal overlap of anterior teeth. This relationship causes the mandibular anterior teeth to track downward from this area of centric contact as they move toward the incisal edges of their maxillary opponents during protrusive and lateral excursions (Fig. 3.11).

Importance of incisal guidance is to provide a discluding influence for teeth in nonfunctional posterior segments.

v. *Condylar guidance* refers to the path that the horizontal rotational axis of the condyles travels during normal mandibular opening. Three components of condylar guidance influence the articulation of teeth.

a. *Contour of articular eminence of the temporal bones*: Articular eminence is the surface of temporal bone that slopes downward and

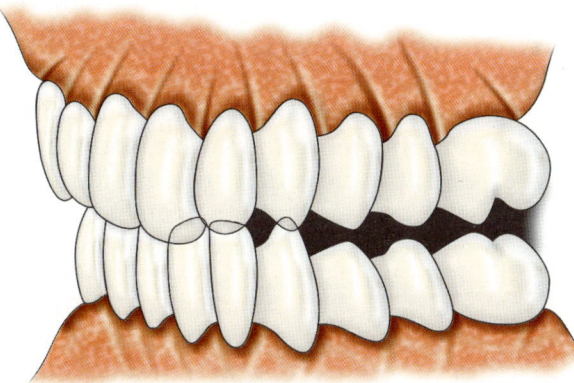

Fig. 3.11: Canine and incisor guidance (Working tooth guidance involving canines, central and lateral incisors)

forward from glenoid fossa of temporomandibular joint. The inclination of the eminence varies from one person to another and can vary between two sides of the same person. The condyles move downward along the eminence as the mandible moves forward.

This forward movement is called 'Translation'. Both condyles translate simultaneously along their eminences in protrusive functional movement.

In lateral functional movements, the condyle on the nonfunctional side translates forward along the eminence while the condyle on the working side rotates in its fossa. If the contour of eminence causes this translating condyle to move downward, this results in separation of posterior teeth on 'non-functioning side' of arch.

b. *Bennett shift*: It is the lateral bodily shift of mandible towards the working side in function and occurs to some extent in most patients during lateral functional movements. The amount and the timing of lateral shift influence the pattern of tooth contact during lateral excursion. The direction and travel of mandibular posterior cusps is influenced by amount and timing of Bennett shift.

c. *Inter-condylar distance*: It is the distance between the condyles. The inter-condylar distance affects the path of lateral functional movement of mandible since it determines the location of vertical axis of rotation in relation to mandibular arch. The farther the condyles are from mid-saggital plane, the more anterior is the path of lateral excursion and vice versa.

vi. *Cusp angle* is the angle made by the slopes of the cusp with a plane that passes through the tips of the cusps and is perpendicular to the line bisecting the cusp.

vii. *Plane of occlusion* is an imaginary surface that touches the incisal edges of incisors and tips of occluding surfaces of posterior teeth. This surface is not flat but curved.

viii. *Curve of spee* refers to the anteroposterior curvature of occlusal plane of posterior teeth, when a line is drawn from the tip of the mandibular canine along the tips of buccal cusps of mandibular posterior teeth (Fig. 3.12).

The greater the curve of spee, the more the posterior aspect of occlusal plane is in line with the translatory path of condyle, hence less will be the discluding influence of posterior guidance. This may cause nonfunctional contact in lateral and protrusive movements. The combined discluding influence of posterior guidance and anterior guidance must exceed the influence of the curve of spee to avoid undesirable nonfunctional contacts. Since posterior guidance is fixed and anterior guidance is usually determined before developing restorations for posterior teeth, the arc of curve of spee must be controlled so that lateral and protrusive nonfunctional contacts are eliminated in natural dentition.

According to *Thielemann's* formula,

$$\text{Balanced occlusion} = \frac{CG \cdot IG}{CS \cdot CA \cdot PO}$$

where,

CG : condylar guidance
CA : cusp angle
IG : incisal guidance
PO : plane of occlusion
CS : curve of spee

The cusp angle and the incisal guidance can be altered by occlusal adjustment in artificial teeth. This formula is used in artificial teeth, its use in natural dentition is limited.

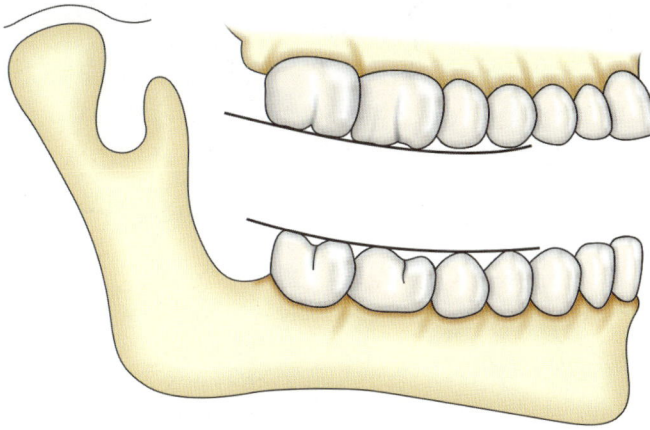

Fig. 3.12: The curve of spee

ix. *Curve of Wilson* refers to the transverse curvature of occlusal plane of posterior teeth, when a line is drawn from cusps tips of one side to the cusps tips of the other side (Fig. 3.13).

OCCLUSAL DESIGNS/SCHEMES

There are four basic designs or schemes of occlusion. The common features of all these designs or schemes of occlusion is that there is a simultaneous contact of the posterior teeth at closure.

The features of individual designs or schemes are as follows:
1. Bilateral balanced occlusion
2. Mutually protected occlusion
   a. Canine protected occlusion
   b. Group function occlusion (unilateral balanced occlusion)

Bilateral Balanced Occlusion

Bilateral balanced occlusion is not used as frequently today as it has been in the past. It is largely a prosthodontic concept which dictates that a maximum number of teeth should contact in all excursion positions of the mandible. This is particularly useful in complete denture construction, in which contact on the nonworking side is important to prevent tipping of the denture. Subsequently, the concept was applied to natural teeth in complete occlusal rehabilitation. An attempt was made to reduce the load on individual teeth by sharing the stress among as many teeth as possible. It was soon discovered, however, that this was a very difficult type of arrangement to achieve. As a result of the multiple tooth contacts that occurred as the mandible moved through its various excursion, there was excessive frictional wear on the teeth.

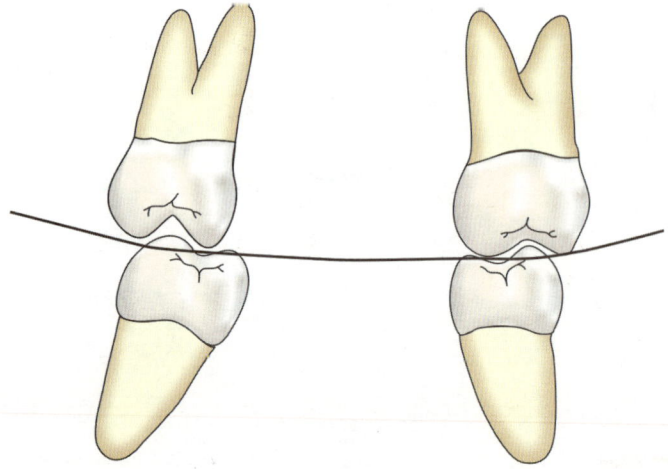

Fig. 3.13: The curve of Wilson

Mutually Protected Occlusion

Mutually protected occlusion (canine-protected occlusion) is also known as *organic occlusion*. A few authors observed that in many mouths with a healthy periodontium and minimum wear, the teeth was arranged so that the overlap of the anterior teeth prevented the posterior teeth from making any contact on either the working or nonworking sides during the mandibular excursion. This separation from occlusion was termed *disclusion*. According to this concept of occlusion, the anterior teeth bear all the load and the posterior teeth are disoccluded in any excursive position of the mandible. The desired result is an absence of frictional wear.

It is an occlusal scheme in which the posterior teeth prevent excessive contact of the anterior teeth in maximum intercuspation, and the anterior teeth disengage the posterior teeth in all mandibular excursive movements.

Features of Mutually Protected Occlusion

- In intercuspal position primary occlusal load is absorbed by posterior teeth (Figs 3.14A to C).
- Anterior teeth contact lightly and do not bear the load.
- During protrusion the overjet and overbite should cause disocclusion of the posterior teeth (Figs 3.15A and B).
- During lateral excursion the overjet and overbite relationship of the contacting teeth on working side should cause disocclusion of teeth on nonworking side (Figs 3.16A to C).
- On the working side either the canines (canine protected) or the canines, premolars and molars may be in contact (group function).
  a. *Canine protected occlusion:* The theory of canine protected occlusion is based on the impression that the canine tooth is the most appropriate tooth, which guides the mandibular excursion (Fig. 3.17).
     It is a form of mutually protected articulation in which the vertical and horizontal overlap of the canine teeth disengage the posterior teeth in the excursive movements of the mandible.
  b. *Group function occlusion:* Group function Occlusion (unilateral balanced occlusion), is a widely accepted method of tooth arrangement in restorative dental procedures today. This concept has its origin in the work of Schuyler and others who began to observe the destructive nature of tooth contact on the nonworking side (Fig. 3.18).

Therefore, unilateral balanced occlusion calls for all teeth on the working side to be in contact during

Occlusion

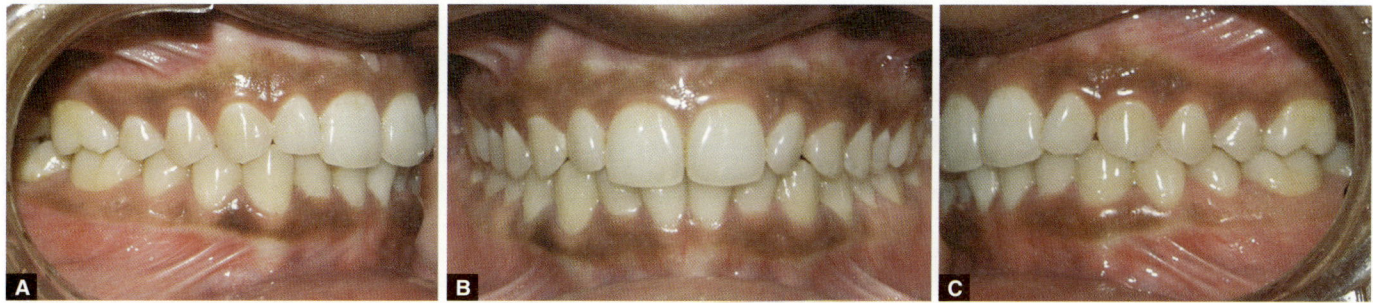

Figs 3.14A to C: Intercuspal positions

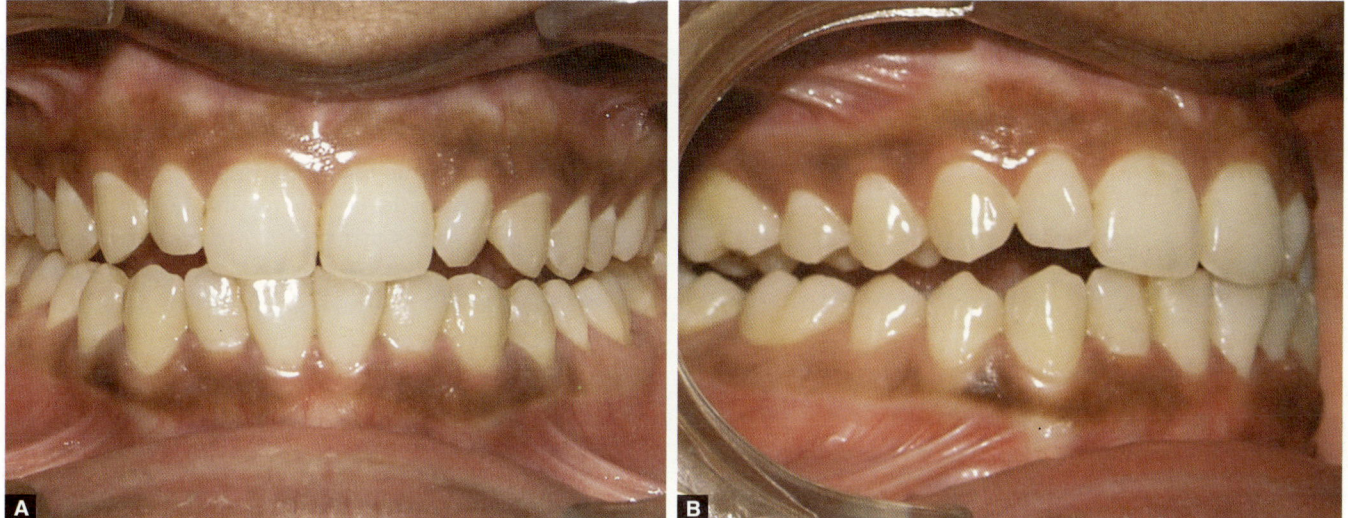

Figs 3.15A and B: **(A)** Protrusive movement; **(B)** Disocclusion of posterior teeth in protrusive movement

lateral excursion. On the other hand, the teeth on the nonworking side are contoured to be free of any contact. The group function of the teeth on the working side distributes the occlusal load. The absence of contact on the nonworking side prevents those teeth from being subjected to the destructive, obliquely directed forces found in nonworking interference. It also saves the centric holding cusps, i.e., the mandibular buccal cusps and the maxillary lingual cusps, from excessive wear. The obvious advantage is the maintenance of the occlusion.

OCCLUSION AND RESTORATIVE DENTISTRY

Analysis of Occlusion Prior to Restoration

Prior to restoration on any tooth, it is imperative for the restorative dentist to examine and analyse the pre existing occlusion. The occlusion can best be examined by consultation, physical examination and analysis of occlusal functions. Further analysis can be carried out using articulators. A diagnosis of the disturbances in occlusion, if any should be eliminated and made prior to the restoration of the teeth.

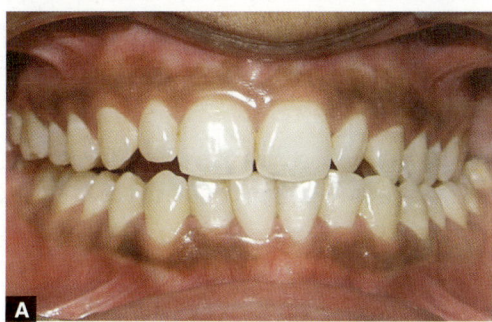 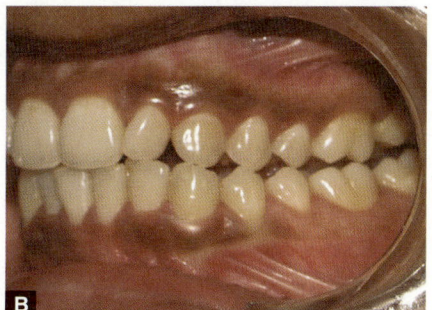 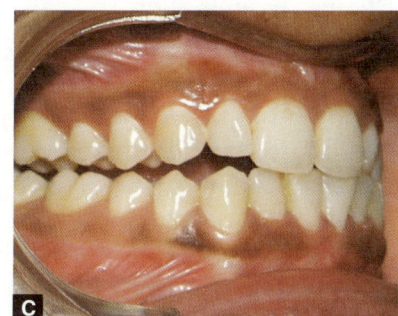

Figs 3.16A to C: **(A)** Left lateral movement; **(B)** Working side contacts; **(C)** Disocclusion on non working side

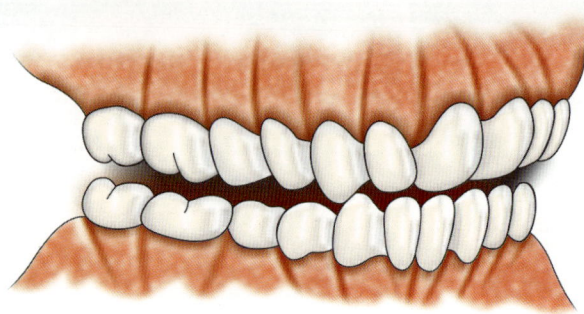

Fig. 3.17: Canine guidance (working tooth guidance involving canines)

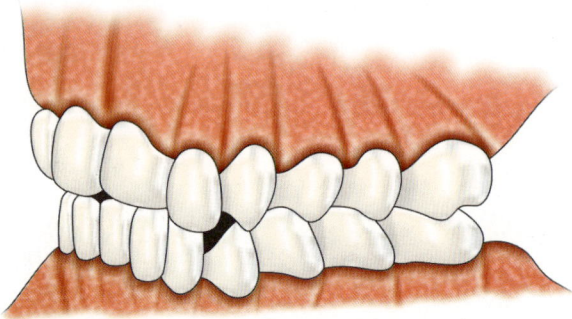

Fig. 3.18: Group function guidance (working tooth guidance involving canines, premolars and molars)

Building a rapport with the patient during the initial conversation in a congenial atmosphere is important. The objective is to recieve accurate information from the patient regarding occlusal disharmony. Certain questions, which can lead to initial diagnosis are:
- Any difficulty in chewing.
- Clicking of teeth or joints during chewing.
- Any difficulty in opening the mouth.
- Any para functional habits such as nail biting, clenching, grinding, etc.
- Bleeding gums while chewing.
- Discomfort with the previous restorations, if any.

The information assimilated from the history will help us in making a preliminary diagnosis of occlusal prematurities or Temporo mandibular joint problems, if any.

Clinical Examination

Care must be taken to assess the oral hygiene status and the health of the periodontium. It is also important to observe the missing, carious and filled teeth. The clinical examination should also include the observation of the following:
- The pattern of occlusal wear.
- Malposition of individual tooth like tipping of teeth.
- Interferences, if any in the cusp-fossa or cusp-ridge relationship.
- Presence of plunger cusps and/or open contacts.
- Tilting, supra eruption or malposition of teeth.
- Periodontal conditions of teeth to include–tenderness, hypermobility or pathological migration.

The information obtained from the clinical examination should be further examined in the light of radiographic examination and the study of diagnostic casts.

The intra oral radiographs or panoramic radiograph will depict the changes in the alveolar bone structure and will also reveal the information regarding bone loss.

The examination of the study casts will help us in gathering information about the morphology of the teeth, intra and inter arch relationship. It will also help us in observing the presence of wear facets, tipping of teeth, supra eruption, migration, open contacts and the presence of plunger cusps

The ideal dynamic relationships are not present in a significant proportion of the population and yet they do not have signs and symptoms of disorder. Adaptation within the stomatognathic system is important. The adaptive capacity may be reduced with age, illness and/or stress. Thus in some individuals, a minor occlusal disturbance (tilted teeth), which previously was a physiologic response might become pathological. Generally, in the absence of any signs or symptoms of trauma from occlusion, prophylactic removal of non ideal contacts is not advisable. These non ideal contacts do have the potential to become interferences, which may require occlusal adjustments at a later date.

In the absence of any signs and symptoms of trauma from occlusion, the restorations of the teeth should be in harmony with the patient's existing maximal intercuspal position. While restoring cases of full mouth rehabilitation, the maximal intercuspal position should be made to coincide with the centric relation of the patient.

Articular Analysis

The occlusal contacts in maximal intercuspal position and during functional or non functional movements are difficult to be examined intra orally. Even when the lips are parted, only the labial and buccal aspects of the teeth are visible and not the lingual aspect of the teeth. Casts mounted on articulator which simulates mandibular movements will help us in examining the occlusion from all aspects.

Let us first study the types of articulators, process of articulation and its significance in restorative dentistry.

Articulators and Articulation

Restoring the occlusion satisfactorily is the basis of treatment in almost every branch of dentistry. The

Occlusion

poorly restored teeth can lead to iatrogenic problems. Many a times, ignorance or poor knowledge of occlusion leads to flat restorations or cuspless restorations. Such restorations affect the health and function of the underlying periodontium and the stomatognathic system. The cuspal occlusion directs the forces of mastication along the long axis of the tooth. The proprioception of the teeth satisfactorily restored will help in regulating the mandibular movements.

Cast and ceramic restorations need elaborate fabrication procedures, which cannot be performed intra-orally. Articulators in such situations simulate patient in the absence of a patient.

"An articulator is a mechanical device, which represents the temporomandibular joints and the jaw members to which maxillary and mandibular casts may be attached to simulate jaw movements."

An articulator has an upper member and a lower member to which the maxillary and the mandibular casts are attached using dental plaster.

Articulation is defined as "the static and dynamic contact relationship between the occlusal surfaces of the teeth during function."

Based on the design of the articulator, the movement between the upper and lower members of the articulator can range from a simple hinge movement to simulation of mandibular movements.

Articulators can also be broadly classified as Arcon and Non-Arcon articulators based on the attachment of the condylar elements to either the lower or upper member of the articulator. When the condylar elements are attached to the lower member, the articulator is called as Arcon articulators and when it is attached to the upper member, it is called as Non-Arcon articulator.

The term Arcon is derived from the first two letters of ARticulator and the first three letters of CONdyle. The movement of the Arcon articulators are similar to the movements of mandible, since the condylar elements are attached to the lower member of the articulator.

Examples of Arcon articulator: Hanau H2, Hanau wide vue, Panadent, etc.

Examples of Non-Arcon articulator: Hanau H, Trubyte, Dentatus, etc.

Types of Articulators

a. *Hinge articulator:* The hinge articulator is basically a cast holder. Only opening and closing movements are possible. There is no possibility of lateral or protrusive movements. Its application is limited to restoration of a single tooth in an otherwise dentate arch. Such an articulator cannot be used for diagnostic purposes.

b. *Plane line and mean value articulator:* Mean value articulators permit a limited degree of protrusive and lateral movements based on the mean values. Normally the condylar guidance of articulator is set at 30° and the Incisal guidance at 15°. These articulators are best suited for fabricating individual crowns or a three unit fixed partial dentures. Fig. 3.19

c. *Semiadjustable articulator:* The semiadjustable articulator is routinely used in restorative dentistry. (Figs 3.20A and B) These articulators accept a facebow transfer to relate the maxillary cast to the hinge axis. Facebow correctly position the maxillary cast spatially in three dimensions by way of the third reference point (orbital plane).

These instruments simulates condylar pathways by using average or mechanical equivalents for all or part of their motion. The horizontal and lateral condylar guidances of the semiadjustable articulators can be programmed using interocclusal record obtained from the patient.

Advantages

- Orients the maxillary cast to the hinge axis of the articulator as it is in the patient's mouth.

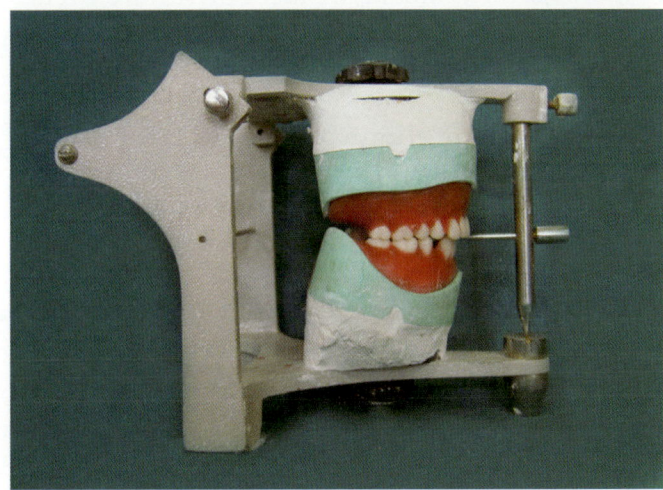

Fig. 3.19: Mean value articulator

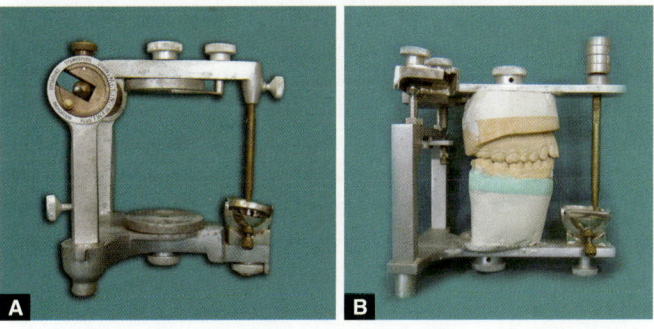

Figs 3.20A and B: **(A)** Hanau semiadjustable articulator; **(B)** Whipmix semiadjustable articulator

- Transfers the retruded path of closure or centric relation.
- Simulates the condylar guidance as it is in the patient.
- Approximate lateral shifts.
- Incisal guide table can be adjusted.

Limitations

- The path traced by the condylar from centric relation to protrusion is curvilinear, where as the protrusive interocclusal record helps us in obtaining a straight path between centric relation and protrusion.
- Arbitary facebow does not locate the true hinge axis. It helps us only in the approximation of the retruded hinge.

d. *Fully adjustable articulators:* These articulators require pantographic tracing to customize the articulator for the individual requirements. These instruments apart from being expensive, are also technique sensitive and therefore are not routinely used for restorative purposes.

Pantographic tracing includes the use of six styli and tracing tablets attached to the maxilla and the mandible by means of facebow and clutches attached. The mandibular position and pathways recorded on the tracing tablets are transferred onto an articulator.

In order to eliminate the time-consuming procedure of transferring the tracings to the articulator, Denar developed the pantronic, an electronic pantograph which provides a computer print out of numerical condylar measurements.

e. *Stereographic or fossa moulded:* These instruments utilize the records from pantographic tracings to customise the condylar guidances using autopolymerising acrylic resins. The engravings of the acrylic is used to simulate the mandibular movements. Swenson TMJ instruments is one such example of this type of articulators.

The Facebow Records

The relationship and the orientation between the terminal hinge axis and the maxilla differs from one individual to another. If this relationship between the terminal hinge axis and the maxilla is transferred from the patient to the articulator, the movements of the articulator, after customising the condylar guidances will closely simulate the mandibular movements.

An instrument which is used to transfer this relationship between the maxilla and the terminal hinge axis from the patient to the articulator is called a facebow (Figs 3.21A and B).

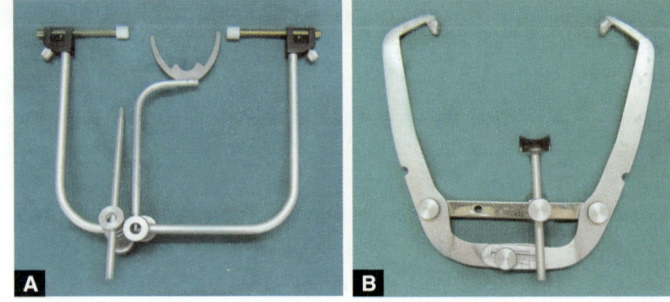

Figs 3.21A and B: **(A)** Hanau facebow; **(B)** Whipmix facebow

A Facebow is *a caliper like device to record the spatial relationship of maxillary arch to some anatomic reference points or point and then transfer this relationship to an articulator; it orients the dental casts in the same relationship to the opening axis of the articulator.*

Facebows can be broadly grouped as arbitrary facebows and kinematic facebows. Arbirtary facebows are used to transfer the orientation relation from the patient to the articulator. Kinematic faceow is used to record the true hinge axis.

The bitefork of the kinematic facebow is attached to the mandible and using the hinge movements of the mandible, the terminal hinge axis can be located. Kinematic facebow is used only when true hinge axis needs to be located for diagnostic restorative procedures.

Arbitary location of the hinge axis is adequate for transferring the orientation relation for most of the restorative procedures. The arbitrary hinge axis is located 13 mm anterior to the tragus on a line drawn from the center of tragus to the outer canthus of eye. This point is called Beyron's point (Fig. 3.22).

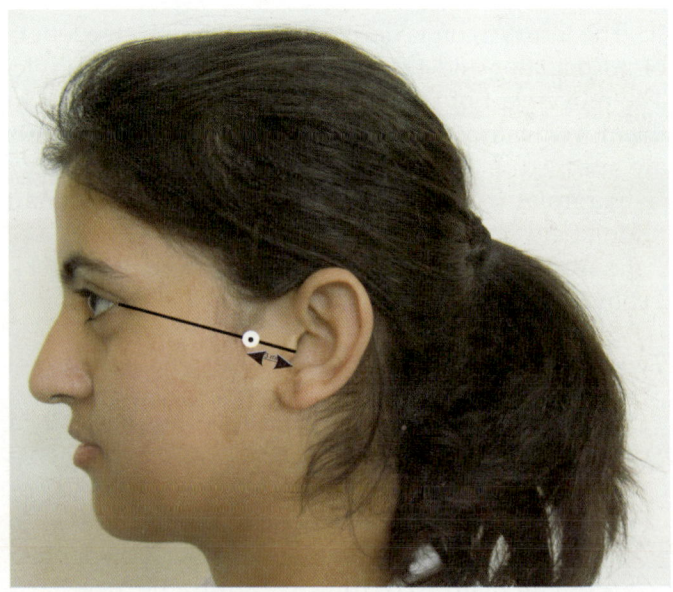

Fig. 3.22: Beyron's point

Occlusion

The facebows have a condylar rod element or an ear piece and a bitefork screwed to each other by a vertical rod and thumbscrews. The condylar element or the earpiece is placed at external auditory meatus. The bitefork is related to the maxillary arch through an impression of the occlusal surfaces. The relationship between the condylar elements/earpiece and the bitefork is recorded and transferred onto the articulator. The maxillary cast is then placed on the bitefork and is attached to the upper member of the articulator to complete the transfer of orientation relation.

Facebows normally use orbitale or nasion as the third point of reference to orient the occlusal plane in its sagittal relationship to the horizontal plane (Figs 3.23A and B).

Articulation of Casts

After mounting the maxillary cast onto the articulator using a facebow transfer, the mandibular cast is then related to the maxillary cast using an interocclusal record. An interocclusal record made in centric relation is used to mount the mandibular cast onto the articulator for diagnostic purposes and to examine the occlusal contacts in centric relation position.

In the absence of any signs and symptoms of trauma from occlusion or temporo mandibular joint disturbances, an interocclusal record made in maximal intercuspal position is used to mount the mandibular cast onto the articulator to develop the occlusal morphology of the restorations.

Mounting the casts on a semi-adjustable articulator using a facebow transfer and an interocclusal record are mandatory to refine the occlusion in lateral excursions and whenever there is a need to alter the vertical dimension on the articulator (Fig. 3.24) When

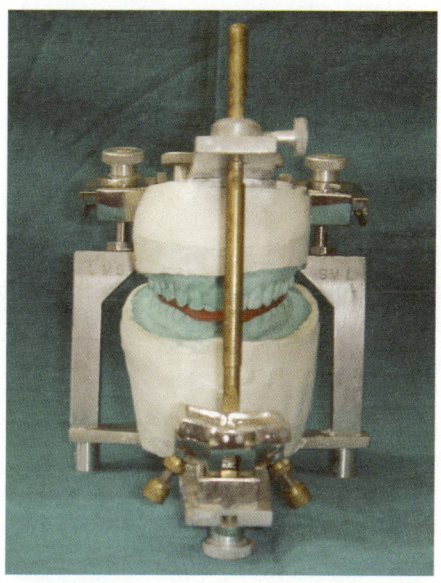

Fig. 3.24: Cast along with interocclusal record mounted on articulator

occlusion needs to be developed in a static relationship, the maxillary and the mandibular casts can be mounted on a simple mean value articulator using only an interocclusal record.

Interocclusal Records

Interocclusal records are used to relate the mandibular casts to the maxillary casts in retruded contact position or in maximal intercuspal position. Interocclusal records can be used to relate the mandile to the maxilla in a protrusive or lateral excursive position to customise the condylar guidances.

The interocclusal records should be made in a material which is dimensionally stable and can actually relate the mandibular and the maxillary casts.

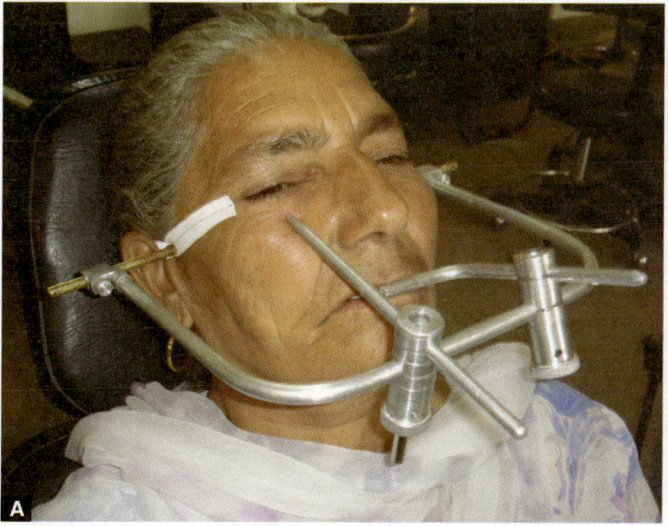
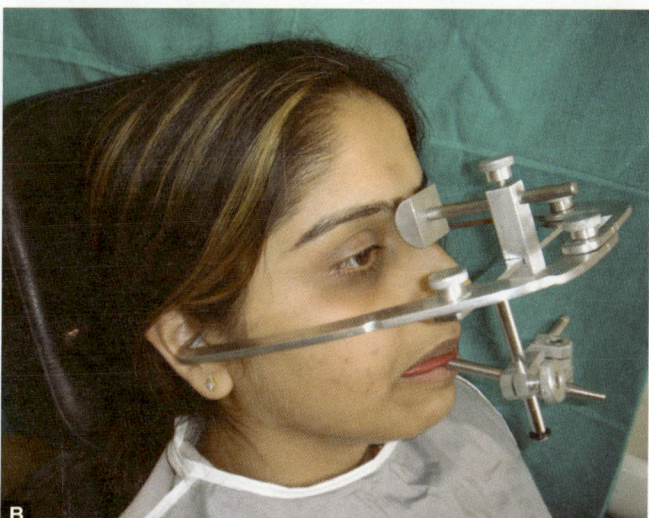

Figs 3.23A and B: (A) Hanau facebow recording (orbital reference point); (B) Whipmix facebow recording (nasion reference point)

The ideal interocclusal record material should have the following properties:
- The material should be soft and mouldable.
- The material should not displace the soft tissues or teeth.
- The material should not guide the mandibular movements
- The material should be dimensionally stable.

Some of the examples of the interocclusal recording medium are alu wax, bite registration wax, hard baseplate wax and impression plaster.

The interocclusal recording material is manipulated according to the manufacturers instructions and is then used to make the interocclusal record in the desired mandibular position (Fig. 3.25). The set interocclusal record can then be used either to mount the cast or to customise the condylar guidances of the articulator. To ensure the accuracy of the mounting a shimstock can be used to verify whether the intra oral occlusal contacts coincides with the occlusal contacts on the articulated casts.

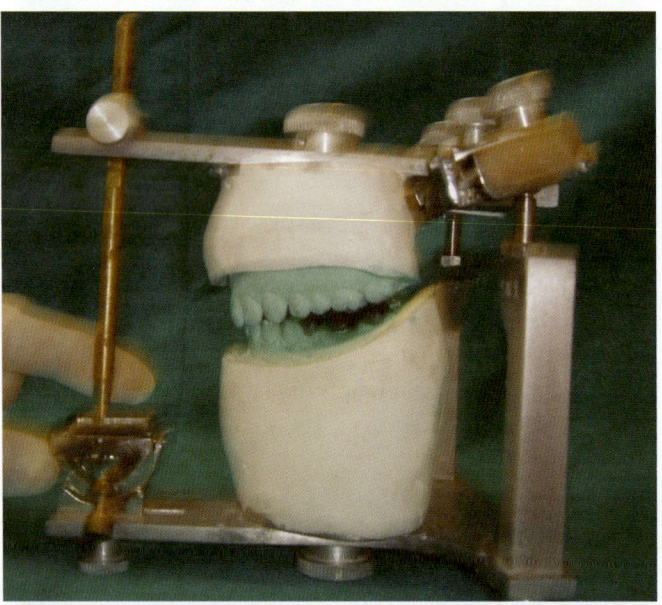

Fig. 3.25: Adjusting interocclusal records during mandibular movements

The type of interocclusal records, articulators and potential interferences with various types of restorations are depicted in Table 3.1.

Occlusal Records for Restoring a Single Posterior Tooth

The interocclusal record is made covering only the prepared teeth with the unprepared teeth in occlusion. The stepwise procedure is:

- The hard baseplate wax is softened in warm water.
- Two sheets thickness of hard baseplate wax is cut to cover the width and length of the prepared tooth/teeth. The cut and softened wax is placed over the prepared teeth. The mandible is guided into the intercuspal position.
- Allow the wax to return to the mouth temperature. Cool it with air-water spray and remove it from the mouth.
- Examine the interocclusal record and if further refining is required, it can be relined with zinc oxide eugenol paste.

Now the interocclusal record is ready for relating the cast and mounting it to an articulator (Figs 3.26A to C).

Occlusal Records for Restoring all Posterior Teeth in a Single Arch

When all the posterior teeth in a single arch is to be restored, the occlusion can be developed in centric relation. The procedure is as follows:

- Establish the vertical dimension of occlusion before the tooth preparation.
- An interocclusal record can be made with two sheets thickness of hard baseplate wax or any other suitable interocclusal recording medium.
- Soften and place the wax over the prepared teeth.
- Guide the mandible into centric relation.
- Allow the wax to return to the mouth temperature. Cool it with air-water spray and remove it from the mouth.
- Examine the interocclusal record and if further refining is required, it can be relined with zinc oxide eugenol paste.

Table 3.1: Type of interocclusal records, articulators and potential interferences with various types of restorations

Type of restoration	Inter-occlusal records	Articulators	Potential interference
Single anterior unit	MIP	Mean value articulator	Protrusive RCP
Single posterior unit	MIP	Mean value articulator	Protrusive lateral RCP
Multiple anteriors	MIP Protrusive	Semiadjustable articulator	Protrusive lateral RCP
Multiple posteriors in one arch	MIP, protrusive, lateral	Semiadjustable and facebow transfer	Protrusive lateral minimal RCP
Multiple posteriors in both arches	Protrusive, lateral	Semiadjustable and facebow	Protrusive lateral minimal RCP transfer or fully adjustable

Occlusion

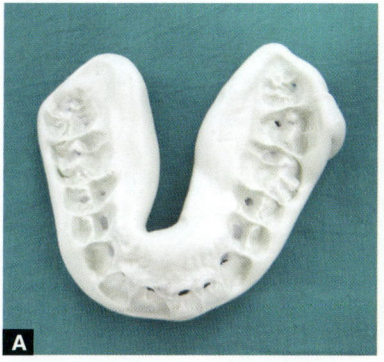 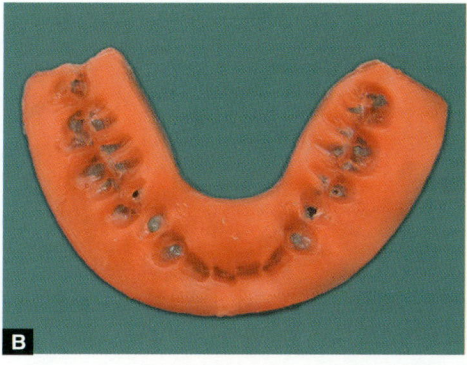 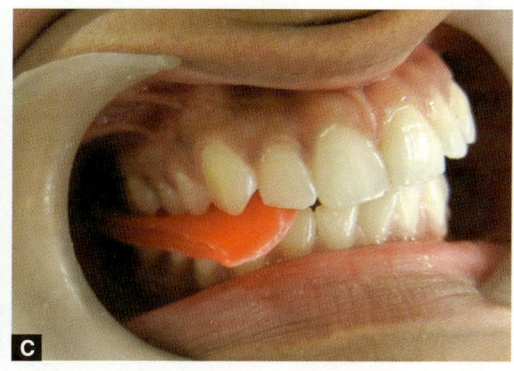

Figs 3.26A to C: (A) Interocclusal records made of silicone registration material **(B)** Interocclusal records made of wax **(C)** Interocclusal records made of wax (Clinical)

- In a partially edentulous arch when there are insufficient number of teeth to support an interocclusal record, wax partial occlusal rims can be used to support the interocclusal recording medium.

Reasons for Restoring the Normal Anatomical form of an Individual Tooth

- The correct relationship with adjacent teeth will give the best support against masticatory stresses, promote deflection of food through the embrasures and prevent food impaction.
- The correct relationship with opposing teeth during mastication will prevent deflective occlusal contacts, which might lead to pain, periodontal damage and fracture of teeth or restoration.
- The correct buccolingual contour will allow deflection of food over the free gingiva, thus protecting the periodontal tissues.
- Will help in maintaining oral hygiene easily.
- Will contribute for esthetics

Consideration for Restoring Individual Tooth

All the dental procedures must be aimed at improving the functional and esthetic relationship between the maxillary and mandibular teeth by closely adhering to the occlusal concepts everytime a dental procedure is performed.

- All the restorations should be in harmony with the occlusion and should contribute for the health of the stomatognathic system.
- The restoration should not introduce any premature contacts and embrasures of these restorations should be optimally placed so as to prevent caries and periodontal problems (Fig. 3.27).
- During the restorative procedures the outline of the procedure should be planned to retain the natural crown contours and guide the developement of occlusal morphology of the restorations.
- The intact buccal and lingual surfaces of the crown guide the accurate contouring of the axial surface of the restoration and help preserve the gingival health.
- Complete coverage restoration and onlays should be preferred only when the occlusal morphology needs to be re established as in grossly destructed teeth.
- Knowledge of normal occlusal contacts of maxillary and mandibular teeth before beginning the tooth preparation is essential to reproduce the normal contacts or to modify the unfavorable contacts (Fig. 3.28).
- Before beginning the tooth preparation examine the occlusal contacts and determine if they should be included or excluded in the outline form. Occlusal contacts should not fall on the restoration-tooth interface.
- The principle of establishing tripod contacts or tripodism can be easily developed on cast restorations fabricated by indirect technique. Tripod contacts are desirable from the point of providing retention and stability of the restoration (Fig. 3.29). However carving a tripod contact intra orally is difficult while placing a restoration. A few authors have advocated the establishment of a single point contact at the bottom of the fossa as an alternative to tripodism (Fig. 3.30).

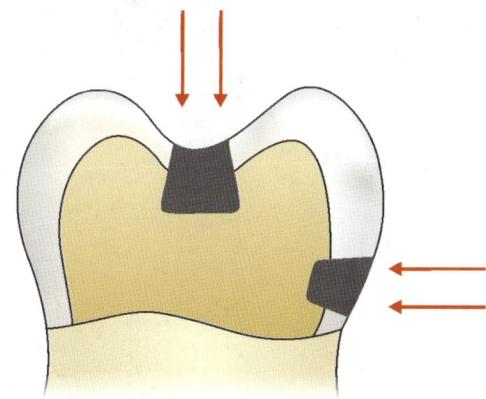

Fig. 3.27: Natural contours guiding the morphology of restorations

Operative Dentistry

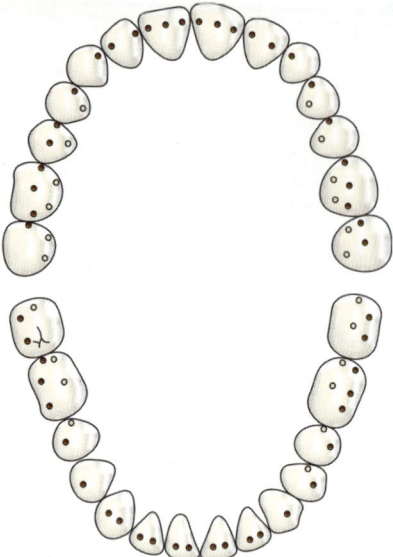

Fig. 3.28: Normal occlusal contacts

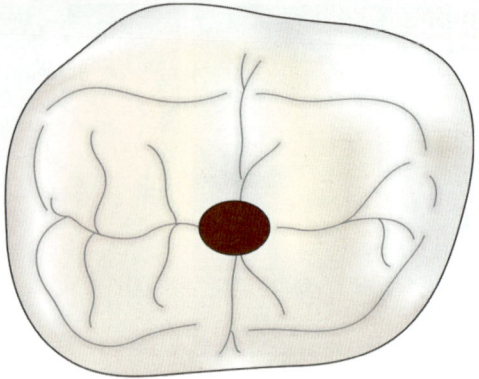

Fig. 3.30: Single point contact

physiologic functions of temporomandibular joint. Occlusal adjustments being irreversible, should be carefully planned. Occlusal prematurities can be adjusted using slow speed handpiece and a small diamond point. After each adjustment, a check of each adjustment should be made. Selective grinding for occlusal adjustments should avoid rendering the cusp tips and should be preferably corrected by modifying the opposing slopes or fossae (Fig 3.32).

History

The history elicited should help us in gathering important information regarding occlusal disharmony.

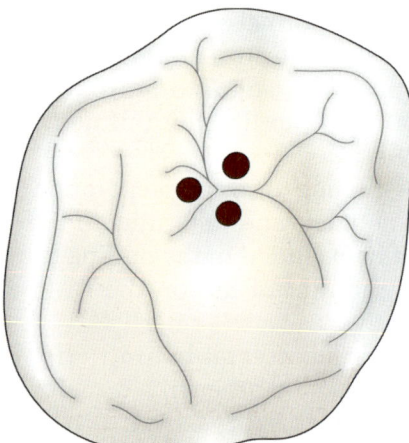

Fig. 3.29: Tripod contacts

- Having established the occlusal contacts, it is mandatory for the restorative dentist to see that the contacts are in harmony with the protrusive and lateral excursive movements (Figs 3.31A and B).

Occlusal Adjustments Prior to Restoration

Occlusal adjustments are done to eliminate the deflective occlusal contacts that interfere with

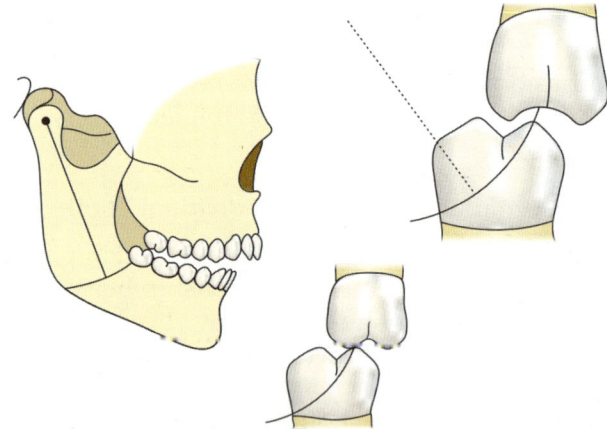

Fig. 3.32: Selective grinding carried along the fossae and slopes of the cusps

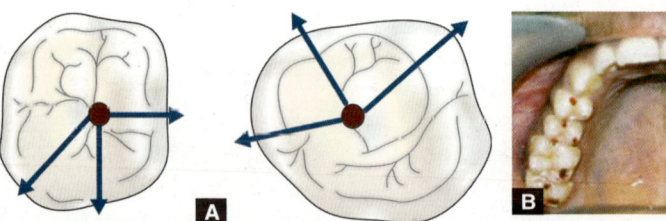

Figs 3.31A and B: (A) Restoration in harmony with excursive movements; (B) Visualization of occlusal contacts

Occlusion

Radiographic Examination

The intraoral radiographs and/or panoramic radiograph will help us in observing the changes around the tooth structure and the alveolar bone.

Articulated Casts

Evaluation of occlusion on study casts can be made only when:
  i. The casts are mounted on a semi-adjustable articulator with facebow transfer.
  ii. The condylar guidances of the articulator is customised.

Clinical Examination

Judicious clinical examination will help us in observing the signs and symptoms of non-physiological occlusion.

Evaluation of Traumatic Tooth Contacts

The traumatic tooth contacts can be primary or secondary.

Primary occlusal trauma: Tooth mobility due to excessive occlusal load despite the presence of intact periodontium

Secondary occlusal trauma: Tooth mobility due to periodontal breakdown in the presence of normal occlusal load.

Procedure for Occlusal Examination

1. Patient's co-operation and feedback is of great help in examining the occlusion and locating the contacts that need adjustments.
2. Wipe the articulating surfaces dry using gauze wipes, as the markings will be clearly visible when teeth are dry.
3. Occlusal contacts or interferences during excursive movements can be identified by:
   - Visual inspection
   - Use of articulating paper
   - Shimstock

Signs and Symptoms of Traumatic Tooth Contact

A tooth in traumatic contact may exhibit one or more of the following clinical features:
- Cracked/ fractured teeth
- Root resorption
- Pulpal hyperemia
- Pulpitis
- Degenerative pulpal changes
- Tooth mobility
- Fremitus
- Fractured restoration
- Alveolar/Periodontal pain
- Large wear facets
- Flaring of anterior teeth/Pathological migration

Elimination of Premature Contacts

Identifying and eliminating the premature contacts is generally referred to as selective grinding.

Objectives of Selective Grinding

- To achieve a stable non-traumatic occlusal contact relationship between maxillary and mandibular teeth in maximum intercuspation/centric occlusion and in all functional excursive positions.
- To provide stability of temporomandibular joint in maximum intercuspation/centric occlusion.
- To improve structural and functional relation of the dentition.
- Bringing occlusal forces within limits of tolerance of the periodontium.
- To permit condyle disc complex to move and function normally or within the physiological limits of tolerance.
- To permit neuromuscular system to function within the adaptive potential of the patient.
- To reduce the effects of parafunctional activities of the patient.
- To improve esthetic needs of the patient.

Occlusal Adjustment Procedures

The simplest treatment that accomplishes the treatment goals is generally the best and the treatment should never begin until the end result is visualised.

Armamentarium: (Fig. 3.33)
- Hand piece(slow speed/high speed).
- Green stones.
- White stones.
- Rubber wheel.
- Articulating paper.
- Paper holding forceps.
- Gauge wipes.
- Green wax sheets.
- T-Scan system.

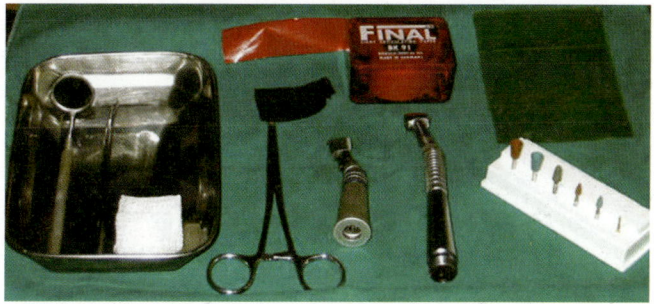

Fig. 3.33: Armamentarium

Preparation of Patient

- Explain the purpose of the occlusal adjustment. Make the patient aware of the changes that takes place during and after the procedure.
- After the initial adjustment the occlusion will feel more comfortable and stable. The occlusion will be re-evaluated after two weeks and that during this period, mobile teeth may become firm and muscles may relax. The occlusion may change slightly after the correction, hence the need for re-evaluation and refinement.

Simulation of Occlusal Corrections on Articulated Study Casts

Occlusal corrections in the patient's mouth should always be preceded by identification and elimination of the occlusal prematurities on the articulated casts.

Mark the casts for adjustment using the articulating paper.

Make the necessary changes on the casts following the guidelines of correcting the natural dentition.

Sequence of Occlusal Adjustments Clinically

For most of the restorative procedures, occlusal prematurities in maximal intercuspal position and excursive movements from there on should be eliminated. Simulate the occlusal corrections carried out on the diagnostic cast in the patient's mouth by the following procedure:

- Shorten extruded teeth.
- Reduce the plunger cusp.
- Correct the prematurities of rotated, mal positioned or tilted teeth.
- Round off the sharp line angles and point angles of teeth.
- Create an ability to voluntarily tap into maximal intercuspal position with patient's head in an upright position.

Elimination of the Slide from Centric Relation to Maximal Intercuspal Position

Identify the anterior component to the slide and eliminate the interference by correcting the distal inclines of the maxillary teeth and the mesial inclines of the mandibular teeth. As a general rule widen the fossae or embrasure areas at the occluding cusps. Do not grind the fossae depth or the cusp tips if it can be avoided (Fig. 3.34).

Elimination of Protrusive Interferences

Interferences during protrusive movements can be eliminated by correcting the distal inclines of the maxillary teeth and the mesial inclines of the mandibular teeth (Fig. 3.35).

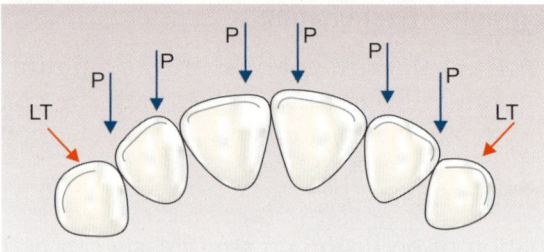

Fig. 3.34: Elimination of interference in anterior guidance

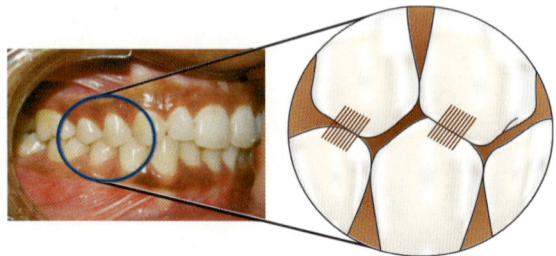

Fig. 3.35: Elimination of protrusive interference

Elimination of Retrusive Intereferences

Interferences during retrusive movements can be eliminated by correcting the mesial inclines of the maxillary teeth and the distal inclines of the mandibular teeth (Fig. 3.36).

Elimination of Working Side Prematurity

Interferences on the working side can be eliminated by following the BULL rule. The palatal inclines of the upper buccal cusps and the buccal inclines of the lower lingual cusps can be modified to eliminate these interferences (Fig. 3.37).

Elimination of Non Working side Prematurity

These contacts pose special problem as they occur on the supporting cusps. However, their elimination is indicated, as they are associated with an increased risk of bone loss, TMJ dysfunctions and mobility. The grinding of palatal cusp tip and may further lead to re-establishment of the interferences as the upper molar may tip down to re-establish contact in ICP (Fig. 3.38).

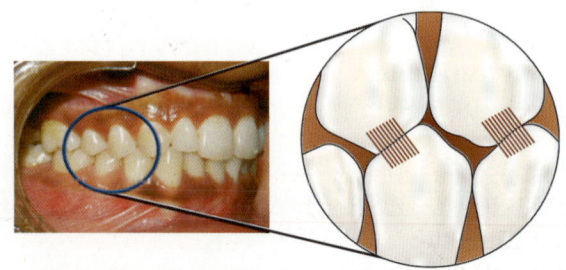

Fig. 3.36: Elimination of retrusive interference

Occlusion

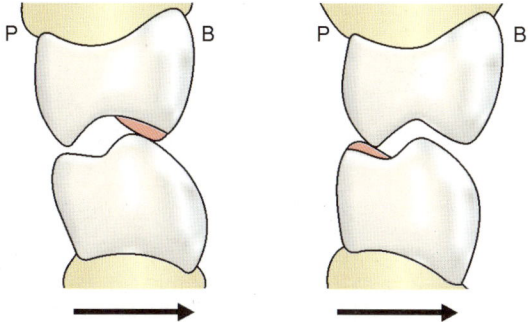

Fig. 3.37: Elimination of working side prematurity

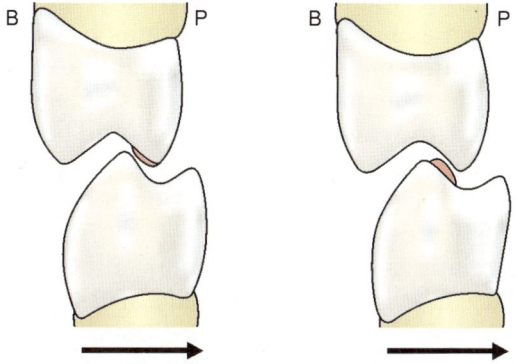

Fig. 3.38: Elimination of non working side prematurity

Protrusion and Posterior Contacts

The interferences in the protrusive movements can be eliminated either by modifying the cuspal inclines of the posterior teeth or by increasing the steepness of the anterior guidance. The steepness of the anterior guidance can be increased or decreased by modifying the palatal inclines of the maxillary incisors.

Eliminating the prematurities of the posterior tooth during protrusion can be achieved by following the DUML rule- Distal facing slopes of the maxillary teeth and the mesial facing slope of the mandibular teeth.

T-Scan System

For years, dental occlusal analysis has been largely a matter of guesswork for dentists. Articulation paper, waxes, pressure indicator paste, etc. were all dentists had to assess and balance the occlusal forces. Most of these methods are not sensitive enough to detect simultaneous contact, and none measure both biting time and force. Tekscan met the challenge by developing the *T-Scan* system. Recently T scan III has been used.

The T-Scan system is a valuable tool that aids in the diagnostic process of analyzing a patient's bite to show what is and what is not functioning properly. When a bite is unstable it can cause pain, broken restorations, gum disease, tooth loss, headaches and TMJ disorder.

The ultra-thin, reusable sensor, shaped to fit the dental arch, inserts into the sensor handle, which connects into the USB port of your windows based PC or laptop and making it easy to move from one operatory to another. Evaluating occlusal forces is as simple as having a patient bite down on the sensor while the computer analyzes and displays timing and force data in vivid, full-color 3-D or 2-D graphics. Vivid graphics make seeing the balance of the bite easy to determine and adjust. The *T-Scan* comes with a full-featured Patient File Management system, which makes storing patient records and tracking occlusal recordings simple. Data can be printed to provide valuable documentation for patient files, patient education or insurance claims.

Benefits

- Easy to use
- Easy to interpret
- Improved clinical results
- Determine premature contacts
- Minimize destructive forces
- Expand your practice in a wide range of applications
- Do not rely on patient feel
- Provide instant documentation
- Use as a patient education tool
- Save time by preventing remakes

Occlusal Consideration During Tooth Preparation

The intact buccal and lingual surfaces of the crown guide the accurate contouring of restoration and help preserve gingival environment. Hence conservative preparation should be planned to avoid losing the guidance from the natural contours of the teeth. Complete coverage restorations on onlays are indicated only when the cusps are severely damaged, fractured or when the occlusal morphology needs to be modified.

The biological width of the periodontium is normally about 2.0 mm from the crest of the alveolar bone. The health of the periodontium can be maintained by not encroaching on the biological width of the tooth.

During tooth preparation adequate amount of the tooth material should be reduced to provide sufficient bulk of the restorative material of choice. The cervical areas should not be over-contoured. Particular care is to be exercised at the line angles where the depth of the shoulder or chamfer is usually inadequate leading to over contouring.

The over-contouring varies from individual to individual and also from one tooth to another in the same individual. The shape of the embrasures should be reproduced as in the functional occlusion. The facial and axial surface should be recontoured in the final restoration only if the existing contour and embrasure do not protect against food impaction.

To protect the functional cusp and improve the structural durability of the restoration, the outline form of the inlays and onlays should not be placed on the occluso buccal line angle for the mandibular posterior teeth and occluso palatal line angle for the maxillary posterior teeth. In such cases the outline form can be extended beyond the functional cusp to include them in the preparation

The depth of the occlusal preparation will vary depending upon the choice of the restorative material. For cast metal restorations the functional cusps are reduced by about 1.5 mm and the non functional cusps are reduced by about 1.0 mm. In case of metal ceramic restorations the functional cusps are reduced by about 2.0 mm and the non functional cusps are reduced by 1.5 mm.

To provide adequate retention for the complete veneer restorations the occlusogingival length of the preparation should be atleast 4.0 mm. In case of short crowns the retention of the crown can be increased by placing grooves and boxes on the axial surfaces.

The adequacy of the occlusal reduction can be ascertained by wax check bites or by making a check cast.

A double or triple thickness of hard baseplate wax is softened and placed on the prepared tooth and the patient is asked to close the teeth into occlusion. The wax is cooled intra-orally and checked under light to determine the adequacy of the preparation.

An alginate impression of the prepared tooth and the adjacent teeth is made using a sectional tray. The impression is then casted using quick setting plaster. This check cast is then occluded with the study cast of the opposing arch to ascertain the adequacy of the tooth preparation.

Examining the provisional restoration under light will also help us in determining the adequacy of the occlusal preparation.

Anterior Restorations

The anterior teeth usually occupy the space in the oral cavity where the forces of the perioral musculature and the tongue is neutralised. While restoring or replacing the anterior teeth, care should be taken to see that they are not moved away from this position.

The horizontal and vertical overlap of the anterior teeth and the anterior guidance should be examined prior to the restoration of the anterior teeth (Fig. 3.39). The anterior guidance varies from one individual to another depending upon the type of occlusion and the jaw relation. Unless warranted they should not be altered while restoring the anterior teeth.

Canines play an important role in both canine protected and group function occlusion. Hence care should be taken to retain the existing guidance or change it as a part of the treatment plan.

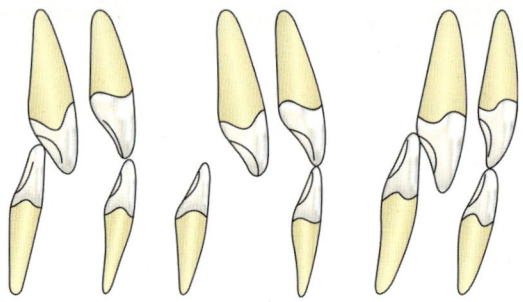

Fig. 3.39: Incisal guidance

Anterior guidance should provide smooth even contacts on as many anterior teeth as possible from Maximal Intercuspal position through the excursion, disoccluding the posterior teeth. If a single tooth is to be restored, the existing guidance should be retained. When all the anterior teeth are to be restored, some changes in incisal guidance and position of teeth can be made if necessary.

The relationship of mandibular anterior teeth to maxillary anterior teeth, especially in cases of class II division I malocclusion, touches the dentogingival junction. In such cases the mandibular incisors can be kept short to prevent trauma from occlusion.

The canine has a favourable crown/root ratio for absorbing occlusal forces. Its root configuration will also provide greater surface area and better proprioception than the adjacent teeth.

The location of the canines, in the anterior part of the oral cavity also makes them suitable for easily correcting the guidance if necessary.

The preparation of the canines must provide adequate bulk of the material to prevent overcontouring of the restoration. For a metal ceramic restoration about 1.5 mm should be reduced on the labial side and about 1mm on the lingual side is usually adequate. However, care should be taken to provide additional bulk of the material in cases of deep bite to increase the structural durability.

While restoring the canines into canine guided occlusion, care must be taken to see that there is disocclusion of the posterior teeth during lateral excursions. While restoring the incisors similar care should be taken to provide adequate space for the bulk of the material and to prevent the overcontouring of the teeth. they should also be restored to provide a harmonious anterior guidance.

Posterior Restorations

Most of the teeth requiring indirect restorations are posterior teeth. Before preparing the posterior teeth for indirect restorations, the existing occlusal scheme should be examined meticulously. In most of the situations occlusion can be developed in the existing maximal intercuspal position.

Occlusion

However, before planning the posterior restorations, we must take into consideration the following:
- Ascertain the stability of the intercuspal position.
- Determine the anterior tooth contact.
- Determine the adequacy of the existing vertical dimension of occlusion.
- Determine the evenness of the plane of occlusion
- Anticipated design of the tooth preparation.

Hindrances that may be caused in developing a harmonious occlusal scheme by the cusps of malpositioned teeth, supra erupted teeth or tilted tooth should be corrected before the tooth preparation.

Using an articulating paper identify the cuspal contacts in the maximal intercuspal position and its movements into excursive movements. In case of intracoronal restorations, these contacts can either completely be included or excluded from the outline form of the restorations (Fig. 3.40).

In case of extracoronal restorations these contacts should be meticulously reproduced in the restoration.

The occlusal contacts located on the cuspal inclines or on the slopes of the ridges are undesirable because they create a deflective force on the tooth. Occlusal contacts should be placed such that the cusps should make a tripod contact with the opposing fossa or a point contact at the bottom of the fossa. Such contacts helps in directing the occlusal forces along the long axis of the tooth which is conducive to the health of the periodontal ligament (Fig. 3.41).

The choice of the posterior tooth restorations between amalgam and complete veneer restorations depends upon the amount of remaining tooth structures and the clincal length of the crown. Complete veneer restorations are preferred over amalgam restorations whenever the amalgam restorations are large, has modifications, has an occlusal isthmus wider than half of the occlusal table or has repeatedly failed.

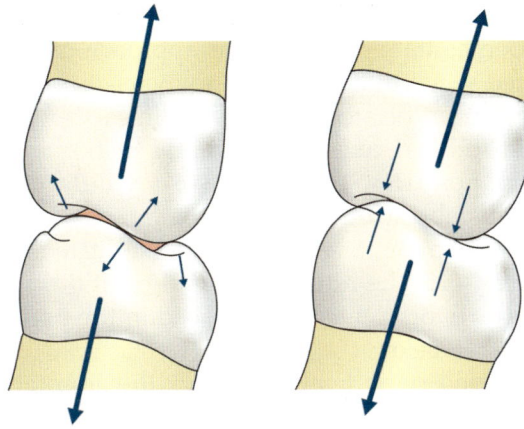

Fig. 3.41: Resultant forces

Restoring Small Number of Units

All restorations either single or multiple units must be in harmony with the planned occlusal scheme. Both an articulating paper and a shimstock can be used to verify the occlusal contacts of the teeth to be restored and the adjacent teeth at the time of try in.

The occlusal contacts both in Maximal intercuspal position and there on, into excursive movements should be in harmony with the planned occlusion. When a distal most tooth in an arch is to be prepared, it is important to accurately record the occlusal relation. Autopolymerising acrylic resin copings can be used to verify the occlusal contacts of the prepared teeth intra-orally and to verify the same on the articulated casts. The thickness of the coping can also be measured to verify the adequacy of the teeth preparation.

Restoring Posterior Single Quadrant

When the posterior teeth in any quadrant are lost, there is a tendency for the opposing teeth to supra-erupt, leading to uneven occlusal plane. The occlusal plane should be corrected prior to the placement of the restorations to prevent occlusal prematurities.

Impressions of the complete arches should be made to ensure that the occlusal contacts of the contralateral side helps us in maintaining the stability of the occlusal contacts. The interocclusal records can then be made to transfer the occlusal relationship of the casts onto an articulator.

Restoring Multiple Units in the Same Arch

When restoring multiple units in a single arch, the occlusion can be developed in the Maximal intercuspal position. Alternatively when restoring all the teeth in

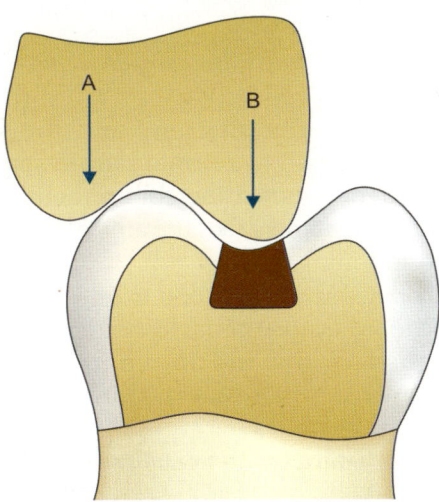

Fig. 3.40: Outline form (A) contact area excluded (B) contact area included

a single arch, the occlusion can be developed in the Retruded contact position. This approach can also be followed when there is a need to increase the vertical dimension, associated with short clinical crowns.

Interocclusal records are made in the retruded contact position, the casts are articulated on a semiadjustable articulator using a facebow transfer.

Provisional restoration are then fabricated to be in harmony with the retruded cuspal position.

These restorations can be placed in the patient for about 4–6 weeks.

Reviewed periodically to check the adaptation of the patient to the new occlusal scheme.

Feeling of comfort, stability and lack of TMJ dysfunction indicates adaptation to the new occlusal scheme.

Premature loss of one or few provisional restorations indicate lack of occlusal harmony or poor retention. Make the necessary corrections to eliminate the cause and place the provisional restorations again. When the patient is adapted to the new occlusal scheme, definitive restoration can then be fabricated to restore the occlusion.

Reasons for Modifying the Occlusal Table

The occlusal table is formed by the sum total of occlusal surfaces of all the posterior teeth. However, in reality, the occlusal table also includes areas beyond the palatal surfaces of upper teeth and the buccal surfaces of lower teeth.

In certain cases this table needs to be modified or made narrower, which leads to:

- *Reduction of force*: When the occlusal table is made narrower, lesser force is applied over the same to undergo masticatory functions. Force is transmitted to all structures underlying the occlusal table, which include the restoration, the tooth structure and the periodontium.
- *Reduction of the effect of force*: The direction in which the applied force is transmitted is governed by muscular activities and the area on which the force is applied. However, the effect of the force may be modified by altering the surface at which the force is applied, thus altering the direction of resolved components.
- *Reduction of torque*: The tendency to rotate may be reduced by altering the point of application of the force relative to the fulcrum. The point of application of the force may be altered by modifying the occlusal table which indirectly depends upon the design of the cavity and the restoration.
- *Facilitation of oral hygiene and reduction of soft tissue biting*: Oral hygiene may be improved and cheek biting can be eliminated by altering the occlusal table.

Role of Contact Areas

Human teeth are designed in such a way that they contribute significantly to their own support as well as supporting the arch. Each tooth assumes the same responsibility in providing support that a brick assumes as a part of a wall. This arrangement relieves the supporting bone of much responsibility and the forces can be dissipated smoothly. A break in the continuity of the line of the contact areas throws additional responsibility on the periodontal membrane and alveolar bone, which they are not designed to sustain. The teeth move into positions, which the supporting tissues find intolerable and eventually lead to breakdown of the supporting tissues. Interproximal contacts aid in shunting the food towards the buccal and lingual areas and thus prevent the food from pushing in between the teeth and thereby impinging on gingival tissues, which could predispose to periodontal problems and/or dental caries.

Good restorative dental procedures must reproduce the proper contact areas. Restorations with contact areas which are flat, open, improperly placed, rough or poorly polished will lead to failure. A slight frictional movement of teeth always occurs between the interproximal surfaces of teeth during physiologic movement; and with time the contact point becomes broad resulting in a wider contact area. If the teeth remained in contact with each other merely by contact points, they would eventually be forced out of dental arch in either a buccal or lingual direction whereas with a wider contact between teeth, this is not likely to occur. The opposing interproximal surfaces of restorations must be hard in order not to flow, flatten, wear or become abraded with use.

Hazards of faulty contacts: Faulty contacts are always detrimental to underlying periodontium.

The types of faults and their consequences (Table 4.2) are as follows:

I. *Too broad contact, buccolingually or occlusogingivally, leads to:*
   - Change in tooth anatomy and the shape of interdental col. The normal saddle-shaped area is broadened. Since the col epithelium is non-keratinized, it increases the area of susceptibility to periodontal disease.
   - Improper shunting of food in buccal and lingual directions because of narrow embrasures, hence the chances of food impingement into the contact area is increased resulting in inefficient mastication.

II. *Too narrow contact, buccolingually or occlusogingivally, leads to:*
   - Food impaction vertically and/or horizontally on col area;

- Wide buccal and lingual embrasures in which normal oral hygiene measures may not gain access predisposing to greater food retention and plaque accumulation in embrasure areas.
III. *Contact placed too occlusally* will result in a flattened marginal ridge at the expense of occlusal embrasure.
IV. *Contact placed too bucally or lingually* will result in a flattened restoration at the expense of buccal or lingual proximal wall.
V. *Contact placed too gingivally* will increase the depth of occlusal embrasure at the expense of the size of contact area or at the expense of broadening or impinging upon interdental col.
VI. *Loose contact* creates continuity between embrasures and interdental col, leading to food impaction.

Role of Contours

All tooth crowns exhibit contours in the form of convexities and concavities which should be reproduced in a restoration.

- *Facial and lingual convexities*: Convex contours on the facial and lingual surfaces of the teeth afford protection and stimulation to the supporting structures during mastication. They direct the food towards the buccal vestibule, palate or tongue while stimulating the surrounding soft tissue by gentle massage rather than irritating it. Overcontoured curvatures can create a favourable environment for the accumulation and growth of cariogenic and plaque bacteria at gingival margin, apical to the height of contour. This further results in chronic inflammation of gingiva.
- *Facial and lingual concavities*: Concavities occlusal to the height of contour whether they are present on anterior teeth or posterior teeth, are involved in occlusal static and dynamic relations, as they determine the pathways for mandibular teeth into and out of centric occlusion. Deficient or dislocated concavities can lead to premature contacts during mandibular movements, which could inhibit the physiologic capabilities of these movements. Excessive concavities can invite extrusion, rotation or tilting of occluding elements into non-physiologic relation with opposing teeth.
- *Proximal contours adjacent to the contact area*: Proximal curvatures adjacent to the contact area form 'V' shaped spillway spaces called embrasures. Embrasures serve as pathways for the passage of food, which is returned to the occlusal surfaces by the movement of the facial tissues and the tongue. Food is prevented from accumulating on the occlusal surface. Occlusal embrasures prevent food impaction into the contact area. All occlusal, buccal, lingual and gingival embrasures should be restored. Too narrow embrasures predispose teeth and supporting structures to heavier stresses. Too wide embrasures offer little protection to the underlying soft tissue.

The readers are advised to consult Chapter 4 for further studies on contacts and contours.

Role of Marginal Ridges

The marginal ridges play an important role in withstanding and dissipating the occlusal stresses. The correct form of marginal ridge compatible with the adjacent tooth and also with its own surroundings is important during carving of posterior restoration. The absence of marginal ridge, or marginal ridge with improper height can lead to altered dissipation of forces subsequently damaging the underlying periodontium. The details as how these forces act on marginal ridges and how the altered marginal ridges deviate the forces are given in Chapter 10.

Relationship Between Toothwear and Restorative Materials

Occlusal forces lead to wear of enamel. The wear is, however, very slow if occlusal forces are appropriately transmitted to underlying bony tissues. The pattern of wear varies individually depending upon various factors. Non-uniform wear of opposing teeth is quite common when one teeth is restored with a restorative material whose wear resistance is different as compared to that of enamel. Very rarely, the wear resistance of a restorative material equals the wear resistance of enamel.

At present, no restorative material is available which wears at the same rate as enamel or as enamel and dentin at later stages. Differential wear can result in localization of occlusal loads with subsequent failure of restorative materials or development of deflective contacts with mandibular repositioning and an effect on a distant tooth.

Hypothetically, if two restorative materials, which wear at a slower rate than the natural teeth are placed so as to oppose each other in a dentition undergoing wear, the restorations will produce occlusal interferences at a later stage.

Non-wearing materials opposing each other can lead to natural teeth wear during contact in lateral and protrusive movements. Conversely, if the materials wear faster than the teeth, the opposing cusp might over-erupt into the worn material. In lateral excursion this cusp might then come in contact with an opposing cusp and if weakened by previous caries can lead to fracture.

Whether or not Compensation for Loss of Occlusal wear occurs?

Murphy investigated the compensatory mechanisms associated with advanced tooth wear. He reported that 50% compensation resulted from continuous eruption (in the form of cementum apposition with root lengthening and differential alveolar bone deposition with reduction in socket depth). A 10% compensation resulted from general bone growth and 40% remained uncompensated as loss of occlusal face height. He postulated that the compensatory mechanisms occurred independently to those of wear, so that occlusal face height remained constant of wear.

Occlusal interferences can develop through differential wear patterns and unmatched compensatory mechanisms. The clinician must appreciate that he is faced with a dynamic situation and not a set of static study casts. He can shape and regulate the form of occlusal surfaces of teeth and restorations so that he can determine surfaces of teeth and restorations, which contact during activities such as mastication, swallowing and bruxism. The advantages of this approach are:

- The direction of stresses through the strongest portions of the restorations and remaining tooth structure can be arranged.
- The effects of occlusal interferences developing from differential wear can be minimized.
- It is possible to maintain the partially restored dentition by means of periodic adjustment.

Since wear defects are not repaired automatically, the dentist should replace and maintain the configuration of teeth in accordance with the functional activities.

Modes of Recording Occlusal Relations for Indirect Restorations

For fabrication of indirect restorations, the occlusal relations are to be recorded so as to reproduce the same on the pattern and the casting. The occlusal relations are simulated on the articulators and the relations during various movements of the mandible are recorded. It has been demonstrated that subjects close their jaws from the rest position to the intercuspal position (ICP) along a habitual path of closure. An altered ICP and mandibular path of closure can be caused by deflecting contacts resulting from restorations, tooth loss, tooth movements or differential wear.

Modes of Recording and Reproducing Mandibular Movements

Physical manipulation of the mandible for occlusal records:
A. The first stage for any occlusal recording is to place the mandible in centric relation. Certain relation can be verified by noting the following points:
   - The condyle is in the superior most position within the fossa. This can be achieved by physically guiding the mandible upwards, while manipulating it backwards from its habitual location. This act should continue until no further upward movement of mandible occurs.
   - The mandible in the centric relation position moves in a pure rotating arc. This can be verified by rotating the mandible up and down in very short arcs.
   - Muscles should be in complete harmony with each other.
   - There should not be any tooth contact at this position.
B. The second stage is to locate centric occlusion. The patient is asked to bite while the operator guides and supports the horizontal position of mandible.
C. The third stage defines lateral excursions, which start from centric occlusion. Supporting pressure is applied at the angle of the mandible on the working side to keep the condyle seated within its fossa. Guiding hand support may be necessary on the non-working side during the medial drop of mandible. The mandible should be guided until the cuspid on the working side is edge to edge and ready to disclude. This stage should be done twice, once for each side.
D. The fourth stage is the protrusive movement. This also starts from centric occlusion and the patient is asked to guide the teeth forward. There should be superio-anterior guiding with light supporting pressure at the angle of mandible while the patient is protruding it. The movement should be exercised until reverse overlap occurs or edge to edge relation is acquired anteriorly.

Transferable Records

These records are usually used for fabricating restorations outside the mouth. They are mainly fashioned in two steps. First step is making the record intraorally in a fairly non-distortable material. The second step involves transferring the information on the material to the articulator. The articulator movements create the same effect on the restoration as the movements of the mandible. The extraorally fabricated restoration then becomes a physiological replaced part in the stomatognathic system.

Both static and the dynamic relations are to be recorded and transferred to the chosen articulator.

A. Static Relationship Transferable Records

These records capture the relationship of the maxillary and mandibular teeth at border locations of the mandibular movement path. They are only transferable to semi-adjustable articulator which is capable of moving from one border location to another with a standard path in between.

These records are also used to correlate upper and lower casts at centric relation or centric occlusion in any type of articulator (hinge, semi-adjustable or fully adjustable).

Facial records are used for centric occlusion, when interocclusal recording is difficult or may create errors. Modified zinc oxide eugenol, impression plaster, silicon rubber base impression material or autopolymerizing acrylic resin can be used to make the recording. The patient's mandible is guided and manipulated to centric relation and then to centric occlusion where the patient is asked to close his teeth forcibly. The paste of the recording material is then flowed over the facial surfaces, covering the canine, premolars and sometimes the mesiobuccal cusp of molars. It should be flowed in the facial embrasures to temporarily lock in them. After setting, the material is removed in facial direction. Any type of articulator can be used to transfer this record to the articulator.

- *Use of hinge articulator:* This is indicated when the occlusion is stable and with adequate holding cuspal elements on both the sides. The only record needed for hinge articulator is the facial centric occlusion record. The opposing cast is occluded to the mounted cast via facial record and the cast then attached to the articulator.
- *Use of semi-adjustable articulator:* Here a facebow record is needed. This is a record capturing the relationship of maxilla to the cranium. For these, three reference points are necessary - one in each direction at the cranial part of stomatognathic system. Joining these three chosen points create a plane close to hinge axis.

A wax carried in special bite-fork is indented with maxillary teeth at three or four reference points and the impression represents the maxilla. Creating the assembly having these four point contacts will formulate interface-bow record. This assembly is attached to the articulator. After fitting the upper cusps of cast into indentations, the cast is attached to the arms of articulator with non-expanding gypsum. The facebow is removed and the upper cast is correlated with lower cast using following steps:

- A centric relation record is used to join the upper and lower casts.
- Held at this relationship, the lower cast is attached to the lower arm of the articulator with a non-expanding gypsum.
- After setting of gypsum, left condylar path controlling screws are loosened.
- The right excursive records are put between the casts and the left condylar path component of articulator are moved until they are steady and in contact with each other and same is done for right condylar path.
- Next protrusive excursive records are made.
- Holding the relationship, the incisal guidance is adjusted according to cast's anterior teeth, overjet, overbite and lateral disclusion capability.

B. Dynamic Relationship Transferable Records

a. Functionally generated path

These techniques capture the effects of the dynamics of mandibular movements as they are performed. The stereo-graphic record thus created is transferred to a 'verticulator' or similar device where it will impart its con-figuration on opposing restorations. Functionally generated path (F.G.P) interocclusal record is useful when checking occlusal clearances, especially in areas difficult to visualize, such as in the central groove or the lingual cusp regions.

To make a F.G.P. interocclusal record, first dry the preparation free of viable moisture. Then lightly press a portion of softened, low fusing inlay wax over the prepared tooth (teeth) and immediately request the patient to close and slide the teeth in all directions.

During the mandibular movements, observe to verify that:

- The patient moves in right lateral, left lateral and protrusive movements.
- The adjacent unprepared teeth are in contact with opposing teeth.
- The wax in the cavity is stable.
- Carefully remove the wax. Hold it across the light and note the degree of light transmitted.

With experience one finds that light is a good indicator of thickness of wax. An alternative method is to use wax callipers or to section the wax to verify its thickness. Insufficient thickness calls for more reduction in the indicated area before proceeding.

Such records give the lab-technician some information how to form occlusal surfaces and position occlusal contacts on the restoration but supply no data on how these structures and contacts might function during mandibular movements.

If information is desired in the laboratory about the pathways of cusps during mandibular movements then a registration must be made of the opposing teeth and their functional paths by:

i. Making FGP interocclusal record which will be used in the lab to make a cast of the functional pathways of cusps ("functional core"); or
ii. Making full arch impressions and mounting the casts properly on semi-adjustable articulator.

The FGP interocclusal record works well when one or two teeth are prepared whereas full arch casts are preferred when more than two prepared teeth are involved. FGP inter-occlusal records can register the interactions of anterior guidance, horizontal condylar guidance, cusp inclines and occlusal contact positions.

The use of full-arch casts mounted on a semi-adjustable articulator is highly recommended when restoring a large portion of the patient posterior occlusion with cast metal restorations.

b. Pantograph and fully adjustable articulator

The pantograph in addition to recording the border locations of the mandible, also accurately locates the exact path travelled by the mandible from one terminal location to another. These paths are recorded in saggital, horizontal and coronal planes.

In most situations of single tooth restorations it is not necessary to locate the exact hinge axis of the mandibular movements. However, in situations where vertical dimension of the teeth is to be changed by restorations or complete mouth rehabilitation, the hinge axis should be located and marked on the side of face.

c. Stereographic tracing and fully adjustable articulators

In most of the adjustable articulators the components of anterior guidance can be mechanically imitated by parts of the articulator. After mounting the upper and lower casts, bring them to centric occlusion. Move the upper and lower anterior teeth apart, then adjust the amount of overjet. Move the upper arm posteriorly and upward to any edge to edge relation, then adjust the overbite. Move the upper arm laterally and on the working side adjust the lateral wing of the anterior guidance to touch the pin at the most lateral border location. Repeat for other lateral location.

Non-transferable Records

Such records are used only for diagnostic or verifying purposes. The technique includes introducing a marking ribbon between the dried mandibular and maxillary teeth while manipulating the mandible into one or more of previously described positions. The interferences so noted during markings are recorded.

The following one or all features are important and should be noted before a final restoration.

- Uneven, non-symmetrical attrition of occluding teeth.
- Supra-eruption, tilting, rotation or bodily movements of a tooth.
- Undercontoured (overcarved) occluding restoration leading to occlusal and possibly lateral displacement of opposing cuspal elements.
- Periodontal diseases facilitating tooth movement, especially laterally.
- Insufficiently restraining cusp-fossa or cusp-marginal ridge relationship allowing repositioning of teeth.
- Plunger cusps against marginal ridges separating them or the same cusp against one side of tooth tilting it laterally.

Final Checking of the Casting for Occlusion

When the proximal contacts have been adjusted and the casting is satisfactorily seated on the tooth, ask the patient to close in maximum intercuspal position (ICP) and inspect the unprepared adjacent teeth to see if there is any space between opposing wear facets. Usually the patient can indicate correctly if the casting needs occlusal adjustment, however the dentist should verify the occlusal relationship objectively.

After drying the teeth, insert a strip of articulating paper and request the patient to close and tap the teeth together in intercuspal position several times. Remove the paper, and examine it by holding it up towards the light for evidence of any areas of penetration caused by the restoration. Any holes can be matched with heavy markings on the castings and there will be shiny, metal colored spots in the centre of the marks. Such heavy contacts should be reduced with suitable abrasive stones while carefully observing the following fundamental concepts for equilibration of occlusion.

- The space observed between opposing wear facets of adjacent unprepared teeth is an indication of the maximum amount of vertical reduction of the casting required.
- Often the 'high' occlusal contacts are too broad and extend onto cusp or ridge slopes. In such cases, grind away the most incorrect portion of the incline contact (a deflective contact) leaving the most correct portion intact.
- Occlusal contacts in maximum ICP should be composed of supporting cusp tips placed against flat or smoothly concave surfaces (or fossae) for stability. The force vector of occlusal contacts should be one that parallels the long axis of the tooth. Contacts on inclines tend to deflect the tooth and are less stable. The use of articulating paper and stone is continued until:
- The heavy markings are no longer produced;
- The contacts on the restoration have optimal position and form;
- There is an even distribution of contacts on the casting and adjacent teeth.

Care must be observed not to over-reduce the occlusal contacts.

In the final phase of equilibration, the strength of occlusal contacts can be tested by using thin plastic sheet (0.0053µ thick) as a feeler guaze. Test the intensity of occlusal contacts of the casting and the adjacent unprepared teeth to see if they hold the sheet equally.

Once the occlusal contacts have been adjusted in intercuspal position, check the contacts during lateral mandibular movements.

Lateral working (functional) contacts on the casting are marked by inserting a strip of articulating paper over the quadrant with the casting and having the patient close in intercuspal position. Then, sliding the teeth towards the side of the mouth where the casting is located.

Contacts between the lingual inclines of the maxillary palatal cusps and facial inclines of mandibular facial cusps should remain only if they are passive and a group function pattern of occlusion is desired.

Nonfunctional, non-working contacts on a restoration can be marked by inserting a strip of articulating paper over the teeth with the castings and having the patient close in intercuspal position and then sliding the teeth laterally toward the opposite side. In a normal arrangement of teeth, contacts that might occur during a non-working pathway are positioned on the facial inclines of the maxillary palatal cusps and the lingual inclines of the mandibular facial cusps. These non-working contacts must be removed with a suitable stone.

Now examine the casting for interferences in protrusive mandibular movements using the articulating paper. The areas that may have to be adjusted to prevent contact are the distal inclines of the maxillary cusps and mesial inclines of mandibular cusps.

Finally, interferences that occur on the casting between centric relation and intercuspal position are identified and corrected. Most patients have a small discrepancy between centric relation and maximum intercuspal position. Such a 'skid' is considered normal for most patients, but the operator should be sure that the casting does not have premature contact between centric relation and intercuspal position. Once the teeth have been marked in centric relation, observe the teeth to be sure that the casting does not have premature contacts in centric relation, and that it does not exacerbate any centric relation–intercuspal position skid. If it does, the mesial inclines of maxillary cusps and distal inclines of mandibular cusps will be the areas that need adjustment.

Various features of an optimum occlusion which should be achieved in any occluding restoration are as follows:

1. There should be no tooth contact at the early stage of centric relation.
2. The mandible should arc along a hinge axis from centric relation to centric occlusion. Any interfering tooth parts within this arcing that create a translatory movement should be eliminated.
3. In the early stages of centric occlusion towards complete intercuspation, there may be forward movement of mandible. However, there should not be any lateral, medial or backward movement of mandible (with the teeth) when moving from centric relation to centric occlusion. Any cuspal incline contributing to this latter 'skid' should be eliminated.
4. At centric occlusion, the holdings cusps should be of sufficient height to be in positive contact with their opposing counterparts. Such an arrangement preserves the vertical dimension of the teeth maintaining the stomatognathic system.
5. At centric occlusion, the holding markings should be symmetrical in magnitude and extent on all holding cuspal elements of both sides.
6. When maximum intercuspation is achieved, there should not be any further movement of mandible or the teeth.
7. Holding cusps occluding with more than one tooth or eccentrically occluding with opposing teeth should not move opposing teeth in a nonaxial direction. This is accomplished by broadening the contact of the cusps with opposing teeth to minimize tipping or wedging.
8. In centric occlusion, the incisal edges of lower incisors should be located at the gingival side of the lingual concavity of the upper incisors, preferably with a flat horizontal shelf or plane. This plane will enhance the holding capability of the lingual concavity keeping the inter-relationship conducive to optimum occlusion.
9. In lateral excursion of the mandible, there should not be any tooth contact on the non-working side of mandible.
10. In lateral excursion of mandible, the holding cusps of the working side should have a valley like space on the opposing teeth (grooves or occlusal embrasures). This is to facilitate their non-interfering passage during lateral excursion. These valleys should have the right depth, right inclination of their surrounding walls and the right direction to allow the smooth passage of the holding cusps, and to be symmetrical to and in harmony with the nature of condylar movements in three dimensions at that side.
11. The disclusion should start posteriorly and end by the cuspid's disclusion.

12. The disclusion path should be perfected so that the optimum direction along the lingual surface of the upper cuspid and the working inclines of the non-working cusps is achieved.
13. Marked contact areas during lateral excursion should be the same when going out of centric and back into centric.
14. During protrusive excursions of mandible there should not be any tooth contact posteriorly.
15. Cuspids should be involved at least in the initial stages of the protrusive movement of mandible.
16. Protrusive contact markings should be evenly distributed and symmetrical on all teeth involved.

Occlusal equilibration of existing dentition should be performed before performing extensive restorative procedures; that will involve a change of occluding surfaces of multiple teeth. If symptoms of facial myodysfunction, temporomandibular joint dysfunction or dysfunction of any part of stomatognathic system are present: such problems should also be dealt with before eliminating occlusal interferences.

It is preferable to mount upper and lower casts in an adjustable articulator and put the articulation through all possible movements. The interferences recorded on the cast are noted and removed in patient's teeth.

The occlusion on the fabricated restorations is simulated in such a way that the restorations are in harmony with the stomatognathic system. Though this is quite a difficult procedure and also time consuming, yet the importance and advantages of establishing functional occlusion in a restoration warrant all clinicians to spend time and utilize expertise on occlusal principles. Occlusal forces set limits on the choice of the material and often guide the design of the preparation. With periodontally compromised teeth, the occlusal planning to minimize non-axial forces lies in the restoration itself. The clinician should keep in mind that virtually all restorations are affected by occlusal forces and ignoring these may lead to treatment failures.

FULL MOUTH REHABILITATION

Full mouth rehabilitation entails the performance of all the procedures necessary to produce a healthy, esthetic, well functioning, self maintaining masticatory mechanism.

Full mouth reconstruction is basically a set of procedures that are aimed at correcting a compromised occlusion. Discrepancy between the retruded contact position and maximal intercuspal position beyond the physiological limits of tolerance can lead to various neuromuscular disorders. Correcting this discrepancy not only restores proper function, but also helps in enhancing the esthetics of the patient.

The main reasons to advocate full mouth rehablitation are:
When there is evidence of:
 i. Periodontal breakdown
 ii. Temporomandibular joint disturbances
 iii. Mutilated occlusion.

Many theories and philosophies of occlusal rehablitation have been developed, few of the widely accepted are as follows:

PMS Philosophy–Pankey Mann Schyler

This approach is not so much a technique as it is a philosophy of treatment that organises the reconstruction of an occlusion into a sequence of goals that must be fulfilled. The emphasis of this technique lies in establishing the anterior guidance initially to be followed by establishing the posterior occlusion. The sequence of reconstruction is as follows:

- Restoration of mandibular anteriors
- Restoration of maxillary anteriors
- Restoration of mandibular posteriors
- Restoration of maxillary posteriors.

Twin table Technique–Sumiya Hobo

This technique has been introduced for developing molar disclusion by the use of two incisal tables. Molar disclusion is determined by the cusp shape factor and the angle of hinge rotation. It is a relatively uncomplicated technique and does not require special equipment. The final prosthesis by the use of the twin table technique results in a restoration with a predictable posterior disclusion and anterior guidance in harmony with the condylar path.

Twin stage procedure–Hobo and Takyama

This procedure considered cusp angle to be the most reliable reference for developing occlusion. The other two determinants, incisal guidance and condylar guidance accorded less importance in this procedure.

Gnathological Concept–Harvey Stallard

The first and oldest philosophy is that of gnathology which is based on a belief that the temporomandibular joints hinge on an axis of rotation in the glenoid fossa of the skull. All occlusion is guided and brought together to a finally tuned order, determined by the axis of the jaw joint rotation. The emphasis was on occlusion and joint position.

Despite these, a single, universally applicable occlusal treatment philosophy, which is scientifically proven does not exist. Many of the current rehablitative philosophies have their roots in empiricism. Hence it is important to recognize the limitations in some of these philosophies possessing sufficient understanding of occlusion. Hence full mouth rehablitation should be prescribed only when there is a definite indication for the same, as the changes brought about by the procedures are irreversible. Further reading is necessary to understand the concepts and techniques of full mouth rehablitation before applying these techniques practically.

BIBLIOGRAPHY

1. Castro, J.J., Keogh, T.P., Cadaval, R.L. and Planas, A.J.: A new system for the transferral of the occlusal morphology in posterior direct composite resin restorations. J. Esthet. Dent: 9, 311, 1997.
2. Christensen, G.J.: Now is the time to observe and treat dental occlusion. J.A.D.A. 132, 100, 2001.
3. Danveniza, M.: Full occlusal protection- theory and practice of occlusal therapy. Aust. Dent. J. 46, 70, 2001.
4. Delong, R., Sanik, C. and Pintado, M.R.: The wear of enamel when opposed by ceramic system. Dent. Mater.: 5, 266, 1989.
5. Dylina, T.J.: Occlusion problems. Dent. Today. 20, 8, 2001.
6. Gray, R.J., Davies, S.J.: Occlusal splints and temporo-mandibular disorder: why, when, how? Dent. Update 28, 194, 2001.
7. Gross, M.D.: Occlusion in Restorative Dentistry – Technique & Theory. Churchill Levingstone: 124, 1982.
8. Guichand, P., Mafart, B.: Evolution of occlusion, past and present time. B.D.J. 191, 2, 2001.
9. Hughes, H.J. and Meyers, G.E.: Practical aspects of occlusion in restorative dentistry. Aust. Dent. J.: 17, 4, 284, 1972.
10. Jantarat, J., Palamara, J.E., Messer, H.H.: An investigation of cuspal deformation and delayed recovery after occlusal loading. J. Dent. 29, 363, 2001.
11. Jenat, T., Lundquist, S. and Hedegard, B.: Group function or canine protection. J.P.D.: 91, 403, 2004.
12. Leibenberg, W.H.: Occlusal index-assisted restitution of esthetic and functional anatomy in direct tooth colored restorations. Quint. Int.: 27, 81, 1996.
13. Lipp, M.J.: Temporomandibular symptoms and occlusion. A review of the literature & concepts. Ny. State Dent. J.: 56, 58, 1990.
14. McCullock, A.J.: Making occlusion work: 1. Terminology, occlusal adjustments and recording. Dent. Update: 30, 150, 2003.
15. McCullock, A.J.: Making occlusion work: 2 Practical consideration. Dent. Update: 30, 211, 2003. Trushkowsky, R.D. and Burgess, J.O.: Complex single tooth restorations. D.C.N.A.: 46, 341, 2002.
16. McIntyre, F.M. and Jureyda, O.: Occlusal function. Beyond centric relation. D.C.N.A. 45, 173 Jan. 2001.
17. Milicich, G., Rainey, J.T.: Clinical presentations of stress distribution in teeth and significance in operative dentistry. Pract. Perio. Aesth. Dent. 12, 695, 2001.
18. Mulrooney, R.: Debating the science of occlusion. J. Can. Dent. Asso. 67, 247, 2001.
19. Parker, M.W.: The significance of occlusion in Restorative Dentistry. D.C.N.A.: 37, 341, 1993.
20. Ramfjord, S.P.: Is it really necessary to record jaw movements? Quint. Int.: 13, 187, 1982.
21. Small, B.W.: Location of incisal edge position for esthetic restorative dentistry. Gen. Dent. 48, 396, 2000.
22. Small, B.W.: The importance of contact and embrasures and their effect on periodontium. Gen. Dent. 48, 239, 2000.
23. Trushkowsky, R.D. and Burgess, J.O.: Complex single tooth restorations. D.C.N.A.: 46, 341, 2002.
24. Warren, K. and Capp, N.: A review of principles and techniques for making inter-occlusal records for mounting working casts. Int. J. Prosthodont.: 3, 341, 1990.
25. Watt, D.M.: Classification of occlusion. Dent. Pract.: 25, 305, 1970.
26. Watt, D.M. and Nakabayashi, Y.: Study of a classification of occlusion. J. Oral Rehabil.: 5, 101, 1978.
27. Wise, M.D.: Occlusion and restorative dentistry. B.D.J.: 143, 45, 1977.

4
Periodontal Restorative Interface

Microbial plaque is undoubtedly the primary etiological agent in periodontal disease. Nevertheless, other factors do contribute to gingival inflammation and subsequent loss of periodontal attachment. The production of plaque is not as important as the retention of plaque on and around the tooth surfaces. This retention increases manifolds in case of calculus deposits, poor margins of the restorations and perhaps the mere presence of a dental restoration.

The outer surface of a restoration is of significance from periodontal aspects. Proper contact, contour, occlusion, marginal adaptation and surface finish are as important to periodontics as to restorative dentistry. These factors influence the course and direction of masticatory forces, the deflection of food bolus and the collection and retention of deposits and/or food debris. Therefore, it is mandatory to have thorough knowledge of the anatomy and morphology of the teeth to be restored and also the techniques leading to restoration of proper cavosurface margins. Thus, all dental restorations should comply with established requirements for periodontal physiology and health with regard to both surface and functional characteristics. The operative dentist should always take care of the health of periodontium during all restorative procedures.

DENTOGINGIVAL UNIT

The dentogingival unit and its epithelial and connective tissue covering can be studied as follows (Figs 4.1 and 4.2):

a. *Gingiva:* It is composed of free gingiva and attached gingiva. The attached gingiva is bound to the cementum and the underlying bone by means of supra-alveolar connective tissue and lamina propria. If restorative procedures are to invade the gingival crevice, approximately 5.0 mm depth of gingiva is involved out of which, 2.0 mm is free gingiva and 3.0 mm is attached gingiva.

A second dimension of gingival tissue to be evaluated is thickness. The clinician, along with taking

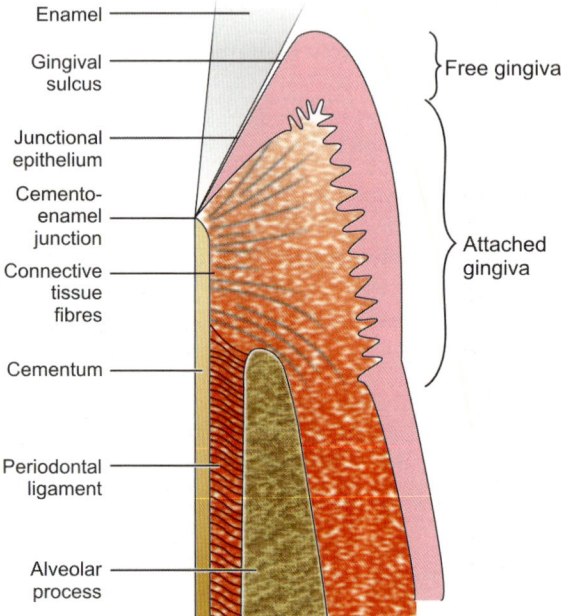

Fig. 4.1: Normal periodontium

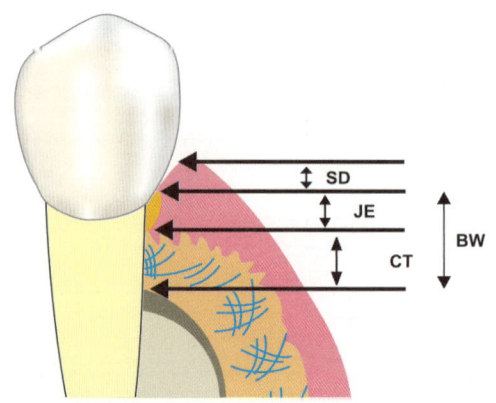

SD : Sulcular Depth
JE : Junctional Epithelium
CT : Connective Tissue
BW : Biological Width

Fig. 4.2: Dentogingival unit (gingiva, gingival sulcus and biological width)

care of the vertical dimensions of the gingiva, should also care for the thickness of the gingiva to tolerate intra-crevicular restorative procedures. The clinical test suggests that if a periodontal probe can be seen through the free gingival margin, the ability of that keratinized tissue to support a restoration is doubtful. In case where sufficient thickness of gingival tissue is not present, the margins of the restorations may induce apical migration of the gingiva.

b. *Gingival crevice:* The gingival crevice lined with crevicular epithelium, extends from the free gingival margin to the junctional epithelium. Two parameters of gingival crevice are important, one is its depth and the other is its circumference. Normally, the depth of the gingival crevice varies from 2.0–3.0 mm. Depth of the crevice can be excessive or inadequate for restorative dentistry. Excessive crevicular depth is pathognomonic of periodontal disease and restorative procedures should be avoided in such cases. For preparing intracrevicular margins in a tooth, a minimum depth of 1.5–2.0 mm is essential so that the margins are covered by free gingiva. If the crevice depth is less and clinician attempts to place margins of the restoration apical to gingival margin, there is a chance of permanent damage to junctional epithelium and underlying connective tissue. Circumferential aspect of crevice must also be understood. In healthy gingiva, there is hardly any space separating the epithelial lining of crevice from tooth surface. While restoring a tooth with full coverage restoration, care must be taken to avoid distension which may occur by qualitative or quantitative violation of circumferential aspect of crevice. Quantitative violation is when excessive material is being placed within the crevice, e.g. overhanging margins of the crowns. Qualitative violation is defined as poor adaptation and roughness of margins of the restoration. Such a violation results in both mechanical irritation of crevicular epithelium and also harbours the microbial flora.

c. *Biological width:* It is also known as Buffer zone, soft tissue cuff, subcrevicular attachment complex, etc. Biological width is defined as combined dimension of the supra-alveolar gingival connective tissue and the junctional epithelium. Average measurements for epithelial attachment and connective tissue attachment have been found to be 0.97 mm and 1.07 mm respectively, thus biological width equals approx. 2.0 mm. A restoration that impinges upon biological width will result in progressive periodontal disease. The margin of restoration should be more than 2.0 mm coronal to alveolar crest.

Encroachment into this space is prevalent amongst restorative dentists as they attempt to place a margin sub-gingival rather than intra-crevicular. The final position of the proposed gingival margin, which is dictated by existing restoration, caries or retention features, must be estimated to determine whether crown lengthening procedures are required or not before restoration to be given. Biological widths vary according to type of tooth which progressively increases from anterior to posterior teeth.

Anterior teeth – 1.75 mm
Premolars   – 1.97 mm
Molars   – 2.08 mm

Restored teeth have wider biological width than non-restored due to longer epithelial attachment around restored teeth. The population variation is depicted in Table 4.1.

PRESERVATION OF PERIODONTIUM

The preservation of healthy periodontium is the most significant factor in long-term prognosis of restored teeth. The health of periodontium depends on the following features of teeth.

Contour

The buccal and lingual surfaces of teeth possess some degree of convexity and afford protection along with stimulation to the supporting structures during mastication. The convexity is generally located at the cervical third of the crown on facial surfaces of all the teeth and lingual surfaces of incisors and canines. The lingual surfaces of posterior teeth have their height of contour in the middle third.

Table 4.1: Population variation and biological width		
85% population	*13% population*	*2% population*
Sulcus –1.0 mm. Normal alveolar crest relation with cemento-enamel junction	Alveolar crest and epithelial attachment (EA) are more apical in relatively normal relation, but with long EA	Alveolar crest and epithelial attachment are more coronal in position, but with short epithelial attachment
Least chances of biological width violation, when margins of the restoration are placed subgingivally	Less chances of biological violation, when margins of the restoration are placed subgingivally	Avoid subgingival margins

This type of curvature determines the direction in which the food would be pushed cervically during mastication. Normal tooth contours shunt food towards the buccal vestibule and tongue or palate in such a way that the passing food stimulates the intervening tissue rather than irritating them (Fig. 4.3).

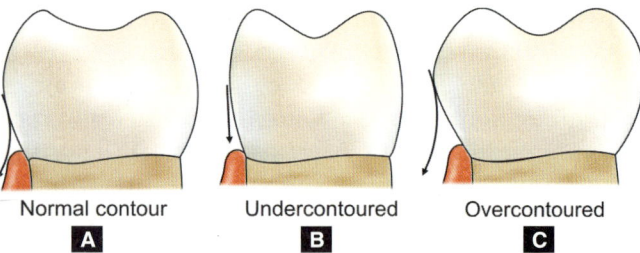

Fig. 4.3: Buccal and lingual curvatures (arrows showing passage of food during mastication)

Clinical Implications

- If the curvatures are over contoured, the supporting tissues usually receive inadequate stimulation by passage of food.
- Under-contoured curvatures may result in trauma to the attachment apparatus.
    i. *Over-contouring:* Over-contouring of restorations is a much greater hazard to periodontal health than lack of contour since both supragingival and sub-gingival plaque accumulation may be enhanced by such restorations. Commonly, porcelain fused to metal crowns are over contoured because of inadequate facial reduction. Such an over contour interferes with the sealing cuff effect of gingiva against the tooth and the self-cleansing mechanism of gingival sulcus.
    ii. *Under-contouring:* The proximal crown contours are generally flat or concave. This provides adequate embrasure space for the interdental gingiva and allows room for plaque removal. The transitional line angle (the area between the proximal surface and the facial or lingual surface) is also generally flat or concave to form the opening for the embrasure space and house the interdental tissue. The transitional line angle is an important consideration in tooth preparation and full crown restorations. If improperly restored, it will adversely affect the gingiva.

Height of Epithelial Attachment

The height of normal gingival tissue, mesially and distally on approximating teeth is directly dependent upon the heights of epithelial attachment on these teeth. Normal attachment follows the curvature of cementoenamel junction if the teeth are in proper alignment and contact (Fig. 4.2). The extent of curvature depends upon:

- The height of contact area above the crown crevice
- Diameter of the crown buccolingually

Crowns of anterior teeth, which are narrower and longer, show the greatest curvature (Fig. 4.4A). Because the crowns of canines distally function as posterior teeth, the curvatures of cementoenamel junction are 1.5–2.0 mm in this regions as compared to the mesial curvature that is 2.5 mm. In premolars and molars, the contact level is apical in relation to the total crown length, consequently these teeth do not have high periodontal attachments interproximally (Fig. 4.4B).

Therefore, proximal surfaces of anterior teeth must be carefully prepared for receiving any restoration. The curvatures of posterior teeth are less critical. The height of attachment must be ascertained by careful probing or by continuous observation of landmarks during operation.

Proximal Contact Areas

Proximal contact areas are areas on proximal surfaces of tooth crowns where a tooth touches the adjacent tooth when the teeth are in proper alignment.

Importance

- Stabilizes the tooth within the alveolus and the arch by providing combined anchorage to all the teeth in either arch. The anterior component of force is transmitted through intact proximal contacts. Missing proximal contacts or deflected forces of occlusion through malpositioned contacts may cause displacement of the teeth and create abnormal forces on the periodontium.
- Helps prevent food impaction.
- Protects the interdental papillae by shunting food towards buccal and lingual areas.

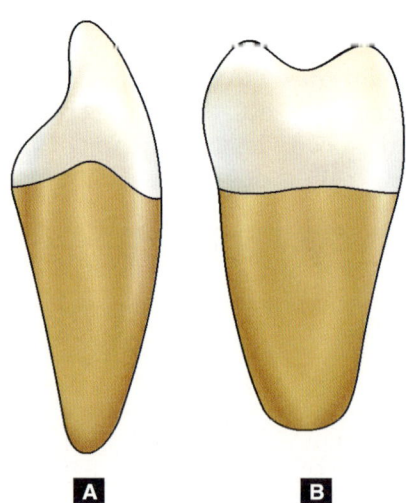

Figs 4.4A and B: Cervical curvatures as found on **(A)** Anterior tooth and; **(B)** Posterior tooth

Location

Proximal contact areas should be considered in two aspects:
- Labial/buccal view showing cervicoincisal or cervicoocclusal location of contact (Figs 4.5A and B).
- Incisal/occlusal view showing labiolingual location of the contact (Figs 4.6A and B).

A generalization may be established in locating contact areas faciolingually. Anterior teeth will have their contacts centered labiolingually, whereas posterior teeth will have their contacts slightly buccal to the centre of buccolingual width. The narrower dimension lingually rather than facially causes wide embrasures lingually compared with facial embrasures in all teeth except in maxillary posterior teeth where the vice versa is true.

Methods of Testing a Contact Area

Pass the dental floss gingival of the contact from facial to lingual or lingual to facial direction. The two ends are then held parallel in occlusal direction. This measures the faciolingual width of contact. Without

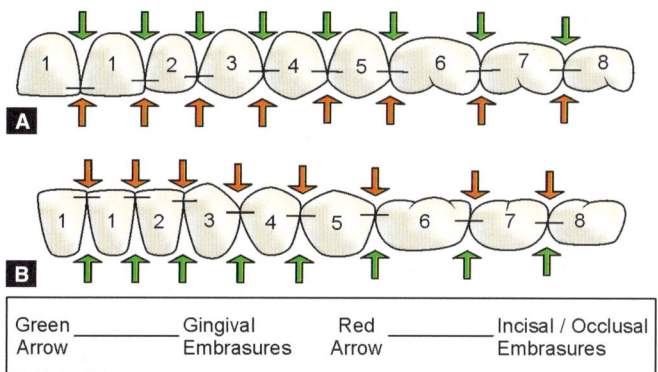

| Green Arrow | Gingival Embrasures | Red Arrow | Incisal / Occlusal Embrasures |

Figs 4.5A and B: Proximal contact areas (cervico-occlusal view) and gingival and incisal/occlusal embrasures. **(A)** Maxillary teeth; **(B)** Mandibular teeth

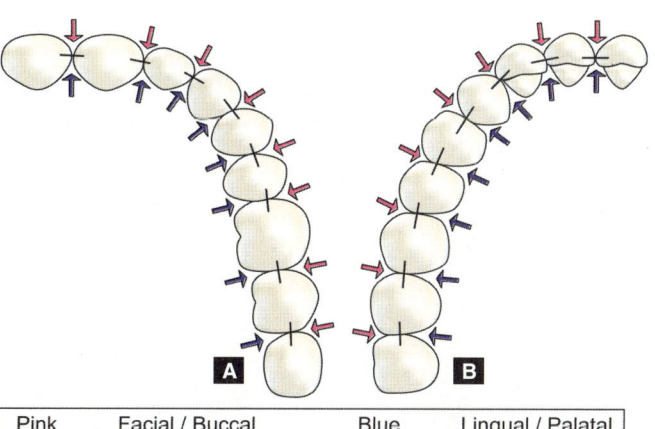

| Pink Arrow | Facial / Buccal Embrasures | Blue Arrow | Lingual / Palatal Embrasures |

Figs 4.6A and B: Proximal contact areas (labio-lingual view) and facial and lingual/palatal embrasures. **(A)** Maxillary teeth; **(B)** Mandibular teeth

removing the floss, the two ends are now held parallel in facial direction. This measures the occlusogingival width of the contact.

In either position, if the parallel strands are more than 1.5-2.0 mm apart, the contact is too broad.

Hazards of faulty reproduction of contact size and location in restorations are given in Table 4.2.

The correct contour cervico-occlusally and faciolingually is shown in (Figs 4.7A and B) respectively.

A case of poor contact between the restored surfaces of mandibular first and second molars was rehabilitated by giving full crown mandibular first molar, creating proper contact and contour of the restoration (Figs 4.8A and B).

Embrasures/Spillways

These are V-shaped spaces that originate at the proximal contact area between adjacent teeth and are named according to the direction towards which they radiate (Figs 4.5 and 4.6).

These embrasures are facial, lingual, incisal/occlusal and gingival. These embrasures are continuous with each other as well as with interproximal spaces.

Functions

- Serve as spillways for escape of food during mastication; therefore the force being brought to bear on the teeth is also reduced. Food is returned to the occlusal table by movement of the facial tissues and tongue.
- Prevents forcing the food into the contact area. When teeth are attrited and occlusal embrasures are lost, food is easily forced through the contact area.

The size and location of contact area determines the size of embrasure spaces. Too large and too small embrasures provide little protection to the supporting structures.

Occlusal Surfaces

Occlusal surfaces should be designed to direct the masticatory forces along the long axis of teeth. Anatomy of occlusal surface should provide well-formed marginal ridges and occlusal spillways to prevent interproximal food impaction.

Marginal ridges are elevated rounded ridges that form the mesial and distal margins of occlusal surfaces of premolars and molars and mesial and distal margins of lingual surfaces of incisors and canines.

Importance of Marginal Ridges

i. In general
  - Maintain balance of teeth in the arch
  - Prevent impaction of food interproximally
  - Help in efficient mastication

Table 4.2: Hazards of faulty contact size and location

Type	Hazards
Broad contact faciolingually	• Interproximal tissue is over-protected and will not receive proper stimulative massage from excursion of food • Extra breadth of contact prevents food from scouring the embrasures
Broad contact occlusogingivally	• Sticky foods are likely to be held • Encroaches upon gingival tissue • If proximal caries occurs, it will be farther gingivally
Contact too far gingivally	• Creates a wider space between the two proximal surfaces in an occlusal direction. Sticky foods are likely to become packed into this space and eventually force the teeth apart • Impinges upon the interproximal tissue
Contact too far incisal/occlusal	• Frequently observed in amalgam restorations • Crest of gingiva is far from contact and predisposes the proximal surface to caries • Prevents food from being pushed into embrasures
Contact too far buccal/lingual	• Buccal/lingual embrasures are narrow, produce inefficient mastication
Loose contact	• Food lodgement in open contact area develops gingival problems and caries

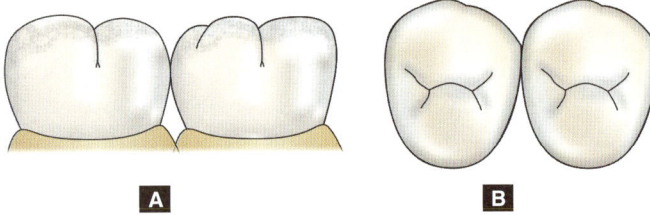

Figs 4.7A and B: Correct contour. **(A)** Cervico-occlusally; **(B)** Faciolingually

ii. In restorative dentistry
- It is imperative to have a marginal ridge of proper dimensions, i.e. compatible with the dimension of the occlusal cuspal anatomy, creating a pronounced adjacent triangular fossa and producing an adjacent occlusal embrasure.
- A marginal ridge should always be restored in two planes; bucco-lingually and cervicoocclusally.

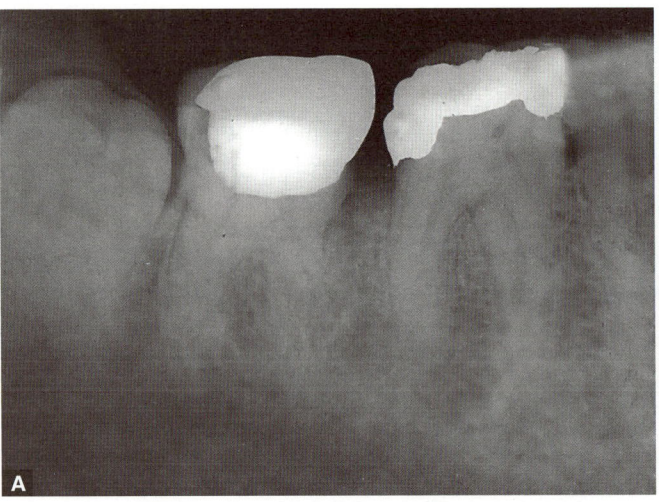
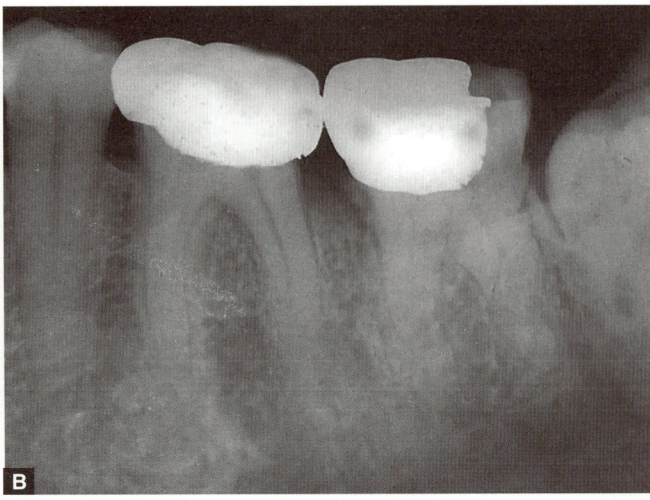

Figs 4.8A and B: (A) No contact; (B) Rehabilitation of contact and contour

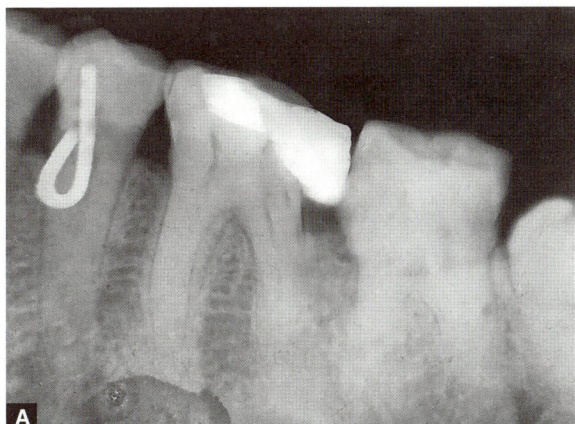
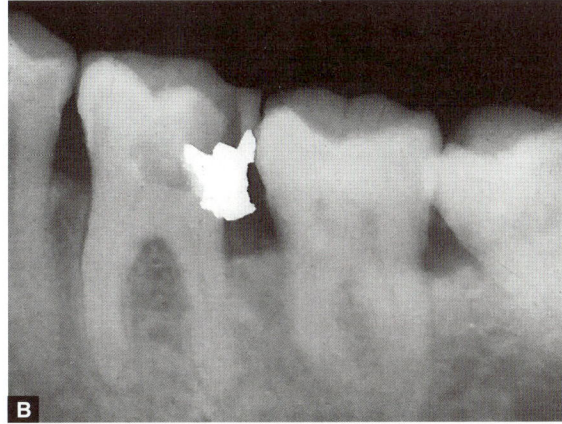

Figs 4.9A and B: Overhanging margins

- Adjacent marginal ridges should be compatible in height.

Margins

The restoration must blend at its margin into the tooth structure without catches. On guiding a sharp explorer over the margin, one should be aware of not passing from tooth to restoration. Composites or plastic fillings seldom permit satisfactory gingival margins. Overhanging margins lead to inter-proximal bone loss. Poor margins will invite plaque retention and tend to harbor micro-organisms (Figs 4.9A and B).

The stepwise rehabilitation procedure of a case in which a single inlay was given in adjacent proximal surfaces of maxillary first and second molars is shown in Figs 4.10A to I.

Surface Finish and Texture

The surface of restorations should be as smooth as possible to limit plaque accumulation. Roughened tooth and restoration surfaces especially in the sub-gingival region result in increased plaque accumulation and increased gingival inflammation.

In clinical situations, porcelain, highly polished gold, and highly polished resin all result in similar plaque accumulation.

Threshold for surface roughness = 0.2 mm; above which bacterial adhesion will be facilitated.

However, further smoothing does not have additional effect

Surface free energy and surface roughness are the two factors influencing plaque growth, latter predominates.

TRAUMA FROM OCCLUSION

At rest position, the teeth are apart and no occlusal forces are applied to them. During mastication the forces applied to the teeth are relatively small. The periodontal ligament fibers are arranged in a definite pattern and most of the fibers are arranged in oblique fashion, which are best suited to tolerate and transmit the vertical forces to the supporting bone. The remaining groups of fibers dissipate the stresses in other directions. Mastication usually does not produce trauma as the teeth touch but minimally. Trauma usually results when teeth are occluded at times other than during chewing. Non-masticatory forces/parafunctional forces viz. clenching, bruxism, etc. which produce traumatic forces. The forces generated by mastication may have different effects than those generated by habits. Since a habit means frequently repeated action, the occlusal forces are sustained over an extended period of time. Therefore the parafunctional forces are significant in the etiology of occlusal trauma.

The tooth when subjected to the forces of occlusion tries to accommodate them, which depends upon the adaptive capacity of the periodontium of an individual. However, various factors like magnitude, direction, duration and frequency of force effect the periodontium that varies in different persons and in the same person at different times. When the occlusal forces exceed the adaptive capacity of the periodontium, tissue injury results. This tissue injury is termed as 'trauma from occlusion'. These excessive occlusal forces not only affect the periodontium but also cause painful spasms in masticatory musculature, temporomandibular joint, dysfunction, excessive tooth wear and injury to the pulp tissue. There are various other terms used to define trauma from occlusion viz. occlusal trauma, periodontal traumatism, overload, etc.

Etiology

The occlusal relationships which produce trauma are as follows:
- Uneven occlusal wear (especially when metal restorations are there on occlusal surface)
- Mesial drifting and tipping caused by loss of adjacent teeth

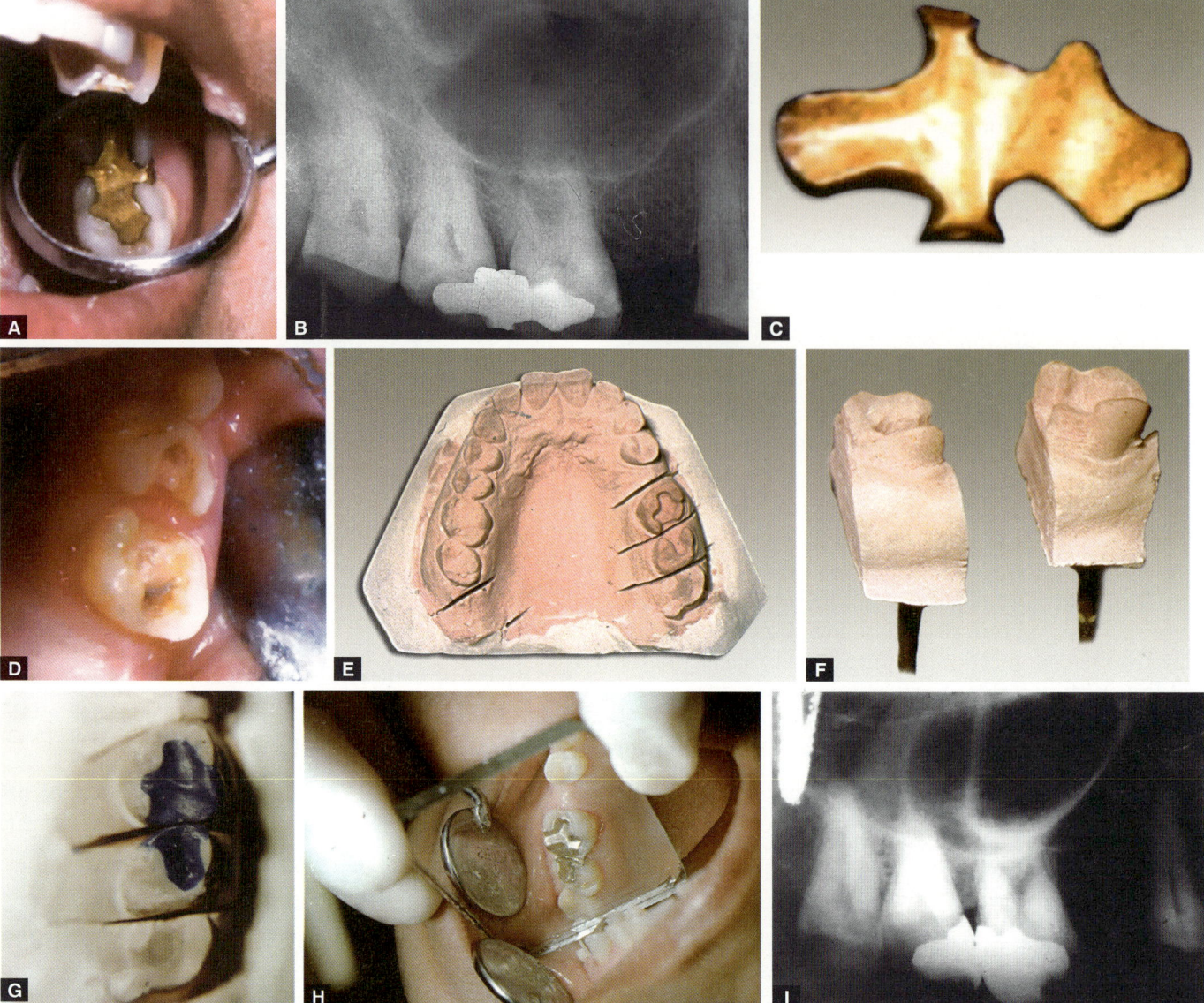

Figs 4.10A to I: Stepwise rehabilitation procedure of a case in which single inlay was given in adjacent proximal surfaces of maxillary first and second molars. **(A)** Joined inlay in maxillary first and second molar; **(B)** Radiograph showing the joined inlay; **(C)** Inlay removed; **(D)** Modified cavity preparation, with cusp reduced; **(E)** Die showing the preparation; **(F)** Individual dies; **(G)** Pattern making; **(H)** Complete restoration; **(I)** Proper contact and contour as shown in the radiograph

- Altered clinical crown/root ratio due to periodontal diseases.
- Teeth serving as abutments for malfunctioning prosthesis (clasped teeth, crowned teeth for cantilever bridges, etc.)
- Excessive overbite relationships
- Habit patterns, e.g. bruxism, clenching, tongue thrusting, etc.

According to Glickman, trauma from occlusion may be acute or chronic. Acute trauma from occlusion develops when there is a sudden change in occlusal force, e.g. biting on a hard object, high restorations or prosthetic appliance which interferes or alters the direction of occlusal forces on the teeth resulting in tooth pain, sensitivity to percussion, increased tooth mobility. The acute trauma from occlusion subsides by shifting the position of teeth, by orthodontic means, natural wearing of teeth or by corrective means like occlusal adjustment.

Chronic trauma from occlusion is a more frequent finding which develops due to gradual changes in occlusion, produced by tooth wear, drifting movement, extrusion of teeth; bruxism, clenching or an acute condition may develop into a chronic condition.

a. *Primary trauma from occlusion*: When alterations in occlusal forces is the primary etiologic factor in periodontal destruction.

For example, insertion of high filling/prosthesis, drifting/extrusion of teeth, orthodontic movements of teeth into functionally unacceptable positions

b. *Secondary trauma from occlusion*: When adaptive capacity of tissues to withstand normally well-tolerated occlusal forces is impaired by bone loss due to inflammation. For example, in patients of chronic periodontitis

Clinically, the physiologic occlusion is manifested in two forms:
- Vertical loading
- Horizontal loading

Vertical Loading

In this form, the applied occlusal force is exerted along the long axis of the tooth. The pressure of stress on the periodontal membrane is greater at the apex than along the sides.

Horizontal Loading

In this form, the applied occlusal force is exerted in a direction oblique to the long axis. There will be compressural stress on the periodontal membrane in the gingival third of the side away from the point of application of force and in the apical third on the side of application of force.

In both vertical and horizontal loading, the occlusion pressure on the tooth is balanced by the resistance of the periodontal tissues.

Torques or rotational forces cause both tension and pressure. Under physiologic conditions they cause bone formation and bone resorption respectively. However, torques injure the periodontium if they exceed the adaptive capacity of periodontium.

As already discussed, there are two ways in which traumatic occlusion may be produced.
- By excessive stress and strains on the teeth
- By weakening of the supporting structures of teeth

Effects of Occlusal Disharmony

The effect of traumatic occlusion depends on the following factors, however, the effect varies in different teeth and in different individuals:
- The magnitude of force
- The direction of force
- Duration of force
- Frequency of force
- Tissue resistance of the patient

The effects of occlusal disharmony can be:
- Discomfort in the region of the temporomandibular joint
- Food impaction
- Abnormal habit
- Pain in and around teeth with improper restorations
- Pulpal disturbances
- Facial pain of obscure origin
- Periodontal abscess
- Cheek biting
- Sensitivity of occlusal/incisal surfaces of teeth due to their abnormal wear
- Mobility of teeth
- Gingival recession
- Pericementitis
- Bruxism
- Unilateral mastication
- Restricted excursion of the mandible resulting in insufficient wear
- Extreme excursions of the mandible resulting in excessive wear
- Migration of upper and lower teeth

Diagnostic Signs of Trauma from Occlusion

Following signs are of diagnostic importance for trauma from occlusion:

Clinical Signs

- Progressive or increased tooth mobility
- Abnormal wear of teeth
- Cheek biting
- Bruxism
- Sharply demarcated linear depressions in the alveolar mucosa, parallel to the long axis of the root and overlying the septal bone

Radiographic Signs

- Widening of periodontal space (Fig. 4.11)
- Thickening of lamina dura (Fig. 4.12)
- Vertical/angular bone loss (Fig. 4.13)
- Rarefaction of bone (Fig. 4.14)
- Condensation of bone (Fig. 4.15)
- Hypercementosis (Fig. 4.16)
- Root resorption (Fig. 4.17)
- Furcation invovlement (Fig. 4.18)

Keeping in view the deleterious effects of trauma from occlusion, the occlusal adjustment is mandatory

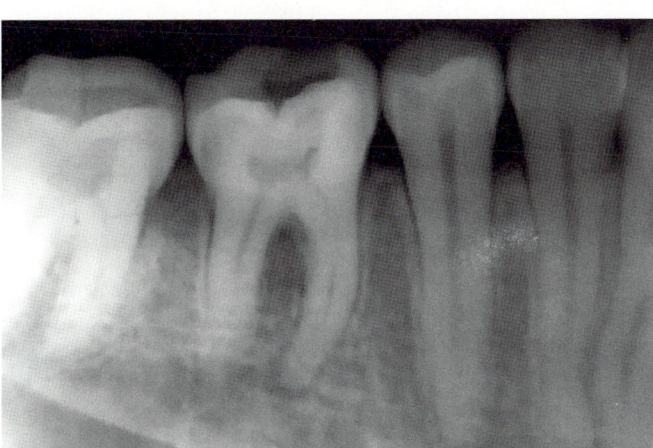

Fig. 4.11: Widening of periodontal ligament space

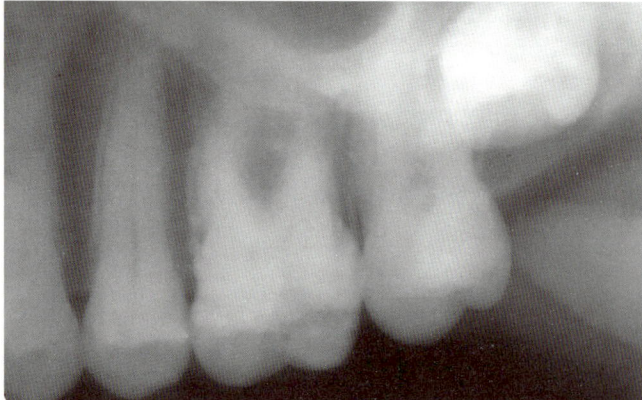

Fig. 4.12: Thickening of lamina dura

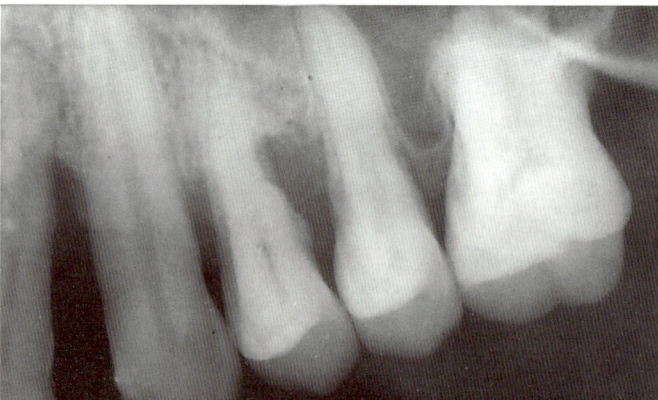

Fig. 4.13: Angular bone defect

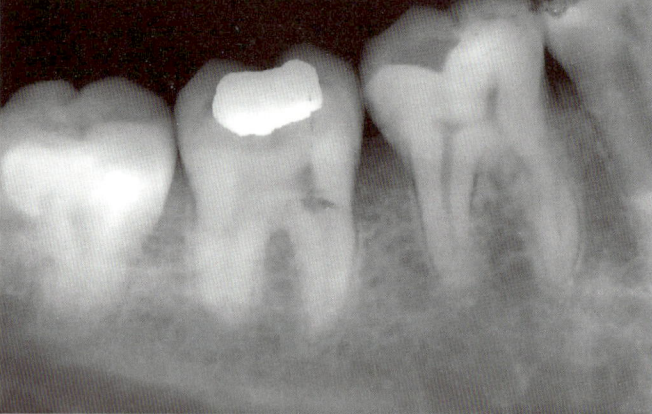

Fig. 4.14: Rarefaction of bone

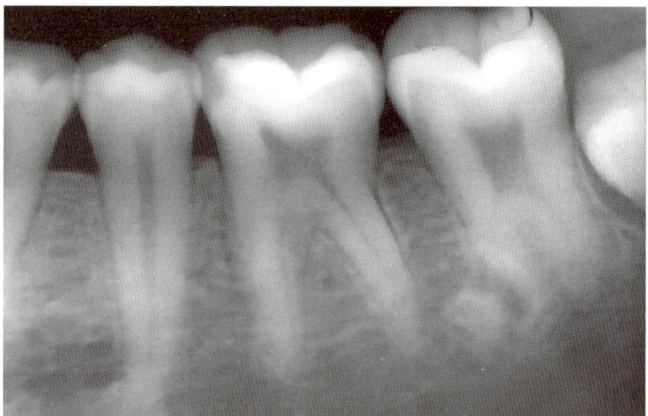

Fig. 4.15: Condensation of bone

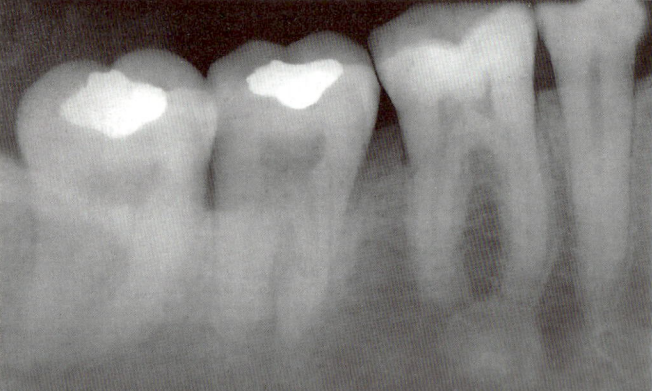

Fig. 4.16: Hypercementosis

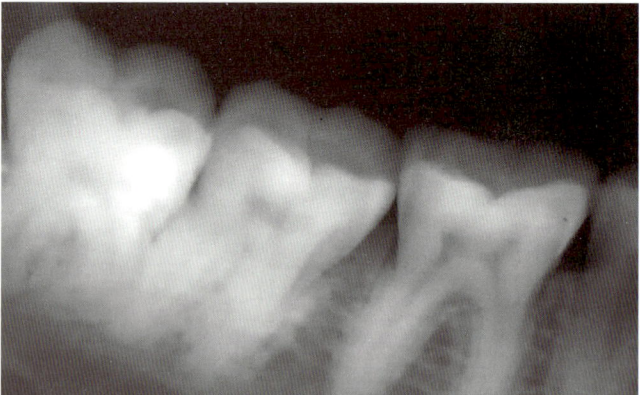

Fig. 4.17: Root resorption

to create functional relationships favourable with the periodontium. In this, all the opposing teeth make simultaneous contact with their antagonists both in normal and functional relations of the jaw. This can be achieved by various means:
- Reshaping of teeth by grinding
- Restorative measures
- Tooth movement
- Extraction of teeth
- Orthognathic surgery

The objective of occlusal therapy is to achieve therapeutic occlusion that may not conform to the

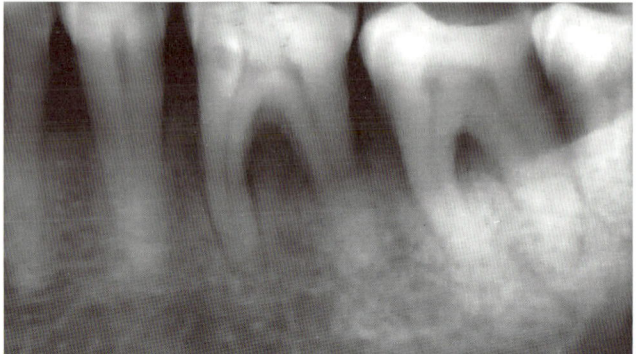

Fig. 4.18: Furcation involvement

concept of ideal occlusion. The basic objectives of any occlusion therapy are:
- Establishment or maintenance of a stable, reproducible intercuspal position.
- Freedom of movement to and from intercuspal position.
- Development of occlusion not noticeable to the patient.
- Maintenance of newly established occlusal scheme over a reasonable period of time. The therapist must evaluate and decide whether the teeth will maintain the occlusal relationship or require some adjunctive aid such as splinting.
- Establishment of an occlusion with acceptable phonation, mastication and esthetics.

Aims of Occlusal Equilibration

The functional aims of occlusal equilibrium include the improvement in the following:
- Masticatory function
- Temporomandibular function
- Musculature function
- Comfort
- Esthetics
- Phonetics
- Tissue stimulation (relative to the age of the patient)
- Prevention or relief (or both) of trauma
- Oral sanitation
- Elimination of food impaction

Diagnosis of Premature Contacts

It is important to find out many supracontacts or prematurities of teeth. Multiple products and procedures have been tried for this to identify and mark the supracontacts or prematurities viz. study casts, roentgenograms, palpation, visual examination, patient's tactile response on closure of teeth, impression on wax and articulating paper markings.

It is advisable to determine occlusal equilibration by as many methods as possible, as depending on only one of the above means will not be certain.

i. *Study casts:* Study casts are of great help in keeping record of the case or in planning occlusal equilibration. They are useful to note the lingual relationships between the teeth for better understanding and analysis of all occlusal factors present. Thus areas of food impaction, plunger cusps, abnormal wear of the teeth, facets and abnormal overbite can easily be observed in study casts.

ii. *Roentgenograms:* Roentgenograms are useful adjuncts in diagnosing lesions of the teeth, periodontal space, lamina dura and alveolar bone changes. Bitewing films aid in diagnosing areas with food impaction. Radiographically, signs of trauma from occlusion include; increased width of the periodontal space and thickening of lamina dura along the lateral aspect of the root, in the apical region and in furcation areas. There is vertical/angular bone loss in interdental septum, condensation of the alveolar bone and root resorption.

iii. *Palpation:* This method, known as fremitus test, is best used on upper teeth to determine movement in such teeth when the teeth are in premature centric occlusion. The ball of the index finger is rested lightly against two adjacent upper teeth at a time and the patient is asked to repeatedly open and close in centric occlusion. A tooth in premature centric occlusion will be felt to move when its antagonist makes contact with it.

iv. *Visual examination:* To know interceptive contacts in centric occlusion, the patient is advised to firmly close the jaw in centric occlusion. Careful observation reveals a slight movement of the tooth in interceptive contact. The gingiva investing the root of a tooth bearing excessive stress may be blanched in some patients.

v. *Patient's tactile response:* Patient is asked to slightly open and close the jaw until the first point of occlusal contact is felt. The patient will feel the bouncing on a single portion of a tooth if there is an interceptive contact. But operator should not rely on first response. For final diagnosis, more investigations are needed.

vi. *Impression on wax:* Impression on wax has been used to determine the areas of interceptive contacts. This method is most reliable to measure prematurities in centric relations. 26 gauge green or pink wax is used. Make wax strips, which can cover occlusal surfaces of teeth. Before taking impressions soften the wax in warm water. After it has been uniformly softened, place the wax strips over the occlusal surfaces of teeth. Ask the patient to bite in it very slowly till he feels the first contact. Take out the impression and chill the wax in ice cold water and examine it against light. Presence of premature contacts is observed as perforation. In order to confirm we must take two to three records. If there is uniform perforation then either the wax was too soft, or patient has closed the mouth firmly.

If thick wax is used and the patient is unable to close the mouth, there will be no records over the wax.

These wax records are transferred on models and perforations are marked on study models with pencil.

vii. *Articulating paper markings:* Articulating papers are very useful for recording interceptive contacts both in the centric and lateral excursions or eccentric relations. Thick easily marking articulating papers should be used. In order to differentiate centric relations (CR) from eccentric relations (ER), use two colors of articulating papers, i.e. red and blue, say red for centric relations and blue for eccentric relations. For better markings, the teeth must be dried and loose teeth should be supported by splints. Place the articulating papers on teeth and ask the patient to bite first in centric relations using red articulating paper and then in eccentric relations using blue articulating paper.

Patient is asked to open and close the mouth repeatedly. When prematurity exists, the marking will appear as a lighter area surrounded by a darker zone on the tooth, which should be grounded. It is advisable to reduce prematurity in centric relations and then in eccentric relations.

Common sources of error are:
- Smudges may mark more of the tooth surface than is actually in contact.
- Some teeth may show markings inadvertently.

To overcome the above errors, always confirm with more than one method.

Occlusal Adjustment by Grinding

Occlusal adjustment by grinding is a procedure where selective reduction of occlusal areas is done to eliminate injurious occlusal forces and to provide functional stimulation for the preservation of periodontal health. Basic idea is to:

i. Eliminate the undesirable occlusal prematurities obstructing the closure of cusps in the fossae, which are responsible for excessive occlusal forces on the periodontium

ii. To create stable mandibular position

It is not simply a matter of grinding down the premature contacts that will create flattened planes which will further disrupt the occlusion, so it is a planned procedure which should be done in stepwise manner restoring and preserving the anatomy of teeth at a particular age. The steps are as follows:
- Grooving
- Spheroiding
- Pointing

a. *Grooving* consists of restoring the depth of the developmental grooves, which have been made shallow by occlusal wear. It is carried out by a tapered cutting tool until a desired depth is achieved.

b. *Spheroiding* consists of reducing the prematurities while restoring the original tooth contour. This is done with a light paint brush stroke, gradually blending the area of prematurity with the adjacent tooth surface. A special effort is made to preserve the occlusal height of the cusps.

When the teeth are flattened by wear, the buccolingual diameter of the occlusal surface is increased. The objective is to restore the bucco-lingual width of occlusal surface to normal dimensions.

c. *Pointing* consists of restoring cups point contours and is done by reshaping the tooth with rotating cutting tools.

At each recall, the occlusion should be analyzed; since occlusion is dynamic and may need minor adjustment every time.

BIBLIOGRAPHY

1. Bwenett, R.R., Diaz, R., Waldrop, T.C. and Hallmon, W.W.: Clinical perspective of periodontal and restorative interaction. Compendium.: 15, 644, 1994.
2. Gomes, S.C., Miranda, L.A., Soares, J. and Oppermann, R.V.: Clinical and histological evaluation of the periodontal response to restorative procedures in the dog. Int. J. Period. & Restorative Dent.: 25, 39, 2005.
3. Jokstad, A.: Clinical trial of gingival retraction cords. J. Prosth. Dent.: 81, 258, 1999.
4. Kamenova, J.: Treatment of occlusal traumatic symptoms using low-power laser irradiation. J. Oral Laser Irradiation: 4, 29, 2004.
5. Kancyper, S.G. and Koka, S.: The influence of intracrevicular crown margins on gingival health: Preliminary findings. J.P.D.: 85, 461, 2001.
6. Kataoka, S. and Mutobe, Y.: In harmony with nature:Periodontium and esthetics. Quint. Int.: 1, 13, 2001.
7. Keogh, T.P. and Bertolotti, R.L.: Crating tight, anatomically correct interproximal contacts. D.C.N.A.: 1, 83, 2001.
8. Leon, A.R.: The periodontium and restorative procedures: A critical review. J. Oral Rehab.: 4, 105, 1977.
9. Padbury, Jr. A., Eber, R. and Wang, H.L.: Interactions between the gingival and the margins of restorations. J. Clinical Perio.: 30, 379, 2003.
10. Paolantonio, M., Dercole, S., Perinetti, G., Tripodi, D., Catamo, G. and Serra, G.: Clinical and microbiological effects of different materials on the periodontal tissues adjacent to subgingival class V restorations. J. Clinical Period.: 31, 200, 2004.
11. Prato, G.P., Rotundo, R., Cortellini, P., Tinti, C. and Azzi, R.: Interdental papilla management: A review and classification of the therapeutic approaches. Int. J. Period. & Restorative Dent.: 24, 246, 2004.
12. Schatzle, M., Lang, N.P., Boysen, H., Burgin, W. and Loe, H.: The influence of margins of restorations on the periodontal tissues over 26 years. J. Clinical Period.: 28, 57, 2001.
13. Yap, U.J. and Oug, G.: Periodontal consideration in restorative dentistry. 1: Operative Considerations. Dent. Update: 21, 413, 1994.

Dental Caries

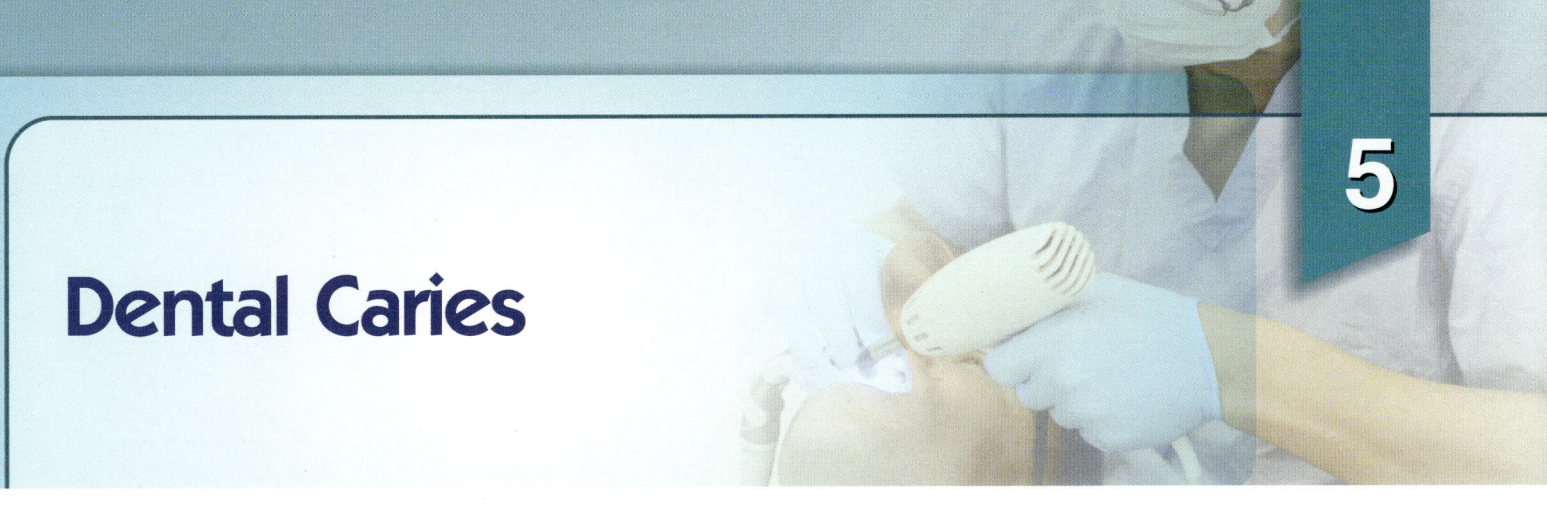

Nature has provided us teeth to perform the functions of cutting, grinding and admixing food with saliva. The hard enamel cover along with the periodontal ligament can withstand forces of mastication. The unique character of tooth is that it is comprised of two tissues of different embryological origin; ectodermal enamel, and mesodermal dentin. Enamel is acellular, avascular and has no nerve supply. It is incapable of any natural defense mechanism based on cellular activity. As the tooth erupts, it is open to complex environment.

Dental caries is the most prevalent disease of mankind. It is strange that the hardest tissue of the body the enamel, which is indestructible otherwise, can disintegrate in the oral environment. *Caries* (Latin meaning 'dry rot') implies slow disintegration that may affect any of the biological hard tissue as a result of bacterial action. This action may affect bone, causing 'bone caries'. Usually such disintegration affects enamel, dentin and cementum (*the tooth*); that is why the term 'dental caries' is most common.

The pattern of dental caries is not uniform even within large countries like India, America or China. This may be because of several important variables that affect caries such as diet, trace elements and other related factors. Different types of caries may have the same etiology; however, the susceptibility of different surfaces of teeth varies. The attack of caries and its severity also varies from individual to individual.

In the recent past, decline in caries prevalence has been reported. It is reported that in the United States alone the mean DMFS for children in the age group 5–12 years declined from 7 to 4, though this much decline is not evident in developing countries. Since 80% of the children reside in underdeveloped countries, it is obvious that preventive measures must be undertaken for these children to improve their oral health.

DEFINITIONS

In simple terms, dental caries can be defined as *the irreversible, slow progressing decay of hard tissues of the tooth*. It is a local disease, which involves destruction of hard tissues of the teeth by metabolites produced by oral micro-organisms

It is defined as *the microbial disease of the calcified tissues of teeth, characterized by demineralization of the inorganic portion and destruction of organic substance of the tooth.*

According to WHO, caries is defined as *a localized post eruptive, pathological process of external origin involving softening of the hard tooth tissue and proceeding to the formation of a cavity.*

CLASSIFICATION OF CARIES

The prevalence of caries is definitely dependant on age pattern and even sex.

Dental caries can be classified according to three major factors:
A. According to morphology of teeth
B. According to severity and progress of lesion
C. According to age

A. According to Morphology of Teeth

According to morphology of teeth, the caries is categorized into following four types:
a. *Pit and fissure caries*: Caries occurring on anatomical pits and fissures of all the teeth. This is also referred to as Class-I caries (Figs 5.1, 5.2).
b. *Smooth surface caries*: Caries occurring on smooth surfaces of the teeth. This is also referred to as Class–II caries (Figs 5.1, 5.3, 5.4)
c. *Root caries*: Caries occurring at the cementoenamel junction or cementum. This occurs predominantly in the older age when there is gingival recession (Figs 5.5, 5.6, 5.7).
d. *Linear enamel caries*: Caries occurring on the labial surfaces of anterior teeth. This is also known as 'Odontoclasia'. The caries occurs at neonatal zone because of trauma at birth or metabolic disturbances.

B. According to Severity and Progress of Lesion

According to severity and progression of lesion, the caries is categorized into following five types:

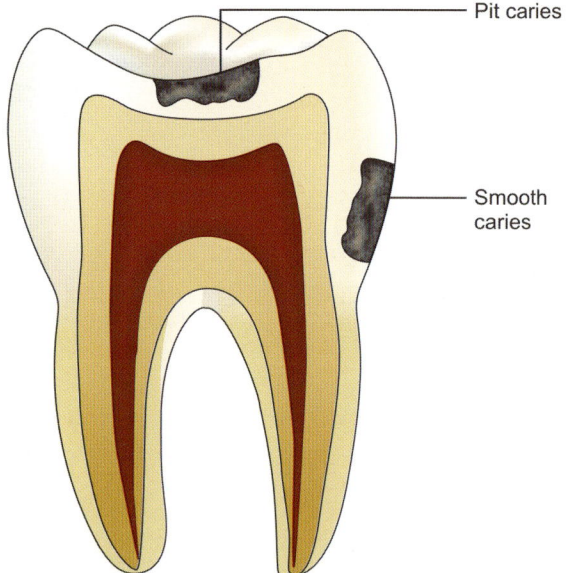

Fig. 5.1: Caries in the pits and fissures and on smooth surface (diagrammatic representation)

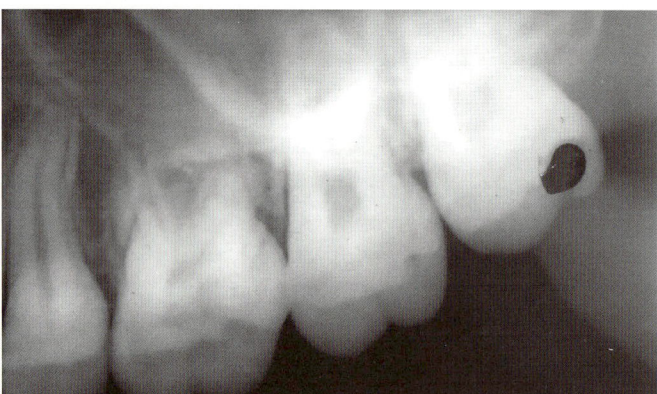

Fig. 5.2: Caries in the pit and fissure (as seen in radiograph)

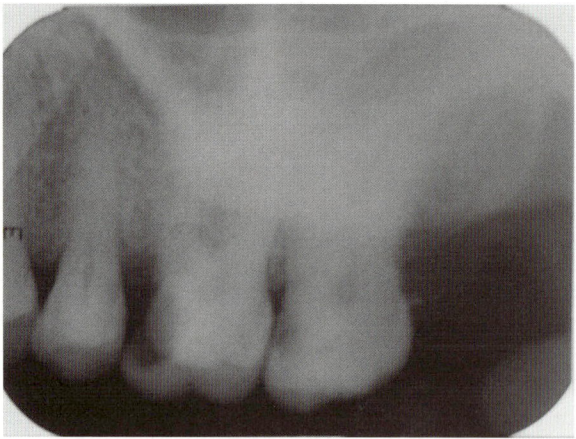

Fig. 5.3: Caries on smooth surface (as seen in radiograph)

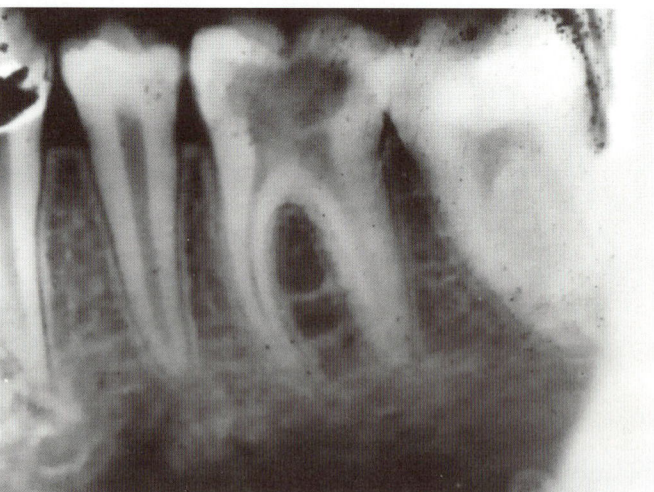

Fig. 5.4: Caries on the smooth surface—buccal surface (as seen in radiograph)

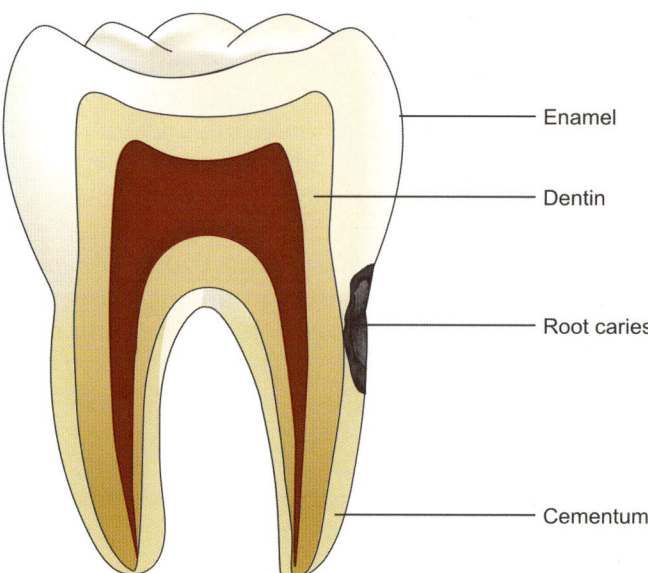

Fig. 5.5: Root surface caries (diagrammatic representation)

a. *Incipient caries*: Incipient caries appears as a white opaque region on any tooth surface. The white opacity is because of surface demineralization of enamel. The incipient lesion can undergo remineralization thereby reversing the process.

b. *Rampant caries*: It is the sudden and rapid onset of caries involving at least two teeth and two surfaces. A caries increment of ten or more new carious lesions over a year is characteristic of rampant caries.

c. *Arrested caries*: Any carious lesion, usually an incipient, may become arrested, if there is a change in oral environment. The arrested caries, clinically appears as a dark brown pigmentation with smooth surface. This is referred to as 'Eburnation', derived from Latin word, which means arrested caries. It can be on occlusal as well as on proximal surfaces.

d. *Recurrent caries*: It occurs at interface of tooth and restorative material. It may be due to defective cavity preparation/restoration leading to microleakage.

e. *Radiation caries*: The radiotherapy of oral cancer lesions may lead to xerostomia, subsequently development of caries, known as radiation caries.

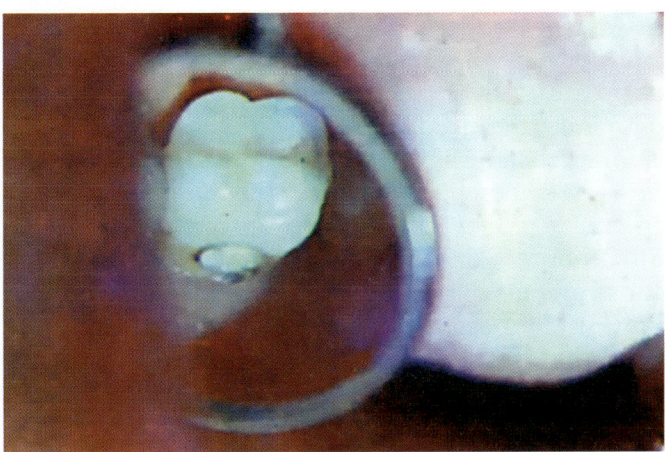

Fig. 5.6: Root surface caries (clinical)

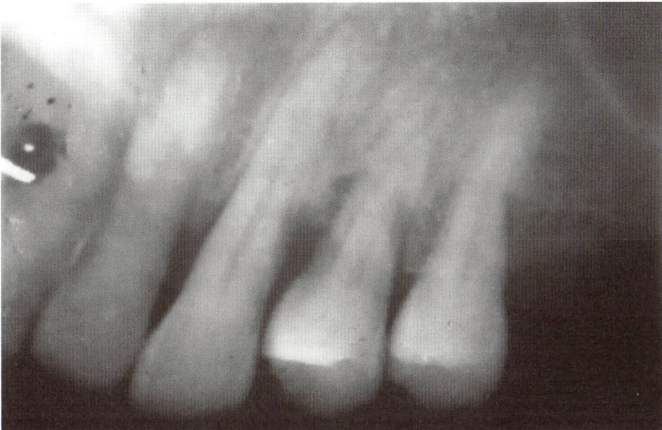

Fig. 5.7: Caries on the cementoenamel junction (as seen in radiograph)

C. According to Age

According to age, the caries is categorized into following three types:

a. *Nursing bottle caries*: In early infancy period, bottle fed babies develop caries usually on maxillary incisors. The prolonged breast-feeding especially at night can also result in such caries.
b. *Adolescent caries*: Caries attack during adolescent period is characterized as adolescent caries.
c. *Geriatric caries*: Caries which occurs in older adults is referred to as geriatric caries. Usually caries of cementum falls under this category.

ETIOLOGY OF DENTAL CARIES

Dental caries is a multifactorial disease. The process by which a tooth can be destroyed easily in oral cavity, which is indestructible otherwise, is very difficult to understand. Till today, no single theory can explain the phenomenon of caries. The caries does not fall into any of the pathological lesions of oral cavity. The caries is not inflammatory in origin nor is it degenerative in nature and neither it is a neoplasm. Dental caries is a local disease, which involves destruction of hard tissues of tooth by metabolites produced by micro-organisms.

Evidence for caries has been found in *Homosapiens* since Palaeolithic times. Numerous references to dental caries, including early theories of caries have been documented. The possible theories are:

The Worm Theory

The earliest reference of tooth decay appeared around 14th century B.C. According to concept of that time, the cause of caries was thought to be invasion of 'worms' into teeth. The association of systemic disease and teeth was probably obtained from writings of a physician around 668 B.C. The physician had mentioned that the inflammation in his arms and legs was due to tooth and that it must be extracted.

The Humoral Theory

Galen hypothetized that the dental caries was produced by the action of acids along with corroding humors. The four recognized humors of the body were blood, phlegm, black bile and yellow bile. The imbalance in these humors resulted in the disease process. Certain authors such as Hippocrates favoured this concept and added that accumulated debris around the teeth helped in corroding action.

Chemical Theory

Robertson (1835) proposed that acids (formed by fermentation of food particles) cause dental decay. The exact nature of acids and the exact mechanism of their formation were not known. Different postulates were suggested. One, putrefaction of protein gave rise to ammonia, which was subsequently oxidized to nitric acid. Another postulate was that the food was decomposed to sulphuric acid. Till then, the activity of bacteria was not recognized.

Parasite Theory

Erdl (1843) described filamentous parasites in the membrane of tooth surfaces. Dental caries was thought to develop as a result of infiltration and decomposition of enamel cuticle (surface protein membrane on the enamel).

Acidogenic Theory

Miller (1889) propagated the concept of acid formation in the oral cavity and attributed the synthesis of acid to the action of micro-organisms. He was of the view that micro-organisms of the oral cavity, by secretion of enzymes or by their own metabolites degrade the carbohydrates into acids. The acids formed were recognized as lactic acid, butyric acid, etc. The carbohydrate content of food lodged onto the tooth surface is the source of acid production. The acid demineralized the enamel surface. After the disintegration of enamel, the organisms along with acids penetrate dentinal tubules leading to dissolution of dentin. The proteolytic enzymes finally digest the organic part.

Three factors are recognized in Miller's observation.
a. Micro-organisms responsible for the caries process.
b. Carbohydrate substrate over the tooth surface.
c. Production of acids initially and protein degradation subsequently.

He summarized his theory as 'Dental decay is a chemicoparasitic process consisting of the dissolution of the hard inorganic and the soft organic part'. In case of enamel, since it consists mainly of inorganic constituents, the second stage is missing.

A few authors presented experimental evidence implicating acids and bacteria as the causative agent of caries. A specific micro-organism, *Leptothrix buccalis* was observed in dentinal tubules, giving the idea that the acids and micro-organisms collectively dissolved the organic part.

Miller was of the view that no single species of micro-organisms were capable of producing acids and digesting proteins. His work was confirmed by the following facts:
- Acid was present in the deeper carious lesions.
- Several micro-organisms of oral cavity were capable of producing acids.
- Lactic acid was identified in carbohydrate saliva combined mixtures.
- Different micro-organisms had the potential to invade enamel and dentin.

Drawbacks

Though Miller's theory is relevant; however, following points were not clear and need explanation:
- The caries on the smooth surfaces of teeth.
- Particular type of micro-organism could not be isolated, which is responsible for particular acid.
- The phenomenon of arrested caries.
- Certain populations exhibit less caries despite of consuming enough carbohydrates.
- Caries of un-erupted/impacted teeth.
- The carious dentin, if left under a filling continues to decay.

Proteolytic Theory

Gottlieb (1944) was of the view that instead of decalcification of inorganic part, as suggested in Miller's theory, the initial action is due to the proteolytic enzymes attacking the lamellae, rod sheaths, tufts and walls of tubules etc, i.e. all organic components. The yellow pigmentation, which he observed with dental caries was attributed to the pigments produced by proteolytic organisms. Caries is initiated at a slightly alkaline pH produced by the proteolytic activity liquefying the organic matrix of enamel. Once the inorganic part sets free after the dissolution of organic part, these salts are dissolved subsequently by acidogenic bacteria. He was of the view that the staphylococci play a vital role in initiating proteolytic activity.

Later *Pincus* (1949) also maintained that the initial process in caries was the proteolytic breakdown of the dental cuticle. The organic membrane was found on all the teeth followed by destruction of the prism sheaths. The loosened prisms then fell out mechanically. He proposed that the Nasmyth's membrane and the enamel proteins (mucoproteins), which are acted upon by the sulphatase enzyme of the bacilli yielding sulphuric acid.

Drawbacks

- Enamel is a highly mineralized tissue. Though enamel contains 1.0 to 1.5% organic matrix out of which 0.6% is protein, initiation of caries with breakdown of this small percentage of protein is highly questionable.
- The sulphatases of gram-negative bacilli which are considered to dissolve the mucoitin sulfate of enamel have not been found in abundance in experimental studies. Moreover, enzyme systems capable of attacking keratin have also not been demonstrated.
- This theory, by and large, lacks experimental support.

Proteolysis Chelation Theory

Schatz et al. (1955) hypothesized that the microbial degradation of organic component by proteolysis followed by dissolution of inorganic part by the process of chelation lead to caries. The word 'chelate' refers to compounds that are able to bind metallic ions such as calcium, iron, copper, zinc, etc. by valence bonds. The proteolysis chelation theory considers dental caries to be bacterial destruction of organic component of enamel and the breakdown products of these organic components to have chelating properties and thereby dissolve the minerals in the enamel even at the neutral/alkaline pH. A variety of agents such as amino acids, amines and peptides, etc. are the breakdown products of organic components of enamel and dentin which can act as chelates.

Drawbacks

- Since the enamel contains very little amount of organic component (1%), can such dissolution

produce sufficient amount of chelates to disintegrate the rest of inorganic enamel (96.6%), is doubtful.
- Although chelation is an accepted biological phenomenon, its role in caries initiation is yet to be established.

Summary analysis of evidence supporting the three main theories of dental caries: Acidogenic theory, Proteolysis theory and Proteolysis chelation theory is given in Table 5.1.

Bioelectric Phenomenon

The mechanisms involved in production of electric voltages are basically piezoelectric effect (voltage produced by physical deformation of bone crystals), ion pump and membrane potential (involved in nerve activity), fuel cells (difference in electron concentrations where high and low redox potentials exist in close proximity with each other). Enamel surfaces of teeth and adjacent structures could develop electrical voltages

Table 5.1: Summary analysis of evidence supporting three main theories of dental caries

Factors studied	Acidogenic	Proteolysis	Chelation
A. Clinical	+	–	–
i. Site of cavities (caries occurs at places where fermentable carbohydrate food is retained on tooth surfaces)	The localization of cavities is confirmed by various authors supported by our clinical experience	No evidence only proteolysis would account for localization and since carbohydrates are used for bacterial energy in preference to protein, proteolysis will be delayed in areas where carbohydrates are retained	No evidence why chelation account for localization
ii. Diet and caries High incidence of caries found in persons using high carbohydrate diet	+ Clinical studies have established the relationship of caries and carbohydrates. Elimination of diet, which forms acids in mouth has been shown to reduce caries Fluorides increase the resistance of enamel to decalcification to acids and hence reduce caries	– No similar association exists in relation to attack by proteolysis. No such studies reported Increased resistance by adding zinc chloride was not approved	– No similar association exists in relation to chelation. No such studies reported effect of fluoride on keratance lacks scientific support
iii. Animal studies Caries detected in animals when fed on carbohydrate diets and prevented by agents which inhibit fermentation	+ Agents such as iodoacetic acid and dicalcium phosphate reduce caries in animals	– Doubtful questionable evidence given	– No studies
B. Mechanism of destruction i. Destruction of inorganic part has been shown both in-vivo and in-vitro	+ Decalcification by acid production has been proved	± (doubtful) No mechanism has been established to show how proteolysis will destroy the calcified tissues	± (doubtful) The keratin in enamel is dissolved by mouth organisms thereby forming chelating agents which dissolve enamel. Evidence reported that the total keratin changed into chelating compounds can dissolve only 1% of calcium in enamel so not convincing evidence to produce detectable caries

(Contd.)

Table 5.1: Summary analysis of evidence supporting three main theories of dental caries (*Contd.*)

Factors studied	Acidogenic	Proteolysis	Chelation
ii. Destruction of organic part has doubtful evidence in all the three theories	± Since organic portion is fragile, it disintegrates as decalcification takes place	± Proteolytic agents destroy human enamel protein is partially supported by scientific evidence	± It was only presumed that oxygen uptake was observed when proteolytic bacterium culture grew in human enamel. But actual organisms were not isolated from enamel. The uptake of oxygen by enamel was as good as auto-respiration
C. Histology of caries	+	Doubtful	−
i. Destruction of enamel is accompanied by loss of calcific material and the organic portion persists	Different zones found in caries in enamel can be explained by acid theory	Bacteria penetrate along the organic tracts in enamel but preteolysis does not explain different zones	No evidence
ii. Appearance of radiolucent area in X-rays	+ Radiolucency seen in radio graphs because of loss of calcium	− No support	− No support
iii. Increase of nitrogen and loss of specific gravity and hardness	+ Loss of inorganic material and persistence of organic material occurs in initial stage which accounts for increase of nitrogen and loss of specific gravity and hardness	− No evidence reported	− No evidence
D. Bacteriology	+	−	Doubtful
i. Isolation of appropriate bacteria from enamel caries	Bacteria producing acid from fermentable carbohydrates is isolated from caries sites	No evidence	Doubtful keratolytic organisms have not been isolated from initial enamel caries but found in deeper cavities
ii. Presence of necessary bacteria in oral cavity	+ Bacterial flora capable of producing decalcifying acids always present in the oral cavity and on the tooth surface	+ Proteolytic types such as Actinomyces bovis, Strepto coccus mitis are generally present in the oral cavity	Doubtful
iii. Bacterial antagonists reduce caries	+ Certain bacterial antagonists such as iodoacetic acid, penicillin, etc. reduce caries in animals and man	No Evidence	No Evidence

by one or all the following: Bony crystalline structures, Enamel that may act as ion permeable membrane and an intensely layered bacterial system (the plaque).

The reduction of pH by bacterial activity coupled with the voltage produced is responsible for inducing demineralization of tooth enamel.

Dental plaque may act as an electrical fuel-cell. The back of the plaque (tooth side) is found to be more electronegative, as compared to the front. The addition of small amounts of glucose solution, contacts and stimulates the front of this bacterial mat, which now becomes highly electronegative. As substrate penetrates past the surface, there is concurrent shift in potential, until the back and front of the bacterial mat are at the same negativity till finally the tooth region of the plaque becomes strongly electronegative with respect to the front. The electrical energies on the order of those developed by plaque will decalcify sound tooth structure. This electrical activity is intensely stimulated by the presence of sugar.

Thus decalcification occurring because of electrical energies does indicate that there might be bioelectric phenomena involved in dental decay.

Levine's Theory

Levine (1977) hypothetized 'see-saw' mechanism in which there is movement of minerals from saliva/plaque to enamel and vice versa (Fig. 5.8). The mechanism emphasized that the demineralization and remineralization of enamel is a continuous process. If in a given interval of time, more ions leave the enamel than enter, then there is a net demineralization, which amounts to the start of the carious process. It has been proved that the passage of ions is not a one way process and that ions are constantly being exchanged between enamel and plaque. At times, the chemical conditions at enamel-plaque interface may favour outward movement of ions and at other times the situation may be reversed. This delicate balance of ions is dependent on many factors. The three most important factors responsible are:

i. pH of plaque.
ii. Calcium and phosphate ion concentration at the interface.
iii. Fluoride ion concentration

If the pH falls below 5 (the critical pH), may be during carbohydrate intake, mineral ions are liberated from the hydroxyapatite crystals of the enamel surface and diffuse into plaque. Within 20 minutes, the salivary buffers neutralize the acid. At this stage, the plaque is supersaturated with ions. Some of the ions are lost and others are deposited onto the enamel. With such repeated episodes, overall demineralization occurs which may lead to caries. For this phenomenon to occur, actual mineral ion concentration of saliva is important. If free calcium and phosphate ions are higher in the saliva because of the dietary and other sources, there would be a greater tendency of ions to move from plaque to enamel. Reverse would be true if ion concentration in saliva is low. Another factor, which plays an important role in 'see-saw' mechanism is fluoride. Fluoride favours movement of ions from plaque to enamel. The initial deposit appears to be in the form of calcium fluoride. Fluoride concentration, as low as 5.0 ppm, can tilt the 'see-saw' in enamel's favour.

Bandlish's Theory

Bandlish emphasized role of attrition and plaque in caries etiology. He hypothetized that oral fluids protect the enamel by providing a protective covering. Attrition makes the fissures wider and removes the superficial layer of the enamel along with the initial carious lesion, if present. The new layer of enamel becomes protective again with the help of oral fluids. In areas where the oral fluids, cannot reach (e.g. contact areas), enamel cannot be made protective against the carious attack.

Organic acids produced by the bacterial fermentation of the carbohydrate cause surface demineralization of the enamel. At this stage the bacteria do not penetrate the intact enamel surface. The demineralized products are redeposited into the enamel during the process of remineralization. Caries occurs only if there is more demineralization and less remineralization.

Caries starts at the contact area where the protective action of oral fluids is not there, i.e. the perimeter of the contact area. Smaller the area, more is the perimeter/unit area; as the area becomes large, the perimeter/unit area falls. Similarly smaller the contact area more the perimeter per unit area, as the contact area becomes more (may be physiologic or with attrition), the perimeter/unit area falls. The effect of acid attack depends upon the perimeter/unit area.

Greater the perimeter, stronger is the attack. As the length of the perimeter/unit area falls with increase

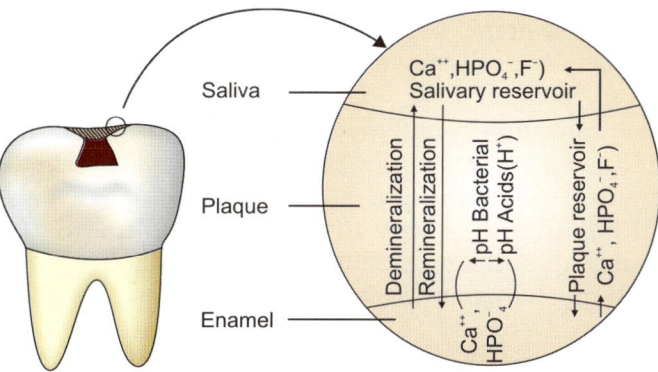

Fig. 5.8: Levine's ionic see-saw theory of dental caries

in size of the contact area, the carious lesion progress faster in a smaller contact area, if other conditions are kept constant.

Dr. Bandlish was of the view that meticulous contact through brushing and cleaning reduces caries not by removing plaque but by removing some part of enamel (Figs 5.9A and B).

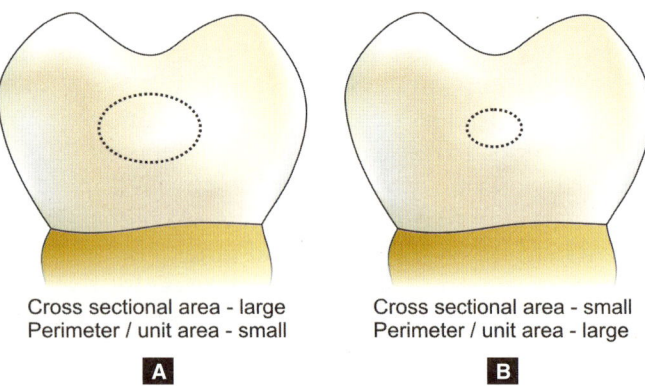

Figs 5.9A and B: Progression of caries is faster in tooth B as compared to tooth A

It is suggested that gradual recession of active enamel lesion to a larger extent is a result of surface wear. Plaque acts as a reservoir of minerals and with its buffering capabilities helps in maturation of enamel surface, thereby reducing caries.

The approximal surfaces gain the beneficial effect of oral fluids during functional movement of teeth. During the bucco-lingual movement of teeth there is more movement at the occlusal border of the contact area and less at the cervical border (Less movement nearer the fulcrum). Where there is more movement there is less incidence of caries, where there is less movement there is more incidence of caries. Accordingly, the cervical border of the contact area is more prone to caries.

In case of occlusal caries, caries starts at places where there is least attrition and least plaque, i.e. where contact of two or more enamel surfaces occurs like in fissures and at cusp tips. He suggested that pits and fissures are not usually full of plaque as the general belief is, but there is only little plaque in the functioning pits and fissures. It is not the depth of a fissure, which is important but the narrowness of the fissure, which makes it more caries prone. Maximum enamel caries occurs in a fissure where the two walls of a fissure either meet or come close to each other. The plunging action of masticatory forces helps to pump the oral secretions into the occlusal fissure of the teeth. The masticatory forces also help to pump the oral secretions into the region of contact area. Food consumption habits are changing. Since less fibrous and softer food is consumed more, the masticatory forces are reduced. The reduced masticatory forces do not force oral secretions into the unprotected areas thereby making these areas more prone to caries.

The convexity of the adjoining surfaces is one of the factors, which affects the incidence or intensity of caries. The more the convex surface, the smaller is the contact area - the less the convex surface, the larger is the contact area. When there is contact between two surfaces of varying convexities the contact area on the more convex surface is smaller. Accordingly, the caries incidence is higher in more convex surfaces. The above mentioned concept of convexities when applied to the caries incidence of different adjacent surfaces seems to be correct except in the case of the contact between the first permanent molar and second premolar. Mesial surface of the first permanent molar is less convex still this surface is more prone to caries. The reason could be that some caries might have been initiated during the period the first molar remained in contact with the second deciduous molar.

According to this concept attrition and plaque must be regarded as defense mechanism against caries.

Systemic Theory

The systemic theory of dental caries highlights the significance of body's own inflammatory response and disturbance of oxidant-antioxidant balance in the internal environment of cells that lead to initiation and progression of caries. It states that in dental caries, the acidic environment primarily erodes the enamel and secondarily triggers an inflammatory response in the dentin layer of the tooth. Similar to the process of periodontal disease, where bacterial toxins initiate the body's own matrix metalloproteinases (MMPs) to break down the periodontium, the collagen matrix of the dentin also is lysed by endogenous MMPs such as collagenase. Essentially, both dental caries stimulated by acid and periodontal disease stimulated by bacterial toxins share a common pathway of oral bacteria initiating a host inflammatory response. This is a significant departure from the concept of the oral bacteria's MMPs creating the dentinal breakdown as recognized in Miller's acidogenic theory.

The systemic theory conceptualizes that all body parts constantly move between states of health, disease, and disease, based on oxidative stress, neutralization by anti-oxidants and the corresponding inflammatory response. A similar reaction takes place in the periodontal tissues and teeth. Nourishment, by either blood supply or fluid flow, replenishes nutrients and antioxidant reserves in cells. The body has mechanisms to regulate hormones and fluid flows. Dentinal fluid flow is regulated by the endocrine portion of the parotid gland, which receives signals from the hypothalamus. Free radicals, specifically Reactive oxygen species (ROS) produced in the mitochondria of the hypothalamus increase with elevated blood glucose. Minimizing the effect of free radicals on the hypothalamus with antioxidants can avoid down-regulation of the parotid hormone, maintaining centrifugal dentinal fluid flow. Excessive MMPs release causing carious process is prevented, and dentinogenesis is enhanced.

A high-sucrose diet affects the tooth from outside by enabling oral bacteria to produce acid and from inside by reducing the dentinal fluid flow. Antioxidants can shield the dentition by decreasing the effects of acid erosion, by minimizing the effect of ROS in the hypothalamus, and by replenishing tissue inhibitors of metalloproteinases in the dentin. Increasing fruit and vegetable intake and nutritional supplementation may prove beneficial in preventing and controlling caries process.

CONTRIBUTORY FACTORS IN DENTAL CARIES

Dental caries is a multi factorial disease. It is reasonable to assume that tremendous variations in caries incidence exist because of a number of factors affecting caries. Basically caries occurs when there is interaction of four principle factors; the host, the microflora, the substrate and the time. All the four factors should be favourable, that is a susceptible host, cariogenic oral flora and a suitable substrate for a sufficient length of time. Diagrammatically, these factors can be portrayed as four circles overlapping each other (Fig. 5.10). Caries occurs in the centre when all the factors are favourably acting.

The four factors contributing to caries process are explained below:

1. The host factor
   A. Tooth
      a. Morphology and position in the arch
      b. Chemical nature
   B. Saliva
      a. Composition
      b. pH
      c. Antibacterial properties
      d. Quantity and viscosity
2. Microflora
3. Substrate or diet
   a. Physical nature
   b. Chemical nature
4. Time

The Host Factors

A. Tooth

a. *Morphology and position in the arch:* Tooth morphology is recognized as an important factor for initiation of caries. Deep pits and fissures make the tooth susceptible to caries because of food impaction and bacterial stagnation. That is why the occlusal surfaces are more prone to caries. The most susceptible teeth are the mandibular first molars amongst the permanent teeth, closely followed by maxillary first molars, then mandibular and maxillary second molars and so on.

Irregularities in the arch form, crowding and overlapping of the teeth also favour the development of caries. Partially impacted third molars are more prone to caries and so are the buccally/lingually placed teeth.

b. *Chemical nature:* The inorganic constituents, such as dicalcium phosphate dihydrate, and fluoroapatite, etc. make the enamel resistant to caries attack. It has been established that surface enamel is more caries resistant than the subsurface enamel. The surface enamel has more minerals and more organic matter and relatively less water. In addition, certain elements such as fluoride, chloride, zinc, lead, etc. accumulate more on the surface enamel than the subsurface enamel.

With the passage of time, teeth become more resistant to caries because of decrease in permeability and increase in nitrogen and fluoride content. The increase in concentration of fluoride at the subsurface is because of ingestion of fluoride with age. It is hypothetized that under practical limits, higher the fluoride concentration of water, the lower the prevalence of caries.

B. Saliva

a. *Composition:* The flow of saliva affects the oral environment vis-à-vis, the dental caries.

The composition of saliva varies considerably. The concentrations of inorganic calcium and phosphorus show considerable variations within

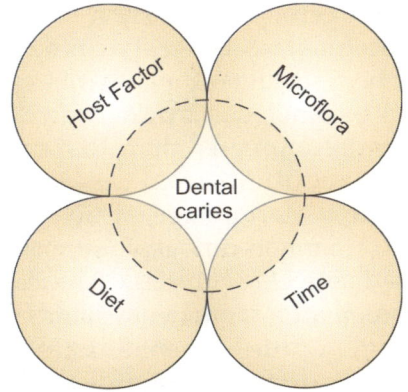

Fig. 5.10: Modern theory of dental caries

resting and the stimulated saliva. Caries prone individuals have low calcium and phosphorus levels. The organic component of saliva has been studied in relation to dental caries. The caries immune persons exhibit greater ammonia content in saliva. The higher ammonia content in saliva retards the plaque formation and neutralizes acid formation. Urea and amino acids have no effect on dental caries. A variety of enzymes, such as amylase and ptyalin have been isolated from saliva. They do help in degradation of starches but their role in caries inhibition is questionable.

b. *pH:* The pH of saliva shows great variations as compared to pH of blood. The pH at which any particular saliva ceases to be saturated with calcium and phosphorus is referred to as the 'critical pH'. Under normal conditions the critical pH is 5.5. Below this value, the inorganic material of the tooth may dissolve. The normal pH of resting saliva is 6-7. A 'buffer' is a component that tends to maintain a constant pH. A fall in buffer capacity of saliva leads to increase in caries incidence.

c. *Antibacterial properties:* The antibacterial properties of saliva have a definite relation with caries incidence. Lysozyme, an antibacterial agent present in saliva, can inhibit airborne and water-borne micro-organisms in the oral cavity, but its role in caries inhibition has not been established. Lysozyme activity in saliva has been found to be greater in caries free children than the caries-susceptible ones. Salivary peroxide is also considered antibacterial; however, no significant correlation has been found between caries resistant and caries susceptible subjects. Antibodies like secretory IgA and IgG against specific bacteria have been reported in human saliva. Specific antibodies against *Streptococcus mutans* have been isolated. Patients with immune dysfunction tend to have more caries than normal.

d. *Quantity and viscosity:* The quantity and viscosity of saliva has definite influence on caries incidence. Human beings suffering from decreased flow of saliva or lack of salivary secretions (xerostomia) usually experience increased rate of dental caries (For example: Sjogren's syndrome, sarcoidosis, diabetes, etc.) However, cariogenic substrate is required for initiation of caries even if salivary secretions are lacking or minimum.

The caries susceptibility increases in patients following radiation therapy of oral cavity. Under decreased salivary flow and subsequently decreased buffering capacity there occurs alteration in the microflora, which favours the growth of more aciduric yeasts.

Certain drugs influence salivary flow, and in turn result in rampant caries. Drugs, which may lead to xerostomia, include anti-depressants and anti-histamines, etc.

Physiological xerostomia occurs in all human beings during sleep. The most important time for plaque removal is before sleeping to avoid caries.

Microflora

It is established that micro-organisms are mandatory for caries. As early as Koch's postulates, it was observed that bacteria played a definite role in caries initiation. The following factors further prove the role of bacteria in caries:

i. Caries will not occur in the absence of micro-organisms.
ii. Caries can occur in animals even if kept on single type of bacterial growth.
iii. All oral organisms are not cariogenic, but histologically majority can be isolated from carious enamel and dentin.

It has been proved that caries is a bacterial infection; however, the cariogenicity of micro-organisms is variable. It has been established that all acid producing organisms are not cariogenic. The role of micro-organisms varies at different sites as follows:

a. *Occlusal caries:* It is established that different organisms display some selectivity as regard their preference of tooth surface. There are differences in occlusal caries and root caries and also in smooth surface caries and pit and fissure caries. *Streptococcus mutans* is considered to be the significant micro-organism playing a vital role in initiation of caries. The main etiological micro-organism in occlusal and pit and fissure caries is the *Streptococcus mutans* because of the following properties:

- It ferments mannitol and sorbitol (synthesized insoluble polysaccharide from sucrose)
- The Mutans streptococci are lactic acid formers which easily colonize on tooth surface
- They are more aciduric than other streptococci. Few of these properties have also been shown by non-cariogenic strains such as Enterococci, Streptococcus faecalis, etc. Two properties, which make them separate from other Streptococci are (i) acid accumulation by *Streptococcus mutans* is substantially greater than that of other oral Streptococci (ii) *Streptococcus mutans* contains lysogenic bacteriophage, which has not been isolated from non-cariogenic strains.

b. *Cemental caries (Root Caries):* The caries at the exposed cementum or cementoenamel junction are known as root caries or senile caries. It can occur at any tooth surface but mandibular molars are most susceptible. The organisms involved in root caries are different from those in other smooth surface lesions. Predominantly *Actinomyces viscosus* have been isolated. Other species of Actinomyces such as *A. naeslundii* and *A. nocardia,* etc. have also been isolated. Exact strains, which produce root caries is not definite but certainly the bacterial flora is different in root caries as compared to occlusal caries.

c. *Deep dentinal caries:* The flora of deep dentinal caries is different. The predominantly present microorganisms are lactobacilli which account for one third of the oral flora. Certain gram-positive anaerobes and filaments are also present such as Eubacterium, Actinomyces, Bacillus, etc.

Substrate or Diet

'Diet' refers to the customary food and 'nutrition' means the assimilated portion of diet, which affects the metabolic process of body. Diet has shown to influence caries. The following dietary factors play role in caries production:

A. Physical Nature

It has been established that the physical nature of diet indirectly affects caries. The diet of primitive man consisted of raw food, which led to attrition and also help in cleansing the debris; thereby, less incidence of caries. Modern diet includes refined foods and soft drinks, which helps collection of debris predisposing to more caries. Further, it is observed that the mastication of food reduces the number of microorganisms. Mechanical rubbing and cleaning definitely has role in caries reduction.

B. Chemical Nature

The nutrients present in meals have definite role in caries process. The main ingredient, carbohydrate, is accepted as one of the most important factor. Only refined carbohydrates are effective in caries production; however, following factors also affect:
 i. Type of carbohydrate (monosaccharides, disaccharides or polysaccharides)
 ii. Frequency of intake
 iii. Time of stagnation

It has been established that sugar given in solution form, is much less capable of producing caries than the same amount of sugar incorporated in food. Also, caries activity is higher when sugar is administered in the form of sticky food, which tends to remain on the surface of teeth. However, when dextranase was incorporated in water, it led to reduction in caries activity.

The vitamins do have significant effect on dental caries incidence. Vitamins A, C and K rarely have any effect on caries production; however, Vitamin B deficiency may exert a caries protective influence on teeth since vitamin B is essential in growth of oral acidogenic flora. They also serve as components of co-enzymes involved in glycolysis. Vitamin D is necessary for the normal development of teeth. Malformation especially hypoplasia and an increase caries incidence has been reported in Vitamin D deficiency cases.

Certain minerals such as calcium, phosphorous and trace elements influence dental caries processs. The role of calcium and phosphorous is controversial. That caries is inhibited by high doses of calcium could not be established. Lower doses of calcium during infancy and intrauterine life can lead to poor calcification of teeth, whereby caries progress becomes easier. It is observed that caries incidence is significantly higher in persons residing in seleniferous areas and decrease in dental caries incidence with increasing vanadium concentration.

Fluoride in various forms also inhibits caries. It is believed that dietary fluoride is relatively unimportant compared to fluoride in the drinking water because of their metabolic unavailability.

Following factors of diet are responsible for dental caries:
 i. Roughness
 ii. Palatability
 iii. Eating and drinking pattern
 iv. Retention and clearance of diet
 v. Age

Time

The frequency to which teeth are exposed to cariogenic (acidic) environments affects the likelihood of caries development. After intake of meals or snacks containing sugars, the bacteria in the mouth metabolize them resulting in production of acids as by-products which decrease pH and lead to dissolution of inorganic content of the tooth. It takes around two hours to return the ph to normal and remineralise the tooth surface through the buffering capacity of saliva. Since teeth are vulnerable during these periods of acidic environments, the development of dental caries relies greatly on the frequency of these occurrences.

THE HISTOPATHOLOGY AND CHEMICAL EVENTS IN CARIES PROCESS

The histopathology and chemical events in caries process vary in enamel, dentin and cementum. Arrested caries also present a different picture. For convenience, the individual events are described.

I. Caries of Enamel

The first sign of enamel caries is seen as a white spot, which appears because of loss of translucency of the affected area. On drying, the area becomes comparatively rougher than the adjacent areas. Many a times, these incipient lesions get mineralized and appear as brown pigmented areas. Histologically, if the lesion has invaded two thirds of the enamel, it becomes evident radiographically. A caries lesion on the smooth surface of enamel is conical in shape with its broad base on enamel surface and the tip on the dentino-enamel junction. When it reaches dentino-enamel junction, it spreads laterally along the junction thereby undermining enamel (Fig. 5.11). In case of fissures, the lesion starts at the adjoining lateral walls. Light microscopy studies of caries of enamel have revealed four distinct zones starting from the advancing front of the lesion. These zones are:

i. 'Translucent zone' which is the advancing front of the lesion.
ii. 'Dark zone' separating the translucent zone from the body of the lesion.
iii. 'Body of the lesion', which is markedly radiolucent.
iv. Surface layer.

   i. The *translucent zone* is the advancing front of the caries. This is visible under longitudinal sections when the teeth are examined in a clearing agent having refractive index similar to that of enamel such as quinoline or balsam. The layer (1% pore volume as compared to 0.1% of normal enamel) admits quinoline giving overall translucent appearance. The preferential removal of inorganic salts (1.2% loss of minerals) is evident whereas removal of organic material is not seen in the translucent zone.
   ii. The *dark zone* exhibits approximately 6% loss of minerals per unit volume of enamel. It shows a positive birefringence in polarized light while normal enamel has negative birefringence. Birefringence is the property of resolving a beam of polarized light into two rays at different velocities. Light passing through this zone causes the brown discoloration of the dark zone.
   iii. The *body of the lesion* is positively birefringent. Microbial analysis indicates reduction of 24% minerals per unit volume compared to normal enamel. This is the largest zone, which exhibits enhanced Striae of Retzius. The pore volume is 25% in the centre of the zone and 5% towards the periphery. An increase in bound water and organic content follows due to ingress of bacteria and saliva.
   iv. The *surface layer* is approximately 20–100 μm thick; it is thinner in active lesion and thicker in inactive ones. Partial demineralization (10% mineral loss) takes place in this layer along with broadening of prism sheaths. Minute pathways do exist in surface layer, which are, however, not detectable by light microscopy.

The ultra-structural changes in enamel as seen under electron microscope reveal that initially there is a scattered destruction of individual apatite crystals. The progressive dissolution of crystals results in broadening of the inter-crystalline spaces so that small areas become filled with amorphous material. This causes the enamel crystals to assume hairy appearance in a longitudinal view. It has also been suggested that there is a higher concentration of carbonate in the crystal centre. Carbonate is preferentially dissolved in an acidic medium. As the number of dissolved crystal increases, the densely calcified tissue becomes progressively more porous; with increase in porosity the crystal arrangement gets disorganized. Eventually, with the diffuse destruction of the apatite crystals, numerous bacteria can be observed invading the enamel lesion.

Chemical Nature of Enamel Caries

Enamel is composed of long thin crystallites of hydroxyapatite surrounded by organic matrix and water. Enamel also contains 2-4% carbonate and about 1.0% of other metals incorporated into the crystal structure. These, apatite, carbonated crystals are about 40nm in diameter. The protein and lipid together with a large proportion of water form the diffusion channels, which help in enamel demineralization or remineralization. Apatites crystals are readily soluble in acids. Before dissolving apatite crystals, the acid must diffuse to the crystal surface through the porous matrix, which surrounds the crystals. It has been shown that the rate of dissolution in weak acid is

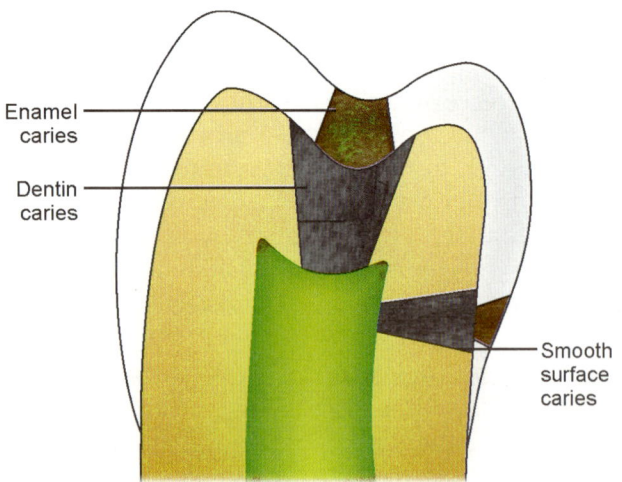

Fig. 5.11: Progress of caries in the pit and fissure and on smooth surface

directly proportional to amount of carbonate present in the crystals. The fluorides may reduce the acidic reaction. During early caries, preferential loss of carbonate and magnesium occurs. However, remineralization of this loss produces a less soluble crystalline material, which incorporates less carbonates. The core of the enamel crystals, probably contain carbonate rich material, which could explain the preferential dissolution of the central portion of crystal. The weak acids produced by plaque bacteria can exist in an un-ionized form in equilibrium.

The initial rate of reaction depends on how rapidly the hydrogen ions reach the enamel crystal surface. The rate of dissolution is affected by diffusion of the undissociated acid into the enamel as well as the concentration of hydrogen ions. This rate is governed by their presence in solution, of the reaction products such as calcium phosphate and fluoride. These products have the capacity to precipitate, dissolve and reprecipitate. So an equilibrium eventually exists which maintains the surface layer but with some loss of minerals. To sum up:

- If subsurface dissolution continues and repair cannot keep pace with mineral loss, this leads eventually to a more extensive damage to crystal structure and cavitation.
- Dissolution of mineral salts, further exposes the organic matrix of enamel and dentin to proteolytic enzymes of the oral flora.
- Protein in enamel is acid soluble and is lost in early stage.

II. Caries of Dentin

When the carious lesion penetrates enamel, it spreads laterally along the dentino-enamel junction. The lesion then invades dentin along the dentinal tubules. The pattern of invasion is depicted as cone shaped lesion with its base at the dentino-enamel junction and apex towards the pulp. The histopathological changes in caries have been divided into following zones; starting from surface these are:

 i. Zone of decomposed dentin
 ii. Zone of bacterial invasion
 iii. Zone of demineralization
 iv. Zone of dentinal sclerosis or hypermineralization
 v. Zone of fatty degeneration of Tome's fibers

All these zones may not be evident in all the carious lesions. In case of acute caries, there occurs a rapid decomposition and demineralization (all these zones may not be evident). The noticeable change in carious dentin is the zone of bacterial invasion. The dentin tubules are distended giving a dilated appearance. Areas in dentin can be seen which are characterized by focal confluence and breakdown of a few dentinal tubules. Earlier, these areas were known as *'liquefaction foci'* (a misnomer, because these distentions are filled with bacteria and not liquid). A deep dentinal carious lesion, progressing slowly, leads to the formation of sclerotic zone beneath the demineralized area. The increase in concentration of calcium and phosphate in sclerotic dentin is possibly by a specific odontoblastic action. Beneath the sclerotic dentin, the odontoblasts may deposit a layer of reparative dentin or secondary dentin. The caries progression tends to be slower in older adults than in young individuals because of generalized dentinal sclerosis with aging. In the earlier stages of caries where only a few tubules are involved, micro-organisms may be found in these tubules. These micro-organisms are known as *'Pioneer Bacteria'*. It has been observed that each tubule usually has only one type of bacteria.

Caries involvement of secondary dentin is slower because the dentinal tubules are fewer in number and more irregular in their course. Sometimes at the junction of primary and secondary dentin, the caries spreads laterally creating a separation between the two layers.

III. Caries of Cementum

The cemental caries is usually seen where there is gingival recession. Clinically, the lesions appear as saucer shaped cavities. Other than carious lesions, erosion, abrasion and idiopathic resorption can affect cementum. The micro-organisms involved in root caries, chiefly Actinomyces, appear to invade cementum either along Sharpey's fibers or between bundles of fibers.

The dentin involvement of cemental caries is similar to that of dentin involvement in coronal caries. There may be sclerotic response, either partially or completely, occluding the tubules with mineral crystals. The period of tissue destruction may alternate with period of reprecipitation of mineral crystals. Since the dentinal tubules are more in coronal dentin than in root dentin, the caries progression may be slower in roots.

IV. Arrested Caries

Arrested caries implies absolute slow progress or no progress of active carious lesions. The conditions under which the arrest of an active lesion occurs are still not very clear. An arrested dentinal lesion differs from an active lesion by its darker pigmentation, absence of visible bacteria within the tubule and impermeability to dyes and isotopes. Three layers are identified in an arrested lesion:

 i. A narrow surface layer, brown in color and leathery in consistency.

ii. The widest layer in the lesion, dark brown in color and hard in consistency.
iii. Sclerotic layer is very hard, white and often harder than normal dentin.

In the most superficial layer, occasional bacteria are present. The peritubular zone is partially absent. In contrast to the surface layer of active lesions, this area is more dense and seems to contain more mineral. The dense condensation at the surface, forms a narrow, homogenous calcified border approximately 2.0-5.0 um in width. The main bulk of arrested carious lesion consists of deeply pigmented and hard dentin. Almost all the tubules in the area contain bacteria. Under this layer, there occurs a bacteria-free zone of almost normal appearance and corresponds to deep calcified layer.

The main features of the deep sclerotic zone are the highly calcified contents of the tubules. No bacteria are observed in either the sclerotic zone or the normal dentin below.

One of the major characteristics of an arrested lesion is its higher degree of mineralization. The possible ways by which the accumulation of minerals occurs can be:

- Remineralization of the surface layer (calcium and phosphate are absorbed from saliva).
- Reprecipitation of dissolved apatite (the minerals dissolved by bacterial acids in the upper demineralized layer reprecipitate to form large apatite crystals).
- Sclerosis by intratubular calcification and obliteration of tubules of deeper layers (the minerals are mediated by odontoblastic processes through blood supply).

The other characteristic is the change in bacterial morphology. In the arrested lesions, the bacterial bodies are coalesced into homogenous masses, which could be the sign of degeneration and disintegration. The bacterial bodies present in the arrested lesion are probably degenerated and non-viable. The third characteristic is the deep pigmentation. The degenerated bacteria or the degradation products of their proteins and nucleic acids are the possible source of pigmentation. Bacteria are very rarely observed in the deeper portions of both the layers of arrested lesion. The underlying affected but bacteria-free layers can remineralize.

Histopathology

The histopathology of arrested caries in described in three zones:
i. The inner barrier (the surface formed as a result of tubular sclerosis in the area between carious and sound dentin).
ii. The outer barrier (formed by a highly mineralized surface)
iii. The mineralized zone (an area extending from the outer barrier towards the root canal in the demineralized dentin).
   i. The *inner barrier* is the surface formed due to tubular sclerosis. The degree of tubular sclerosis is directly related to the arrest of progress of caries. The permeability of dentin is reduced, thereby the diffusion of acids and proteolytic enzymes from carious dentin do not reach pulp. The formation of inner barrier usually depends upon the integrity of odontoblast layer in the pulp. However arrested lesions also occur in the absence of functional pulp.
   ii. The *outer barrier* blocks the diffusion of bacterial metabolism products into dentin. Certain crystals, independent from odontoblastic processes are found in dentinal tubules near the surface.
   iii. The *mineralized zone* or the remineralization depends upon the degree of bacterial invasion and the integrity of tissue. The zone of bacterial penetration is separated from the zone of advancing demineralization by a mineralized band located below the surface. It is established that the conversion from an active to arrested lesion is associated with the influx of ions thus preventing further demineralization of dentin. However, it is not clear whether the conversion is based only on mineral deposition at surface of lesion or complete remineralization of the body of the lesion.

SECONDARY CARIES

The caries around a restoration is termed as secondary caries. It is also known as *'recurrent caries'*. The caries may be present at surface enamel surrounding the restoration or extend underneath it along the margins. The caries on the opposing tooth surface in contact with the restoration is termed as 'contact caries'. The main etiological factor for secondary caries is marginal leakage around the restorations. It is most unfortunate that all restorations leak, the degree however varies. It has been observed that in cases where the width of the marginal defect is less than 50 mm, the risk for secondary caries is low. Other reasons, which may (though less likely) predispose to secondary caries is ditching or fracture of the restoration at the edges. Secondary caries around silver amalgam and cast restorations is shown in Figs 5.12A and B. A rough surface of the filling coupled with poor oral hygiene may retain more plaque, subsequently the acids, which can diffuse into the microspaces adjacent to the cavity walls. Also, an improper cavity preparation where fissures are left untouched renders the tooth susceptible to secondary caries (Fig. 5.13B). The formation of secondary carious lesions may be higher in unpolished than in polished enamel surfaces. Radiologically a thin radiolucent line is seen under the restoration (Fig. 5.14).

Epidemiology of Secondary Caries

The literature is not sufficient as regards prevalence and location of secondary caries.

Goldberg et al. (1981) reported 19.8% occlusal, 9.7% mesial, 14.9% distal, 11.8% lingual; 23.9% buccal secondary caries and in total 17.7% surfaces showed recurrent caries in 914 restored teeth.

Eriksen et al. (1986) in their study of 1694 Class II restorations found 5.5% to be affected by recurrent caries; 4.9% recurrent caries was observed with amalgam restorations; 4.3% with composite restorations and 1.3% with gold restorations.

Espelid and Tveit (1991) classified secondary caries as S-1 (initial caries lesion characterized by discoloration only), S-2 (lesions characterized by softness and/or cavitation in enamel), and S-3 (lesions with cavitation on the root surfaces). Their observations were 89.7% S-3 lesions, 58.5% S-2 lesions and 73.3% S-1 lesions. They, however, did not specify the status of the occlusal caries.

Pimenta et al. (1995) in their study on amalgam restorations showed that 47.16% surfaces were non-ditched with caries while 54.94% were non-ditched without caries. Further, 58.82% were ditched with caries and 41.18% were ditched without caries.

Mjor (1998) in his study after examining secondary caries at different locations under different materials observed secondary caries in 3.8% Class I amalgam restorations, 0.4% Class.I composites, 4.3% glass-ionomer and 4.3% unspecified. In Class II restorations, amalgam showed 90% gingival caries, 5% occlusal and 10% other sites. Similarly, composite and glass-ionomers showed 75% and 80% gingival, 8% and 10% occlusal and 15% and 10% on other surfaces.

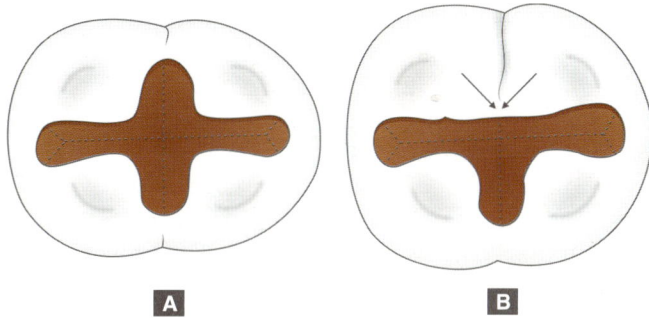

Figs 5.13A and B: **(A)** Proper cavity preparation; **(B)** Improper extension of cavity can predispose to secondary caries

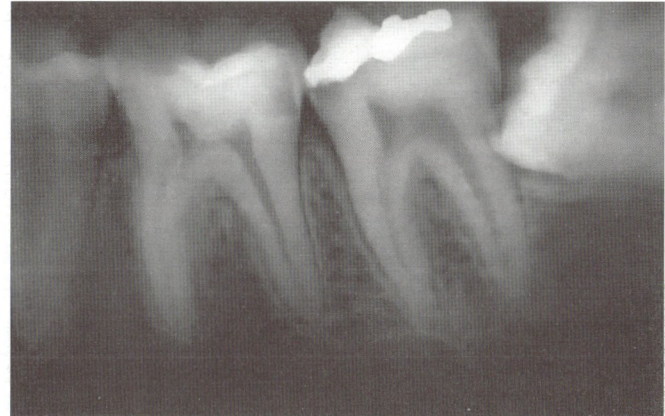

Fig. 5.14: A thin radiolucent line seen under the restoration in radiograph

Microbiology

Secondary caries, like primary caries, is believed to be caused by action of acids produced by bacteria. In a way secondary caries resembles pit and fissure caries. It requires an environment simulating pits and fissures where a storehouse for nutrients is available and micro-organisms can survive and colonize.

The three common organisms seen to be associated with secondary caries are Mutans streptococci, Lactobacilli and Actinomyces viscosus. However, no single species can be ascertained in its cause and the

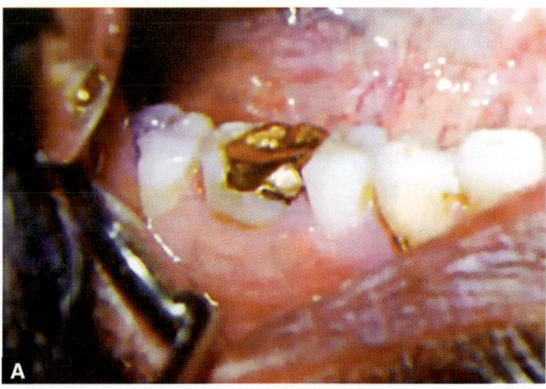
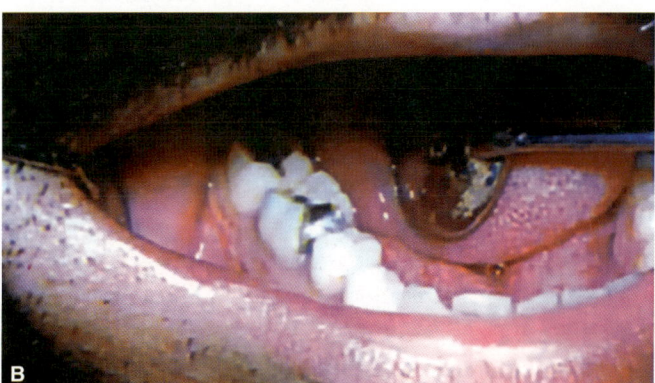

Figs 5.12A and B: Secondary caries around. **(A)** Cast restoration; **(B)** Amalgam restoration

number and type of organisms vary with different lesions. The presence of significant numbers of these bacteria in dentin of secondary caries indicates their role in the formation and development of secondary carious lesions.

Predominance of Streptococci and other types of gram +ve cocci have also seen found in vivo from failed restorations. Mutans streptococci and Lactobacilli have been found to increase in significant numbers in the dentin of teeth restored with amalgams having marginal defects wider than 40 μm. In case of secondary caries, restorative material definitely affects the activities of these micro-organisms. The type of restorative material influences qualitatively and quantitatively the microflora in the lesion; e.g. gamma-2 free amalgams can inhibit the metabolic activity of micro-organisms due to release of copper. Release of fluorides from the restorative materials may also have protective effects.

The micro-organisms found in the secondary dentinal lesions are of same nature as encountered in advanced dentinal lesions or of root dentinal lesions. Dentin is decalcified at pH 5.7 or below and most of the micro-organisms as discussed are capable of lowering the pH below this value. The inference can be that recurrent dentinal caries may be caused by a variety of micro-organisms, which can gain access to the dentin. Though Mutans streptococci and Lactobacilli are cariogenic, other less acidogenic bacteria could also be involved in the causation of recurrent dentinal caries.

Histopathology

Secondary caries may reveal an 'outer lesion' or a 'cavity wall lesion' or both. When a tooth is restored, the surrounding tooth structure is considered in two planes: the outer tooth surface and the cavity wall. The *'outer lesion'* refers to one which forms on the outer surface of the tooth; whereas, the *'wall lesion'* occurs on the walls of the cavity (Fig. 5.15). The outer lesion is considered as a result of primary attack; whereas, wall lesion is because of leakage at the tooth-restoration interface. The penetration of hydrogen ions plays a key role in the process of demineralization. The hydrogen ions may penetrate along the microspaces (The diffusion, capillary forces and differences in electrical potential between the tooth surface and the filling can lead to penetration of hydrogen ions into the microspaces).

The progress of outer lesion results in a cavity on the superficial tooth structure bordering the restoration. The wall lesion, however, can occur deep along the cavity walls. The outer lesion and a greater part of the wall lesion is seen to be bordered by a positive (dark) zone. In the outer lesions of enamel,

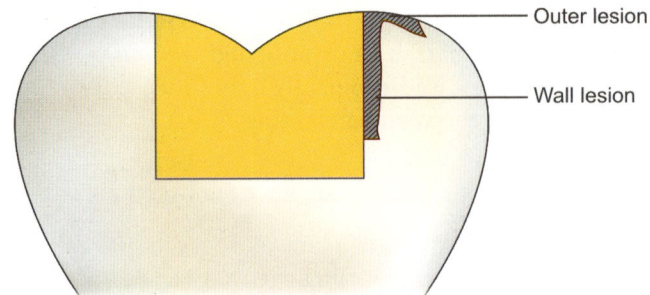

Fig. 5.15: Secondary caries under a restoration-outer lesion and wall lesion

lesions revealing >5% spaces are higher than lesions revealing <5% spaces, approximately in the ratio 4.2: 1.43. On the other hand, the opposite is true for the cavity wall lesions of enamel, i.e. lesions revealing <5% spaces are higher than lesions revealing >5% spaces, approximately in the ratio 3: 1. Lesions that correspond to less than 5% of spaces are visible only by polarized light whereas those corresponding to more than 5% of spaces are observable because of their radiolucent appearance also.

In the dentin, the wall lesion under polarized light shows a phenomenon indicative of demineralization, as the conventional carious process. Four types of variations have been commonly reported in the cavity wall lesions of dentin which can be:

a. Superficial demineralization of the cavity wall.
b. Subsurface demineralization without visible changes of the wall surface.
c. Subsurface demineralization with increased radiopacity of the surface layer. The radiopacity may be a result of reprecipitation of mineral ions from the underlying demineralized area or because of the deposition of mineral ions from amalgam, especially tin ions, in the surface of the dentin wall.
d. Alternating zones of increased radiopacity and radiolucency. The following layers can be distinguished:
   i. Towards the cavity-a narrow layer of highly increased radio-opacity.
   ii. A narrow layer of highly increased radiolucency.
   iii. A narrow layer representing same degree of radio-opacity as the intact dentin.
   iv. A broad radiolucent dentin,
   v. A broad layer of increased radiopacity.

Possibly, release of ions from a cement base or from amalgam material may have contributed to the radiopacity of layer 1, but the other layers may be a result of the alternations of demineralization and reprecipitation.

Caries in the dentin follows dentinal tubules, while in the cementum, caries proceeds preferentially along the Sharpey's fibers.

Differentiating Secondary Caries with Residual Caries

It is emphasized that residual caries left during cavity preparation must be differentiated from secondary caries. In case of residual caries, the demineralized areas are non uniformly divided whereas in secondary caries the area displays a fairly constant width in its course along the curvature of the cavity wall. It is very difficult, rather not possible to accept that the well defined uniform width of demineralization in secondary caries might be due to incorrect excavation of caries or cavity preparation.

The wall lesions of secondary caries and the damage caused to cavity walls during preparation procedures (burns) should also be differentially diagnosed. Wall lesions appear translucent while burns appear opaque under ordinary light. Wall lesions show grey fluorescence of low intensity under ultraviolet light while burns show white fluorescence of high intensity. Microradiographically, the wall lesions are radiolucent while burns are radio-opaque.

BIBLIOGRAPHY

1. Acevedo, A.M., Ray, M.V., Socorro, M. and Rojas-Sanchez, F.: Frequency and distribution of Mutans Streptococci in dental plaque from caries-free and caries-affected Venezuelan children. Acta. Odont. Latinoam.: 22, 15, 2009.
2. Ardu, S., Perroud, R. and Krajei, I.: Extended sealing of interproximal caries lesions. Quint. Int.: 37, 423, 2006.
3. Bandlish, L.K.: Attrition and plaque defense mechanism of teeth. The Probe 23, 67, 1981.
4. Bibby, B.G., Gustafson, G. and Davies, G.N.: A critique of three theories of caries attack. Int. Dent. J.: 8, 685, 1958.
5. Bratthall, D. and Hansel, P.G.: Cariogram: a multifactorial risk assessment model for a multifactorial disease. Comm. Dent. Oral Edpidem.: 33, 256, 2005.
6. Brazzelli, M., McKenzie, L., Fielding, S., Fraser, C., Clarkson, J. and Kilonzo, M.: Systemic review of the effectiveness and cost effectiveness of Heal Ozone for the treatment of occlusal pit/fissure caries and root caries. Health Tech. Assess.: 10, 80, 2006.
7. De Carvalho, F.G., Silva, D.S., Hebling, J., Spolidorio, L.C. and Spolidorio, D.M.: Presence of mutans sptreptococci and Candida spp. In dental plaque/dentine of carious teeth and early childhood caries. Arch. Oral Biol.: 51, 1024, 2006.
8. Gonzalez-Cabezas, C.: The chemistry of caries: Remineralization and demineralization events with direct clinical relevance. Dent. Clin. North Am.: 54, 469, 2010.
9. Gonzalez-Cabezas, C., Gregory, R.L. and Stookey, G.K.: Distribution of three cariogenic bacteria in secondary carious lesions around amalgam restorations. Caries Res.: 33, 357, 1999.
10. Ismail A., Tellez M., Pitts,N., Ekstrand K., Ricketts D., Longbotton C., Eggertsson,H., Deery C., Fisher J., Young,D., Evans, W.: Caries management pathways preserve dental tissues and promote oral health. Community Dentistry and Oral Epidemiology: 41, e12-e40, 2013
11. Kidd, E.A. and Fejerskov, O.: What constitutes dental caries? Histopathology of carious enamel and dentin related to the action of cariogenic biofilm. J.D.R.: 83, C35, 2004.
12. Kidd, E.A.M., Toffenetti, F. and Mjor, I.A.: Secondary caries. Int. Dent. J.: 42, 127, 1992.
13. Marsh, P.D.: Dental plaque as a biofilm: the significance of pH in health and caries. Compend. Contin. Educ. Dent.: 30, 76, 2009.
14. Klinke, T., Kneist, S., deSoet, J.J., Kublisch, E. and Foster, A.: Acid production by oral strains of Candida albicans and Lactobacilli. Caries Res.: 43, 83, 2009.
15. Malhotra A. and Hegde M: Medical management of dental caries: a change in therapeutic approach. International Research Journal of Pharmacy: 4,1,2013
16. Marza-leona, M., Paivi, R., Sirkha, J., Ansa, O. and Matti, S.: Childhood caries is still in force: A 15 year follow-up. Acta. Odont. Scand.: 66, 189, 2008.
17. McIntyre, J.M., Featherstone, J.D.B. and Fu, J: Studies of dental root surface caries.1: Comparison of natural and artificial root caries lesions. 2: The role of cementum in root surface caries. Aust. Dent. J. 45, 24 & 97, 2000.
18. Mjor, I.A. and Toffenetti,F: Secondary caries: A literature review with case reports. Quint. Int. 31, 165, 2000.
19. Nguyen, T., Tsang, P., Shi, W. and Qi, F.: Dental caries and chemical warfare within the mouth. J. Calif. Dent. Assoc.: 33, 947, 2005.
20. Ozer, L. and Thylstrup, A.: What is known about caries in relation to restorations as a reason for replacement? A Review. Adv. Dent. Res.: 9, 394, 1995.
21. Russell, R.R.: Changing concepts in caries microbiology. Am. J. Dent.: 22, 304, 2009.
22. Schupbach, P., Lutz, F. and Guggenheim, B.: Human root caries: Histopathology of arrested lesions. Caries Res.: 26,153, 1992.
23. Shimotoyodome, A., Kobayashi, H., Tokimitsu, I., Hase, T., Inoue, T., Matsukubo, T. and Takaesu, Y.: Saliva-promoted adhesion of Streptococcus mutans MT8148 associates with dental plaque and caries experience. Caries Res.: 41, 212, 2007.
24. Sikri,V and Sikri,P: Secondary caries - A dilemma. J. Cons. Dent. 3, 5, 2000.
25. Simmonds, R.S., Tompkins, G.R. and George, R.J.: Dental caries and the microbial ecology of dental plaque: a review of recent advances. NZ. Dent. J.: 96, 44, 2000.
26. Ten Cate, J.M.: Remineralization of deep enamel dentin caries lesions. Aust. Dent. J.: 53, 281, 2008.
27. Takahashi, N. and Nyvad, B.: Caries ecology revisited: Microbial dynamics and the caries process. Caries Res.: 42, 409, 2008.
28. Takahashi, N. and Nyvad, B.: The role of bacteria in the caries process: Ecological perspective. J. Dent. Res.: 90, 294, 2011.
29. Tanzer, J.M., Thompson, A., Wen, Z.T. and Burne, R.A.: Streptococcus mutans: fructose transport, xylitol resistance and virulence. J.D.R.: 85, 369, 2006.
30. Tinanoff, N.: Association of diet with dental caries in preschool children. Dent. Clin. North. Am.: 49, 725, 2005.
31. Westerman, G.H., Hicks, M.J., Flaitz, C.M. and Powell, G.L.: In vitro caries formation in primary tooth enamel: role of argon laser irradiation and remineralizing solutions treatment. J.A.D.A.: 137, 638, 2006.
32. Whitaker, E.J.: Primary, secondary and tertiary treatment of dental caries: a 20 year case report. J.A.D.A.: 137, 348, 2006.
33. Wright J.: defining the role of genetics in etiology of dental caries: J. Dent. Res. 89,11,2010

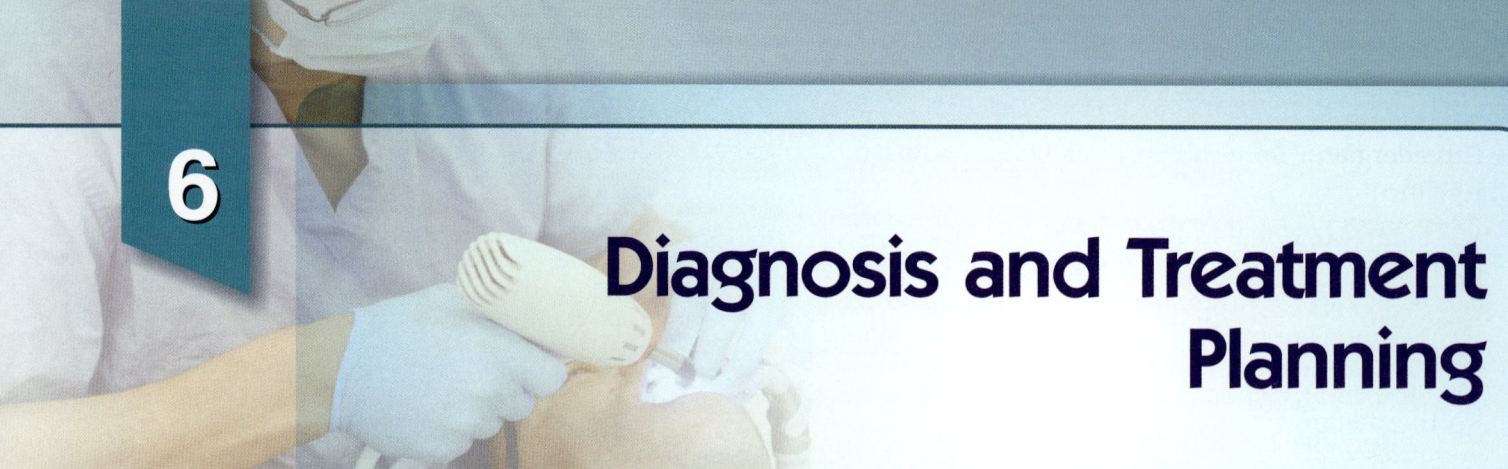

6. Diagnosis and Treatment Planning

One of the primary goals of operative dentistry is to provide functional stomatognathic system along with pleasing esthetics. Such a goal can be achieved only with sound foundation, which in any treatment regime is 'proper diagnosis'. 'Diagnosis' is a vast subject in itself; however, in operative dentistry, the diagnosis is restricted to dental caries along with diseases of the surrounding periodontium. Quite often, dental problems are diagnosed by the patients and the dentist is dictated to treat the same accordingly. The role of dentist is to make the patient aware of all the ailments in detail. Prior to any treatment plan, the dentist must arrive at a proper diagnosis, which should be made clear to the patient. The treatment plan is then finalized in accordance with the patient's demand and requirement keeping in view the oral health, awareness towards dentistry, physical well being and last but not the least the economic condition. Once mutual understanding is reached, treatment can be executed instructing the patient regarding the maintenance phase.

Definition

Diagnosis literally means the determination and judgement of variations from the normal. *It is defined as the utilization of scientific knowledge for identifying a diseased process and to differentiate it from other diseased processes.*

Diagnostic process may not be able to depict the true relation of the diagnostic test, which is carried out to diagnose the clinical problem; however, it provides a varying degree of certainty. Usually the test is interpreted as positive or negative and hence the disease is either present or absent. However in certain cases, the diagnostic tools are misleading, i.e. the test can be positive in the absence of disease (false positive) or negative in the presence of disease (false negative).

Diagnostic tests are usually assessed in terms of specificity and sensitivity. *'Specificity' refers to the ability of the test or observation to clearly differentiate one disease from the other.* Specificity is the ability to rule out the lesion when it is truly absent. *'Sensitivity' refers to the ability of a test or observation to detect the disease whenever it is truly present.* The sensitivity and the specificity of a test should be considered when the decision has to be made as to which test should be preferred for a particular disease.

It is well known that diagnosis starts the moment patient enters the clinic. Patient's overall assessment, way of dressing, neatness of clothes, gait and general well-being should be noticed at the first instance. Excitement and apprehension on the face of the patient should also be observed. By this time the patient is socially and psychologically assessed.

HISTORY OF THE PATIENT

History of the patient includes thorough conversation with the patient prior to any check up. It includes personal, family, medical and dental history. Conversation is an art. We must learn how to converse and to excavate patient feelings. One must be a good listener. First, don't ask any question. Let the patient feel comfortable and reveal his/her problems in detail. Second, during conversation, the dentist should be very attentive; he should not indulge in cross talking with the assistant or the nurse. Let there be one to one conversation. Once the patient feels comfortable, other questions can be asked.

Personal and Family History

Personal and family history includes patient's personal habits, awareness towards oral health, awareness towards general health along with the financial background. Attitude of parents and grandparents towards oral care is equally important. Certain conditions, which are likely to be inherited, should be explored by asking a series of questions and other conditions related to the socio-economic status of the family should also be noted.

Medical History

The detailed information regarding childhood diseases and treatment taken, history of X-radiations and allergies is important prior to start of any dental treatment. Certain cardiac abnormalities and systemic diseases demand less strenuous procedures while requiring prophylactic antibiotic cover. Physiological changes associated with aging also influence dental treatment. Certain medicines, which reduce salivary flow and/or alter the basic defense mechanisms of the body, and that have direct or indirect influence on the dental procedures should be noted. Other enquiries which should not be missed are; any allergy to drugs, past history of drugs taken, presence of anaemia, asthma, diabetes, arthritis, hepatitis, epilepsy, bleeding disorders, cancers, pregnancy, etc.

Dental History

Dental history includes getting information about the patient's awareness towards dentistry, any previous visits to dentists and any systemic medicines taken. Any allergy to local anaesthetics and local antiseptics should also be noted. Past treatment of any tooth and its complication, if any, has an important impact on the treatment plan.

Chief Complaint

The patient's chief complaint is a symptom or a group of symptoms, which the patient describes in his/her own words. The patient should be encouraged and guided to discuss all aspects of his ailment. Such information is necessary to determine and plan the treatment. Most commonly, the chief complaint is 'pain'; though it can be esthetic problems due to discolored or malaligned teeth, fractured teeth, etc. Immediate alleviation of pain is mandatory, whenever there is a complaint of pain. The cause of pain, its onset, duration, character and the related factors should be assessed and the required treatment given. The complete history should always be taken whatever the chief complaint may be.

CLINICAL EXAMINATION

After conversing with the patient in detail, the dentist arrives at some preliminary diagnosis. This is followed by a clinical examination of the oral cavity. The oral cavity is visually examined, thoroughly palpated, and if need be, percussion tests are undertaken to reach at some conclusion. Thorough examination of the anteroposterior relationship of the jaws, noting lateral and protrusive movements of the mandible and hearing for clicking sounds in the temporomandibular joint are also important. Inspection and palpation of the lips, labial and buccal mucosa, cheeks, palate, oropharynx, floor of the mouth and tongue are carried out in sequence and the recordings are noted.

Examination of the Orofacial Soft Tissues

The examination of the orofacial soft tissues requires a systematic approach. First, examine the submandibular glands and cervical lymph nodes for abnormalities in size, texture, mobility and sensitivity to palpation. Second, palpate the masticatory muscles for pain and tenderness. Then start in one area of the mouth and follow a routine pattern of visual examination and palpation proceeding from the cheeks, vestibule, mucosa, lips, lingual and facial alveolar mucosa to the palate, tonsillar area, tongue and the floor of the mouth.

Examination of the Gingiva

The examination of the gingival color, form, level of attachment and depth of gingival sulcus may reveal variations from the normal. These variations in an otherwise normal oral cavity are indicative of systemic diseases. Certain local conditions like improper restorations usually aid in gingival and periodontal problems. Before undergoing any operative procedure, periodontal health should be restored. Adequate post treatment time should be allowed for healing and tissue regeneration. Healthy and inflamed gingiva are shown in Figs 6.1A and B.

Examination of the Teeth

The examination of teeth includes:
  i. Number, form and morphology
 ii. Color
iii. Restorations
 iv. Proximal relationships (contact and contour)
  v. Attrition, abrasion and erosion
 vi. Occlusion
vii. Fractures
viii. Vitality of tooth
 ix. Carious lesions

  i. *Number, form and morphology:* The number of teeth is more relevant during young age especially during mixed dentition period. The development of teeth and availability of space should be watched closely. Also look for congenitally missing and supernumerary teeth (Figs 6.2A and B). Panoramic radiographs are helpful in assessing the number and form of teeth. The total number of teeth present at any particular age is also indicative of the patient's interest in dental care and accordingly aids in devising a suitable treatment plan. The form of teeth should be noted. Teeth can show microdontia or macrodontia, gemination, concrescence, dens in dente, amelogenesis imperfecta, dentinogenesis imperfecta, etc. Morphology of the teeth, many a times, is indicative of a systemic disease; for example, mulberry molars in syphilis. The

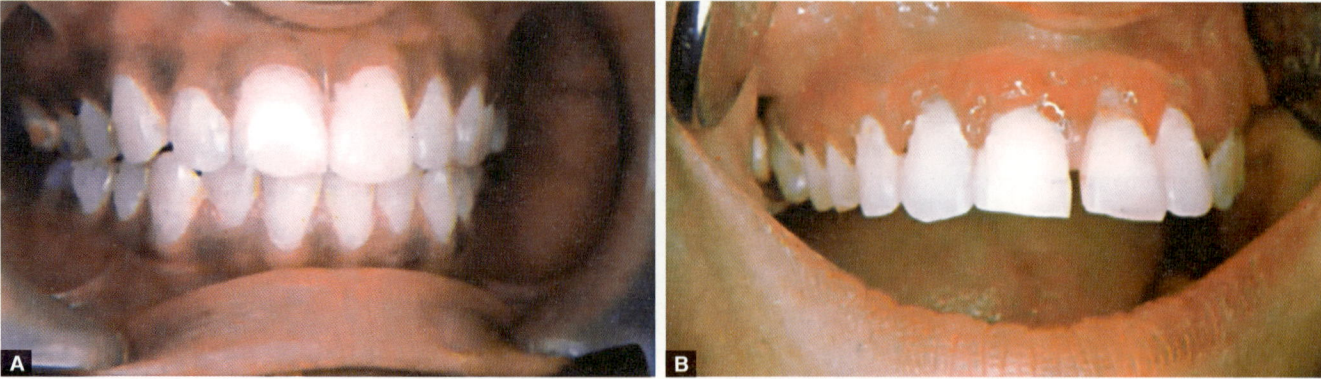

Figs 6.1A and B: **(A)** Protusive movement; **(B)** Disocclusion of posterior teeth in protusive movement

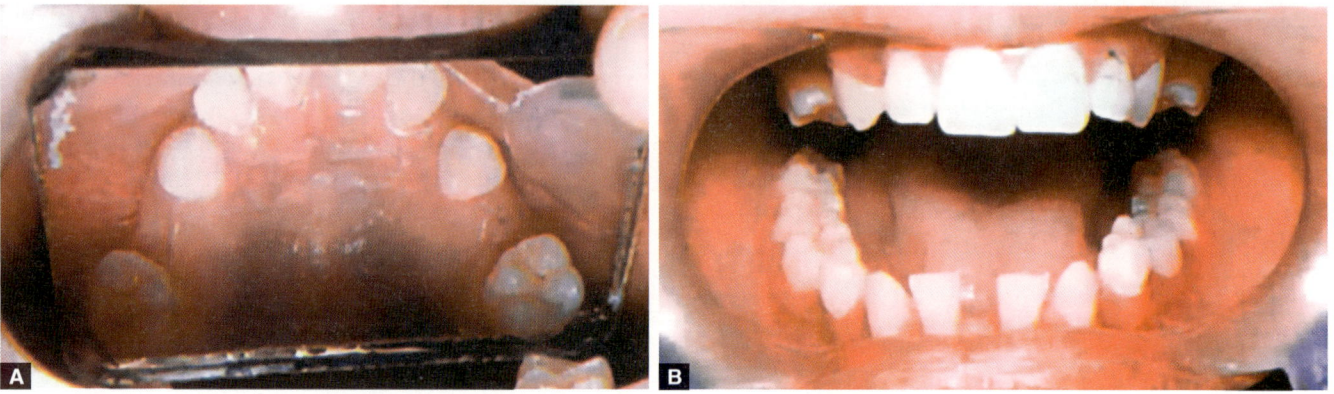

Figs 6.2A and B: **(A)** Maxillary premolars missing; **(B)** Mandibular lateral incisors missing

operative dentist, may need to change the 'square' type molar to proper shape so as to avoid periodontal problems. Certain morphological changes also occur in hypoplastic teeth, which are of great importance during restorative procedures.

ii. *Color:* Color is gaining importance these days with the advent of esthetic restorative materials. Abnormal tooth color is indicative of certain systemic diseases. Non-vital teeth or teeth in which the pulp is undergoing necrosis also exhibit altered color. Teeth with systemic diseases like erythroblastasis foetalis and congenital porphyria also show abnormal color. Other conditions in which there may be seen a color change are amelogenesis imperfecta, dentinogenesis imperfecta, fluorosis and intake of tetracycline during pregnancy and infancy (Figs 6.3A and B). If any localized change is visible in color of enamel such as opacity it may be

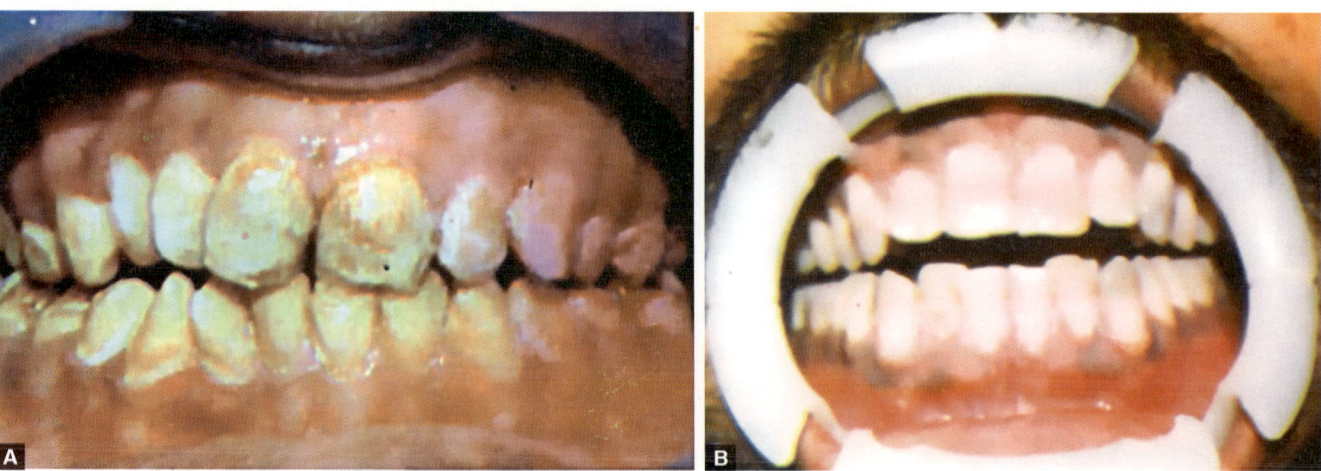

Figs 6.3A and B: **(A)** Fluorosis; **(B)** Tetracycline stains

indicative of initiation of caries process or hypoplastic area.

iii. *Restorations:* The restorations present, if any, should also be evaluated. The following features should be noted:
   - Number of restorations present.
   - Restorative material used.
   - Extent of the restoration.
   - Fractured restorations.
   - Marginal ditching or secondary caries.
   - Discolored restorations.
   - Stained margins of the restoration
   - Anatomical contours.
   - Overhanging restoration.
   - Voids
   - Marginal ridge incompatibility

iv. *Proximal relationships (Contacts and contours):* Maintenance of proper contact between two teeth and their exact location is of utmost importance in restorative dentistry so as to protect and stimulate the underlying interdental col. Loose contacts lead to food impaction, thereby leading to periodontal problems (Fig. 6.4A). Conversely, very tight contact deteriorates the periodontal ligament of both the teeth; the one, which is restored, and the other adjacent to it.

Restoration of proper contour of the proximal, buccal and lingual surfaces and embrasure areas of the restored and adjacent teeth are one of the major concerns in operative dentistry. Over contoured and under contoured restorations are harmful to the underlying periodontium; may lead to secondary caries, etc. Improper facial and lingual contours invite plaque accumulation leading to thickening of gingival margins and other periodontal problems. Many a times, the contour of natural teeth needs to be improved so as to achieve optimal periodontal health. During restoration of proximal lesions, care should be taken to have the proper form of embrasures (Fig. 6.4B). If it is not feasible with one restorative material, other restorative materials may be tried.

v. *Attrition, abrasion and erosion: Attrition* is the wear of enamel due to masticatory forces, which may be physiologic due to aging or pathologic due to bruxism (Fig. 2.2). *Abrasion* is the loss of tooth surfaces usually associated with mechanical means when continued for longer duration (Fig. 2.2). Cervical abrasions are most commonly associated with faulty tooth brushing and using hard brushes. *Erosion,* on the other hand is the loss of enamel and then dentin subsequent to acidic dissolution or at times idiopathic (Fig. 2.3). The etiology of erosion should be looked for, since continuous erosion leads to failure of restoration. Erosion can affect any tooth surface, especially more prevalent in labial surfaces of anterior teeth and buccal surfaces of posterior teeth.

Various restorative materials are available for restoring these lesions; however, care should be exercised to avoid overextension of these materials into the gingival sulcus.

vi. *Occlusion:* Maintenance of functions and esthetics is the major goal of operative dentistry. Improper occlusion leads to many problems like periodontal problems, muscle tenderness, temporomandibular joint dysfunctions, etc. Such a situation may be seen in under filled cavities and when improper occlusal contacts like premature contacts exist.

Type of occlusion has its impact in planning the type of restoration. Premature contacts and excessive stresses during lateral movements of

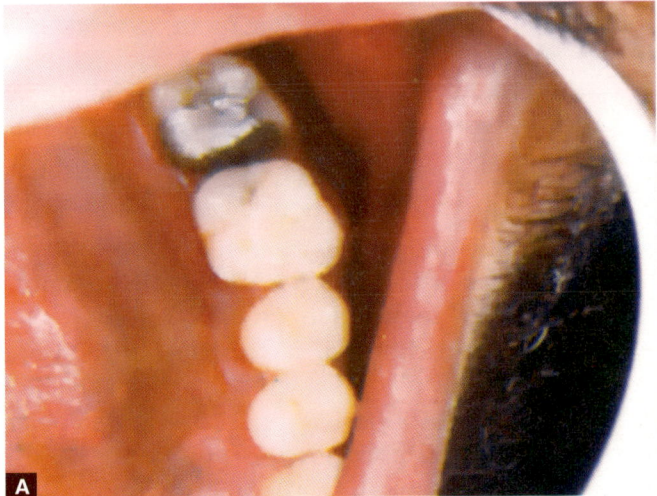
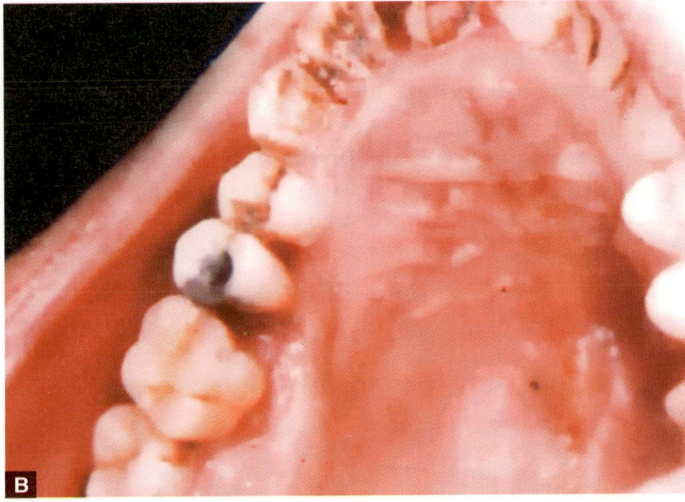

Figs 6.4A and B: (A) Open contact; **(B)** Improper embrasure

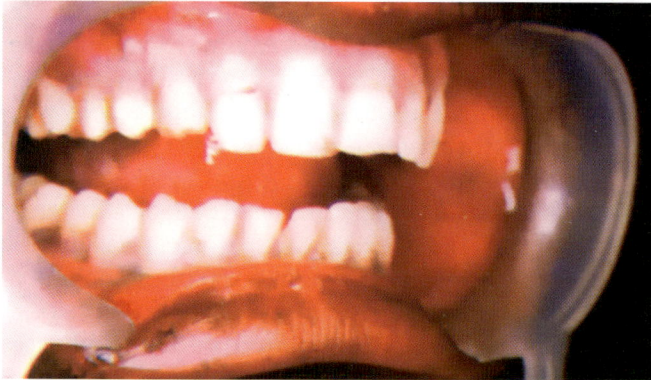

Fig. 6.5: Fractured maxillary lateral incisor

mandible should be noted and corrected before planning for the future restorations.

vii. *Fractures* Fractured teeth, partial or complete, should be noted during routine examination (Fig. 6.5). Cusps weakened by underlying carious process or large restorations in a tooth may fracture under various masticatory stresses. Such fractures normally do not result in pulp exposure. Use of pins for a restoration also creates internal shear stresses, which may invite complete/incomplete fractures of the tooth. Complete fracture of only crown or along with the roots is evident with most of the large mesio-occluso-distal restorations.

Occasionally, only fracture lines are present which may or may not extend up to the underlying pulp. This is known as 'Cracked tooth syndrome'. Patients can present with symptoms such as sensitivity to biting pressure, thermal sensitivity or even lancinating pain, which cannot be correlated with the local findings and the radiographs. Though transillumination is the best method of diagnosing cracks, patient's awareness and the clinical experience of the operator are mandatory to diagnose cracks in early stages. One should remain suspicious of cracked tooth until and unless diagnosed.

viii. *Vitality of tooth:* The restorative treatment plan depends upon the vitality of tooth (pulp vitality). Pulp vitality tests are important tools in our diagnostic armamentarium, since these tests not only determine the vitality of the tooth, but also the pathological status of the pulp. More so, the treatment plan is greatly influenced by these tests.

Pulp vitality tests are of the following types:

A. Thermal tests
   a. Cold test
   b. Heat test
   c. Laser

B. Electrical tests
C. Measurement of surface temperature of the tooth.
   a. Thermographic cholestric liquid crystals
   b. Time temperature graph
   c. Hughes Probeye camera
D. Laser Doppler flowmetry
E. Pulse oximetry
F. Dual wave spectrophotometry
G. Optical reflection vitalometer
H. Photoplethysmography

(For details, the reader is advised to refer 'Essentials of Endodontics' – by Vimal K Sikri)

ix. *Carious lesions:* The diagnosis of carious lesions has traditionally been limited to 'cavitation'. In the recent past, the tactile/visual approach of diagnosing caries was considered sufficient. However, cavitation is the late event in the carious process, which is preceded by a wide-ranging period of subsurface demineralization. Before subsurface demineralization, the possibility of other changes in the oral environment should be diagnosed. Therefore, early detection of incipient carious lesions and the caries activity processes prior to tooth destruction are the primary goals of an effective diagnosis and treatment planning.

No single test has been developed which can be considered as an absolute test for caries diagnosis. The concept of diagnosis of caries prior to its occurrence has gained importance. Individuals are identified according to their 'caries risk' levels. Certain tests are undertaken which foretell the person's susceptibility or risk to caries. These are known as *caries activity tests*.

CARIES RISK ASSESSMENT

'Caries susceptibility' refers to the inherent tendency of the host and the target tissue (the tooth) to be affected by the caries.

Caries risk assessment is the procedure to predict the future caries development before the classical onset of disease.

Factors affecting evaluation of caries risk:

- Morphology and chemistry of teeth (arrangement and number of teeth, occlusal relations, retentive areas, enamel maturation, etc.).
- Biological and chemical factors (localization and composition of plaque, microbial activity, etc.).
- Salivary factors (buffering capacity, immunological factors, oral clearance, etc.).
- Diet (frequency, amount and quality of carbohydrates taken, intake of fluorides, etc.).

- Epidemiology (family caries experience, caries experience in deciduous teeth).
- Systemic conditions (diseases that may influence oral health).

Risk assessment of caries done by:
- Dental saliva pH indicator
- Plaque check pH kit
- Saliva check buffer
- Clinpro caries diagnosis L-pop
- Caries risk assessment tool
- Traffic light matrix model

Clinpro caries diagnosis L-pop measures the lactic acid production and evaluates the microbial flora of the mouth by sampling the microflora of the tongue.

American Academy of Pediatric Dentistry (AAPD) classifies risk in infants, children and adolescents (AAPD Caries risk assessment tool). This tool was based on following factors: (Table 6.1)

a. Clinical conditions
b. Environmental characteristics
c. General health conditions

A traffic light matrix (TL-M) model offers a systematic approach to the assessment of all the risk factors which contribute to caries activity. Information is gathered and used to produce a risk profile from which a patient centered treatment regime can be developed. The model is based on the fact that the caries process is multifactorial and it will be driven by changes to one or more aspects of the overall oral environment. The concept of using the colors red, yellow and green in a traffic light color system to convey the different levels of risk has been used previously in both dentistry and health education. The traffic light is the first element of this system and it builds on the existing risk assessment models as well as including an assessment of patient motivation and lifestyle activities. It does not attempt to predict caries

Table 6.1: AAPD caries risk assessment tool

Caries-risk indicators	Low risk	Moderate risk	High risk
Clinical conditions	• No carious teeth in past 24 months • No enamel demineralization • No visible plaque; no gingivitis	• Carious teeth in past 24 months • Area of enamel demineralization • Gingivitis	• Carious teeth in past 12 months • More than 1 area of enamel demineralization (enamel caries "white-spot lesion") • Visible plaque on anterior (front) teeth • Radiographic enamel caries • High titers of mutans Streptococci • Wearing dental or orthodontic appliances • Enamel hypoplasia
Environmental characteristics	• Optimal systemic and topical fluoride exposure • Consumption of simple sugars or foods strongly associated with caries initiation primarily at meal times. • High caregiver socioeconomic status • Regular use of dental care in an established dental home	• Suboptimal systemic fluoride exposure with optimal topical exposure • Occasional (i.e., 1-2) between meal exposures to simple sugars or foods strongly associated with caries • Midlevel caregiver socioeconomic status (i.e. eligible for school lunch program or SCHIP) • Irregular use of dental services	• Suboptimal topical fluoride exposure • Frequent (i.e., 3 or more) between meal exposures to simple sugars or foods strongly associated with caries. • Low-level caregiver socioeconomic status (i.e., eligible for Medicaid) • Active caries present in the mother • No usual source of dental care
General health conditions		• Children with special health care needs • Conditions impairing saliva composition/flow	

incidence but rather it acts as an early warning system that alerts the clinician to the presence of risk factors that are capable of changing the oral environment. The TL-M model allocates a threshold value for each risk category. If the information elicited from questioning or by clinical testing yields results which exceed the predetermined threshold values the model alerts the clinician to a possible problem. The model investigates sixteen risk factors and scores a red light, yellow light or green light for each risk factor depending upon predetermined criteria. The system uses a specially designed form to record risk factors and the test can be carried out either by a dentist or an auxillary who has been trained to collect the data.

The second element of the TL-M model is matrix (Table 6.2). This is designed as a means of assessing the patient's present disease status and attitude to maintaining their own dental health. It is a very useful measure of the patient's ability or willingness to comply with treatment directives. Attitude towards dental health is scored as A, B or C on the vertical axis of the grid and the current disease status is scored as 1, 2 or 3 and is recorded on the horizontal axis.

Table 6.2: Matrix component of traffic light matrix model

	Disease status		
Attitude	1	2	3
a			
b			
c			

1. No current disease
2. Need for repair or maintenance
3. Active disease

a. Yes
b. May be
c. No

The sixteen risk factors, grouped under five headings used in the TL-M model are:

Saliva
- Ability of minor salivary glands to produce saliva
- Consistency of unstimulated saliva
- pH of unstimulated saliva
- Stimulated saliva flow rate
- Buffering capacity of stimulated saliva

Diet
- Number of sugar exposures per day
- Number of acid exposures per day

Fluoride
Past and current exposure

Oral Biofilm
- Differential staining
- Composition
- Activity

Modifying Factors
- Past and current dental status
- Past and current medical status
- Compliance
- Lifestyle
- Socio-economic status

CARIES ACTIVITY TESTS

Caries activity tests are primarily undertaken to evaluate the susceptibility of the individual towards caries. 'Caries activity' refers to the increment of active lesions (new and recurrent) over a period of time. Caries activity is the measure of the speed of progression of caries lesion. Caries activity tests measure the degree to which the local environmental challenge (for example, dietary and related effects on microbial growth) favours the probability of initiation of caries.

The tests are based on the hypothesis that oral micro-organisms and fermentable carbohydrates are causative agents in dental caries and the retention of carbohydrates in oral cavity favour growth of micro-organisms.

Use of Caries Activity Tests

For clinicians
- To determine the need for caries control measures.
- To determine optimal time for expertise restoration.
- Aid in determining the results of the preventive measures undertaken.
- Orthodontists can be cautioned during the treatment.

For research workers
- Aid in selection of cases for the study of caries.
- Helps in screening of patented therapeutic agents.
- Serves as an indicator of period of exacerbation.

Caries activity tests help
- Identify high risk individual/groups
- Determine the need of preventive regimes for particular individual/groups.
- Ensuring low level of caries activity before extensive restorations
- Monitor the effectiveness of oral health education programs

Ideal requirement of caries activity tests
- Should have sound theoretical basis
- Should be accurate as regards duplication of results
- Should be simple and inexpensive
- Should be less time consuming

The routinely used tests are:

Diagnosis and Treatment Planning

A. Lactobacillus Count Test

This test is of a historical interest only and is limited mainly to research. It basically evaluates lactobacilli bacteria in the saliva quantitatively. Their number increases with increased consumption of carbohydrates.

Procedure

The patient is asked to chew paraffin before breakfast and the saliva is collected in a bottle. A 1:10 dilution is prepared by pipetting 1.0 ml of this saliva sample into 9.0 ml tube of sterile saline solution. This is shaken and 1:100 dilution is made by pipetting 1.0 ml of 1.10 dilution into another 9.0 ml tube of sterile salt solution. The 0.4 ml of each solution dilution is spread on the surface of an agar plate. The plates are labeled and incubated at 37°C for 3-4 days. A count of number of calories is made by using quebec counter.

It is observed that the bacterial count up to 1000 is unimportant; between 1000-5,000 is indicative of slight caries activity; between 5,000–10,000 is moderate caries activity and count over 10,000 is associated with high caries activity (Table 6.3).

Table 6.3: Number of lactobacilli and caries activity

Number of lactobacilli		Caries activity
0-1000	+	Little or no caries
1000-5000	+	Slight caries
5000-10000	+ +	Moderate caries
10, 000 and more	+ + +	Marked caries

Advantages
- Simple
- Useful for screening larger groups

Disadvantages
- Inaccurate for predicting onset of caries
- Does not exclude the possibility of growth of other aciduric micro-organisms
- Complex equipment required
- Growth of colonies takes longer time
- Counting of colonies is tedious
- Results take several days
- Costly

B. Snyder Test

Snyder introduced a relatively simple colorimetric test for the estimation of relative number of lactobacilli in the saliva. The test has been widely used as a diagnostic tool as well as to evaluate the patient's acceptance of dietary changes or preventive measures designed to reduce dental caries.

Method

Saliva is collected as is given in lactobacillus test. A tube of snyder glucose is melted and then cooled to 50°C. 0.2 cc of collected saliva is pipetted into 10 ml of medium and is incubated at 37°C for 72 hours. Rate of color change is indicative of the caries activity.

Glucose agar medium with bromocresol green
+
0.2 ml of saliva
↓
Incubated at 37°C

Color changes in		
24 hrs.	48 hrs.	72 hrs.
Yellow	Yellow	No color change
Marked caries susceptibility	Definite caries activity	Caries inactive

Advantages
- This test is easier and an acceptable method of educating people.
- Color changes can be noted easily as compared to the counting of bacteria.
- Cost effective

Disadvantages
- Cannot predict the extent of expectancy of caries with any reliability for one individual.
- Color change might not be clear
- Measures acidogenic potential; salivary organisms may not be representative of those in plaque
- Time consuming

C. Salivary Reductase Test

It is one of the recent tests adopted to evaluate the caries activity. It measures the activity of the enzyme reductase in salivary bacteria. The saliva is collected as mentioned earlier and mixed with a dye - Diazoresorcinol. The change of color is noted in 15 minutes.

Advantages
- No incubation required
- Time saving (quick results)

Disadvantages
Results vary with time after food intake and after brushing

Color Changes

Blue — Non conducive
Orchid — Slight caries activity

Red — Moderate caries acitivity (High caries activity if color changes to red prior to 15 miutes)
Colorless — Highly conducive

D. Alban Test

The use of this test is recommended because of its low cost, simplicity, diagnostic values and motivational values. This test eliminates the need for melting the medium as the medium used is soft and allows easy penetration of saliva and acids. Also the procedure is simple as the patient expectorates directly into the tubes that contain the medium.

Method

60 gms of Snyder test agar is placed in one litre of water and boiled over low or medium heat. When adequately melted, the molten agar is distributed in tubes, each tube containing 5.0 ml of the test medium. The tubes should be allowed to cool before storing them in the refrigerator. This procedure prepares the tubes along with the test medium and is ready to be used when desired.

For the actual testing, the patient is asked to expectorate directly into the tube such that sufficient amount of it is present to cover the surface of the test medium. A funnel facilitates the collection of saliva. The tubes are labelled and incubated at 37°C for 4 days. Observations are made for the color change (bluish green, pH 5.0 to definite yellow, pH 4 or less) and the depth of color change. According to Alban, the volume of saliva, the time of day at which the saliva is collected and the proximity of this time to the time of eating does not significantly affect the results.

Advantages
• Simple and inexpensive
• Ideal for motivation and education

Disadvantages
• More armamentarium required
• Color change evaluation might be subjective

Scoring is done as given below:

No color change	–
Color change beginning at the top of medium	+
One half color change from top to bottom	+ +
Three fourths color change from top to bottom	+ + +
Total color change to yellow	+ + + +

The final recording after 72 or 96 hours of incubation is carried out as follows:
- Readings negative for the entire incubation period are labelled 'negative'.
- Reading are labelled 'positive' irrespective of the degree of positivity.
- Slower change or less color change compared to the previous test is labelled as 'improved'.
- Faster change or more pronounced change compared to the previous test is labelled as 'worse'.
- When readings are identical compared to the previous test, it is labelled as 'no change'.

E. Fosdick's Calcium Dissolution Test

The acid formed when patient saliva is mixed with glucose and powdered enamel incubated at 37°C is used for four hours to evaluate the amount in milligrams of powdered enamel dissolution.

Saliva is stimulated by chewing gum (paraffin is avoided because glucose is needed for the test; in case paraffin can't be avoided, additional glucose is added). Part of saliva so collected is analyzed for calcium content. The rest is kept in a tube containing 0.1 gm of powdered enamel for four hours at body temperature. After that it is analyzed for calcium content. The caries activity is directly proportional to enamel dissolution.

Disadvantages
• Complex test
• Accurate measurements difficult
• Costly

Dewar, later modified the test measuring pH of the saliva-glucose-enamel mixture (Instead of calcium dissolution, only pH is measured).

F. Ora Test

The Ora test evaluates the oral microbial level. It is based on the role of oxygen depletion by micro organisms in expectorated milk samples. In normal conditions the bacterial enzyme, aerobic dehydrogenase transfers electrons or protons to oxygen. Once oxygen gets utilized by the aerobic organisms, methylene blue acts as an electron acceptor and gets reduced to leucomethylene blue. This reflects the metabolic activity of the aerobic organisms.

In this test 10 ml of sterile milk is rinsed in the oral cavity for 30 seconds and the expectorate is collected. 3.0 ml of this milk is transferred to a tube and 0.12 ml of 0.1% methylene blue is added. The tubes are observed every 10 minutes for any color change and also the time of initiation of color change. The higher the infection lesser is the time taken for the change in color reflecting higher oral microbial level.

Diagnosis and Treatment Planning

Advantages

- Not-toxic, simple and inexpensive
- Trained personnel not required
- Can also monitor gingival inflammation
- Good for motivation and education
- Cost effective

Disadvantages

- Lack of specificity (does not identify a specific group of micro-organisms in a specific disease).
- Does not differentiate between onset and progress of caries.
- Positive signs can be obtained with other infections of oral cavity.

G. Swab Test

It is preferably used in young children, since no collection of saliva is necessary. The basic principle is of snyder test. The oral flora is taken by swabbing the buccal surface of the teeth with a cotton applicator. It is then incubated in the medium. The change in pH following 48 hours incubation period is evaluated on pH meter.

Advantages

- No collection of saliva required
- Predict caries increment, particularly in children

H. Streptococcus Mutans Level Test

The test measures the number of *Streptococcus mutans* colony forming units (CFU)/unit volume of saliva by culturing the plaque samples from discrete sites (occlusal/proximal) for detecting and quantifying *Streptococcus mutans* on the teeth. Tongue blades/wooden spatulas are used to collect the samples of organisms. These are then pressed against *Streptococcus mutans* selective mitis salivarius bacitracin agar. The agar plates are incubated at 37°C for 48 hours in CO_2 gas.

The test is interpreted as:

Level of *Streptococcus mutans* > 100/ml of saliva = Unacceptable

Advantage

Frequency of isolation of *Streptococcus mutans* is high prior to initiation of lesions.

Disadvantages

- *Streptococcus mutans* tend to be located as specific sites
- Shelf life of plates is one week; so not convenient for chairside tests.
- Difficult to distinguish between carrier state and cariogenic infection.

I. Salivary Buffer Capacity Test

Salivary buffer capacity test can be quantitated using either pH meter or color indicator. The test measures the quantity of acid in milliliters required to lower the pH of saliva through an arbitrary pH interval (say from pH 6.0 to 7.0) or the amount of acid/base necessary to bring color indicators to their point.

Ten milliliter of stimulated saliva is collected at least one hour after eating. 5.0 ml of this is taken in a beaker. The pH of saliva is adjusted at 7.0 by addition of lactic acid or base. Lactic acid is further added until pH 6 is reached. The amount of lactic acid needed to reduce the pH from 7.0 to 6.0 is a measure of buffer capacity. The number is converted to milliequivalent per liter.

There is an inverse relationship of buffering capacity of saliva and caries. The saliva of individual having sufficient number of carious lesion frequently has lower acid buffering capacity then the saliva of those who are relatively caries free.

Advantage

Simple and effective

Disadvantage

May not correlate adequately with caries activity.

J. Streptococcus Mutans Dip-slide Method

These tests comprise Dentocult SM and Cari Screen SM.

These tests classify salivary samples according to estimates of Streptococcus mutans colonies growing on modified mitis salivarius agar.

Procedure A (Dentocult SM)

- The patient is asked to chew paraffin wax for five minutes and the resultant stimulated saliva is collected.
- Saliva is poured over agar coated slide, totally wetting the surface, and excess is allowed to drain off.
- Slides are dried for 10–15 minutes, bacitracin disks are placed in middle of the inoculated agar.
- A CO_2 tablet is inserted in the tube containing the slide, which is then incubated for 48 hours.
- A zone of inhibition 10-20 mm in diameter is formed around each bacitracin disk.
- S. mutans appears as blue colonies growing within the zone of inhibition.
- The colony density is compared with a model chart.

Procedure B (Cari Screen SM)

- Bacitracin tablet is placed in buffered diluents and allowed to dissolve completely.

- The patient is asked to chew paraffin wax for 15-20 seconds swallowing the saliva.
- While continuing to chew the wax the patient expectorates approx. 1.0-2.0 ml of stimulated saliva directly into diluents vial, which is then capped and gently mixed by repeated inversion.
- The dip slide coated on both sides with MSB agar (without bacitracin), is then immersed for few seconds in the buffered diluent containing bacitracin and patient's saliva.
- A CO_2 tablet is placed in the empty dip slide vial, and 2 drops of water are added.
- The dip slide is replaced in its vial and cap is securely tightened.
- The vial is placed upright for 48 hours at 37°C in an incubator and then allowed to stand at room temperature overnight.
- The colony density on agar is compared with a reference colony density chart.
- This test correlates strongly with actual laboratory methods of quantifying S. mutans by standard culturing.
- The S. mutans colonies can be recognized when viewed through a magnifying lens by their opaque, highly convex appearance and irregular shape.

K. Streptococcus Mutans Replicate Technique

This technique localize *Streptococcus mutans* colonies on tooth surface using a solid impression matrix composed primarily of sucrose and commercial gum base.

Procedure

- Imprint of tooth surface to be sampled is obtained by pressing the matrix against it.
- Matrix is washed for several seconds in water to remove non adherent cells and saliva.
- Matrices are placed in liquid broth and incubated at 37°C overnight and examined directly for overgrowth of S. mutans colonies at specific sites.

CARIES DIAGNOSIS

Several methods are being employed for diagnosing caries. The process of *caries diagnosis* involves *assessing the caries risk of an individual and applying different diagnostic methods*. Each method uses either one or all of the following:
- Assessment of environmental conditions such as pH, salivary flow and salivary buffering
- Determination of bacterial activity
- Identification of subsurface demineralization

Other factors viz. age, gender, fluoride exposure, general health and oral hygiene should also be considered.

DIAGNOSTIC TOOLS

1. Visual
2. Tactile
3. Radiographic
    a. Conventional
        i. Intraoral periapical
        ii. Bitewing
    b. Xeroradiography
    c. Modified radiographic techniques
        i. Digital enhancement
        ii. Computer image analysis
        iii. Subtraction radiography
        iv. CBCT
4. Electric resistance (Electrical conductance and impedance)
5. Optical detection
    a. Optical caries monitor
    b. Fiberoptic transillumination (FOTI)
    c. Digital imaging fiberoptic transillumination (DIFOTI)
    d. Ultraviolet illumination
    e. Transillumination with near infrared light
    f. Laser induced fluorescence
    g. Quantitative laser fluorescence (QLF)
    h. DIAGNOdent
    i. Infrared fluorescence
6. Endoscopy/videoscopy
7. Dyes
8. Recent advances/newer techniques
    a. CO_2 Laser
    b. Terahertz imaging
    c. Multiphoton imaging
    d. Optical coherence tomography
    e. Infrared thermography
    f. LED technology (Midwest caries ID)
    g. Alternating current impedance spectroscopy (Carie Scan)
    h. Frequency domain infrared photothermal radiometry and modulated luminescence
    i. Magnetic resonance imaging (MRI)
    j. Ultrasonic imaging

1. Visual

Visual examination includes looking for cavitation, surface roughness, opacification and discoloration. The teeth are cleaned and dried with compressed air and illuminated under adequate light source. The examination takes about ten minutes. Problem with using this method is that discoloration of the pits and

Table 6.4: Visual scoring system

Score	Inference
0	No or very slight change in enamel transparency after drying
1	Opacity not visible on wet surface but distinct on drying
2	Opacity distinctly visible without drying
3	Localized breakdown in opaque enamel along with gray discoloration of dentin
4	Cavitation in enamel exposing the dentin

fissures may be a universal finding in normal healthy adult teeth, which may be mistaken for the presence of caries (Table 6.4).

2. Tactile

Tactile examination includes determining roughness or softness of the tooth surface with a sharp explorer. Both penetration and resistance to removal of an explorer tip (catch) have been interpreted as an evidence of demineralization. However, one needs to determine how effective is probing.

Probing of the fissures and smooth surfaces for diagnostic purposes is an age-old diagnostic aid. But in the recent past, probing has been criticized and questioned because of several reasons viz:

a. May transmit cariogenic bacteria from one site to another.
b. May produce irreversible traumatic defects in potentially remineralizable enamel.
c. May not be able to add any information to the visual examination
d. Mechanical binding of an explorer tip in a fissure may not be because of caries but because of other causes like:
   i. Shape of the fissure
   ii. Sharpness of an explorer: A sharp explorer has a diameter of 200 microns at its tip and pressing this tip with forces parallel to the blade may actually push the tip into enamel
   iii. Force of application: Heavy probing pressure may cause sticking of the probe tip into enamel fissures

Dental floss and tooth separators are also employed to detect proximal caries. After the tooth has been thoroughly cleaned, floss is inserted through the contact area and dragged occlusally against one proximal surface. If it shreds, one can suspect a proximal cavity. One disadvantage when using floss is that overhanging restorations on the proximal side also give us the same features. Tooth separators and wedges basically aid in visually detecting the proximal caries by separating the teeth.

International Caries Detection and Assessment System (ICDAS)

International caries detection and assessment system (ICDAS) is an improved version of visual/tactile method of detecting caries. WHO probe, which is a ball-ended sphere presenting 0.5 mm in extremity, has been used to evaluate presence of discontinuities/microcavitations in enamel.

ICDAS is a two-digit identification system (X-Y). First the status of the surfaces is recorded as unrestored, sealed, restored or crowned. After that a second code is used (Y). This code evaluates the visual changes in the enamel to evaluate the visual changes in the enamel to extensive cavitation. The description is given in Table 6.5.

Since enamel is thin in deciduous teeth as compared to permanent teeth, ICDAS cannot properly distinguish the lesion of outer and inner enamel of deciduous teeth.

The system has provided high sensitivity and specificity for proximal caries in in-vitro conditions;

Table 6.5: ICDAS scoring criteria

Score	Criteria
0	No or slight change in enamel translucency after 5 seconds air drying
1	First visual change in enamel (seen after prolonged air drying) or change in confines of pits and fissures
2	Distinct visual change in enamel
3	Localized enamel breakdown in opaque enamel (no signs of dentin involvement)
4	Underlying dark shadow from dentin
5	Distinct cavity with visible dentin
6	Extensive distinct cavity with visible dentin, involving more than half the surface

however, the sensitivity has been low for proximal caries in vivo. Other additional features need be added to improve sensitivity on these surfaces.

The system is being used for caries lesion activity assessment. The caries activity assessment is based on the knowledge of clinical appearance of the lesion coupled with tactile sensation when ball-ended WHO probe is moved across the tooth surface.

The system also reflects theoretical concepts regarding the caries process. Caries activity assessment and the ICDAS when used together can estimate the depth/severity of caries activity, which are all fundamental prerequisites for the diagnosis and management of the individual lesion (Table 6.6).

Nyvad's System

Nyvad's system is another option for activity assessment of caries lesions. According to this system, score can be attributed to all observed characteristics of the lesion, eventually classifying the lesion as inactive or active. If the lesion presents at least one feature compatible to an active lesion, the operator classify the lesion as active. The system uses plaque is as an indicator for caries lesions activity and standard probes to assess roughness (Table 6.7).

Nyvad index is also used to assess depth of lesion in primary teeth. The methodology used in Nyvad's system is modified to include uses of prophylaxis and WHO probe for inspection.

Table: 6.6: Caries lesion activity assessment used after evaluation with ICDAS

Criteria	Activity score
Visual appearance ICDAS score 1, 2 (brown lesions)	1
Visual appearance ICDAS score 1, 2 (white lesions)	3
Visual appearance ICDAS score 3, 4, 5, 6	4
Plaque stagnation area (along the gingiva around contact area, entrance of pits and fissures and cavities with irregular borders)	3
Non-plaque stagnation area (flat pit and fissures)	1
Surface texture rough or soft surface on gentle probing	4
Surface texture smooth or hard surface on gentle probing	2

Table 6.7: Nyvad's system

Score	Category	Criteria
0	Sound	Normal enamel translucency and texture (slight staining allowed)
1	Active caries (surface intact)	Enamel surface is whitish/yellowish; opaque with loss of luster; feels rough; covered with plaque generally. No clinically loss of tooth substance; lesion extending along the walls of lesion (fissures intact)
2	Active caries (discontinuity of surface)	Same criteria as in score 1. Localized surface defect in enamel only. No undermining of enamel
3	Active caries (cavity)	Enamel/dentin cavity easily detectable with naked eye; cavity surface leathery/soft on gentle probing. (may and may not pulpal involvement)
4	Inactive caries (intact surface)	Enamel surface white/brown/black. Enamel shiny and feels hard and smooth when the tip is moved gently across the surface. No clinically detectable loss of tooth substance. Intact fissure morphology.
5	Inactive caries (surface discontinuity)	Same criteria as in score 4. Localized surface defect in enamel only. No undermined enamel of softened floor detectable with explorer.
6	Inactive caries (cavity)	Enamel/dentin cavity easily visible with naked eye. Surface of the cavity appear shiny and feels hard on probing. No pulp involvement
7	Filling (sound surface)	
8	Filling and active caries	Caries lesion may be cavitated or non-cavitated
9	Filling and inactive caries	Caries lesions may be cavitated or non-cavitated

Diagnosis and Treatment Planning

Caries Risk Assessment Using Classification and Regression Trees (CART)

Classification and regression trees (CART) is being used to identify patients at high or low risk of caries. This is one method of determining, using decision tree technique to classify data. It provides a set of rules that can be applied to an unclassified dataset to predict important factors involving caries risk.

Sensitivity and specificity are statistical measures of the performance of the binary classification test. Sensitivity measures the proportion of actual positives which are correctly identified; whereas, specificity measures the proportion of negatives. For caries risk assessment, the following parameters for each patient were considered : age, number of decayed, missing and filled teeth (DMFT), level of cariogenic bacteria such as streptococcus mutans and lactobacilli, the flow rate and buffer capacity of saliva.

The Treatment Decision-making Process

The dentist should classify the teeth according to the severity scores using, for example, the ICDAS. Thereafter, the activity of lesions must be evaluated and a score assigned for each specific surface, classifying each surface as an active or inactive caries lesion. A decision-making tree based on this evaluation can help the dentist make decision (Flow chart 6.1).

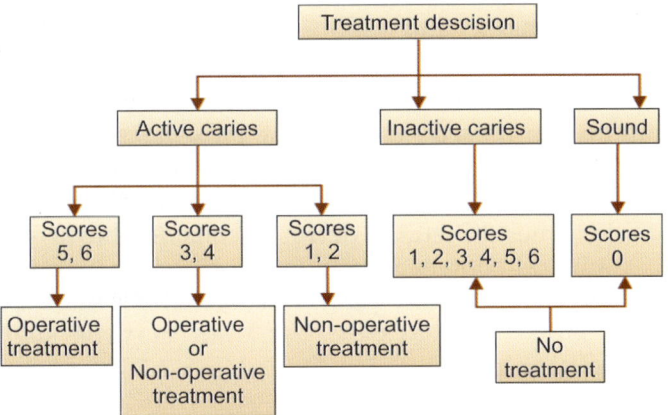

Fig. 6.6: Decision-making tree for dental caries lesions to be used after examination using ICDAS and lesions activity assessment

If a site is classified as sound (score 0) or with ICDAS scores 1 to 6 with inactive lesion, no treatment is necessary for caries management. Aesthetic or functional rehabilitation could be considered, but no treatment is necessary to arrest caries progress, because these lesions have already been arrested. When the surface is classified as active, non-cavitated caries lesions (ICDAS scores 1 or 2), non-surgical treatment is needed to avoid progression of the lesion to a more severe condition (cavitation).

If the tooth surface is classified as ICDAS score 5 or 6 and the lesion is active, usually surgical treatment is recommended in an attempt to reduce the progression of the caries lesion and provide conditions for the dentin-pulp reaction.

In active caries lesions classified as ICDAS score 3 or 4, either non-surgical or surgical treatment can be considered. A bitewing radiograph can aid the clinician in choosing between non-surgical and surgical approaches, because radiography will give better information about lesion depth and proximity to the pulp. In proximal surfaces, caries lesions not evident to visual inspection could be better detected using the adjunct bitewing radiographic method. If the lesion on the radiographic image is restricted to the enamel and is active, non-surgical management is the best choice. If the lesion reaches the middle third or more of the dentin, surgical treatment usually is the best option because most of these lesions are cavitated. On the other hand, if the radiographic image indicates an initial dentin caries lesion (the outer third of dentin), the dentist should check for the presence of cavitation to decide which non-surgical or surgical treatment is necessary. Here, temporary separation with orthodontic rubbers would be helpful. As an alternative for clinicians, Nyvad's system can be used instead of ICDAS. Here, the treatment decision is made in a similar way to that described for ICDAS.

3. Radiographic Methods

Radiographic examination has great value in the detection of those carious lesions which are not readily determined by clinical examination, especially the smooth surface caries on the proximal sides. The carious process leads to demineralization of the affected area of the tooth and that area appears radiolucent on the radiograph. Radiographs do have certain limitations; therefore, the combination of clinical examination along with the radiographic aid is considered mandatory for diagnosing caries.

Problems encountered with the radiographic method are:

- Overlapping of approximal contacts
- False diagnosis due to over-estimation of lesion depth which may appear to be increased due to change in angulation
- Occlusal lesions, many a times, become imperceptible because of solid buccal and lingual cusps.
- Radiolucency on radiograph cannot be judged whether that is because of caries or resorption or any other defect.

- It is a two-dimensional image of a three-dimensional object. Because of this, sometimes interpretation becomes difficult.
- A superficial demineralization on the buccal and lingual surfaces may be imaged on the radiograph as an approximal carious lesion.
- Fracture of one lingual cusp may appear as radiolucent approximal cavity.
- Tilt of maxillary lateral incisors appears as caries on the mesial side of the lateral incisors.
- Cervical burnout areas may mimic cervical caries.

Despite of these problems, radiographs are a boon to the profession and with the advent of newer techniques, many of these problems have been sorted out.

The following methods are used in routine:

A. Conventional Radiography

Conventionally, two types of techniques are usually employed. These include *intra-oral periapical radiography* and *bite-wing radiography* (Figs 6.7A and B). Others like occlusal radiographs (Fig. 6.7C), and panoramic radiographs are important but rarely employed in the detection of caries. Panoramic views are employed for having a broader view of the oral cavity. Moreover, the panoramic technique utilizes intensifying screen, which may hamper the finer details; whereas, the occlusal technique does not determine the angulation of a tooth in that particular arch.

Periapical radiographs are primarily useful for detecting changes around the roots and in between the teeth. The paralleling technique is superior to bisecting technique for detecting caries in both anterior and posterior teeth. Bitewing radiographs are important to detect incipient lesions at the contact points. With this technique, approximately eight teeth in one radiograph can be visualized as regard incipient carious lesions, cervical margins of the restoration, alveolar crest height, lamina dura as well as the size of the pulp chambers.

Radiographic Appearance of Caries

i. *Occlusal caries:* Radiographs are usually ineffective for the detection of occlusal caries until it reaches the dentin. Once in dentin, the classical radiographic change is a broad based thin radiolucent zone in the dentin with little or no change apparent in the enamel.

A further significant manifestation of advanced occlusal caries in dentin is a band of increased opacity between the carious lesion and the pulp chamber. The white band represents the calcification within the primary dentin, which will not be evident in buccal caries.

The extensive lesions are evident in the radiograph as a large hole or a cavity in the crown of the tooth.

Limitations of radiographic interpretation of occlusal caries are:

- Caries in enamel becomes more difficult to detect because of superimposition of adjacent enamel over the fissures.
- Lesions involving buccal grooves of molars are superimposed over the occlusal area and can simulate occlusal lesions.
- A thin radiolucency at the dentino-enamel junction in occlusal caries, many a times, considered as normal difference of radiolucency in enamel and dentin.
- Difficult to distinguish between occlusal caries and the internal resorption.

ii. *Interproximal caries:* Since the proximal surfaces of posterior teeth are often broad, the loss of small amount of mineral content (incipient lesions) becomes difficult to detect. A considerable loss of mineral content is mandatory before it becomes visible on a radiograph. The actual depth of the lesion is always deeper than may be seen radiographically.

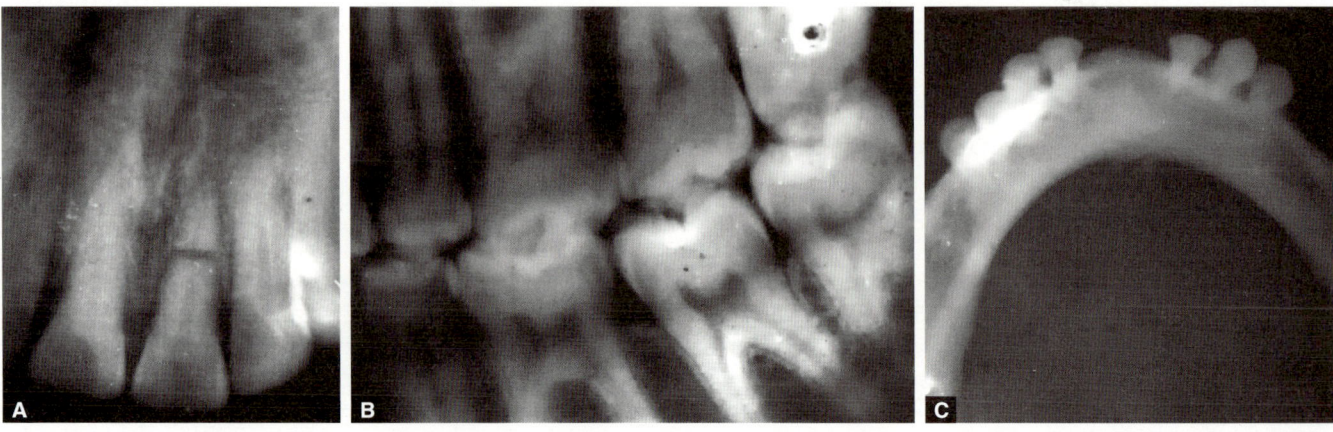

Figs 6.7A to C: **(A)** Intra-oral periapical radiograph; **(B)** Bite-wing radiograph; **(C)** Occlusal radiograph

With the utilization of fluorides and other preventive techniques, it is observed that the lesion develops slowly which may take more than a year before it becomes evident on the radiograph. The white chalky appearance is first evident on the outer surface of enamel between the contact point and the height of the free gingival margin. The caries susceptible zone is a 1.0 to 1.5 mm broad zone below the contact point, which may enlarge with the receding gingiva. Radiographically, a small radiolucent notch is evident below the contact area. Magnifying glasses can be used to evaluate these incipient lesions.

With the advancing lesion, the radiographic image is like a diffuse triangle with the base at the surface of the tooth. Once the lesion crosses the dentino-enamel junction and invades into the dentin, the lesion appears as another triangle with the base at dentino-enamel junction. Collectively, these may appear as two triangles with their bases facing towards the external surface. Involvement of the dental pulp by the carious process is usually difficult to predict from its radiographic appearance. Clinical examination is mandatory to confirm whether pulp is involved or not.

Posterior bitewing radiographs are preferably utilized to detect interproximal caries. Recurrent caries at the cervical margins is best observed in bitewing films, since the central ray is directed along the plane of the cervical areas. Bitewing radiographs are useful in monitoring and evaluating the progress or arrest of dental caries. Care should be taken to standardize the positioning, exposure time and the processing conditions. The use of ionizing radiations are never without hazards, so all efforts should be made to minimize radiation exposure. Radiation dose can be reduced by collimation of the X-ray beam, ensuring that the timer is functioning accurately and use of E and F-speed films, etc.

iii. *Root caries:* Root caries, also known as cemental caries or senile caries, involves cementum of exposed root surfaces. *Root caries is defined as the soft progressive lesion of the root surfaces usually having ill-defined saucer-like appearances.* These are usually observed within 2.0 mm area of cement-enamel junction. An exposed root surface is always at an increased risk of developing caries. Root caries has been classified into four grades of severity:

Grade I : Incipient
Grade II : Shallow, less than 0.5 mm depth with pigmentation
Grade III : Deep lesions, more than 0.5 mm depth
Grade IV : Pulpal involvement

Polishing and recontouring of the defect followed by fluoride application can be helpful in preventing the initial lesions. Diagnosis of root caries is not difficult, except in cases where the lesion is on interproximal surfaces adjacent to deep periodontal pockets. Since root caries progresses more rapidly than enamel caries, early diagnosis becomes mandatory, otherwise it may lead to pulpal involvement. Such teeth are even difficult to treat endodontically.

iv. *Secondary caries: Caries that occurs adjacent to the restorative material is known as secondary caries or recurrent caries.* It is established that secondary caries is the major cause of failure of restorations and is eight times more common than the primary lesions. Diagnosis of secondary caries is usually dependent on the clinical examination as the radiographs may not be helpful until the lesion is in advanced stage. There is no clinical parameter, which distinguish between active and inactive lesions. Other problems in diagnosis of secondary caries are:

- Lesions on the occlusal surface, between restoration and enamel, cannot be visualized until reached to an advanced stage. Discoloration of margins as an evidence for secondary caries may not a definite parameter as discoloration can be due to extrinsic stains or corrosion products also.
- Radiographs can diagnose the cervical portion of the interproximal lesions, which is a prime site for secondary caries, but careful comparison with the previous radiographs is a must before concluding. Similarly, radiolucency under composite restorations may be deceptive because the bonding agents are also radiolucent.
- It is often difficult to differentiate between secondary caries and caries which has been left during restorative procedures [residual caries].

Probing, by and large, should be avoided for diagnosis of secondary caries; however, gentle probing can be recommended. In the anterior part of the oral cavity, transillumination is preferred for the diagnosis of discolored dentin, especially under tooth-colored restorations.

B. Xeroradiography

In this technique the image is recorded on an aluminium plate coated with a layer of selenium particles. These selenium particles are given a uniform electrostatic charge and are stored in a unit called *'conditioner'*. When X-rays are passed on to the film, it causes selective discharge of the particles. This forms the latent image and is converted to a positive image by a process called *'development'* in the processor unit. The main characteristics of xero-radiographic technique are the ability to have both positive and negative prints together. When positive current is applied to the film, negative particles are attracted and when negative current is applied, positive particles are attracted.

Xero-radiography is twice as sensitive as conventional D-speed films. The phenomenon of *'Edge enhancement'* is possible with this technique. *Edge enhancement means differentiating areas of different densities especially at the margins or edges.*

Xero-radiography was considered to be superior, but recent studies have indicated that these are comparable to E-speed films of conventional radiography for diagnosing caries.

Disadvantages of this technique are:
- The electric charge over the film, many a times, causes discomfort to the patient since the humid environment of oral cavity acts as a medium for flow of current.
- Exposure time varies, as manufacturers do not indicate the exact thickness of the plate.
- The process of development can't be delayed and is to be completed within 15 minutes. Although xero-radiography technique seems to be promising, but features of edge enhancement, etc. were soon taken over by fast developing digital imaging systems.

C. Modified Radiographic Techniques

i. *Digital enhancement:* Computers are now widely used for diagnostic purposes. A digital image is an image formed and represented by a spatially distributed set of discrete sensors and pixels. When viewed from a distance, the image appears continuous, but closer inspection reveals individual pixels. Digital image is an image that is recorded with non-film receptors.

There are two types of non-film receptors for recording digital images.
- The digital image receptor (DIR) which collects the X-rays directly (Direct digital imaging)
- Video camera for forming digital images of a radiograph (Indirect digital imaging)

Digital image receptor works on a charged couple device (CCD), which is electronically connected to a computer. CCD is a semiconductor made up of metal oxides such as silicon that is coated with x-ray sensitive phosphorous. The CCD is sensitive both to x-rays and visible light. The intraoral DIR is placed in the oral cavity instead of the x-ray film. The image area is limited by the size of the CCD present in the digital image receptor. Once the image is captured by the CCD, (like an image of silver halide crystals in an X-ray film) it can be stored in the computer memory for image processing and can be displayed for viewing (Fig. 6.8).

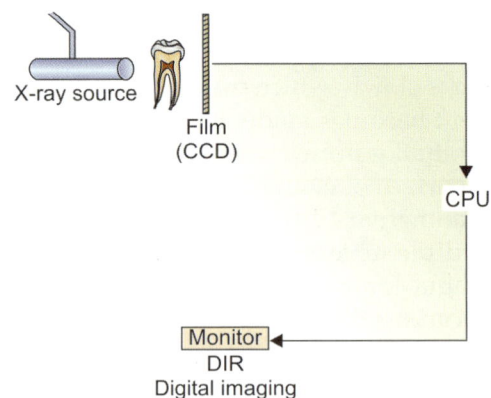

Fig. 6.8: Diagrammatic representation of digital imaging

The examples of digital radiography systems along with their image receptor size are:
- Radio-Visio-Graphy (RVG) (Trophy -Japan)   19 × 28 mm
- Flash Dent (Villa - Italy)   20 × 24 mm
- Sens-A-Ray (Regam - Sweden)   17 × 26 mm
- Vixa (Gendex - Italy)   18 × 24 mm

Advantages
- Darkroom is not required, instant image is viewed.
- The quality of image is consistent.
- Super resolution.
- Greater exposure latitude.
- Elimination of the hazards of film development.
- Radiation dose is decreased.
- Capability for tele-transmission.

Disadvantages
- The life expectancy of CCD is not fixed
- Patient's discomfort
- Temporary image retention
- Slower speed

Conventional film radiographs may provide insufficient density and contrast in the area under suspicion for a carious lesion. Contrast can be enhanced by digital mode up to 70%. It has also been observed that digital method is 50% more sensitive in detecting occlusal caries as compared to conventional films.

ii. *Computer image analysis:* The observer variations in the interpretation of radiographs are well known. The computers made it possible to use automated procedures which may overcome the shortcomings of human eye. Softwares have been developed for automated interpretation of digital radiographs in order to standardize image assessment. These programs are based on the "expert system" which contains facts about the pathologic conditions. The clinician enters the patient's data and the programme compares the patient's data with the basic knowledge of the pathology. This programme displays the possible diagnosis, and even inform the possibilities of other ailments. The system can suggest the need for additional tests to improve the reliability of the diagnostic outcome.

Automated analysis provides sensitive and objective observations, which may also permit the detection of small lesions that otherwise, may not be visible to naked eyes. Different features of teeth in intraoral as well as extraoral radiography can be recognized. Applications have been developed to support the interpretation of angular periodontal bone defects and to quantify carious lesions.

Advantages
- Automated analysis may provide sensitive and objective observation of smaller lesions which otherwise are not perceptible to naked eye.
- It is possible to monitor the lesion.
- Quantification of small lesions is possible.

Disadvantages
- There is always a need for standardization of exposure geometry.
- Sensitivity is higher but specificity is lesser.
- Time consuming and less economical.

iii. *Subtraction radiography:* Subtraction radiography is a technique by which structured noise is reduced in order to increase the detectability of changes in the radiographic pattern. The structured noises are the images, which are not of diagnostic value and interfere in routine interpretation of radiographs.

Subtraction images can be obtained from photographic and electronic methods. The disadvantages of these methods such as; inability to produce correct projection geometry and improper density and contrast led to use of digital substraction radiography.

Digitization is achieved by taking a picture of the radiograph using high quality video camera. This is fed to a computer-imaging device, termed as *digitizer*. Two standardized radiographs produced with identical exposure geometry are used. The first one is the '*Reference Image*' and the subsequent images are for comparison. The reference image is displayed on the screen. Then the subsequent images are superimposed

The difference between the original and the subsequent images will show as dark bright areas, which can be interpreted readily. One should remember that digitization does not increase the information available in the original radiograph. Only it turns the image into a form, which can be read by the computer.

It is established that approximal carious lesions are clearly visible by digital subtraction method. Subtraction radiography is also considered superior to conventional film radiography for detecting recurrent caries. It is also useful in detecting the progress of re-mineralization and de-mineralization patterns of dentinal caries.

The assessment of alveolar bone height in determining the progression of periodontal disease has been one of the major uses of subtraction digital radiography. It is demonstrated that digital subtraction radiography is 90% accurate in detecting as little as 5% mineral loss of bone; whereas 30–60% of the mineral content of the bone has to be lost before a radiographic lesion could be seen on a conventional radiograph. The minimal thickness of bone that can be detected under optimal conditions has been found to be 0.12 mm. For all these observations, correct projection geometry is mandatory.

iv. *CBCT:* The application of cone beam computed tomography CBCT in dental caries diagnosis has not been widely studied. The investigation to apply in caries diagnosis stems from its numerous advantages when compared to all current forms of x-ray imaging. CBCT utilizes the least amount of radiation to obtain a diagnostic image.

4. Electric Resistance (Electrical Conductance and Impedance)

It is established that sound tooth enamel is a good electrical insulator due to its high inorganic content. Enamel demineralization results in increased porosity of enamel. Saliva fills these pores and forms conductive pathways for electric current. The electric conductivity is directly proportional to the amount of demineralization. Electric resistance is measuring the electrical conductivity through these pores.

Since saliva is a better electrical conductor than enamel tissue, the conductivity increases with increase of demineralization. Electrical resistance is also measured during controlled drying. By drying the tooth surface, the resistance is determined by the tooth structure, avoiding electrical conductance by saliva. The higher values indicate well-mineralized tissue, whereas low values indicate demineralized tissue. The electrical conductivity of a tooth changes with demineralization even when the surface remains macroscopically intact.

The electrical impedance values between each portion of tooth and mucous membrane is depicted in Fig. 6.9.

Operative Dentistry

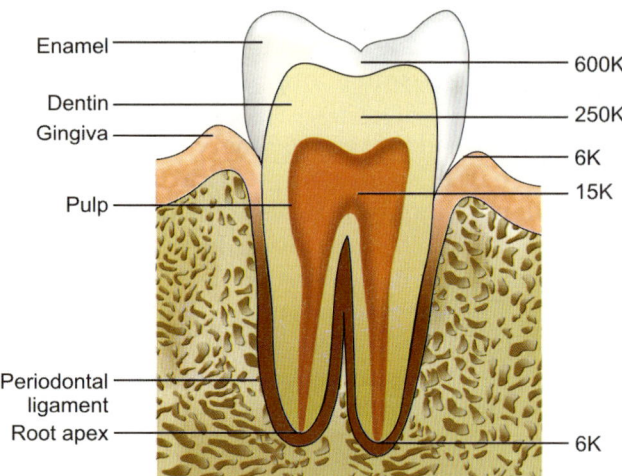

Fig. 6.9: Electrical impedance values between each portion of the tooth and the oral mucosa

Advantages
- Very effective in detecting early pit and fissure caries.
- It can monitor the progress of caries during caries control programme.

Disadvantages
- It can only recognize demineralization and not caries specifically. The hypomineralization areas, may be of developmental origin or carious origin, will give similar type of readings.
- Presence of enamel cracks may lead to false positive diagnosis.
- A sharp metal explorer is utilized which is pressed into the fissure causing traumatic defects.
- Separate measurements are required for different sites making full mouth examination quite time consuming.

Devices using electrical conductance property are:
- AC ohmmeter
- Caries meter- L
- Vanguard electronic caries detector
- Electronic caries monitor
- Electrical impedance tomography
- Electrochemical impedance spectroscopy

i. *AC ohmmeter:* AC ohmmeter, though not in use these days, utilizes 500 Hz alternating current of frequency, to detect variation in electrical resistance at different areas of tooth. A dental explorer with 0.1 mm tip is placed over the tooth site and another metal sheet is kept in contact with cheeks, contralateral to the tooth to be measured.

ii. *Caries meter-L:* The caries meter-L, manufactured by two companies, G-C International Corp., Belgium and Onuki Dental Co. Ltd., Japan is a painless and safe modality for evaluating changes in mineral contents (Fig. 6.10). It works on the principle of electrical conductivity. Sine waves of 400 Hz are utilized to measure currents for the caries meter. The electrical impedance is indicated by four colored lights: Green, yellow, orange and red. The inference can be drawn by change in color, subsequently the treatment decision (Table 6.8).

iii. *Vanguard electronic caries detector:* The Vanguard electronic caries detector, manufactured by Massachusetts manufacturing corporation, USA, overcame the inconsistency in the flow of air. The probe tip is placed centrally in the fissure and the superficial saliva is removed while taking the reading (in caries meter-L, the fissures are moistened with saliva). The measured conductance is converted to ordinal scale from 0 to 9. The readings are inversely related to the resistance and indicate increasing degrees of demineralization.

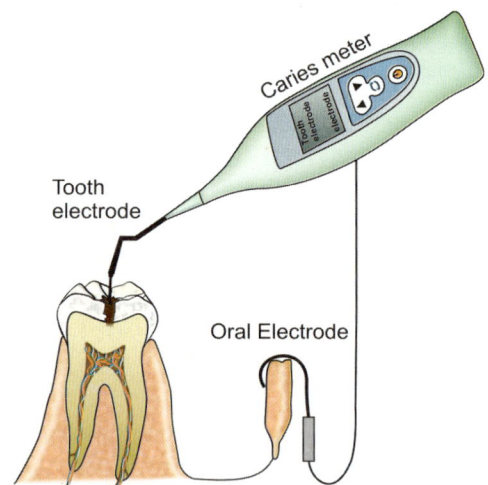

Fig. 6.10: Electronic caries detector

Table 6.8: Colors, inference, impedance values and treatment options			
Color	Impedance values	Inference	Treatment options
Green	600 kΩ	Healthy tooth (no caries)	No treatment required
Yellow	Between 250 and 600 kΩ	Enamel caries	Observe for sometime: Use preventive methods
Orange	Between 15 and 250 kΩ	Caries extending into dentin	Remove caries and restore
Red	Below 15 kΩ	Caries invading tooth pulp	Root canal treatment

Diagnosis and Treatment Planning

iv. Electronic caries monitor (ECM): Electronic caries monitor employs a single fixed frequency (21 Hz, 23 Hz and 25 Hz) alternating current measuring the electric conductivity of tooth.

The initial design is close to the Vanguard caries detector. The electrical probe is placed onto the tooth site and the reference electrode on the lips. The ECM readings can be seen on a screen in front of the device, which may vary in a range of about –1.00 to 13.00 (precisely –0.70 to 13.20), representing increasing electrical conductance. A higher reading means more decay (Table 6.9).

Table 6.9: Clinical interpretation of ECM values

Range	Clinical interpretation
–1.0 to 1.0	Sound enamel
1.01 to 3.00	Incipient caries
3.01 to 6.00	Enamel caries (up to DEJ)
6.01 to 8.00	Dentinal caries
8.01 to 13.00	Deep dentinal caries

The performance of ECM has been reported to be moderate; could not be correlated with histological lesion depth and also the reproducibility was insufficient. Three modified models ECM II, III and IV have also been introduced. These types vary in their display of results and their options for measurement techniques. No obvious improvement could be observed with these newer models.

v. Electrical impedance tomography: Electrical impedance tomography (EIT) is based on the principle of electrical impedance. Unlike caries meter, which uses fixed frequency, EIT uses a range of frequencies and provide information on capacitance and impedance.

vi. Alternating current impedance spectroscopy (CarieScan): The alternating current impedance spectroscopy is used to quantify caries at an early stage. This device involves passing of an insensitive level of electrical current through the tooth to identify the presence and location of the decay. The response waves are measured and the impedance is calculated by a transfer function relationship of the applied voltage and the acquired current. The CarieScan as claimed is not affected by optical factors such as staining or discoloration of the tooth; it provides a qualitative value based on the disease state rather than the optical properties of the tooth. The device is indicated for the detection, diagnosis, and monitoring of primary dental caries on occlusal and accessible smooth surfaces, which are not clearly visible to the human eye. It cannot be used to assess secondary caries, the integrity of a restoration, root caries, and the depth of an excavation.

5. Optical Detection

A. Optical Caries Monitor

Optical caries monitor is a non-destructive method to quantify light scattering in bulk dental enamel and early carious lesions. Light scattering by enamel has been shown to be caused mainly by the crystals in relation to their immediate environment. Light incident under 45° in a collimated beam enters the sample and scattered forwards, sidewards and backwards. Light emerging from the illuminated spot is collected by the fiberoptic head. When scattering is weak, collected flux is low whereas when scattering is strong (carious enamel), collected flux is high.

B. Fibre Optic Transillumination (FOTI)

Fibre optic transillumination (FOTI) works under the principle that since a carious lesion has a lowered index of light transmission, an area of caries appears as a darkened shadow that follows the spread of decay through the dentin. Fibre Optic Trans Illumination was initially designed for the detection of proximal caries.

Fiberoptic consists of a halogen lamp and a rheostat to produce a light of variable intensity. The 150-watt lamp generates a maximum light intensity of 4000 lx at the end of 2.0 mm diameter cable. Two attachments are used: a plane mouth mirror mounted on a steel cuff and a fiberoptic probe of 0.5 mm diameter so that it can be placed in the embrasure region. It produces a narrow beam of light for transillumination. The rheostat is set to give a light of maximum intensity. For examination, the tip of the probe is placed in the embrasure immediately beneath the contact point of the proximal surface to be examined either on the buccal or lingual surface depending on the tooth. The marginal ridge is viewed from the occlusal surface.

A shadow extending to the dentino-enamel junction beneath the marginal ridge may be evident if there is a break in the integrity of the enamel of marginal ridge.

Advantages
- No hazards of radiations.
- Simple and comfortable for the patients.
- Lesions, which cannot be diagnosed radiographically, can be diagnosed by this method.
- Not time consuming.

Disadvantages
- Permanent records are difficult to maintain as can be kept in radiographs.
- It is subjected to intra and inter observer variations.
- Difficult to locate the probe in certain areas.

C. Digital Imaging Fiberoptic Transillumination (DIFOTI)

Digital imaging fiberoptic transillumination was developed in an attempt to reduce the perceived shortcomings of FOTI by combining FOTI and a digital CCD camera.

Images captured by the camera are forwarded for computer analysis. The use of the CCD allows instantaneous images, projected and can be compared for clinical changes between several images of the same tooth over time. In addition, illumination and other conditions that may affect the quality of the image can be more easily controlled. DIFOTI has been approved by the FDA for the detection of incipient, frank and recurrent caries. It instantly creates high resolution digital images. It enables dentists to confirm the presence of decay that can't be seen radiographically, visually or through use of an explorer. Any operator can take DIFOTI image in three seconds or take a full mouth set of images in a matter of minutes.

D. Ultraviolet Illumination

Ultraviolet (UV) light has been used to increase the optical contrast between the carious region and the surrounding sound tissue. The natural fluorescence of tooth enamel, as seen under UV light illumination is decreased in areas of less mineral content such as in carious lesions, artificial demineralization or developmental defects. The carious lesion appears as a dark spot against a fluorescent background. The method is still not been developed into a quantitative method.

Advantages
More sensitive than the visual-tactile method.

Disadvantages
- The carious lesion and the other defect with demineralization appear same.

E. Transillumination with Near Infrared Light

Transillumination of dental enamel with near-infrared light is a promising non-ionizing imaging method for detection of early caries lesion. Dental enamel is highly transparent in near infrared at 1300 nm. Increased mineral loss leads to increased scattering and absorption. Caries thus appear as dark regions because less light reaches the detector.

F. Laser Auto Fluorescence (LAF)

The visible light has been used as the light source for the detection of smooth surface and fissure caries at an early stage. The tooth is illuminated with a broad beam of blue green light of 488 nm wavelengths from an argon ion laser and the fluorescence observed in the 540 nm range. This fluorescence of enamel occurring in the yellow region (540 nm) is observed through a yellow high pass filter to exclude the tooth scattered blue light. Demineralized areas appear dark in this region. Healthy tooth fluoresces differently from that of carious tissue impregnated with fluorescent dyes. Demineralized tissues absorb dyes like Fluorol TGA, Sodium fluorescein etc and fluoresce strongly. This is referred to as *dye enhanced laser fluorescence*.

Recently, a quantified version of laser fluorescence has been developed. In this technique a micro camera is used to capture the real image. A computer screen displays the real images of the teeth under examination.

Advantages
- Convenient and a relatively fast method.
- Carious lesions can be detected and their mineral loss measured. Natural lesions with a diameter of less than 1.0 mm and a depth of 5–10 mm have been detected and measured with this technique.
- Preventive measures can be evaluated.
- It is suitable for quantifying mineral loss around different restorations.

G. Quantitative Laser Fluorescence (QLF)

The basic fundamental for the application of light induced fluorescence in detecting carious lesions and quantifying mineral loss are based on this concept. QLF caries detection system relies on the fluorescence signal observed when teeth are exposed to blue light (λ- 488 to 514 nm). This causes sound tooth structure to fluoresce. Carious tooth tissue may also fluoresce, but the disruption of the regular structure of the tooth at this point results in profound scattering and no or little fluorescence is detected. Consequently, sound tooth structure fluoresces at $\lambda > 520$ nm, whereas carious tooth tissue appears dark.

Earlier, Argon ion laser emitting blue green light (λ–488 nm) was used. This source produces diffuse monochromatic light (Light of a characteristic wavelength) and when a tooth is exposed to this light source, fluorescence of the enamel occurring in the yellow wavelength is observed (540 nm) through a yellow high pass filter to exclude tooth scattered blue green light. Demineralized areas appear as dark spots.

A portable variant of this system was produced, the QLF^{TM} (Fig. 6.11). The system includes measurement probe, control unit and a computer fitted with a frame grabber.

H. DIAGNOdent Caries Detector

This is a commercial development of laser fluorescence and a variant of the QLF system (Fig. 6.12).

The control unit consists of an illumination device with imaging electronics. The light source is a special arc lamp based on xenon technology. The light from this lamp is filtered using a blue transmitting filter (520 nm). A liquid light guide then transports the blue light to the concerned tooth. A dental mirror provides uniform illumination of the area to be recorded. The recording of fluorescence image is carried out using a yellow transmitting filter (540 nm) positioned in front of a color CCD sensor. The image is digitized by a frame grabber (which converts the analog signals to digital signals) and is available for quantitative analysis with a customized QLF software.

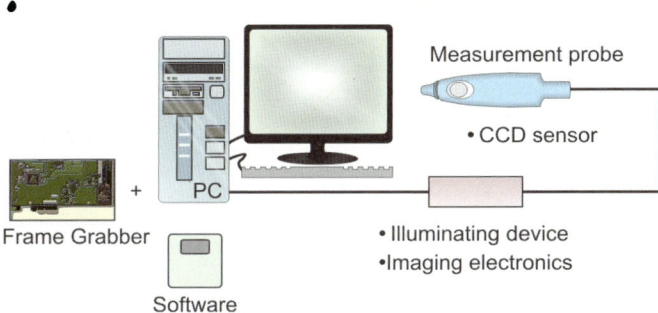

Fig. 6.11: Schematic set-up of the QLF system

Disadvantages

- Only discerns enamel demineralization and can't differentiate between decay, hypoplasia or unusual anatomic features.
- Potential for operator bias as it relies upon a subjective analysis of a stored tooth image.
- Inability to detect or monitor interproximal lesions.
- Limited to measurement of enamel lesions.

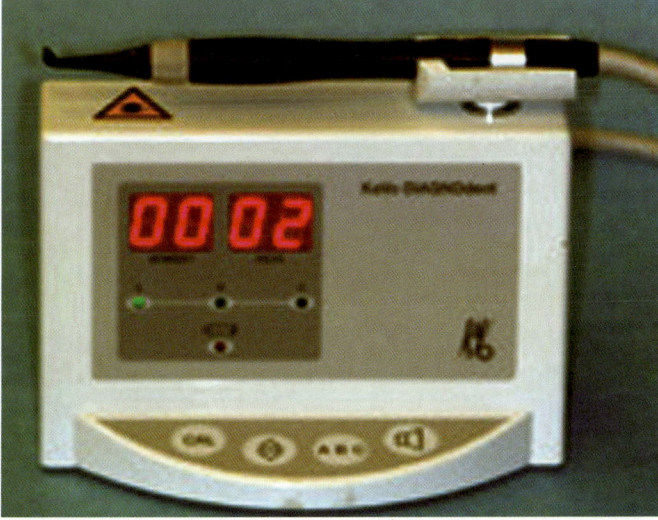

Fig. 6.12: DIAGNOdent

QLF is best suited for longitudinal diagnosis of early lesions of the enamel on accessible smooth surfaces. As the image of the lesion can be stored on computer, it can be reanalyzed and compared with newly acquired images to access the status of a lesion (progression or regression).

Principle of Working

This device makes use of laser autofluorescence technology, but instead of using blue light it uses red light, of wavelength 655 nm, output <1 mW. This red laser light identifies caries as having an increased fluorescence over sound tooth; whereas, blue light as

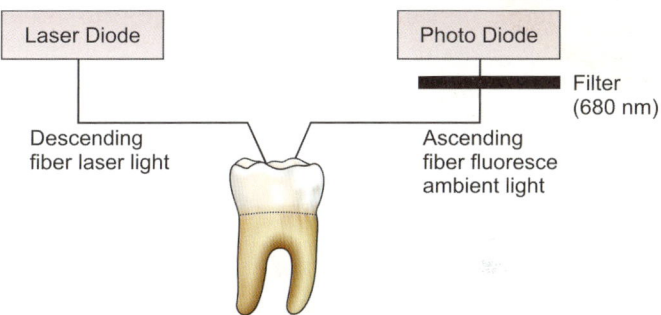

Fig. 6.13: DIAGNOdent working principle

Advantages

- 90% success to diagnose pit and fissure caries.
- Sensitivity (0.92) is more than electronic caries monitor.
- High reproducibility and reliability.
- Easy and quick to use.
- Readily transportable
- Non-invasive and painless.
- Doesn't suffer from operator bias.
- Safe, no x-ray exposure.
- Interactivity engages patient in examination process.
- Promotes minimally invasive treatment.

Disadvantages

- False results with presence of plaque and debris.
- Can't distinguish between hypomineralized and carious structure.
- Readings do not relate to the amount of dentinal decay.
- Can't be used for recurrent caries
- Scientific evidence showing a direct correlation between the numeric diagnodent reading and the severity of disease is lacking.
- When compared with QLF device, QLF rather than merely supplying the arbitrary value characteristic of DIAGNOdent supplies information on the fluorescence loss.

used in QLF system highlights caries as a reduced fluorescence compared to sound tooth (Fig. 6.13). Source of light is a diode laser that emits light at 655 nm wavelength from a fiber optic bundle directed onto the occlusal surface of a tooth. Light is transported to the angulated tip within a central fiber. Around the central fiber, additional fibers are concentrically arranged to collect fluorescent light from dental hard tissues. The reflected and ambient lights are eliminated by a filter.

A photodiode measures the amount of fluorescence light passing through the filter. This signal is finally processed and presented on display as an integer of 0–99 with an audible beep.

In general, values between 5 and 25 indicate initial lesions in enamel and values greater than this indicate early dentinal caries. Advanced dentinal caries yields values greater than 35. At a diagnodent value of about 30, an operative intervention should be considered.

l. Infra-red Fluorescence

In this technique, the tooth is exposed to light (irradiation) with a wavelength of between 700 and 15,000 nm. Barrier filters are used to observe any resulting flouorescence. It has been established that the technique would be able to discriminate between sound and carious enamel and dentin. Further studies are required to determine if the fluorescence signal from exposure to infra-red irradiation is greater than that from other wavelengths. Additionally, there can be potentially damaging effects on the dental pulp due to heating effects from absorption of infra-red irradiation, given the increased penetration and decreased scattering of the longer wavelength.

Specific coherent source of such irradiation have been relatively difficult to acquire, and detection involves the use of infra-red sensitive detectors as charge coupled devices (CCDs) or film.

6. Endoscope/Videoscope

Endoscopic technique is based on observing the fluorescence that occurs when tooth is illuminated with blue light in the wavelength range of 400-500 nm. Difference is seen in the fluorescence of sound enamel and carious enamel. When this fluoresced tooth is viewed through a specific broadband gelatine filter, white spot lesions appear darker than enamel.

Similarly a white light source can be connected to an endoscope by a fiberoptic cable so that the teeth can be viewed without a filter. This technique is referred to as *white light endoscopy*.

It has been established that this technique allows visualization of small carious lesions in the enamel that are difficult to detect with the naked eye. The clinical detection of small carious lesions would greatly facilitate the preventive management modalities.

Additionally, a camera can be used to store the image. The integration of the camera with the endoscope is called a *videoscope*. A miniature color video camera is mounted in a custom-made metal mirror holder. This is designed in such a way that the image of the surface of enamel can be viewed directly over a television screen. The video-tapes are viewed by expert independent examiners who had also examined the teeth visually and by conventional methods.

Advantages
• Magnified image provides better evaluation. • Clinically feasible.

Disadvantages
• Requires meticulous drying and isolation. • Time consuming. • Costly.

7. Dye Penetration Method

Dyes have a widespread use in dentistry (Fig. 6.14). Dyes can visualize a subject from its routine background or if several objects have a similar appearance, coloring by a dye may discriminate between them and allow identification. The observation of the coloring can be qualitative or quantitative. For a qualitative assessment, it is sufficient to observe for color or differentiate colored objects from the noncolored ones. For a quantitative assessment, the intensity of color is to be determined. The total area, which is colored, can be compared with

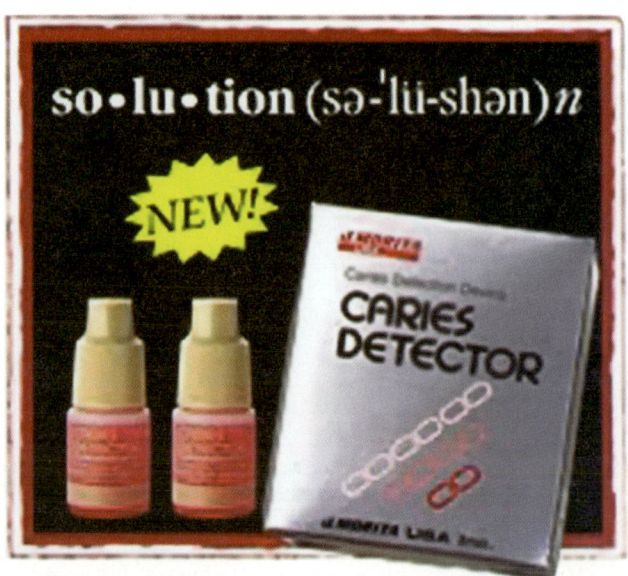

Fig. 6.14: Caries detecting dyes

the uncolored areas. The intensity of color can be determined by absorption or fluorescence. Absorption can be measured by quantitating the decrease of light intensity at a particular wavelength and fluorescence can be measured by quantitating the increase of light intensity at a particular wavelength.

In caries diagnosis, qualitative examination is sufficient; observation of colored dye signifies presence of caries. Dyes should fulfil the following criteria before being recommended for clinical use.
- Should be absolutely safe for intra oral use.
- Should be specific and stain only the tissues it is intended to stain.
- Should be easily removed and not lead to permanent staining.

A. Dyes for Detection of Carious Enamel

Various dyes have been tried to detect carious enamel, each having some advantages and disadvantages.

'*Procion*' dyes stain enamel lesions but the staining becomes irreversible because the dye reacts with nitrogen and hydroxyl groups of enamel and acts as a fixative.

'*Calcein*' dye makes a complex with calcium and remains bound to the lesion. 'Fluorescent dye' like Zyglo ZL-22 has been used in-vitro, which is not suitable for use in-vivo. The dye is made visible by ultraviolet illumination.

'*Brilliant blue*' has also been used to enhance the diagnostic quality of fiberoptic transillumination.

Use of dyes for diagnosing enamel lesions cannot be used clinically as yet. If possible it will allow lesions to be visualized at an early stage and thus allow remineralization procedures to be carried out early in the treatment plan.

B. Dyes for Detection of Carious Dentin

Histopathologically, carious dentin is divided into two layers - outer layer of decalcification, which is soft and cannot be remineralized and the inner decalcified layer, which is hard and can be remineralized. Dyes have been tried to differentiate between these two zones of dentin caries. *0.5% Basic Fuchsin in propylene glycol* has proved to be successful for the purpose.

Basic fuchsin dye was considered to be carcinogenic; therefore it has been replaced by *acid red and methylene blue*. Methylene blue is also slightly toxic so acid red is preferred.

Quantification is not necessary because the dye is only used to identify carious dentin.

Modified Dye Penetration Method

'The Iodine penetration method' for measuring enamel porosity of the incipient carious lesions is being used. Potassium iodide is applied for a specific period of time to a well-defined area of the enamel and thereafter the excess is removed. The iodine, which remains in the micropores, is estimated and that indicates the permeability of enamel. Applying this method for caries diagnosis remains a complicated procedure, because for each type of acid attack, a separate calibration under the same condition is needed.

8. Recent Advances/Newer Techniques

A. Carbon Dioxide Laser

Radiation of wavelength 10.6 µm - the most commonly used for CO_2 lasers, is strongly absorbed by water to the extent that it can be vapourized instantaneously. The fact that most biological tissues contain large quantities of water makes them vulnerable to destruction by irradiation from a laser beam of such a wavelength. The water in tissue is vapourized leaving a residue of carbon based material.

Philosophy underlying application of carbon dioxide lasers as a diagnostic tool is based on assumption that subsurface layer of early carious lesion has more organic content when compared with adjacent sound enamel. Photo-vaporization by a CO_2 laser of this organic material in the incipient carious lesion will leave a carbonized residue, which will appear black.

At low power levels and short interaction times, the inorganic substance of sound enamel with a minimum water content will be much less affected by CO_2 laser beam.

B. Terahertz Imaging

This method of imaging uses waves with terahertz frequency ($=10^{12}$ Hz or a wavelength of approximately 30 µm). This wave-form is short enough to provide reasonable resolution but long enough to prevent serious loss of signal due to scattering (Fig. 6.15).

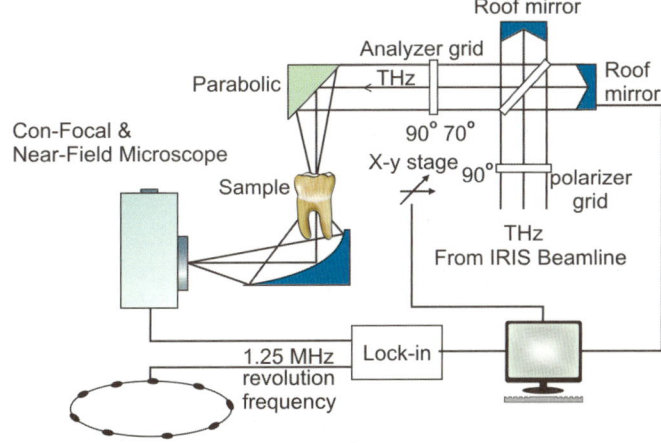

Fig. 6.15: Schematic diagram of the THz scanning

Advantages
• Relative transparency of human tissue to terahertz rays. • Low powers used for imaging (~ 1 μW). • Use of non-ionizing radiation. • No alteration of electrical charge to the tissues examined. • Adverse thermal effects are unlikely • Low signal-to-noise ratio for facilitates extremely clear imaging.

Disadvantages
• The complexity of the laser source • Precise manipulation mandatory • Care is required in image interpretation, since terahertz waves are strongly absorbed by water, a potential complication in the oral cavity. • High cost

For an image to be obtained by terahertz irradiation, the object is placed in the path of the terahertz beam. Alternatively, the terahertz beam can be scanned over the surface of an object. It is also possible to record terahertz images using a CCD detector. Dental applications for this technique have been limited but promising. Longitudinal sections through three teeth have demonstrated increased terahertz absorption by early occlusal caries and an apparent ability to discriminate dental caries from idiopathic enamel hypo-mineralization. Work is in progress to image intact teeth with early carious lesions.

C. Multi-photon Imaging

Infra-red light (λ = 850 nm) has been used for multiphoton imaging of teeth. In conventional fluorescence imaging (QLF), a single 'blue' photon is used to excite a fluorescent compound in the tooth. In the multiphoton technique, two infra-red photons (with half the energy of the blue photon) are absorbed simultaneously. Ultra-short pulses (100 fs) of 850 nm laser light are generated at 200 MHz. The average beam power is in the multiwatt range. By scanning a focused beam, one can record, from the focal plane, the fluorescence resulting from two-photon excitation. If the focal plane is then changed, through the enamel toward the dentin, a series of optical sections can be created. With this technique, sound tooth tissue fluoresces strongly, whereas carious tooth tissue fluoresces to a much lesser extent. In practice, by using motors with micron accuracy, one can move the plane of focus through the tissue and record the sectional images from the tooth to form a 3-D image. Caries will appear as a dark form within a brightly fluorescing tooth. To highlight the diseased tissue, the image may be displayed in its negative form so that caries appears bright within a dark tooth.

Multi-photon imaging is able to collect information from carious lesions up to 500 microns in depth. Currently, the technique has been performed only on extracted teeth and the large and complex laser equipment required to produce such an image will require many years to develop into a clinically usable form.

Advantages
• Provides 3-D image. • A non-invasive method. • Low risk of phototoxicity to the pulp due to low average speed of laser power used. • Enhanced depth of penetration due to longer incident wavelength used. • Possibility of quantifiable measurement of mineral loss, as function of fluorescence loss, from a carious lesion in three dimensions.

D. Optical Coherence Tomography (OCT)

This is an imaging technique that is capable of providing two-dimensional or three-dimensional images of subsurface tissue. The differences in scattering or polarization between sound and carious enamel can be exploited. Laser light of wavelength such as 840 to 1310 nm is used. It passes into tissue and the emerging light is detected in relation to its phase, which is a measure of the distance that it has travelled.

The reflectivity of the tooth tissue decreases with demineralization. The percentage change in reflectivity of the tissue can be quantified as a measure of the change in mineral status of the tissue following demineralization.

OCT systems use super luminescent diodes as a light source.

The changes in signal are related to the degree of scattering and possibly the degree of mineralization. OCT has also been used to assess the restoration-tooth interface. This could have implications for the non-invasive diagnosis of secondary caries. As with all optical methods, it is likely that uptake of stain will confound the technique.

E. Infrared Thermography

Thermal radiation energy travels in the form of waves. It is possible to measure changes in thermal energy when fluid is lost from a lesion by evaporation. The thermal energy emitted by sound tooth structure is compared with that emitted by carious tooth structure. It is a method of determining lesion activity rather than a method of determining the presence or absence of a lesion. The method described by Kaneko *et al.* (1999) uses indium/antimony thermal sensors, which can detect temperature changes in the order of 0.025°C. With a constant flow of air over the surface of the tooth, the change in temperature of the lesion is compared with that of the surrounding sound tooth structure. The source-to-sensor distance is 20 cm, and the time taken to capture the data for a lesion is up to 2 min.

F. LED Technology (Midwest Caries I.D)

The midwest caries I.D. uses infrared and red light emitting diodes (LEDs) and a fiber optic to distribute light to the observed area present at the probe tip. A second fiber optic collects light from the observed area to a photo detector that measures returned collected light. This photo detector then transmits the signal to a microprocessor that compares signal levels with defined parameters. When the result is positive, the processor deactivates the third green LED and pulses at a higher intensity than the red LED. When the detection is negative (i.e. healthy tooth area), the green LED is dominant resulting in a green illumination when healthy structure is detected and red illumination when caries are detected. A buzzer also beeps with different frequencies to indicate the intensity of demineralization detected. Midwest Caries I.D. cannot be used on composites or amalgams but can be used to check the marginal ridges of occlusal amalgams. If the probe is tipped at too much of an angle when checking for approximal caries, total surface light reflection can occur giving a false positive. Opaque artifacts (plaque, calculus, and organic plug) can cause false positives.

G. Alternating Current Impedence Spectroscopy (CarieScan)

This device is based on the technology of alternating current impedance spectroscopy and involves the passing of an insensitive level of electrical current through the tooth to identify the presence and location of the decay. The frequency domain is based on a sinusoidal signal applied to a sample at known amplitude and frequency. The response wave form is then measured and the impedance calculated by a transfer function relationship of the applied voltage perturbation and acquired response current. CarieScan is not affected by optical factors such as staining or discoloration of the tooth; it provides a qualitative value based on the disease state rather than the optical properties of the tooth. The device is indicated for the detection, diagnosis, and monitoring of primary coronal dental caries (occlusal and accessible smooth surfaces), which are not clearly visible to the human eye. It cannot be used to assess secondary caries, the integrity of a restoration, dental root caries, and the depth of an excavation within a cavity preparation. For assessment of caries, while tufted sensor brush contacts the tooth surface being examined, a soft tissue contact, which is a disposable metal clip that is placed over the lip in the corner of the patient's mouth, connects to the CarieScan via a soft tissue cable to complete the circuit. During measurement, a green color display indicates sound tooth tissue, while a red color indicates deep caries requiring operative treatment and a yellow color associated with a range of numerical figures from 1 to 99 depicts varying severity of caries, which may require only preventive care.

H. Frequency-domain Infrared Photothermal Radiometry and Modulated luminescence

It is a dual probe technique which combines the advantages of PTR (Photo thermal radiometry) and LUM (modulated luminescence). The combined technique of PTR and LUM outputs four signal channels simultaneously: amplitudes and phases of photothermal and luminescence waves generated in response to harmonic laser source excitation.

PTR has depth profilometric ability: it can penetrate and yield information about an opaque or highly scattering medium beyond the range of optical imaging. The laser-intensity modulation-frequency dependence of the penetration depth of thermal waves make it possible to perform depth profiling of materials. Thus, the PTR signal consists of both surface and subsurface responses of dental tissue and can distinguish between caries, stains and white spots.

The fluorescence technique (LUM) monitors radiative emission variation between optically excited healthy and carious fluorophores.

Advantages

- It is a depth profilometric technique while other photonic based technologies are not.
- It is sensitive to changes in both optical and thermal properties of the sample
- It has the highest signal dynamic range in detecting very early demineralization
- It is a diagnostic tool which combines both specificity and sensitivity
- It is reliable and non-invasive.

I. Magnetic Resonance Imaging

This technique uses a moderated magnetic field in the same way as MRI, as developed from NMR (Nuclear Magnetic Resonance). In the laboratory, the technique has been found to be capable of producing highly accurate three-dimensional reconstructions of teeth and lesions of caries as confirmed by histological investigations. This technology is however, not available for clinical application.

j. Ultrasonic Imaging

Ultrasonic imaging was introduced for detecting early carious lesions in smooth surfaces. The demineralization of natural enamel is assessed by ultrasound pulse echo technique. It is observed that there is a definite correlation between the mineral content of the body of the lesion and the relative echo amplitude changes.

The ultrasonic probe is used which sends longitudinal waves to the surface of the tooth and also serves the function of receiving the waves. Initial white spot lesions, which extend only upto enamel, produce no or weak surface echoes. The sites with visible cavitation produce echoes with substantially higher amplitude. The method is a potential alternative to radiographic diagnosis of caries on the approximal surfaces. It is also more sensitive than visual-tactile method; however, it is not a quantitative method.

The benefits of caries diagnosis are further reinforced by understanding the following facts:

- Combination of more than one diagnostic tool is recommended for diagnosis purposes.
- Each diagnostic tool has some limitations at different level of severity. Optimizing the conditions used in the clinical situation would help minimize the limitation.
- Diagnosis of caries activity is more important than caries severity.
- Diagnosis of presence/absence of caries is part of the overall management process. The operator is to choose the treatment modalities.

BIBLIOGRAPHY

1. Aido, M., Stookey, G.K. and Zero, D.T.: Ability of quantitative light induced fluorescence (QLF) to assess the activity of white spot lesions during dehydration. Am. J. Dent.: 19, 15, 2006.
2. Amaechi, B.T.: Emerging technologies for diagnosis of dental caries: The road so far. J. Applied Phy.: 105, 1, 2009.
3. Ando, M., Cabeza, C.G., Isaacs, R.L., Ekert, G.J. and Stookey, G.K.: Evaluation of several techniques for the detection of secondary caries adjacent to amalgam restorations. Caries Res.: 38, 350, 2004.
4. Angmar-Mansson, B. and ten Bosch, J.J.: Optical methods for detection and quantification of dental caries. Adv. Dent. Res.: 1, 14, 1987.
5. Angmar-Mansson, B. and ten Bosch, J.J.: Advances in methods for diagnosing coronal caries - A review. Adv. Dent. Res.: 7, 70, 1993.
6. Ansari, G., Beeley, J.A., Reid, J.S. and Foye, R.H.: Caries detector dyes – an in-vitro assessment of some new compounds. J. Oral Rehab.: 26, 453, 1999.
7. Anttonen, V., Seppa, L. and Hausen, H.: Clinical study of the use of the laser fluorescence device Diagnodent for detection of occlusal caries in children. Caries Res.: 37, 17, 2003.
8. Bab, I.A., Fuerstein, O. and Gazit, D.: Ultrasonic detector of proximal caries. Caries Res.: 31, 322, 1997.
9. Baca, P., Parejo, E., Bravo, M., Castillo, A. and Liebana, J.: Discriminant ability for caries risk of modified colorimetric tests. Med. Oral Path. Oral Cir. Buccal.: 1, 978, 2011.
10. Bader, J.D., Shugars, D.A. and Bonito, A.J.: A systemic review of the performance of methods for identifying carious lesions. J. Public Health Dent.: 62, 201, 2002.
11. Baelum, V.: What is an appropriate caries diagnosis? Acta. Odontologic. Scand.: 68, 65, 2010.
12. Bamzahim, M., Aljehani, A. and Shi, X.C.: Clinical performances of diagnodent in the detection of secondary carious lesions. Acta Odont. Scand.: 63, 26, 2005.
13. Braga, M.M., Mendel, F.M. and Martignon, S.: In-vitro comparison of Nyvad's system and ICDAS II with lesion activity of occlusal caries lesions in primary teeth. Car. Res.: 43, 405, 2009.
14. Braga, M.M., Ekstrand, K.R., Martignon, S., Imparato, J.C.P., Ricketts, D.N.J. and Mendes, F.M.: Clinical performance of two visual scoring systems in detecting and assessing activity status of occlusal caries in primary teeth. Car. Res.: 44, 300, 2010.
15. Braga, M.M., Mendes, F.M. and Ekstrand, K.R.: Detection activity assessment and diagnosis of dental caries lesions. Dent. Cl. North Am.: 54, 479, 2010.
16. Crawley, D.A, Longbottom, B.E., Ciesla, C.M., Arnone, C., Wallace, V.P., Pepper, M: Terahertz pulse imaging: A pilot study of potential application in dentistry. Caries Res. 37, 352, 2003
17. Danowska, H.M.A., Planchaert, A.J.M., Suliborski, S. and Verdonschot, E.H.: Reliability and validity issues of laser fluorescence measurements in occlusal caries diagnosis. J. Dent.: 30, 129, 2002.
18. Grondahl, H.G.: Digital radiology in dental diagnosis: a critical review. Dentomaxillofacial Radiology: 21, 198, 1992.
19. Gungor K, ErtenH, Akarslan ZZ, Celik I and Semiz M: Approximal carious lesions depth assessment with insight and ultraspeed films. Oper. Dent. 30, 58, 2005
20. Haak, R., Wicht, M.J., Hellmich, M., Grossman, A. and Woack, M.J.: The validity of proximal caries detection using magnifying visual aids. Caries Res.: 36, 249, 2002.
21. Hall, A. and Girbin, J.M.: A review of potential new modalities for caries lesions. J.D.R.: 83 (spl. Issue), 689, 2004.
22. Harase, Y., Araki, K. and Okano, T.: Accuracy of extraoral tuned operative computed tomography (TACT) for proximal caries detection. Oral Surg., Oral Med., Oral Pathol.: 101, 791, 2006.
23. Hausen, H.: Caries prediction – state of the art. Comm. Dent. Oral Epidem.: 25, 87, 1997.
24. Hintze, H. and Wenzel, A.: Clinical and laboratory radiographic caries diagnosis - A study of the same teeth. Dentomaxillofacial Radiology: 25, 115, 1996.
25. Hintze, H., Wenzel, A., Danielsen, B. and Nyvad, B.: Reliability of visual examination, fibre optic transillumination and bite wing radiography and reproducibility of direct visual examination following tooth separation for the identification of cavitated carious lesions in contacting approximal surface. Caries Res.: 32, 204, 1998.

26. Ito, A., Hayashi, M., Hamasaki, T. and Ebisu, S.: Risk assessment of dental caries by using classification and regression trees. J. Dent.: 39, 457, 2011.
27. Jablonski-Momeni, A., Ricketts, D.N.J., Stachnin, V., Heinzel-Gutenbrunner, R.M.M. and Pieper, K.: Occlusal caries: evaluation of direct microscopy versus digital imaging used for two histological classification systems. J. Dent.: 38, 204, 2009.
28. Karlsson, L.: Caries detection method based on changes in optical properties between healthy and carious tissue. Int. J. Dent.: 1, 2010.
29. Karlsson, L. and Tranarus, S.: Supplementary methods for detection and quantification of dental caries. J. Laser Dentistry: 16, 8, 2008.
30. Kielbassa, A.M. Current challenges in caries diagnosis. Quint. Int.: 37, 421, 2006.
31. K. Markowitz, RM Stenwall, M. Graye. The effect of distance and tooth structure on laser fluorescence caries detection. Oper. dent 2012, 37-2, 150–180.
32. Lussi, A., Hibst, R. and Paulus, R.: DIAGNOdent: An optical method for caries detection. J. Dent. Res.: 83, C80, 2004.
33. Lussi, A., Imwinkelrid, S., Pitts, N.B., Longbottom, C. and Reich, E.: Performance and reproducibility of a laser fluorescence system for detection of occlusal caries in vitro. Caries Res.: 33, 261, 1999.
34. Meller, C., Heyduck, C., Tranaeus, S. and Spleeth, C.: A new in vitro method for measuring caries activity using quantitative light induced fluorescence. Caries Res.: 40, 90, 2006.
35. Mendes, F.M., Ganzerla, E. and Nunes, A.F.: Use of high powered magnification to detect occlusal caries in primary teeth. Am. J. Dent.: 19, 19, 2006.
36. Mjor, I.A.: Clinical diagnosis of recurrent caries. J.A.D.A.: 136, 1426, 2005.
37. Nair, M.K., Tyndall, D.A., Ludlow, J.B. and May, K.: Tuned Aperture Computed Tomography and Detection of Recurrent Caries. Caries Res.: 32, 23, 1998.
38. Nishimura, M., Oda, T., Keviyo, N., Matsumura, S. and Shimono, T.: Using a caries activity test to predict caries risk in early childhood. J.A.D.A.: 139, 63, 2008.
39. Nyvad, B.: Diagnosis versus detection of caries. Caries Res.: 38, 192, 2004.
40. Pitts B and Ekstrand K.: International Caries Detection and Assessment System (ICDAS) and its International Caries Classification and Management System (ICCMS) – methods for staging of the caries process and enabling dentists to manage caries. Community Dentistry and Oral Epidemiology 41,1,2013
41. Pitts, N.: ICDAS – an international system for caries detection and assessment being developed to facilitate caries epidemiology, research and appropriate clinical management. Comm. Dent. Health: 21, 193, 2004.
42. Pretty, I.A.: Caries detection and diagnosis: Novel technologies. J. Dent.: 34, 727, 2006.
43. Pretty, I.A., Ellwood, P.G., Davies, R.M., Worthington, H.W. and Ellwood, R.P.: The effect of illumination and focal distance on light induced fluorescence images in vitro. Caries Res.: 40, 73, 2006.
44. Reich, E., Marrawi, F. Al, Pitts, N. and Lussi, A.: Clinical validation of a laser caries diagnosis system. Caries Res.: 32 (abs. 89), 297, 1998.
45. Roberts-Thomson, K. and Stewart, J.F.: Risk indicators of caries experience among young adults. Aust. Dent. J.: 53, 122, 2008.
46. Rock, W.P.: The diagnosis of early carious lesions: a review. J. Pediat. Dent.: 3, 1, 1987.
47. Rouhonen M, Palo K and Alander J.: Spectroscopic Detection of Caries Lesions. Journal of Medical Engineering: 161090, 2013.
48. Steinberg, S.: Adding caries diagnosis to caries risk assessment. The next step in caries management by risk assessment (CAMBRA). Compendium: 30, 522, 2009.
49. Stookey, G.: Should a dental explorer be used to probe suspected carious lesion? No-use of an explorer can lead to misdiagnosis and disrupt remineralization. J.A.D.A.: 136, 1526, 2005.
50. Tam, L.E. and Mc Comb, D.: Diagnosis of occlusal caries: Part II. Recent Diagnostic Technologies. J. Can. Dent. Assoc.: 67, 459, 2001.
51. Tranacus, S., Shi, X.Q. and Angmar-Mansson, B.: Caries risk assessment, methods available to clinicians for caries detection. Comm. Dent. Oral Epidem.: 33, 265, 2005.
52. Tyndall, D.A. and Rathore, S.: Cone beam CT diagnostic applications: caries, periodontal bone assessment and endodontic applications. Dent. Cl. North Am.: 52, 825, 2008.
53. Virajslip, V., Thearmontree, A., Aryatawong, S. and Paibonwarachat, D.: Comparison of proximal caries detection in primary teeth between laser fluorescence and bitewing radiography. Pediat. Dent.: 27, 493, 2005.
54. Wenzel, A., Pitts, N., Verdonschott, E.H. and Kalsbeek, H.: Developments in radiographic caries diagnosis - A review. J. Dent.: 21, 131, 1993.
55. White, G.E., Tsamtsouris, A. and Williams, D.L.: Early detection of occlusal caries by measuring the electrical resistance of the tooth. J. Dent. Res.: 57, 195, 1978.
56. Yaniholu, F.C., Ozturk, F., Hayran, O. and Analoni, M.: Detection of natural white spot caries lesions by an ultrasonic system. Caries Res.: 34, 225, 2000.
57. Young, D.A. and Featherstone, J.D.: Digital imaging fiberoptic transillumination, F-speed radiographic film and depth of approximal lesions. J.A.D.A.: 136, 1682, 2005.
58. Zakim, C.M., Taylor, A.M., Ellwood, R.P. and Pretty, I.A.: Occlusal caries detection by using thermal imaging. J. Dent.: 38, 788, 2010.
59. Zandona, A.F., Santiago, E., Eckert, G., Fontana, M., Ando, M. and Zero, D.T.: Use of ICDAS combined with quantitative light induced fluorescence as a caries detection method. Caries Res.: 44, 317, 2010.

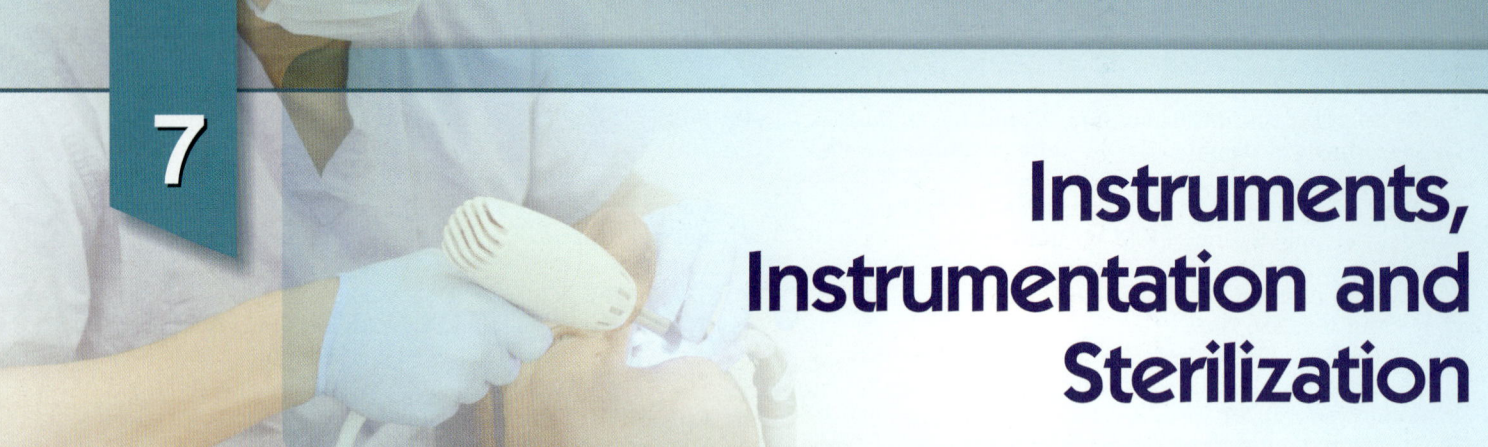

7. Instruments, Instrumentation and Sterilization

In order to properly prepare a cavity, the tooth tissues, enamel and dentin must be excised with specific instruments in an efficiently ordered sequence. The hardness of enamel makes it very difficult to excise, shape and refine the tooth. Also, most cavity preparation requires the use of both rotary and hand instruments. Rotary burs or diamonds are used for gross reduction, creating angulation and final refinement of the cavity preparation. The hand cutting instruments are used to produce intricate details of the cavity preparation and to insert and finish the restorative material.

With the evolution of tooth reduction methods, today most of the cavity preparation is performed with the air turbine handpiece. The regular speed rotary and hand instruments account for only a small portion of the tooth reduction, probably less than 10%, but hand cutting instruments are still an integral part of any dental armamentarium. In the use of hand cutting instruments, there is no vibration, pressure or pain element as compared to high speed instruments.

HAND CUTTING INSTRUMENTS

Modern hand instruments, when properly used, produce beneficial results that are advantageous to both the operator and the patient. It should be noted that certain results can be satisfactorily achieved only with hand instruments.

The standardization of the design of hand cutting instruments by the manufacturers has been helpful to the practitioner. All instruments are identified by a nomenclature and number that describes the size, design and common clinical usage.

The proficiency and quality of the clinical treatment depend on the proper selection and use of the cutting instruments; therefore, the nomenclature and design of the operative instruments must be mastered and an adequate number of sharp and sterile instruments should be available for each clinical procedure.

Metals used in the Manufacture of Hand Instruments

Carbon steel: It is an alloy made by the addition of a small percentage of carbon to iron. It is capable of being hardened, softened and tempered. Its melting point is approximately 1500–1600°C. There are two varieties of steel:
 i. Soft
 ii. Hard

Soft steel contains 0.5% or less of carbon while *hard steel* contains from 0.5–1.5%, carbon. Other ingredients are manganese 0.2%, silicone 0.2% and the rest is iron (91.4–91.6%).

Heat Treatment of Steel

Two heat treatments namely hardening heat treatment and tempering heat treatment are given to steel to obtain maximum benefits.

In hardening heat treatment, steel is heated to full cherry-red color, approximately to 1500°F (815°C) in oxygen-free environment, then immediately plunged into cold water or oil. The hardening heat treatment hardens the alloy but makes it brittle and brittleness is directly proportional to the amount of carbon present.

In tempering heat treatment, steel is reheated for 1 hour at 350°F (176°C) and then plunged in cold salt water/slightly acidulated water/oil/mercury. Tempering relieves the strain, decreases brittleness and increases toughness.

Stainless Alloys

a. *Stainless steel*: It is composed of carbon 0.6–1.0%; chromium 18% and iron 81–81.4%. It is extremely hard but requires very careful and precise heat treatment during manufacture. The resistance to staining of these alloys is attributed to the formation of a thin coating of transparent oxide on their surface, therefore it must be kept highly polished at all times to prevent corrosion. It loses a sharp edge on repeated usage easily as compared to carbon steel, so is used for handle, shank and part of blade.

b. *Monel metal*: A natural alloy of nickel, copper and iron, Monel metal contains approximately nickel 67%, copper 28%, and iron 5%. It is markedly resistant to acids and superheated steam.

c. *Nichrome*: Nichrome contains chiefly nickel 60–80%, chromium 12–20% and iron 0-2.6%. It can be subjected to high degrees of temperature, does not oxidize easily and does not maintain a sharp edge.

d. *Stellite*: This product is available in several grades and consists chiefly of cobalt 65–90%, chromium 10–35%, with small quantities of tungsten, molybdenum, iron or nickel. Its chief characteristics are hardness, strength, density, high melting point, maintenance of cutting edge and resistance to action of acids.

e. *Tarno*: It is made up of popular chromium alloy and is used for manipulation of the cements.

Design Characteristics of Hand Cutting Instruments

A hand instrument consists of the following essential parts (Fig. 7.1):

Handle or shaft: It is mostly straight and octagonal in cross-section, and may be serrated to increase friction for hand gripping.

Handles are available in various sizes and shapes. Large, heavy handles are not conducive to delicate manipulation; therefore most instrument handles are small in diameter and light. Most hand instrument handles are a continuation of the shank. If the shank and blade are separate from the handle and intented to be screwed into it, the instrument is known as a *conesocket instrument*. The advantage with the cone-socket instrument is that, if the working end is broken, it may be easily replaced incurring less expense. The disadvantage is its tendency to loosen at the joint.

Shank: It connects the shaft with the blade or working point. It usually tapers from its connection with the shaft to where the blade begins. Any angulation in the instrument can be placed at the junction of shaft and shank.

Blade/Nib: The working end of cutting instrument is called the *blade* whereas working end of the non-cutting instrument such as condenser is called a *nib* (Figs 7.2A to F). The working surface or end of nib is called a *face*. It begins at the angle where the shank is terminated.

Cutting edge: It is the working part of the instrument. It is usually in the form of a bevel with different shapes.

Blade angle: It is defined as the angle between the long axis of the blade and the long axis of the shaft (Fig. 7.3).

Cutting edge angle: It is defined as an angle between the margins of the cutting edge and the long axis of the shaft (Fig. 7.3).

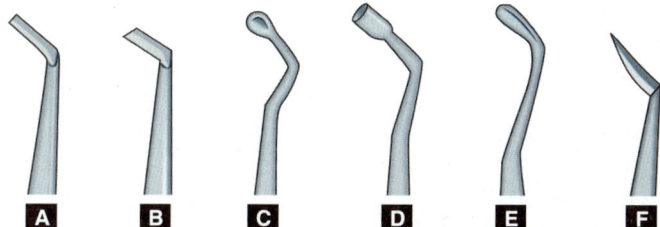

Figs 7.2A to F: Characteristic blades/nib of; **(A)** Hatchet; **(B)** Hoe; **(C)** Excavator; **(D)** Condenser; **(E)** Plastic instrument; **(F)** Carver

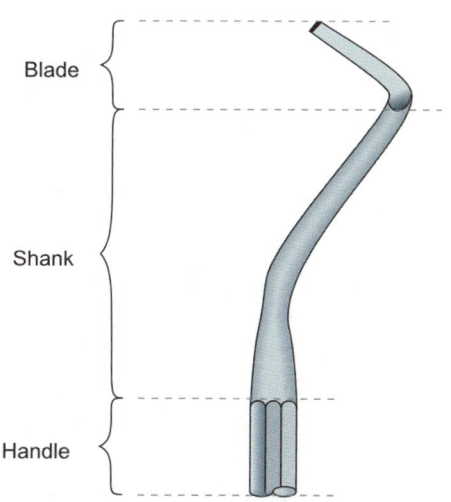

Fig. 7.1: Part of a hand instrument

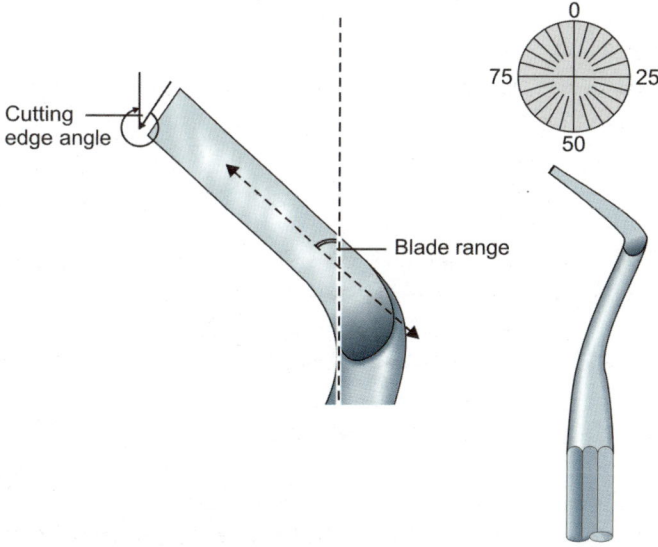

Fig. 7.3: Biangle hatchet showing blade angle and cutting edge angle

The main principle of cutting with hand instruments is to concentrate forces on a very thin cross-section of the instruments at the cutting edge. Thus the thinner this cross-section, the more the pressure that is concentrated and the more efficient instrument will be.

Instrument Nomenclature

Dr. G.V. Black established a nomenclature for hand instruments, similar to the biological classification.

1. *Order:* Purpose of instrument, e.g. excavator or scaler.
2. *Suborder:* Position or manner of use, e.g. push, pull.
3. *Class:* Form of working end, e.g. hatchet, chisel.
4. *Subclass:* Shape of the shank, e.g. monangle, binangle.

Naming of the instruments usually moves from 4 to 1, e.g. a binangle hatchet push, excavator. In most cases, the suborder describing the position or manner of use is variable and non-specific; and for practical purpose it is usually omitted.

Instrument Formula

Dr. G.V. Black gave an instrument formula that describes the dimension and angulation of the hand instruments.

The basic formula consists of three units whose measurements are based upon the metric system:

The *1st figure* represents the width of the blade in tenths of a millimeter.

The *2nd figure* represents the length of the blade in millimeters.

The *3rd figure* represents the angle which the blade forms with the axis of the handle. This angle is expressed in 100th of a circle or centigrades.

These three measurements are sufficient for describing a great percentage of instruments. However, for instruments with their cutting edges at an angle other than a right angle to the long axis of the blade, a *fourth unit*, cutting edge angle, is added to the basic three-unit formula. This additional number represents the angle formed between the cutting edge and the long axis of the handle. It is placed in the second position of the formula, i.e. before the length of the blade. For example a gingival marginal trimmer has a 4 unit formula.

Direct and Lateral Cutting Instruments

Direct Cutting: It is one in which the force is applied in the same plane as that of the blade and handle. It is called a *single plane instrument*. Even if they may have two or more curves or angles in their shank, all are in the same plane as the handle (Fig. 7.4). They can be used in direct and lateral cutting, provided that they are contra-angled.

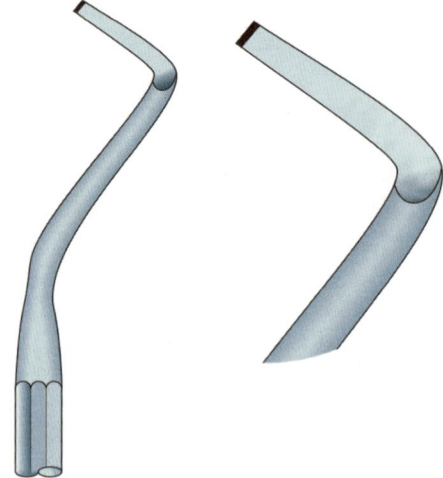

Fig. 7.4: Binangle hatchet with cutting edge in the plane of the instrument

Direct cutting instruments are made either Left or Right by placing a bevel on one side of the blade. If the instrument is held with the cutting edge down and pointing away from the operator, and bevel is on the Right side, it will be a Right-sided instrument. If the bevel is on the Left, it will be a Left-sided instrument (Fig. 7.5).

Lateral cutting instruments: These are the instruments in which the force is applied at a right angle to the plane of the blade and handle. These usually have a curved blade and are called *double plane instruments*. They have an angle or curve in a plane perpendicular to that of the handle. These can be used only in the lateral cutting.

Lateral cutting instruments are made Left and Right, by having the curve or angle which is at a right angle to the principal plane, either on the Right or Left. Holding the instrument with its blade down and

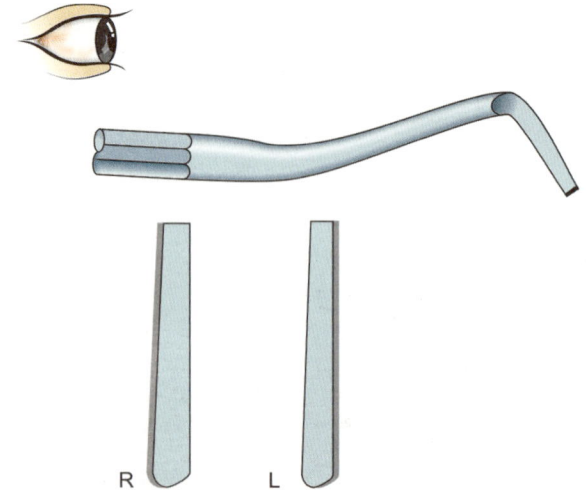

Fig. 7.5: To determine bevel (R, L) hold the instrument with primary cutting edge pointing down and away

cutting edge pointing away, the instrument having that curve of the blade directed to the right is a right instrument and similarly so for the left.

Contra-angling: In many instruments, shank has bends at one or more points to angle the blade relative to the long axis of the handle. The extent of this arrangement depends on the length of the blade and the degree of angulation in the shank. Accordingly, the working point is moved out of line with the axis of the handle. If the working point is moved out of line with the axis of handle, the instrument will be out of balance in lateral cutting motion, and force will be required to keep the instrument from rotating in the hand.

For eliminating this problem, instruments are designed to have one or more angles in the shank, placing the working point within 3.0 mm from the axis of the handle. This principle of design is called *contra-angling*.

The length of the blade required is determined by the depth of the cavity and the blade angle is determined by the accessibility requirements. Greater angles are required as we move posteriorly and in incisal portions of proximal cavities in anterior teeth. So, in addition to balance, contra-angling will provide better access and a clear view of the operating field.

Single bevelled instruments: Instruments which have a bevel on only one side of the instrument blade are known as *single bevelled instruments*. The instrument is held such that the instrument blade faces downwards and away from the operator.

If these are regularly bevelled on the side away from the shaft, they are called *"distally bevelled"*. If these are bevelled on the side of the blade towards the shaft, they are called *"mesially bevelled"*.

If the bevel is on the right side of the instrument blade, it is a *right-sided instrument* and if the bevel is on the left side of the instrument, it is a *left-sided instrument*.

When these types of instruments have no angle in the shank or an angle of 12.5° or less they are used in push (direct cutting) and scraping motions. If this angle in the shank exceeds 12.5°, the instruments could be used in pull (distally bevelled) and push (mesially bevelled) motions (Figs 7.6A to C).

Bi-bevelled instruments: Instruments which have two bevels on the opposing side of the instrument blade which meet together to form the cutting edge are called *bi-bevelled instruments*, e.g. ordinary hatchet.

Triple-bevelled instruments: Bevelling the blade laterally, together with the end, forms three distinct cutting edges in a triple bevelled instrument, e.g. angle former.

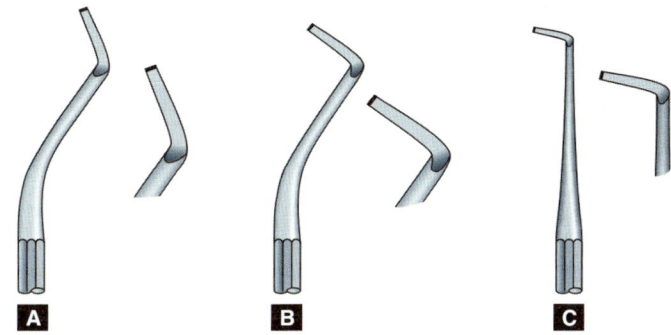

Figs 7.6A to C: Transition from chisel; **(A)** to hoe; **(B and C)** by increasing blade angulation

Circumferentially bevelled instruments: These are usually double-planed instruments where the blade is bevelled at all peripheries, e.g. spoon excavator.

Single-ended and double-ended instruments: Single-ended instruments are confined to only one specific function; while double-ended instrument incorporates the right and left or mesial and distal forms of the instrument in the same handle.

Single-plane instruments with no angle in the shank have the potential for five cutting movements—vertical, right, left, push and pull.

A right-left single-plane instrument with one or more angles in the shank will have four potential cutting movements; which are-vertical, push, pull, right or left. For the mesially and distally bevelled single-planed instruments the four movements are vertical, right, left and push or pull, depending upon the location of the bevel.

Classification of Instruments

A. *Chisels*
   a. Straight
   b. Monangle
   c. Binangle
   d. Triple angle

B. *Excavators*
   a. Hoe
   b. Spoon
   c. Cleoid-Discoid

C. *Modified form of chisels*
   a. Hatchet
   b. Gingival margin trimmer
   c. Angle former
   d. Wedelstaedt chisel

D. *Miscellaneous*
   a. Dental probes
   b. Knives
   c. Dental files

A. Chisels

These are instruments designed after ordinary carpenter's tools and are intended for planing and cleaving. These are characterized by a blade that terminates in a cutting edge formed by a one-sided bevel. Cutting edge of a chisel is at right angle to the shaft (Figs 7.7A to D).

There are following types of chisels available.
a. *Straight chisel*: These have a straight blade in line with the handle and shank. The cutting edge is on one side only (Fig. 7.8B).
b. *Monangle chisels*: In these, the blade is placed at an angle to the shaft. It may be mesially (Standard) or distally (Reverse) bevelled (Figs 7.9A and B).
c. *Binangle chisels*: These have two angles between the shaft and the blade. It may be mesially or distally bevelled (Fig. 7.10 and 7.8A).
d. *Triple-angle chisels*: These have three angles in the shank and are usually used to flatten pulpal floor. It may also be mesially or distally bevelled.

B. Excavators

Excavators are used for excavation and removal of caries and sharpening or refinement of the internal parts of the cavity preparation.

Types

a. *Hoe*: A hoe is a descriptive term given to a form of chisel in which the angle of the blade more nearly approaches a right angle, i.e. 25 centigrade. It is a single-planed instrument, which can be distally bevelled or mesially bevelled and used with pull motion (Fig. 7.6 and 7.8E).
Application: These are used for cutting mesial and distal walls of premolars and molars.

Both hatchets and hoes are used to remove harder varieties of caries as well as to give form to the internal parts of the cavity preparation.
b. *Spoon*: In these, the cutting edge is ground to a semi-circular circumferential bevel and sharpened to a thin edge. These are available in pairs with the blade of one curved to the right, and the blade of the other curved to the left. The spoon excavators are double-planed instruments with right or left cutting movement only (Fig. 7.11).
Application: Used for removal of decayed dentin.
c. *Cleoid-Discoid*: It is similar to the spoon excavator, except that the blade resembles a claw, hence the name 'cleoid'. It is used in carving amalgam and excavating decay from areas of difficult access.

C. Modified Forms of Chisels

These are designed to perform specific functions:
a. *Hatchet*: Hatchets are used for splitting or cleaving undermined enamel in proximal cavities and on buccal and lingual walls where it is not possible to use a chisel. The smaller sizes are primarily used in anterior teeth and larger sizes are mainly used in posterior teeth (Fig. 7.8C).
b. *Gingival margin trimmer (G.M.T.)*: It is a modified form of hatchet (Fig. 7.8D and F). A few distinct

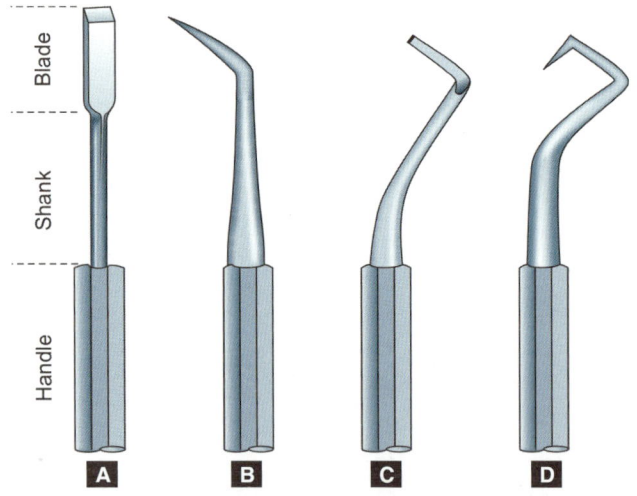

Figs 7.7A to D: (A) Straight chisel; (B) Monoangled instrument-face away from the axis of the handle; (C) Binangled instrument-face close to the long axis of the handle and; (D) Triple-angled instrument

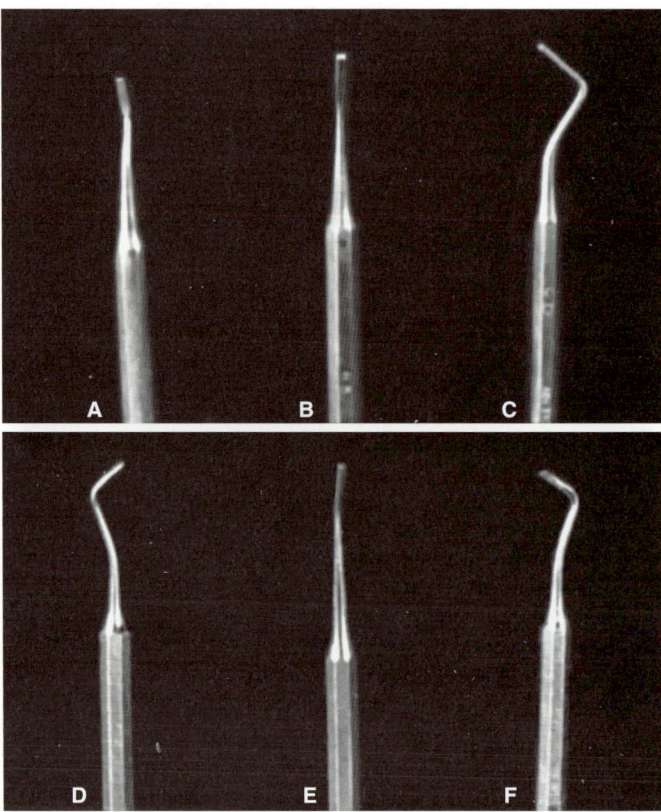

Figs 7.8A to F: Instruments. (A) Binangled chisel; (B) Straight chisel; (C) Enamel hatchet; (D) GMT; (E) Hoe; (F) GMT

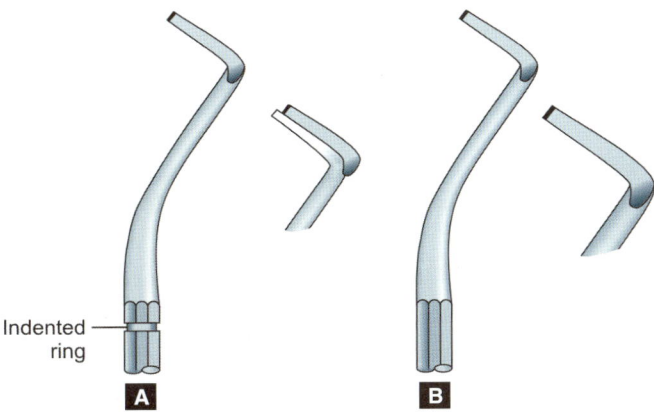

Figs 7.9A and B: (A) Reverse bevel cutting edge; (B) Standard bevel cutting edge

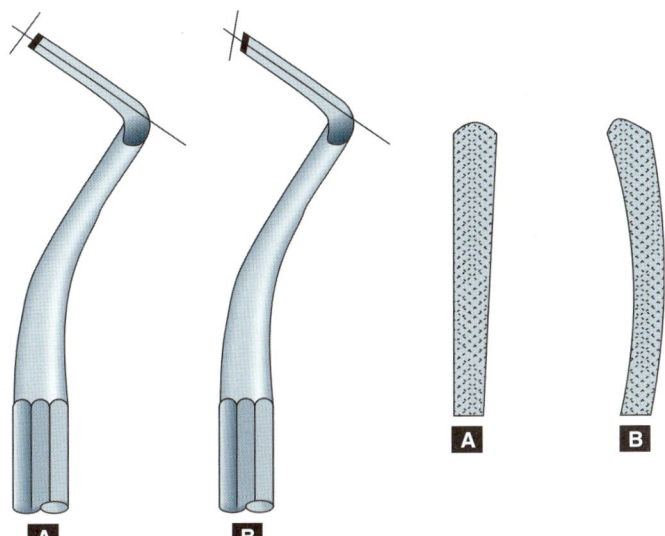

Figs 7.12A and B: Enamel hatchet. (A) Compared with gingival margin trimmer (B)

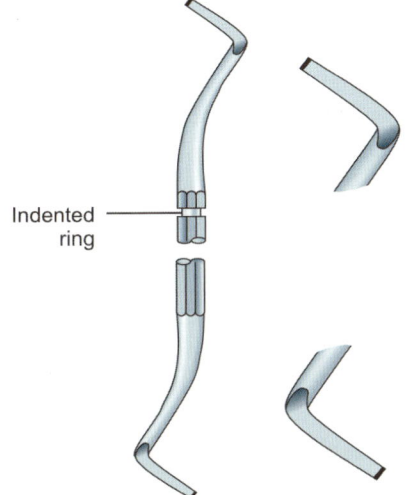

Fig. 7.10: Binangled chisel

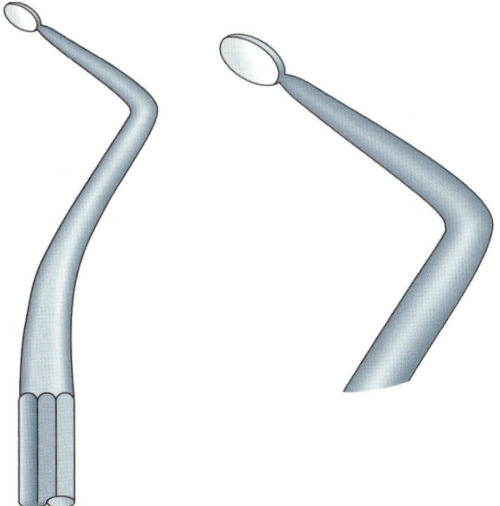

Fig. 7.11: Spoon excavator

modifications of the basic hatchet design are noted as:

   i. Cutting edge of a hatchet is at a perpendicular angle to the axis of the blade while cutting edge of a gingival margin trimmer is at an angle other than a perpendicular angle (G.M.T.) to the axis of the blade (so a 4-unit formula).

  ii. Hatchet has a straight blade, the blade of a G.M.T. is curved (Figs 7.12A and B).

 iii. Hatchet is a single plane instrument while G.M.T. with curved blade is a double plane instrument, so is primarily a lateral cutting instrument. It is paired with Right and Left sided bevels.

 iv. There are two pairs of these instruments, consisting a set of four. In a given size each pair has a right and left bevelled instruments. The cutting edges of one pair make an acute angle with that edge of the blade furthest from the handle. These are distal gingival margin trimmer. A typical distal GMT is the 10-95-6-12, the second number in instrument formula may vary from 95 to 100. The cutting edge of other the pair makes an acute angle with that edge of the blade nearer to the handle. These are mesial gingival margin trimmer. A typical mesial GMT is the 10-80-12, the second number in instrument formula may vary from 75 to 85.

GMT is used for creating a proper bevel at the gingival cavosurface margin and to bevel axiopulpal line angle in class II cavity. Distal GMT is used for distal surface and the mesial GMT is used for mesial surface. It is also used for trimming the margins of various walls of cavity preparation.

It is used for forming sharp angles in internal parts of the cavity preparations.

c. *Angle former*: It is a modified form of chisel. In this instrument, the primary cutting edge is sharpened

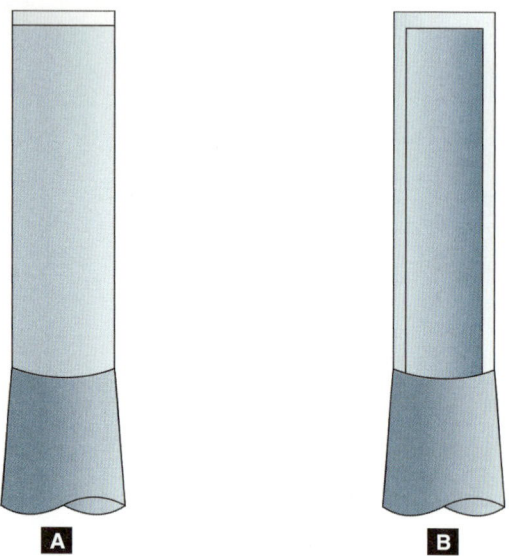

Figs 7.13A and B: Transition from chisel **(A)** To angle former **(B)** (by angling primary cutting edge)

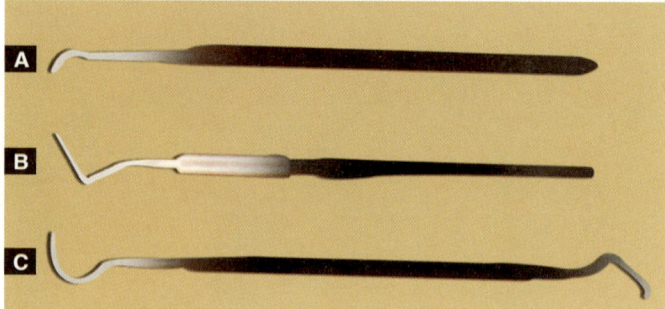

Figs 7.14A to C: Instruments. **(A)** Naber's probe; **(B)** Graduated probe; **(C)** Explorer

at an angle to the axis of the blade. The angle of cutting edge to the blade axis is usually 80–85° (4 unit formula). Blade of the angle former is bevelled on the sides also, to form three cutting edges. The acute cutting angle being directed to the right or left makes the angle former a paired instrument. Right of the pair is identified by an indented ring. It is a single plane instrument (Figs 7.13A amd B).

It is used to accentuate line and point angles in the internal outline form. It is frequently used in cavity preparation for cohesive gold to establish retention form.

d. *Wedelstaedt chisel*: It is like a straight chisel, but with a slight vertical curvature in its shank. It is bevelled on one side only which can be placed mesially or distally.

It is used for cleaving undermined enamel and for shaping walls. They are single planed instruments, with three cutting motions; vertical, right and left. The mesially bevelled can be used in push movements and the distally beveled can be used in pull motions.

D. Miscellaneous

a. *Dental Probes:* Various types of probes are available, these can be straight, curved or graduated (used in periodontology) (Figs 7.14A to C).
b. *Knives:* Nibs of these instruments carry knife-edged faces on one of their sides only. The knives known as finishing knives, amalgam knives are made in various sizes and shapes.

They are used for trimming off excess filling material on the gingival, facial or lingual margins of a proximal restoration or trimming and contouring the surface of a class V restoration.

Knives for specific purposes
Wilson's Knife: In this, the nib is in a plane at perpendicular angle to that of the shaft, so that it can be introduced interproximally for use.

Stein's Knife: It has a trapezoidal nib and is used mainly for direct gold restorations for contouring and margination.

c. *Dental files*: Nib in files can be foot-shaped, hatchet shaped or parallelogram shaped with serrations. If the serrations are directed away from the handle, it is a push file and if the serrations are directed towards the handle, it is a pull file.

These are used for smoothening of margins; if knives and carvers are not sufficient to produce the requisite cavosurface margins at the gingival end, files can be used to achieve above said requisite.

Instrument Grasps

It is more than just a manner of holding the instrument and must be taken quite seriously otherwise bad habits may be acquired that result in loss of operating efficiency and accumulation of unnecessary strain on the operator.

Fundamentally there are four grasps used with hand instruments, which are as follows:

1. *Pen grasp*: It is similar to the method of holding a pen, except that the pulps of the thumb, 1st and 2nd fingers contact the instrument, while the tip of the 3rd and 4th fingers are placed on the adjoining teeth (as rests).

The position of 2nd finger is important for good control and thrust to the instrument. This way, due to greater length of the 2nd finger, the application point for the force will be near the working point of the instrument.

2. *Inverted pen grasp*: This is similar to the pen grasp, but the hand is rotated so that the palm is facing upwards. It is usually used in upper teeth. Not used too frequently, but on certain occasions, depending on the area of operation, type of instrument used

and position of the point and operator, modifications of the inverted pen grasps are used.

3. *Palm and thumb grasp*: It is similar to the method of holding a knife, when cutting a piece of wood. The handle is placed in the palm of the hand and grasped by the four fingers, while the thumb rests on an area other than that being operated on. A supporting rest provided by the thumb is necessary because digital control is somewhat insufficient.

   This grasp is used when the thumb must rest at some point distant from the operating site. It may be useful on maxillary teeth particularly the right side, when working from the right rear chair position.

4. *Modified palm and thumb grasp*: When it is feasible to rest the thumb on the same tooth being operated or on a tooth immediately adjacent, the modified palm and thumb grasp may be used.

   The handle of the instrument is held between the pulps of the thumb and the 1st and 2nd fingers. The 3rd and 4th fingers are about half closed; they contact the handle under the 1st joint of each finger and press the handle against the distal area of the palm.

   It provides greater freedom of movement and delicacy of control may be obtained.

Rests: Rests are used to steady the hand during operating procedures and these also act as guards when thrust force is applied.

Whenever feasible, the rests should be on the arch being operated on and preferably on the same quadrant. The closer the rest areas are to the operating area, the more reliable they are. In some instances, it is impossible to secure a rest on tooth structure, and soft tissues must be used. Such rests as well as those distant to the tooth being operated upon, do not afford a reliable rest.

Guards: Guards are finger positions of the hand opposite the one using the instrument, to steady the parts being operated on and to protect them from injury in case the instrument accidentally slips off the working surface.

These should be used particularly when adjacent teeth are not available as rests or when rests must be obtained on soft tissues or on the opposite arch.

Sharpening of Hand Instruments

Instruments are dulled by repeated contact with tooth tissues and by frequent sterilization. Use of instruments with dull cutting edges cause more pain, prolong operating time, reduce quality and preciseness in cavity preparation and also make control difficult. Therefore, it is essential that all cutting instruments be sharp.

Sharpening is done by reducing the bulk of the metal at the cutting edge, following the original configuration of the bevel.

There are many types of sharpening instruments which include stationary oilstones, e.g. Arkansas stones, mechanical sharpener, diamond hone and stones that are used in the handpiece. In the use of any sharpening equipment, there are several basic principles that should be followed:

1. Do not sharpen dirty instruments.
2. Establish the proper bevel angle (usually 45–60°) and the desired angle of the cutting edge to the blade before placing the instrument against the stone and maintain these angles while sharpening.
3. Use a light stroke or pressure against the stone to minimize frictional heat.
4. Use a rest or guide whenever possible.
5. Remove as little metal from the blade as possible.
6. Lightly hone the unbevelled side of the blade after sharpening to remove the fine bur that may be created.
7. Keep the sharpening stones clean and free of metal cuttings.

Stationary stone technique: The size of the Arkansas oilstone should be at least two inches wide and five inches long. Before using, a thin film of light oil should be placed on the working surface. Stone should be laid on a flat surface and should not tilt while sharpening. Instrument should be grasped with a pen grip, to avoid its rotation or change in angles while sharpening. To ensure stability during the sharpening strokes, third and fourth fingers are used as rest and guide along a flat surface to prevent rolling or dipping of the instrument.

Mechanical techniques: While using reciprocating honing sharpener (mechanical sharpener) the blade should be placed against the steady rest and the proper angle of the cutting edge to the blade should be established before activating the motor.

Handpiece stones are used chiefly for instruments with curved blades, especially for the inside curve of the blades. The handpiece should be run at a slow speed and instrument should be held lightly against the stone with a pen grasp and third and fourth fingers should be used as rests. With this method of sharpening, care must be exercised not to throw oil from the stone as it is being used.

ROTARY CUTTING INSTRUMENTS

The term 'rotary instruments' in dentistry refers *to a group of instruments that turn on an axis to perform a work such as cutting, abrading, burnishing, finishing or polishing tooth tissues or a restoration.* While majority

> **Advantages of hand cutting instruments**
> - They are self limited in cutting enamel, i.e. they will not cut sound enamel, but cut only enamel undermined by loss of dentin.
> - They can remove large pieces of undermined enamel quickly, thus saving time and effort.
> - No vibration or heat accompanies the cutting, making it painless and with no adverse effects on the tooth tissues.
> - Most efficient means of precise cutting, especially when cutting is needed adjacent to important anatomy.
> - Create smoothest surface of all cutting instruments.
> - Have the longest life span, as can be re-sharpened.

of the cutting procedures earlier employed for cutting enamel and dentin used hand instrumentation, nowadays the bulk of the tooth tissue removal is accomplished using rotary instruments.

The early instruments were used to break away enamel undermined by caries and to scoop out carious dentin. The history of the early development of rotary instruments is incomplete. The development and evolution of rotary equipment is a continuous process. There are two types of rotary instruments, i.e. Handpiece and Dental burs. Dental handpieces are classified according to the driving mechanism.

Dental Handpieces

1. Gear Driven Handpiece

The three conventional designs of handpieces are straight handpiece, contra-angle and prophylaxis angle. Rotary power is transferred to the straight handpiece by a belt that runs from an electric engine over a series of pulleys and a three piece extension cord arm. Rotary cutting instruments are inserted into a chuck at the front of the handpiece. The desired angle handpiece is attached over the front end of the straight handpiece for operation. Rotary power is transferred from the straight handpiece by a shaft and gears inside the angle section.

Conventional handpieces are designed to operate at speeds under 5000 rpm. A long sheathed contra-angle helps to reduce vibration. By the use of several speed increasing transmissions it is possible to obtain speeds of 100,000 rpm with a gear driven angle that has an automatic lubricating system.

Gear driven handpieces are very versatile, being capable of a wide speed range and use. All operative procedures can be accomplished with this type of equipment. However they function best at low speed because of so many moving parts with metal to metal contact. High torque is available at all speeds. Proper maintenance is of utmost importance to prevent excessive heat, vibration and wear within the handpiece.

2. Water Driven Handpiece

In 1953, a hydraulic driven turbine handpiece was reported to operate satisfactorily at 60,000 rpm. Two years later the first commercial model called a Turbojet became available. Improved units have both straight and angle handpieces which will operate at speeds upto 100,000 rpm. The turbojet is designed as a compact mobile unit and only electricity is needed to operate it. The soundproof cabinet contains a motor, water pump, water reservoir and the necessary plumbing for circulating the water. Water is conveyed to and from the handpiece by a co-axial type tubing (tube inside a tube). The small inner tube carries water under high pressure to rotate a turbine in the handpiece head and the larger outer tube returns the water to the reservoir. From here it is recirculated over and over. The handpiece is extremely quiet and has the highest torque of any turbine angle handpiece.

3. Belt Driven Handpieces

A belt driven angle handpiece called the Page-Chayes became available in 1955 and was the first angle handpiece to operate successfully at speeds above 100,000 rpm. All gears were eliminated by having a small belt run inside the handpiece sheath over ball bearing pulleys in the angle sections. The rotary cutting instrument has a 1/6 inch shank held in the handpiece by friction grip.

Improved models of the belt driven design are the Page-Chayes 909 and the Twin 909. The Twin 909 is a complete unit having two engines and a foot control. Rotary power is transferred to either handpiece by a separate single belt which runs the handpiece and has smooth transition of speeds between 1500 and 180,000 rpm.

Belt driven angle handpieces are relatively free of maintenance problems because the bearings have factory sealed lubrication. They have a history of excellent performance and great versatility.

4. Air Driven Handpieces

In the latter part of 1956, the first clinically successful air driven turbine handpiece became available with free running speeds of approximately 300,000 rpm. A small compact unit consists of a handpiece, control box, foot control and various connector hoses. When the foot control is activated, compressed air flows through the control box and is carried by a flexible hose to the back of the handpiece. From here the air is directed to the head of the handpiece and is blown against the blades of a small turbine to produce rotation while the greater part is exhausted at the back of the handpiece or returned to the control box. The rotary instrument's 1/6 inch shank is held by friction grip. The speeds drop from 300,000 rpm to 160,000 rpm with a lateral workload of 1¾ ounces. The reason is that air turbines have low torque and will stall at lateral workloads of 4½-5½ ounces. This is an excellent safety feature since excessive pressure cannot be applied to rotary instrument.

Speed Ranges and Uses

Low/Conventional speed : Below 6000 rpm
High/Intermediate speed : 6000-100,000 rpm
Ultra/Super speeds : Above 100,000 rpm

Low Speed

It is used for excavating caries with round burs, refining cavity preparations, using sand paper disks, marginating gold restorations and polishing procedures.

High Speed

It can be used for cavity preparations but not as effectively as ultra speeds. A large selection of specifically shaped instruments is required. Many finishing procedures such as the placement of retentive grooves and bevels are best performed at high speeds. This speed range is preferred where vision is poor or a more positive sense of touch is needed as a guide or both.

Ultra Speed

At speeds above 100,000 rpm smaller more versatile cutting instruments are used. This speed range is desirable for such operations as bulk reduction, obtaining outline form and removing metal restorations. Some cavity preparations may be completed entirely at ultra speeds, but usually the operator will use lower speeds for finishing touches.

Common Features of Rotary Instruments

Despite of a great variation that is seen among rotary cutting instruments, they have certain design features in common which are the (1) shank, (2) neck, and (3) head (Figs 7.15A and B).

Shank: The shank is that part of the rotary instrument that fits into the handpiece, accepts the rotary movement from the handpiece and controls the alignment and concentricity of the instrument. The three commonly seen instrument shanks are:
- Straight
- Latch type
- Friction grip

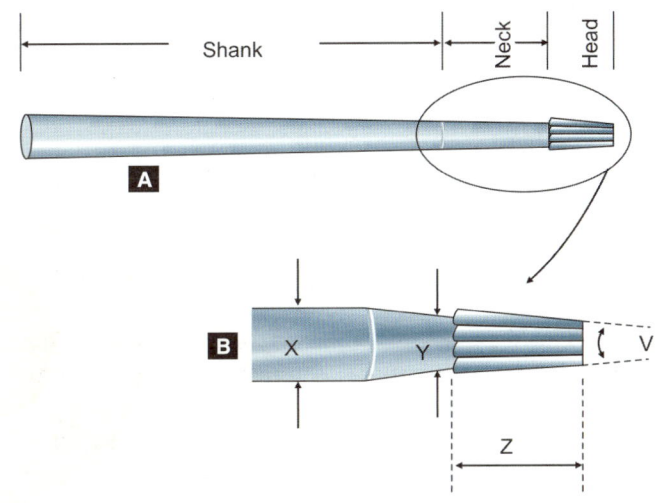

Figs 7.15A and B: (A) Parts of a rotary cutting instrument; **(B)** Enlarged view shows (x) shank diameter (y) neck diameter (z) head length and (v) taper angle

Straight handpiece shank is a simple cylinder. It is held in the handpiece by a metal chuck. However because of its long length, its access to posterior region of the mouth is difficult and is mostly used for finishing and polishing completed restorations extra orally.

Handpieces that use latch type instruments have a metal tube within which the instrument fits very closely. The posterior portion of the instrument shank is flattened on one side so that it fits into a D-shaped socket at the end of the bur tube. These are retained by a latch that slides into the groove found at the shank end. Their short length allows easy access to posterior regions of the mouth and is primarily used at low and medium speeds for finishing procedures.

Friction grip shank is a simple cylinder which is held in the handpiece by friction between the shank and a plastic or metal chuck. Dimensional accuracy of the shanks is important in these instruments, because even a minor variation in shank diameter can cause changes in performance and difficulty with insertion, retention and removal. The overall length is smaller than the latch type instruments, thus improving access to posterior regions. These are designed to be used at high speeds.

Neck: The neck is the intermediate part of the instrument that connects the shank to the head. It tapers from the shank diameter to a smaller size adjacent to the head, and its size should be so adjusted that it allows greatest possible visibility and manipulation. The neck dimensions hence may be a compromise between the need for a large cross-section to provide strength and a small cross-section to improve access and visibility. It's main function is to transmit rotational and translational forces to the head.

Head: The head is the working part of the instrument whose cutting edges perform the desired shaping of the tooth structure. The heads of instruments show great variations in design and construction. Based upon their head characteristics, the instruments can be bladed or abrasive. Heads can vary in their material of construction, size and shape.

Dental Burs

Bur is defined as a rotary cutting instrument with cutting heads of various shapes and two or more sharp edged blades, used as a rotary grinder. It is used for various purposes such as finishing restorations, surgical removal of bone and tooth preparation. The earliest burs were hand made. Machine made burs were introduced in 1891, which were made of steel. Later on the carbide burs replaced the steel burs.

Composition

Depending upon their composition, dental burs can be classified into two types: stainless steel burs and tungsten carbide burs. Steel burs are cut from steel blank parallel to the long axis of the bur. The bur is then hardened and tempered to a Vicker's hardness number of 800. Steel burs however perform well only at low speeds and dull rapidly at high speeds or when cutting enamel. Once dulled, their cutting effectiveness is reduced thereby increasing heat production and vibration.

Tungsten carbide burs on the other hand are obtained by alloying in which complete fusion of the constituents does not occur. The tungsten carbide powder is mixed with powdered cobalt/nickel under vacuum. A partial alloying of the metals takes place. A blank is then formed and the bur is cut from it with a diamond tool. The Vicker's hardness number of this type of bur is in the range of 1650–1700. Carbide burs were introduced in 1947 and have largely replaced steel burs for cavity preparation. These perform better than steel burs at all speeds and their superiority is greatest at high speeds. Carbide is harder than steel and therefore does not dull rapidly. However, carbide is also more brittle and more susceptible to fracture when subjected to a sudden blow.

In most of the modern burs, a combination of the two is used. The carbide head is attached to a steel shank and neck by welding or brazing. This combines the advantages of the two, in one. Substitution of steel in the shank and neck permits the manufacturer more freedom in design of the instrument and also reduces the cost of construction. A major drawback with the use of these burs is that steel necks bend, in comparison to carbide necks which fracture under sudden stress. A bur that bends even slightly produces increased vibration and over cutting as a result of increased run out.

Classification

There are various systems for the classification of burs.
1. According to their mode of attachment to the handpiece, they can be classified as latch type or friction grip type.
2. According to their composition, they can be classified as stainless steel burs, tungsten carbide burs or a combination.
3. According to their motion, they can be classified as right or left bur. A right bur is one which cuts, when it revolves clockwise and a left bur is one which cuts when revolving anticlockwise.
4. According to the length of their head, they can be classified as long, short or regular.
5. According to their use, they can be classified as cutting burs or those used to finish and polish restorations.
6. According to their shapes, they can be classified as round, inverted cone, pear shaped, wheel shaped, tapering fissure, straight fissure, end cutting, etc.

Bur Shapes

The term *'bur shape' refers to the contour or silhouette of the bur head*. The basic head shapes are the round, inverted cone, pear, straight fissure, tapering fissure and end cutting (Figs 7.16A to F).
a. *Round bur*: A bur with a spherical head is a round bur. It is used for initial tooth preparation, removal of caries, extension of the preparation and for the placement of retentive grooves.
b. *Inverted cone bur*: A bur with a rapidly tapering cone head whose small end of the cone is directed towards the bur shank. It is used for establishing wall angulations and providing undercuts in cavity preparations.
c. *Pear shaped bur*: A bur with a slightly tapering cone with the small end of the cone directed towards the

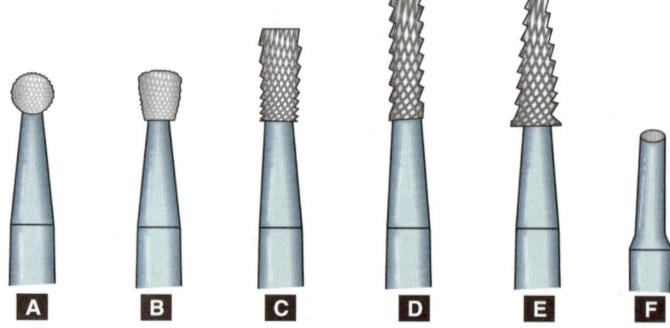

Figs 7.16A to F: Different shapes of commonly used dental burs. **(A)** Round; **(B)** Inverted; **(C)** Pear; **(D)** Straight fissure; **(E)** Tapering fissure; **(F)** End cutting

bur shank. It is used in class I cavity preparations for gold foil. A long length pear bur is advocated for cavity preparations for amalgam.

d. *Straight fissure bur*: A bur with the head shape of an elongated cylinder. It is used for amalgam cavity preparations.
e. *Tapering fissure bur*: A bur with a tapering cone head with the small end of the cone directed away from the bur shank. It is used for inlay and crown preparations.
f. *End cutting bur*: This bur is cylindrical in shape, with just the end carrying the blades. It is used for carrying the preparation apically without axial reduction.

Bur Sizes

The original numbering system for the burs was developed by SS White Dental Manufacturing Company in 1891. In this system the burs were grouped by 9 shapes and 11 sizes. The ½ and ¼ designations were added later with the introduction of smaller sized instruments (Table 7.1). Crosscut burs were indicated by adding 500 to the equivalent non crosscut size, e.g. no. 56 bur with crosscuts was designated as 556. Similarly, an end cutting bur was indicated by adding 900 to the equivalent size. There was a general uniformity in this system for about 60 years.

Changes gradually occurred over time without actually disrupting the system. Certain sizes vanished and the new ones were introduced in 1955 and are still being used though rarely (Table 7.2).

Modifications in the Bur Design

Modifications in the bur design were seen with the introduction of high speed hand pieces. The three other major changes included:
- Reduced use of crosscuts
- Extended heads on fissure burs
- Rounding of the sharp tip angles

Crosscuts are notches present on the blade of the instrument to obtain adequate cutting effectiveness at low speeds (Fig. 7.17). At higher speeds they tend to produce unduly rough surfaces, so many of the

Table 7.1: Original bur head sizes (Adapted from SS White Dental Manufacturing Company)

Head shapes	Head diameter in mm											
	0.5	0.6	0.8	1.0	1.2	1.4	1.6	1.9	2.1	2.3	2.5	2.8	3.0
Round	1/4	1/2	1	2	3	4	5	6	7	8	9	10	11
Wheel		11½	12	13	14	15	16	17	18	19	20	21	22
Cone		22½	23	24	25	26	27	28	29	30	31	32	33
Inverted cone		33½	34	35	36	37	38	39	40	41	42	43	44
Bud		44½	45	46	47	48	49	50	51	52	53	54	55
Straight fissure (flat end)		55½	56	57	58	59	60	61	62				
Straight fissure (pointed end)		66½	67	68	69	70	71	72	73				
Pear		77½	78	79	80	81	82	83	84	85	86	87	88
Oval		88½	89	90	91	92	93	94	95				

Table 7.2: Standard bur head size (carbide & steel) (Adapted from SS White Dental Manufacturing Company)

Head shapes	Head diameter in mm												
	0.5	0.6	0.8	1.0	1.2	1.4	1.6	1.9	2.1	2.3	2.5	2.8	3.0	3.3
Round	1/4	1/2	1	2	3	4	5	6	7	8	9	10	11	
Wheel			11½	12		14		16						
Inverted cone			33½	34	35	36	37	38	39	40				
Plain fissure			55½	56	57	58	59	60	61	62				
Round crosscut					502	503	505	506						
Straight fissure crosscut				556	557	558	559	560	561	562	563			
Tapered fissure crosscut					700	701	702	703						
End cutting fissure					957	958	959							
Round finishing					A	B	C	D		200	201		202	203
Oval finishing										218	219		220	221
Pear finishing										230		231	232	
Flame finishing					242	243	244	245	246					

Operative Dentistry

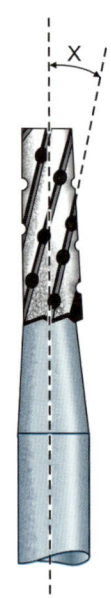

Fig. 7.17: Cross-cut bur, lateral view: (x) spiral angle

crosscut burs designed to be used at low speeds have now been replaced by equivalent non crosscuts burs to be used at high speeds.

With the use of high speeds, carbide fissure burs have been introduced that have extended head lengths, two to three times the normal length of similar diameter. Such a design is not practical at low speeds using a brittle material such as carbide.

The third major change of rounding of the sharp tip corners was made by *Markely and Sockwell*. Sharp angles in the bur head can result in areas of increased stress concentration in the teeth and increase their tendency to fracture. Rounding of the sharp angles enhances the strength of the tooth and also the instrument lasts longer because there are no sharp corners to chip and wear.

Although many new bur sizes and shapes have increased the nomenclature of burs in current use, the number actually required for use in the clinics has reduced. Most commonly used burs are listed in Table 7.3.

Design of a Dental Bur

The actual cutting action of a bur takes place at the edge of the blade present on the bur head. The bur head consists of uniformly spaced blades with depressed areas in between them (Fig. 7.18). These depressed areas are called as the *flute or the chip spaces*. The number of blades on a bur is usually even because even numbered blades are easy to produce in the manufacturing process. The blades on a cutting bur are usually 6 to 8 to 10 and those on a finishing bur are usually 12 to 40. The greater the number of blades, smoother is the cutting action at low speeds. At high speeds, no more than one blade cuts effectively at any one time.

Blade: The projection on the bur head is known as the *blade or the tooth*. This terminates in the cutting edge. It has two surfaces: *the blade face/rake face* and *the blade back/flank/clearance face*. Rake face is the surface of bur blade on the leading edge and clearance face is the surface of the bur blade on the trailing edge.

Rake angle: The rake angle is the most important design characteristic of a bur blade. *It is the angle between the rake face and the radial line (line connecting the centre of the bur and the blade)*. Accordingly, it can be a positive, negative or a zero rake angle (Figs 7.19A to C). A rake angle is negative when the rake face is ahead of the radial line. It is said to be positive when the rake face trails the radial line. A zero rake angle

Table 7.3: Key dimensions and names of recommended burs				
Manufacturer's	*ADA size no.*	*Shape*	*Head diameter (mm)*	*Head length (mm)*
¼	¼	Round	0.50	0.40
½	1/2	Round	0.60	0.48
2	2	Round	1.00	0.80
4	4	Round	1.40	1.10
33S	–	Inverted cone	0.60	0.45
33.5	33.5	Inverted cone	0.60	0.45
169	169	Tapered fissure	0.90	4.3
169	169L	Elongated tapered fissure	0.90	5.6
329	329	Pear normal length	0.70	0.85
330	330	Pear normal length	0.80	1.00
245 =	330L	Pear elongated length	0.80	3.00
271 =	171	Tapered fissure	1.20	4.0
272 =	172	Tapered fissure	1.60	5.0

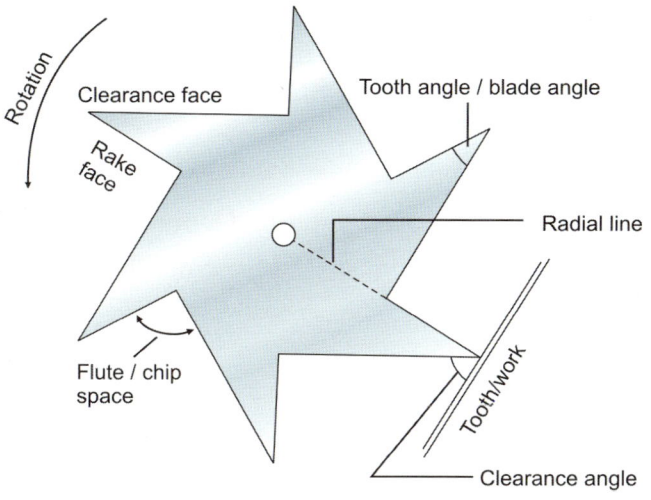

Fig. 7.18: Cross-section of a bur

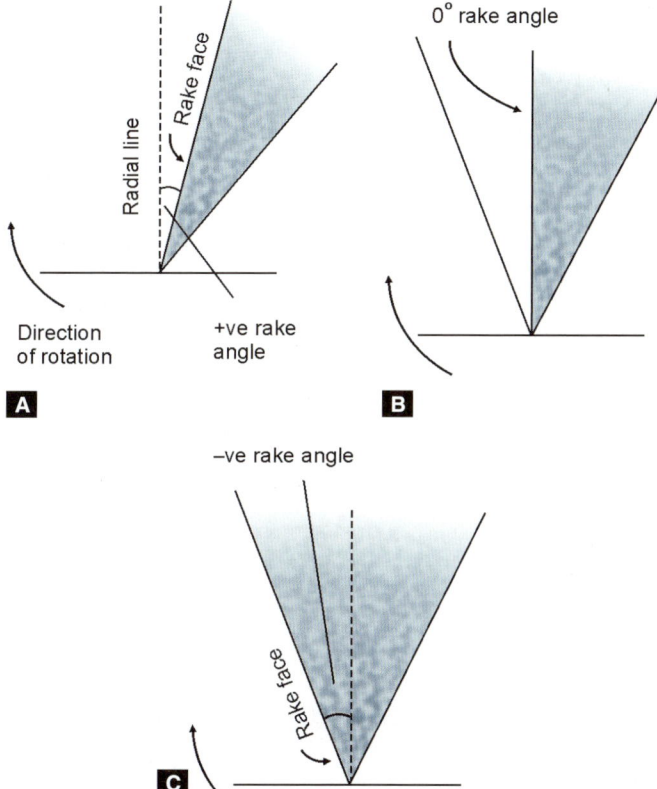

Figs 7.19A to C: **(A)** Positive rake angle; **(B)** Radial rake angle; **(C)** Negative rake angle

also known as the radial rake angle is seen when the rake face and the radial line coincide with each other.

Land: The plane surface immediately following the cutting edge is called the land (Fig. 7.20).

Clearance angle: The angle between the clearance face and the work (e.g. tooth) is called the clearance angle. If a land is present on the bur, the clearance angle is divided into two: primary clearance angle, i.e. the angle between the land and the work and a secondary

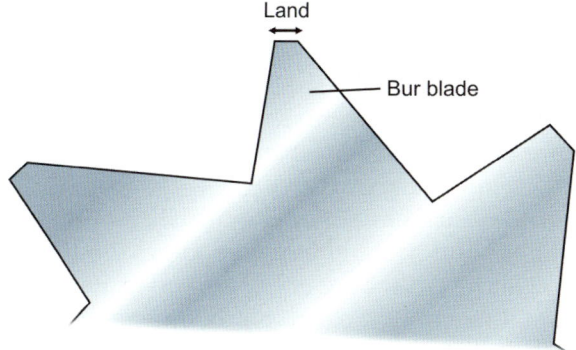

Fig. 7.20: Bur blade with a land

clearance angle, i.e. the angle between the clearance face and the work. If the clearance face is curved, then it is known as the *radial clearance* (Figs 7.21A and B).

Blade angle/tooth angle: It is the angle between the rake face and the clearance face. In case a land is present, it is the angle between the rake face and the land.

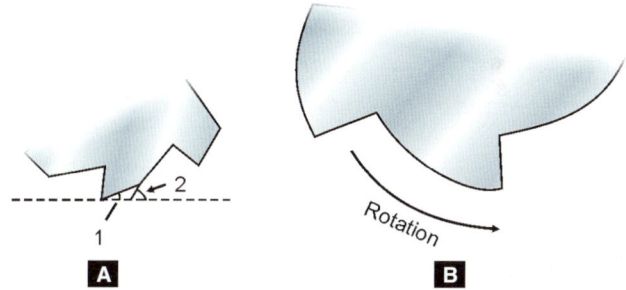

Figs 7.21A and B: **(A)** A land on the bur blade divides the clearance angle into two: (1) primary clearance angle and (2) secondary clearance angle; **(B)** Bur with a curved clearance face is known to have a radial clearance

Factors Influencing the Cutting Effectiveness and Efficiency of a Bur

A large number of factors govern the cutting effectiveness and efficiency of a bur which are as follows:

1. Rake Angle, Clearance Angle and Blade Angle

The more positive the rake angle, the greater is the cutting efficiency of the bur. However, a positive rake angle also has two major drawbacks. (1) It reduces the bulk of the bur blade, as a result the bur tooth can easily curve, flatten or even fracture during use. (2) A positive rake angle produces a chip that is larger and tends to clog the flute space whereas a negative rake angle produces a chip that is smaller and moves away from the blade.

The clearance angle eliminates friction between the cutting edge and the work and prevents the bur from digging excessively into the tooth structure. An increase in the clearance angle, however reduces the blade angle, thereby decreasing the bulk of the bur blade.

Increasing the blade angle reinforces the cutting edge and reduces the chances of the blade edge to fracture. Carbide is brittle, hence requires greater edge angles to minimize fracture.

Carbide burs have blades with slightly negative rake angle and a blade angle of approximately 90°. Their clearance faces are either curved or have a land to provide a small clearance angle near the cutting edge and a greater clearance space.

2. Neck Diameter

A neck that is too small in diameter will result in an instrument unable to resist lateral forces. A large neck on the other hand may interfere with the visibility and restrict access to coolants. As the head of the bur increases in length and diameter, the movement exerted by the lateral forces also increases and the neck needs to be larger.

3. Spiral Angle and Crosscuts

Burs with small spiral angles are preferred at high speeds as small angles produce more efficient cutting (Fig. 7.17).

Crosscuts are notches in the blade edges to increase the cutting effectiveness at low and medium speeds. The greater the length of a blade, greater is the force required to initiate cutting. Crosscuts tend to reduce the total length of the bur blade that is cutting at any one time. This increases the force per unit area and thereby reduces the pressure required to initiate cutting.

As each crosscut blade cuts, it leaves ridges of tooth structure in place of the notches. Because the notches in the two succeeding blades are not in line, ridges left by one blade are removed by the other at low and medium speeds. However, at high speeds, it is usually only one blade that cuts effectively, leaving behind the ridges and hence a rough surface.

4. Concentricity and Run-out

Concentricity is a direct measurement of the symmetry of the bur head. It measures how closely a single circle can be passed through the tips of all the blades. It is an indication as to whether one blade is longer or shorter than the others. It is only a static measurement.

Run-out, on the other hand is a dynamic measurement of the maximum displacement of the bur head from its axis of rotation while the bur runs. The average clinically acceptable run-out is 0.023 mm. Run-out occurs if the head is not in line with the axis of the bur, if the bur neck is bent and even if the bur is not held straight in the handpiece. Run-out tends to increase the vibrations of the bur and also removes excessive amount of tooth structure. Tooth removal with run-out is inefficient, inaccurate and heat generating. Run-out is more important clinically compared to concentricity.

5. Heat treatment

Heat treatment is used to harden a bur made of soft steel. This process preserves the cutting edge and hardens the bur to increase its life. Carbide burs do not require heat treatment.

6. Influence of Load

Load is the force exerted by the operator on the tool head and not the pressure induced in the tooth during cutting. It has been estimated to be in the range of 1000–1500 gms (2-3 pounds) for low rotational speeds and from 60–120 gms (2-4 ounces) for high rotational speeds. The cutting effectiveness of the bur is reduced when the load applied is below the minimum required and also is reduced when the load applied is above the maximum required.

7. Influence of Speed

At a given load, the rate of cutting increases with the rotational speed but not in direct proportion. The rate of cutting is more at speeds above 30,000 rpm than that below this speed. However, it has been found that at speeds greater than 1,50,000 rpm the rate of cutting is nearly the same as at still higher speeds. There is also a minimum rotational speed for a given load below which the tool will not cut.

8. Number of Teeth or Blades

The number of teeth in a dental bur are usually limited to 6–8. Since the external load applied is distributed among the blades, decreasing the number of blades increases the force on one blade and also increases the size of the chip removed. This tends to reduce the clogging tendency since the flute space becomes larger. However, a major drawback with burs having less teeth is that the tendency for bur tooth wear is more and the cutting life is reduced. Also, a fewer number of bur teeth increases the tendency for vibration.

A fissure bur with straight flutes also produces less temperature rise than one with spiral flutes. This may be due to the formation of large chips with the use of a straight fluted bur. Large chips carry away more heat compared to smaller chips.

Polymer Burs

Recently, a novel concept of bur material was proposed with the idea of removing only the infected dentin and not the affected dentin. The SS White (USA) introduced polymer bur (Smart Prep) which has a unique flute design, constructed from a medical grade polyether-ketone-ketone (PEKK) with particular hardness and wear resistance. This enables the bur to remove only soft caries-infected dentin, leaving the caries-affected dentin intact. The bur usually works in slow speed (500–800 rpm) and quickly dulls when encounters the highly calcified caries-affected dentin. The polymer burs are single use, self-limiting instrument, which wears away rather than cutting sound dentin. The operator can feel the resistance of the healthy dentin. The polymer burs elicit no pain, therefore, can be effectively used without anesthesia.

Abrasive Instruments

Abrasive instruments constitute the second major category of rotary cutting instruments. The head of these instruments consists of small angular particles of a hard substance held in a matrix of softer material. This softer matrix that holds the particles together is also called as the *binder*. Different materials used for a binder are ceramic, metal, rubber, shellac, etc. Rubber and shellac wear away easily and hence are used for delicate abrasion like finishing and polishing.

Cutting occurs at a large number of points, where the hard particles protrude from the binder. As the instrument is used, the particles are wrenched away from the binder and new particles then replace the older ones thereby providing a continuous supply of particles. This increases the life of the instrument. Furthermore, the abrasive should be so distributed that the surface of the tool wears away evenly. The wide spacing between the particles prevents the packing or clogging of the resultant debris.

Abrasive instruments can be grouped into diamond abrasives and other abrasives. Diamond instruments have great clinical impact in operative dentistry because of their long life and great effectiveness in cutting enamel and dentin and hence shall be discussed in detail. Other abrasive instruments include use of silicon carbide, boron carbide, aluminium oxide, garnet and sand for producing grinding wheels, discs or stones, etc.

Diamond Abrasive Instruments

Diamond instruments for dental use were introduced in 1942 and became quite popular because of their superior performance. Their preference over tungsten carbide burs is based on their greater resistance to abrasion, lower heat generation and longer life. Diamond instruments consist of three parts: a metal blank, powdered diamond abrasive and a bonding material (Fig. 7.22).

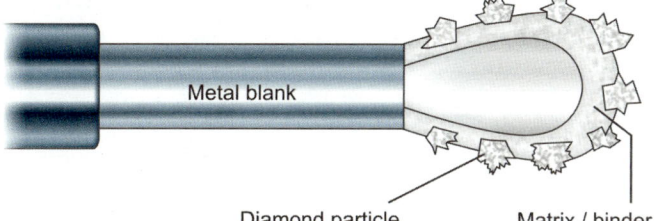

Fig. 7.22: Schematic diagram of dental diamond instrument

The metal blank resembles a bur without blades. Like any other rotary instrument it has the same three essential parts: head, neck and shank. The head of the blank is slightly smaller than the final dimensions of the instrument head. The shape and size of the metal blank controls the shape and size of the finished instrument.

The abrasive diamonds may be natural or synthetic that are crushed to a powder of desired particles, in size and shape. These are manufactured in multiple layers by electrodeposition, sintering or microbrazing and provide a continuous regeneration of the cutting surface as wear occurs.

The bonding agent serves the purpose of holding the abrasive particles together as well as attaches the particles to the metal blank. Ceramic and metals are the most commonly used bonding agents for diamond instruments.

Classification

The various classification systems employed for the burs also hold true for the diamond abrasive instruments. In addition, the latter may also be classified on the basis of the average particle sizes of the abrasive, i.e.
- Coarse grit diamond burs (125–150 μ particle size)
- Medium grit diamond burs (88–125 μ particle size)
- Fine grit diamond burs (60–74 μ particle size)
- Very fine grit diamond burs (38–44 μ particle size)

Head Shapes and Sizes

Diamond instruments are available in a variety of shapes and sizes that correspond to the burs except for the smallest diameter burs (Fig. 7.23). Because of the presence of an abrasive layer on the underlying metal blank, the smallest diamond instrument cannot be as small in diameter as the smallest burs. For a given size and shape, there are as number of further divisions and subdivisions, thereby expanding the list of available abrasive instruments in comparison to the burs. It is also possible to give them any specialized shape for which a blank can be easily manufactured, whereas it would be impractical to cut blades on a similar specialized shape in a bur.

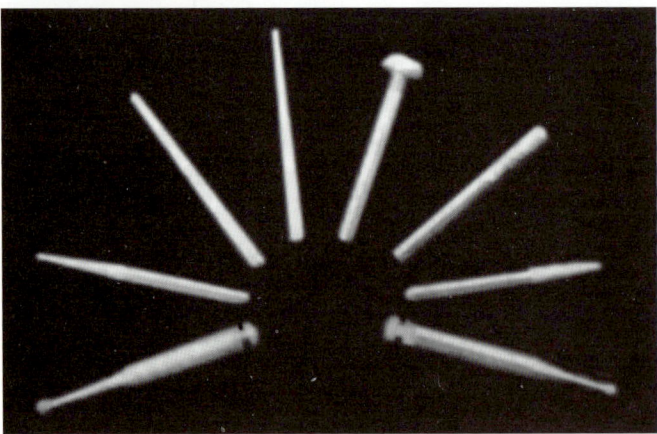

Fig. 7.23: Diamond instruments of varying shapes

Due to the lack of any standard and uniform nomenclature for diamond instruments, it becomes necessary to select them visually to obtain the desired shape and size; and mention the catalogue number when describing it.

Factors Influencing the Abrasive Efficiency and Effectiveness

The clinical performance of diamond abrasive instruments depends upon a number of factors, few of which are cited below:

1. *Size of the abrasive particles*: The larger the size of the particles, deeper is the penetration on the surface of the work; hence rapid removal of material occurs with coarse grit burs compared to medium or fine grit burs. However, Siegel et al (1996) found no statistically significant difference in the cutting efficiencies of coarse and medium grit burs from the same manufacturer.
2. *Shape of the abrasive particles*: The abrasive particles should be irregular in shape for greater efficiency. Irregular particles will present a sharp edge whereas round smooth particles or cubical particles will present a flat face to the work. Hence, the former cuts better.
3. *Density of the abrasive particles*: Density of the particles refers to the number of abrasive particles per unit area. In instruments with high density the particles are closely spaced whereas in those with low density the particles are widely spaced. Therefore, at constant loads, a greater force will be exerted on each particle of the substrate, when the particles are widely spaced increasing the grinding efficiency. Coarse grit burs have a low density compared to fine grit burs.

   In a study conducted by Grajower et al (1979), it was found that the grinding rate of the burs with particles densities higher than 60 diamonds/mm^2 remained constant after four minutes of use whereas it continued to decrease for burs with lower densities. The low density burs may have decreasing grinding rate because of the deeper penetration of their diamonds into enamel causing early particle dislodgement.
4. *Hardness of the abrasive particles*: For the bur to be efficient, the hardness of the abrasive particle should be greater than the hardness of the work on which it is to be used. Only then can the abrasive indent the surface and remove the material.
5. *Clogging of the abrasive surface*: Clogging of the spaces between the particles by grinding debris effects grinding because this partially blocks the penetration of the abrasive particles into the surface. Clogging is enhanced when the particles are close together and if 'undercuts' are present on the protruding part of the particle. Use of coolants during grinding may wash away the debris and prevent clogging. Hence cleaning is always recommended after each use of bur.

   Microscopic observations suggest that debris accumulation may be more detrimental to cutting efficiency than are wear and diamond chip loss from the bur surface.
6. *Speed and pressure*: The same factors are involved here as discussed with the bladed burs. Proper speed and pressure are the major factors determining the life of a bur. The usual cause of failure of abrasive instruments is when excessive pressure is applied on to them to increase their cutting rate at inadequate speeds. This results in the loss of diamonds decreasing their cutting efficiency.
7. *Miscellaneous*: These include many uncontrolled operating parameters like individual dental techniques, differences in dental hard tissues, rotation speed, turbine air pressure, differences in handpieces, etc. Lateral stresses on the bond between the abrasive particles and the instrument increase with the velocity of the particles, their penetration into the substrate and the resistance of the substrate to abrasion. Also, lateral forces are larger if the crystal particles are oriented with facets parallel to the ground surface or perpendicular to the direction of motion than with sharp cutting edges in that direction.

Disposable Diamond Abrasives

The Centres for Disease Control and Prevention clearly state that all dental instruments that penetrate soft or hard tissues or come into contact with the oral tissues must be sterilized after each use to prevent cross contamination (Fig. 7.24). However, for dental burs, the multistep debriding, cleaning and sterilization procedures are time consuming. The

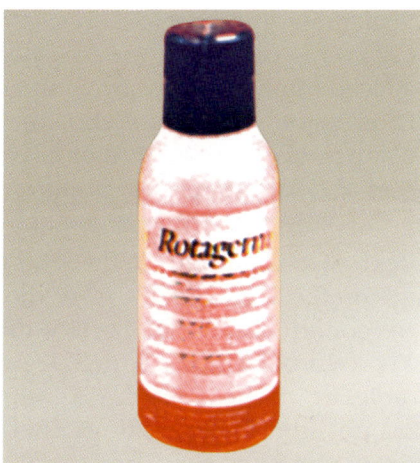

Fig. 7.24: Solution used for disinfection and cleaning of burs

"single patient use" or disposable diamond bur is a recent introduction that minimizes the risk of cross contamination of blood-borne pathogens at an equal cost. Some of the disposable diamond burs are marketed as Cobra, Monosteryl, Neo, Patriot, SS White and Spring. The disposable burs have an added advantage that a new, sharp cutting instrument is provided for every patient.

Siegel et al (1996) in their study measured the cutting experiences of 15 types of conventional and disposable round and tapered diamond burs. The results showed comparable cutting efficiencies between the two; and hence the use of disposable burs could reduce the risk of clinical cross infection.

Other Abrasive Instruments

Many types of abrasive instruments other than the normally used diamonds are used in dentistry. They are used for shaping, finishing and polishing restorations both in the clinic and in the laboratory. The cutting surfaces of the head are composed of abrasive particles held in a continuous matrix of softer material. They can be of two types: moulded abrasives and the coated abrasives.

Moulded abrasive instruments have heads manufactured by moulding or pressing a uniform mixture of abrasive and matrix around the roughened end of the shank. The abrasive is distributed throughout the matrix such that new particles are exposed by continual wear. Rigid moulded instruments have rigid polymer or ceramic as their matrix. These are used for grinding and sharpening procedures. Soft moulded instruments use flexible matrix materials, such as rubber to hold the abrasive. These are used for finishing and polishing procedures. The mounted heads are termed as points or stones. Unmounted discs or wheelstones are also available that can be attached to a mandrel with a screw.

Coated abrasive instruments are mostly discs which have a thin layer of abrasive cemented to a flexible backing. This allows the instrument to confirm to the surface contour of a tooth or restoration. Unlike the moulded instruments, coated abrasives have to be discarded once they wear off. They are used in the finishing of enamel walls of cavity preparations as well as finishing of restorations.

Materials: The matrix materials are usually resins or rubber. A rubber matrix provides a flexible head on instruments and is used for polishing. A harder, nonflexible rubber matrix is often used for silicon carbide discs. The abrasive may be either sintered to the matrix or resin bonded.

The abrasives used may be natural or synthetic including silicon carbide, aluminium oxide, garnet, quartz, pumice, cuttle bone, etc.

Different Methods of Cutting

Cutting can be measured in terms of effectiveness and efficiency. *Cutting effectiveness is the rate of removal of tooth structure in mm/min or mg/sec.* Effectiveness does not include side effects such as heat or noise. *Cutting efficiency is the percentage of energy which produces cutting.* Cutting efficiency is decreased when some amount of energy is wasted as heat or noise. Increase in rotational speed increases both effectiveness and efficiency but also associated with it are disadvantages like more heat, noise and vibration.

Rotary instruments can cut by two mechanisms, bladed cutting and abrasive cutting *Blade cutting refers to the use of a bladed instrument or cutting by any instrument in a blade like fashion.* For the blade to cut, it must be sharp, have higher hardness and modulus of elasticity than the material being cut and be applied with force. The sheared segments form a distorted layer that moves up the rake face until it breaks or until the blade disengages from the surface as it rotates. These chips then accumulate in the clearance space between the flutes until they are washed away or removed by centrifugal force.

A lot of heat is produced with the use of these bladed burs. Distortion of the tooth structure which occurs ahead of the blade produces heat. Frictional heat is also produced by the chips rubbing against the rake face and that of the blade tip against the cut surface of the tooth.

Abrasive cutting or grinding the use of bonded or coated abrasive instruments for removing small particles of the substrate. Grinding instruments contain randomly arranged abrasive particles that are very sharp and tend to have large negative rake angles.

When these instruments are used on ductile substrates, some part may be removed as chips and some part may flow laterally around the cutting tip forming ridges. Repeated deformation produces work hardening and finally the distorted material becomes brittle, breaks off and is removed. This type of cutting is less efficient than that of a blade and hence burs are preferred for cutting ductile materials such as dentin. Abrasive instruments are most efficient when used to cut brittle materials such as enamel.

Cutting with Burs or Diamonds

Advantages

- It is a familiar and well known procedure.
- Precision is obtained, i.e. margins are clearly identifiable.
- It is easy to control the cutting.
- The practitioner has tactile perception of the extent of cutting.
- Debris can be removed by water and use of suction.
- Practitioner's vision while cutting is relatively good.

Disadvantages

- Cutting with these instruments usually causes pain.
- Vibration caused by cutting usually cracks or fractures tooth structure.
- Noise produced with their use is objectionable.
- Constant use and sterilization can cause them to breakdown.
- Dull burs produce lot of heat and potential pulp damage.
- Overcutting is easy if the operator loses control or the patient moves inadvertently.

Patient and Operator Positions

Along with the discussion of cutting instruments, instrument grasps and manipulation, the position of the dental chair and patient and the position the operator assumes when working should be considered. The knowledge of patient and operating position is essential for the welfare of both the patient and the operator.

The dentist should maintain proper position and posture during treatment because (i) it has a definitive bearing on the correct performance of his operations, (ii) it affects the comfort and cooperation of the patient (iii) it influences the health of the operator, the operator is less likely to get strain, fatigue, be more efficient and less chances of getting musculoskeletal disorders.

Position of Dental Chair and Patient

The adjustment of dental chair is an important consideration. If the chair is incorrectly placed the accuracy, exactness and precision necessary to the performance of the operation are lessened and the patient is placed in an unnecessarily, uncomfortable position. Thus not only the cooperation of the patient is lost but also actual interferences may be established.

McGhee et al (1956) states two important reasons for placing the patient correctly in the dental chair:

1. Comfort of the patient: When the patient is sitting comfortably, he will relax more readily and his confidence in the operator grows more quickly–two conditions which are extremely desirable.
2. Proper position for operating: This is for the benefit of the operator. The operation can be completed more accurately, swiftly and easily when access to the field of operation is good.

   Modern dental chairs are designed to provide total body support and comfort in any position. These chairs rely on raising, lowering and letting the backrest or the entire chair for position accommodation. The letting of backrest only causes sliding of the patient in the chair which does not happen when both the backrest and seat are moved together in the recent programmable chairs.

While seating the patient in the chair the following points should be kept in mind in relation to dental chair:

- Before the patient is brought into the operatory to be seated any mobile equipment or moveable appliances should be moved out of the way to afford the patient direct access to the chair and without twisting, turning, bending, stooping, etc. to get himself seated.
- The height should be low, the backrest upright and the armrest adjusted to allow the patient to get into the chair. After patient is seated the armrest is positioned to its normal position.
- The adjustable headrest cushion or on articulating headrest attached to the chair back is positioned to support the head and elevate the chin slightly away from the chest. In this position neck muscle strain is at a minimum and swallowing is easiest. The chair is then adjusted to place the patient in recline position.
- The patient should be lowered to position that places the treatment site as close as to the dentist's elbow level as possible.
- The chair design should provide access and maximum working area to the operator.
- It should be placed at convenient position with adjustable control switches.
- The chairs equipped with programmable operating positions are preferred. To improve

Instruments, Instrumentation and Sterilization

infection control, chair with a foot switches for patient positioning are recommended.

The most common patient positions for restorative dental procedures are (i) upright position (ii) almost supine (iii) recline 45 degree however, the choice of patient position varies with the operator, the type of procedure and the area of mouth involved in the operation.

In almost supine position, the patient's head, knees and feet are approximately at same level. Patient head should not be lower than the feet except in case of when the patient is in syncope (Fig. 7.25).

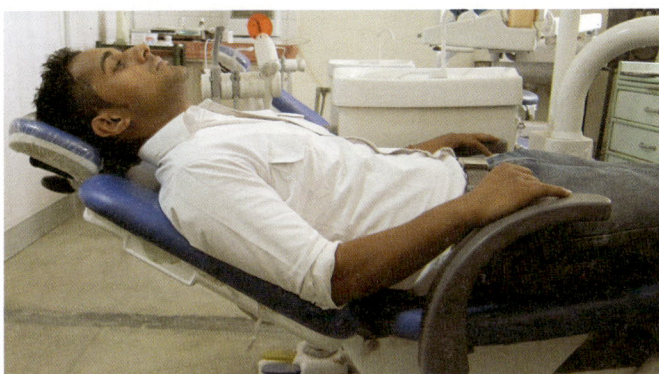

Fig. 7.25: Supine position

In reclined 45 degree position the chair is reclined at 45 degree. Consequently, mandibular occlusal surfaces are almost at 45° to the floor (Fig. 7.26).

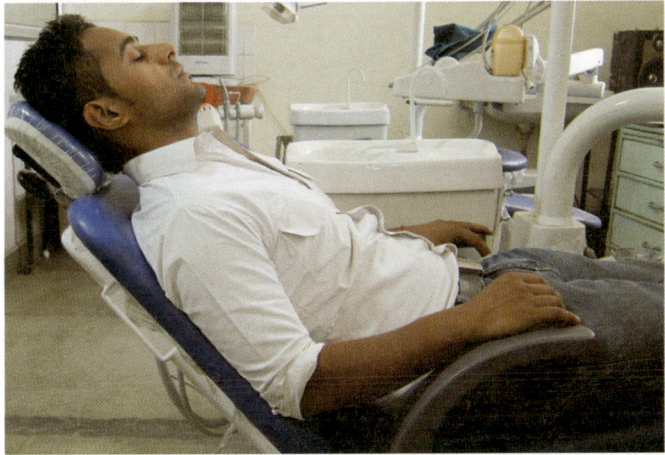

Fig. 7.26: Recline position

As a rule, when operating in the maxillary arch the maxillary occlusal surfaces should be oriented approximately perpendicular to the floor and the mandibular arch the mandibular occlusal surfaces should be almost at 45° to the floor.

After the operation is completed the chair should be brought back to the upright position and chair height should be lowered so that the patient can leave the dental chair easily, gracefully and preventing undue strain or loss of balance.

Operating Positions

Fundamental operating positions may be explained by the location of the operator in relation to patient position. For right-handed operator there are essentially three positions–right front, right and right rear and the extent reverse should be applied for the left handed operators. A four position direct rear has also been used for certain areas of the mouth. For better understanding, sitting positions of operator are related to the clock. In this clock concept, an imaginary circle is drawn over the dental chair, keeping the patient head at the centre of the circle. Then the numbering to circle is given similar to clock with the top of the circle at 12 o' clock. Accordingly, the operator's positions (right-handed operator) can be 7 o'clock (right front), 9 o'clock (right), 11 o'clock (right rear) and 12 o'clock (direct rear). For left handed operator it can be 5 o'clock (left front), 3 o'clock (left) and 1 o'clock (left rear). All of these positions may also be used for the standing positions of the operator.

Right front Position

The operator assumes a position next to the chair arm and direct access to the teeth. This position facilitates examination and work on (i) mandibular anterior teeth, (ii) mandibular posterior teeth on right side and (iii) maxillary anterior teeth. The pen grasp is the fundamental grasp for this position. To increase ease and visibility, the patient's head may be turned towards the operator.

Right Position

Here the operator sits exactly right to the patient (Fig. 7.27) . This position is convenient for working on (i) facial surfaces of maxillary right posterior teeth,

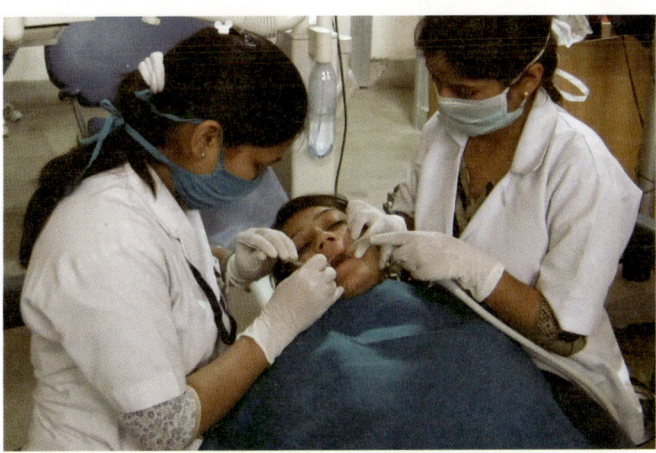

Fig. 7.27: Right position

(ii) Facial surfaces of mandibular right posterior teeth and (iii) the occlusal surfaces of the mandibular right posterior teeth. The pen grasp is used from this side.

Right Rear Position

This is the position of choice for most operations. Most areas of mouth are accessible from this position either using direct or indirect vision. Here the operator is behind and slightly to the right of the patient (Fig. 7.28). The left arm is positioned around the patient's head when working from this position the areas included are (i) Palatal and incisal (occlusal) surfaces of maxillary teeth, and (ii) Mandibular teeth especially on the left side. Direct vision may be used on these teeth, however, the use of mirror will improve the visibility with the reflection of light and retraction.

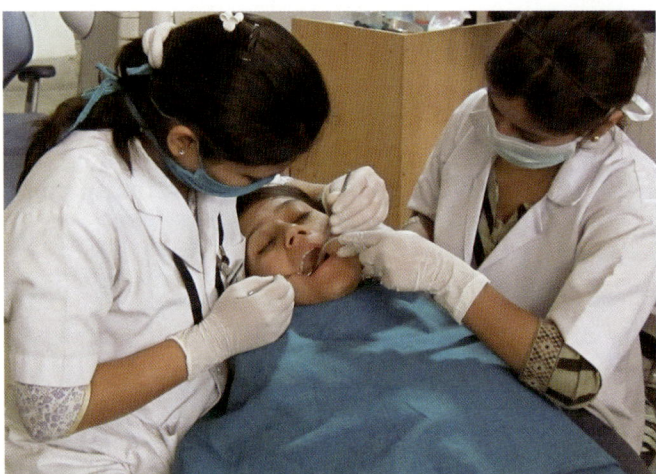

Fig. 7.28: Right rear position

Direct Rear

This position has limited application. Here the operator sits directly behind the patient and looks down over the head of the patient during procedure. This position is used for operating on lingual surfaces of mandibular anterior teeth. In the maxillary arch some direct vision but mainly mirror is used for the preparation (Fig. 7.29).

Operating Stools

There are various varieties of the stools available for dentist and assistant in the market. The features required for operating stools should be : (i) It should be on casters for mobility (ii) be sturdy and well balanced, (iii) The seat should be round, well padded with smooth cushion edges and adjustable up and down (iv) The backrest should be adjustable forward, backward as well as up and down along with full back support. The assistant's stool should have a foot ring for footrest. Operator stools do not have a footrest.

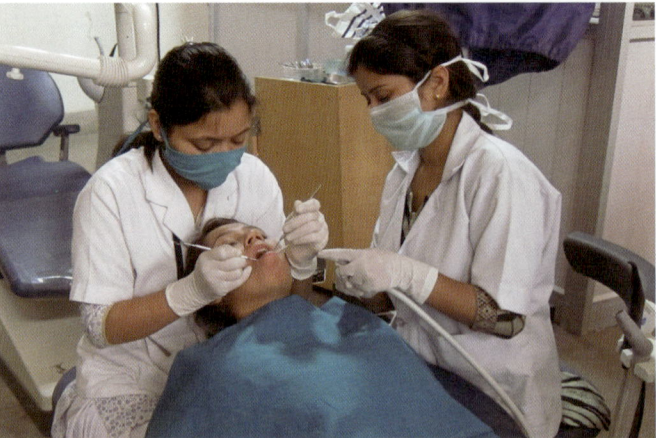

Fig. 7.29: Direct rear position

Some operator and assistant stools have backrest with curved extensions that offer additional body support. Comfortable, well-designed stools help to reduce tension and fatigue.

Position and Operator

Dental practice is a sedentary occupation and frequently produces great strain on the physical and nerve forces of its devotees. Every effort should be made to eliminate unnecessary strain and to keep the natural forces of the body at the highest state of efficiency through adopting correct posture at the chair avoiding eyestrain and eliminating all deteriorating forces likely to reduce nerve power and physical endurance. Usually sitting position is preferred in modern dentistry to relieve stress on operator's legs and support his back.

The correct position of operator for examining and operating the teeth may be described as follows:
- The operator should sit back on the cushion, using the entire seat and not just the front edge. The upper body should be positioned so that the spinal column is straight or bent slightly forward and supported by the backrest of the steel.
- The back and chest are held in upright position with the shoulders squared to promote circulation and proper breathing. Position that create any unnecessary curvature of the spine or slumping of the shoulders should be avoided.
- The thighs should be parallel to the floor and lower legs perpendicular to the floor. Feet should be flat on the floor. If the seat is too high, its front edge will cut off circulation to the user's legs. This ideal position cannot be maintained at all times, however, it should be used as much as possible.
- Operator should breathe deeply slowly and naturally through nose avoiding inhaling the patient's breath or exhaling into patient's face.

- The points of bodily contact with the patient should be as few as possible. Dentist should not rest forearms on the patient's shoulders and hands on the face of the patient.
- Proper working distance, similar to that for book reading should be maintained during dental procedures. This will lead to increased cooperation and confidence.
- When the patient is properly positioned, the distance between eyes of the dentist and working field should be 12″-14″, however, small, detailed or inaccessible tooth preparations may require closer proximity for adequate visibility.
- Dentist should not use patient's chest as instrument trolly.
- Patient's head can be rotated backward, forward or from side-to-side for operator's ease, access and visibility while doing work. Sacrificing good operating posture should be avoided.
- Operator should leave left hand free during most of dental procedures for retraction using mouth mirrors or fingers of left hand.
- Operator when operating for an extended period, change in position for a short time reduces muscle strain and lesser fatigue.

Position of Assistant

- The selected position for the assistant is essentially the same as for the operator, except that the stool is 4 to 6 inches high for maximal visual access.
- Assistant should sit as close as possible to back of the patient's chain with feet directed towards the head of the chair and in erect position with parallel thighs and feet firmly placed on foot support ring at the base of the assistant stool. These positions can be adjusted according to specific needs.
- The instrument tray should be placed towards the head of the patient's chair and positioned to allow easy access to the instruments and materials. When properly seated, both the operator and assistant will be able to provide service for at least 8 hours a day with a minimum of strain and fatigue over a period of many years.

Instrument Exchange

For right handed dentist there are four zones of working area, i.e. (i) Operator's zone (lies between 7 o'clock to 12 o'clock), (ii) Assistant's zone (between 2 to 4 o'clock), (iii) Static zone (between 12 to 2 o'clock) and (iv) Transfer/exchange zone (between 4 to 7 o'clock). The transfer of instrument between the operator and assistant should occur in the exchange zone below the patient's chin and several inches above the patient's chest. Instrument should not be exchanged over the patient's face.

All instruments and materials are located in the assistant's zones. Static zone is a non-traffic area where other equipments can be placed when an object or material is heavy or dangerous if held near the patient's face, it should be passed through the static zone.

To increase efficiency, and reduce stress and fatigue of dentist and assistant there should be cooperation from both side. The assistant should know the sequence of treatment steps and have the required instruments and materials ready at the proper time. Assistant should be ready to pass the next instrument and receive the used one in a smooth motion. The assistant should take the instrument from the operator rather than operator dropping in assistant's hand. Instrument should be arranged in orderly fashion for comfortable exchange.

Magnification

Another important aspect of the restorative procedure for increasing efficiency and visibility is magnification of working area. Several types of magnification devices, i.e. Loupes, surgical telescopes, and bifocal eye glasses are available which increases visibility and provides protection to eye from injury.

STERILIZATION OF INSTRUMENTS

The importance of aseptic techniques using sterilized instruments, disinfectant solutions, etc. coupled with other barriers, has long been emphasized. Unless the instruments and equipments are properly sterilized, a variety of saliva and blood-borne pathogens can easily travel from patient to patient. Thus it becomes mandatory for dental personnels to employ effective methods of sterilization and infection control to deliver quality healthcare.

Terminology

Sterilization: Sterilization is defined as the process by which an article, surface or medium is freed of all living micro-organisms either in vegetative or spore state.

Disinfection: Disinfection is the removal or destruction of any micro-organism capable of causing infection.

Three levels of disinfections are differentiated depending on the type and form of micro-organisms destroyed:

i. ***High level disinfection:*** A process that can kill some, but not necessarily all bacterial spores. It is tuberculocidal, and if the disinfectant is capable of destroying bacterial spores, it is labeled sporicidal.

ii. ***Intermediate level disinfection:*** A process that is capable of killing *mycobacterium tuberculosis*, HBV and HIV. It may not be capable of killing bacterial spores.

iii. ***Low level disinfection:*** A process that kills most bacteria, some fungi and some viruses. It does not kill *M. tuberculosis* or bacterial spores.

Antisepsis: Antisepsis is a measure used to prevent infection by inhibiting growth of micro-organisms in wounds or tissues. An antiseptic is an agent that inhibits the growth of micro-organisms on living surfaces.

Categorization of Dental Instruments and other Commonly used Items

The instruments have been categorized depending on their contact with different tissues to determine what type of sterilization or disinfection is required.

The categories are as follows:

1. ***Critical items:*** Instruments which touch sterile areas of the body or enter the vascular system and those that penetrate the oral mucosa, e.g. curettes, burs, files and scalpels. Because of their potential for harboring micro-organisms, dental handpieces must also be sterilized. Instruments in this category must be sterilized and stored in appropriate packages. Single use items must be properly discarded.
2. ***Semi-critical items:*** Instruments which touch mucous membranes but don't penetrate tissues come under this category. This includes amalgam condensers, saliva ejectors, etc. These items should be sterilized; however if this is not feasible, high-level disinfection or disposal is required.
3. ***Non-critical items:*** This includes those items that don't come in contact with the oral mucosa but are touched by saliva or blood contaminated hands while treating patients. Such items include light switches, countertops and drawer pulls or cabinets. These areas should be properly disinfected.

The relation between type of item and its decontamination is tabulated in Table 7.4

Processing of instruments and equipments prior to sterilization includes cleaning, rinsing, drying and packaging of instruments and assessment of sterilization unit through chemical and biological indicators before the instruments are being sterilized.

PRESOAKING AND CLEANING

Presoaking of contaminated instruments keeps them wet until a thorough cleaning can be done. This prevents drying of blood, saliva and debris on instruments and facilitates cleaning.

Manual Cleaning/Hand Scrubbing

- Use stiff nylon cleaning brushes
- Use only neutral pH detergents
- Brush delicate instruments carefully and if possible, separate them from general instruments.
- Make sure that the instrument surfaces are visibly clean and free from stains and tissues
- Heavy utility gloves should be worn while processing contaminated instruments

Mechanical Devices

Ultrasonic Cleaner

Ultrasonic cleaning systems (Fig. 7.30) fare better than hand scrubbing as they can remove even dried blood and saliva. Moreover, this allows instruments to be cleaned with minimal chance of exposure to body fluids through cuts and punctures and hence, is safer.

Chemicals in the Ultrasonic Bath Solution

- Alkaline Phosphatase Enzyme
- Buffer (7.0–10.0 pH)
- Glycine
- De ionized water
- Magnesium chloride
- Phosphatase substrate
- Potassium chloride
- Potassium phosphate (monobasic)

Table 7.4: Relation between type of item and its decontamination

Disposable items	Non-critical items	Semi-critical items	Critical items
Dispose	Clean ↓ Low level disinfection ↓ Dry and store	Clean ↓ High level disinfection or sterilization ↓ Dry and store	Clean ↓ Sterilization ↓ Dry and store

Instruments, Instrumentation and Sterilization

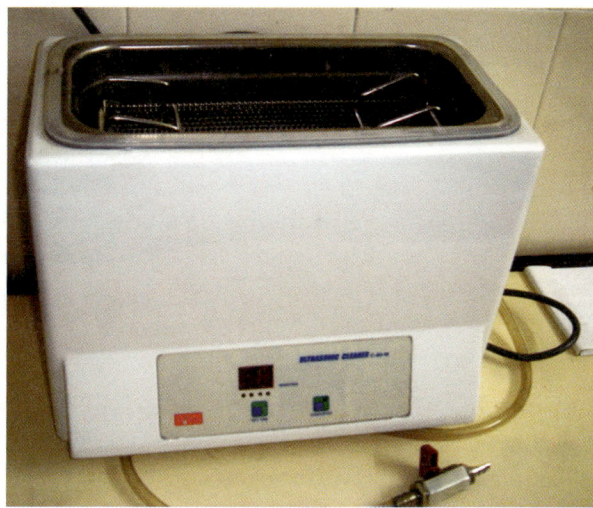

Fig. 7.30: Ultrasonic cleaner

- Sodium chloride
- Sodium hydroxide (10N)
- Sodium phosphate, dibasic
- Zinc chloride

An ultrasonic cleaning device should provide fast and thorough cleaning without damage to instruments, have a lid, a well designed basket and an audible timer and be engineered to prevent electronic interferences with other electronic equipment and office communication systems.

Washer Disinfector

This is an upcoming method for cleaning and disinfection. Physical cleaning due to high flow of water, in terms of both volume and pressure, spraying over all items results in effective mechanical cleaning. Temperature is maintained to a point below 45°C to avoid any protein coagulation during the flushing stage.

Disinfection Stage

It is the heat disinfection process, wherein temperature of water is elevated gradually to almost its boiling point.
a. Initial microbial activation phase (temperature 45°–52°C); endospores germinate and enter negative phase.
b. Microbial inactivation phase (temperature 85°–95°C); pathogenic micro-organisms are inactivated or killed. Spores already entered into germinative phase are also killed here (indirectly sporicidal).

Requirements of Detergent Used in Washer Disinfector

- Anti-lipid action at high temperature
- Anti-protein action at low temperature
- Enzymatic action

- Likewise temperature, contact time is also a crucial factor. Lower disinfection temperature requires longer contact times (disinfection phase)

Disadvantages

The problem lies in maintaining the disinfection as the products are obtained in a wet and unwrapped state.

Enzyme Cleaners

Enzymes are powerful tools for cleaning reusable instruments. A properly selected enzyme cleaner can facilitate much of the pre cleaning work and improve effectiveness. The key to effectiveness, however, is the selection of the proper enzymatic product.

Enzymes accelerate the chemical reactions of the biological processes and are very specific in their catalytic behavior such that a protease will work only on proteins. Some enzymes are even more specific and will work on specific proteins while others will work on a broad spectrum of proteins, e.g. Klenzymer cleaners.

Since the enzymes normally used in instruments cleaning formulations do not attack metals; they are well suited for cleaning many reusable devices.

Other Ingredients

Many other compounds are put into the cleaning product to enhance effectiveness, stability and fragrance or color.

For a surgical cleaning process, Protease formulas have been optimized to attack the proteins normally found in medical soils. For surgical procedures that result in fatty soils, such as orthopedic surgery, a Lipase formula (such as Adi-enzyme) for instrument cleaning is best.

Disadvantages

- Corrosion, rust, discoloration, swelling, staining and loss of elasticity are just a few of the problems that can be caused by use of incompatible enzyme compounds.
- Enzyme cleaner contains proteins in the form of enzymes. If these cling to instrument surface, they can interfere with terminal sterilization process by hiding bacterial contamination. Chemical residues may not be removed in the sterilization process, so the next patient will be exposed to the cleaning product.

PACKAGING

After cleaned instruments have been rinsed and dried, they are to be packaged in functional sets before sterilization. This packaging protects the instruments from contamination after sterilization and before use at chair-side. A variety of packaging materials are available, with self-sealing, paper-plastic, peel pouches being the most convenient (Table 7.5).

METHODS OF STERILIZATION

The classification of sterilizing agents is tabulated in Table 7.6.

A. PHYSICAL METHOD

Heat

Dry Heat

Dry heat kills by protein denaturation, oxidative damage and the toxic effect of elevated levels of electrolytes. Examples are tabulated in Table 7.6.

Table 7.5: Sterilizing method of packaging material	
Sterilizing method	*Packaging material*
Steam	Paper/plastic pouches, Nylon type plastic tubing, sterilization paper, wrapped cassettes, thin clothes
Chemical vapour	Paper/plastic pouches, sterilization paper
Dry heat	Dry heat type nylon plastic tubing, sterilization paper

Thermal death time: The minimum time required to kill a suspension of organisms at a predetermined temperature in a specified environment.

Table 7.6: Classification of sterilizing agents		
Physical	*Chemical*	*Radiation*
Dry Heat	**Chemiclave alcohols**	**Non-ionizing**
• Flaming/Burning	• Ethanol	• Infrared
• Hot air oven	• Sopropanol	• Microwave
• Glass bead sterilizer	**Aldehydes**	
• Hot salt sterilizer	• Formaldehyde	
• Microwave	• Gultaraldehyde	
	• Ortho-phthaldehyde	
Moist Heat	**Phenols**	**Ionizing**
• Temperature below 100°C (Pasteurization)	• Cresol	• Gamma rays
• Temperature at 100°C (Boiling)	• Chlorophenol	• Ultraviolet
• Steam at atmospheric pressure (Steaming)	• Carbolic acid	
• Steam under pressure (Autoclave)		
	Chlorhexidine	
Filtration	**Halogens**	
• Diatomaceous earth	• Chlorine	
• Asbestos pads	• Iodine	
• Porcelain membranes	**Dyes**	
Cold	• Aniline	
Desiccation	• Acridine	
Sunlight	**Metallic agents**	
	• Mercurial compound	
	• Surfacine	
	Gases	
	• Ethyleneoxide	
	• Formaldehyde	
	• Betapropiolactone (BPL)	
	Miscellaneous	
	• Plasma gas sterilization	
	• Performic acid	
	• Superdioxide water	

i. *Flaming/burning:* The instruments like scissors, tweezers, scalpels, needles, etc. are usually sterilized by this method. The instrument to be sterilized is dipped in alcohol (3 parts of ethyl alcohol and 1 part formalin) and passed over the flame 2-3 times. It is not considered an effective method of sterilization (Fig. 7.31)
ii. *Hot air oven:* Hot air oven can be used to sterilize glassware, forceps, scissors, scalpels and swabs. *Cotton, rubber instruments, gloves, etc. cannot be sterilized.*

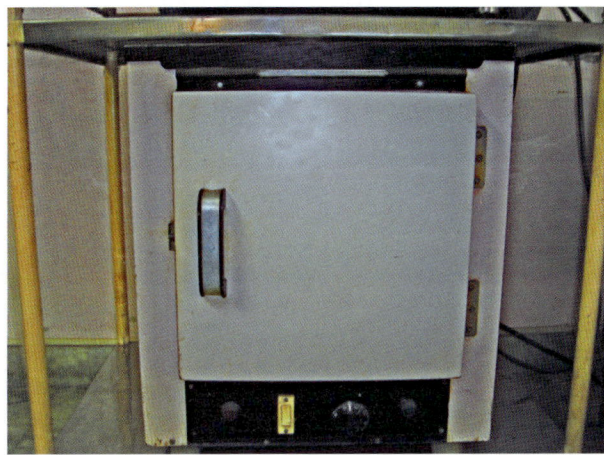

Fig. 7.32: Hot air oven

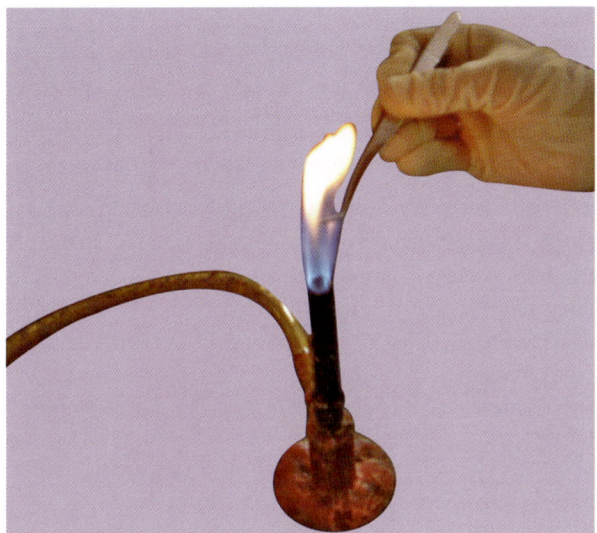

Fig. 7.31: Flaming

The recommendations for conventional hot air oven holding period temperatures are:

150°C two hours (cutting instruments)
160°C 45 minutes for unwrapped and 60 minutes for wrapped instruments.
170°C 18 minutes
180°C 7.5 minutes
190°C 1.5 minutes

The oven must be cooled slowly for about two hours before operating the door. Hot air is a bad conductor of heat and its penetrating power is low. The oven must be fitted with a fan for even distribution of air and elimination of air pockets. It should not be overloaded and the materials should be so arranged as to allow free circulation of air in between (Fig. 7.32).

New 'Rapid Heat-transfer units' are being used:
- The Cox unit by Alpha Scientific
- The Guardian 2000 by Dentronix

iii. *Glass bead sterilizer:* It is a heat transfer device using glass beads as a medium to sterilize instruments. Glass beads should be less than 1.0 mm in size because larger beads are not effective in transferring heat due to large air spaces between the beads. The instruments to be sterilized are immersed into the heated-up glass beads (temperature 218°C-280°C) and left for a specific period of time (Fig. 7.33).

The time specified for each instrument:
- Root canal instruments : 5 seconds
- Absorbent points (butt end first) and cotton pellets: 10 seconds
- Long handled instruments, tips of cotton pliers, blades of scissors : 5 seconds

iv. *Hot salt sterilizer:* Hot salt sterilizer uses table salt in place of glass beads and molten metal as heat transferring agent. It is used to sterilize absorbent points broaches, files, reamers and other root canal instruments.

The instruments desired to be sterilized are put into the sterilizer and left for a period of time, specific for

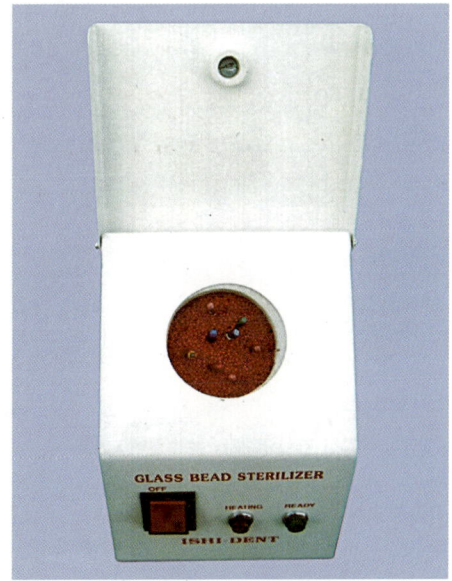

Fig. 7.33: Glass bead sterilizer

that instrument. Hottest part of the salt bath is along the outer rim, starting at the bottom. Immerse instrument at least a quarter inch below salt's surface and in the peripheral area. It consists of a metal cup in which table salt is kept at a temperature of 425°F–475°F (218°C–246°C).

Advantages
- Use of table salt (readily available)
- Table salt does not cling to the wet instruments, as glass beads and molten metal do.
- Cost effective

Both glass bead sterilizer and hot salt sterilizer are considered to be an auxiliary method of sterilization only, as they have been proved inefficient in killing spores.

v. *Microwave sterilization:* Microwave energy has been utilized in the past as a means of sterilizing food products, etc. Microwave sterilization of dental instruments could not become popular because the metals are heated slightly by microwaves, unless they happen to be magnetic. An auxiliary heat source is required that should be capable of direct interactions with the microwaves in order to produce heat, which in turn will sterilize the instruments. The metallic instruments, under microwave develop a corona discharge or arc, which can melt the instrument tips, if placed together.

The microwaves have been used to vaporize the liquid sterilant and the instruments are exposed to either vaporized sterilant alone or both the microwave and the vaporized sterilant. The instruments are placed in a pressurized atmosphere. Alternatively instruments can directly be exposed to microwaves in microwave oven. The drawbacks of this procedure are (i) the instruments need to be rotated three-dimensionally (ii) microwave absorbers are required within the oven to prevent arcing.

Advantages of Dry heat
- Maintenance of sharp edges of the cutting instruments. Practically, dry heat is the best method for sterilization of burs.
- No corrosion of instruments.
- Less expensive than steam autoclaves.
- Industrial forced draft ovens usually provide a larger capacity at a reasonable price.
- Rapid cycles possible at high temperature.
- Packs are dry after cycle.

Disadvantages of Dry heat
- Prolonged sterilization time is required because of poor heat conduction by air and poor penetration properties of dry heat.
- High temperature may damage more heat sensitive items such as rubber or plastic goods.
- Sterilization cycles are prolonged at lower temperatures.
- Heavy loads of instruments, crowding of packs and heavy wrapping easily defeat sterilization.

Caution
- Instruments should be pre-dried
- Instruments should not be added during the sterilization cycle.

Moist Heat

Moist heat kills by denaturation and coagulation of protein. The advantage of steam lies in the latent heat liberated when it condenses on a cooler surface, raising the temperature of that surface. In a complete moisture free atmosphere, bacteria are most resistant to heat (because oxidation of cell contents requires much higher temperatures than that needed for coagulation of proteins).

Following procedures are usually employed:

i. *Temperature below 100°C:* It is used for pasteurization of milk. Either 63°C for 30 minutes (holder method) or 72°C for 15–20 seconds (flash process) followed by cooling rapidly to 13°C or lower. All non-sporing pathogens are destroyed. Vaccines or non-sporing bacteria are heat inactivated at 60°C for one hour in vaccine baths. Serums or body fluids containing coagulable proteins can be sterilized by heating for one hour at 56°C in water bath on several successive days. *Staphylococcus aureus* and *streptococcus faecalis* require 60 minutes at 60°C; 80°C for 5–10 minutes destroy the vegetative forms of all bacteria, yeasts and moulds. Poliomyelitis virus requires 60°C for 30 minutes and Hepatitis virus in serum requires 60°C for 10 hours.

ii. *Temperatures at 100°C:* Vegetative bacteria are killed almost immediately at 90–100°C but not spores (Fig. 7.34). Hard water for boiling should not be used and sterilization can be promoted by the addition of 2.0% sodium bicarbonate to water. Material should be immersed in water and boiled for 10–30 minutes without opening the lid of sterilizer. Time periods up to 24 hours may be necessary to kill bacterial spores and even this prolonged time will not kill many viruses. For this reason, boiling water is not recommended for sterilization of tissue penetrating instruments.

Instruments, Instrumentation and Sterilization

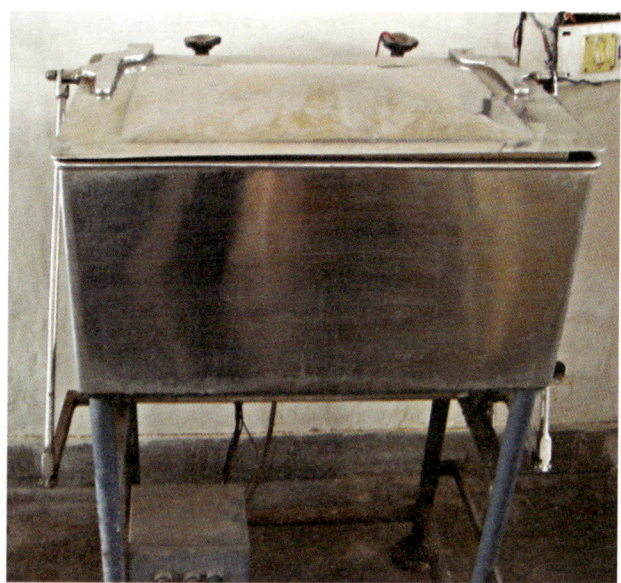

Fig. 7.34: Sterilization by boiling

iii. *Steam at atmospheric pressure:* An exposure of 90 minutes usually ensures sterilization. In case of steamer, the instruments are in touch with steam only. It consists of a vertical metallic container having a perforated tray in the middle. The water is filled under it, which boils and produces steam. The steam at 100°C cover the instruments in the middle tray and sterilizes them.

iv. *Steam under pressure (Autoclave):* The principle of autoclave is that, water boils when its vapour pressure equals that of the surrounding atmosphere. Saturated steam has greater penetrating power. When steam has greater penetrating power, it condenses to water and gives up its latent heat to that surface. The large reduction in volume sucks in more steam to the area and the process continues till the temperature of that surface is raised to that of the steam. The condensed water ensures moist conditions for killing the microbes.

The recommendations for temperature and holding period are:

121°C–15 minutes at 15 lbs pressure
136°C–Three minutes at 30 lbs pressure for unwrapped and 5–12 minute for wrapped instruments. Instruments should be removed only after drying completely as wet packages are considered non-sterilized.

Articles that can be sterilized in the autoclave include most culture media, saline and other articles not damaged by high temperatures viz. syringes, needles, dressings, sponges, gowns, rubber gloves, tubing, aprons, etc. (Figs 7.35A to C).

Autoclaving is damaging for almost all high speed dental handpieces. Without prior treatment of oil emulsion, burs are also destroyed in autoclaving. Instead of steam, chemical vapours of various alcohols, acetone, formaldehyde can be used at 126.6°C. These vapours are less corrosive to instruments than steam.

Flash Sterilization (Rapid Cycle Autoclave)

Flash sterilization is a modification of conventional high vacuum steam sterilization, used for carrying out in-patient sterilization or rapid chairside sterilization of critical devices. Instruments are placed unwrapped at 132°C for 3-4 minutes at 27–28 lbs pressure. The sterilization time may vary with the type of sterilizer and the type of item (i.e. porous vs non porous items)

Uses

- It is considered acceptable for processing precleaned instruments that cannot be packaged, sterilized and stored before use.
- It is also used when there is insufficient time to sterilize an item by the preferred package method.
- Flash sterilization, can be used to carry out in patient sterilization of dental handpieces and instruments. But, it is not considered as effective as the routine packaged sterilization and thus should not be used for reasons of convenience, as

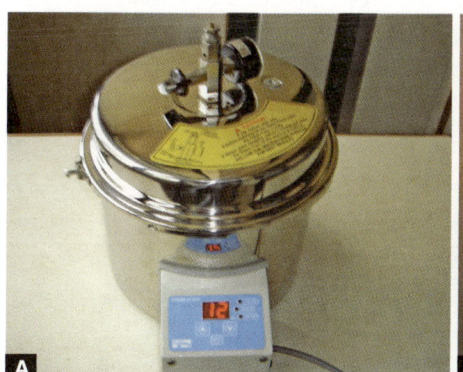 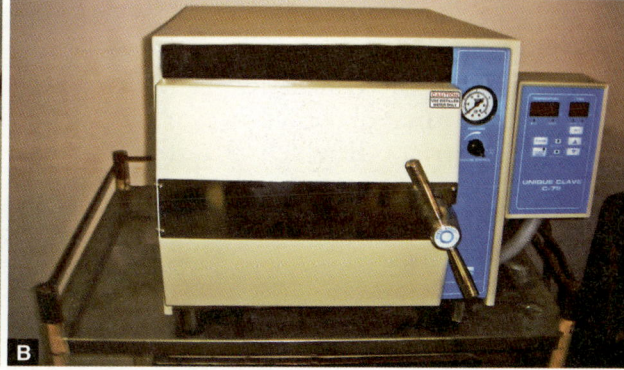 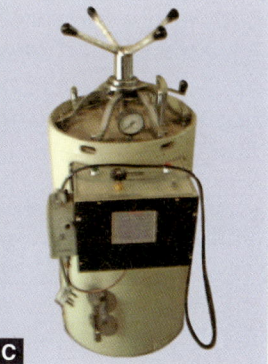

Figs 7.35A to C: Various types of autoclaves

an alternative to purchasing additional instrument sets or to save time.

Precautions while Operating the Steam Sterilizers

i. The valve should first be turned to the 'off' position. Steam should then be allowed to dissipate from the sterilizer until it is safe to open the door.
ii. Once the goods have been sterilized, they can be removed from the chamber. However, they must not be placed on a cold surface because the heat within the pack will condense upon contact with the surface and moisten the pack, leading to its contamination.

Advantages of Autoclaves

- Most rapid and effective method for sterilizing cloth packs and towel packs. Other methods are not suitable for processing cloth packs.
- Good penetration of heat.

Disadvantages of Autoclaves

- Heat sensitive items like plastic and rubber can't be autoclaved.
- Autoclave tends to rust carbon steel instruments and burs.
- Steam appears to corrode the steel neck and shank portions of some diamond instruments and carbide burs. To avoid or minimize the corrosive action of steam on metals, ammonia, dicylohexyl ammonium nitrite or cyclohexylamine and dicylamine or 2.0% sodium nitrite can be used.
- Instruments removed from the chamber are wet which increases the turn around time of sterilization.

Filtration

The method is not used in dentistry, though it is used for sterilizing fluids, which cannot be heated.

Cold

This method is used to retard microbial growths in foods and to preserve biological materials. It acts by (i) increasing the viscosity of the proteins (ii) impeding the diffusion of toxic products from the cell (iii) increasing enzymatic activity (iv) formation of ice crystals within and outside the bacterial cell which mechanically ruptures the cell. Temperatures around 0°C have more inhibitory effect than sub-zero temperature.

Desiccation

This method is unreliable and is only of theoretical interest.

Sunlight

The microbicidal activity of sunlight is mainly due to the presence of ultraviolet rays in it. It is responsible for spontaneous sterilization in natural conditions. Sunlight is not sporicidal, hence it does not sterilize.

B. CHEMICAL METHOD

The chemical agents used for disinfection act in various ways:

- Protein coagulation
- Disruption of cell membrane
- Removal of free sulphydryl groups which are essential for functioning of the enzymes
- Substrate competition

A good disinfectant is one that is non-corrosive, readily available, relatively pleasant flavor, nonirritating to breathe, effective on most microorganisms and economical. The levels of activity of various chemicals for disinfection are tabulated in Table 7.7.

Office disinfection procedures involve using a liquid chemical at room temperature to kill microorganisms on submerged instruments or operatory surfaces. If the chemical is not sporicidal (for example– iodophores, synthetic phenolics, phenols, alcohol/ phenolics, sodium hypochlorite, glutaraldehyde) it is called disinfectant and can be expected to achieve only disinfection.

If the chemical is sporicidal, it is called a sterilant (2% or 3.2% concentration of glutaraldehyde) and may be expected to achieve sterilization, but only after 10 hour contact time on pre-cleaned items.

Unfortunately, the level of microbial killing, achieved by use of liquid chemical disinfectants or sterilants in the office can't be routinely verified as can be done with heat sterilizers through spore testing.

Table 7.7: Chemicals for disinfection

Level	Use	Examples
Low level	Surfaces without blood	Some phenolics and iodoforms
Intermediate level	Surfaces with blood	Alcohol, chlorines, phenolics, iodoforms
High level	Immersion	Glutardehyde, strong peroxides, o-phthaldehyde

Antiseptics are used preoperatively to cleanse the skin of the patient and also the hand and arm of surgical personnel. Some antiseptics can be used as disinfectant, but their ability to inhibit the growth of micro-organisms may not be as efficient as an agent specified for use as a disinfectant only.

Factors Affecting Germicidal Activity

1. Effective concentration of agent.
2. Time of exposure–there is a relationship of time to temperature, kind and number of organisms, type of material to be disinfected, presence of organic matter.
3. Temperature–increased temperature results in increased lethal activity.
4. pH–Some chemical agents have more activity in acidic pH (anionic detergents) and some in basic pH (cationic detergents).
5. Presence of contaminants–some agents combine with organic matter and become ineffective.

Chemical Vapour Sterilizers (chemiclave)

These sterilize instruments using chemical vapours. The active chemical ingredients include 72.38% ethanol and 0.23% formaldehyde (vaposteril). The water content is below 15% level, above which rust, corrosion and dullness of metal occurs.

The chemical vapour sterilizers are basically meant for instruments which cannot be heated beyond 132°C and instruments prone to rust.

The sterilization cycle of the chemiclave is at 132°C at 20 pounds pressure for 25–30 minutes. This ensures total sterilization. Instruments can be sterilized in both wrapped and unwrapped state in 20 minutes. The main advantage of these chemical sterilizers is that instruments do not corrode nor are they blunted. This method is a popular mode of sterilization in endodontic offices.

However, penetration of the chemical vapours is not as effective as that of steam in the autoclaves.

Advantages
• Fast turn-around time.
• Protection of carbon steel instruments from rust or corrosion.
• Availability of dry, immediately usable instruments.

Disadvantages
• Items sensitive to elevated temperature will be damaged.
• Bad odour is released when chemicals are heated.
• Limited availability of apparatus and high cost.

Caution
• Load only dry instruments.
• Check the door gasket for leaks to avoid frequent sterilization monitoring failures.

Alcohols

Ethyl alcohol and isopropyl alcohol are the most frequently used chemical disinfectants. It is used mainly as skin antiseptic and act by denaturing proteins. There is no action on spores or viruses. It is generally used at a concentration of 60–70% in water. Ethyl alcohol, on standing, oxidizes to acetic acid and acetaldehyde, which are corrosive to metals. Isopropyl alcohol is a better fat solvent, more bactericidal and less volatile than ethyl alcohol. Methyl alcohol is effective against fungal spores and is used for treating cabinets and incubators affected by them. Alcohol is found poorly effective against all micro-organisms and not at all effective against spore formers and is not an accepted method for disinfection of surfaces and instruments.

Aldehydes

i. *Formaldehyde:* It is active against amino groups in the protein molecules. In aqueous solutions it is markedly bactericidal, sporicidal and virucidal. Formaldehyde gas is used for sterilizing instruments and heat sensitive catheters, fumigating wards, sick rooms and laboratories. Clothing, bedding, furniture and books can also be disinfected. The irritant vapour can be nullified by exposure to ammonia vapour after disinfection is completed.

ii. *Glutaraldehyde:* It is similar to formaldehyde, but less toxic and less irritant to eyes and skin. It can be used to treat corrugated rubber anaesthetic tubes and face masks, plastic endotracheal tubes, metal instruments and polythene tubing. Glutaraldehyde will kill bacterial spores, fungi and perhaps all viruses by alkylation. Prior to patient exposure, instruments must be thoroughly rinsed with sterile water to remove the compound. Disinfection occurs in 10–30 minutes (Fig. 7.36). A plethora of glutaraldehyde preparations exist today and various types of preparations capable of sterilization are:
   – 2% acidic, 60°C for one hour
   – 2% alkaline, at room temperature for 10 hours
   – 2% alkaline, at room temperature for 6.75 hours with phenolic buffer
   – 2% neutral, at room temperature for 10 hours.

Gultaraldehydes are generally not recommended for sterilization because of the instability of activated

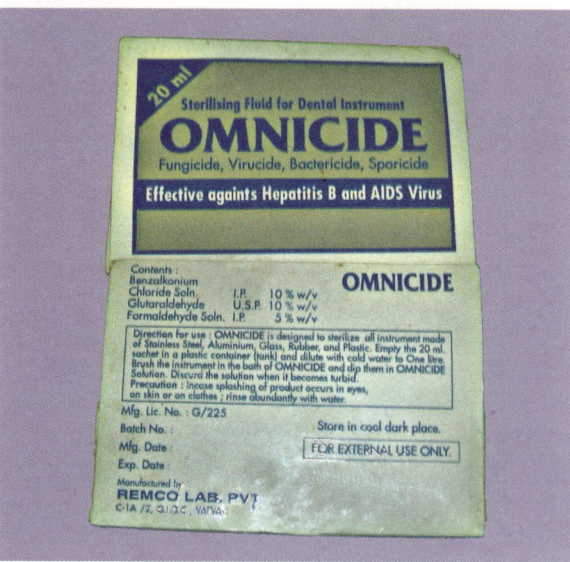

Fig. 7.36: Aldehyde disinfection

solutions, problems of dilution and inability to monitor sterilization.

Disadvantages
• Corrosion of easily oxidized metals
• Need for fresh solution for each sterilization/ disinfection process.

iii. *Ortho-phthaldehyde:* OPA is a disinfectant solution, available in 0.55% active OPA concentration with excellent microbicidal activity. It presents with various advantages when compared with glutaraldehyde:
1. Shorter processing time
2. Non irritant to eyes and nasal passages
3. Excellent stability over a wide range of pH (3–9)
4. Weak; barely perceptible odour.

Disadvantages
• It tends to stain proteins gray; thus needed to be handled with caution, avoiding exposure to skin.
• Higher cost.

Dyes

The Aniline and Acridine dyes are used as skin and wound antiseptics. Both are bacteriostatic in high dilution. Aniline dyes are effective against gram-positive organisms, inhibited by organic matter. Acridine dyes are also effective against gram-positive organisms but very little effected by organic matter. If impregnated in gauze they are slowly released in a moist environment.

Disadvantages
• May discolor surfaces.
• Must be prepared daily.

Halogens

Chlorine and iodine are the most widely used halogens.

Chlorine in aqueous form, is used as disinfectant of water supplies, swimming baths, food and dairy industries. Chlorine is most commonly used as hypochlorites. It is markedly bactericidal and has got a wide spectrum of activity against viruses. Organic chloramines are used as antiseptic for dressing wounds.

Chlorine dioxide: The chlorine dioxide compounds disinfect instruments and operatory surfaces in one to three minutes when used correctly. The solution requires no rinsing and leaves no residue after use. There are no special handling or disposal requirements. Solutions can sterilize items in six hours at room temperature. The substance has been reported to be non-toxic, nonirritating and non-sensitizing.

Sodium hypochlorite: It is more suitable for surface disinfection than for instrument sterilization because of its highly corrosive action on metals. Dilution of 1:5 to 1:1 are generally recommended. On surfaces, sodium hypochlorite is virucidal, bactericidal and tuberculocidal. Disinfection can occur in 3-30 minutes depending upon the amount of debris present. It is the least expensive of the surface disinfectants.

Disadvantages
• Corrosive factor.
• Solution tends to be unstable and should be prepared daily.
• Strong, unpleasant odour.
• Plastic chair covers have a tendency to crack after prolonged use.

Iodine: Iodine in aqueous and alcoholic solutions has been used as skin disinfectant. It is an active bactericidal and moderately active against spores and viruses.

Iodophors (iodine mixed with a detergent): Iodophor is a broad spectrum disinfectant, i.e. effective against a host of pathogens including HBV, *M. tuberculosis*.

One of the inherent advantages of the compound is slow release of elemental iodine to enhance the bactericidal activity. A surfactant carrier keeps a surface moist to protect the iodophor during this release and the action may continue even after the surface appears dry.

The most effective dilution for hard surface iodophors is one part iodophor concentrate to two third part of soft or distilled water. Hard water inactivates the iodophor. Biocidal activity occurs within 30 minutes.

Iodophors also have an in-built color indicator. When the solution is fresh, an amber color is present. With age, the solution changes to light yellow, indicating the loss of iodophor molecules. The iodophor compound is to be used solely as a disinfectant. Its sporicidal capabilities have not been shown.

Disadvantages
• Vapour toxicity
• Hand and eye irritation
• Expensive
• Discoloration of some metals

Phenols

Phenols are the oldest disinfectants. Their effect is due to their cell membrane damaging capacity causing lysis. Low concentrations precipitate proteins and membrane bound oxidases and dehydrogenases are inactivated. It is a powerful microbicidal agent. None of the phenolic comounds are sporicidal at room temperature, but they are active against many viruses, fungi and bacteria.

Phenolic compounds are often used for disinfection of walls, floors or other surfaces that do not come into contact with body tissues.

Disadvantages
They may cause damage to some plastics and they do corrode certain metals such as brass, aluminium and carbide steel (Corrosive effect is neutralized by mixing them with sodium bicarbonate).

Chlorhexidine (Hibitane) is a relatively non-toxic skin antiseptic, active against gram-positive organisms and fairly effective against gram negative ones. Aqueous solutions are used in the treatment of wounds.

Surface Active Agents

These are widely used as wetting agents, detergents and emulsifiers. They are often classified into anionic, cationic, non-ionic and amphoteric groups. The cationic surface active agents are important antibacterial agents. They act on phosphate groups of cell membrane, causing the membrane to lose its semi-permeability, subsequently, cell proteins are denatured.

Cationic agents in the form of quarternary ammonium compounds are bactericidal, active against gram-positive organisms and to a lesser degree gram-negative organisms. They also act on spores and most viruses, e.g. Cetyl trimethyl ammonium bromide (cetavlon or cetrimide) and benzalkonium chloride. Anionic agents (soap) and organic matter reduces their efficacy.

Anionic compounds (soap) have moderate activity. Soaps from saturated fatty acids are more active than those from unsaturated fatty acids.

The amphoteric compounds are active against a wide variety of gram-positive and gram-negative organisms and some viruses.

Metallic salts: Salts of mercury, silver, copper are used as disinfectants. They are protein coagulants and combine with sulphydryl groups of cell enzymes. Mercuric chloride is highly toxic as compared to organic compounds (thiomersal, phenyl mercury nitrate and mercurochrome), which are used as mild antiseptics. Copper salts are used as fungicides.

Surfacine: It is a new antimicrobial agent with a persistent activity (upto 13 days) that may be used on animate or inanimate surfaces. It incorporates a water soluble antimicrobial compound (silver iodide) in a surface-immobilized coating (polyhexamethylenebiguanide). Micro-organisms contacting the coating accumulate silver until the toxicity level is exceeded; dead organisms eventually lyse and detach from the surface. It can be applied on the surface by brushing, dipping or spraying without prior surface treatments. Though tested to show broad spectrum activity, it is still to be released by FDA.

Peracetic acid: Peracetic acid in aqueous solution is an effective germicide against the wide spectrum of micro-organisms, however, it is corrosive. In concentration of 1.0 mg/litre and 40% or higher relative humidity, it is sporicidal within 10 minutes.

Oils

Hot oil baths have been used to sterilize metallic instruments. The oil can reach a temperature of 175°C and after instruments reach that temperature, 15 minutes of submersion is necessary for sterilization. To ensure temperature conversion of the instruments, often one hour or more of submersion is used.

Gases

Ethylene Oxide

It has a boiling point of 10.7°C. This is considered a highly penetrating, inflammable and explosive gas. It is rendered non-inflammable for hospital use when

mixed with carbon dioxide or fluorinated hydrocarbon such as freon. The features regarding ethylene oxide are:
- Its action is due to its power of alkylating the main carboxyl, hydroxyl and sulphdryl groups in the protein molecule. It also reacts with DNA and RNA.
- It is toxic which includes autogenecity and carcinogenecity; thus all items sterilized by this method must be aerated following exposure.
- It is used for sterilizing heart-lung machines, respirators, sutures, dental equipments, books, clothing, glass, metal and paper surfaces, plastics and food-stuffs, etc.

Method: Goods are placed in a chamber where they are exposed to the gas for a certain period of time according to manufacturer's instructions. Usual exposure time ranges from 1¾ to 12 hours. Humidity and temperature are critical factors in the destruction of micro-organisms during gas sterilization. The chamber is generally maintained at 40% to 80% humidity, temperature ranging from 50°C to 60°C and gas concentration between 200–800 mg/dl.

Caution: The oil can defeat sterilization, so handpieces should be cleaned but not oiled before ethylene oxide sterilization. The cost of the equipment and long sterilization time make this method impractical.

Advantages
• Preferable for materials sensitive to heat. • Complete penetration

Disadvantages
• Time of sterilization and ventilation is long • It is toxic, carcinogenic, flammable and explosive. • It needs an aeration period after the process due to formation of ethylene chlorohydrin.

Formaldehyde

It is used for fumigation of operation theatres by adding 150 gm of potassium permangnate to 280 ml. formalin for an average room. Heat resistant vessels should be used. The doors should be sealed and left un-opened for 48 hours. It is less popular than ethylene oxide because of its odour.

Advantages
• Preferable for materials sensitive to high heat. • No need for ventilation of materials after sterilization.

Disadvantages
• Toxic and carcinogenic. • Cannot be used for the sterilization of liquids.

Betapropiolactone (BPL)

It has a boiling point of 163°C. It is a gas of low penetrating power with rapid biocidal action but also has carcinogenic activity. In the concentration of 0.2%, it is used for sterilization of biological products. The BPL is capable of killing all micro-organisms and is very active against viruses.

Miscellaneous

Plasma Sterilization

Plasma is basically an ionized gas. Plasma sterilization is fast evolving into a promising alternative to standard sterilization techniques. It uses a technique, which involves UV irradiation, photo desorption and chemical etching. The spores are made up of atoms like carbon, oxygen, hydrogen, nitrogen and the like. The radicals react with these atoms to form compounds like carbon dioxide which can be subsequently flushed out. When the organism loses such atoms that are intrinsic to its survival, it dies.

Advantages
• The process is carried out usually at room temperature and hence poses no dangers associated with high temperature (unlike autoclaves). • It does not involve any chemical and hence non toxic (unlike ethylene oxide) • Time of treatment is fast and of the order of one minute or less. • It is versatile and can sterilize almost any material and any shape.

Disadvantages
• Not a proper method for the sterilization of liquids

Performic Acid

A new liquid sterilant that uses performic acid that is produced, by using of two components solutions of hydrogen peroxide and formic acid. It is fast acting against spore forming bacteria and is being used in an endoscope-reprocessing system marketed as Endoclens.

Superdioxide Water

It is a new disinfectant containing hypochlorous acid at a concentration of approximately 144 mg/L and free chlorine radicals. It is stated to be non-toxic to biological tissues and non-corrosive to metallic instruments with a broad spectrum activity.

C. RADIATION METHOD

Non-ionizing Radiations

The non-ionizing radiations consist of rays with wavelength longer than those of visible light. These rays by and large are absorbed as heat:

i. *Microwave sterilization:* Explained on page 134.
ii. *Infra-red radiation:* The heat generated by these radiations and subsequently oxidation leads to killing of micro-organisms. The five to ten minutes exposure is sufficient to completely sterilize all the equipments. The infra-red rays can also be used for monitoring the sterilized instruments.

Ionizing Radiations

The ionizing radiations can be (i) particulate or (ii) electromagnetic. The particulate radiations are cathode rays having high energy electrons. These are usually used in treatment of cancers.

The electromagnetic radiations are of short wavelength (UV-rays, γ-rays and cosmic rays). Ionizing radiations are highly lethal to DNA and other vital cell constituents. There is no appreciable increase in temperature and the process may be referred as 'cold sterilization'.

i. *Ultraviolet radiations:* The bactericidal range of ultraviolet wavelength is 240–280 nm. The rays are absorbed by protein and nucleic acid of the organisms. A chemical reaction is set within the cell, which leads to its death. These rays are basically used to clean the surface environment minimizing the bacteria. The air, water and the surroundings are sterilized by this method. Ultraviolet radiation is used to disinfect enclosed areas such as entryways, hospital wards, operation rooms, virus laboratories for storage and maintenance of previously sterilized materials UV rays have much lower energy and poor penetrability as camp and to x-rays (Fig. 7.37).

ii. *Gamma rays:* Gamma rays are formed with the self integration of Co-60 or Ce-137. It is a useful method for industrial sterilization of heat sensitive products. The source of gamma rays (Co-60) is housed within a reinforced concrete building with 2 m thick walls. Articles being sterilized are passed through the irradiation chamber on a conveyer belt and move around a raised source. Gamma radiation easily reaches all parts of the object to be sterilized due to its high penetration ability. The items can be pre-packed in hermetically sealed packages, impermeable to micro-organisms, before sterilization. Consequently, the sterile shelf life of these supplies is practically indefinite, i.e. up to the point of use. The sterilizing effect is instantaneous and simultaneous in the whole of target. These radiations are measured in radians. Usually 2.5 megarads are required to effect sterilization.

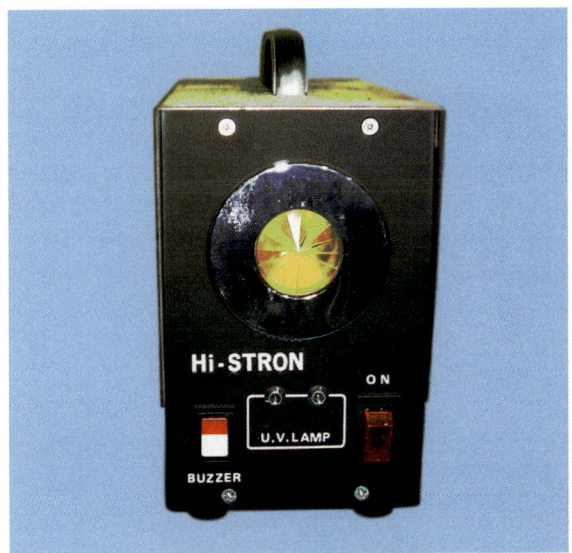

Fig. 7.37: Ultra violet unit

iii. *E-beam radiation:* E-beam irradiation method is attracting more attention recently for the sterilization of medical devices and has many advantages like being safe, having no emission and high speed processing. It is very similar to gamma irradiation as being an ionising energy but the difference is its high dosage rates and low penetration. Another difference is the use of e-beams which has a source of electricity producing high charge of electrons. These electrons can be continuous or pulsed and generated by e-beam accelerators. Electron absorption by the product to be sterilized is the mechanism of the e-beam sterilization and that causes a change in the chemical and molecular bonds and the destruction of DNA chain of the reproducing cells of the bacteria on the material. The process is cost effective but the construction of the e-beam sterilization institution is expensive.

CAUSES OF STERILIZATION FAILURE

Many a time, despite using the best available sterilizing unit, the sterilization is not achievable. The killing of the micro-organisms fails when the sterilizing agent does not make the proper contact for the proper time. Usual procedural errors are responsible for such a menace.

Recommended sterilization procedures for commonly used articles			
Instruments	I Choice	II Choice	III Choice
Metal instruments	Moist heat	Dry heat	Chemical
Surgical burs	Moist heat	Dry heat	Chemical
Surgical handpieces	Moist Heat	Chemical	—
Air rotor handpieces	Moist Heat	Chemical	—
Air rotor cord	Gas	—	—
Micromotor cord	Gas	—	—
Rubber tube suction	Moist heat	Chemical	Gas
Cautery tip	Gas	Chemical	—
Mouth mirror	Moist Heat	Chemical	Dry heat
3-way syringe	Moist Heat	Chemical	Dry heat
Glass slab	Gas	Chemical	Chemical
Sutures	Gas	Chemical	—
Needles	Moist heat	Dry heat	Chemical
Gauze, Gloves	Moist heat	—	—
Suction tip	Moist heat	Dry heat	Chemical
Light cure tip	Moist heat	Chemical	Dry heat
Drapes, Gowns	Moist heat	—	—

The common causes can be:
1. *Improper cleaning:* The instruments should be thoroughly cleaned before sterilizing. Dental materials, blood or even saliva may not allow the sterilizing agent to reach at the site. Preferably the cleaning should be done with detergent; alternatively wash in running water.
2. *Improper placement:* The instruments to be sterilized should not be packed tightly, or one above the other. Appropriate space should be there between the instruments so as to allow the sterilizing agent reach all the surfaces.
3. *Improper timings:* For proper sterilization, the sterilizing agent should contact the surface of the instrument for a given period of time depending upon the unit, which is used and the instrument/object, which are sterilized. The sterilizing time includes safety factor time, which ensures the total killing of microorganisms.
4. *Malfunctioning of the unit:* Sometimes the unit, which is used for sterilization may have manufacturing defect, which leads to failure. For example during autoclaving, the pressure and/or the temperature displayed may not be correct and the operator believes the false readings.

CONTROL OF STERILIZATION

It becomes mandatory for the operator to check the appropriateness of sterilization, i.e. whether the required temperature is achieved or the object is free of microorganisms. This can be done by recording cycle time, temperature and cannot be taken as surety of sterilization. Similar tapes are also designed, which indicate the penetration of steam under pressure.

The following tests can be carried out:

i. *Autoclave tape:* The tape is impregnated with a dye and the color white is changed to brown or black depending upon the temperature achieved. This test is only an indication of the temperature and cannot be taken as surety of sterilization. Similar tapes are also designed, which indicate the penetration of steam under pressure.

ii. *Thermocouple:* The thermocouple probes are designed specifically to monitor the temperature and the time during sterilization. The probes can be inserted into the article to be sterilized and the potentiometer indicates the temperature and the time.

iii. *Microbial tests:* In this test, a particular species of bacteria (usually *Bacillus stearothermophilus* for steam and chemical vapour, *Bacillus subtilis* for dry heat and ethylene oxide) is used as a test organism. Paper strips impregnated with around one million bacterial spores are dried and put along the object to be sterilized. After sterilization process is over, the strips are then incubated for 5–7 days. Though this method is perfect to test sterility, but practically not suitable because of the time lapse for knowing the exact status of the sterilization.

iv. *Chemical indicators:* Certain chemical agents when put to certain temperature and for particular time lead to color change, which shows the sterilization achieved. The chemical shows red for danger; orange for caution and green for complete sterilization. Different types can be used for steam sterilizers and for autoclaving.

CLEANING AND DISINFECTION OF HANDPIECES

The dental handpiece and turbine due to constant contact with oral fluids are contaminated on both external and internal surfaces. Micro-organisms are even capable of forming biofilms on the internal surface of handpieces and waterlines. Contamination of the internal parts of the dental handpiece may originate from saliva aspirated during treatment of patients or from the air and water supply of dental units where micro-organisms may build up in biofilms.

A range of microbiological flora has been identified in dental unit waterline samples by use of morphological and biochemical characteristics.

This holds a potential to infect healthy dental patients. Therefore, sterilization of handpiece is must. Rinsing out water lines of the unit with Tween 80 and Ponceau 4R dye gives a marked reduction in microorganisms. Hydrogen peroxide in a concentration of 3% is also helpful in reducing the flora but these cannot replace autoclaving.

Steam Sterilization

Steam sterilization of handpieces is one of the routinely used methods. The cleaning and lubricating is performed as prescribed by the manufacturer.

General Steps

1. Leave the handpiece attached to the hose after treatment and wipe away visible debris from the handpiece. Operate the air/water system for 20-30 seconds to flush the water and air lines with the vacuum line or a sink, container or absorbent material.
2. Remove the handpiece from the hose and clean the outside thoroughly. Use ultrasonic cleaning only when recommended by the handpiece manufacturer.
3. Clean/lubricate internal portions as directed by the manufacturer. Reattach to the air/water system and blow out excess cleaner/lubricant with a vacuum line or sink, container or absorbent material. Depending on the handpiece, it is to be lubricated before and after sterilization.
4. Wipe away excess lubricant from the outside. If using fiberoptic handpieces, clean the lubricant from the fiberoptic connecting interface as directed by the manufacturer.
5. Follow the manufacturer's instructions for the type of heat sterilizer (e.g. steam, autoclave, chemical vapour) and maximum temperature that can be used. Package the handpiece in the proper bag for the type of sterilizer being used and heat process following the sterilizer instructions.

Cleaning the fiberoptics with detergent solution or any other suitable organic solvents may prove useful. For handpieces with a metal-bearing turbine, the handpieces and the sheath is cleaned with running water and detergent. See manufacturer's directions for further cleaning and lubrication before and after sterilization. Cover the handpiece in a sheath and autoclave.

Chemical Vapour Pressure Sterilization

This method works well with ceramic-bearing handpiece, however, chemicals may impair functioning of others.

Ethylene Oxide Gas Sterilization

The Ethylene oxide gas is commonly used for handpieces. Internal and external cleaning is important so as to facilitate ethylene oxide gas to penetrate the handpieces. However, oil left in the handpieces can impair sterilization.

The ethylene oxide exposure for at least 12 hours is required for an effective sterilization of handpieces.

Dry Heat Sterilization

It is generally not recommended for sterilization of dental handpiece. The dry heat disinfection process is under evaluation for handpieces.

A device, which combines flushing, lubrication and autoclaving has been marketed commercially as 'Sterimax.'

CLEANING, DISINFECTION AND STERILIZATION OF BURS

Most of the times, burs bathe in patients' saliva and blood, and as they are heavily contaminated, the use of single-use burs is advocated.

Several options exist in handling contaminated dental burs prior to sterilization.

1. Decontaminate at chairside with wet guaze using a disinfectant before transport.
2. Place in an ultrasonic cleaner or washer disinfector using separate bur holder.
3. Use disposable burs/diamonds.
4. Hand scrub under a solution (last option).

For Autoclave sterilization, burs can be protected from rusting by keeping them submerged in a small amount 2.0% sodium nitrite solution.

1. Add 20 mg of sodium nitrite crystals in 1 L of distilled water to prepare 2.0% sodium nitrite (not nitrate) solution.
2. After ultrasonic cleaning, rinse the burs and place them in a small glass or metal beaker with a perforated lid.
3. Fill the beaker with fresh nitrite solution ensuring complete submersion of burs.
4. Autoclave with a normal sterilization cycle.
5. Fluid from the container is discarded through the perforated lid and burs are transferred to a sterilized bur holder or tray using a sterile forceps.
6. Before use, if needed, rinse off burs with sterile water to wipe away any sterile residue left on burs.

INFECTION CONTROL

The last few decades have brought about considerable changes in the practice of general dentistry. Infection control has been one of the most significant areas of change.

Most dentists have accepted 'universal precautions' as their standard of care for minimizing the risks of cross-infection between their patients and their office personnel. The new CDC recommendation emphasizes the use of 'standard precautions' (which replaces the term 'universal precautions') for the prevention of exposure to and transmission of not only blood borne pathogens, but also other pathogens encountered in oral health care settings. The essence of universal precautions/standard precautions is the placement of body fluid impermeable barriers between health care personnels and their patients' potentially infectious body fluids and use of methods to reduce injury and accidents involving sharp, body fluid contaminated instruments.

Universal use of gloves, masks, protective eyewear, overgarments, plastic barriers, etc. provide a professional health care environment.

ENVIRONMENT OF DENTAL OPERATORY

In order to understand the problem of microbial contamination that faces dentistry, it is necessary to examine the dental treatment environment.

Mircobial exposures to the dental operatory involve both air-borne contamination and digital contamination of surface.

- *Air borne contamination:* Aerosols, spatter.
- *Digital contamination:* Barrier protection of personnel and equipment, and other methods of avoiding direct contact with various surfaces are required to avoid digital contamination.
- *Cross infection:* Among hospital patients and personnel, cross-infection and the routes of transmission come directly under the scrutiny of physicians, nurses and infection control personnel. However, in the dental settings, evidence of oral or systemic cross-infections is much more difficult to obtain because such patients may have contacted infections elsewhere, before or after having a dental treatment. Patients infected usually are not aware of the source of their infection. Infection outbreaks are usually detected in personnel only when they occur in clusters as recognized by oral health workers during epidemiological studies.
- *Patient vulnerability:* Although infection risks for dental patients have not been investigated as properly as for hospital patients, they appear to be less vulnerable. Since infection control practices are routinely used, transmission of infection from dental patients is rare.
- *Personnel vulnerability:* When dental personnel experience exposure to saliva, blood and possible injury from sharp instruments, they are more vulnerable to infections if they have not used the proper protective barriers.

Infection control procedures have helped in reducing risks in dental offices, as well as inculcating confidence in both patient and the personnel.

Control of Infectious Diseases

The infection control in dentistry involves protection of patients and members of dental team from different kinds of infectious diseases so that the dental practice is made safer. The procedures for infection control are designed to kill or remove microbes or to protect against contamination. Because microbes cannot be seen, it is usually difficult to determine if a given procedure is carried out in bacteria-free environment or not. One must follow *'infection control assurance'*, i.e. taking all steps necessary to ensure the desired results.

Objectives

The following goals have been suggested for infection control programme.
- Decrease the number of pathogenic microbes to the level where normal body resistance mechanisms can prevent infection.
- Break the cycle of infection from dentist, assistant and patient and eliminate cross-contamination.
- Treat all patients and instruments as though they could transmit an infectious disease.
- Protect patients and personnel from infection and protect all dental personnel from the threat of malpractice.

Patient Evaluation

The identification of patients with transmissible diseases and of those belonging to high-risk groups is essential before evaluation begins. A thorough medical history should be obtained and reviewed. The medical history serves the following purposes:
- To detect any recognized illness that requires medical diagnosis and treatment.
- To identify any infection or high risk that may be important to a person exposed during examination or treatment.
- To manage the infected patients.
- To follow adequate infection control procedures, bearing in mind that general history-taking is not capable of detecting all infectious persons.

The medical history should be updated at subsequent visits. Specific questions should be asked regarding medications, current and recurrent illness, unintentional weight loss, lymphadenopathy, oral soft tissue lesions, other infections and history of hepatitis or any allergic reactions. Since the medical history and examination can't reliably identify all patients with blood borne pathogens, blood and body fluid precautions should be consistently used for all patients. The concept stresses that all patients should be assumed to be infectious for HIV and other blood-borne pathogens and the same infection control procedures should be used for all patients, i.e. universal precautions.

METHODS FOR INFECTION CONTROL

Immunization

Vaccines play an important role in the infection control process; Hepatitis B is a major health hazard for dental health care personnel. Because of this risk, ADA Council on Dental Therapeutics and CDC have recommended that all dental personnel involved in patient care receive the Hepatitis B vaccine.

Many blood borne pathogens exist for which there is presently no vaccine, including HIV and non-A/non-B hepatitis. Proper infection control procedures are therefore recommended to prevent transmission of such pathogens.

Transmissible Diseases of Concern to Dental Surgeons and Auxiliaries
• Hepatitis (type A, B, non-A/non-B) • Acquired immune deficiency syndrome (human immunodeficiency virus) • Syphilis • Gonorrhea • Influenzas • Acute pharyngitis • Pneumonias • Tuberculosis • Herpes • Chickenpox • Infectious mononucleosis • Rubella • Mumps

Groups at High Risk of contacting Hepatitis B

• Health care personnel
• Selected patients and patient contacts
  – Patients and staff in hemodialysis units and hematology/oncology units
  – Patients requiring frequent or large-volume blood transfusions or clotting factors (i.e. hemophiliac patients)
  – Residents and staff of institutions for the mentally handicapped
  – Household and sexual contacts of persons with persistent hepatitis B antigen
    Newborns of hepatitis B surface antigen carrier mother
• Populations with high incidence of the disease
  – Alaskan natives
  – Indo-Chinese refugees
  – Haitian refugees
  – Native Pacific Islanders
  – Sub-Saharan Africans
• Morticians and Embalmers
• Blood Bank and plasma bank workers
• Prisoners
• Use of illicit injectable drugs
• Frequent travellers

Personal Barrier Technique

Both OSHA (Occupational Safety and Health Agency) and CDC (Centre for Disease Control) have recommended the following:

A. Hand Washing

The recommended hand washing procedure begins with a thorough initial scrubbing of all surfaces of the nails, fingers, hands and lower arms with an antimicrobial preparation. All jewellery must be removed. Care should be taken to avoid the use of a stiff bristle brush, which will cause abrasions and lacerations to the skin and nail area. The initial scrubbing should be accomplished with a soft, sterile brush or a disposable sponge in three latherings, each followed by a one or two minute rinse with cool to luke warm water.

The water should flow from fingertips to the elbow and not run back towards the area previously rinsed. Using a separate paper towel for each hand, drying should begin at the fingers moving to the hands and then to the surfaces of the arms.

A shorter hand washing procedure may be followed for the rest of the day. Hands must be washed between the patients before gloving. The rationale for hand washing after gloves is that gloves become perforated during use and bacteria enter beneath the gloves and multiply rapidly. Washing hands before gloving reduces the skin microbial flora and helps prevent the irritation by waste products of bacterial growth under the gloves.

Hand cleansers containing a mild antiseptic like 3% PCMX (P-chloro, meta-xylenole) or chlorhexidine are preferred to control consistent pathogens and to suppress over growth of skin bacteria.

B. Gloves

Gloves provide the patient with protection from contamination of micro-organisms on the practitioner hands and protect dental health care workers from contamination by patients' blood and saliva. Gloves need to be changed between patients and are not to be washed with detergents at any time. Gloves should be inspected periodically during patient care and torn or punctured gloves should be removed as soon as possible.

Criteria for selection of gloves include:
- Lowest possibility of manufacturing defects
- Well-fitting
- Good tactile sensitivity
- Do not cause hypersensitivity
- Do not become tacky after wetting
- Resistant to wearing
- Conducive to glove powder
- Taste and odour not offensive
- Reasonable cost

Gloves used in dentistry are of four types:
  i. *Sterile surgical gloves:* These gloves assure a fit of high quality, however they are expensive.
  ii. *Latex gloves:* These are not commonly used in dentistry. They are adversely affected by alcohols, sterilizing/disinfecting solutions, soaps and detergents. Washing latex gloves with soaps or detergents brings lipids to the surface resulting in their becoming tacky or sticky.
  iii. *Vinyl gloves:* They are sometimes referred to as 'overgloves'. These are used when intraoral procedure has to be interrupted for a brief time, e.g. to answer a telephone call or briefly examine another patient. Following washing and drying of gloved hands, the overgloves can be slipped over the regular examination gloves and removed when work with the initial patient is resumed.
  iv. *Heavy utility gloves:* These should be worn when handling contaminated sharp instruments because they are wear resistant. Certain utility gloves (Nitrite types) can be washed, sterilized, disinfected and reduced and are tear resistant. It is recommended that gloves should not be reused. Double gloves may be indicated for patients with known infectious diseases, such as Herpes, HBV and HIV. Gloves that have been contaminated with an infectious entity should be sterilized before being discarded. Boxes of gloves should be stored away from sunlight in tightly closed, heavy plastic bags to minimize oxidation.

C. Face Masks

The face mask is an important barrier providing protection from inhalation of aerosols, generated by high speed handpiece and air water syringes and also prevent spatter from patients' mouth and splashes of contaminated solutions and chemicals from contacting the mucus membrane of mouth and nose. Face masks may be composed of glass or synthetic fiber, paper, cloth, foam or other synthetic materials. The fiber type mask is considered to be more efficient in filtering bacteria. Effective face masks should provide a minimum filtration of 95% of 3 m particles and should have ability to block aerosols as well as larger particles of blood, saliva and oral debris. A properly fitting mask should:

- Fit comfortably around the entire periphery of face
- Not leak air out of the sides
- Not touch lips or nostrils
- Not irritate skin
- Provide breathing effectively
- Not cause fogging of protective eyewear

Masks with highest filtration are rectangular, folded types used for surgeries. Dome-shaped masks are adequate barriers against spatter and are considered to prevent HBV and HIV infection. To best protect against aerosols, edges of the rectangular mask are pressed close around the bridge of nose and face. Masks should be grasped only by the string or band at the sides or back of head to remove it.

Face masks should be changed once per hour or between each patient contact or whenever it becomes moist or visibly soiled.

The outside of masks should not be touched as it significantly decreases the filtration capability of mask.

D. Protective Clothing

The general recommendations for clinical wear include reusable or disposable gowns and laboratory coats or uniforms with long sleeves, high neck and long knee length. Head covers are also recommended during procedures that result in splashing blood or other body fluids as hair can trap heavy contamination and if not washed thoroughly, can be rubbed back from a pillow onto the face at night.

The gowns should be changed at least daily and should be changed immediately if soaked or spattered with blood or other contaminants. The reusable garments should be placed in bags marked with a 'bio hazard' symbol. Laundering can be effectively accomplished with a high temperature (60°C to 70°C) wash cycle with normal bleach followed by machine drying (100°C or more). Cool water containing 50 to 150 ppm of chlorine can also be used. This method has been found to be effective in killing the AIDS virus.

Shoes should be changed at the office or kept out of reach of small children at home because they are in constant contact with saliva and blood splatter that settle on the floor.

functions should be controlled from a foot switch to avoid possible contamination by use of hand operated switches.

The greatest potential for cross-contamination in a dental chair is from chair mounted controls. The finger-operated switches normally have cracks and crevices, which are impossible to clean and disinfect. Electrical switches are particularly susceptible to corrosion when contacted by liquid disinfectants. Plastic sheaths should cover switches.

The headrests should be covered by disposable covers. Arm slings tend to trap debris and must be carefully cleaned prior to disinfection.

D. Operator Stool

Disinfection of operator stool is important.

Adjustment of the height of the stool is usually accompanied by grasping a lever located under the stand. Covering the lever with plastic sheath will control cross-contamination.

The seat material should be of vinyl plastic, particularly when maximum asepsis is required. Cleaning and disinfecting porous seat covering may be accomplished with soap and water.

E. Cabinet

The cabinets should be minimally used. The materials and equipment should be stored out of the treatment room and brought in only when needed for a particular procedure.

The cabinets should be made of materials that will withstand repeated cleaning and disinfection. Work surfaces should be disinfected for each patient. Other surfaces should be disinfected weekly.

F. Utility Items

Generally supply of water, compressed air, suction, etc. are often located in one room. The air-conditioned room should have excellent air circulation with an exhaust to the outside.

A potential source of physical and microbial contamination is often the main water supply. Preventive measures for water systems include use of a water sediment filter and softening and/or deionization of the incoming water supply, which will help prevent clogging of water passages in dental equipments.

Suction pumps are usually so designed as to have smooth flow of water and air for proper operation. The sediment trap on incoming line is a real source of contamination. The trap should be located in a well lighted and accessible area. The trap should be disassembled and flushed with copious amounts of water to remove all sediments, plaque and debris collected in the cup.

The air exhaust should be routed outside and not allowed to empty into the adjacent room.

The air compressor intake filter must be positioned in an area of clean, cool and dry air. Care must be taken so that the intake filter is cleaned and replaced on a regular schedule. The outgoing air supply line should be routed through air filter with a filtration capacity of 0.01μ.

Air compressor tank must be drained daily to ensure that a build-up of water in the tank is not allowed. This water is a source of serious microbial contamination.

G. Dental Unit Water Lines

It has been established that the dental unit water system is contaminated.

Contaminated oral fluids may be drawn back into turbine chamber of handpiece by negative pressure created or may be retracted into the water lines. While dental units have anti retraction valves, these valves do fail. The retraction should be checked periodically by observing the tip of waterline proper. If a drop of water "hangs" on tip, retraction is not occurring. If the water is drawn back into the line, retraction is proper.

Inherent water system contamination

The dental unit water lines become colonized with micro-organisms including bacteria, fungi and protozoa which form the biofilm. The micro-organisms in the biofilm produce a protective polysaccharide matrix that serves as a reservoir which can amplify the number of micro-organisms in water used for dental treatment. These micro-organisms exit through dental handpiece or air water syringe. This matrix, which can be 30-50 μ thick, affords the biofilm flora resistance to antimicrobial agents. Because of this resistance to antimicrobial agents, the biofilm is difficult to remove.

Bacterial growth in biofilms on the inner walls of dental unit water lines is a universal occurrence. The bacteria may include a variety of species, which can increase infection risk to immuno-compromised persons.

The ADA recommends that infection control measures be established and followed such that dental unit treatments should contain <200 CFU/ml (colony forming unit/ml). The regulatory standard for safe drinking water is <500 CFU/ml in water used as coolant/irrigant for non-surgical dental procedures.

Improving dental unit water quality

The dental waterlines should be flushed at the beginning of the day to decrease the microbial load. However, this doesn't affect biofilm in the waterline or improve the quality of water used during dental treatment. Therefore, the recommended value of <500 CFU/ml is usually not achieved. The effective methods include self contained water systems combined with chemical treatment, in-line water systems combined with chemical treatment, in-line microfilters and combinations of these treatments. The water containing <500 CFU/ml of bacteria in a self-contained water system will not eliminate bacterial contamination if biofilms in the water system are not controlled. Removal of dental waterline biofilm requires use of chemical germicides.

The blood and saliva with micro-organisms can enter the dental water system during patient treatment. Dental devices that are connected to the dental water system and that enter the patients' mouth should be operated to discharge water and air for a minimum of 20-30 seconds after each patient. This procedure is intended to physically flush out blood and saliva that might have entered the turbine, air or waterlines. The majority of recently manufactured dental units are engineered to prevent retraction of oral fluids. Even with anti retraction valves, flushing for a minimum of 20-30 seconds after each patient is recommended.

Sterile irrigation solutions

Sterile solutions are used as a coolant/irrigant in the performance of oral surgical procedures where a greater opportunity exists for entry of micro-organisms into the vascular system and other normally sterile areas. Conventional dental units can't deliver sterile water even when equipped with independent water reservoirs because the water bearing pathway can't be reliably sterilized. Delivery devices preferably disposable products should be used to deliver sterile water.

H. Saliva Ejectors

Back flow from low-saliva ejectors occurs when the pressure in the patient's mouth is less than that in the evacuator. The micro-organisms present in the line usually get retracted into the patients' mouth. This back flow can be a potential source of cross-contamination. Furthermore, it has been established that gravity pulls fluid back toward the patients' mouth whenever a length of suction tubing holding the tip is positioned above the patient's mouth or during simultaneous use of other evacuation.

The suction tubings should be smooth and even on both internal and external surfaces. A few systems are available with removable tubings, which may be heat sterilized; however, most systems need disinfection procedures.

Tubings for handpieces, scalers, air/water syringes and other instruments are difficult to maintain in an aseptic condition. The tubings should be straight, not coiled, smooth on the outer surfaces preferably made of non-absorbent materials.

Miscellaneous items

Cameras, light curing units, lasers, air abrasion units and, etc. are some miscellaneous items that must be protected against contamination. They are used in operatory and can't be sterilized or even readily disinfected. Clear plastic bags of suitable size should be used covering these items.

FUTURE DEVELOPMENTS

The researchers are working hard to improve the sterilization and asepsis properties of the dental equipment. Molded, seamless components are being designed and manufactured for all types of treatment equipment. Noncontact controls are being popularized for achieving better asepsis.

The switches are so designed which can be disinfected easily and are operated with the back of hand.

The future will provide increased value of remote control modules to remove unnecessary components from the treatment vicinity. The instrument control modules will be replaceable by the operator.

The internal and external surfaces of fluid and air hoses will be completely smooth to discourage collection of micro-organisms. The custom fitted barrier materials for asepsis will be utilized in routine. The use of disposable equipments and staff gowns, etc. will continue to increase.

BIBLIOGRAPHY

1. Allen K.L., Salgado T.L., Janal, M.N. and Thompson, V.P.: Removing carious dentin using a polymer instrument without anaesthesia versus a carbide bur with anaesthesia. J.A.D.A.: 136, 643, 2005.
2. Bartoloni J.A., Charleton D.G. and Flint, D.J.: Infection control practices in dental radiology. Gen. Dent., pp. 264, 2003.
3. Bonsor S.J. and Pearson G.J.: Current clinical applications of photo-activated disinfection in restorative dentistry. Dent. Update: 33, 147, 2006.
4. Chrinstensen G.J.: Air abrasion tooth cutting. State of the art. J.A.D.A: 129, 484, 1998.
5. Dahlin T.: Efficient and high quality cavity preparation. Quint. Int.: 5, 20, 1982.
6. Eames W.B., Nale, J.L.: A comparison of cutting efficiency of air-driven fissure burs. J. Am. Dent. Assoc.: 86, 412, 1973.

7. Eames W.B., Reder, B.S. and Smith, G.A.: Cutting efficiency of diamond stones. Effect of technique variables. Oper. Dent.: 2, 156, 1977.
8. Glenner R.A.: Hand cutting instruments. J. History of Dent.: 43, 81, 1995.
9. Grajower R., Zeitchick, A. and Rajstein, J.: The grinding efficiency of diamond burs. J. Prosthet. Dent.: 42, 422, 1979.
10. Henry, E.E. and Peyton, F.A.: The relationship between design and cutting efficiency of dental burs. J. Dent. Res.: 33, 281, 1954.
11. Janota M.: Use of SEM for evaluating diamond points. J.P.D.: 24, 88, 1973.
12. Katoh Y., Sunico, M., Medina, III V, Shinkai, K.: Newly developed diamond points for conservative operative procedures. Oper. Dent.: 26, 76, 2001.
13. Kellett M. and Hollbrook, W.P.: Bacterial contamination of dental handpieces. J. Dent.: 8, 249, 1980.
14. Klein R.C., Party, B.E. and Gershey, E.L.: Virus penetration of examination gloves. Biotechniques: 9, 196, 1990.
15. Kolstad R.A.: How well does the chemiclave sterile handpieces? J.A.D.A.: 129, 985, 1998.
16. Larsen T., Anderson, H.K. and Fiehn, N.E.: Evaluation of a new device for sterilizing dental high speed handpieces. O. Surg., O. Med., O. Path.: 48, 513, 1997.
17. Lewis D.L., Arens, M. and Appleton, S.S.: Cross contamination potential with dental equipment. Lancet: 340, 1252, 1992.
18. Lloyd L., Burke, F.J.T. and Cheung, S.W.: Handpieces asepsis: A survey of attitudes of dental practitioner. B.D.J.: 178, 23, 1995.
19. Malmstrom H.S.: Chaves Y and Moss M.E.: Patient preference: conventional rotary handpieces or air abrasion for cavity preparation. Oper. Dent. 28, 667, 2003.
20. Martin M.V. and Bartzokan C.A.: The boiling of instruments in general dental practice: a misnomer for sterilization. B.D.J.: 159, 18, 1985.
21. Martin M.V.: The significance of the bacterial contamination of dental unit water system. B.D.J.: 163, 152, 1987.
22. McDowell C., Baumgartner, L. and Vermilyu, S.: Durability of dental burs following multiple sterilization cycle. Gen. Dent., pp.485, 1989.
23. McDowell Russell, A.D.: Antiseptics and disinfectants: Activity, action, and resistance. Clin. Microbiol. Rev.: 12, 147, 1999.
24. Meritt R.: Low energy lasers in dentistry. B.D.J.: 172, 90, 1992.
25. Meskin L.H.: HIV update: misinformation persists. J.A.D.A.: 130, 1260, 1999.
26. Miller C.H.: Sterilization and disinfection: what every dentist needs to know? J.A.D.A.: 123, 46, 1992.
27. Morrant G.A.: Burs and rotary instruments: introduction of a new standard numbering system. B.D.J.: 147, 97, 1979.
28. Morrison A. and Conrod, S.: Dental Burs and endodontic files: Are routine sterilization procedures effective ? J.C.D.A.: 75, 39, 2009.
29. Parker H.H. and Johsnon, R.B.: Effectiveness of ethylene oxide for sterilization of dental handpieces. J. Dent.: 23, 113, 1995.
30. Pederson E.D., Stone, M. and Ragain, J.C.: Biofilms in dental-unit waterlines. Scientific review of Issue Impacting Dentistry, 1, 1, 1999.
31. Pilcher E.S. Tietge, J.D. and Draughn, R.A.: Comparison of cutting rates among single-patient-use and multiplepatient-use diamond burs. J. Prosthodont.: 9, 66, 2000.
32. Pinto, L.S., Peruchi, C., Marker, V.A. and Cordeiro, R.: Evaluation of cutting pattern produced with Air abrasion systems using different tip designs. Oper. Dent.: 26, 308, 2001.
33. Rohrer M.D. and Bulard, R.A.: Microwave sterilization. J.A.D.A.: 110, 194, 1985.
34. Rutala A.W. and Weber, D.J.: New disinfection and sterilization methods emerging infectious diseases, 7, 348, 2001.
35. Rutala A.W. and Weber, D.J.: Guideline for disinfection and sterilization of prior-contaminated medical instruments. Infection Control and Hosp Epidemio: 31, 107, 2010.
36. Scully C., Porter, S.R. and Epstein, J.: Compliance with infection control procedures in a dental hospital clinic. B.D.J.: 173, 20, 1992.
37. Siegel S.C., Von Framhofer, J.A.: Dental cutting: the historical development of diamond burs. J.A.D.A.: 129, 1198, 1998.
38. Siegel S.C. and Von Fraunhofee, J.A.: Assessing the cutting efficiency of dental diamond burs. J.A.D.A.: 127, 763, 1996.
39. Sockwell C.L.: Dental handpieces and rotary cutting instruments. Dent. Clin. North Am.: 15, 219, 1971.
40. Tate, W.H., Goldschmidt, M., Ward, M. and Grant, R.L.: Disinfection and sterilization of composite polishing instruments. Am. J. Dent.: 8, 270, 1995.
41. Watson T.F. and Cook, R.J.: The influence of bur blade concentricity on high speed tooth cutting interaction: a video rate confocal microscopic study. J.D.R.: 74, 1749, 1995.
42. Watanabe T., Miyazaki M. and Moore, K.: Influence of polishing instruments on the surface texture of resin composites. Quint. Int.: 37, 61, 2006.
43. Wesson M.D. and Thornton J.D.: Eye protection and occlusal complication in the dental office. Gen. Dent., pp.19, 1989.
44. Whitworth M.: A comparison of discontamination methods used for dental burs. Brit. Dent. J.: 197, 635, 2004.
45. Williams J.F., Johnston A.M., Johnson, B., Huntingon, M.K. and Mackenzie, C.D.: Microbial contamination of dental unit water lines. J.A.D.A.: 124, 59, 1993.

8
Matrices, Retainers and Wedges

Human teeth are designed in such a way that the individual tooth contributes significantly to their own support as well as collectively the teeth in the arch support the stomatognathic system. Each tooth is attached in the alveolar bone socket with fine periodontal fibers. These fibers act as cushion and this arrangement relieves the supporting bone of much responsibility and lessens the mass of bone that would otherwise be required. A break in the continuity of the tooth contacts throws an additional responsibility on the periodontal membrane and alveolar bone, which they may not be able to sustain.

Failure to respect and preserve these relationships will not only cause premature failure of the restoration but also periodontal problems as well as initiation of caries around the adjacent tooth structure. A clear understanding of this interproximal relationship will help the clinician to preserve these structures in a much better manner. To achieve an ideal contact, a clinician should have adequate knowledge of the ideal tooth forms. For example:

- A perfect triangular interproximal space between two adjoining teeth. This space gradually widens out to the labial/buccal and lingual surfaces to form the embrasures.
- Interproximal embrasures are extending on all the four sides, i.e. occlusal, gingival, buccal/labial and lingual having definite shape around each contact area.
- The base of the triangular shaped interproximal space is located at the alveolar border, while the apex is at the point of contact. Reverse is true for other embrasures, the apex is always at the contact and the base towards the outer surface.
- Anterior teeth usually exhibit marble contacts with less pronounced embrasures.

These ideal conditions are frequently marred by the stresses incident to time, wear, local irritants, configuration disturbances, and imperfectly performed dental operations. The most important function of proximal contact is the protection of the interdental papillae. On anterior teeth where the papillae form cone-like projections, properly placed point contacts are necessary. A broader buccolingually contacting area is required on bicuspids because the crests of the papillae broaden out in this region. Similarly, as we move distally, the widest contacting area is required on molars because they have the widest interproximal papillae. Improper configuration of the proximal area may:

 i. cause displacement of teeth bucally, lingually, mesially or distally.
 ii. exert a lifting force on the tooth when placed too high occlusally.
 iii. disturb the axial relationship of the teeth, resulting in trauma.
 iv. cause rotation of the teeth.
 v. cause injury to the investing structures by excessively opening or closing the contact and interproximal embrasures.
 vi. disturb the coordination of the inclined planes and cusps, causing defective occlusal contacts.
 vii. cause vertical or horizontal food impaction.

TOOTH SEPARATION

Many a time prior separation of the teeth is necessary to restore a proper contact. The separation is also helpful in many other situations like:

- For examination of interproximal spaces
- For preparation of cavities
- For insertion and polishing of restorations
- For removal of foreign bodies, such as fruit seeds, fragments of toothpicks, or bone sequestrums, etc.

Two methods are generally employed for accomplishing separation:

- Slow separation
- Rapid or immediate separation

Slow Separation

In this method, the teeth are slowly and gradually forced apart inserting certain materials between them. The advantage of slow separation is that the repositioning occurs physiologically without injuring periodontal ligament fibers. The disadvantage of this method is that the procedure is time consuming and may require many visits.

Materials used for slow separation are base plate, gutta-percha, orthodontic wire, wood or rubber. Gutta-percha may be used in case of adjoining proximal cavity of posterior teeth. Soften the gutta-percha with heat and pack into the cavity overfilling at the proximal side. The material is kept in position for a week and can be renewed, if necessary, until separation is accomplished.

Copper wire usually used for orthodontic purpose can also be passed beneath the contact. The two ends are brought occlusally, twisted together, trimmed and tucked inwards to avoid catching the soft tissues. The wire can accomplish separation in 48 hours.

Rapid or Immediate Separation

This is the most valuable and frequently used method.

The rapid separator should carefully be applied and skillfully handled to produce desired results. Such a method is useful and more advantageous over slow separation method. Though, the method is quick and useful in clinical conditions, yet it may rupture the periodontal ligament fibers and also rapid separation induces pain at the site. The rapid or immediate separation is achieved following two principles, viz. Wedge principle and Traction principle.

The separation by *'Wedge principle'* is accomplished by the insertion of a pointed wedge shaped device between teeth in order to create space at the contact area. The more the wedges move facially or lingually the greater will be the separation. This separation is brought about by mechanical device (Elliot separator) along with wedges.

a. ***Elliot Separator:*** Occasionally, it is desired that separation be obtained for a short while, as the stability necessary for long operations is not required. In this case, the wedge principle is desirable. The Elliot separator is one such example. During its application, care must be exercised to prevent slipping. This type of separation is useful in examining a proximal surface or in final polishing of the contact point after all other contouring has been completed (Fig. 8.1).
b. ***Wedges leading to separation include:***
   i. Wooden wedges
   ii. Metal wedges

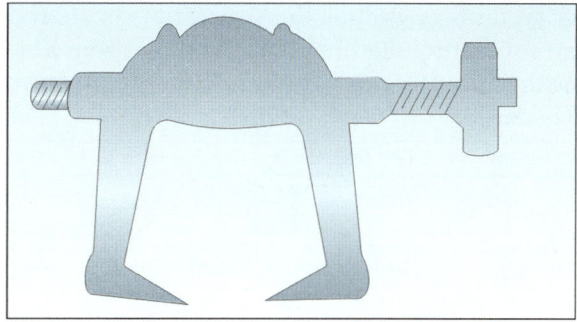

Fig. 8.1: Elliot separator

   iii. Silver wedges
   iv. Celluloid or plastic wedges
   v. Medicated wood wedges

The separation by *'Traction principle'* is always accomplished with mechanical devices, which engage the proximal surfaces of the teeth to be separated by means of holding arms. These are mechanically moved apart, creating separation between the clamped teeth.

Examples of separators, which work on traction principle, are:

a. Non-interfering true separator
b. Ferrier double bow separator
c. Ivory adjustable separator
d. Perry separator
e. Woodward separator
f. Parr's Universal separator
g. Dentatus-Nystrom separator

The first and second types of separators are still being used, others are mentioned here for academic purpose only.

a. ***Non-interfering true separator:*** This device is indicated when continuous stabilized separation is required during the dental operation. Its advantage is that the separation can be increased or decreased after stabilization, and the device is non-interfering (Fig. 8.2).
b. ***Ferrier double-bow separator:*** With this device, the separation is stabilized throughout the operation.

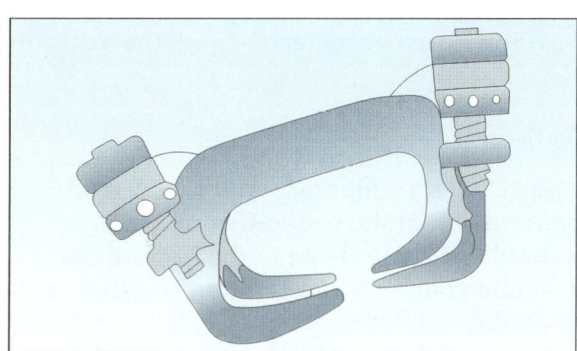

Fig. 8.2: Non-interfering true separator

Its advantage is that the separation is shared by the contacting teeth, and not at the expense of one tooth, as with the previous type of instrument (Fig. 8.3).

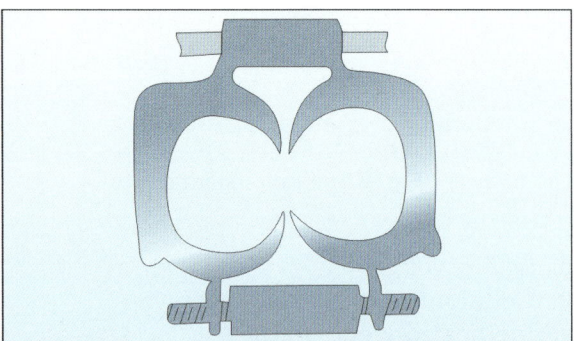

Fig. 8.3: Ferrier double bow separator

MATRICES

The word matrix is derived from the Latin word 'Mater' which means 'Mother'. It was introduced in the year 1871 by *Dr. Louis Jack*.

The matrix is a device used to contour a restoration to simulate that of a tooth structure, which it is replacing.

Ideal requirements of a matrix are:
- It should be inserted easily and should be sufficiently rigid to retain the contour given to it so that it can be transferred to the restoration.
- It should not adhere to or react with the restorative material.
- It should resist the condensation pressure.

Matricing is the procedure, whereby a temporary wall is created opposite to axial walls and surrounding areas of tooth structure that were lost during preparation. The matrix should possess the exact three-dimensional contour (including the contact area) of the future restoration. Not only should it be immobile while the material sets but also it should not react with it. On the other hand it should be easily removable after hardening of restorative material without compromising the created contact and contour or characteristics of the restorative material.

Objectives

- It must act as a temporary wall of resistance during introduction of the restorative material.
- It should provide shape to the restoration.
- It should confine the restoration within acceptable physiological limits.
- It must assist in isolating the gingiva and rubber dam during introduction of the restorative material
- It must help in maintaining the dry operative field thereby preventing contamination of the restoration.

CLASSIFICATION OF MATRICES

Matrices are classified in two ways; one is based on mode of retention and second is based on transparency. The first two are based on modes of retention and the next two are based on transparency.

- Mechanically retained matrices
- Self-retained matrices
- Non-transparent matrices
- Transparent matrices

Materials used as matrices include stainless steel, cellulose acetate (cellophane), cellulose nitrate (celluloid) and polymer materials. Matrix system is mostly formed of two parts: a *band*, which is made of metal, polymeric material or celluloid (Figs 8.4A, B) and a *retainer*. Matrices are commonly supplied as strips of different dimensions. They may be 0.001" (0.025 mm) or 0.002" (0.05 mm) thick. The width of the matrix band may be 1/4", 3/8", 5/16" or 1/8".

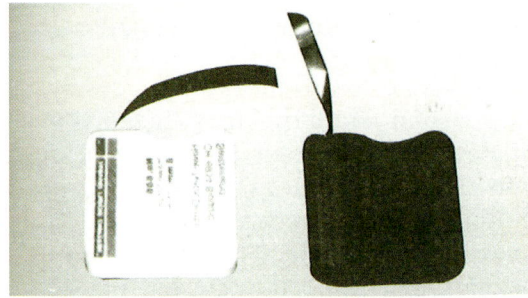

Fig. 8.4A: Stainless steel and plastic matrices

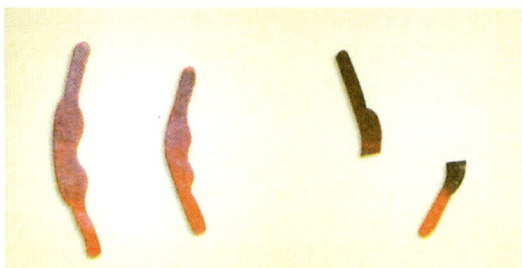

Fig. 8.4B: Matrices

Matrices for Class II, MOD and Complex Restorations

Early mechanical matrices were the Miller's matrix, Woodward's screw matrix and the loop matrix (Figs 8.5A, B and C). These matrices were not flexible and their insertion around the tooth was difficult. However, they led to separation of teeth. The other major disadvantage was that the contact and contours were lost once they were drawn onto the teeth. This

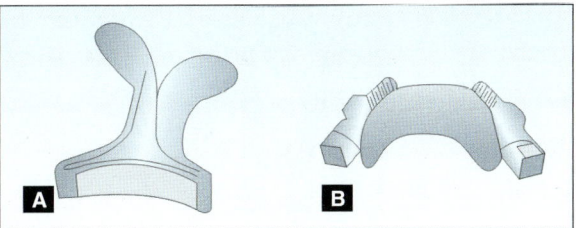

Figs 8.5A and B: (A) Miller clamp matrix **(B)** Woodward's screw matrix

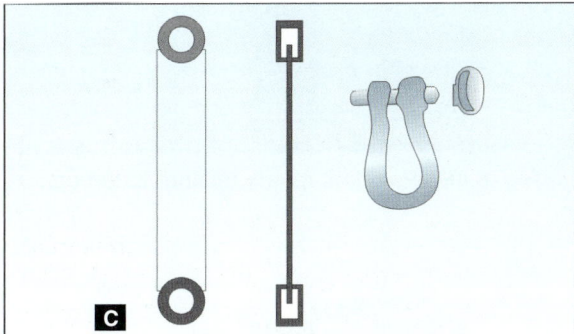

Fig. 8.5: (C) Loop matrix

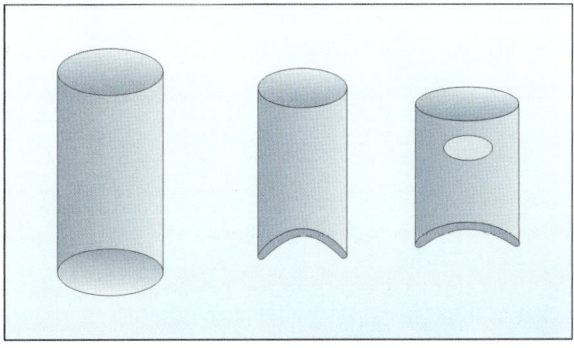

Fig. 8.6A: Copper band matrix

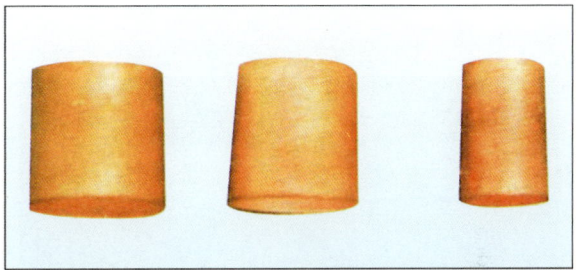

Fig. 8.6B: Copper band

led to the advent of stainless steel matrices of 0.002-inch thicknesses to be screwed with the help of retainers. The disadvantages of early matrices were eliminated since the new matrices could be contoured according to the contour of the tooth to be restored.

Recently, the demand for rigid type of matrix has been increased because of the use of condensable restorative materials. Such matrices can better withstand the forces of condensation.

A few authors are of the opinion that the matrix be held without the use of retainers, only wedges are sufficient. The rationale is that the retained matrices usually produce straighter proximal areas and matrix held with only wedges produce better contours and contacts.

For MOD preparation and complex restoration, a continuous matrix band is indicated. Such a matrix band may be retained with a mechanical holder and may be ligated. Copper bands can be used for such purposes. These can be trimmed with scissors, smoothened and placed onto the teeth. These can be kept there till the restoration sets. These are mostly used with silver amalgam restorations involving more than two surfaces (Figs 8.6A and B).

Sectional Matrix System

For Class II resin composite restoration, the use of sectional matrix systems and separation rings to obtain tight proximal contacts is recommended. The sectional matrix system and separation rings are made up of nickel-titanium alloy to create a consistent force to separate teeth and then return to their original shape after use, helping to deliver a tight gingival seal and anatomically shaped restoration. Some of the commercially available systems are-

   i. Palodent Plus Sectional matrix system (Fig. 8.7A)
  ii. Composi–Tight 3D sectional matrix system (Fig 8.7B)
 iii. Triodent V3 Ring matrix system (Fig. 8.7C) etc.

The technique for the placement of the Palodent Plus sectional matrix is as follows (Figs 8.8A to E):

1. Place a matrix band that most closely approximates the occluso-gingival height of the tooth. The band should be oriented with concave edge towards the occlusal margin of the tooth.
2. Insert wedge.
3. Apply the 3D –ring retainer. Hold the ring retainer with the ring placement forcep and place it over the wedge.

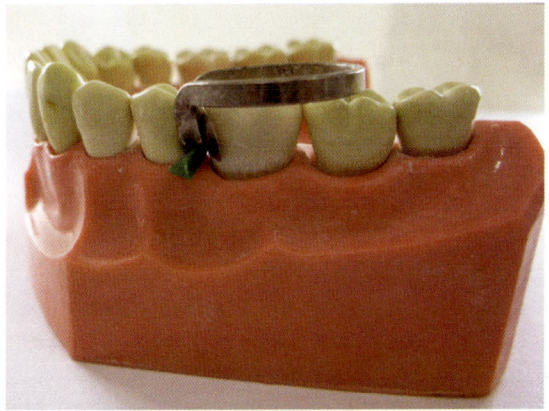

Fig 8.7A: Palodent Plus sectional matrix system

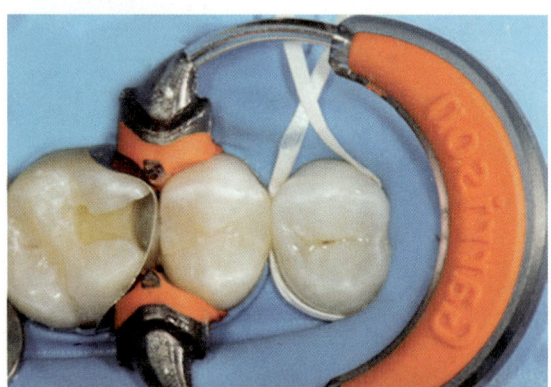

Fig. 8.7B: Composi Tight 3D sectional matrix system

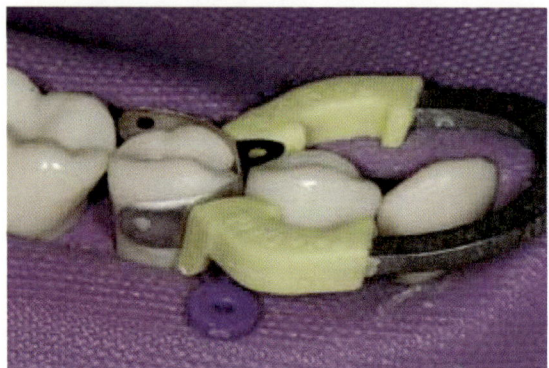

Fig. 8.7C: Triodent V3 ring matrix system

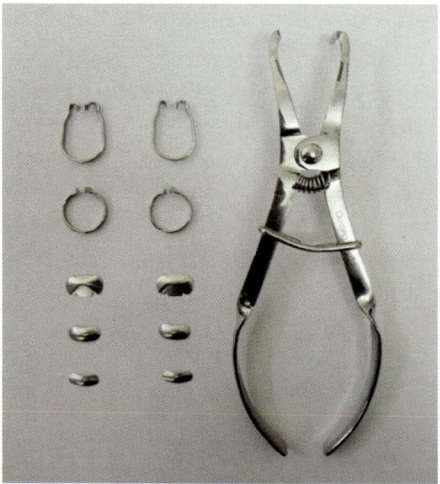

Fig. 8.8A: Components of palodent sectional matrix system

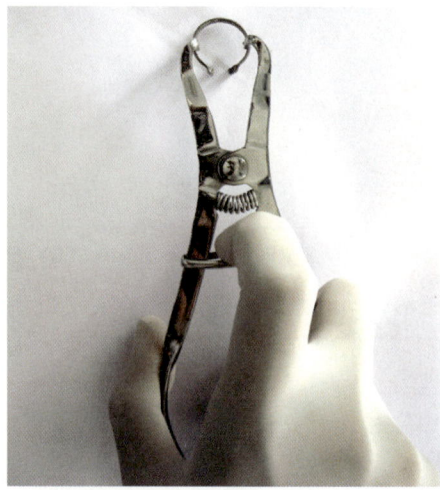

Fig. 8.8B: Palodent matrix retainer in forceps

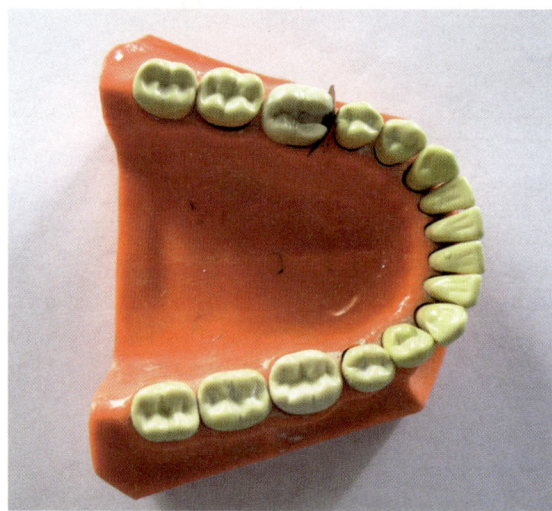

Fig. 8.8C: Palodent matrix band placed

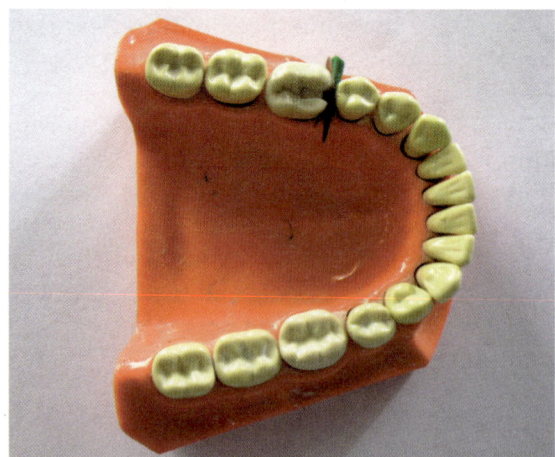

Fig. 8.8D: Palodent matrix band with wedge placed

4. Burnish the band in the desired contact area against the adjacent tooth and make sure there is no springback of the band.
5. Restore the cavity as desired.
6. Remove the ring, wedge and band. Removal of the ring and band may require the need of forcep.

MATRICES FOR CLASS III DIRECT TOOTH-COLORED RESTORATIONS

These are usually transparent plastic matrix strips. For silicate cements they are usually celluloid strips and

Matrices, Retainers and Wedges

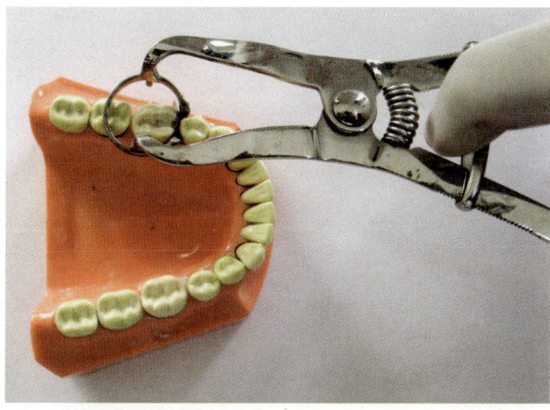

Fig. 8.8E: Palodent retainer holding the band

for resins they are cellophane strips. Mylar strips may be used for either material.

The suitable plastic strip is burnished over the end of a steel instrument, e.g. handle of a tweezer, to produce a 'belly' in the strip. This will allow for a curvature, which, if properly contoured and designed, will reproduce the natural proximal contour of the tooth (Figs 8.9A and B).

In distal surface of canine, since the fixation of retainer is difficult, a metal band is moulded into "S" shape and stabilized using wedges and/or impression compound (Fig. 8.10).

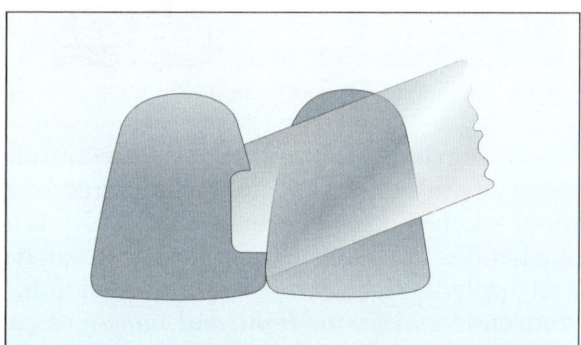

Fig. 8.9A: Matrices for class III cavity preparation

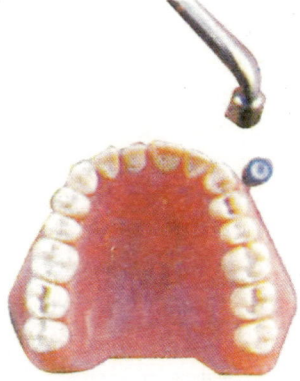

Fig. 8.9B: Plastic matrix applied around left maxillary canine on model

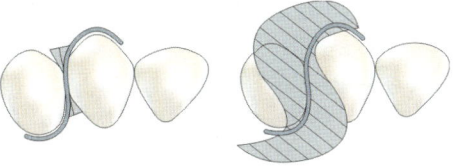

Fig. 8.10: 'S' shaped matrix for distal surface of canine

MATRICES FOR CLASS IV PREPARATIONS FOR DIRECT TOOTH-COLORED RESTORATIONS

A suitable plastic strip is folded and molded into L shape. One side of the strip is cut so that it is as wide as the length of the tooth. The other side is cut so that it is as wide as the width of the tooth. The strip, with a wedge in place, is adapted to the tooth. It is important that the angle formed by the fold of the strip approximates the normal corner of the tooth and supports the matrix on the lingual surface, which is held by the forefinger of the left hand. The cavity is then filled to slight excess, and one end of the strip is brought across the proximal surface of the filled tooth. When this is completed, the other end of the strip is folded over the incisal edge. The matrix is held with the thumb of the left hand.

Prefabricated matrices are also available, or it can be fabricated to suit the required restoration. Commonly available matrices are:

i. *Aluminium foil incisal corner matrix*: These are 'stock' metallic matrices shaped according to the proximo-incisal corner and surfaces of anterior teeth (Fig. 8.11). They can be adapted to each specific case. This type of matrix cannot be used for light cured resin material.

ii. *Transparent crown form matrices*: These are 'stock' plastic crowns, which can be adapted to tooth anatomy (Fig. 8.11). In bilateral class IV preparations use the entire crown form but in a unilateral class IV cut the plastic crown incisogingivally into two halves and use only the side corresponding to the location of the preparation (Fig. 8.12).

iii. *Anatomic matrix*: Prior to preparing the teeth (tooth), a study cast for the affected tooth or teeth

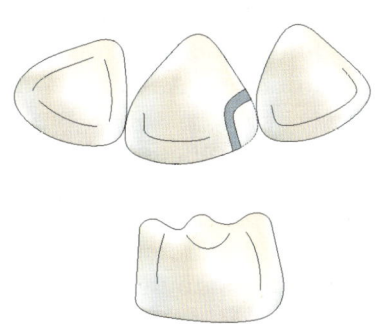

Fig. 8.11: Matrices for class IV cavity

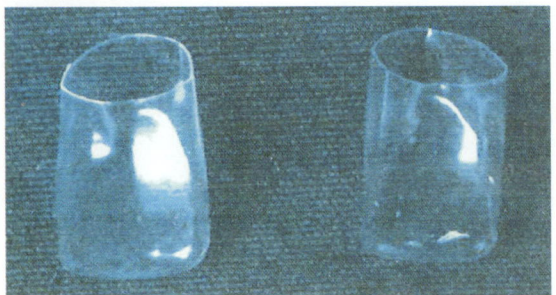

Fig. 8.12: Transparent celluloid crowns

together with at least one intact adjacent tooth on each side is made. It is preferable, especially in multiple involvements where the restoration(s) is (are) part of the disclusion mechanism, to make full arch study models and mount them in centric occlusion.

The defective areas are restored on the study model in a fairly heat resistant material (plaster, acrylic resin, blocking compound, plasticine, etc.) to the appropriate configuration. A plastic template is then made for the restored tooth or teeth on the model using a combination of heat (to thermoplastically soften the template material) and suction (vacuum) consequently to draw the moldable material onto the study model. The template is trimmed gingivally to fit the tooth or teeth and adjacent periodontal architecture. It should seat on at least one unprepared tooth on each side. The matrix should be vented by perforating the corners of its part corresponding to the future restoration. The restorative material is inserted into the preparation, and then the matrix is filled with the material and inserted over the prepared and partially filled tooth, ready for curing.

MATRICES FOR CLASS V PREPARATIONS FOR DIRECT TOOTH-COLORED RESTORATIONS

The matrices for class V restorations are also available as prefabricated or the same can be fabricated outside the oral cavity to suit the required restoration. The commonly available matrices for class V restoration are:

i. *Prefabricated plastic matrices:* These are available in different sizes and can be utilized with light cure restorations. A handle is also provided to hold the matrix in place till the material sets (Fig. 8.13). The clinical application of this matrix is shown in Fig. 8.14.

ii. *Aluminium or copper collars for non-light colored restorations:* Aluminium or copper bands are preshaped according to the gingival third of the buccal and lingual surfaces. They can be adjusted to each specific case so that the band will cover

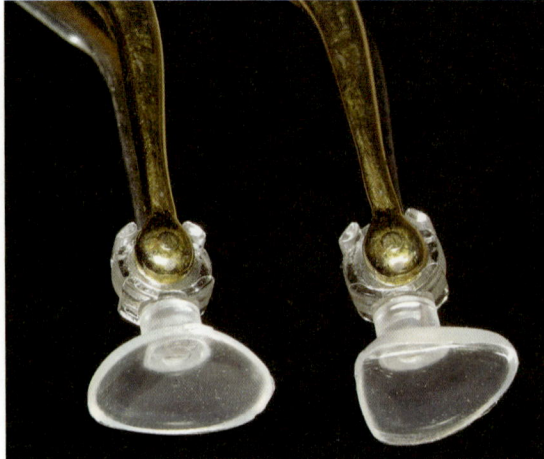

Fig. 8.13: Prefabricated plastic cervical matrices

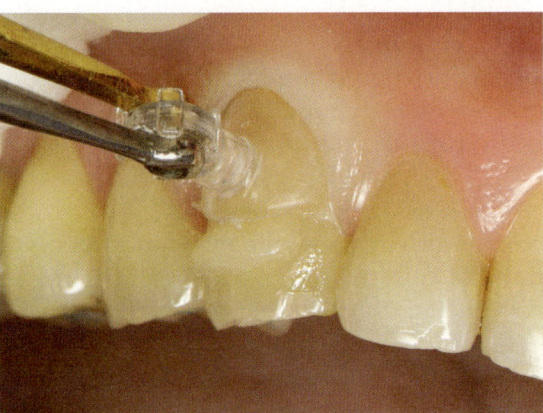

Fig. 8.14: Adaptation of cervical matrix to a Class V cavity

1.0–2.0 mm of the tooth surface circumferential to the cavity margins. They are then mounted on the tip of a softened stick of compound, which is used as a handle. Fill the cavity with restorative material and apply the adjusted collar onto the tooth.

iii. *Anatomic matrix for light and non-light cured, direct tooth-colored materials:* Anatomic matrix can be fabricated as for class IV cavities. The study models for the defective tooth or teeth with at least one intact tooth on each side is made. After restoring the defects on the model, a plastic template is prepared, as described before. The template is cut mesio-distally, keeping its occlusal (incisal) portion and the facial and lingual parts where the defects are. It is then trimmed gingivally and used as a matrix for applying pressure and keeping the restorative material while being cured.

MATRIX RETAINERS

Matrix retainers are gadgets used to retain the matrix bands in position. Some matrices do not need any special mechanical devices to hold them in position. Some matrices may require simple retainers like wires, silk thread, dental floss and impression compound. Some matrices need special mechanical retainers.

a. **Mechanical retainers:** Various types of mechanical retainers used are as follows:

   i. *Nystrom's retainer:* The shape of the slot ensures a 20°–30° inclination of the retainer in relation to the band. The narrowest part of the slot always faces the gingiva. Twisting of the band because of interference with the lip or the front teeth is thus avoided. In order not to traumatize the gingiva an angulation of the edge has been made.

   ii. *Ivory Matrix Holder No. 1 and 8:* Both these retainers are used to hold the matrix to provide a wall for the proximal surface. Ivory Matrix Retainer no. 8 provides bands for encircling entire crown of the tooth. This is suitable for both class II cavities and for mesio-occluso-distal cavities. Since the matrix metal is thin enough, it will pass through the contact of the uncut side in the building of class II amalgam restorations (Figs 8.15A, B). The application of these retainers is shown in Figs 8.16A, B.

   iii. *Steele's Siqveland Self-Adjusting Matrix Clamp:* It is so built that it will form two diameters of the band at the same time; larger diameter for the occlusal end and smaller for the gingival end. Anatomic adaptation is possible without wedges, although additional support at the gingival area is not contraindicated. The band follows the tooth contour without impinging on the gingival tissue. Its principle is that of a movable slide which holds and tightens the band in the required position (Fig. 8.17).

   iv. *The Tofflemire Universal Dental Matrix Band Retainer:* Tofflemire (Fig. 8.18) is the most recent development, presenting a number of advantages. Besides being very stable and of sturdy construction, it permits the easy removal of the holder from the band, facilitating carving and final removal of the band (Fig. 8.15C). Operating instructions are as follows:

   1. Turn the knurled nut (B) to the right until the diagonal slot (C) is about ¼ inch from the inner end of the retainer.
   2. Hold the knurled nut (B) from rotating while the knurled nut (A) (at the end of the spindle) is turned a like number of turns in the opposite direction (left), until the point of the spindle clears the diagonal slot channel for the reception of the free ends of the matrix band.

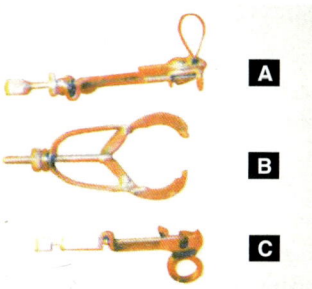

Figs 8.15A to C: Retainers from top to bottom **(A)** Ivory No. 8 **(B)** Ivory No. 1 **(C)** Tofflemine

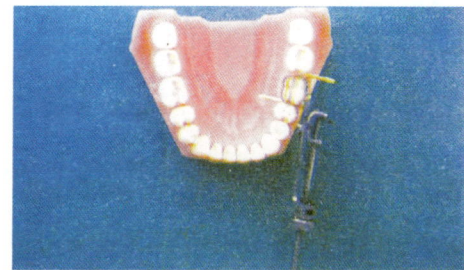

Fig. 8.16A: Application of Ivory No. 8 retainer and band

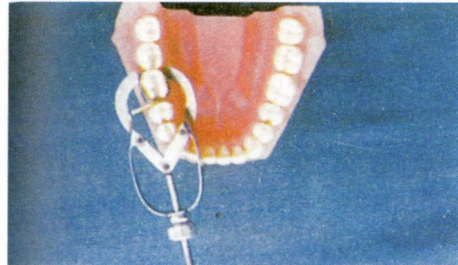

Fig. 8.16B: Application of Ivory No. 1 retainer

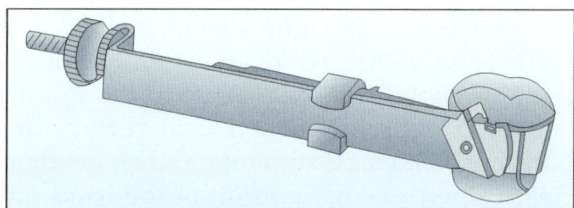

Fig. 8.17: Siqveland matrix retainer

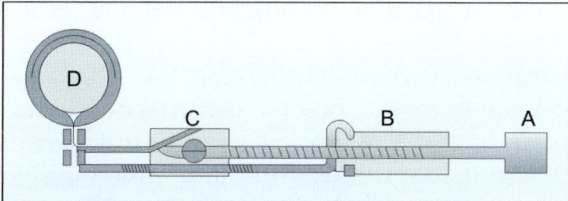

Fig. 8.18: Tofflemire matrix retainer

   3. Insert the 'occlusal edge' of whichever type of matrix band (D) is decided upon in the diagonal slot (C). The preshaped loop, thus formed, is placed in the guide channel

selected in such a manner that the metal arch of the guide channel serves as an occlusal 'stop' and materially aids the carrying of the band over the contour of the tooth.

The folded type of band is particularly well suited for teeth having an exaggerated axial contour, such as bell-crowned, posterior adult teeth, and primary molars; the curved type of band is well suited for the average, moderately contoured, posterior teeth and the straight band is applicable to all other teeth having moderately slight or less than average contour.

Fitting Band to the Teeth

- Guide the band gently over the tooth, using the retainer as a carrier. Should the loop be too small to pass over the contour of the tooth, turn the knurled nut (B) a turn or two to the left, and the loop will be enlarged automatically to the size needed. Conversely, the loop is decreased in size, or tightened around the tooth, by turning the knurled nut (B) to the right. Avoid over tension in tightening the knurled nut (B), thereby eliminating needless breakage of bands.
- After completing the condensation of the amalgam, and after initial setting, do the preliminary carving. The retainer is then removed from the band without disturbing the band at this time. This is accomplished by holding the knurled nut (B) steady while the knurled nut (A) is turned a few turns to the left, thereby permitting the retainer to slip off the band.
- The band is then removed carefully from each contact point, one at a time, in the following manner: support the occlusal surface of the freshly condensed restoration, then gently ease each interproximal portion of the band out of its inclined plane by using a lateral rotation motion rather than an occlusal traction motion. The application of Tofflemire retainer is shown in Fig. 8.19.

b. **Automatrix:** Automatrix, also known as roll-in band matrix is a disposable system where band and retainer are constructed as one unit. Bands of different lengths, widths and thicknesses are available (Fig. 8.20) (length: 4.7 to 7.9 mm and thickness: 0.38 to 0.05 mm). The matrix along with the tightening device is shown in (Fig. 8.21). Although the auto matrix system is intended for use where cavity preparations are extensive, the instability of this system renders it less suitable. Furthermore, proper contour and proximal contact may be difficult to achieve. The auto matrix system is primarily useful in patients who cannot tolerate retainers and in patients with partly erupted teeth where the height of the tooth provide insufficient support for the retainers.

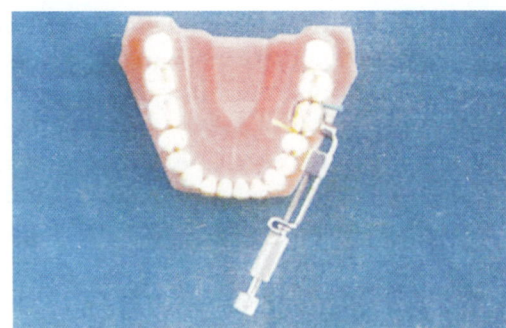

Fig. 8.19: Application of Tofflemire retainer and band

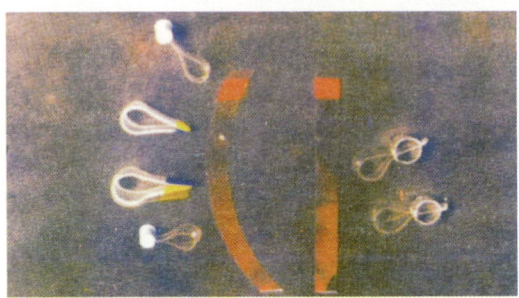

Fig. 8.20: Automatrix system

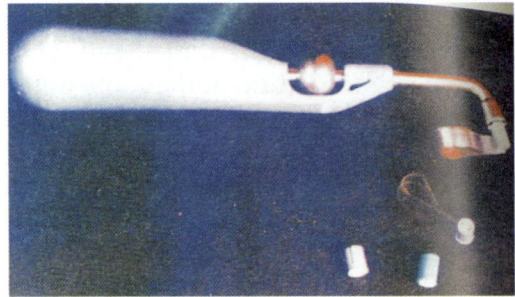

Fig. 8.21: Tightening device for automatrix

WEDGES

Wedges are the third component of the matrix system. However, judging from numerous radiographs of proximal amalgam fillings, little attention seems to have been paid to this important step in the treatment. Overhangs are reported in up to 50 percent of all restorations. The condensation pressure necessary for proper gingival adaptation of the amalgam especially those made from lathe-cut or admixed alloys, leads to surplus of material if wedging is neglected. However, amalgams made from spherical alloys may pose even greater problem in terms of overhangs. This is due to the high plasticity and small particle size of these amalgams.

Wedging serves the following purposes:
- Prevents surplus amalgam being forced into the gingival crevice.
- Assists in contouring the cervical part of the proximal surface
- Separates the teeth to compensate for the thickness of the matrix band such that proximal contacts is reestablished when the band is removed
- Stabilizes the matrix

Wedges are made of wood or plastic. Wooden wedges are preferred because:
- They are easy to trim with a scalpel and they adapt well to the tooth surface.
- When properly shaped they remain stable during condensation.
- Wooden wedges can be cut from toothpicks

In general a wedge must be triangular or trapezoidal in cross-section (Fig. 8.22). The width of the base should be slightly larger than the space between the tooth to be restored and the neighbouring tooth in order to separate the teeth. Occlusally however the wedges must not be too thick as this may influence the proximal contour. If the wedge is not high enough only point contact between the wedge and the band is achieved. This may lead to poor contour or displacement of the wedge during condensation. Loss of contact point may occur if the cross-sectional height of the wedge is too large. A uniform tapering of the wedge is needed in order to render sufficient and even contact throughout the proximal embrasure. A piece of cotton roll may compensate for discrepancies between root surface and matrix band caused by concavities of the root surfaces.

The decision as to whether the wedge should be inserted buccally or lingually is made after inspecting the cavity preparation with the appropriate band in place. This reveals where maintenance of gingival contact is most needed. The location of the retainer often dictates the direction of insertion. In general, the wedge is inserted from the lingual, as this embrasure is normally larger in size. However, since the lingual wedge will interfere with the tongue, it is preferred from the buccal side. In case of maxillary teeth, placement of wedge is preferred from palatal side. In no case, the wedge should be inserted from both the sides (Figs 8.23A and B). If the wedge is inserted from both the sides, it might leave some space just below the contact area leading to overhanging of silver at that area. During insertion, care should be taken to ensure that the wedge is apically positioned in relation to the gingival cavity wall.

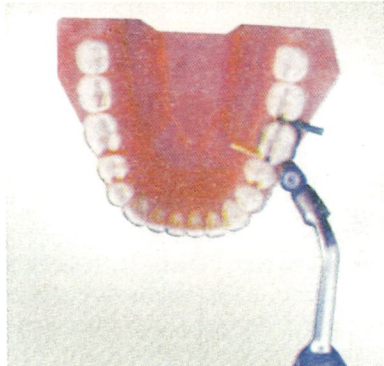

Fig. 8.23A: Placement of wedges

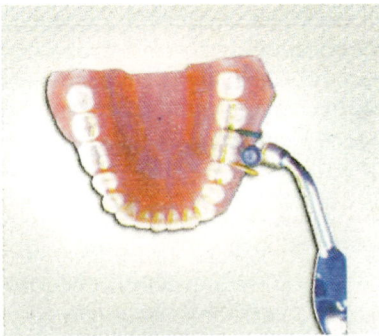

Fig. 8.23B: Placement of wedges

If the wedge is significantly apical of the gingival margin, a second, usually smaller wedge may be 'piggy-backed' on the first wedge. 'Piggy-back' wedging is particularly useful in patients with recession of interproximal tissue level.

The gingival wedge should be tight enough to prevent any possibility of an overhang of restorative material in at least the middle two thirds of the gingival margin.

Occasionally, a concavity may be present on the proximal surface gingivally of the contact and extending as fluting onto the root (e.g. mesial of the maxillary first premolar). A gingival margin located in this area will be similarly concave. To wedge a matrix band tight against such a margin, a second

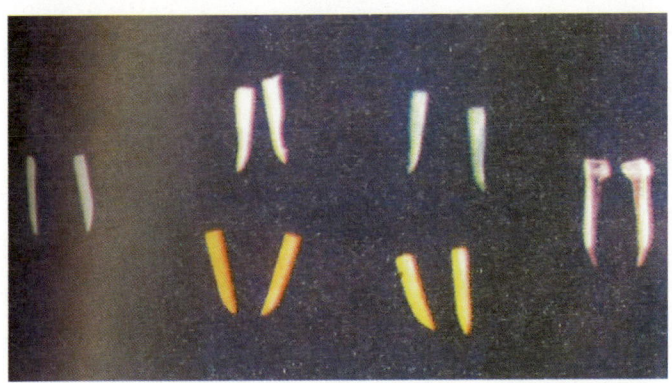

Fig. 8.22: Different shapes and size of wedges

pointed wedge can be inserted between the first wedge and the band by wedge wedging. The wedging action between the teeth should provide enough separation to compensate for the thickness of the matrix band. This will ensure a positive contact relationship after the matrix is removed following the condensation and initial carving of the restoration.

The clinician should have an adequate knowledge of the anatomical and functional aspects of contacts and contours so as to reproduce them with ideal restorative materials. Extensive knowledge about the matricing serves as a guide to reproduce near to normal contacts between teeth, which in turn help to maintain the oral cavity in sound health.

BIBLIOGRAPHY

1. Alhouri, N., Watts, D.C., McCord, J.F. and Smith, P.W.: Mathematical analysis of tooth and restoration contour using image analysis. Dent. Mater.: 20, 893, 2004.
2. Brackett, M.G., Contreras, S., Contreras, R. and Brackett, W.W.: Restoration of proximal contacts in direct Class II resin composites. Oper. Dent. 31, 155, 2006.
3. Cenci, M.S., Lund, R.G., Pereira, C.L., De carvalho, R.M. and Demarco, F.F.: In vivo and in vitro evaluation of Class II composite resin restorations with different matrix systems. J. Adhes. Dent. 8, 127, 2006.
4. Chan, D.C.N.: Custom matrix adaptation with elastic cords. Oper. Dent.: 26, 419, 2001.
5. Cunningham, P.J.: Matrices for amalgam restorations. Aust. Dent.J. 13, 139, 1968.
6. Denehy, G. and Cobb, D.: Impression matrix technique for cusp replacement using direct composite resin. J. Esthet. Restor. Dent.: 16, 227, 2004.
7. Dunn, W.J., Davis, J.T. and Casey, J.A.: Polytetrafluoroethylene (PTFE) tape as a matrix in operative dentistry. Oper. Dent.: 29, 470, 2004.
8. Farah, J.W. and Powers, J.M.: Packable composites: sectional matrices. Dent. Advisor: 16, 2, 1999.
9. Hamilton, J.C.: Posterior Class II composite restoration utilizing a custom occlusal matrix. Pract. Period. Aesthet. Dent.: 11, 371, 1999.
10. Harrington, W.G., Moon, P.C., Crockett, W.D., Shepard, F.E: Reinforced matrices for pin amalgam restorations reduce microleakage. J.P.D. 41, 622, 1979.
11. Ireland, E.J.: Evaluation of a new matrix band and wedge for amalgam preparations having lingual or facial extension. Gen. Dent.: 33, 434, 1985.
12. Kaplan, I., Schuman, N.J.: Selecting a matrix for class II amalgam restoration. J.P.D. 56, 25, 1986.
13. Kucey, B.K.: Matrices in metal ceramics. J.P.D. 63, 32, 1990.
14. Loomans, B.A., Opdam, N.J., Roeters, F.J., Bronkhorst, E.M., Burgersdijk, R.C. and Dorfer, C.E.: A randomnized clinical trial on proximal contacts of posterior composites. J.Dent. 34, 292, 2006
15. Len Boksman: Matrix Systems and the Class II Composite Resin. Oral Health: 23–34, 2010
16. Mamoun, J.S. and Ahmed, M.: Amalgam matrix for class II and class V preparations connected at the proximal box. J.A.D.A.: 137, 186, 2006.
17. Medlock, J.W., Re, G.J.: Contoured mylar matrices. J.P.D. 51, 364, 1984.
18. Meyer, A.: Inadvertent deformation of amalgam matrices. Gen. Dent. 26, 51, 1978.
19. Meyer, A.: Proposed criteria for matrices. J. Can. Dent. Asso.: 53, 851, 1987.
20. Qualtrough, A.J.E. and Wilson, N.H.F.: The history, development and use of interproximal wedges in clinical practice. Dent. Update: 3, 66, 1991.
21. Qualtrough, A.J, Wilson, N.H.: Matrices: their development and use in clinical practice. Dent.Update 19, 284, 1992.
22. Rajstein, J., Tal, M.:Astudy of the contour and external surface of class V composite fillings. J. Oral. Rehab. 6, 21, 1979.
23. Roberts, G. J.: Matrices for the acid etch and composite technique. J. Dent. 4, 190, 1976.
24. Schaffer, J. L.: Use of retainerless matrices for restorative binding. Dent. Surv. 53, 36, 1977.
25. Shennib, H.A., Wilson, N.H.: An investigation of the adequacy of interproximal matrices commonly used with posterior composite restoratives. J. Dent. 14, 84, 1986,
26. Woodmansey, K.F.: Replacing compound with resin composite for quick and efficient matrices. J.A.D.A.: 129, 1601, 1998.

Isolation of the Operating Field

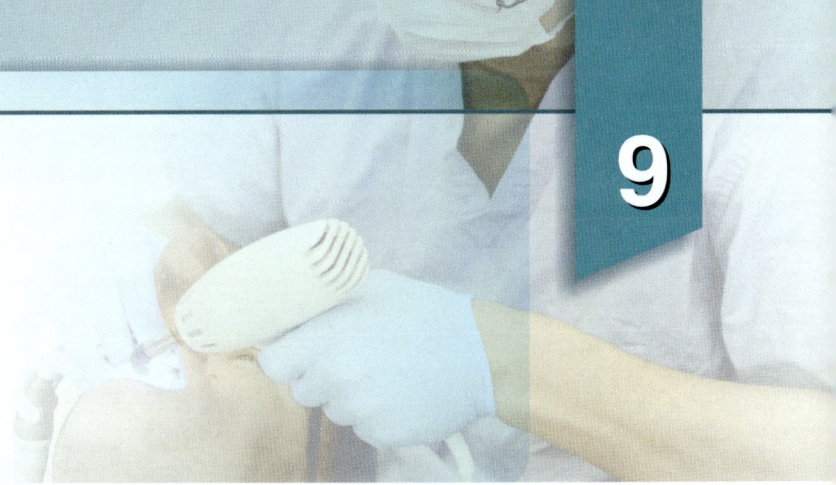

Any operative procedure necessitates the need for adequate control over the operating field. It is imperative that there should be proper moisture control, good accessibility and visibility as well as adequate room for instrumentation around the working area. Such an environment is necessary for easy manipulation and insertion of restorative materials. *Isolating the working area* includes *isolation from moisture* like saliva, blood and gingival crevicular fluid and *isolation from the soft tissues* like lips, cheeks, gingiva and tongue. A number of methods can be employed either singly or in combination to obtain this isolated environment. Isolation hence shall be studied under two heads:

- *Isolation from moisture*
- *Isolation from the soft tissues*

ISOLATION FROM MOISTURE

Various aids available for this purpose are:
A. *Direct methods*
  1. Rubber dam
  2. Cotton rolls and cotton roll holder
  3. Gauze pieces
  4. Absorbent wafers
  5. Suction devices
  6. Gingival retraction cord
B. *Indirect methods*
  1. Comfortable position of the patient and relaxed surroundings
  2. Local anaesthesia
  3. Drugs
      i. Anti-sialogogues
      ii. Anti-anxiety drugs
      iii. Muscle relaxants

A. DIRECT METHODS

Rubber Dam

Dr. S.C. Barnum, introduced the use of rubber dam in dentistry in 1864. It is undoubtedly one of the best methods for providing isolation from saliva and soft tissues but is not very widely used probably because it is thought of as a time consuming, cumbersome and an uncomfortable procedure. However once mastered, the stigmas attached with the use of rubber dam are easily overcome.

Purpose

- Isolation of the operating site from moisture, i.e. saliva, sulcular fluid and blood.
- Re traction of the soft tissue, i.e. cheeks, lips, tongue and minimally, gingiva.
- Increases accessibility and visibility to the working area.
- Improves efficiency of the operator as intermittent expectoration and rinsing by the patient is avoided.
- Improves properties of the dental materials and hence the final outcome of the restoration.
- Protection of the patient and the operator. The patient is protected against accidental aspiration of instruments, debris, medicaments or irrigating solutions. Protects against soft tissue injury when using rotary instruments. Additionally, both the patient and the operator are protected against any cross infection.
- Reduces patient chatter.

Use of rubber dam should be avoided in:

- Asthmatics and mouth breathers as they may not tolerate the dam.
- Partially erupted and malpositioned teeth that may not receive a retainer easily.
- Rare cases when the patient simply does not allow placement of a rubber dam because of psychological reasons.

Armamentarium

A rubber dam kit should have the following items in it:

a. **Rubber dam sheets:** Available in the form of rolls from which square sheets can be cut or individual

Fig. 9.1: Rubber dam sheets

sheets are also available (Fig. 9.1). These may have the following characteristics:

Size: 5" × 5" or 6" × 6" square

Thickness:
Thin – 0.0063"
Medium – 0.008"
Heavy – 0.010" (Provides better retraction of soft tissue and are more resistant to tearing)
Extra heavy – 0.012"
Special heavy – 0.014"

Color: Available in several colors, but green and blue colors are preferred because they provide good contrast with the surroundings. Rubber dam sheet has a shiny side and a dull side. The dull side should face the operator so as to reduce any light reflected from it.

b. **Rubber dam clamps**: Also known as retainers, these are used to secure the dam to the teeth that are to be isolated (Fig. 9.2). These also minimally retract the gingival tissue, which is especially useful when preparing and restoring class V cavities. A retainer has 2 jaws connected by a bow. On each jaw are present 2 prongs which means that there are 4 prongs in a clamp and each prong rests on the mesial/distal line angle of the tooth to be clamped. A prong should not extend beyond the angle of the tooth otherwise it would interfere with the placement of a wedge or matrix band and also may cause gingival trauma. Certain retainers have prongs that are inverted, i.e. directed gingivally. These are more convenient to use on partially erupted teeth or when additional soft tissue needs to be retracted.

Two types of retainers are:

i. *Winged retainers*: These retainers have wing like projections on the outer aspect of their jaws. Hence they provide extra retraction of the rubber dam from the field of operation. The wings are passed through the punched hole in the dam and then the dam and the retainer placed together onto the concerned tooth. After placement, the dam is slipped carefully over the wings onto the tooth.

ii. *Wingless retainers*: These have no wings on their jaws, i.e. they are smooth on their outer aspect. The retainer is first placed on the tooth and the dam then stretched over the clamp onto the tooth.

Several clamps are available in various sizes and shapes. The larger clamps are used for adult patients and the smaller ones (pedodontic clamps) for children. There can be universal clamps for mandibular molars, maxillary molar clamps, bicuspid clamps, double bow clamps for anterior teeth (Fig. 9.2).

New clamps

Tiger clamp
- These are clamps with serrated jaws
- For partially erupted and structurally compromised teeth

Silker-Glickman clamp (S-G clamp)
Extended wings allow for rubber dam placement around teeth with minimal tooth structure

Haller clamp
- Holding of the tongue and cheek
- Fixation of cotton rolls
- Retraction of the gingiva
- Dryness of the field work
- Keeps operating field dry in all tasks of adhesive dentistry
- Possible to work without assistance
- Improves the optical impression (Cerec)

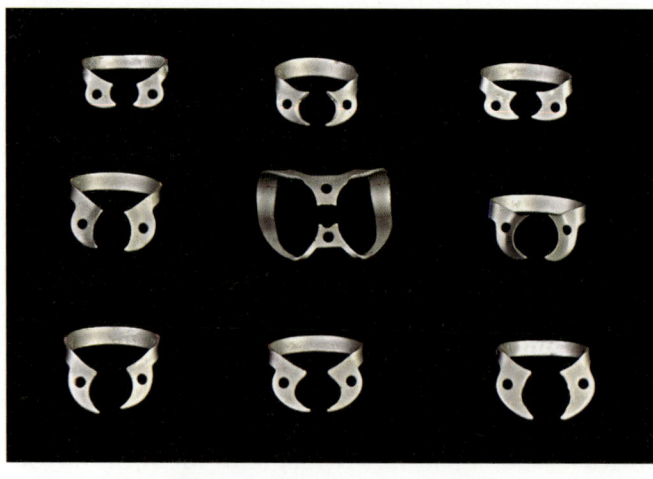

Fig. 9.2: Rubber dam clamps

Isolation of the Operating Field

- Improved relative dryness when rubber dam is not required
- Quality improvement

Cushee clamp

- Increases patient comfort through eliminating contact of steel clamp with gingiva and tooth enamel.
- Enhances rubber dam seal to limit leaking from above or below dam.
- Helps protect natural tooth structure and delicate, costly restorations.
- Reduces clamp slippage.

c. **Rubber dam retainer forceps:** It is a forcep that holds the retainer and facilitates its placement and removal from the tooth (Fig. 9.3).

d. **Rubber dam holder:** Also known as the rubber dam frame, it holds the borders of the dam and positions it. The frame is U shaped and could be an adult or pedodontic one made of metal or plastic. The metal one is known as the *Young's frame*. Plastic frame is useful when a radiograph is to be taken without removing the frame (Fig. 9.4). The frame has minute projections on its outer surface where the dam is secured. An additional two hooks may be present on the sides of the frame where the neck strap may be optionally attached. The frame is preferably placed beneath the dam rather than above it.

New frames

Nygaard ostby frame
- Radiolucent nylon frame
- Polygonal in shape
- Also known as shark mouth

Articulated frame
- Foldable metal frame
- Developed to facilitate endodontic radiography

Derma frame
- Pliable metal rubber dam frame.
- Can be bent to take radiographs and for patient comfort while retaining the dam in place.

Safe – T – frame
- New rubber dam frame design.
- Easier to use with a more secure fit.
- Replaces the conventional one piece frame with a two piece frame design.

e. **Rubber dam punch:** It is a punch for making holes in the dam and is characterized by a rotating metal disc, which bears five or six holes of different sizes, and a sharp pointed plunger (Fig. 9.5). When the handles of the punch are pressed, the plunger should rest in the center of the hole. If not, the plunger tip would get damaged and its cutting ability ruined. This is commonly seen as an incompletely cut hole. The holes are of different sizes according to the size of different teeth. Use the particular hole suggested for that particular tooth, otherwise a tight seal will not be possible or the dam may tear during its placement.

f. **Rubber dam template/stamp:** Both have positions of the teeth marked on them and are used to transfer them to the rubber dam sheet for the holes to be punched (Figs 9.6A and B).

g. **Dental floss:** A strand of dental floss (Fig. 9.7) should be tied around the retainer before it is carried into the oral cavity. This is a safety measure to prevent accidental aspiration of the clamp should it slip. Floss should be passed through both

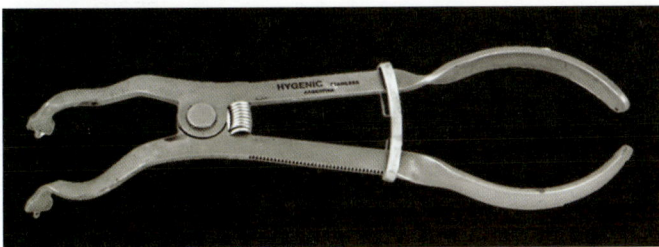

Fig. 9.3: Clamp forceps

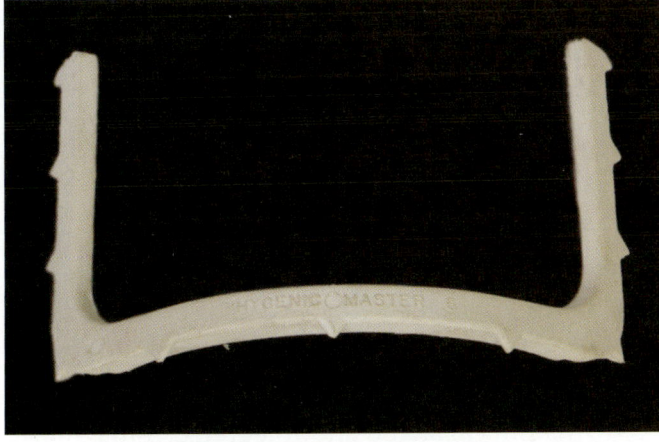

Fig. 9.4: Rubber dam frame

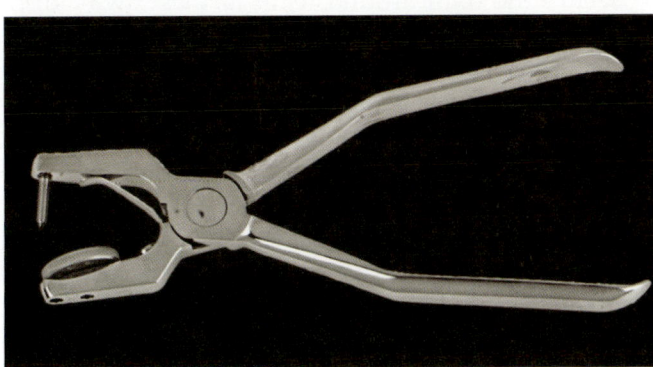

Fig. 9.5: Rubber dam punch

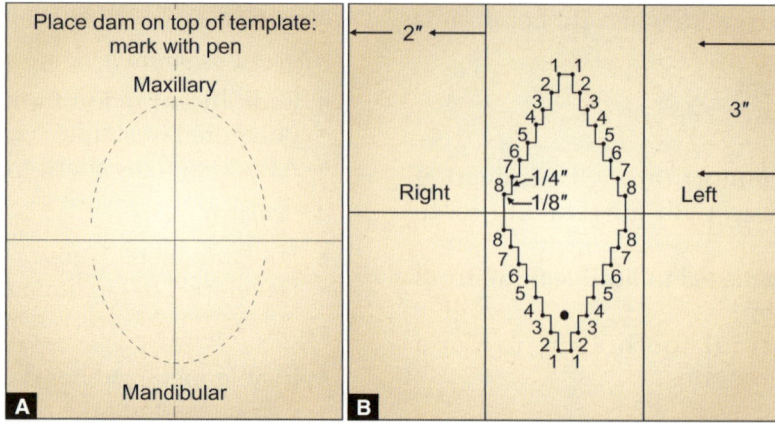

Figs 9.6A and B: **(A)** Rubber dam template (as provided by the manufacture); **(B)** Rubber dam template (self-made)

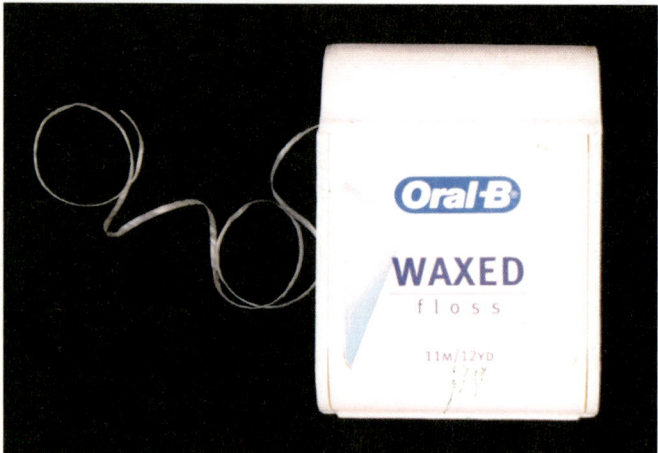

Fig. 9.7: Dental floss

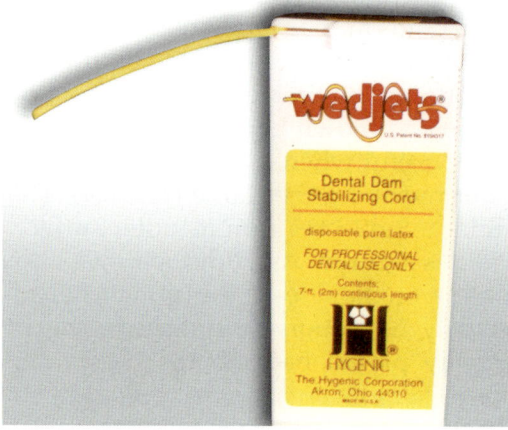

Fig. 9.8: Stabilizing cord

the holes in the jaws and around the bow of the clamp. In case of a fracture involving the bow both parts of the clamp can then be retrieved together. The floss should be adequately long, say twelve inches so that the strand hangs out of the mouth for a sufficient distance. Dental floss may also be used for passing the rubber dam sheet through interproximal contact and also to serve as a retainer in place of conventional clamps.

h. *Wedjet:* This is an elastic cord generally used to secure the dam around teeth farthest away from the clamp (Fig. 9.8). It can also be used to push the dam through the interproximal contact and also in some places as a retainer instead of a clamp.

i. *Lubricant:* A lubricant aids in passing the dam over the tooth. It is applied on both sides of the dam in the area of punched holes. Lubricants may be commercially available or ones like soap, vaseline, shaving cream, etc. can also be employed. Vaseline or petroleum jelly should also be applied on the patient's lips and corners of the mouth to avoid constant irritation from the rubber dam and cracking of the skin.

New Rubber Dam

Instidam

- Compact design fits outside the patients mouth. Non-threatening and comfortable to the patient.
- Built-in flexible frame, with pre punched hole off-center by ½ inch.
- Pre punched hole helps eliminate tearing and additional holes may be punched of necessary.
- Made with translucent natural latex that is very stretchable, tear resistant and provides easy visibility.
- Radiographs may be taken without removing the dam by bending the instidam to the side.
- Produces minimal pull on clamp.
- Single use only.

Handidam

- It is a pre framed rubber dam.
- Easy to put on the patient and saves time.

Optra dam

- Anatomical shape and integrated frame makes placement fast and easy by one person (Fig. 9.9).

Isolation of the Operating Field

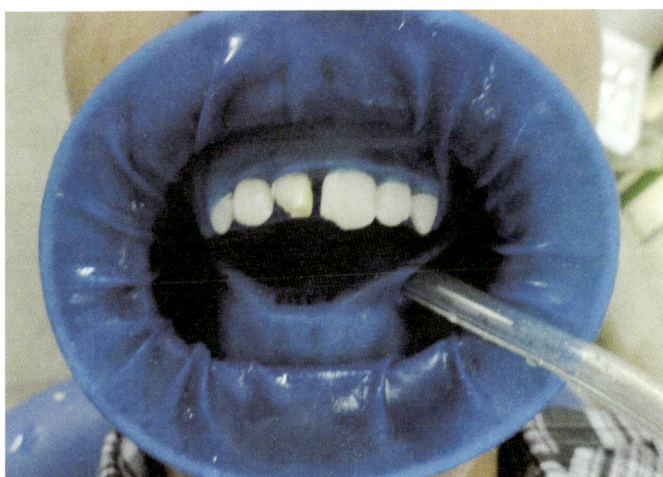

Fig. 9.9: Optra dam

- Flexible in all directions, hence comfortable for patient for long time periods.
- Both arches are fully exposed and provides much easier access to a considerably enlarged treatment field and a completely dry field is achieved simultaneously.
- No metal clamps are required.
- The most outstanding features of Optra Dam include a patented anatomical shape as well as high flexibility in all directions.
- Can be kept in place while x-rays are being taken.
- Available in two adult sizes – Regular and small.

Optidam
- 3-D anatomically contoured frame and dam design, allows easy placement, and accommodates anatomical variations in the mouth; dramatically reducing hand fatigue and improving patient comfort.
- Minimal tension on the clamp due to the design.
- Powder free dam – contains no cornstarch or talc powder, reducing the chance of air borne particles that can cause an allergic reaction.
- Available in anterior and posterior versions.
- Preformed dam with raised lab design which ends tooth marking and hole punching.
- Anatomical frame – 3 – D Thermoplastic frame is safe to autoclave at 134°C for 3 mins.

Liquid Dam
- It is a resinous material applied on the gingival aspect of the tooth surface prior to power bleaching or other procedures requiring intraoral protection
- This does not produce heat when cured and remains flexible after curing

Supplementary Aids for Retention

Low fusing impression compound is occasionally used to supplement the retention of the retainer on the tooth. It is especially useful when coronal tooth structure is not adequate.

Rubber Dam Application

Rubber dam undoubtedly is one of the best methods for providing isolation from saliva and soft tissues.

Remember the following points during rubber dam application:
- When using rubber dam, isolate at least three teeth at a time. Single tooth isolation is usually not recommended except in certain cases when root canal treatment is to be performed.
- For working on central incisors, lateral incisors or on mesial aspect of canines, isolation is done from first premolar to first premolar of the opposite side. Isolation in the anterior area may not require the use of retainers. The use of supplemental aids of retention may suffice.
- For working on the distal aspect of canines and premolars, isolate two teeth posteriorly and punch holes until the opposite lateral incisor anteriorly.
- For working on the molars, isolate till the posterior most tooth on the same side and till the lateral incisor on the opposite side.
- Spacing between two holes in the dam should be adequate (approximately ¼th"). If inadequate spacing is present between the holes, there are chances that the rubber dam sheet will move to the mesial or the distal of the papilla, thereby exposing and injuring the gingiva as well as not providing proper isolation. This also increases the chances of tear of the dam. If the holes are overspaced, rubber dam will bunch in between the teeth thus interfering with the operative procedure.
- When cervical retainer is to be applied, the hole for particular tooth is punched a little facial to the arch, so as to accommodate for the extension of the dam gingivally. The heavier sheet is used when extra retraction is required.
- When thin sheets are used, the holes punched should be of the smaller size so as to obtain proper fitting around the tooth.

Procedure

Stepwise procedure of rubber dam application is as follows. Different areas isolated by rubber dam is shown in Figs 9.10A to D.

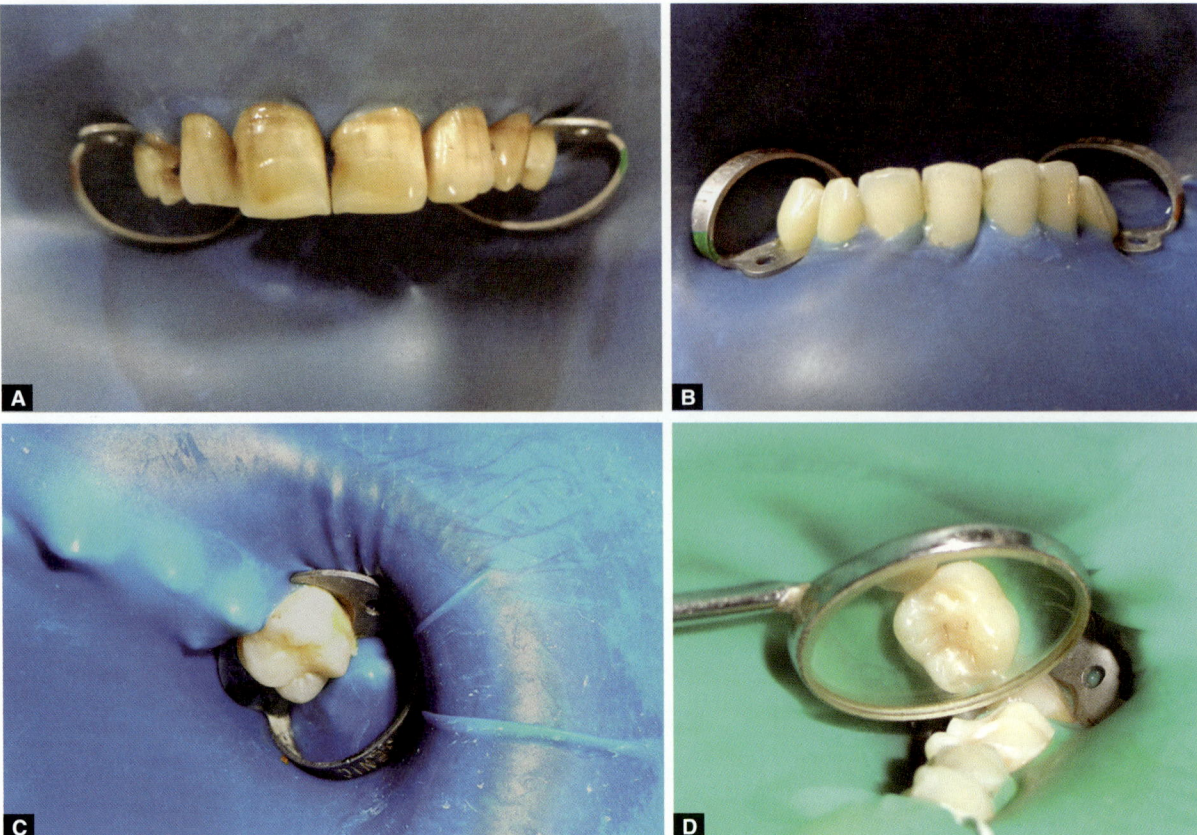

Figs 9.10A to D: **(A)** Upper anterior teeth isolated by rubber dam; **(B)** Lower anterior teeth isolated by rubber dam; **(C)** Maxillary first molar isolated by rubber dam; **(D)** Lower posterior teeth isolated by rubber dam

- Attain a comfortable patient position. Check for any debris or calculus around the teeth. Remove them before proceeding for placement of the rubber dam. If rubber dam is to be placed around a tooth, which is restored with a proximal restoration or a crown, check for any overhanging margins or sharp edges with the help of a dental floss. These are first corrected before proceeding to avoid any rubber dam tear.
- Check for tightness of the proximal contacts by passing the floss obliquely from buccal or lingual. This way the floss is prevented from snapping through the contact and traumatizing the gingiva. Very tight proximal contacts would not allow the passage of rubber dam hence one should consider some other form of isolation in such cases. However, minimally tight contacts that are difficult to floss can be wedged apart to allow the passage of rubber dam.
- Select a rubber dam clamp depending on the type of the tooth to be isolated. A suitable clamp is one, which has all its four prongs resting on the four line angles of the tooth. It should be stable without hurting the surrounding tissues and the restoration. A clamp forcep is used to seat the clamp onto the tooth first on the lingual cervical region then onto the buccal cervical region. Before trying the clamp onto the tooth, dental floss is tied around it. The length of the floss should be such that it hangs outside the mouth for a sufficient distance. Check for the stability of the clamp by pressing against the bow. Minute instability may be overcome by using impression compound to stabilize the clamp. Often the prongs may require grinding to improve stability.
- Take a rubber dam sheet. Punch a hole on its upper right corner or mark it with 'R' for identifying the patient's right side. The sheet is then placed on a template and the position of the holes marked on it with a pen. However with a template, only fixed positions can be obtained. When considerable variations are required the dam can be centred on the teeth to be isolated and the positions marked.
- A lubricant is then applied on both sides of the punched hole to facilitate the passage of dam over the tooth. The patient's lips and corners of the mouth are also coated with a lubricant.
- The rubber dam is now placed on the tooth. Its placement can follow different patterns like:
    i. First place wingless clamp on the tooth. Stretch the lips of the appropriate hole in the rubber

dam sheet and then slide it over the bow and jaws of the clamp and around the cervical of the tooth.

ii. Place the wingless clamp and the rubber dam together around the tooth. For this the rubber dam is passed over the bow of the clamp. The clamp forceps engages the holes in the jaws beneath the dam and is used to place the clamp along with the dam over the tooth. The dam is then stretched and slid over the jaws onto the cervical of the tooth.

iii. Use winged clamp. Both the clamp and the dam can be placed together. For this the rubber dam is passed over the bow. The clamp forcep engages the holes in the jaws and is used to place the clamp along with the dam over the tooth. The dam is then stretched and slid onto the cervical of the tooth.

iv. First place the rubber dam on the tooth and then secure it in position by placing a winged or wingless clamp.

- Make sure that the floss exits from the cheek side of the patient.
- The rubber dam should be cautiously passed through the contact. It should always pass in a single thickness. For this the rubber dam sheet is stretched at the lips of the hole faciolingually and the sheet held obliquely at the contact with its edge pointing gingivally. First try and insert the sheet without a floss. The floss aids in slipping the edge of the dam along the tooth. It may require multiple attempts before the sheet is completely passed through the contact. Once it has passed through the contact, the contact is sufficient to hold the sheet back. Never place floss wholly on the rubber dam as it will create a double thickness of the sheet in that area.
- The rubber dam is similarly passed around each tooth one by one, until the desired number of teeth have been isolated.
- The rubber dam is then bunched in one hand and with the other hand a napkin drawn over the bunched portion onto the face.
- The rubber dam is unfolded and spread neatly. Slowly and steadily the dam is hooked to the projections on the frame while making sure there are minimal folds in the dam. The frame can be placed either above or below the dam but preferably beneath the dam.
- The edges of the rubber dam around the holes are then inverted into the gingival sulcus to obtain a proper seal around the tooth. For this an air-blast is used to dry the dam and the tooth in the concerned area and edges inverted with a spoon excavator or an explorer tip.

- When any operative procedure is being carried out, a low volume evacuator tip may be passed through an extra hole made in the dam into the lingual sulcus and allowed to remain there throughout the procedure. A high volume evacuator tip on the other hand is placed above the rubber dam for intermittent suctioning throughout the procedure.
- On removal of the rubber dam, first pull the dam away from the tooth and cut all the inter-septal rubbers with a pair of sharp scissors. Then the retainer is removed from the tooth using a retainer forceps. The dam and the frame are then simultaneously removed from the oral cavity. The patient's lips and corners of the mouth are wiped of the lubricant with a napkin. Ask the patient to rinse and check for any shreds of rubber dam that may have been separated and left behind. Gently massage the gingiva surrounding the tooth especially around the clamped tooth.

Cotton Rolls and Cotton Roll Holder

Cotton rolls are not only moisture absorbents but also aid in minimally retracting the soft tissues from the operating field. These generally are isolation alternatives when rubber dam application is not practical or possible. When used in association with profound anaesthesia, absorbents provide acceptable dryness for procedures like examination, impression taking, cementation, sealant placement, topical fluoride application, etc. Use of a saliva ejector and cellulose wafer along with cotton rolls further control salivary flow.

The removal and placement of cotton rolls is basically carried out by the operator's assistant. He should continually remove drenched cotton rolls and insert dry ones.

Loose cotton can either be rolled manually into a cotton roll or prefabricated cotton rolls are also available (Fig. 9.11). Prefabricated rolls are more compact and can absorb a greater amount of moisture.

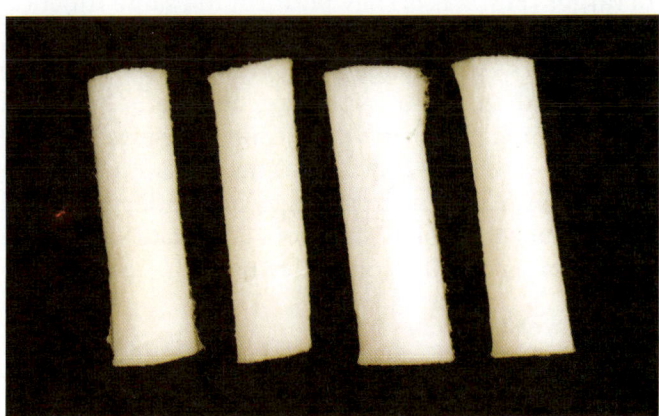

Fig. 9.11: Prefabricated cotton rolls

They are available in varying diameters and lengths. They are usually available in no. 2 (small) and no. 3 (medium) sizes. The surface of the cotton roll can be smooth or woven to improve their compactness.

Cotton rolls can be placed into position and stabilized with commercial holding devices known as cotton roll holders. The disadvantage with the use of cotton roll holders is that they have to be removed from the mouth for changing the cotton rolls. The advantage is that they provide slightly more retraction of the cheeks, lips and tongue thus improving accessibility and visibility of the working area.

For isolation in the maxillary anterior area, small sized rolls are placed on either side of the labial frenum and for mandibular anterior area, in the lingual sulcus along with one cotton roll on either side of the mandibular labial frenum.

The maxillary posterior teeth are isolated by inserting a cotton roll in the adjacent vestibule. This will not occlude the parotid duct opening, hence a cheek pad or cellulose wafer is additionally laid over this area of the cheek. Such placements are aided by the use of saliva ejectors to remove saliva from the lingual sulcus.

The mandibular posterior teeth are isolated by inserting one cotton roll in the buccal vestibule usually the medium sized roll and the larger one between the teeth and the tongue.

In the lingual sulcus even two cotton rolls can be used, one inserted to the depth of the sulcus and the other one laid above it. Cheek pads should be applied and use of saliva ejector in the opposite lingual sulcus aids in completing the isolation.

Avoid removing dry cotton rolls. They should be slightly moistened before removal to prevent the pulling of the epithelial covering of the mucosa along with it.

Gauze Pieces

Gauze sponges may be supplied in pieces of 2" × 2" or larger (Fig. 9.12). They perform the same function as cotton rolls and are generally used for isolating larger areas. Additionally, they may be used as throat screens when minute instruments are being used without rubber dam or when indirect restorations are being inserted, so as to avoid accidental aspiration (Fig. 9.13). Also gauze sponges are better tolerated by the delicate tissues, are more acceptable and have less chances of adhesion to dry tissues.

Absorbent Pads/wafers

Absorbent pads are generally made up of cellulose and hence are also called as *cellulose wafers* (Fig. 9.14). They may be available in different shapes to fit various

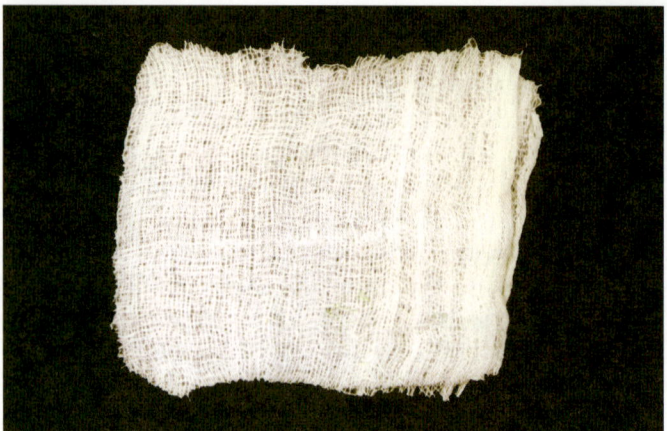

Fig. 9.12: Gauze piece - 2" × 2"

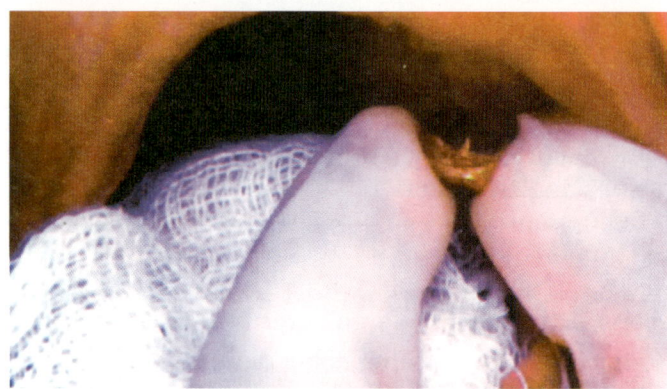

Fig. 9.13: Throat screen used to prevent accidental ingestion/aspiration

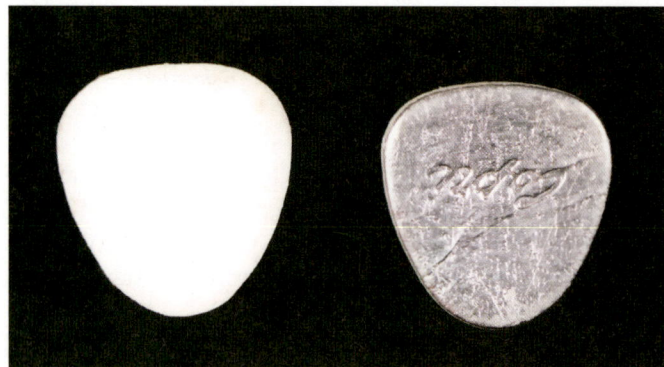

Fig. 9.14: Cellulose wafers/cheek pads

locations in the mouth. Most commonly they are used inside the cheeks to cover the parotid ducts. These are more absorbent than the cotton rolls or gauze pieces.

Evacuation Systems

Vacuum systems are generally of two types: high vacuum evacuation system which is generally operated by the dentist and/or the dental assistant. The other one is the low vacuum evacuation system which is attached to the saliva ejector and may remain in the mouth during the operative procedure. The high vacuum evacuation system is usually stronger than the low vacuum evacuation system.

A. High Volume Evacuators

When using a high speed handpiece, both air and water emerge from the head of the handpiece to wash the working area and to act as a coolant for the bur and the tooth. High volume evacuators are preferred to remove this collected moisture and debris in the mouth because low volume saliva ejectors are slow at work and poor at clearing solids (Fig. 9.15). A practical test for determining the efficacy of a high volume evacuator is the ability of the evacuator tip to clear 150 ml of water in approximately one second.

The high volume evacuator tips are usually made up of disposable plastic or autoclavable metallic tips. The tip is usually bevelled and is placed intermittently in the mouth during the operative procedure by the dental assistant. The evacuator tip is placed as near as possible to the tooth being prepared but it should not interfere with the operator's access or vision. Also it should not be positioned so close to the handpiece head that air water supply is diverted away from the rotary instrument. The tip of the evacuator should be placed distal to the tooth being prepared. For ease of manipulation, the assistant holds the evacuator tip in his right hand and the air water syringe in his left hand.

High volume evacuation has the following *advantages*:
 i. Removes shavings of tooth and restorative material as well as other debris from the working site
 ii. Toxic material is readily removed
 iii. Decreases treatment time as intermittent rinsing and washing is avoided

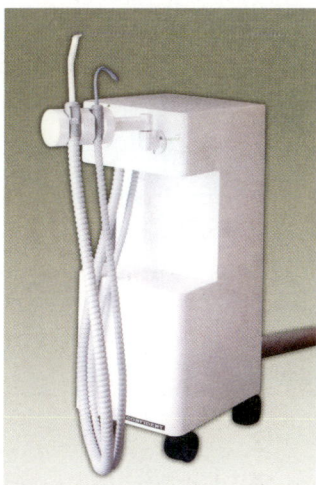

Fig. 9.15: High volume evacuator and saliva ejector

B. Low Volume Evacuators

Low volume evacuators are basically saliva ejectors which are meant to remove the saliva that collects on the floor of the mouth. These can be left in the mouth during the operative procedure. They are available with disposable plastic tips (Fig. 9.16) or autoclavable metallic tips (which should have a rubber end to prevent irritation to the delicate tissue). They may be shaped by bending with fingers and are most often used along with cotton rolls, cheek pads and rubber dam.

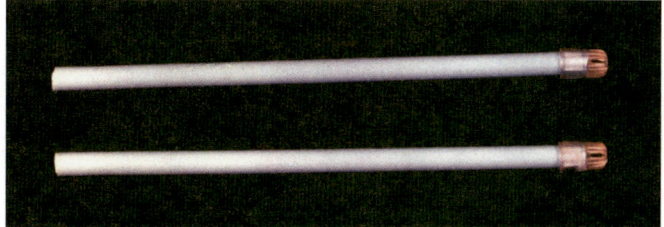

Fig. 9.16: Disposable plastic suction tips

Saliva ejectors should be placed with their tips on the floor of the mouth, directed backwards and not directly in contact with the tissues. This is to prevent aspiration of the delicate mucous membrane into the holes of the tip and their getting traumatized by the vacuum energy. Preferably place a cotton roll or gauze piece beneath the tip when you are using one. Avoid pushing the saliva ejector during instrumentation as this could damage the soft surrounding tissues. When using it along with the rubber dam, the saliva ejector can be passed through a hole punched in the rubber dam into the sulcus or directly beneath the rubber dam into the sulcus.

Gingival Retraction Cord

These are readymade cotton or synthetic fibers woven in the form of cords. Various types of cords e.g: braided, non-braided, plain or impregnated are available in different sizes (Figs 9.17A and B). The plain cords may be impregnated with chemicals before or after their insertion into the sulcus. Some cords are wrapped in resin wire to make them more compact and immobile. These cords are inserted in the gingival sulcus to keep the moisture and gingiva away from the tooth surface for certain procedures like making the impression of a cavity or subgingival tooth preparations.

Gingival retraction cord is used when the use of rubber dam is not practical or appropriate. Its use should be accompanied by other isolation methods. It should not be used for the displacement of gingival tissues when the later are swollen/inflamed. Only

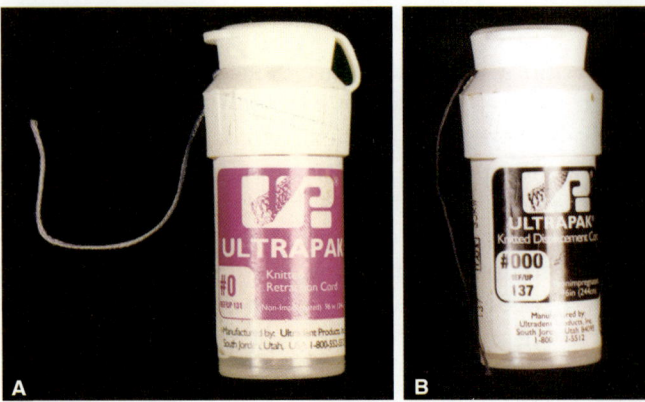

Figs 9.17A and B: (A) Knitted retraction cord, #0 size; **(B)** Knitted retraction cord, #000 size (Ultrapak)

healthy gingiva returns to its original position after removal of the retraction cord.

A properly impregnated cord causes:
- Displacement of the free gingiva laterally by few tenths of a millimeter thus opening the sulcus,
- Apical positioning of the gingival crest although no attempt is made to force the gingival retraction cord apically,
- Transient dehydration of the gingiva and
- Decreased bleeding (when the cord is impregnated with a vasoconstrictor like adrenaline or a styptic like Hemodent).

A gingival retraction cord:
- Provides improved access and visibility.
- Protects gingiva from abrasion during cavity preparation.
- Restricts excess restorative material from pushing into the sulcus.
- Everts gingival tissue thus exposing margins of the cavity.

Placement of the Retraction Cord

1. Insert cord only after anaesthetizing the area.
2. Choose cord that can be gently inserted into the sulcus without causing ischaemia.
3. The diameter of the cord should be such that it does not blanch the tissue nor is inadequate in applying pressure. If several cords have to be inserted, start with the smallest diameter one followed by the larger ones.
4. Length of the cord should be such that it extends 1.0 mm beyond the gingival width of the cavity or extends around the whole circumference of the tooth.
5. Avoid putting the ends interproximally. The ideal location is at the axial angles of the tooth, where the interdental col has its maximum height thus creating a better grip and stabilization on the packed cord.
6. The packing instrument should be blunt, hatchet or hoe-shaped preferably with a serrated face. Several instruments in different sizes should be available so as to fit different locations within the same sulcus. A cowhorn explorer or plastic instrument can also be used for the same purpose. Whatever instrument is used, the cord should be packed slowly and progressively.
7. Use forces that are directed laterally and angulated slightly towards the tooth surface. Apical pressure may seriously damage the junctional epithelium.
8. In shallow sulcus or when there is thin free gingiva, there may be difficulty in stabilizing the cord in place. Here, after inserting one end of the cord, stabilize it with a blunt instrument while the rest of the cord is packed.
9. Never remove the cord dry otherwise it may adhere to the dry epithelium and on pulling cause its abrasion and profuse bleeding.
10. Immediately after removal check for pieces of gingival retraction cord that may have been torn and left in the gingival environment.
11. The cords can be left in place if they do not interfere with the circumferential tie and are immobile.
12. For healthy healing of the periodontium, any substance irritating the gingiva should be removed and efficient plaque control measures followed.

New Gingival Retraction Materials

Expa Syl
- Gingival retraction paste available from Kerr Dental products.
- Soft clay based material.
- Effective and tissue friendly product, designed as an alternative to retraction cord placement for hemostasis.
- Can be used for:
  - Crown and bridge impressions
  - Impressions for indirect restorations.
  - Impressions for veneers.
- Kinder on the periodontal ligament fibers when compared to retraction cord placement.
- Does not cause excessive trauma to soft and delicate tissues.

Method of Placing

In areas where fluid control is needed, place soft cotton pellets over the area. The expa syl material is expressed and then condensed with gentle finger pressure. Cover the area with gauze and allow the patient to close the mouth while keeping the area dry and isolated. Wait for 2–3 minutes; heavy bleeding – longer time around 5–7 minutes.

Magic Foam Cord

- Non hemostatic gingival retraction system from Coltene whaledent.
- It is an expanding poly vinyl siloxane material.
- Designed for fast and easy retraction of the gingival sulcus.
- Non traumatic method of gingival retraction when compared to retraction cord placement.
- There is no need for pressure or packing of the material.
- Effortless removal, comes – off in one piece. There is no need for extensive rinsing of the sulcus for removing residue or hemostatic chemicals.
- Comfortable to the patient.

Method of Use

Magic foam cord material is syringed around the crown preparation margins and a comprecap is placed to reportedly maintain pressure. After 5 mins the cap and foam are removed and the tooth is ready for final impression.

Disadvantages
• Relatively expensive material. • Intra oral tips are too large to adequately inject the material into the sulcus. • Hemostasis must be achieved prior to using magic foam cord significantly reducing clinical efficiency.

B. INDIRECT METHODS

All the above mentioned measures are helpful in eliminating the collected moisture and saliva directly from the oral cavity. However, there are measures that actually reduce the amount of salivation and hence aid in isolation indirectly. These are:

1. ***Comfortable and relaxed position of the patient:*** The patient should be comfortably seated in the dental chair. At no time should he be tensed. Moreover, the surroundings should also be pleasant and relaxing. All these features as well as a comforting attitude of the dental staff reduce the anxiety levels of the patient and aids in reducing salivation.
2. ***Local anaesthesia:*** Using a local anaesthetic helps in reducing the discomfort associated with the treatment in addition to controlling moisture by decreasing salivation. Making the patient comfortable, less anxious and less sensitive to stimuli helps in producing a lower salivary flow thus helping in moisture control. Another advantage is the vasoconstriction caused by the local anaesthetic (containing vasoconstrictor) which helps in reducing haemorrhage at the operating site.
3. **Drugs:** Drugs can reduce salivation but are rarely indicated. These include antisialogogues, antianxiety agents, sedatives, etc.
    i. *Antisialogogues*: Premedication may be indicated using an anticholinergic agent to depress salivation. Atropine can be given half an hour before the appointment, but should be avoided in patients with high ocular pressure or with cardiovascular problems.
    ii. *Antianxiety agents and barbiturate sedatives*: Premedication with these drugs is quite helpful in apprehensive patients, for example, Diazepam or Barbiturates, 24 hours before the appointment. Because of psychological dependence on these drugs, these should be given only for short periods and to selected patients.
    iii. *Muscle relaxants*: may also be tried.

ISOLATION FROM THE SOFT TISSUES (SOFT TISSUE MANAGEMENT)

During any operative procedure adequate care should be taken to protect the soft tissues surrounding the tooth, which include the cheeks, lips, tongue and gingiva. Also, in order to aid in proper cavity preparation, subsequent impression procedures and restoration, soft tissue should be excluded from the operating site. Various methods of isolating soft tissues are as follows:

Retraction of the Cheeks, Lips and Tongue

Various devices employed for the retraction of cheeks, lips and tongue include:
- Rubber dam (most efficient)
- Cotton rolls and holder
- Tongue guards
- Tongue depressors
- Cheek and lip retractors
- Mouth mirrors

- Rubber dam and cotton rolls for retracting soft tissues have been discussed earlier.
- Tongue guards basically protect against injury to the tongue. They create a wall between the tongue and the operating field. They can be made of plastic (usually disposable) or metal (autoclavable).
- Tongue can be manipulated and protected by using a tongue depressor which lowers the tongue so as to avoid interference during any operative

procedure. Also cheek retraction can be readily accomplished with it. Disposable wooden tongue depressors are quite popular.
- Cheek and lip retractors usually fit around the upper and lower lips including the corners of the mouth and help in pulling them backward and outward exposing the facial surfaces of maxillary and mandibular teeth. Some of these devices fit only one lip. These are used mainly for photographic purposes and when working on anterior teeth (Fig. 9.18).

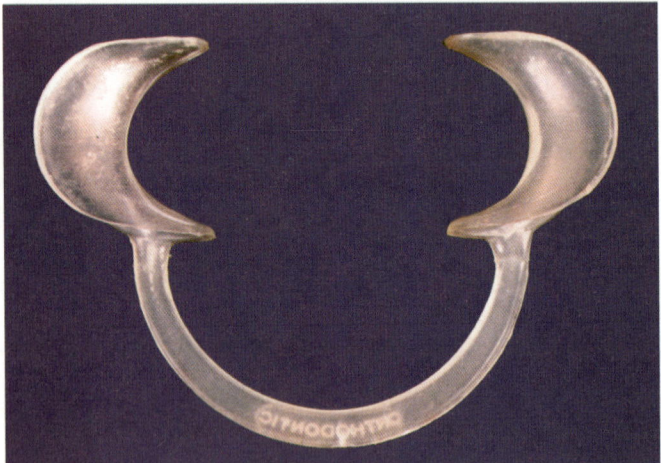

Fig. 9.18: Cheek and lip retractor

Retraction of the Gingiva

There are four means of accomplishing gingival retraction and are frequently used in combination.
- Physico-mechanical means
- Chemical means
- Electrosurgical means
- Surgical means

1. Physico-mechanical Means

This involves mechanically forcing the gingiva away from the tooth surface both in the lateral and the apical direction. It should be used only when the gingiva is healthy with a very good vascular supply and there is a definite zone of attached gingiva apical to the free gingiva. Bone support should be sufficient without signs of resorption. Any one of these techniques can be used:

a. *Rubber dam*: Use of heavy, extra heavy and special heavy weight rubber dam sheets provide a modest mechanical displacement of the gingival tissue. Additionally use of a No. 212 cervical retainer (Ferrier W.I. clamp) also helps in gingival retraction. However, it is not applicable in every case especially where the cervical extension is severe.

b. *Gingival retraction cords or rolled cotton twills* introduced into the gingival sulcus not only aid in isolation against gingival fluid seepage but also produce apical and lateral deflection. Results are obtained in 30 minutes or less. These methods are used when a rubber dam is not used.

c. *Wooden wedges* placed interdentally depress the gingival tissue.

d. *Charbeneau* has referred to the use of *cotton twills combined with fast setting Zinc oxide eugenol cement* in the gingival sulcus to provide retraction. It is an effective and a conservative method but also time consuming. The method involves mixing Zinc oxide eugenol to a thin creamy consistency and rolling cotton into appropriate lengths of twills (about the diameter of the dental floss) along with this cement. The rolls are thoroughly dried with a paper towel to remove excess liquid and gain a compactness. The operative field is dried and isolated and the twills then placed into the base of the gingival sulcus. Care should be taken that these twills are compressed laterally rather than apically. The pack is held in position because of the fast setting Zinc-oxide eugenol cement. The pack should remain in position for a minimum of 48 hours to be effective, but should not be placed in the gingival sulcus for longer than seven days. Extended periods of placement can result in loss of periodontal attachment and is therefore not recommended.

e. *Gutta-percha or eugenol packs* have also been used for the purpose of gingival retraction.

2. Chemical Means

This is the most popular technique for gingival retraction. Generally, the chemicals used are as follows:

a. *Vasoconstrictors*: These cause vasoconstriction and consequently reduce the blood supply of the area, decrease haemorrhage, tissue fluid seepage and hence the size of the free gingiva. Included in this category are epinephrine and nor-epinephrine. The disadvantages associated with its use are:
- Causes rapid transient elevation in blood sugar and blood pressure if applied directly to the abraded gingiva, hence contraindicated in cases of hypertension, diabetes, hyperthyroidism, drug sensitivity, heart patients, etc.
- Produces local ischemia which is injurious to the gingiva.

b. *Astringents and styptics*: These include biologic fluid coagulants and tissue coagulants. *Biologic fluid coagulants* coagulate blood and tissue fluids locally thus creating a surface layer which seals against blood and sulcular fluid seepage. These are quite

safe to use as they do not induce any systemic effects. Examples are:
- Alum (100%)
- Aluminium potassium sulphate (10%)
- Aluminium chloride (15–25%)
- Tannic acid (15–25%)

Tissue coagulants coagulate the superficial surface layer of sulcular and gingival epithelium as well as the leached fluids thus producing a temporarily non permeable film for underlying fluids and blood. Unlike biologic fluid coagulants, surface tissue coagulants if used for prolonged periods or in excessive amounts and concentration can cause ulceration, local necrosis and changes in the dimension and contour of the free gingiva. Examples are: Zinc chloride and Silver nitrate.

These chemicals can be carried to the operating site by following means:
 i. *Cords:* The main advantage with the use of cords as a carrier is that these do not stick to the affected tissues. The major disadvantage is the difficulty in inserting these cords into the sulcus.
 ii. *Cotton rolls:* Loose cotton can be drawn into rolls of desired diameter and then introduced into the gingival sulcus. These may be impregnated with chemicals before or after insertion. Their advantage over cords is that they can be compacted easily because of their looseness, produce adequate widening of the trough and cause more shrinkage because of the ability to hold more chemical. Their disadvantage is that superficial sulcular epithelium may get incorporated into the cotton which may be pulled off thus causing haemorrhage and seepage once the roll is removed.
 iii. *Cotton pellets:* Cotton pellets can be used to carry chemicals to the already inserted retraction cord or cotton rolls. They may be left in place to provide a continuous supply of chemicals.

3. Electrosurgical Means

Electrosurgical means of gingival tissue management is usually used when access to the working area is not available by the more conservative methods. Its major advantage over surgical method of gingival tissue management is that it causes minimal haemorrhage and the angle between the electrode and the handle can be adjusted as per the requirements.

Principle

Alternating electric current is passed through an apparatus to substantially increase its frequency (60–120 to million or more per second). The current at this extremely high velocity passes through the body without inducing shocks. This energy is concentrated at tiny electrodes producing extremely localized tissue changes which can be limited to the superficial 2-3 cell layers.

Four actions can be seen depending on the amount of energy produced:
a. *Cutting:* Extremely precise cutting is possible without inducing any bleeding and with minimal tissue involvement and after effects. This is possible when minimal energy is produced by controlled use.
b. *Coagulation:* Because of the greater heat generated, there occurs surface coagulation of tissues, oozed fluids and blood. Overdose leads to carbonization.
c. *Fulguration:* Because of still greater energy used and heat generated, fulguration has deeper tissue involvement. It is always associated with carbonization and may have comparatively more after effects.
d. *Desiccation:* It is the most dangerous action because of the uncontrolled and unlimited nature. Causes massive destruction of the tissues both in depth and width.

Cutting is the most commonly employed action while coagulation is less commonly employed. The differences in the energy produced depends on electric variables like shape and size of the electrode used, energy input and output, frequency of current, conduction, etc.

Certain rules to be followed when using an electrosurgical unit for isolation purposes are:
- The working site should be properly isolated with minimal moisture present. Excess dehydration should be avoided.
- Adequate current should pass at the site of surgery.
- Use only fully rectified, undamped, filtered current with minimum energy output required for cutting action.
- For cutting, unipolar electrode is used with feather touch and rapid intermittent strokes until adequate cutting is done and the required width of the sulcus is obtained. Do not touch the free gingival crest as it can lead to gingival recession. Always cut on the inside walls of the sulcus. Probe or loop type electrodes are the best suited ones.
- For coagulation, bulky unipolar electrodes are used with a partially rectified, partially dampened energy output. The electrode should not touch the tissue but is held very close to it for coagulation to occur.
- After registering the details of the circumferential tie, the involved tissues and surface films are

curretted, creating fresh bleeding. If bone or periodontal attachment has been involved, a suture and periodontal pack should be applied to promote healing.
- During the procedure the following points need to be noted :
  – Do not touch metallic fillings for fear of short-circuiting.
  – Sparks indicate too high energy output.
  – Clean electrode tips with alcohol sponge after each use.

4. Surgical Means

Use a sharp knife to remove interfering and unneeded gingival tissues surgically. Also it is used for placing whole of the periodontal attachment apparatus apically to create a healthy retracted free gingival tissue.

BIBLIOGRAPHY

1. Adams H.: Managing gingival tissues during definite restorative treatment. Quint. Int.: 2, 141, 1981.
2. Akca E.A., Yildirim, E., Dalkiz, M. and Yavuzyilmaz, H.: Effects of different retraction medicaments on gingival tissues. Quint. Int.: 37, 53, 2006.
3. Azzi, R., Tsao, T.F., Carrauza, F.A. and Kenney, E.B.: Comparative study of gingival retraction methods. J. Prosthet. Dent.: 50, 561, 1983.
4. Baharav H., Laufer, B.Z., Langer, Y. and Cardash, H.S.: The effect of displacement time on gingival crevice width. Int. J. Prosthodont.: 10, 248, 1997.
5. Barghi N. Knight, G.T. and Berry, T.G.: Comparing two methods of moisture control in bonding to enamel: a clinical study. Oper. Dent.: 16, 130, 1991.
6. Bowles W.H., Tardy, S.J. and Vahadi, A.: Evaluation of new gingival retraction agents. J. Dent. Res.: 70, 1447, 1991.
7. Cochran M.A., Miller C.H. and Sheldrake, M.A.: The efficacy of the rubber dam as barrier to the spread of microorganisms during dental treatment. J. Am. Dent. Assoc.: 141, 119, July 1989.
8. Costello M.R.: Dental dams: The secret tool for infection control. Compend. Contin. Educ. Dent. 27, 196, 2006
9. Donovan T.E., Gandara B.K., Nemetz, H.: Review and survey of medicaments used with gingival retraction cords. J. Prosthet. Dent.: 53, 525, 1985.
10. Forrest W.R. and Perez R.S.: The rubber dam as a surgical drape: protection aginst AIDS and hepatitis. Gen. Den.: 37, 236, 1989.
11. Heling I., Sommer, M. and Kot, I.: Rubber dam – an essential safeguard. Quint. Int.: 19, 377, 1988.
12. Jones C.M. and Reid, J.S.: Patient and operator attitudes toward rubber dam. ASDC J. Dent. Child.: 55, 452, 1988.
13. Kopac I. Cvetke, E.and Mariou, L.: Gingival inflammatory response induced by chemical retraction agents in beagle dogs. Int. J. Proshodont. 15, 14, 2002
14. Mamoun J.: A prosthesis for achieving dry field isolation of molars with short clinical crowns. J.A.D.A.: 133, 1105, 2002.
15. Medina J.E.: The rubber dam – an incentive for excellence. Dent. Clin. North Am.: 255, March 1957.
16. Meechan J.G., Jastak, J.T. and Donaldson, D.: The use of epinephrine in dentistry. J. Can. Dent. Assoc.: 60, 8256, 1994.
17. Meraner M.: Soft tissue management for difficult cervical restorations. Gen. Dent.: 54, 117, 2006.
18. Nelson J.F.: Ingesting an onlay: a case report. J. Am. Dent. Assoc.: 123, 73, 1992.
19. Nemetz E.H. and Seibly W.: The use of chemical agents in gingival retraction. Gen. Dent.: 38, 104, 1990.
20. Peterson J.E., Nation W.A. and Matsson, L.: Effect of a rubber dam clam (retainer) on cementum and junctional epithelium. Oper. Dent.: 11, 42, 1986.
21. Scott A.: Use of an erbium laser in lieu of retraction cord: a modern technique. Gen. Dent. 53, 116, 2005
22. Strydom C.: Handling protocol of posterior composites: Part 3: matrix system. SADJ 61, 18, 2006.
23. Wong R.C.K.: The rubber dam as a means of infection control in an era of AIDS and hepatitis. J. Indiana Dent. Assoc.: 67, 41, Jan./Feb. 1988.

Principles of Cavity Preparation

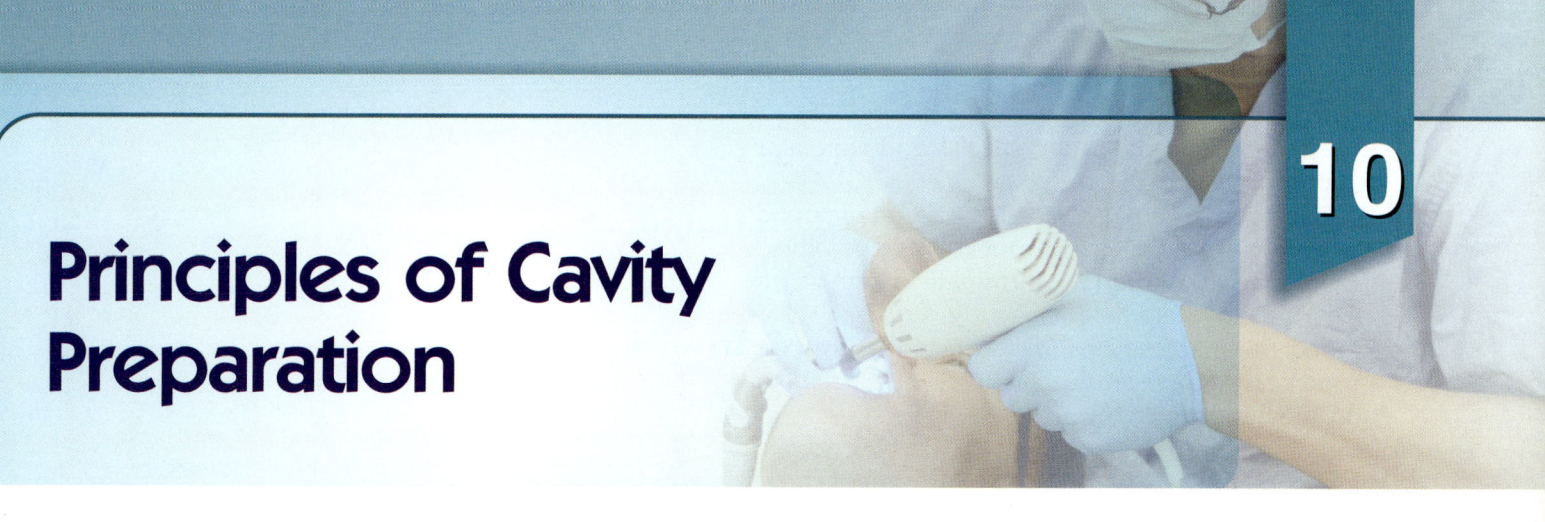

One of the basic phases of operative dentistry is the cavity preparation. The most prevalent and the most common ailment in dentistry – the caries, is frequently confronted by all, especially the operative dentist. Removal of caries and preparing proper foundation for the restorative material is the key to success for any clinician. Therefore, it is mandatory for any operative dentist to be thoroughly apprised with all the fundamentals of cavity preparation.

A cavity in dentistry is defined as *'a defect in enamel, dentin or cementum resulting from the pathological processes, mostly the dental caries'*. Other processes such as abrasion, erosion, etc. can also cause such defects.

Preparation of the cavity includes *'the performance of all mechanical procedures required to remove the carious and affected tissues and to shape the remaining enamel and dentin so as to receive a biologically and mechanically sound restoration'*.

The preparation of a cavity should be carried out in an orderly sequence, following certain principles. *Dr. G.V. Black* suggested six principles for cavity preparation, which by and large are followed, though each principle has been modified keeping in view the advancement in restorative materials. These principles are as follows:

1. Outline form
2. Resistance and Retention form
3. Convenience form
4. Removal of remaining carious dentin
5. Finishing of the enamel walls and margins
6. Toilet of the cavity

Proper cavity preparation is accomplished through systematic procedures based on these principles. For understanding cavity preparation, knowledge of tooth anatomy and its related parts is mandatory. The direction of enamel rods, thickness of enamel at various places, size and position of the pulp, the relation of the crown with the gingival tissue and other related factors must be kept in mind to facilitate proper cavity preparation. The physical and mechanical properties of the restorative materials to be used should also be taken care of during cavity preparation.

OUTLINE FORM

Outline form means carrying the margins of the cavity to the position it will occupy upon completion of the cavity.

Dr. G.V. Black, described outline form as *the area of tooth surface or the enamel margin to be included in the finished cavity.*

This is basically the external outline form. The internal outline form, however, includes the inner dimensions and details of the prepared cavity. In young people, the internal outline form should be prepared carefully as pulp chamber is large and more superficial.

One should visualize the outline form in one's mind before any cutting is started. It prevents over-cutting and over-extension, which often leaves weak remaining tooth structure.

Factors influencing outline form are:
a. Location of the carious lesion
b. Extent of the carious lesion
c. Position of pits and fissures
d. The proximity of the lesion to other defects in the enamel
e. The relationship of adjacent and opposing teeth
f. The relationship of soft tissue
g. Type of restorative material to be used
h. Functional requirements of the restoration
i. Esthetic considerations

Establishing Outline Form for Occlusal Cavities

The outline form for occlusal cavities is controlled by following factors:
a. Extend the cavity margins to sound tooth structure and remove all unsupported enamel.
b. Include all susceptible fissures in the outline form. This phenomenon of 'Extension for Prevention'

was first suggested by *Marshall Ebb* and was later adopted by *Black*.

c. When two cavities have less than 0.5 mm of sound tooth structure between them, they should be joined.
d. Cavity margins should not terminate in high stress areas, such as cusp heights or ridge crests.
e. Extend the margins to allow sufficient access for proper cavity preparation, restoration placement and finishing procedures.
f. Type of material to be used.

Figs 10.1A to D show the outline form for occlusal cavities.

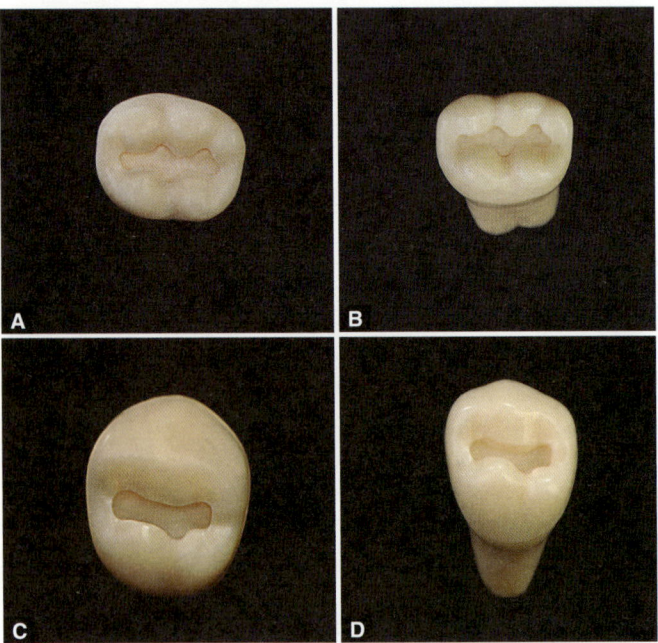

Figs 10.1A to D: (A) Mandibular first molar (occlusal view); **(B)** Mandibular first molar (linguo-occlusal view); **(C)** Mandibular second premolar (occlusal view); **(D)** Mandibular second premolar (linguo-occlusal view)

Establishing Outline form for Proximal Cavities

The outline form for proximal restorations is controlled by the following factors:

a. Position and crest of healthy gingiva, age of the patient vis-a-vis the epithelial attachment and the scope for future gingival recession.
b. Dimensions of contact area in the concerned tooth. The contact area is to be involved and later restored to same configuration.
c. Extent of caries at and around the contact area.
d. Oral hygiene of the patient.
e. Possible forces of mastication which the restoration will be withstanding.
f. Margins should be in self-cleansing areas (Fig. 10.2).

Figs 10.3A and B show the outline form for proximal cavity in posterior tooth and Figs 10.4A and B show the outline form for proximal cavity in anterior tooth.

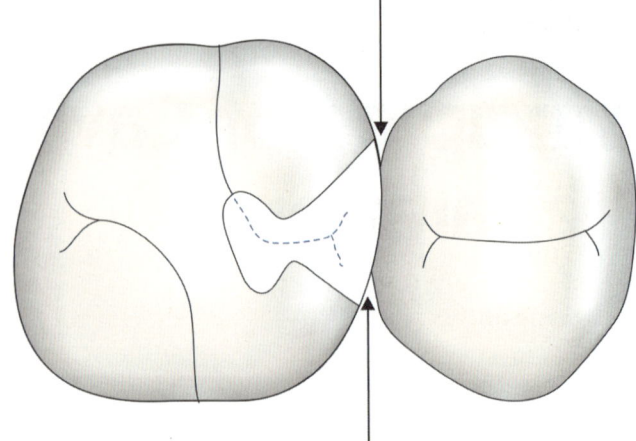

Fig. 10.2: Axial margins should clear the contact area and extend into embrasures for self-cleansing action

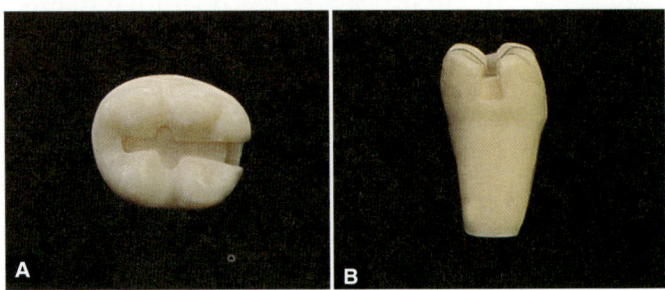

Figs 10.3A and B: 3 Outline form for proximal cavity in mandibular first molar, **(A)** Occlusal view; **(B)** Proximal view

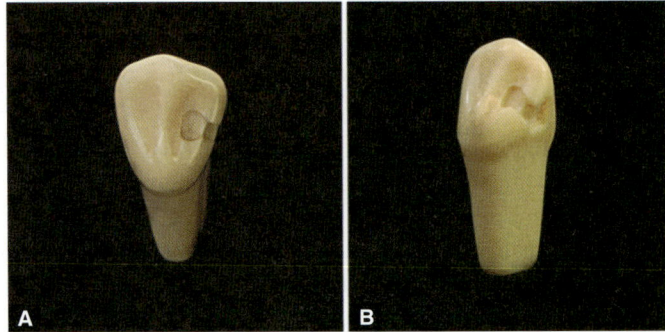

Figs 10.4A and B: Outline form for proximal cavity in maxillary canine, **(A)** Palatal view; **(B)** Mesio-palatal view

Above all, in cases where the decay in dentin has undermined enamel especially under the cusps and up to line angles of the tooth, this decay becomes the controlling factor requiring the removal of all caries along with unsupported enamel. This procedure might lead to the need for cuspal coverage or the cast restoration.

There are no set rules in cavity preparation that cannot be modified; however, these modifications should be within limits so as not to defy the basic principles.

There are certain conditions which may warrant restricted or reduced extension:

Principles of Cavity Preparation

- Proximal cavities
- Root proximities
- Esthetic requirements

Certain conditions may require increased extension:
- Mental or physical handicap patients
- Advanced age of the patient
- When additional resistance or retention is required
- Need to adjust tooth contours

Various authors have questioned the principle of 'extension for prevention'. It has been well established that the gingival sulcus is not bacteria free and studies using disclosing solutions have shown the so-called self-cleansing areas are virtually non-existent. Therefore, there is no need to extend the cavity margins gingivally more than necessary for adequate preparation and finishing. In class II amalgam preparation, the objective of preparation of the occlusal portion is to provide access to the proximal lesion and to remove defective pits and fissures. Access to the proximal surface may be attained by a slot preparation, which is simply a self-retentive proximal box. Authors are of the view that isthmus fracture is related more to improper occlusal contact than to the lack of bulk of the restorative material. The conservative amalgam is subjected to minimal occlusal stress and therefore, the incidence of isthmus fracture is reduced.

Establishing Outline Form for Gingival/Cervical Cavities

The outline form for the gingival/cervical cavities, both in buccal and lingual surfaces is controlled by the following factors:
- Health and position of the gingiva. In young patients the restoration is covered by gingiva, i.e. most of the restorative margins in such patients are kept sub-gingival. However, in older patients, with the recession, the margins can be kept supragingival.
- Forces of mastication, abnormal occlusal contacts and eating pattern of the patient should also be kept in mind while planning cervical cavities.
- Contour of the buccal/lingual surfaces
- Extent of the caries
- Oral hygiene of the patient, vis-à-vis brushing habits, and the quality of brush.

Fig. 10.5 shows the outline form for cervical cavities.

The outline form for root caries is controlled mainly by the site of the lesion, extent of the caries, age of the patient and the oral hygiene. By and large, root caries is managed by excavating the caries and restoring without any injudicious extension.

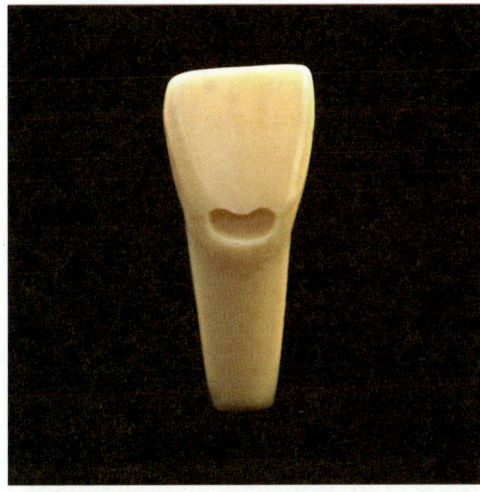

Fig. 10.5: Outline form for cervical cavity in maxillary central incisor

Modifications of Outline Form

The rationale for modifying cavity design reflects the development of new materials, modifications of traditional materials with better physical properties, awareness of patients towards better oral health, coupled with the use of fluorides and improved equipments in the dental office. In occlusal outline form, if the buccolingual intercuspal extension is greater than 2/3rd of the cusp incline, it reduces the strength of the cusps and if lesser than 1.0 mm, results in poor condensation resulting in porosity and poor adaptation of the restoration. In proximal outline form, if the bucco-lingual extension is less than 1.5 mm or the occlusogingival extension is less than 2.0 mm, there is a high probability that cavosurface margins are in contact with the adjacent tooth.

The occlusogingival extension is measured relative to the marginal ridge. The usual mean distance from the marginal ridge to the cemento-enamel junction is 5.0 mm for premolars and 6.0 mm for molars. The ideal gingival extension required is 4.0 mm with 2.0 mm as the range of variation.

The outline form varies with the use of different restorative materials. Both external and internal outline forms are to be modified with the advent of newer restorative materials.

The preparation design for composite restorations differs from that for amalgam in outline form, cavity depth, and in preparation of the enamel at cavosurface margins. Cavities prepared for composite should be shallower and the occlusal outline narrower than for amalgam. The low tensile strength of amalgam dictates bulk placement especially where heavy forces are applied. Amalgam requires a minimal cavity depth of 2.0 mm with an adequately wide isthmus. Composites because of their high tensile strength permit a narrower and shallower isthmus. As composites undergo volumetric shrinkage of 1.5% to 2.0% during polymerization, a minimal cavity outline reduces the tendency for open margins. The proximal outline is similar to that for amalgam. The proximal grooves reduce withdrawal at the gingival margin caused by polymerization shrinkage.

In composites, a short bevel at the enamel margin has been advocated to promote better sealing by etching. Enamel in the proximal wall should be bevelled because prism direction is at right angles to the surface. Occlusal bevels are unnecessary because the prism directions in the zone of the central fossa are inclined towards the fossa. It has been shown that a parallel-sided non-bevelled occlusal section provided excellent sealing against microleakage in comparison with a bevelled margin.

It has always been controversial whether bevel should be given or not in the cavity preparation for composites. The authors who are in favour of beveling advocate that by beveling:

- The surface area is increased and the mechanical retention is improved.
- Marginal adaptability is improved.
- Remove the prismless layer of surface enamel
- Expose the ends of enamel rods for better etching.
- The color matching is improved since the transition from tooth to composite is gradual.

However, those who are not in favour of beveling and favour butt joint state that:

- The orientation of prisms varies in different anatomical sites and beveling each site accordingly will be practically difficult.
- Composite in thin sections are liable to fracture especially at stress bearing areas.
- Optimum strength of restoration is achieved by providing butt joints.

I am of the view that the enamel margin in composite restoration should be bevelled except at the occlusal surface. By beveling labial/lingual surfaces of anterior teeth, color matching is definitely improved. In cases of cervical lesions, bevel should be given only on occlusal/incisal wall and not on cervical wall. Similarly, bevel should be avoided in cervical/gingival cavosurface margins in proximal restorations.

Enameloplasty

It is defined as the procedure of reshaping or recontouring the enamel surface with suitable rotary cutting instruments to remove the shallow areas by rounding or saucering the enamel so that the area becomes cleansable, finishable and allows conservative placement of enamel margins. Enameloplasty does not extend to the outline form. Use of enameloplasty produces smooth union of tooth surface and restorative material (Fig. 10.6).

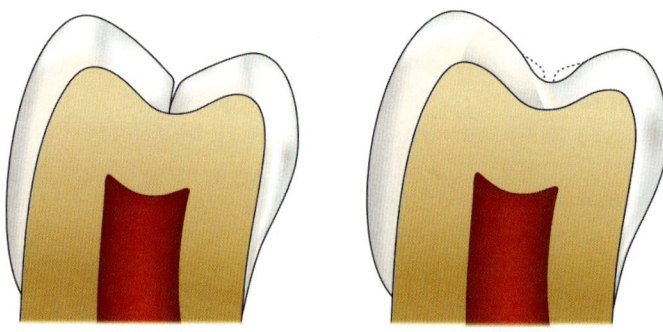

Fig. 10.6: Enameloplasty

Indications

- If 1/3rd or less of enamel depth is involved, fissure may be removed by enameloplasty.
- In case the supplemental grooves extend till the cuspal inclines.
- On shallow fissure that approaches or crosses a lingual or facial ridge.

Cusp Capping

Many a times, during the cavity preparation, due to extent of caries or any other reason, preparation may

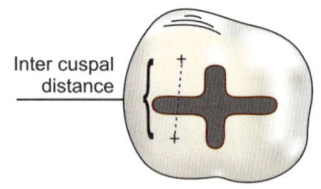
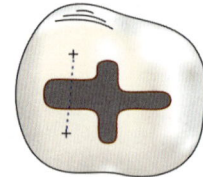
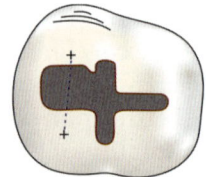

One third of the cuspal incline involved (Cusp Capping not necessary)

One half of the cuspal incline involved (Consider Cusp Capping)

Two Third of the cuspal incline involved (Cusp Capping mandatory)

A   **B**   **C**

Figs 10.7A to C: Protocol for cusp capping

extend on to the cuspal inclines or the intercuspal distance increases which reduces the strength of the cusp. The cusps so weakened are unable to bear the masticatory forces and may fracture. Cusp capping refers to the coverage of the weakened cusp to prevent its fracture (Figs 10.7A to C).

Indications

- If the intercuspal distance is one-third, there is no need of cusp capping
- If the intercuspal distance is one-half, cusp capping can be considered
- If the intercuspal distance is more than one-half, cusp capping is mandatory

Alternatively, the weakened cusp may be reinforced by substituting lost dentin with glass-ionomer cement.

RESISTANCE AND RETENTION FORMS

These are two important features to be taken care of during cavity preparation. These two features are interrelated and interdependent that is why they are considered simultaneously. Few authors have even preferred the term 'retention-resistance form'.

'Resistance form' may be defined as *'that shape and configuration of the cavity that best enables both the restoration and the tooth to withstand occlusal forces without fracture'*. The resistance form is in direct relation to the degree of exposure of the restoration to the occlusion and to the force used in mastication. On an average, a force of 150 lbs is exerted on molars by adults. Greater the occlusal contact, the greater will be the chances of fracture. The amount of the remaining tooth structure and the choice of the material also have an impact on the resistance form.

Features contributing to resistance form are:

a. The cavity should be prepared as a box with a flat floor. Flat floor resists the occlusal stresses, being at right angle to such forces (Figs 10.8 and 10.9). The flat floors can be more than one. Flat floor will help prevent the movement of the restoration

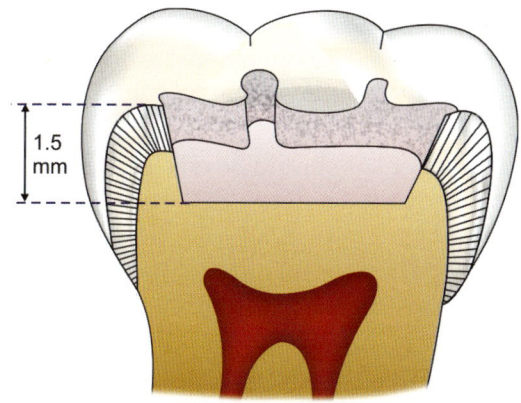

Fig. 10.9: Maintain uniform depth of the pulpal floor

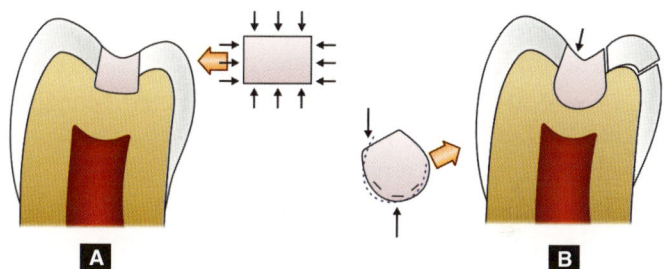

Figs 10.10A and B: Cup shaped cavity preparation leads to tooth fracture

whereas the rounded pulpal floor may allow a non bonded restoration rocking movement producing wedging force, which may result in shearing of tooth structure. (Figs 10.10A and B). Two or three flat seats peripheral to the excavated sites provide better resistance form to the prepared cavity.

b. Cusps and ridges with dentin support should not be undermined. The extension of the external walls of the cavity preparation should be kept as small as possible. When a fissure is cut, the cavity margin should extend to 1/3rd the distance from the central groove to cusp tip (Fig. 10.11).

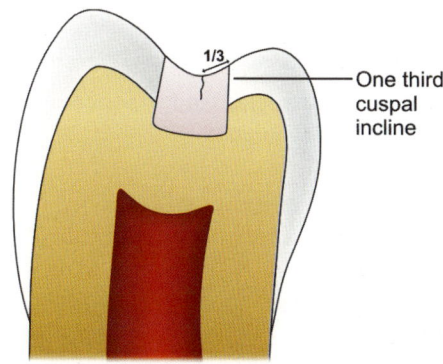

Fig. 10.11: When a fissure is cut, the cavity margin should extend to one-third the distance from the central groove to the cusp tip

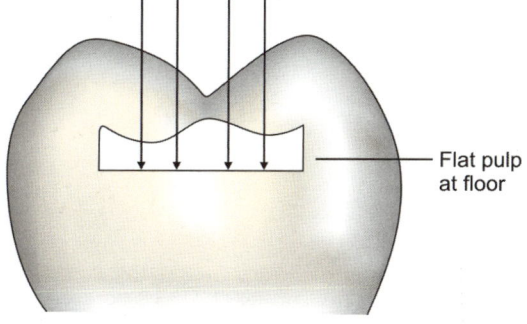

Fig. 10.8: Sectional view of a class I cavity in which flat floor provides resistance form

c. The restorative material should have enough thickness depending upon its respective compressive and tensile strengths to prevent its fracture under load.
d. Weakened cusps should be enveloped or included in cavity form to prevent damage from lateral forces.
e. Rounding/coving of line angles avoids stresses directly on to the tooth, Fig. 10.12 thereby resistance to fracture is increased. The sharp line angles lead to poor resistance form at the cavity-restoration interface (Fig. 10.13).
f. Uniform depth: 1.5-2.0 mm overall depth or 0.2-0.5 mm into dentin.
g. To bond the restorative material to the tooth structure wherever possible.
h. Preservation of cusps and marginal ridge. Marginal ridges should be minimally encroached so as to preserve their strength (Fig. 10.14).
i. All enamel walls must consist of either full length enamel rods on sound dentin or full length enamel rods on sound dentin supported on preparation side by shortened rods also on sound dentin (Fig. 10.15). The enamel rods vary in orientation at different locations within the the tooth. The angulation of enamel rods at occlusal third, middle third and cervical third are depicted in (Fig. 10.16).

The above features make the tooth to better withstand the occlusal stresses. The minimal thickness of amalgam and cast gold to resist fracture is approximately 1.5 mm, though little more depth is required for amalgam to achieve the requisite bulk (Fig. 10.9). However, in composites and glass-ionomers, the depth is not the criteria for achieving resistance form. Porcelain also requires more depth; 2.0 mm occlusal depth is required for porcelain inlays and 1.5 mm for crowns.

'Retention form' may be defined as *'the shape and configuration of the cavity that enables the restoration to be retained in that cavity under all types of tipping and tilting stresses.'*

The retention form usually varies with the type of the material.

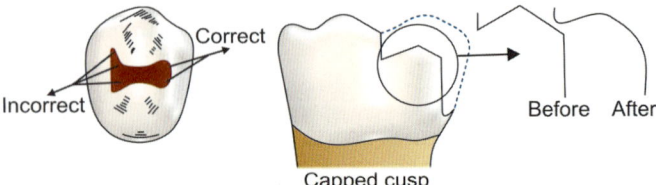

Fig. 10.12: Rounding of external and internal line angles

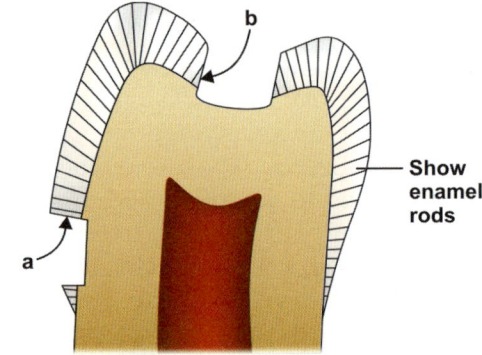

Fig. 10.15: Full length enamel rods on sound dentin (a) and full length and shortened enamel rods on sound dentin (b)

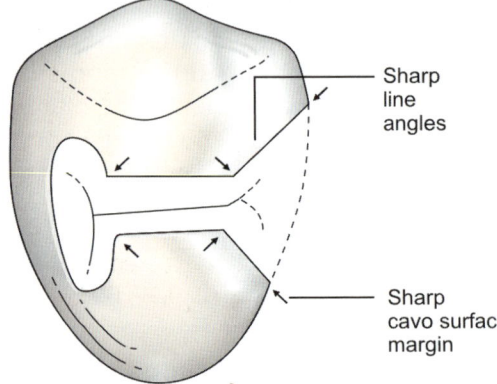

Fig. 10.13: Sharp line angles lead to poor resistance form at the cavity restoration interface

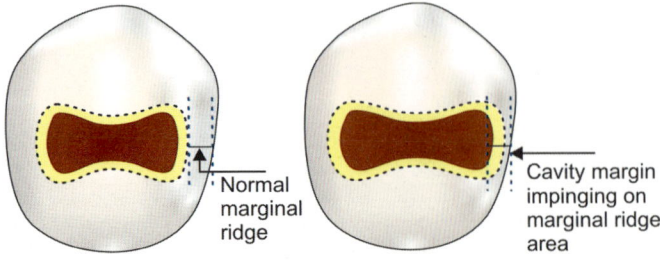

Fig. 10.14: Cavity margin impinging on Marginal Ridge area

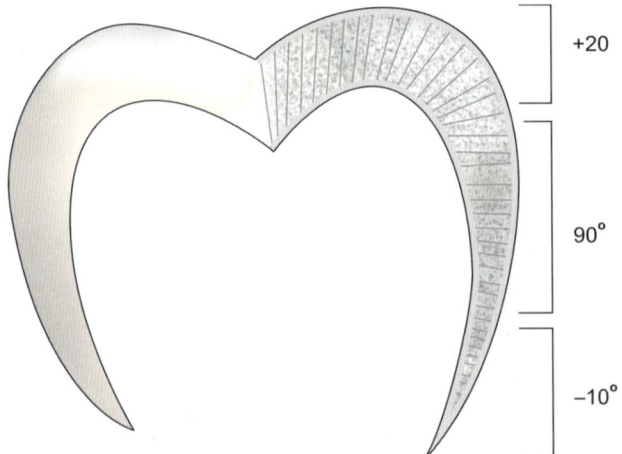

Fig. 10.16: Orientation of enamel rods (longitudinal section)

Features contributing to retention form are:
a. Magnitude of the occlusal forces and the area of the restoration, which will be under the occlusal load.
b. Configuration of the cavity. The total surface area, i.e. both width and depth of the cavity
c. Available height of the cavity walls
d. Amount of remaining dentin

Primarily for silver amalgam, the retention form is achieved by:
 i. Converging the walls occlusally, both for class I and class II cavities
 ii. Occlusal dovetail in class II preparations (Fig. 10.17)
 iii. Slight undercuts can be given in the dentin (Fig. 10.18).
 iv. Adhesive systems in amalgam can bond it micromechanically to the tooth structure and decrease microleakage.
 v. Cavosurface angle of 90 degrees, i.e. butt joint.

For cast restorations the retention form is achieved by:
 i. Parallelism of walls. A slight divergence (2°–5°) can be given for proper withdrawal of the pattern.
    In case the available height of the walls is less, the divergence should be kept minimum. At least one half of the total wall should be kept parallel and the rest can be diverged.
 ii. Occlusal extension is mandatory even if no occlusal caries is present since it prevents tilting. The outline form for the occlusal extension is same as for occlusal cavities (Figs 10.19A and B).
 iii. Reverse bevel at the gingival wall will prevent tipping movements.

In direct filling gold, the restoration is retained by the elastic compression developed in the dentin due

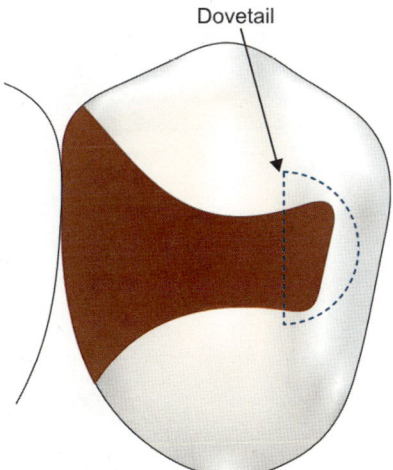

Fig. 10.17: Occlusal dovetail in Class II preparation on maxillary first premolar

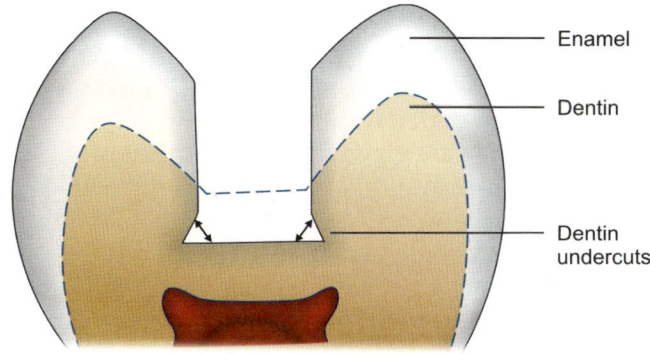

Fig. 10.18: Undercuts in dentinal walls used for providing retention form

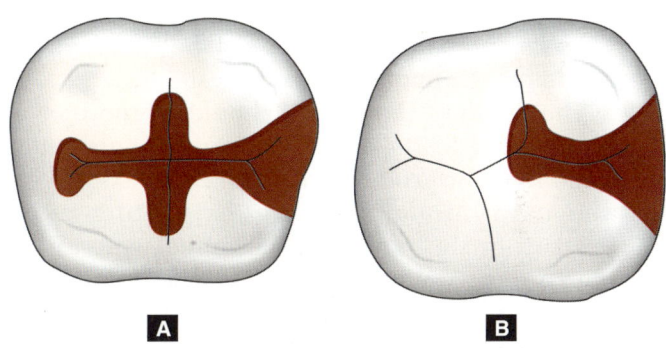

Figs 10.19A and B: Occlusal lock related to the morphology of: **(A)** Mandibular tooth and **(B)** Maxillary tooth

to condensation of the foil and also the starting points prepared in the cavity aid in retention.

In composites, micromechanical bonding helps to achieve the retention form. For this bonding agents are used. The surface area of the cavity and the type of bonding agent, both aid in the retention form. It has been established that the enamel bonding agents can produce bond strength up to 35 MPa, though most of the available bonding agents provide bond strength up to 22–24 MPa.

Despite of providing all these features material wise, many a times, the prepared cavity is not retentive. In such cases, other devices are used which provide extra retention and even reinforce the tooth in certain conditions. All such devices are termed as 'secondary retentive devices', which are as follows:
 i. Slots
 ii. Locks
 iii. Grooves
 iv. Skirts
 v. Pins

 i. *Slots:* Slots are given in dentin to increase the surface area of the preparation and also to have more convergent walls. These are 1.0-1.5 mm deep box type preparations and can be given in occlusal wall or gingival wall or both. Usually the slots are given all along the width of the occlusal/gingival wall. Each slot has four walls, which aid in further retention. Slots can be given with any type of restorative material (Fig. 10.20).

ii. *Locks:* These are given in the proximal box of class II cavity preparation and are indicated mainly for silver amalgam restorations. Though not of much use, the locks are also tried with composites and glass-ionomers.

Locks are usually given in dentin either in the walls of the proximal box or in the occlusal box at the line angles; or axial wall with the proximal wall. These are 0.2-0.3 mm wide and 0.5 mm deep into the dentin (Figs 10.21A and B).

iii. *Grooves*: Grooves are indicated for cast restorations. These are prepared in the walls of the proximal box inside the dentino-enamel junction.

The depth of the groove should be more or at least equal to its width for providing proper retention. The grooves are given at the axiobuccal and axio-lingual line angles, putting more pressure on the buccal and the lingual walls rather than at the axial wall (Fig. 13.9). The grooves are prepared parallel or slightly diverging occlusally for proper withdrawal of the pattern.

The grooves are also given in three quarter and full/half crown preparations (Figs 10.22A, B and 10.23).

Wherever grooves are given care should be taken to place the groove in one plane. More than one groove per wall is rarely indicated and if necessary, can be given keeping proper parallelism and dentin around each groove.

iv. *Skirts:* Skirts are indicated in cast restorations and are the extensions of the proximal box at the line angles of the tooth or even away from it. The margins of the restoration are kept on healthy tooth structure and bevelled. This type of enveloping the walls increases the total surface area of the restoration thereby increasing the retention. In case, the caries has undermined the cusps; the cuspal coverage is considered; which is also a part of the skirt preparation. Skirts can be

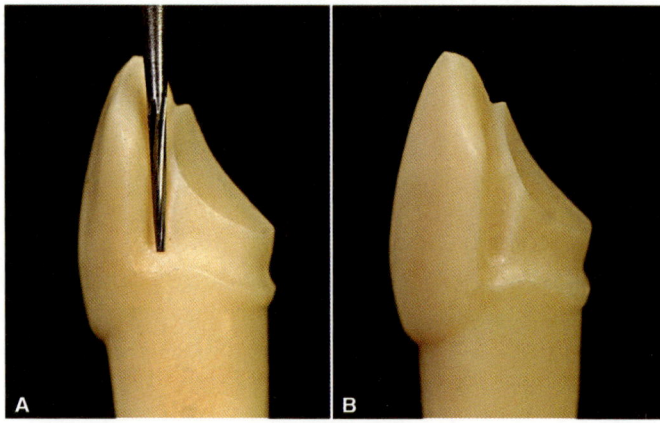

Figs 10.22A and B: (A) Preparation of proximal grooves in 3/4th crown of maxillary canine; **(B)** 3/4th crown with groove (proximal view)

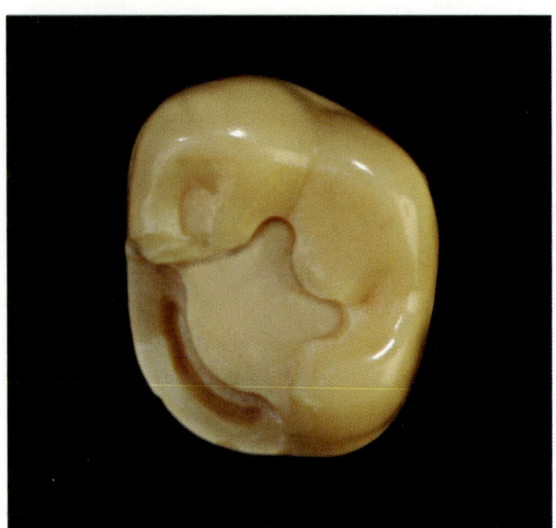

Fig. 10.20: Slot preparation in maxillary second molar

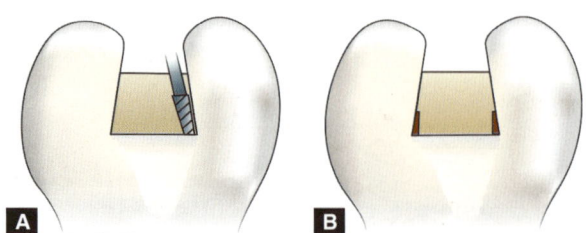

Figs 10.21A and B: Locks in the proximal box **(A)** fissure bur preparing lock at the axio-buccal/lingual line angle **(B)** completed locks

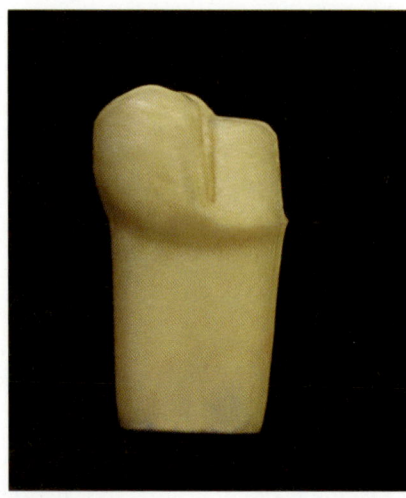

Fig. 10.23: Half crown with grooves (buccal view)

given on one side or both the sides depending upon the extent of the lesions and the required retention in the particular tooth.

v. *Pins:* Various types of pins are available in different shapes and sizes suitable for different situations. Pins provide extra retention and can be used with silver amalgam, composites and cast restoration. The detail regarding use of pins is given in Chapter 14.

CONVENIENCE FORM

This is the form of the cavity, which visualizes lesion more clearly. Convenience form implies that the operator must create sufficient access to the lesion to facilitate visibility and instrumentation in the preparation of the cavity and the insertion of a restorative material. The shape of the cavity is modified so as to have proper access to the lesion, better manipulation during restoration and finally for better finishing and polishing. Mostly this form is required in proximal cavities, in both anterior and posterior teeth, i.e. Class III and Class II cavities (Fig. 10.2).

Features influencing convenience form are:
- Armamentarium to be used
- Location of the cavity margins
- Accessibility for caries removal and pulp protection
- Accessibility for placing restorative material
  - Finishing of the cavity margins
  - Starting points, if any
  - Other retentive areas
- Type of the restorative material to be placed

In class II cavities, access is gained through the marginal ridge of the respective side. Other modalities such as 'tunnel preparation', etc. could not satisfy the restorative criteria for long. In cases of class III cavities, convenience form is mainly through lingual side since labial enamel is to be preserved as far as possible, until and unless the caries dictates gaining approach from the labial side.

In class I and class V cavities, the approach is direct onto the lesion and the convenience form is not difficult to achieve. Diverging of the walls of the cavity in cast restoration is a part of convenience form so as to have proper withdrawal of the pattern. For direct filling gold, starting points are given both at gingival and incisal point angles. The cavity can be widened to facilitate the movement of condenser at this point and other areas of the cavity. Such intentional widening of the cavity is for gaining the convenience form in direct gold restorations.

REMOVAL OF REMAINING CARIOUS DENTIN

It is defined as *'the elimination of any infected carious tooth structure or faulty restoration left in the cavity preparation'*. After preparing the cavity and achieving sufficient resistance and retention forms, i.e. adequate width and depth is maintained according to the requirement of the material, the remaining portion is checked for any left-over caries. The site and location of such caries is important since it will dictate the future modification of the preparation. Caries left on the pulpal/axial wall is excavated thoroughly making the cavity deeper. Preferably 0.75 mm-1.0 mm dentin should always cover the pulp. If caries is still present at the pulpal/axial wall, it should be excavated slowly with hand excavators, even if it leads to exposure. Such exposures are later treated accordingly. Indirect pulp capping, advised by certain authors is not required, if the remaining caries is hard, arrested or unaffected.

In no case soft and infected caries should be left over the pulp. Such residual caries leads to pulpal inflammation and subsequently slow death of pulp. Chemical dyes such as 0.5% Basic fuschin may be helpful in differentiating the infected and the affected dentin. Few authors are also of the view that if some micro-organisms are left untreated and the cavity is filled, these become inactivated and get destroyed. However, it is always advisable to remove all the infected dentin.

In case of children and young pulps, the left over caries is best tolerated. And also, vital pulp is needed for proper root formation. In such cases, remaining caries along the walls of the cavity should be excavated and the extent of such lesions is thoroughly checked. The undermining of enamel so produced can be treated in two ways:

i. The undermined area is filled with glass-ionomers or glass-cermet cements making the configuration of the walls as required.
ii. Cuspal coverage can be considered.

The removal of remaining restorative material needs extra care since the tooth colored restorative materials pose problem for their complete removal. Use of magnifiers and round burs revolving at slow speed is recommended.

Ideal method to remove the hard heavily discolored dentin is the use of round carbide bur in a high speed handpiece with air coolant.

Pulp may be infected by forcing the micro-organisms into the dentinal tubules using excess pressure with spoon excavators, etc.

PULP PROTECTION

Pulp protection, though not taken in principles of cavity preparation, is an important step before final restoration.

The pulpal injuries are usually caused by following factors:

- Heat generated by injudicious cutting
- Restorative materials with good thermal conductivity
- Chemical ingredients of the restorative materials
- Galvanic currents
- Ingress of micro-organisms through microleakage

The underlying pulp is to be protected if the remaining dentin is less. It has been established that the 2.0 mm-2.5 mm remaining dentin is capable of countering external stimuli, therefore procedure for pulp protection may not be required. In case the remaining dentin is less, pulp is to be protected using liners and bases depending upon the amount of dentin left and the restorative material to be used.

'Base' is the material, which is applied over the pulpal/axial wall and act as a substitute for lost dentin. The thickness of the base depends upon the amount of dentin lost. The total bulk (dentin + base) should be at least 2.0 mm. The bases provide mechanical, chemical and thermal protection to the pulp. The materials like zinc phosphate cements, polycarboxylate cements, glass-ionomers, calcium hydroxide and zinc oxide eugenol are used as bases. In case of pulp exposure or very near to pulp exposure, a calcium hydroxide base is preferred below the usual cements (Figs 10.24A and B). This way the application of base can be divided into two steps. However, the recently introduced light cure calcium hydroxide can be given as a total base, since it provides the sufficient strength. Many a times, mild undercuts are given before placing bases, though extra care is to be taken while placing these undercuts.

The base is applied only on the pulpal and the axial wall. The cements are not given on the other walls of the cavity preparation. All cements, by and large, dissolve in oral fluids, the quantity may vary. This dissolution leads to spacing at the tooth-restoration interface leading to microleakage. Therefore, the cements are avoided on the walls which are open to oral environment.

The term 'liner' is used for those materials, which can be applied to a cavity surface in a relatively thin film. The thickness of liners usually does not exceed 0.1 mm. Apart from providing thermal and chemical insulation, the liners fill the minor intricacies between the tooth and the restorative material. All the material

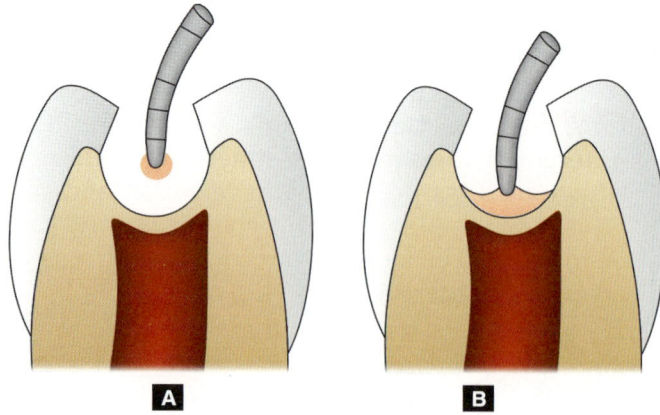

Figs 10.24A and B: (A) Cavity approaching pulp, (B) Application of calcium hydroxide liner

used for bases can be used as liner; however, calcium hydroxide and zinc oxide eugenol are preferred.

CAVITY VARNISH

For shallow cavities, cavity varnish can be applied on the walls especially in silver amalgam and cast gold restorations. However, in composites and glass-ionomers, the application of cavity varnish is avoided.

Cavity varnish is a mixture of copal resin and the organic solvents and on application, the solvents evaporate, leaving a resin layer over the dentin (Fig. 10.25). This seals the dentinal tubules, which leads to better marginal adaptability, especially with silver amalgam till the corrosion products fill the gap. Two coats of varnish are considered sufficient, since varnish is hydrophobic and with single application, 55% wetting is achieved (smear layer over the dentin has moisture). With the second application, 85–90% wetting is achieved which is sufficient to provide the necessary sealing. Dentin bonding agents are also

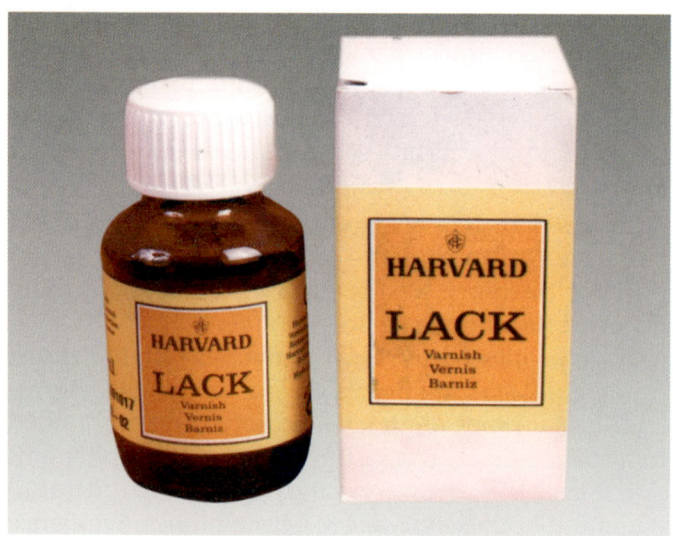

Fig. 10.25: Cavity varnish

recognized as the dentin sealing agents and can be used as substitutes for cavity varnish.

Functions

- Prevents microleakage.
- Reduces post-operative sensitivity by not allowing ingress of fluid from the cavity margin.
- Prevents penetration of toxic materials into the dentin from the restorative material.
- It does not act as an insulator.

FINISHING THE ENAMEL WALLS AND MARGINS

This is the procedure carried out to finish the cavosurface margins and the enamel at the cavity walls in such a way so that the best possible adaptation of the restorative material is achieved.

This procedure creates a smooth junction between restoration and tooth and also provides maximum strength to both the tooth and the restorative material especially near the margins.

Features influencing cavosurface margins

i. Location of the margins vis-à-vis direction of the enamel rods
ii. Type of the restorative material to be used
iii. Degree of smoothness required
iv. Previous restorative material used, if any

Thorough knowledge of anatomy of enamel rods is mandatory for proper finishing of cavity preparation.

- The rods extend full length from dentino-enamel junction to outer enamel surface
- The enamel rods radiate from dentino-enamel junction to the external surface of the enamel.
- In axial sections, occlusally, the rods make a +20° to +30° angle with the long axis of the tooth. In the middle, they are perpendicular and in the gingival third they make an angle of –5° to –10° (Fig. 10.16).
- The rods usually converge toward concave surfaces and diverge toward convex surfaces.

Finishing of enamel margins is carried out almost in every restorative material. In case of silver amalgam, butt end of the cavosurface margins are preferred because of poor edge strength of amalgam (Figs 10.26A). The gingival wall is slightly bevelled, thereby removing the unsupported enamel rods (Fig. 10.27). In gold foil restorations, an ultra short bevel is given at the cavosurface margins. A short bevel is given for cast gold restoration (Figs 10.26B). Beveling, however, is avoided in porcelain, and resin materials. Beveling in composite is controversial as is described earlier. However, labial walls in class III and occlusal walls in class V cavities can be bevelled for proper color matching.

Design of Cavosurface Angle

It should be 90 degree, i.e. butt joint.

i. Due to poor edge strength of amalgam.
ii. It provides strength to both amalgam and tooth structure.

Bevelling of External Walls

Indications

- Cast metal
- Composite restorations (beveling can also be done in case of large restorations)

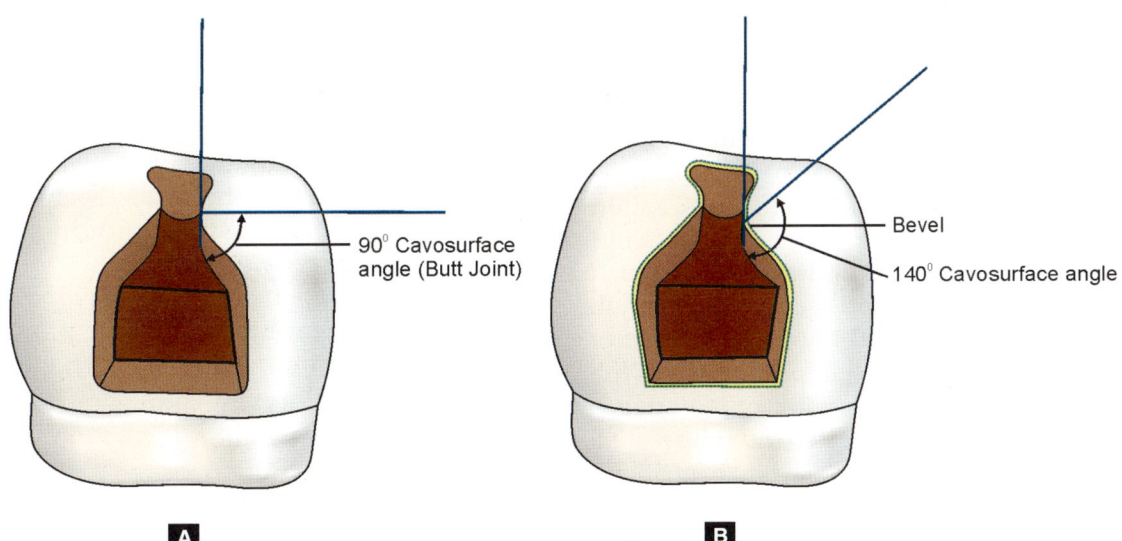

Figs 10.26A and B: (A) 90° Cavosurface angle (Butt Joint) for silver amalgam; (B) 140° Cavosurface angle for cast gold

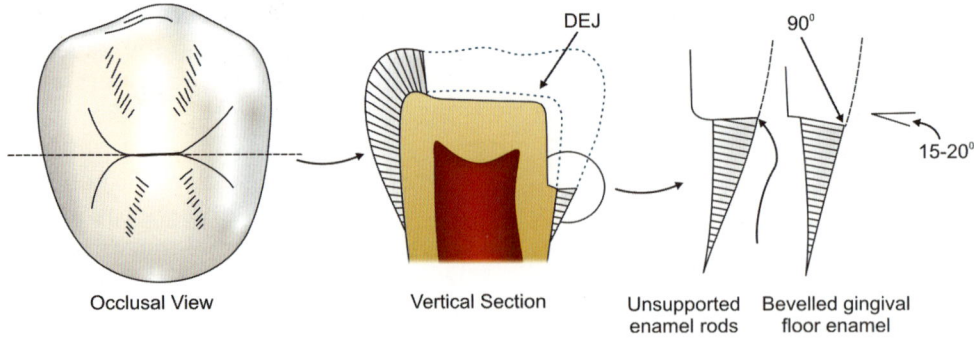

Fig. 10.27: Bevelling the gingival floor in Class II cavity for silver amalgam

Contraindications

- Ceramics
- Silver amalgam (except 15 to 20 degree gingival bevel)

Purposes

- It provides strong enamel margin.
- Marginal seal in undersized casting.
- To burnish marginal metal.
- Adapt gingival margins of the casting.

Degree of Desired Smoothness and Roughness

- Choice of restorative material can decide this
  - For smooth walls - cast metal restorations
  - For rough walls – composite restorations as they increase the surface area of restoration
- High speed to finish enamel
- Plain cut fissure burs produce the finest surface
- Hand instruments, e.g. GMT and enamel hatchet to plain the enamel walls
- Not much smoothness is required in case of amalgam and gold foil

TOILET OF THE CAVITY

This is the final procedure in cavity preparation and consists of removing all debris and cut dentinal chips from the walls of the cavity. Warm water can be utilized along with drying with oil free air. A cotton swab can also be used to sweep out the debris. Mild acidic solutions have been tried but are not of much use (Fig. 10.28). Use of antiseptic solutions, alcohol, etc. should be avoided. The step of *'sterilization of cavity walls'* could not gain much importance over the years mostly because of advent of newer materials.

The overdrying of the cavity with compressed air, etc. is also avoided, especially in composite restorations, the bonding agents are hydrophilic and prefer wet dentin.

The *'conditioning'* of the cavity floor and walls is carried out for glass-ionomer restorations. By using

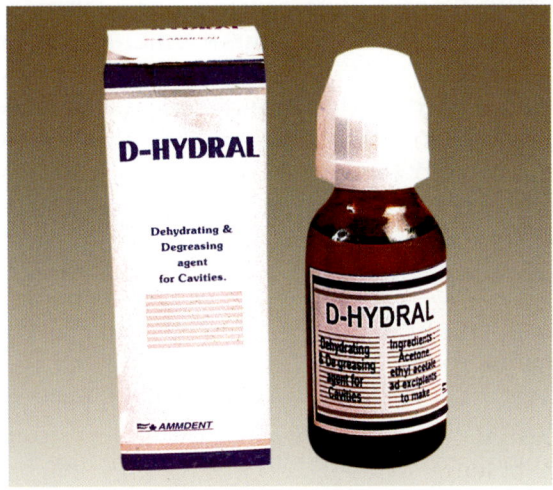

Fig. 10.28: Dehydrating and de-greasing agent for cavity cleansing

mild acids or etchant for 8–10 seconds, the surface calcium is re-oriented and reorganized making it conducive for bonding with glass-ionomer. In case of *'etching'*, the inorganic salts are partially demineralized leading to enamel tags which later help in mechanical union between the tooth and the restorative material. The smear layer is also removed or altered with this phenomenon – the detailed discussion is given in Chapter 16.

After finally cleaning the cavity, extra care should be taken for proper control of the operating field. In no case saliva or moisture should enter in an otherwise clean cavity.

In my opinion, the following steps should be followed in sequence during cavity preparation for successful restoration:

- Planning the cavity preparation
- Initial cavity preparation
- Final cavity preparation
- Finishing the prepared cavity
  a. *Planning the cavity preparation:* Before starting the cutting procedure, spend some time for planning the preparation. The final shape of the cavity is

Principles of Cavity Preparation

anticipated in mind keeping in view the following features:

i. Choice of the restorative material
ii. Extent of the carious lesion
iii. Occlusal contacts
iv. Shape of the contacts, contour and embrasures
v. Age of the patient
vi. Oral hygiene status and patient's awareness towards oral health

With the advancement in adhesive restorative materials coupled with patient's insistence for tooth colored restorations, most of the clinicians are preferring composites as a material of choice for restoring both anterior and posterior teeth. In case of composites, the cavity preparation is kept shallow and narrow since the tensile strength of these materials is good. However, in silver amalgam, the cavity is kept wider and deeper so as to have more bulk of the material. The bulk provides proper resistance to the restoration because of its poor tensile strength.

With the use of cast restorations, the abnormal contacts, contours and occlusal disharmonies can be corrected. These restorations can also be planned for wider cavities involving more than two surfaces of the tooth. Cast restorations especially the full crowns and partial crowns need sufficient surface area and sufficient length of the walls. In case sufficient height is not available, other treatment modalities such as pin restorations should be planned. The placement of margins in cast restorations depends upon the material to be used and the age, vis-à-vis the gingival condition of the patient.

In each case, patient's awareness towards oral health and oral hygiene is very important. In older age, with attrition and gingival recession, care should be taken to restore the tooth in such a way so as to utilize minimum chair time.

b. *Initial cavity preparation:* Once planned for the choice of the restorative material and the extent of cavity margins, the cavity preparation is started using appropriate burs and other instruments. During initial cavity preparation, care is taken to remove all carious lesion, whether undermining enamel or not and whether near or over the pulp. The susceptible pits and fissures should be involved in cavity preparation. Leaving susceptible pits and fissures subsequently lead to secondary caries with all the restorative materials even with composites. The unsupported enamel should be removed.

c. *Final cavity preparation:* After initial cavity preparation, the cavity is checked thoroughly for any remaining caries, unsupported enamel and the depth of remaining dentin over the pulp. The final cavity preparation should be based on the following features:

i. Magnitude of occlusal forces
ii. Available surface area of the tooth
iii. Amount of remaining dentin left over the pulp
iv. Amount of remaining dentin under the cusps and ridges, and also whether these cusps and ridges are working or non-working
v. Extent of caries at the contact areas
vi. Extent of caries at the gingival areas
vii. Whether caries lesions are joining two or more than two surfaces
viii. Age of the patient, esthetic consciousness and extent of gingival recession vis-à-vis the chair time which can be utilized
ix. Finally the economic status

The pattern of occlusal stresses plays an important role in restorative dentistry. Every class of cavity whether anterior or posterior, smaller or larger, will have to withstand the forces during mastication and during various movements of the mandible. The mechanics involved in restorations vis-a-vis occlusion have been described earlier. Care should be taken to manipulate the working cusps and inclines properly. Strength of the working cusps is maintained by filling the undermining enamel with glass-ionomer cements and/or covering the cusps. Remember 3.0 mm of vertical height of walls is required to achieve resistance/retention in cast restorations. In case such a height is less, the other sides of the tooth should be involved to counter the dislodging forces. Finally, if the surface for counter is not sufficient or total vertical height is much less than required, pin restorations can be considered.

Composites and glass-ionomers are usually not given in stress bearing areas, though recent composites and pin-retained composites are showing some promising results. Composites are also being tried in wider cavities and in cases requiring cuspal coverage.

Cervical restorations should be given an extra time for final inspection because the pattern of occlusal forces in different individuals plays a vital role in retaining these restorations in place. The longevity of these restorations, vis-à-vis the marginal leakage and secondary caries also depends upon these stresses. Proper undercuts should be given and if need be, pins can be considered for achieving retention. The extension of lesion at the cementum should be dealt with firmly as this area is more prone to leakage.

After giving final shape to the cavity, bases and liners should be given to make the floor smooth and to protect the underlying pulp. With the advancement in composites and glass-ionomer cements, flat floors may not be the requisite, but protection of pulp is needed with every restorative material. Fast setting zinc oxide eugenol, zinc phosphate cement, glass-ionomer cements and light cure calcium hydroxide can be considered depending upon the need for substituting dentin and the restorative material to be given.

d. *Finishing the prepared cavity:* The final cavity shall be thoroughly washed and cleaned before placing the restoration. Some debris of cements or previous restorative materials or even dentin chips might be clinging to the cavity walls. Washing with normal saline or warm water under pressure is helpful. Squeezing the cavity walls with cotton will further clean the cavity. The cavity should be dried with oil free air and without any pressure. The enamel margins can be smoothened with hand cutting instruments and the cavosurface margins are bevelled depending upon the restorative material to be given. The enamel rods at the gingival direction are to be dealt with cautiously. In case the gingival wall is in cementum, it should not be bevelled.

The finished cavity should be maintained till the completion of final restoration. During the restorative procedures, the cavity is to be protected from saliva, moisture and other contaminants. The final phase of restoration is completed under strict isolation.

Care at each step leads to success of the treatment.

FORCES EXERTED DURING OCCLUSION/MASTICATION AND THEIR RESOLUTION

Various types of forces are exerted on teeth during movement of mandible and also during mastication. Since the tooth surfaces are curved or at an incline, these forces are not only vertical but other types of forces may also be exerting on these surfaces. The tooth, in turn, counteracts these forces with the help of periodontal membrane and alveolar bone.

If the surfaces are flat and perpendicular to the force of mastication, only vertical forces would take part. But in curved surfaces, other forces are also set up and the resulting forces might not be exerted along the long axis of the tooth (Figs 10.29A and B). This phenomenon can be understood by studying the resolution of forces on inclined planes. The cuspal planes are taken as inclined planes.

When a force acts perpendicular to a fixed horizontal surface, the resolving force reacts perpendicular to the surface with an equal and opposite force. If the surface is tilted at an angle to the horizontal, it still reacts at right angle to the surface (Figs 10.30A and B).

Thus, the reaction force no longer opposes the applied force in direction nor is equal to its magnitude. Hence the forces are not in equilibrium when applied on inclined planes.

The equilibrium can be maintained if more than one force is exerted on tooth or the forces are resolved in both directions. Let us discuss how the forces act on cuspal incline planes (Fig. 10.31). AB is a tangent drawn at incline plane or the contact between two cusps. Angle represents the angle made with the horizontal AC by the tangent AB of the cuspal contact. M is the force of mastication and N is the resolving force. M is perpendicular to the horizontal AC and N is perpendicular to the incline plane, tangent AB, H is the horizontal component of the resolving force,

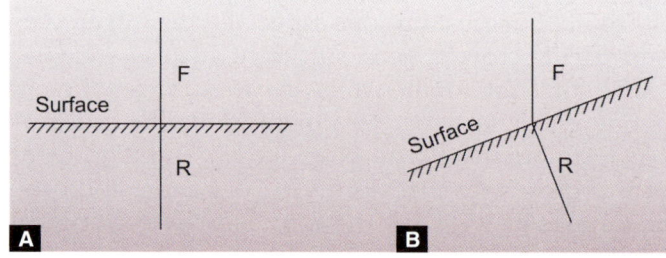

Figs 10.30A and B: Force and its resolution on: **(A)** Horizontal and **(B)** Inclined surfaces

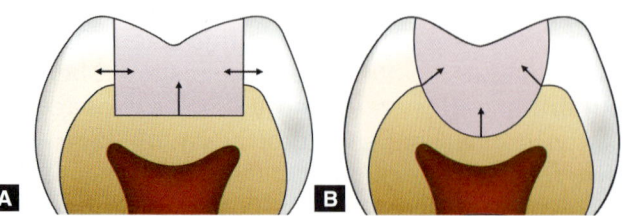

Figs 10.29A and B: Counteraction of occlusal forces: **(A)** Flat floor; **(B)** Curved floor

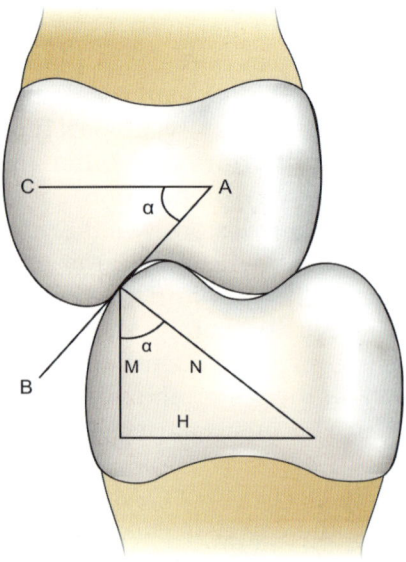

Fig. 10.31: Forces acting on cuspal inclines

Principles of Cavity Preparation

which maintains the equilibrium. As the angle decreases, i.e. incline plane decreases, N and H become shorter and finally merge with M, i.e. equal to zero.

The effect of friction between cusps also plays an important role. Friction is the resistance to a sliding motion of one body over another and the coefficient of friction is the force of friction over normal force.

Many a times, two or more inclined surfaces with slopes facing each other of one tooth contact the buccal and lingual cusps of the opposing tooth or the buccal and lingual cusps and marginal ridges. This condition accounts for the proper balance in occlusion and in case the contact is not normal, it may account for displacements of the restoration or the fracture of the teeth. The effect so produced is termed as wedging effect.

The horizontal components of the normal force are responsible for this wedging effect. These horizontal components set up by inclines are equal and opposite and tend to push the inclined surfaces apart.

Forces Acting on the Tooth

A. *In centric occlusion* forces a, b, c act at three contact points (Fig. 10.32A).

R_{ab} is the resultant of forces a and b. R_{ab} and c are the two adjacent sides of the parallelogram passing through a given point as shown in Fig. 10.32B, then, the resultant is represented by diagonal passing through the same point, i.e. V_{abc}.

H_c is the horizontal component of force c. H_{ab} the horizontal component of force a & b and H_c should be equal for achieving equilibrium that is why R_{abc} and V_{abc} are equal.

B. *During chewing*, when mandible moves from centric occlusion to lateral position, the resultant of forces acting is not vertical but incline laterally (Fig. 10.32C).

During this movement, forces A and B are increased and C is decreased with resultant changes in horizontal and vertical components.

Here we observe that H_{ab} is greater than H_c and the net resultant is H_{abc}. So the net horizontal component is along the direction of a and b. By using triangle of vector addition, the resultant is represented by R_{abc}. The resultant R_{abc} is a thrust inclined buccally on the maxillary teeth and lingually on the mandibular teeth, whose horizontal component is H_{abc}.

C. *During chewing*, when mandible moves from lateral to centric occlusion, the resultant of forces acting is not vertical but inclined medially (Fig. 10.32D).

When tough food is compressed or all cusps are in intimate contact at the three points, the forces a and b are decreased and c is increased with resultant changes in horizontal and vertical components. Since during chewing H_c is greater than H_{ab} and the net resultant is H_{abc}. So the net horizontal component is along the direction of c. By using triangle of vector addition, the resultant is represented by R_{abc} (Figs 10.32D).

The resultant R_{abc} is a thrust inclined palatally on the maxillary teeth and buccally on the mandibular teeth, whose horizontal component is H_{abc}.

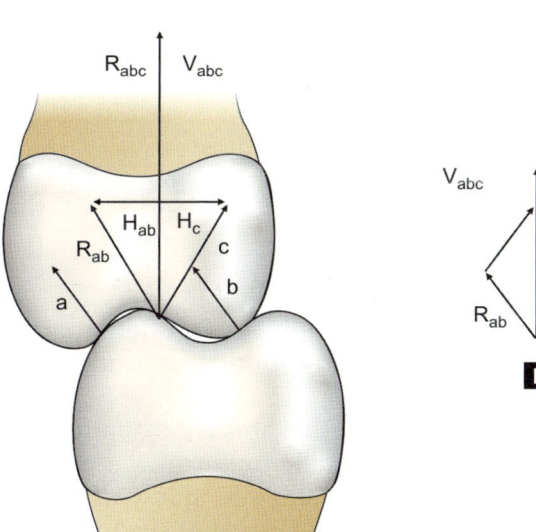
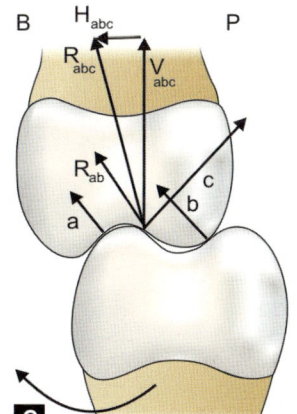
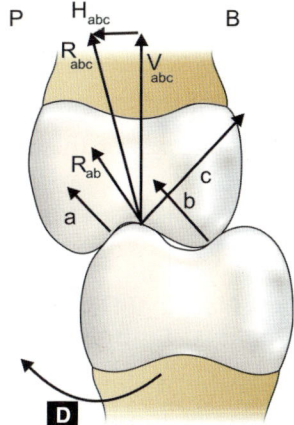

Figs 10.32A to D: **(A)** Forces acting on tooth during centric occlusion; **(B)** R_{ab} and c are the two adjacent sides of the parallelogram; **(C)** Forces acting on tooth during chewing (movement - centric occlusion to lateral); **(D)** Forces acting on tooth during chewing (movement - lateral to centric occlusion)

Mechanical Functions of the Marginal Ridges

1. Normal Marginal Ridge

Forces 1 and 2 act on marginal ridges of teeth A and B respectively. The horizontal component of 1, H_1 and the horizontal component of 2, H_2 counteract each other. The vertical component V_1 and V_2 are resolved normally by the underlying tissues (Fig. 10.33).

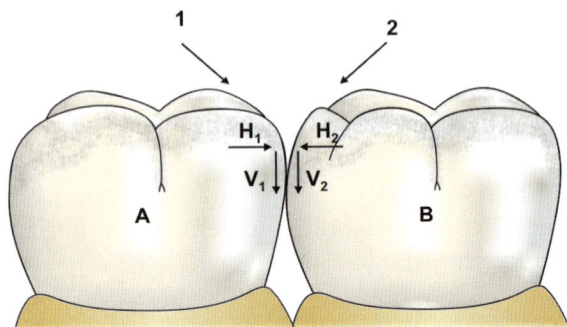

Fig. 10.33: Normal marginal ridge

2. No Marginal Ridge

In Fig. 10.34 tooth B has no marginal ridge. Force 1 and 2 are acting on tooth A and B. The horizontal component of 2, H_2 is missing in the tooth B, because force 2 is mainly directly towards tooth A. Horizontal component H_2 will drift the tooth A apart and the vertical component V_1 and V_2 of both the forces 1 and 2 will help the food impact vertically. The vertical force V_2 will be more than required, there may occur slight tilting of the tooth B. This will further deteriorate the resolution of forces and lead to further food impaction (Fig. 10.34).

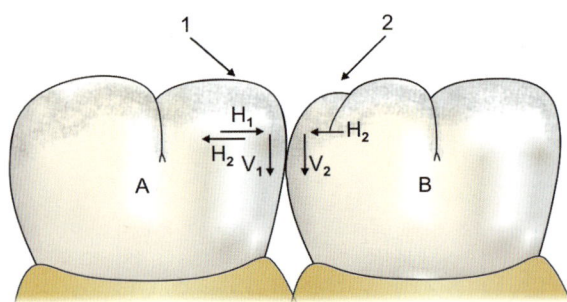

Fig. 10.34: No marginal ridge

3. A Marginal Ridge with a Wider Occlusal Embrasure

In spite of putting optimal pressure on marginal ridges of tooth A and B, the forces 1 and 2 act on adjacent teeth. The force 2 will put pressure on tooth A and force 1 will put pressure on tooth B. This will lead to drifting of both the teeth. The vertical component of forces will wedge the food in between the two teeth (Fig. 10.35).

Similar effect is seen when one marginal ridge is higher than other.

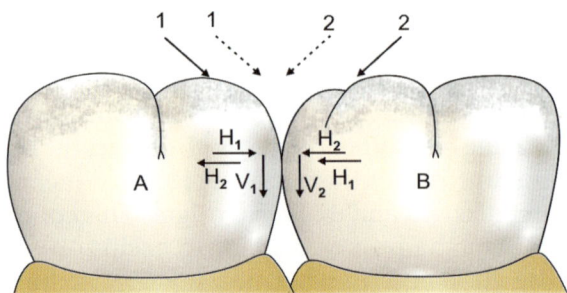

Fig. 10.35: Wide occlusal ebmrasure

4. No Occlusal Embrasure

In totality, the vertical component of forces 1 and 2 will be more concentrated than horizontal components. Though there will not be any vertical impaction of food, the continuous impact of higher concentration of vertical component of forces may lead to changes in alveolar bone after sometime (Fig. 10.36).

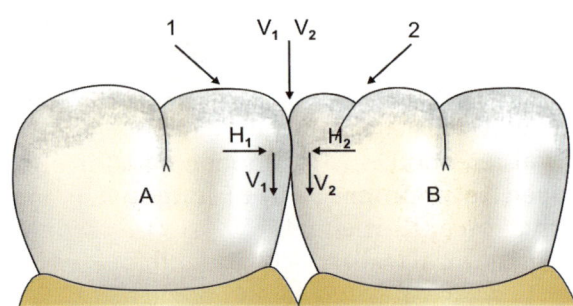

Fig. 10.36: No occlusal embrasure

Vertical Loads and Distribution of Sresses

As the load is applied over the teeth, stresses are distributed both:
i. Parallel to the long axis and
ii. Perpendicular to the long axis.

The force or the load is applied at different areas at a time and the stress distribution depends upon various factors.
- If the cross-section of that area is constant, stress distribution is practically uniform.
- If there is variation in cross-section (such areas are normally termed as prisms), stress varies from point to point, being inversely proportional to area.
- If change of cross-section area is abrupt, greater concentration of stress occurs at that point.

Principles of Cavity Preparation

In vertical loading, there will be shearing stresses in prism in any plane. This shearing stress increases to a maximum at 45° and then decreases to zero at 90°. Therefore, materials that are weaker in shear than in compression or tension rupture in planes at 45° to the axis.

The modulus of elasticity of the material is an important property and should be taken care of. If a cavity is restored with gold inlay or porcelain, the modulus of elasticity varies between the tooth and the restorative material. With the vertical force exerting on both, the compression will be the same for the restoration and the tooth, but since gold/porcelain is much stiffer, they will be highly stressed. Since $S = \delta E$

S (stress) = δ (unit strain) × E (modulus of elasticity)

When the force is applied perpendicular to the prism axis, the resultant resolution is known as beam. Beam can be supported from both the ends (simple beam) and may be supported from one end (Cantilever beam). The MOD preparations are the examples of simple beams whereas MO/DO preparations are the examples of cantilever beam. The retention of the restoration depends upon these beams, although the strength and the deflection of the material also play part.

Moment of force = Force × perpendicular distance

The bending moment is at the axiopulpal line angle, which tends to rotate the restoration out of the cavity. Gingival retention with a moment equal to $F \times L$ is required to counteract this moment. The total retentive force (R) is equal to $F \times L/l$ where l is the depth of the axial wall. If we take depth of the gingival wall (d) into account, then R and d will be in the same direction, so their moment of force is zero. Therefore, the depth of the gingival wall does not take part in retention (Fig. 10.37).

In MOD preparation, the force (F) is divided equally on both the sides. The mesio-distal distance (L) is also divided into two. The moment of force at the midpoint is:

$F/2 \times L/2 = FL/4$

If this moment of force is divided into two (because it is actually acting on both the ends) than the moment of force is FL/8.

Since the beam forms a concave downward curvature between the load and the fixed end, therefore, by sign convention, this end moment is taken as negative.

By equation $R \times l = FL/8$

So $R = FL/8l$

The negative sign is used only in vector form and in magnitude only positive sign is used.

Similarly, as in MO/DO preparation if we take depth of gingival wall (d) into account, then R and d will be in the same direction, so their moment of force remains zero (Fig. 10.38).

It is presumed in MOD preparations that the length of the axial wall (l) is kept equal on both the ends. If there is marked discrepancy between the two ends, the end result may not be the same as is described earlier. Therefore, preferably the length of the two axial walls should be the same.

In cervical/gingival restorations, it has been established that certain forces act on the cervical region, which could destabilize the restoration and even lead to cracks at the cemento-enamel junction.

In functional occlusion, the lingual slopes of buccal and palatal cusps of the maxillary teeth contact the buccal slopes of the buccal and lingual cusps of the mandibular teeth. The forces acting on inclined planes of the occluding cusps consequently lead to transverse stresses. These transverse stresses try to bend the tooth gingivo-occlusally. Since the teeth are firmly held in alveolar socket, these rotations are minimum and counteracted.

In cases where a cavity is cut on the cervical surfaces, depending upon the height of the axial wall, the deflective force is increased. If the restorative materials are not adhesive in nature, a gap can be created at the cervical surface of the restoration on buccal side and occlusal surface on the lingual side.

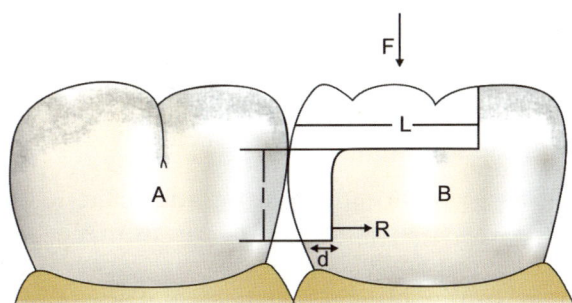

Fig. 10.37: Moment of force in MO/DO preparations

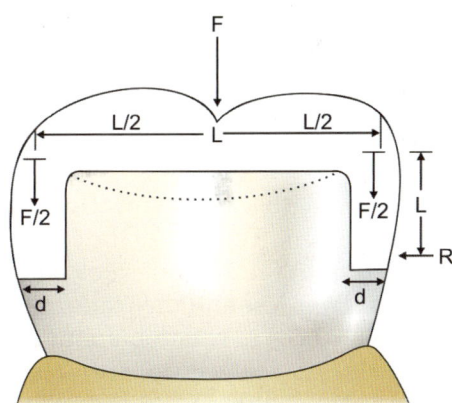

Fig. 10.38: Moment of force in MOD preparation

In Fig. 10.39, buccal cusp of mandibular tooth and palatal cusp of maxillary tooth are in contact. Force (F) is applied at incline plane perpendicular to the tangent of the planes. The horizontal component (H) acts approximately at the centre of the tooth. The vertical component (V) is constant. The deflection is mainly by the horizontal component which depends upon the height of the axial wall (L) and the depth of the occlusal (d_1) and cervical walls (d_2).

Since bending moments depend upon modulus of elasticity, a young tooth may deflect more because of its less modulus of elasticity.

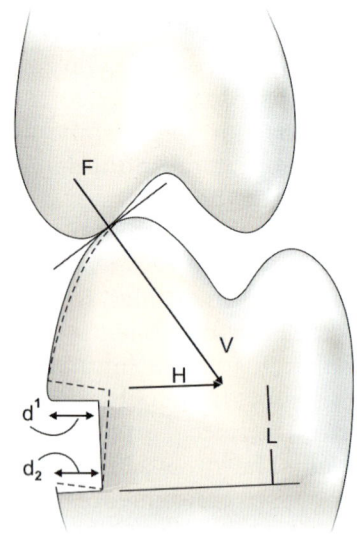

Fig. 10.39: Moment of force in cervical cavities

Application of Stresses and their Distribution in Individual Restorations

Class I Restoration

Class I lesion can be restored with different materials. For restoration with Amalgam, it is recommended to converge the side walls occlusally and to keep the floor flat. In case the floor is not kept flat, the forces will rotate the restoration on both the sides. And also, since the remaining dentin will be less at the center and if the restoration is deep, the forces might fracture the tooth.

The problems with cast restorations are much severe. The movement/rotation of the cast restoration is easy, if the pulpal floor is not kept flat. Since the depth of the cavity is less and the walls are diverging occlusally, the chances of rotation are much more.

Such rotational forces, to some extent are counteracted by adhesive materials such as composites and glass-ionomers.

Class II Restoration

In class II restorations, the stresses, which tend to rotate the restoration (bending stress), mostly act on marginal ridges.

Since the bending stress acting at the axiopulpal line angle increases rapidly as its radius of curvature decreases, the axiopulpal line angle should be well rounded, to increase the strength of the material by increasing the bulk at this point. If the modulus of elasticity of the material differs with that of tooth, the stresses act as on a beam (described earlier). In such cases gingival lock is required to counter the rotation of the restoration.

In MOD restorations, centers of rotation are at the intersection of the neutral planes and not at the axiopulpal line angle. The bending of the occlusal portion is caused as in the other case, by the difference between the total masticatory force and the support given by the pulpal floor of the cavity. Gingival retention and roundening of the axiopulpal line angles are required as in MO or DO cavity.

In cases where the opposing cusps occlude in such a way that one contact point is on a proximocclusal restoration while the other is on tooth structure, there is a tendency to wedge the two apart. To prevent this wedging the occlusal lock is used even though occlusal surface is not involved by caries.

Class III and Class IV Restorations

Since these lesions are not in direct contact with opposing teeth, only transverse stresses play part in dislodging/rotating the restoration.

In such restorations, there is tendency to rotate about an axis approximately parallel to the long axis of the tooth. As incisal retention cannot be made due to thin labiolingual size, so lingual lock is placed on lingual surface. It should be as close to the incisal edge as possible and still be in dentin to reduce the stress in this lingual lock.

In maxillary teeth, force of mastication has labial component, which provides the seating effect on the restoration. In case the labial enamel is not intact, the chances of dislodgement of the restoration will increase. In mandibular teeth, the component of the masticatory force is from the labial to the lingual so chances of dislodgement of restoration are more.

Class V Restoration

The Class V restoration is not subjected to direct occlusal stresses so thought to be free from mechanical problems. But analysis indicates that physical forces putting on occlusal surfaces could result in displacement of the restoration.

It is established that the buccal cusps of mandibular teeth and the palatal cusps of maxillary teeth contact each other during occlusion. The vertical stresses on the teeth lead to transverse stresses and this component of stresses tends to rotate the cervical restoration. The stresses increase with the cusp slopes of the maxillary teeth and the lingual inclines of the mandibular teeth. The mandibular teeth bend more than maxillary teeth. A gap is evident on the cervical/occlusal wall of the cavity and if the depth of these walls is less, the restoration may come out.

BIBLIOGRAPHY

1. Boston D.W.: New device for selective dentin caries removal. Quint. Int.: 34, 678, 2003.
2. De Boever J.A., McCall W.D., Holden S. and Ash M.M.: Functional occlusal forces, an investigation by telemetry. J.P.D.: 40, 326, 1978.
3. Elderton R.J., Jenkins C.B., Marshall K.J., Hooper S.M., Foster L.V., Hooper G.R., Roberts K.: Changing perceptions of the requirements of cavity preparations. B.D.J. 6, 30, 1990.
4. Hess J.C.: Revision of the principles of cavity preparations. Dent. Cosmos 42, 1835, 1974.
5. Hood J.A.A.: Biomechanics of the intact prepared and restored tooth: Some clinical implications. Int. Dent. J.: 41, 25, 1991.
6. Hood J.A.A.: Stress/displacement analysis of a class V restoration in a premolar. J. Dent. Res.: 58, 1210, 1979.
7. Hunt P.R.: Rational cavity design principles. J. Esthet. Dent. 6, 245, 1994.
8. Jokstad A., Mjor, I.A.: Cavity designs for class II amalgam restorations-A literature review and a suggested system for evaluation. Acta. Odontol. Scand. 45, 257, 1987.
9. Kidd E.F.: How 'clean' must a cavity be before restoration? Caries Res.: 38, 305, 2004.
10. Krejc I., Dietschi, D., Lutz, F.U.: Principles of proximal cavity preparation and finishing with ultrasonic diamond tips. Pract. Perioesth. Dent. 10, 295, 1998.
11. Lenon A.M.: Fluorescence aided caries excavation (FACE) compared to conventional method. Oper. Dent.: 28, 341, 2003.
12. Love R.M.: Clinical management of infected root canal dentin. Pract. Perioesth. Dent. 8, 581, 1996.
13. Marinello C., Soom, U. and Schaerer, P.: Tooth preparation in adhesive dentistry. Dent. Today: 10, 46, 1991.
14. Osborne J.W. and Summit, J.B.: Extension for prevention. Is it relevant today? Am. J. Dent. 11, 189, 1998.
15. Pissis P.: The indirect inlay procedure-accuracy and aesthetics: A review of principles. Pract. Perio. Asthe. Dent. 7, 65, 1995.
16. Piva E., Martos J and Dermarco F.F.: Microleakage in amalgam restorations: Influence of cavity cleansers solutions and anticariogenic agents. Oper. Dent. 26, 383, 2001.
17. Re G.J., Pruitt D., Childers J.M., Norling B.K.: Effect of mandibular molar anatomy on the buccal class I cavity preparation. J. Dent. Res. 62, 997, 1983.
18. Rosenstied, E.: The retention of inlay and crowns as a function of Geometrical form. Br. Dent. J.: 388, Dec. 3, 1957.
19. Silva N.R.F.A. Carvalho, R.M. Pegoraro L.F., Tay F.R. and Thompson V.P.: Evaluation of a self-limiting concept in dentinal caries removal. J. Dent. Res.: 85, 282, 2006.
20. Sturdevant J.R., Bader J.D., Shugars D.A. and Steet T.C.: A simple method to estimate restoration volume as a possible predictor for tooth fracture. J.P.D.: 90, 162, 2003.
21. Terklla L.G., Mahler D.B., Eysden J.V.: Analysis of amalgam cavity design. J.P.D. 29, 204, 1973.
22. Woolsey G.D. Matich. J.A.: The effect of grooves on the resistance form of cast restoration. J.A.D.A., 97, 978.1978.
23. Yaman S.D. Yetmez, M. Turkoz, E. and Akkas, W.: Fracture resistance of class II approximal slot restorations. J.P.D.: 84, 297, 2000.
24. Yip H.K. Samaranayake L.P.: Caries removal techniques and instrumentation: A review. Clin. Oral. Investig. 2, 148, 1998.

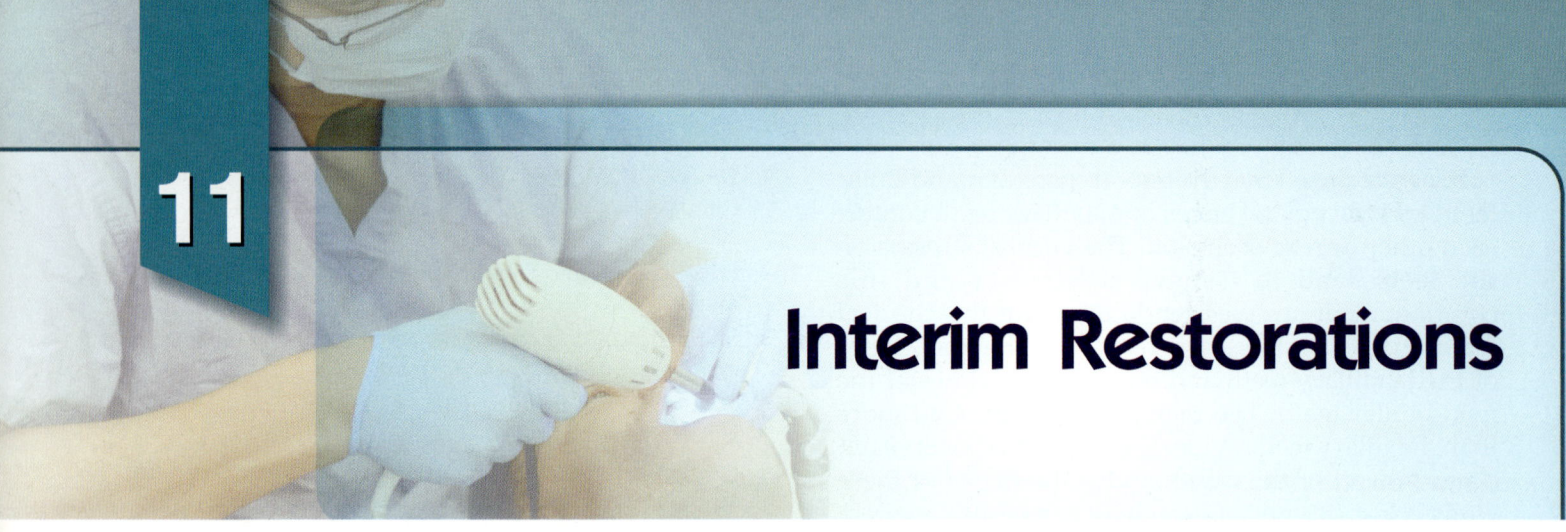

11. Interim Restorations

When confronted with extensive, complex treatment plans, judicious sequencing is vital to both dentist and the patient. The interim restorations or the intermediate restorative materials enhance patient motivation, which lead to successful completion of the chosen treatment plan.

Interim restorative materials are temporary or semi-permanent materials, which are used until a permanent restoration is inserted. The selection of these materials depend on the size of the cavity, its form, the period for which the restoration is required to remain in place and the eventual restoration which is planned to replace it. For small cavity preparations, the temporary material may be introduced without application of the matrix, whereas in large preparations, a matrix is adapted and then the material is inserted. Gross excess is removed before the material has completely hardened. The matrix is removed and the carving is finally completed.

RATIONALE

I. In routine, the operative treatment may not be completed in one visit. In such cases, it is necessary to fill the prepared cavity with an intermediate restorative material during the inter appointment phase. Intermediate restorations allow temporary functioning of the tooth, maintain intra arch relationships, prevent supraeruption and also provide esthetics. Additionally, it allows the pulp dentin organ and periodontium to recover before placement of permanent restoration.

II. In subjects where multiple teeth are affected by acute caries, the infected tooth structure is removed and the defects restored with a temporary material. With this technique most of the infecting organisms are removed and further spread of caries is arrested. Further, the interval between initial treatment and the permanent restoration provides time to assess the patients' compliance with oral hygiene instructions and the progress/arrest of caries activity.

III. Intermediate restorative materials are helpful in teeth with questionable pulpal prognosis. They limit the progress of demineralization in dentin and allow the underlying pulp to heal. These are also used in direct and indirect pulp capping procedures. This allows time for the underlying periodontal organ to heal as well as form a reparative dentin barrier.

The *requisites* of an ideal material for interim restoration are:

- Easy and rapid mixing
- Easy to place in cavity and shape with hand instruments
- Rapid set to ensure stability
- Good strength, especially when used in larger cavities and for full crowns
- High abrasion resistance and low oral solubility
- Dimensional stability (coefficient of thermal expansion should match that of tooth)
- Good marginal sealing
- Easy to remove to facilitate placement of permanent restorations
- Non-irritant to pulp and other oral soft tissues
- Tasteless and odourless
- Acceptable color for use in anterior teeth
- Cheap and readily available

Various interim restorative materials are:

A. *For intracoronal preparation*
   I. Gutta percha
   II. Dental cements
   - a. Zinc-oxide eugenol cement
   - b. Modified zinc-oxide eugenol cement
   - c. Cavit
   - d. Zinc phosphate cement
   - e. Modified zinc phosphate cement
   - f. Zinc silicophosphate cement
   - g. Polycarboxylate cement
   - h. Calcium hydroxide

B. *For extracoronal preparation*
  I. Prefabricated crowns
     a. Celluloid crowns
     b. Polycarbonate crowns
     c. Stainless steel crowns
     d. Aluminium crowns
  II. Indirect acrylic restorations

FOR INTRACORONAL PREPARATION

Gutta-Percha

It is a pure solidified juice obtained by tapping Isonandra Gutta, an evergreen tree of the order Sapotaceae found principally in the Malay Peninsula and Archipelago. Chemically, it consists of a hydrocarbon (pure gutta) $C_{10}H_{16}$, albane ($C_{40}H_{64}O_3$) and guttane, thereby resembling rubber in origin and composition.

For practical purposes, gutta-percha is not used in its pure state but other ingredients are often added such as burgundy pitch, white wax, zinc oxide, calcium oxide, magnesium oxide, carbon, pieselgutta, etc to give it the desirable working qualities (Fig. 11.1). It was introduced in dentistry by Hill (1847), and was famous as Hill's stopping.

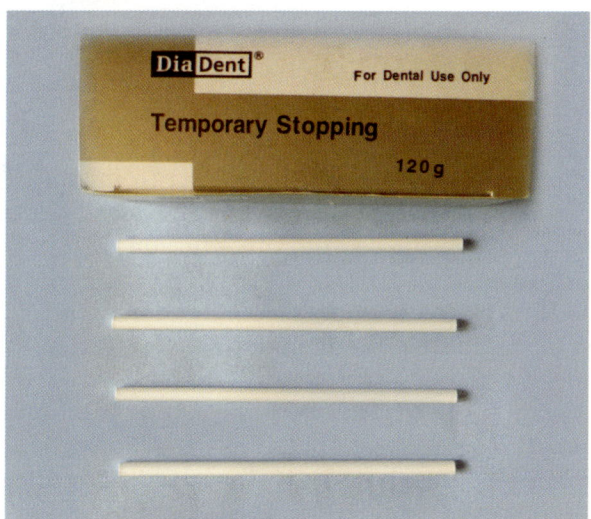

Fig. 11.1: Gutta-percha sticks

Gutta-percha for dental use is supplied in three forms:
- Low heat (softens below 200°F)
- Medium heat (softens within the range of 200°F-210°F)
- High heat (softens within the range of 230°F-240°F)

Manipulation

Before insertion into the cavity preparation, the walls may be slightly moistened with solvents so as to soften

Physical properties
• Pure gutta-percha is almost colorless with a slight pinkish or grayish hue. • It is odourless. • It is slightly elastic and contracts on cooling. • Non-irritating to the soft tissues. • Softens on heating and hardens again on cooling. • Readily soluble in chloroform and partially soluble in eucalyptus oil. • Specific gravity is 0.96-1.0. • Low crushing strength and abrasion resistance. • Ease of insertion and removal when desired.

Disadvantages for use as a restorative material are
• Strength and abrasion resistance are poor. • Excessive shrinkage on cooling with consequent tendency to draw away from the cavity walls during hardening. • When exposed to air, Gutta-percha deteriorates to a hard brittle material because of oxidation. • Becomes porous and disintegrates after some time. • Very high coefficient of thermal expansion (198×10^{-6} °C.) • Higher plastic flow.

gutta-percha minimally and increase its adhesiveness. The material is carefully softened over an alcohol lamp or Bunsen burner. Avoid overheating as it could burn leading to oxidation of its components and hindering its properties. It is then inserted in cavity in pieces or in bulk. It is thoroughly condensed with wet smooth burnisher of suitable size. Remove excess material immediately with a hot, flat spatula or burnisher, trimming towards the margins. Smoothen the surface with slightly warm instrument. Ask the patient to bite and check for occlusion.

Dental Cements

Cements are the most widely used materials for temporary restorative purposes. These consist of a powder and a liquid which when mixed produce a plastic mass, which is inserted into the cavity and allowed to set. The uses of dental cements is given in Table 11.1.

Zinc Oxide Eugenol Cement (ZOE)

Zinc oxide eugenol (ZOE) is the most widely used temporary restorative material. It seems to have been developed from zinc oxychloride cements, which consisted of a powder: 75% zinc oxide and 25% pulverized glass or silica and a liquid: zinc chloride

Table 11.1: Cements employed for intermediary restorations

Cement	Primary use	Secondary use	Pulp response	Anticariogenic potential
Zinc oxide eugenol	Temporary and intermediate restoration Luting agent Thermal insulating base Pulp capping agent	Root canal restoration Periodontal bandage	Mild	
Zinc phosphate	Luting agent for restoration and orthodontic bands	Intermediate restoration Thermal insulating base Root canal restoration	Moderate	
Polycarboxylate	Luting agent Thermal insulating base	Luting agent for orthodontic bands Intermediate restoration	Mild	Yes
Zinc silicophosphate	Luting agent for restorations	Intermediate restoration Luting agent for orthodontic bands	Moderate	Yes
Calcium hydroxide	Thermal base Pulp capping agent	Temporary restorations	Soothing	

and a little borax. They were slow setting, and a notable shrinkage was generally observed. These cements found only limited application, as they disintegrated readily and the products of disintegration were found to be corrosive and irritant to pulp tissue. Earlier workers used to mix zinc oxide powder with creosote and oil of cloves. Later the liquid was replaced with eugenol (Fig. 11.2).

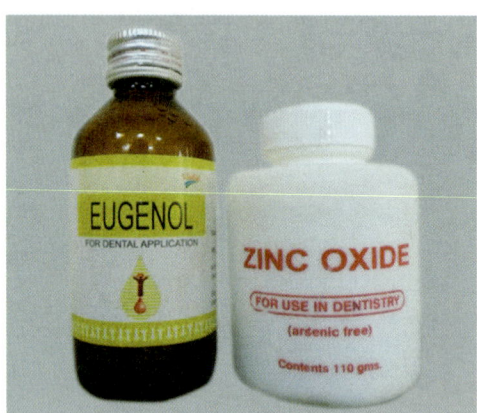

Fig. 11.2: Zinc oxide eugenol

Zinc oxide eugenol offers much better biocompatibility than rest of the dental cements. It is a good insulator and sealer of pulp dentin organ. Additionally, it has an antiseptic effect on microorganisms remaining in dentin, and also has a sedative and anti-inflammatory action on pulp dentin organ. When inserted into the cavity, it has an approximately neutral pH of 7.0. Unfortunately, its strength is not sufficient enough to resist forces of mastication, lacks resistance to wear and has a relatively high solubility in the oral cavity.

Basically there are two types of zinc-oxide eugenol cements available

Type I: ZOE cements used as a base or temporary restoration.

Type II: ZOE cements used as a cavity liner and cementation of appliances.

Zinc oxide eugenol cements differ from zinc oxide eugenol impression pastes in that the latter contains plasticizer like linseed oil, olive oil, mineral oil, etc. which increases its flow.

Early zinc oxide eugenol cement contained, 100% zinc oxide and 100% eugenol. It was easy to mix and place but was hydrolytically unstable and lacked adequate strength. Moreover the setting reaction was quite slow which usually led to distortion. The slow set offered an advantage since large quantity of material could be mixed at the beginning of the day and stored. The physical properties of the cement are given in Table 11.2.

Modified Zinc Oxide Eugenol Cement

To improve upon the working, handling and setting characteristics, various modifications were tried and are still being tried. Improved properties have been achieved by two approaches:

- Partial substitution of eugenol by o-ethoxybenzoic acid (EBA)
- Addition of fused quartz or aluminium oxide or resin polymer to the powder component

Table 11.2: Physical properties of cements used for interim restoration

Cement	Composition Powder	Composition Liquid	P:L ratio	Compressive strength psi (MPa)	Tensile strength psi (MPa)	Solubility (in H₂O) % wt	Film thickness (μm)	Modulus of elasticity (psi)	Setting time (mts)	pH at 24 hrs.	Coeff. of thermal expansion (°C/cm)	Coeff. of thermal conductivity
Zinc oxide eugenol	Zinc oxide 70% Rosin 30% Zinc acetate traces	Eugenol 100%	3:1	800-4000 (6-28)	300 (2.1)	0.04	25	0.03	24 hrs.	7.0	3.98×10^{-4}	35×10^{-5}/°C
EBA-alumina reinforced ZnOE	Zinc oxide 70% Alumina 30%	Ethoxybenzoic acid 62.5% Eugenol 37.5%	4:1	8700-11600 (60-80)	800 (5.8)	0.05	25	0.79	7-9	6.7	—	66×10^{-5}/°C
Polymer reinforced ZnOE	Zinc oxide 80% Polymethyl 20% methacrylate	Eugenol 85% Olive oil 15%	4:1	5400-5800 (37-40) (4.1)	600	0.08	32	0.39	6-9	6.8	—	60×10^{-5}/°C
Zinc phosphate	Zinc oxide 90.2% Magnesium oxide 8.2%, Silica dioxide 1.4%, Bismuth dioxide 0.1%, Misc. 0.1%	Phosphate 54.4% Silica acid Water 36% Others 0.6%	2.5:1 for filling 1.5:1 luting	15000 (104)	800 (5.5)	0.1-0.3	Type I-25 Type II-40	1.96	4-7	Initially 3.5, after 24 hours = 5.5	Dry: 3.11×10^{-4} Wet: 3.88×10^{-4}	—
Polycarboxylate	Zinc oxide 90% Magnesium oxide 10%, Stannous fluoride (traces) or Alumina 30% replaces zinc oxide	40% polyacrylic acid Itaconic acid water	2:1 for filling and 1:1 for luting	8300-14000 (57-99)	900 (6.2)	0.1-0.25	25	0.74	7-9	Initially 1.5, soon = 5.5	—	—
Zinc silico-phosphate	Silica 35% Alumina 25% Zinc oxide 10-20% Fluoride 17% Calcium oxide 1-50%	Phosphoric acid 48% Water 35% Buffers 17%	2.5:1 for filling and 1.5:1 for luting	21000 (145)	1100 (7.6)	0.4	30	—	3.5-4	Initially 1.5 at 24 hours = 5.0	4.38×10^{-4}	—
Resin	Resin matrix, inorganic fillers, organo silanes, photo or chemical initiators and activators	Methyl methacrylate, tertiary amine		10000-25000 (70-172)	—	0-0.01	10-25	0.31-0.46	2-4	—	3.25×10^{-4}	—
Calcium hydroxide				10-27	—	0.4-7.8	—	0.37	2.5-5.5	10-12.3	—	—

I. Resin Reinforced Zinc Oxide Eugenol Cements

The conventional zinc oxide eugenol cements have been modified by the addition of polymeric substances like polymethyl methacrylate to the powder component. The degree of reinforcement appears to be dependent to a great extent upon the particle size and on uniformity of distribution of the resinous and inorganic phases of the powder components.

20% polymethyl methacrylate is usually added to zinc oxide as powder and is mixed with eugenol along with accelerators like zinc acetate and zinc stearate (Fig. 11.3). Thymol or hydroxyquinoline as antimicrobial agents are added in traces.

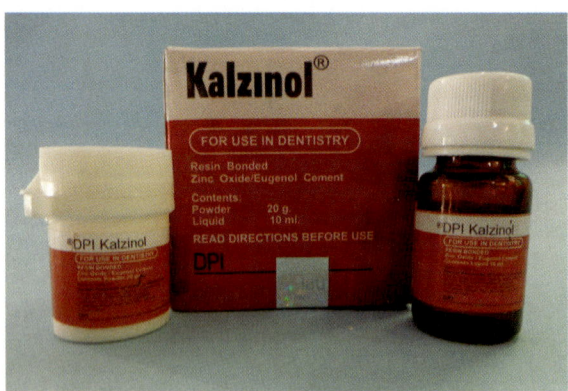

Fig. 11.3: Resin modified zinc oxide eugenol

The constituents of powder and liquid are as follows:

Powder	Weight %
Zinc oxide	80.0%
Polymethyl-methacrylate	20.0%
Zinc stearate	Traces
Zinc acetate	Traces
Thymol	Traces
Liquid	
Eugenol	85%
Olive oil	15%

Resin improves the strength, homogeneity and smoothness of the mix, decreases flow, brittleness and solubility. Resin may physically bond to the other components or react chemically with the eugenol. Zinc stearate acts as a plasticizer and zinc acetate improves the strength of the cement. Zinc stearate and zinc acetate also act as accelerators. Olive oil acts as a plasticizer and masks the irritating effects of eugenol.

II. EBA (Ortho Ethoxy Benzoic Acid) Modified Cement

Ortho Ethoxy benzoic acid as chelate was tried to improve upon the physical properties of zinc oxide eugenol. EBA chelates with zinc probably by forming an ionic complex with divalent metal ions such as Zn^{++} and forms 'zinc benzoate'.

By adding certain fillers and resins, the solubility and disintegration of the cement can be reduced to 1.2%. Fillers viz. quartz, fused quartz, alumina, dicalcium phosphate, lead oxide and mercuric oxide, etc. substantially improve the mechanical properties of the material. Lead oxide and mercuric oxide were found to be toxic, so were discarded soon. The composition is:

Powder: 70% Zinc Oxide and 30% alumina or 70% Zinc Oxide and 30% fused quartz and calcium phosphate

Liquid: EBA-62.5%, Eugenol-37.5%.

Addition of EBA to eugenol and its reaction with zinc oxide resulted in the following properties:
- Increases the amount of powder that can be incorporated to liquid to obtain a mixture of standard consistency.
- Increases compressive, tensile and shear strength. It closely resembles that of zinc phosphate.
- Decreases the setting time only if the EBA concentration is less than 70%. More than 70% EBA increases the setting time sharply.
- The density increases from 2.68 gms/ml for conventional zinc oxide eugenol to 3.31 gms/ml for EBA cement.
- Increases solubility and disintegration characteristics of the products from 0.04% for zinc oxide eugenol to 0.05% for EBA cement.
- The linear coefficient of thermal expansion increased to $60 \times 10^{-6}/°C$ compared to $35 \times 10^{-6}/°C$ for zinc oxide eugenol.
- Addition of EBA does not have any adverse effect on pulp.

In an attempt to reduce solubility, MBA (5-methoxy Benzoic acid) – a more hydrophobic homologue of EBA, was tried. However, it didn't prove favourable and the solubility further increased.

Brauer et al (1983)[7] tried a new modification in which vanillate esters were added in the liquid. The powder consisted of 64% zinc oxide, 30% Al_2O_3 and 6% hydrogenated resin. The liquid contained EBA 87.5% and Hexyl vanillate 12.5% and no eugenol. The new cements exhibited high strengths, low solubility and low disintegration values. Further it eliminated the irritating effects of eugenol and also did not inhibit free radical polymerization of composite and acrylic resins. Additionally they also adhered to non-precious alloys, plastics and composites.

Some zinc oxide cements contain antibiotics and steroids as anti-inflammatory agents. These are used as pulp capping agents and as sealers in root canal therapy. Barium sulphate may be added for radioopacity.

Setting of Zinc Oxide Eugenol Mixtures

Eugenol is a colorless or pale yellow liquid. Eugenol darkens and thickens on exposure to air because of oxidation. It is slightly soluble in water, ethanol and chloroform. One of the conditions necessary for the reaction of eugenol with zinc oxide, is that the organic reactor has a methoxy group ortho to the hydroxyl group in the benzene ring. Among other organic compounds, which possess such a structural formulation are guicacol and methylguicacol and hence react similarly with zinc oxide.

Anhydrous zinc oxide does not react with eugenol. This infers that water is an essential feature in its setting reaction. Conventional zinc oxide eugenol having 2% water takes 24 hours to set whereas the presence of 5% water in the zinc oxide reduces the setting time to about 15 minutes. Different types of Zinc oxide also influence the rate of reaction. Zinc oxide powders decomposed to zinc hydroxide, zinc carbonate and similar salts at temperatures of approximately 300°C appear to be the most active in their reaction. Thus the rate of reaction between zinc oxide and eugenol is dependent on the nature, source and moisture content of zinc oxide, and to the purity and moisture content of eugenol.

Water is an essential initiator of the setting reaction. Thereafter, the reaction gets autocatalytic, as water is the reaction product itself. Two molecules of eugenol react with one molecule of zinc hydroxide to form a zinc eugenolate chelate, $[(C_{10}H_{11}O_2)_2Zn]$.

$$ZnO + H_2O \longrightarrow Zn(OH)_2$$
$$Zn(OH)_2 + 2E \longrightarrow ZnE_2 + 2H_2O$$
$$\text{(Eugenol)} \quad \text{(Zinc eugenolate)}$$

The rate of setting, is influenced by the following:
- A drop of water sharply accelerates the setting reaction but excessive water tends to decrease the same. Humidity generally fastens the setting.
- Additives such as zinc stearate, zinc acetate, magnesium chloride, primary alcohols and acetic acid act as accelerators. Resin also causes an increase in the rate of setting within limits.
- Within limits, greater the ratio of zinc oxide to eugenol, faster is the setting.
- Smaller the particle size of zinc oxide, shorter is the setting time.
- Higher the temperature, shorter is the setting time.

Manipulation

Zinc oxide eugenol is usually available in the powder and liquid form. Mixing can be carried out with a stainless steel spatula over a clean glass slab. Disposable paper pads can also be used. The required amount of powder and liquid as instructed are dispensed onto the slab. The powder in bulk is incorporated into the liquid and thoroughly spatulated. A series of smaller amounts are added subsequently and spatulated. The correct consistency is achieved when the mix is heavy putty like and can be picked up in the fingers without sticking. The heavy mix of cement is rolled into a rope and kept ready for use.

With the plastic instrument, the cavity is filled and the excess is removed carefully. A large cotton pellet saturated with hot water is patted over the entire surface of the cement. The hot water hastens the set of the cement imparting harder surface.

Physical Properties

The physical properties of commonly available zinc oxide cements are given in Table 11.2.

Biological Effects of Zinc Oxide Eugenol

When zinc oxide eugenol is placed in cavities, it is exposed to aqueous media such as saliva and dentinal fluid. Hydrolysis of zinc eugenolate occurs under the effect of water, yielding eugenol and zinc hydroxide. Eugenol thus liberated can diffuse through dentin into the pulp or directly into the saliva.

The release of eugenol is not markedly affected by the ratio of zinc oxide/eugenol mix but depends on the remaining dentin thickness. Binding of eugenol to calcium, forming chelate as well as to the organic matrix especially collagen, slows down the diffusion rate of eugenol through dentin.

The effect of eugenol on pulp is concentration dependent. When exposed to low concentrations, eugenol is protective to the pulp by inducing a sedative and an anti inflammatory effect. These low concentrations can be obtained by diffusion of eugenol from a zinc oxide eugenol filling through a layer of intact dentin. When exposed to high concentrations, eugenol is highly cytotoxic.

Protective Effects of Zinc Oxide Eugenol

Zinc oxide eugenol has been described as a good cavity sealant, prevents leakage and subsequent growth of bacteria. The material has been shown to exert beneficial effects on pulp. These are as follows:
  i. *Bactericidal effect:* Eugenol is bactericidal at relatively high concentrations of 10^2–10^3 mol/L.

This effect is seen in areas of dentin immediately below the zinc oxide eugenol cement, which has high concentration of eugenol. Bactericidal effect is beneficial but these concentrations are toxic to pulp.

ii. *Sedative effect:* At low concentrations, eugenol acts like a local anaesthetic. It decreases intradentinal fluid activity minimizing the sensitivity to hot, cold or sweet. Eugenol also inhibits neural conduction.

iii. *Anti-inflammatory effect:* Eugenol in low doses causes resolution of mild inflammation. It inhibits neutrophil function and chemotaxis, and removes harmful free radicals like superoxide, which are generated by these cells. Eugenol is a potent inhibitor of prostaglandin H-Synthetase, an enzyme essential in the arachidonic acid cycle. As a result both prostaglandins and leukotrienes are inhibited from formation, which are potent mediators of inflammation. In cases of severe inflammation, zinc oxide eugenol is virtually of no use.

Toxic Effects of Zinc Oxide Eugenol

Eugenol is cytotoxic at high concentrations. The toxic effects are as follows:

- It kills bacteria at 10^{-2} to 10^{-3} mol/L concentration. Lower concentrations can inhibit cell respiration and cell division. This may be because of high affinity of eugenol to plasma membranes.
- It irreversibly blocks the conduction of action potentials in the nerve, i.e. neurotoxic effect.
- It stimulates the release of superoxide from neutrophils, causing increased tissue damage.

Cavit

It is a premixed non-eugenol paste used for temporary restorations and cavity bases (Fig. 11.4). It contains zinc oxide, zinc sulphate, calcium sulphate, glycol acetate, polyvinyl acetate, polyvinyl chloride acetate, triethanolamine and red pigments. The exact percentage composition is not confirmed.

The setting reaction is initiated by saliva; and water. Zinc oxide reacts with calcium sulphate and zinc sulphate leading to a set mass. Both Cavit and zinc oxide eugenol are similar in that they set hygroscopically. Cavit sets with continual penetration of water, whereas zinc oxide eugenol undergoes an autocatalytic reaction, which is initiated by water and in which one of the reaction products is water itself. If the premix is spatulated with a little amount of water, the setting reaction is greatly shortened. Because of water sorption, one of the characteristic features of Cavit is a high linear setting expansion of 14.20% during its setting which is almost double that of zinc oxide eugenol, i.e. 8.40%. These hygroscopic properties of Cavit provide better seating into the cavity walls, which accounts for its effectiveness against interface penetration. A minimum thickness of atleast 3.0-3.5 mm of cavit is required to be more effective.

When inserted into dry cavity preparations, Cavit creates a negative pressure, causing aspiration of odontoblasts leading to pain. However, no aspiration is evident when the cavity is moistened with water or eugenol. Resolution of the aspiration, if any, occurs after ten days, thereafter, secondary dentin formation starts.

Cavit is not a satisfactory material for cementation because of its film thickness (91 μ) and hygroscopic expansion. This causes the restoration to rise producing hyperocclusion. Compressive strength of Cavit is approximately 2000 psi, half that of zinc oxide eugenol. pH of both the materials is almost the same, i.e. 6.9-7.0. Antibacterial properties are probably because of zinc oxide and zinc sulphate.

The non-eugenol zinc oxide cement is available in different varieties (Figs 11.5 and 11.6).

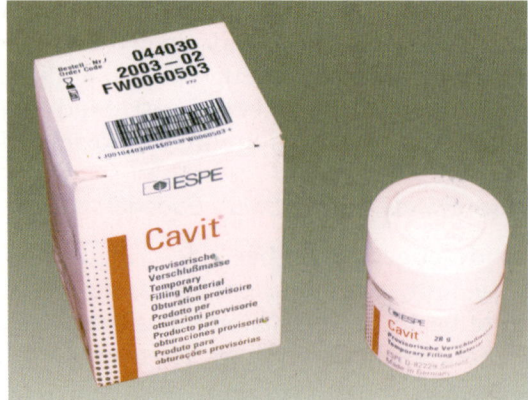

Fig. 11.4: Provisional restorative material (Cavit)

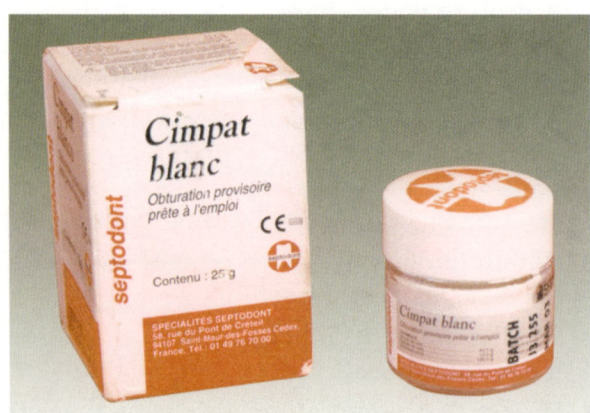

Fig. 11.5: Provisional restorative material (Cimpat blanc)

Interim Restorations

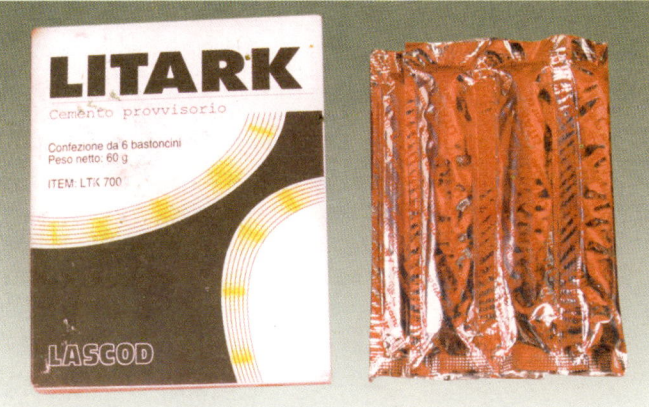

Fig. 11.6: Provisional restorative material (Litark)

Zinc Phosphate Cement

Zinc phosphate cement is one of the widely used materials in dentistry, though its use is declining now because of advent of other modified cements. Introduced by Pierce in 1879, the cement has successfully been used for temporary restorations and as a luting agent (Fig. 11.7). The cement is of two types depending upon the particle size, though the composition of the cements is almost the same.

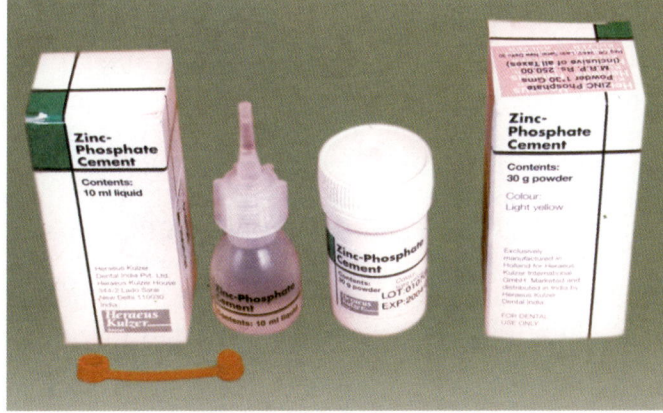

Fig. 11.7: Zinc phosphate cement (powder and liquid)

Type I – cements are fine grained and are capable of forming film of thickness 25 μ or less. They are designed for seating precision appliances.

Type II – cements are medium particle sized and are designed for cementation of appliances other than precision appliances, e.g. orthodontic bands. Also used as intermediate restorations and thermal insulating bases. The film thickness for Type II cements, is 40 μ.

Composition

The composition of routinely used zinc phosphate cement is as follows:

Powder	Weight %
Zinc oxide	90.2%
Magnesium oxide	8.2%
Silicone dioxide	1.4%
Bismuth trioxide	0.1%
Barium oxide	Traces
Barium sulphate	Traces
Calcium oxide	Traces
Liquid	
Phosphoric acid (free acid)	38.2%
Phosphoric acid (combined with Aluminium and Zinc)	16.2%
Aluminium	2.5%
Zinc	7.1%
Water	36.0%

Zinc oxide is the principal ingredient of the zinc phosphate cement powder. Other ingredients are added to control the working characteristics and the final properties of the mixed cement.

Magnesium oxide – reduces the temperature of the calcination process.

Silicone dioxide – acts as a filler and aids in calcination process.

Bismuth trioxide – imparts smoothness to the freshly mixed cement mass but in large amounts may also lengthen the setting time.

Zinc phosphate cement may be prepared in a variety of colors depending upon the calcination process. Commonly, pigmenting substances such as copper oxide, bismuth oxide and magnesium oxide in the concentrations of 1/2000-1/5000 are added to the powder.

The liquid contains water content of $33 \pm 5\%$ (average 36%). The water controls the ionization of the acid, which in turn influences the reaction process of the liquid and powder. A pure phosphoric acid solution containing free phosphoric acid is generally very reactive. Zinc and aluminium buffers are added to reduce its reactivity. Alternatively, the amount of free phosphoric acid is decreased, the process is known as dilution.

Zinc phosphate cement liquid is adjusted by either partial neutralization or dilution. Therefore, the liquid from one manufacturer should not be used with the powder of another manufacturer.

Setting Reaction

When the powder is brought into contact with the liquid, wetting occurs, and a reaction is initiated. The surface of the alkaline powder is attacked by the acid liquid, resulting in an exothermic reaction. The nature of the setting reaction and its products is not very clear.

The set cement is a hydrated amorphous network of zinc phosphate that surrounds unreacted particles of zinc oxide of about 2–8 μ. This hydrated network on drying produces extremely porous cement. The porosity is because of the excess water present in the cement which evaporates. When a higher liquid:powder ratio is used, the number of pores in the set cement increases.

Setting Time

The setting time is 4-7 minutes. At 37°C, the first 60-90 secs. is consumed in the mixing of powder and liquid. Several factors influence the rate of setting of zinc phosphate cement. These are as follows:

Under the Control of the Manufacturer

- The composition and the sintering temperature of the powder.
- The composition of the liquid, i.e. the water content and amount of buffering salts present.
- The particle size of the powder: smaller the particle size, greater the surface area in contact with the liquid and hence rapid is the reaction.

Under the Control of the Operator

- *Powder/liquid ratio:* Working and setting times can be increased, by decreasing the powder/liquid ratio. The procedure is however not acceptable as with a reduction in powder/liquid ratio, there also occurs a decrease in strength and pH of the cement.
- *Rate of powder incorporation:* If all the powder is added at one time, the reaction is very rapid. Introduction of a small quantity of powder into the liquid increases the setting time by reducing the amount of heat generated especially for first few increments.
- *Mixing temperature:* This is the most effective method of controlling setting time. Decreasing the temperature by cooling the glass slab increases the setting time.
- *Spatulation time:* Prolonging the spatulation time destroys the forming matrix. Fragmentation of the matrix needs extra time to rebuild the bulk of matrix.
- *Water contamination or loss of water:* The addition of water decreases setting time and loss of water increases setting time.

Manipulation

To obtain the desired working characteristics and properties of the cement mass, a proper amount of powder should be incorporated into the liquid. Certain precautions should be taken to achieve the desired results.

Mixing Slab

Since combination of powder and liquid is a highly exothermic reaction, it is necessary to dissipate the heat, otherwise the reaction will proceed too rapidly towards completion. A properly cooled glass slab (18–20°C) is one method to dissipate heat. The temperature of the slab should not be lowered around the dew point otherwise water droplets will form and contaminate the mix. Water dilutes the liquid and shortens setting time. A cool slab also allows greater incorporation of powder leading to better consistency and better physical properties.

Powder/Liquid Ratio

A larger powder/liquid ratio greatly improves the properties of the mixed cement, therefore the maximum possible powder should be used to obtain a particular consistency. The powder/liquid ratio for filling is 2.5:1 and for luting cement is 1.5:1.

Care of the Liquid

The liquid of the cement should always be stored in stoppered bottles and exposure to air should be avoided as far as possible. Exposure to air will lead to change in the water/acid ratio, which affects the subsequent setting and working qualities of the cement. The liquid exposed to humid environment, absorbs water from the surroundings; whereas when exposed to dry environment it loses water. When the water content of the liquid is reduced, it is often evident by the formation of crystals on the walls of the bottle, or a general cloudiness of the liquid. This might be because of the precipitation of the buffering salts. Unfortunately, if water is absorbed by the liquid, no change in appearance can be observed. Repeated opening of the bottle over a long period of time undoubtedly alters the water/acid ratio of the remaining liquid. Therefore approximately the last one fifth of the liquid should be discarded. The addition of water causes greater ionization of the phosphoric acid and hence a rapid reaction. The subtraction of water results in a lengthened setting time. For similar reasons, liquid should not be left for a longer time on the slab before mixing.

Mixing Procedure

Mixing is accomplished with a long narrow bladed stainless steel spatula on a cool glass slab. The desired amount of powder is placed on the slab and divided into 6-7 increments. First the smallest increment is incorporated and spatulated over a large area for approximately 15 seconds followed similarly by rest of the increments one by one. The cement is mixed with the spatula held flat on the surface of the slab, moved in a rotary motion. Before moving on to the next increment, achieving a uniform consistency of the preceding mix is important. Completion of the mix usually requires 60–90 seconds.

Mixing over a large surface area on a cooled glass slab allows the heat to be dissipated most effectively. Incorporation of small increments at the start allows partial neutralization of the liquid, hence the temperature rise would not be high. Later on, larger amounts of powder incorporated during the middle of the mixing period, saturates the liquid with the newly forming zinc phosphate. The quantity of unreacted acid is less at this time because of the prior neutralization of the acid. The amount of heat liberated likewise is also less. Finally, smaller increments are added, so that the desired consistency is achieved. Thus the mixing procedures begins and ends with smaller increments, first to obtain slow maturation of the liquid and last to gain a critical consistency.

For manipulation/mixing of zinc phosphate cement, another method known as frozen slab method has also been tried.

In this method, the glass slab is cooled in a refrigerator at 6°C-10°C. No attempt is made to prevent moisture from condensing on the slab, when it is brought to room temperature. The amount of powder incorporated with the frozen slab method is 50 to 75% more than with the normal procedures. The compressive and tensile strengths are not different from those prepared from normal mixes because incorporation of condensed moisture in the mix in the frozen slab method counteracts the higher powder/liquid ratio.

The advantages of this method include substantial increase in working time, approximately four times and a shorter setting time of the mix.

Physical Properties (Table 11.2)

I. Consistency and film Thickness

The consistency of the zinc phosphate cement depends upon the particle size and type of the material as described earlier. Two consistencies are generally utilized:

- *Inlay/luting consistency (Type I)*
- *Base/filling consistency (Type II)*

The luting consistency is described as a consistency in which the cement will string up for at least 1.0-1.5 inch before breaking up.

The filling consistency is a heavy putty like consistency in which on lifting the spatula the extended cement point folds over to form a small loop and does not sink back into the mixture.

Average film thickness for Type I cement = 25 μ
Average film thickness for Type II cement = 40 μ

II. Strength

The compressive strength of zinc phosphate cement is 10,000 psi and the tensile strength is 800 psi, if powder/liquid ratio is 2.5:1 and spatulation time is 45 seconds.

The handling of the cement during its placement is important. If the area is not properly isolated and the cement comes in contact with water permanently, the unreacted phosphoric acid is diluted and leached out resulting in a cement which has a soft, friable and chalky surface.

III. Dimensional Stability

Zinc phosphate cement exhibits a slight initial expansion apparently because of water sorption. This expansion is then followed by a slight shrinkage in the order of 0.04%-0.06% in seven days.

IV. Thermal and Electrical Conductivity

Zinc phosphate cement exhibits a good thermal and electrical resistance. Presence of moisture however reduces its insulating potential.

V. Solubility and Disintegration

According to the ADA specification no. 8, the maximum solubility for zinc phosphate cements should not exceed 0.3%. In the initial stages, if the insufficiently set cement comes in contact with saliva, there occurs a leaching of free (unreacted) phosphoric acid. In order to prevent this from occuring, a high powder/liquid ratio should be used and the cement be allowed to set under isolation until enough interlacing crystals of zinc phosphate are formed to prevent the saliva from getting in and liquid from leaching out. Under acidic conditions, zinc phosphate cements are considerably less durable and show more solubility and disintegration.

Biological Properties

Three minutes after the start of mixing, the pH of zinc phosphate cement is approximately 3.5. The pH increases rapidly approaching neutrality in 24-48 hrs. The pH is lower and remains lower for thin mixes. Therefore, any damage to pulp from acid attack by zinc phosphate cement probably occurs during the first few hours after insertion. Hence in deep cavities pulp protective measures are required.

Modified Zinc Phosphate Cements

i. *Fluoridated cements:* Fluorides, such as stannous fluoride, etc., are added to zinc phosphate powder. The approximate concentration of fluoride is ten percent. Fluoride release continues over a long period and fluoride uptake results in reduced enamel solubility and increased hardness. These cements have a somewhat lower strength and a higher solubility than conventional zinc phosphate cements.

ii. *Copper cements:* Copper cements may consist of a portion of cuprous oxide (red) or cupric oxide (black) added to the zinc oxide powder. Other salts of copper, cuprous iodide (white) and copper siliceous oxide (green) have also been tried. The main object of addition of copper is to render the cements germicidal in the mouth. Silver salts have also been used for the purpose. There is little evidence for any advantage of these cements over conventional cements. Copper and silver are both bacteriostatic, but the longevity of their action is questionable.

Zinc Silicophosphate Cements

These materials are a combination of zinc phosphate cement and silicate cements, also known as silicophosphate cement.

Composition and Setting

The powder consists of a combination of silicate glass and zinc oxide, the latter in minor amounts. The silicate glass contains 13 to 25 percent fluoride. The liquid is similar to silicate liquids containing about 50 percent phosphoric acid, 4 to 9 percent zinc and 2 percent aluminium. Some materials have been labeled 'germicidal' because of the presence of small amounts of mercury or silver compounds. The setting reaction has not been fully investigated but the set cement seems likely to consist of unreacted glass and zinc oxide particles bonded together by an alumino-phosphate gel containing zinc, calcium, aluminium and fluoride ions.

Manipulation

The powder is incorporated into liquid in two or three large increments on a cool glass slab and spatulated to produce a thick paste for fillings or a thin paste for luting.

Three types of cements available are:
Type I: For use as a cementing medium
Type II: For use as a temporary filling material
Type III: For dual use – cementing medium and temporary filling material.

Properties

- Compressive strength of the set cement is appreciably higher than the zinc phosphate cement.
- These materials are tougher and more abrasion resistant than zinc phosphate cements.
- Solubility under clinical conditions is less than that of zinc phosphate cements.
- Better adaptation to the tooth structure.
- Fluoride release is evident.
- The set cement is more translucent than the opaque zinc phosphate.
- The mix is highly acidic and the pH remains low, after setting for prolonged periods of time.

The disadvantage of this cement is higher film thickness and greater potential for pulp irritation.

Polycarboxylate Cements

Polycarboxlyate cements were introduced by *Smith* in 1968. These cements have the strength and manipulative properties comparable to phosphate cements and low irritant potential under suitable conditions. The advantage of this cement is its adhesive qualities and also the anticariogenic properties (Fig. 11.8).

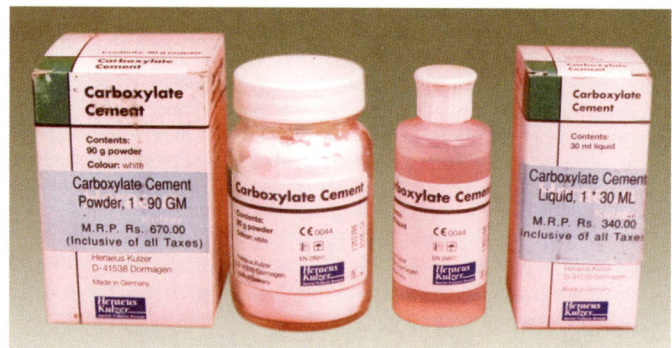

Fig. 11.8: Polycarboxylate cement (powder and Liquid)

Composition

Polycarboxylate cements consist of powder and liquid. The powder is a modified zinc oxide similar to that used in zinc phosphate cements. Stannic oxide may be substituted for magnesium oxide. Other oxides, such as bismuth and aluminium can be added. The powder may also contain small quantities of stannous fluoride, which modify the setting time and enhance manipulative characteristics. It also increases strength. However, fluoride release from these cements is only minimal.

The liquid is an aqueous solution of polyacrylic acid. A copolymer of other unsaturated carboxylic acids, such as itaconic or tartaric acid is also added in minute quantities. The concentration of the polyacrylic acid is approximately 40%. By altering the compositions of the liquid, the setting characteristics and properties of the cement can be modified.

Setting Reaction

The setting reaction involves an acid base phenomenon. The mixing of liquid and powder leads to ionization of the polyacrylic acid. Surface dissolution of the powder particles under the influence of the acid causes it to release zinc, magnesium and tin ions. These ions are transported in the solution as hydrated complexes along with the less tightly bound water.

Zinc may react with 1–4 carboxyl groups, whereas calcium binds with 2 carboxyl groups. The bond is purely ionic and is hydrolytically unstable leading to the loss of zinc and other ions. When an unset cement is placed on a clean calcific surface, it sets through chelation. Poly-acrylic acid additionally forms complexes with proteins, which may further promote its property of adhesion.

Water molecules play an important role in the cement structure. There are both tightly bound and loosely bound waters that correspond to intrinsic and secondary waters respectively.

The H^+ displaces both intrinsic and secondary water, so the free acid is not hydrated. Magnesium ion on the other hand only displaces secondary water, so wherever ionic bonding with this ion is present, a layer of intrinsic water separates the cation and the anion. As the reaction proceeds, the acid continues to ionize to polyanion and creates a demand for water thereby absorbing water from the cement. The hardened cement consists of a hydrated amorphous gel matrix in which unreacted particles are dispersed. The matrix is the 'continuous phase' whereas the unreacted powder is the 'interrupted phase'. The two phases are bound together by the cation depleted portion of the original powder particles. The matrix structure is porous to some extent but has better packing characteristics than zinc phosphate cement.

On the basis of their compositions, polycarboxylate cements are of three types.

Type I: Powder contains 90% zinc oxide and 10% magnesium oxide.

Type II: 30-40% alumina replaces zinc oxide powder.

Type III: The polyacrylic acid is freeze dried and incorporated in the powder. The liquid is the water.

Manipulation

The recommended powder/liquid ratio ranges from 1:1 to 2:1. The higher ratio is for restorative purposes and the lower for luting purposes. Polycarboxylate cement especially the liquid should not be stored in a refrigerator because the low temperature causes the liquid to thicken or lead to gel formation.

Mixing is done on a glass slab or a non-absorbent paper pad. The glass slab is somewhat advantageous as it can be cooled and hence allows extension of the working time. The working time ranges from 3–5 minutes, which can be extended to 10–15 minutes, if the glass slab is chilled to 4°C.

The liquid should be dispensed just before the mixing is to be started because exposure of the liquid to air even for a few minutes results in evaporation of the water, subsequently, increasing the viscosity of the liquid.

Powder is incorporated into the liquid in two or three large increments, using rapid spatulation. The mix should be completed in 30 seconds to allow maximum length of working time. If good bonding to the tooth structure is to be obtained, the cement must be placed on the tooth structure while it is still glossy. A dull surface would indicate insufficient carboxyl groups available for bonding to the calcium in the tooth surface.

The correct consistency for cementation is viscous and will flow back under its own weight when drawn up with a spatula. Polycarboxylate cements have thixotropic properties, that is the viscosity decreases when shear forces are applied as during spatulation or when placing a restoration.

Physical Properties (Table 11.2)

i. *Viscosity:* The initial viscosity of polycarboxylate cements is more than the viscosity of zinc phosphate mix just after mixing. Polycarboxylate cements also exhibit pseudoplastic behaviour.

ii. *Setting Time:* The setting time, for polycarboxylate cements should range within 7–9 minutes from the start of mixing.

iii. *Film Thickness:* The film thickness for these cements is slightly higher than zinc phosphate cements but is well within the clinical limits of 25 μ.

iv. *Strength:* The 24 hour compressive strength for polycarboxylate cements is less than that of zinc phosphate cements. However, the tensile strength of polycarboxylate cements is higher than that of zinc phosphate cements.

v. *Dimensional stability:* Polycarboxylate cements show a linear contraction when setting at 37°C. The amount of contraction ranges from 1% for a wet specimen to 6% for a dry specimen. These contractions are more pronounced than that observed for zinc phosphate cements.

vi. *Bond strength:* Polycarboxylate cements bond to enamel and dentin, which is attributed to the ability of the carboxyl groups in the polymer molecule to chelate to calcium ions in the hydroxyapatite. Because of the higher inorganic component of enamel, bond strength to enamel is greater than the bond strength to dentin.

Bond strength to enamel = 3.45-13.1 MPa
= (500-1900 psi)
Bond strength to dentin = 2.07 MPa (300 psi)

Optimum bonding however requires a clean tooth surface and adequate number of carboxyl groups. The bonding of polycarboxylate cements to gold casting alloy is likewise very important. Sand blasting or electrolytic etching of the gold surface is necessary to obtain a clean surface.

vii. *Solubility and disintegration*: Solubility for polycarboxylate cement varies from 0.10-0.25%. The solubility is because of leaching out of zinc and magnesium ions, the rate however decreases as the cement ages.

Higher powder/ liquid ratio decreases the leaching out of the zinc ions because the setting reaction is faster. Furthermore with the presence of less liquid, less percentage of zinc ions are liberated from zinc oxide.

Biological Properties

The pH of the cement liquid is approximately 1.5. However, the liquid is rapidly neutralized by the powder. Thus, the pH of the cement rises rapidly (5.5) as the setting reaction proceeds, compared to the slow rise in pH of zinc phosphate cements. Also, the larger size of the polyacrylic acid molecule and its binding to calcium and proteins limits its diffusion through the dentinal tubules. Polyacrylic acid is a weak acid and causes minimal movement of the fluid in the dentinal tubules. Additionally, it is biocompatible with the pulp. All these factors make polycarboxylate cement less irritating than zinc phosphate cements.

Calcium Hydroxide

Initially, calcium hydroxide was used only as a pulp capping agent, both in direct and indirect pulp capping because of its higher pH values. It was considered to help in killing bacteria at the site and inducing secondary dentin formation. Because of its favourable properties, it was used as subbase under a cement base especially in deep cavities.

With the improvement in its physical properties, and its compatibility with composites, it is now used as a base and also as an interim restoration. Dycal, the commonly available calcium hydroxide preparation consists of two tubes; one containing base and the other catalyst (Fig. 11.9).

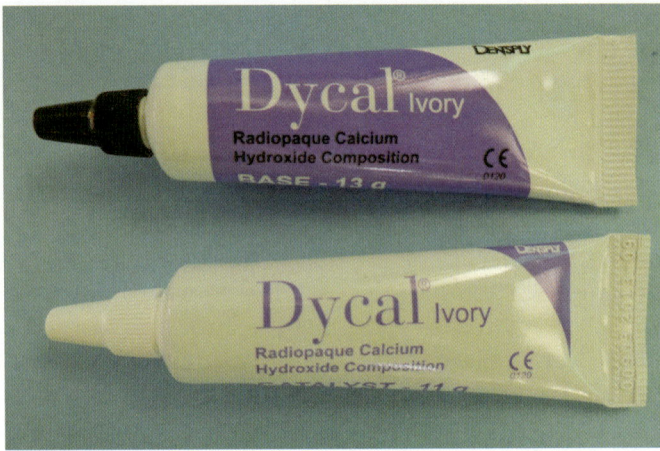

Fig. 11.9: Quick setting calcium hydroxide (Dycal)

The composition is

Base
- Zinc oxide
- Calcium phosphate
- Calcium tungstate
- Iron oxide
- 1,3-butylglycoidisalicylate

Catalyst
- Calcium hydroxide
- Zinc oxide
- Zinc stearate
- Iron oxide
- N-ethyl p-toluene sulfonamide

The base and the catalyst are mixed in the ratio of 1:1 on a clean disposable pad. The setting time is approximately one minute outside the oral cavity. However, it decreases substantially inside the oral cavity because of higher temperature and humidity. Recently light cure calcium hydroxide is also made available. These materials, along with having properties of calcium hydroxide, exhibit better physical properties like better compressive and tensile strengths and less solubility in oral fluids.

The composition is:
- Calcium hydroxide
- Calcium hydroxyapatite
- Barium sulphate
- Certain fluorides
- Resin matrix

The calcium hydroxide preparation is preferably used as an interim restoration in cases where composite is to be used as final restoration. Half of the filling can be removed and the other half can be used as a base under the composite restoration.

These are also used as interim materials in preventive dental care programme. Calcium hydroxide is very effective in cases of rampant caries. The progress of rampant caries is very quick so immediate permanent restoration is not preferred. Progress/arrest of caries can be evaluated before final restoration is given.

FOR EXTRACORONAL PREPARATIONS

Prefabricated Crowns

Various types of prefabricated crowns are available, chiefly among these are aluminium, stainless steel, celluloid and polycarbonate crowns (Fig. 11.10). Crown forms available in anatomic shapes are most effective because of the function and protection they offer to the gingival tissues. Transparent crowns are usually used for anterior teeth and the metal crowns for the posterior teeth. If anatomic crowns are not available, these can be cut according to the contour of the tooth to be restored. The cut edges are smoothened with a mounted stone or rubber tips. Usually these crowns are kept slightly away from the gingival margins, since these may lead to gingival recession at those areas. The patient is instructed to brush carefully so as not to injure the gingival margin.

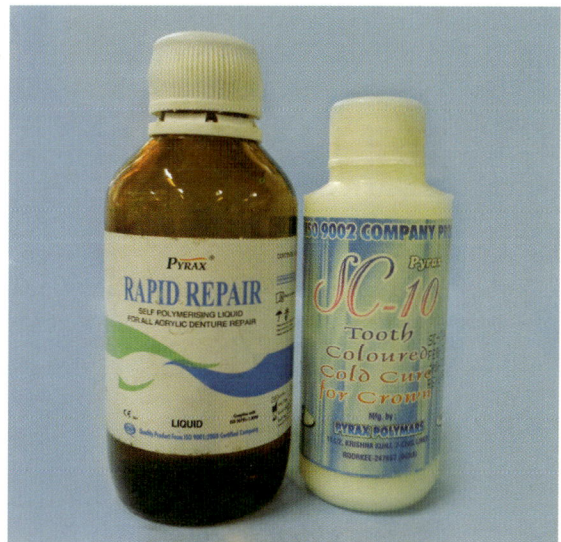

Fig. 11.11: Self-cure acrylic resin—powder and liquid

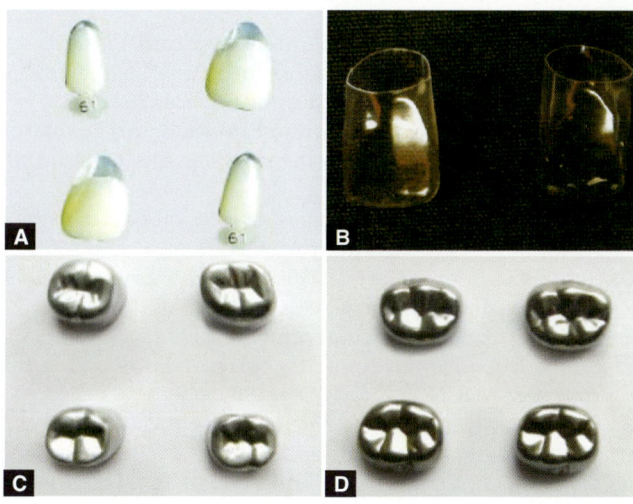

Figs 11.10A to D: Prefabricated interim restorations **(A)** prefabricated polycarbonate crowns, **(B)** prefabricated cellulose crowns, **(C)** prefabricated aluminium crowns, **(D)** prefabricated stainless steel crowns

The crowns are filled with a thin mix of zinc oxide eugenol cement and fixed onto the tooth. The excess cement is wiped out. The patient is asked to bite smoothly and the occlusion is checked. 3% hydrogen peroxide can be used to clean the marginal area of remaining cement.

Indirect Acrylic Restorations

Several resins are being used to make temporary restorations, however self curing acrylic is the widely used material (Fig. 11.11). This fulfills the aims of temporary restorations in providing esthetics and partial function to the restored tooth. Acrylics can be used both directly over the tooth or fabricated outside the oral cavity and then seated. The major drawback of using direct acrylic is that the free monomer and the heat produced during exothermic reaction are harmful to the pulp and the gingival tissues. The disadvantage of indirect method is the time required for fabrication of the restoration. However, the accuracy, appearance and function achieved by this type of restoration strongly favours its use.

Technique

A pre-operative rubber base impression of the arch is taken and stored. In case the tooth to be restored is partially broken or otherwise mutilated, the cast is prepared from the impression and the tooth is build with wax over the cast. A fresh impression is taken from that cast and stored.

The tooth preparation is completed. After gingival retraction, a rubber base impression is taken and a cast is made. The tooth to be restored is coated with cold mold seal. Self cure acrylic resin of the desired shade is mixed in a dappen dish and poured into the tooth impression already stored. The cast is inserted into the impression and kept there for few minutes. The cast and the impression are separated after some time. A temporary crown is ready simulating shape, size and contour of the original tooth. The same is finished, polished and seated onto the prepared tooth along with the zinc oxide eugenol cement. ZOE should not be used if the temporary crown is to be used for a longer time, since eugenol weakens the acrylics. The gingival area is cleaned and the occlusion is finally checked.

Indirect acrylic restorations can also be fabricated over the cast mounted on the articulators, but such restorations may not match the configuration of original tooth and may not be very pleasing.

Interim restorations are mandatory for the protection of pulp and gingival tissues. Along with sealing the cavity preparation, they also provide esthetics and partial functioning of teeth. For extracoronal preparation they stabilize the tooth movement till permanent restoration is given. The time spent for interim restorations adds boon to our clinical practice.

BIBLIOGRAPHY

1. Bansal R.K., Tewari U.S., Singh P. and Murthy, D.V. : Influence of talc on the properties of polycarboxylate cement.
   J. Oral Rehab. : 24, 76, 1997.
2. Behrend D.A.: Temporary protective restorations in crown and bridge work. Aust. Dent. J.: 12, 411, 1967.
3. Braumer G.M., McLanghlin R. and Huget E.F.: Aluminium oxide as a reinforcing agent for zinc oxide eugenolo-ethoxy benozoic acid cement. J.D.R.: 47, 662, 1968.
4. Brauer G.M., Simon L. and Sangermano L.: Improved zinc oxide eugenol type cements. J.D.R.: 41, 1096, 1962.
5. Brauer G.M., Stansbury J.W. and Acgental H.: Development of high strength acrylic resin compatible adhesive cements. J.D.R.: 62, 366, 1983.
6. Burke F.J., Murray M.C. and Shortall A.C. : Trends in indirect dentistry provisional restorations. Dent. Update: 32, 443, 2005.
7. Civjan S. and Brauer G.M.: Clinical behaviour of O-EBAEugenol zinc oxide cements. J.D.R.: 44, 80, 1965.
8. Civjan S., Huget E.F., Wolfhard G. and Waddell L.S.: Characterization of zinc oxide eugenol cements reinforced with acrylic resin. J.D.R.: 51, 107, 1972.
9. Crowell W.S.: Physical Chemistry of Dental Cements. DCNA: 6, 763, Oct. 1983.
10. Deveaux E., Hildelbert P., Neut C., Boniface B. and Romond, C.: Bacterial microleakage of Cavit, IRM and TERM. O. Surg., O. Med., O. Path.: 74, 634, 1992.
11. Gilles J.A., Huget E.F., Stone R.C.: Dimensional stability of temporary restorative materials. O. Surg., O. Med., O. Path.: 40, 796, 1975.
12. Gilson T.D. and Myres G.E.: Clinical studies of Dental Cement – II. Further investigation of the zinc oxide eugenol cement for temporary restorations. J.D.R.: 48, 366, 1972.
13. Gough M. : A review of temporary crown and bridges. Dent. Update : 16, 203, 1994.
14. Gratton D.G. and Aquilino S.A. : Interim restorations. D.C.N.A. : 48, 487, 2004.
15. Grieve, A.R.: A study of dental cements. B.D.J.: 127, 405, 1969.
16. Hammod. BD, Cooper. JR and Lazarchik. DA.: Predictable repair of provisional restorations. J Esthet Restor Dent 2, 19, 2009.
17. Hume W.R.: The pharmacological and toxicological properties of zinc oxide eugenol. J.A.D.A.: 113, 789, 1986.
18. Lui. JL, Setcos. JC and Phillips. RW.: Temporary restorations: a review. Oper Dent 11, 103, 1986
19. Markowitz K., Moynihan M., Liu M. and Kim, S.: Biologic properties of eugenol and zinc oxide eugenol. O. Surg., O. Med., O. Path.: 73, 729, 1992.
20. McComb D.: Comparison of physical properties of commercial calcium hydroxide lining cements. J.A.D.A.: 107, 610, 1983.
21. Meryon S.D., Johnson S.G. and Smith A.J.: Eugenol release and the cytotoxicity of different zinc oxide eugenol combination. J. Dent.: 16, 66, 1998.
22. Murray M.C. Smith P.W., Watts D. and Wilson, N.H.F. : Occlusal registration : science or art ? Int. Dent. J. : 49, 41, 1999.
23. Nejactidanesh F., Lotfi H.R. and Savabi O. : Marginal accuracy of interim restorations fabricated from four autopolymerizing resins. J.P.D. : 95, 364, 2006.
24. Nemkovsky C.E. and Gross M.D. : Transferring provisional restorations to final master casts. J. Oral Rehab. : 21, 157, 1994.
25. Norman R.D., Swartz M.L., Phillips R.W. and Raibley J.W.: Direct pH determination of setting cements 2. The effects of prolonged storage time, powder/liquid ratio, temperature and dentin. J.D.R.: 45, 1214, 1966.
26. Pashley E.L., Tao L. and Pashley D.H.: The sealing properties of temporary filling materials. J.P.D.: 60, 292, 1988.
27. Patras. M, Naka. O, Duokoudakis. S and Pissiotis. A.: Management of provisional restorations' deficiencies: a literature review. J Esthet Restor Dent 24, 26, 2012.
28. Phillips R.W., Swartz M.L. and Rhodes B.: An evaluation of carboxylate adhesive cement. J. Am. Dent. Assoc.: 81, 1353, 1970.
29. Saby B. : Provisionalization as an integral part of esthetic restoration. Oral Health : pp.49, 2002.
30. Servais G.E. and Cartz L.: Structure of zinc phosphate dental cement. J.D.R.: 50, 613, 1971.
31. Smith D.C.: A new dental cement. B.D.J.: 5, 381, 1968.
32. Smith D.C.: Dental cements, current status and future propsects. DCNA: 6, 763, Oct. 1983.
33. Smith D.C.: A review of zinc polycarboxylate cements. J. Canad. Dent. Assoc., No. 1, 22, 1971.
34. Usumez A., Ozturk A.N. and Aykent F. : The effect of dentin desensitizers on thermal changes in the pulp chamber during fabrication of provisional restoration. J. Oral Rehab. : 31, 579, 2004.
35. Wassell. RW, St. George. G, Ingledew. RP and Steele JG.: Crowns and other extracoronal restorations: provisional restorations. Br Dent J 192, 619, 2002.
36. Weaver R.G., Johnson B.E., Cvar J.F. and McCune R.J.: Clinical evaluation of intermediary restorations. J. Dent. For Child.: 39, 189, 1972.
37. Widerman F.H., Eames W.B. and Serene T.P.: The physical and biological properties of Cavit. J.A.D.A.: 82, 378, 1971.
38. Wilson A.D. and Batchelor R.F.: ZnO eugenol cements II. Study of erosion and disintegration. J.D.R.: 49, 593, 1970.
39. Wilson A.D., Clinton D.J. and Miller R.P.: Zinc oxide eugenol cements: IV Micro structure and hydrolysis. J.D.R.: 52, 253, 1973.
40. Wolcott R.B. and Kraske L.M.: A clinical evaluation of temporary restorative material. J.P.D.: 12, 782, 1962.
41. Xie, D. Fadah M. and Park J.G. : Novel amino acid modified zinc polycarboxylates for improved dental cements. Dent. Mater. : 21, 739, 2005.

Silver Amalgam

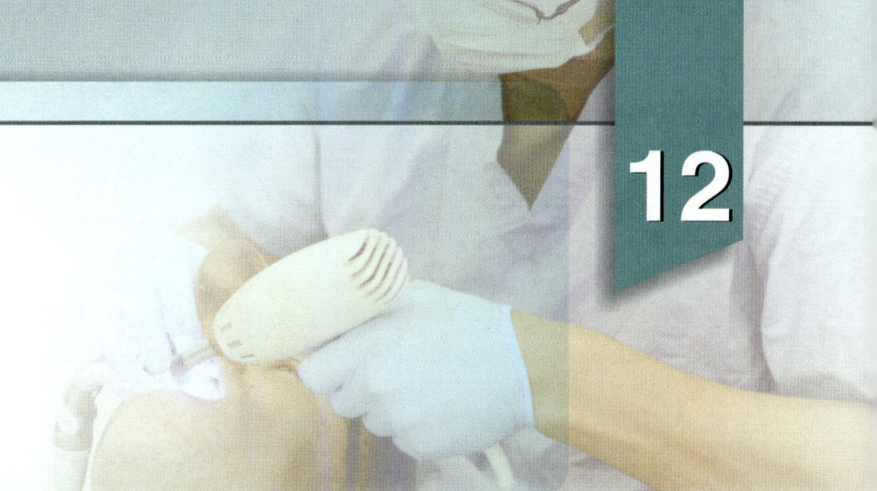

Silver amalgam, undoubtedly, is the most commonly and widely used restorative material. It has withstood all challenges of time and still being used widely despite of the advent of various other restorative materials. When compared with other materials, especially the esthetic ones, the advantages of silver amalgam always surpass the disadvantages, thereby making this material the choice of the operator in routine.

Silver amalgam if properly manipulated produces a restoration, which could provide many years of service. The average life span of silver amalgam is 8-10 years, though early failures have also been reported. 50% of the failures in amalgam restorations are due to faulty cavity preparation and the rest due to faulty manipulation. Therefore, understanding of both is mandatory for achieving optimal success. Secondary caries and fracture, the two major failure signs, are attributed to both poor manipulation and cavity designs.

Advantages

1. Ease of handling: The manipulation of silver amalgam viz. mixing, squeezing and condensing, etc. is very simple and easily understood.
2. Wide range of applications: If esthetics is not a major concern, silver amalgam can be given in any class and any size of the cavity. It can also be used as retrograde fillings.
3. Optimal dimensional changes: The silver amalgam falls within the range of ADA specification no. 1 which permits ± 0.2 percent expansion/contraction during setting.
4. Physical characteristics: Physical characteristics of silver amalgam are comparable to enamel and dentin. The compressive strength, hardness, etc. are within optimal limits.
5. Biocompatibility: Silver amalgam is biologically stable and accepted. Allergic reactions to components of silver alloy have rarely been reported.
6. Economical.

This chapter deals with cavity preparation and proper manipulation of silver amalgam.

Disadvantages

1. Poor esthetics: Even the properly polished silver amalgam restorations are not esthetically acceptable.
2. Marginal degradation or ditching is prominent in low copper or conventional silver amalgams. However, with high copper alloys, marginal degradation or ditching has been minimized.
3. Excessive cavity cutting is required because of its poor edge strength.
4. Tensile strength is less.
5. Silver is a good thermal conductor, so base is required under these restorations.
6. Galvanic current can be produced in association with gold fillings or even in same restoration with non-uniform condensation.
7. Oral lichen planus has also been reported with silver amalgam.

COMPOSITION OF ALLOY

Amalgam is a mixture of mercury, with one or more metals. An alloy is a union of two or more metals. Usually in dentistry, this union is by means of heat. The advantage of alloying metals is that when a new compound is formed, it possesses properties that are not present in single element. Mercury, having the property of dissolving other metals, produces a plastic mass, which has low fusion temperature.

Conventional Silver Alloy

Conventional silver alloy as envisaged by G.V. Black, falls within the range of ADA specification No.1, contains the following:

Silver (Ag)	68–72% (wt %)
Tin (Sn)	25–27%
Copper (Cu)	2–6%
Zinc (Zn)	0–3%

However recently, alloys with copper contents more than 6% and may be upto 30% have been

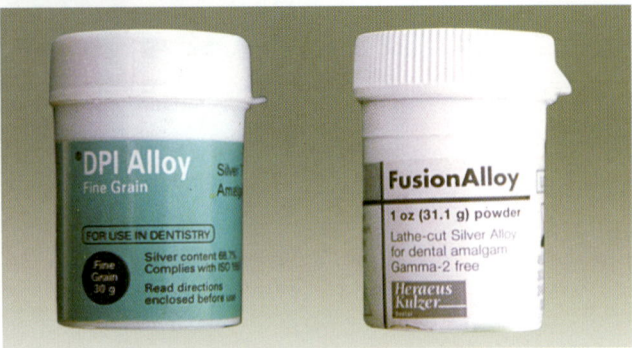

Fig. 12.1: Commercial preparation of low copper (DPI alloy) and high copper silver alloy (Fusion alloy)

introduced with the idea of eliminating γ_2 phase (Fig. 12.1). With the introduction of high copper alloys, wider limits of each constituent have been accepted. Various authors have tried different combination of alloys, using Palladium (Pd), Gold (Au), Cadmium (Cd), Manganese (Mn), Nickel (Ni), and Iridium (Id) with varying success.

An alloy which contains more than 6% copper is referred to as a high copper alloy. High copper alloys came into being with the idea of eliminating γ_2 phase, the phase responsible for corrosion.

The early alloys were admixed alloy having silver copper eutectic and conventional alloy, however later they were modified to make it single composition.

Admixed/Blended Alloy

This alloy is a mixture of two types of particles viz. lathe cut low copper alloy particles and spherical eutectic (silver copper) alloy particles. The content of copper may vary from 9–20%.

Admixed alloys are of following two types:

i. *Type I alloy*: It contains two parts of conventional lathe cut particles and one part by weight of silver copper eutectic alloy. The overall composition is approximately-
   Silver   69%
   Copper   13%
   Tin   17%
   Zinc   1%

ii. *Type II alloy*: It is the reverse of type I alloy, i.e. it contains two parts of spherical silver copper alloy and one part of conventional alloy. The approximate composition is:
   Silver   60%
   Tin   25%
   Copper   15%

Single Composition/All in One Alloy

In this powder, each particle of the alloy has the same chemical composition, that is why they are called single composition alloys.

The copper content in various single composition alloys ranges from 13–30%. These may be of the following types:

i. *Ternary alloys*: The composition can be either silver 60%, tin 25%, copper 15% or silver 40%, tin 30%, copper 30%.
ii. *Quaternary alloys*: Silver 60%, copper 13%, tin 24%, indium 3%.
iii. An alloy similar to (i), but containing particles in spheroidal form (i.e. particles are not perfectly spherical).

EFFECT OF CONSTITUENT METALS ON THE PROPERTIES OF AMALGAM

Silver

- Increases strength: The strength is basically because of unreacted AgSn (γ phase) particles in the matrix. Higher the silver, higher will be the γ-phase.
- Decreases flow. The flow is also because of the unreacted AgSn (γ phase) particles. Higher the unreacted particles, lesser will be the flow.
- Increases setting expansion. This is because of the formation of γ_1 phase, which is AgHg. The volume of γ_1 phase is greater than both Ag and Hg independently.
- Resists tarnish and corrosion.
- Reduces setting time by accelerating the setting process, since the reaction of silver and mercury is very fast.
- It whitens the alloy.

Tin

- Reduces strength: With increase of tin, the AgHg is reduced and SnHg is increased which is a weaker phase.
- It helps in amalgamation since tin has great affinity for mercury. It also controls the fast reaction between silver and mercury because of this affinity.
- Increases setting time.
- Decreases setting expansion. The SnHg phase causes the contraction.
- Reduces the resistance to tarnish and corrosion.

Copper

- Increases strength: The phenomenon of increased strength is the same as of silver. Only AgSn alloys are very brittle and do not show uniform coherence, i.e. why some amount of copper is a must.
- Reduces flow.
- Increases setting expansion. It has been shown that if copper is more than 5% excessive expansion occurs.
- Copper makes the alloy less susceptible to slight imperfections during manipulation by dentists.

Zinc

- It prevents oxidation during manufacturing of alloy.
- Contributes to the cleanliness or workability of silver amalgam during trituration and condensation.
- Responsible for delayed expansion if zinc containing alloys are contaminated with water. The expansion occurs after 3-4 days because zinc reacts with water releasing hydrogen. This hydrogen basically causes expansion.
- Like copper it also makes the alloy less susceptible to imperfection during manipulation by dentists.

MANUFACTURING OF ALLOY

First step in the manufacturing process of conventional alloy is melting together the constituents. The ingot is given a homogenization heat treatment. The temperature varies from 150–400°C. This different homogenization temperature varies from manufacturer to manufacturer and also the type of the particles. In case of lathe cut particles higher temperature treatment is given while in spherical alloy lower temperature treatment is preferred. Following the heat treatment the ingot is reduced to filings. The particles are further reduced by ball milling. From higher temperature, the alloy particles are brought to lower temperature to reduce the internal stresses. This total phenomenon is called the 'Thermodynamic Equilibrium' of the alloy particles. Many alloys supplied these days, however, are not in thermodynamic equilibrium. In case of high copper alloys, which are an admixture of two different alloy powders, no such equilibrium is reached. Various authors are of the view that thermodynamic equilibrium of dental amalgam alloy is not a prerequisite for good amalgam.

ALLOY MERCURY REACTION

The reaction of alloy and mercury, traditionally take Silver and Tin, without taking copper and zinc. The reaction is:

$$AgSn + Hg \longrightarrow AgHg + SnHg + AgSn$$
$$\gamma \qquad\qquad\qquad \gamma_1 \qquad \gamma_2 \qquad \gamma$$

The γ or the AgSn are the unreacted particles. The γ_1 phase is the first phase formed during setting because silver dissolves more quickly in mercury than tin. However, mass transport of mercury into alloy particles might contribute to the formation of new phases equally. After the reaction, the unreacted particles (AgSn) are embedded in a matrix of reaction products with mercury. In conventional amalgams both γ_1 and γ_2 phases form a continuous network. The distribution of γ_2 phase is important, as it is the phase, which is responsible for corrosion of silver amalgam.

The exact formula of the phases γ, γ_1, γ_2 remains controversial. Various authors have described these in different ways and there is hardly any unanimity among them.

A few authors have even challenged the basic formula of γ_1 (AgHg) + γ_2 (SnHg) by showing that the γ_1 (AgHg) contains some tin also. Some amount of copper and zinc might also be there. The γ_2 phase, however, might contain only minute amount of other components. In case of aging amalgam, another phase AgHgSn, i.e. β phase is formed. It has been shown that amalgams remain in a state of non-equilibrium which might be for one year or even more. The percentage of phases in the conventional alloy is AgHg 66.25%, SnHg 6.25%, AgSn 25% and residual Hg 2.5% (Fig. 12.2).

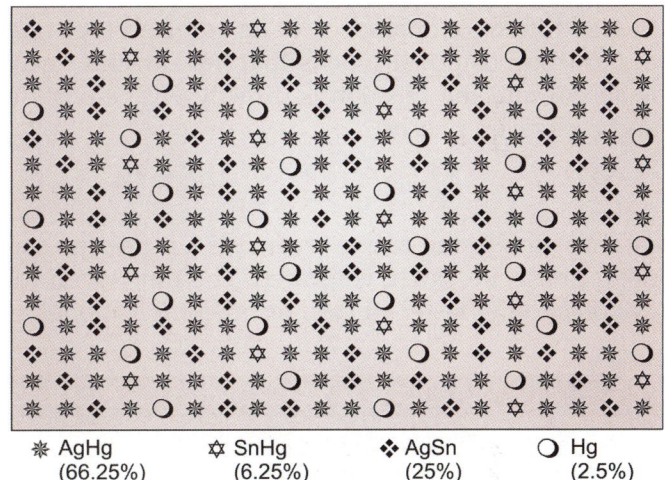

AgHg (66.25%) SnHg (6.25%) AgSn (25%) Hg (2.5%)

Fig. 12.2: Distribution of phases in conventional alloy

In case of high copper alloys the reaction is different. The reaction occurs in two phases. The first phase is equivalent to the one as shown in conventional alloys, i.e.

$$AgSn + Hg \longrightarrow AgHg + SnHg + AgSn$$
$$\gamma \qquad\qquad\qquad \gamma_1 \qquad \gamma_2 \qquad \gamma$$

The second phase is the eutectic of silver copper phase, which are called α_1 and α_2. This type of reaction occurs in admixed type of high copper alloy. In an eutectic, two metal phases are present, which are separated but closely adjacent to each other. Here α_1 is silver rich and α_2 is copper rich. These two along with γ (AgSn) react with mercury and again γ_1 (AgHg) and γ_2 (SnHg) is formed. All the tin does not react with mercury; part of tin reacts with the eutectic α_1 and α_2.

$$AgSn + AgCu + Hg \xrightarrow[\text{mixing}]{\text{After}} AgHg + Sn_7Hg + AgSn$$
$$\gamma \qquad \alpha_1 + \alpha_2 \qquad\qquad\qquad \gamma_1 \qquad \gamma_2 \qquad \gamma$$
$$\ldots + Cu_3Sn + Cu_6Sn_5 + AgCu$$
$$\varepsilon \qquad \eta \qquad \alpha_1 + \alpha_2$$

The reaction goes on. After one week, the SnHg (γ_2) phase reacts completely with the eutectic. The silver forms γ_1 and the tin forms η and ϵ.

$$\underset{\gamma}{AgSn} + \underset{\alpha_1 + \alpha_2}{AgCu} + Hg \xrightarrow{\text{After one week}} \underset{\gamma_1}{AgHg} + \underset{\alpha_1 + \alpha_2}{AgCu} + \underset{\epsilon}{Cu_3Sn} \dots + \underset{\eta}{Cu_6Sn_5} + \underset{\gamma}{AgSn}$$

The reaction is not finished yet. After approximately one year, silver tin phase also vanishes. The tin further diffuses into the silver copper eutectic slowly and forms more of $\alpha_1 + \alpha_2$ phase. The final reaction is:

$$\underset{\gamma}{AgSn} + \underset{\alpha_1 + \alpha_2}{AgCu} + Hg \xrightarrow{\text{After one year}} \underset{\gamma}{AgSn} + \underset{\alpha_1 + \alpha_2}{AgCu} + \underset{\gamma_1}{AgHg} \dots + \underset{\eta}{Cu_6Sn_5}$$

The difference of reaction in an admixed type and the unicompositional type is that the eutectic AgCu is absent and the reaction is directly with silver tin and copper tin phases.

$$\underset{\gamma}{Ag_3Sn} + \underset{\epsilon}{Cu_3SN} + Hg \longrightarrow \underset{\gamma_1}{AgHg} + \underset{\eta}{Cu_6Sn_5}$$

Thus finally the phase formed is Cu_6Sn_5 (η) and no γ_2 phase, i.e. SnHg is formed. The time taken for the reaction is faster in case of unicompositional as compared to admixed type. The comparative analysis of low copper and high copper silver alloys is given in Table 12.1.

CAVITY PREPARATION

Cavity preparation is defined as *'the mechanical removal of caries and shaping the remaining tooth tissues in such a way so that after restoration it can withstand masticatory forces and will be able to prevent subsequent caries'*.

The principles of cavity preparation are described in Chapter 10.

Cavity designs for amalgam restorations are given here.

Class I (Cavities on the anatomical pits and fissures of all the teeth)

The carious lesions occur mostly in occlusal pits and fissures and also the buccal/lingual pits of posterior teeth and lingual pits of anterior teeth.

A. Cavities on the Occlusal Pits and Fissures

In case the caries is present only on occlusal pits and fissures, the outline is planned keeping in mind the features like extent of caries, oral hygiene, caries index

Table 12.1: Comparative analysis of low copper and high copper silver alloys

Low copper	High copper
1. More mercury is required for amalgamation (53.37%). Solubility of tin in mercury is 170 times more than in copper and 17 times more than in silver.	Less mercury is required.
2. Dominant phase is AgHg, i.e. γ_1.	Dominant phase is Cu_6Sn_5, i.e. η.
3. Corrosion due to γ_2 phase is due to formation of tin oxychloride from tin. Dissolution of this oxide or chloride leads to porosity.	Cu_6Sn_5 (η) phase is the least corrosion resistant phase. Corrosion occurs in the form of $CuCl_2 \cdot 3Cu(OH)_2$. Order of corrosion of different phases is: $\underset{\gamma_1}{AgHg} < \underset{\gamma}{AgSn} < \underset{\text{Eutectic } \epsilon}{Ag_3Cu_2} < \underset{\eta}{Cu_3Sn} < \underset{}{Cu_6Sn_5} < \underset{\gamma_2}{SnHg}$
4. Surface tarnish is associated with γ and γ_1.	Surface tarnish is due to copper-rich phases.
5. Low copper alloys can be amalgamated in slow speed and low energy amalgamation.	High copper alloys require high speed and high energy amalgamation because copper has low solubility in mercury as compared to silver and tin.
6. Setting reaction is slow. Early burnishing and finishing is recommended.	Setting reaction is fast. It can be burnished at first not appointment.
7. Low copper amalgam has higher value of creep. The range is between 1-8%.	Creep is much less. (Mostly less than 1% and might be as low as 0.1%.)
8. Compressive strength between one hour and 7 days is 150-350 MPa.	Compressive strength varies between 250–500 MPa between one hour and 7 days especially with unicomposition alloys.
9. Tensile strength in 24 hours is 60 MPa.	Tensile strength is 64 MPa for single composition alloys.
10. Dimensional changes are more in low copper alloy; varies from 10-20 μm/cm.	Much less with high copper alloy; varies from 1–9 μm/cm.

of the patient and choice of the restorative material. After planning the outline form, the surface is cleaned with water and air. A small round bur is used to enter the deepest or most carious pit, moving the bur parallel to the long axis of the tooth crown. When the bur touches the dentino-enamel junction or slightly into the dentin, the straight fissure bur/diamond point is utilized for further preparation. Conventionally, No. 245 (S.S. White) carbide bur is used to obtain convergent cavity form along with rounded line angles. When the pits are equally carious, cavity preparation can be started on any pit. The fissure bur is moved along the fissures maintaining the uniform depth, which is initially 1.5 mm (Figs 12.3A). The preparation at the initial level is kept slightly short of the desired outline form. Again start with the same bur, with a light push-pull motion in the fissures to reduce the facial and lingual walls. This way a flat pulpal floor is created with facial and lingual walls almost parallel. However in teeth with steep cuspal inclines the pulpal floor can be kept according to cuspal heights maintaining uniform depth of the pulpal floor (Fig. 12.3B).

Extension into the marginal ridges dictates slight tilting of the bur (approximately 10 degrees) mesially and distally respectively to create occlusal divergence at mesial and distal marginal ridges respectively. This procedure prevents the undermining of marginal ridges.

The distance of margins of such an extension to the proximal surface must not be less than 1.5 mm in premolars and 2.0 mm in molars. In case the distance is slightly less, the divergence of the walls can be avoided. However, if the said distance is approximately 1.0 mm, the inclusion of proximal surfaces can be considered (Figs 12.4A and B).

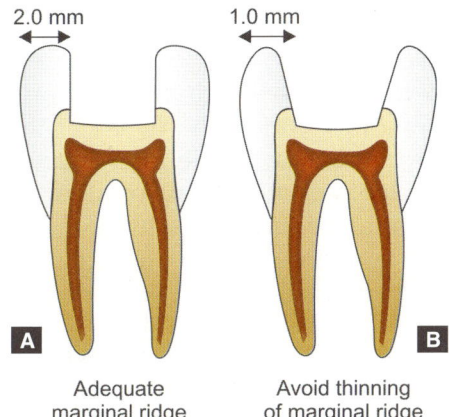

Figs 12.4A and B: Extension of cavity outline along marginal ridge

The buccolingual width of the cavity should be approximately 1.0-1.5 mm or 1/4th of the intercuspal distance. In case, the caries so dictates, the width can be more, but in no case more than half the cuspal inclines should be involved. In case where more than half or 2/3rd cuspal inclines are involved, the covering of cusps become mandatory.

Alternatively, in spite of covering cusps in such circumstances, the undermined carious lesions are excavated from below the cusps and this undermined area is filled with glass-ionomer cement or composite resin. The rest of the cavity is restored with silver amalgam. It has been shown that these teeth exhibit same fracture resistance as the teeth without any undermined cuspal caries.

All the cavity walls should be joined by definite line and point angles, which are kept rounded (Figs 12.5A and B).

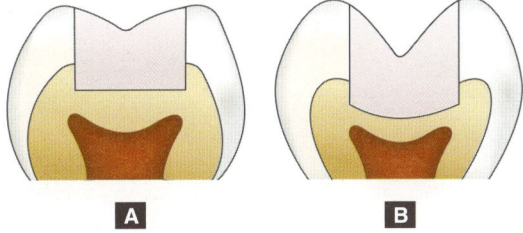

Figs 12.3A and B: (A) Ideal depth for silver amalgam; (B) Modification of pulpal floor when cusps are steep

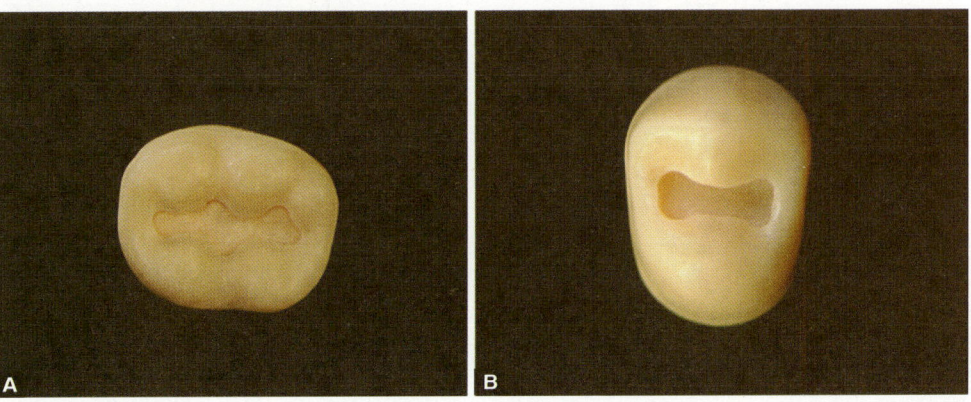

Figs 12.5A and B: (A) Class I cavity preparation in mandibular first molar; (B) Class I cavity preparation in maxillary first premolar

The cavosurface margins are kept at right angle to the cavity walls. This type of butt joint minimizes marginal breakdown of amalgam. No type of bevel or flaring is given, because this produces a feather edge for silver amalgam, which is liable to fracture. However, in teeth with steep cuspal inclines, the butt joint is compromised and the cavosurface margins are kept at an angle less than 90°. The acute angle in such preparation protects the cusps by minimizing the undermining of enamel. The depth of the cavity is placed 0.5 mm below the dentino-enamel junction. This much depth provides bulk of silver amalgam as well as retention because of elasticity of dentin. When the silver is condensed the dentin expands and later contract to make a grip of the restoration. The question arises, if the depth is beneficial both ways (bulk and elasticity of dentin) then why not to extend the cavity 2.0 to 3.0 mm below the dentino-enamel junction. The simple answer is that by doing so the more of dentinal tubules will be in contact with silver amalgam and the alloy being good conductor, leads to sensitivity to hot and cold. It is established that 2.0 to 2.5 mm of remaining dentin is an automatic insulator and the rest can be utilized as an elastic for the benefit of silver amalgam restorations.

The crossing ridges should be preserved as far as possible (transverse ridge and oblique ridge). If the caries involves more than half the planes of these ridges, the total ridge can be involved. Remember loss of crossing ridges is more detrimental for tooth than crossing the marginal ridges.

In cases where the caries or the anatomic contours demand the divergent walls other than mesial and distal marginal ridges, the cavity walls up to dentino-enamel junction is kept parallel and the rest can be divergent. The parallelism in the dentinal walls will provide the requisite resistance and retention form to the restoration.

Many a time, caries extends at one or more points below the otherwise flat pulpal floor. Such carious lesions are either excavated with fine excavators or removed with small round burs. These depressions in the pulpal floor are filled with sedative cement like zinc oxide eugenol or calcium hydroxide. All other features remain the same (Figs 12.6A and B).

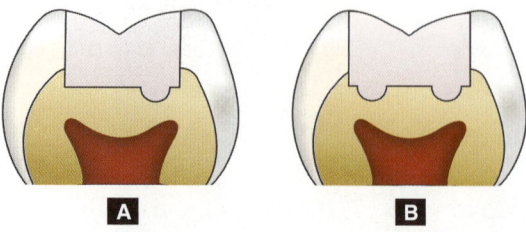

Figs 12.6A and B: **(A)** Localized extension of the cavity at the pulpal floor

Regarding restoration of endodontically treated teeth, the pattern is dictated by the remaining tooth tissue. In case where only the occlusal area is involved, the pulp chamber is cleaned and washed of any remaining root canal filling material. The chamber is filled with bases like zinc oxide eugenol or calcium hydroxide and the pulpal floor is made flat. The undermined carious lesions as well as the undermined enamel rods are removed and the rest of the cavity walls are prepared as described earlier.

B. Cavities on Pits and Fissures on the Occlusal 2/3rd of Buccal and Lingual Surfaces of Posterior Teeth and Lingual Pits of Anterior Teeth

The pits and fissures on the occlusal 2/3rd of the buccal and lingual walls of the posterior teeth can be involved either individually or in association with the pits and fissures on the occlusal surfaces. In case where the pits and fissures of only one surface are involved, facial or lingual, it is necessary to remove the decayed portion and widen it accordingly to remove undermined enamel. The shape is generally oblong or triangular depending upon the extent of caries and the mesiodistal width of the tooth (Figs 12.7 A and B). The walls of the cavity are joined in a continuous fashion. The axial wall is kept flat and the surrounding walls are made slightly convergent towards the cavosurface margins. Preferably the angle between the axial and the surrounding walls is kept acute. The cervical wall is kept following the contour of cemento-enamel function.

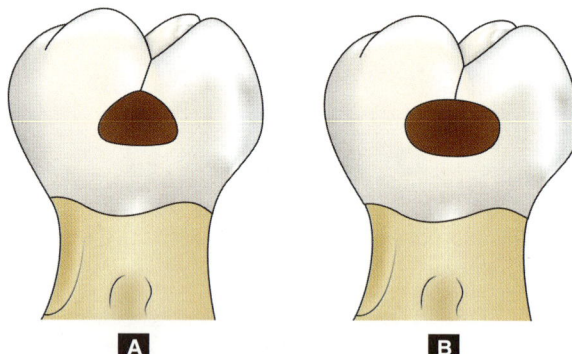

Figs 12.7A and B: (A) Cavities on the buccal pits of posterior teeth: **(A)** Triangular; **(B)** Oblong

Most commonly, the carious lesions at the buccal and lingual sides are connected to the occlusal lesions. This connection may be external or internal. Internal connecting lesions usually undermine the overlying enamel, therefore, have to be involved in cavity preparation.

In such cases, the occlusal portion is prepared as described in Class I. Care is taken to protect the cuspal planes as far as possible, especially, the ones adjacent to the carious grooves., e.g., in case of disto-palatal cusp of maxillary Ist molars, since the cusp is small, the cutting is done more at the expense of the oblique ridge. In case of distal cusp of mandibular first molar, the cutting is done more at the expense of disto-buccal cusp. These precautions will avoid the weakening of cusps.

After preparing the occlusal cavity, keep the straight fissure bur perpendicular to the pulpal floor and move towards the buccal/lingual direction as the caries dictates. Then with the side of tapering fissure bur, the step is prepared, keeping the bur parallel to the buccal/lingual surface of the corresponding grooves (Figs 12.8).

The axial wall so produced will be placed in dentin, 0.5 mm inside the dentino-enamel junction. The gingival wall is made 1.5 mm wide and is extended till termination of the buccal/lingual grooves. The axial and gingival walls of the buccal/lingual box are flattened keeping mesial and distal walls parallel. These two walls, mesial and distal can be kept convergent occlusally in case caries dictates wider gingival walls (Fig. 12.9).

In case where the apical ends of the buccal and lingual grooves are at the same level as the pulpal floor, the buccal/lingual extension will have no steps. Many a times, the pulpal floor can be deeper as compared to the apical end of these grooves, a condition that is called the *reverse step* in the occlusal direction. In these cases, the axial wall is made by the help of base materials as zinc phosphate cement, zinc oxide eugenol and, etc.

The gingival wall in all cases meets the tooth surface at 90° angle. The axial wall makes an obtuse angle with the pulpal floor.

The flat gingival wall along with parallel mesial/distal walls is desirable for proper resistance form. However, for retention form, either occlusal convergence of mesial and distal wall is maintained or retention locks are given. These locks are placed in dentin in both mesio-axial and disto-axial line angles. These locks terminate at the level of pulpal floor.

The cavosurface margins of the box as well as the occlusal cavity are finished with enamel hatchets (Fig. 12.10).

Similarly in case of lingual pits in the anterior teeth, the shape of the cavity can be round or oblong. The depth and walls are kept as in buccal/lingual pit cavity preparation (Fig. 12.11).

Class II (Cavities on the proximal surfaces of posterior teeth)

The carious lesion can be only on proximal side without involving the occlusal area or both occlusal and proximal areas can be involved. The caries on the proximal areas are generally below the contact

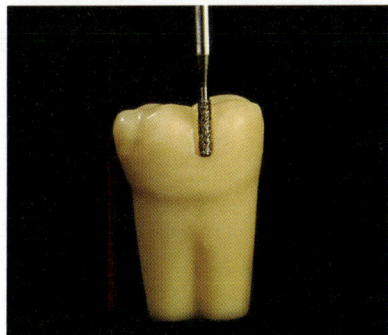

Fig. 12.8: Preparation of lingual wall of Class I buccal complex in mandibular first molar

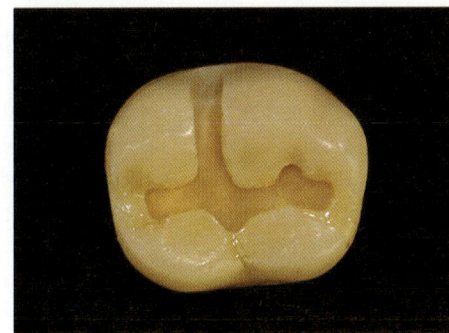

Fig. 12.10: Class I cavity with buccal complex in mandibular first molar

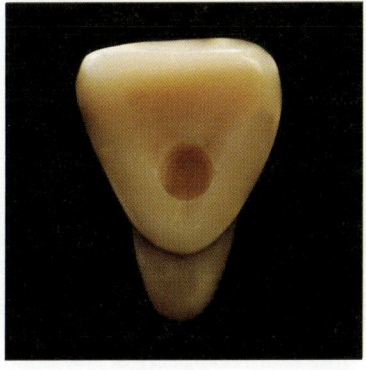

Fig. 12.9: Preparation of mesial and distal walls of buccal complex

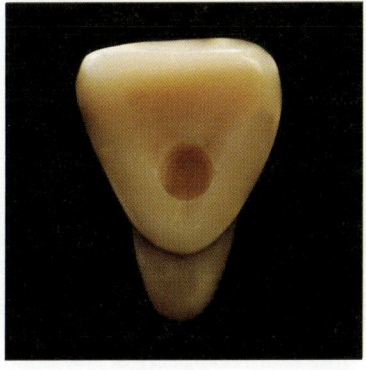

Fig. 12.11: Cavity on the lingual pit of maxillary lateral incisor

point. For gaining access, the occlusal side is to be involved, except in few cases (described later).

The outline form of the occlusal part is the same as described for Class I and the outline form of the proximal box is dictated by various factors viz.:

i. *Extent of caries*: Mostly the caries are around contact areas and the buccal and lingual walls of the proximal box are kept in self-cleansing areas.
ii. *Convexity of the proximal surfaces:* In cases of convex proximal surfaces, the contact area is comparatively smaller and the extension of the cavity preparation will be minimal towards the embrasures.
iii. *Caries and plaque indices*: The more the caries and plaque indices, the more is the need to extend the proximal walls into self-cleansing areas.
iv. *Masticatory loads:* In cases where the masticatory loads are great, the bucco-lingual width of the total preparation is kept minimum possible.

Prepare the occlusal cavity as described earlier, keeping the pulpal floor flat and 0.5 mm into the dentino-enamel junction and maintaining the parallelism of opposing walls. Position the flat fissure bur perpendicular to the pulpal floor and extend towards the marginal ridge of the proximal area to be involved. The flatness of the pulpal floor is maintained at that level too.

The isthmus width should be as narrow as possible and should not be more than 1/4th of intercuspal distance or 1.0-1.5 mm wide.

Hold the bur perpendicular to the pulpal floor and using light motion go deep slightly below the contact point and create a trough. This way, initial axial and gingival walls are created (Figs 12.12A and B). The bur is moved buccally and lingually including the contact area. Care should be taken, if convenient, to leave thin shell of enamel over the preparation to protect the adjacent tooth coming in contact with the bur. Later, this shell can be removed by using enamel hatchets. Alternatively, the adjacent tooth can also be protected by using matrix bands.

The buccal and lingual proximal walls are kept in embrasures and meet the tangent of the respective cavosurface margin at 90° angle (Fig. 12.13).

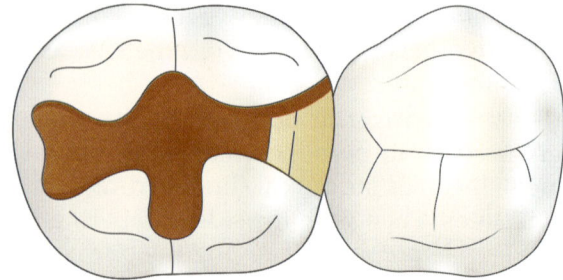

Fig. 12.13: Walls of the proximal box of class II cavity

In case of maxillary teeth, mostly the molars, the contact area is more buccally placed, i.e. the lingual embrasures are larger than the buccal embrasures. In such cases, extending the bucco-proximal wall into the embrasure may lead to excessive cutting of the buccal cusps. To avoid this, a *reverse curve* is made in the buccal proximal wall so as to have sufficient amount of dentin in that area and also to achieve butt joint with the cavosurface margins. This curve is towards the axial wall side and the rest is kept straight. The total wall is not curved, since by doing so the silver amalgam restoration will not be at right angle to the cavosurface margins, thereby weakening the restoration.

Such a curve, though mostly given in maxillary molars, can be given in any tooth where the contact area is deviated or more pronounced on one side.

The marginal trimmers are used to bevel or round off the axio-pulpal line angle. The gingival cavosurface margins are trimmed off of the unsupported enamel. The bucco-gingival and linguo-gingival line angles are also kept rounded (Figs 12.14A and B).

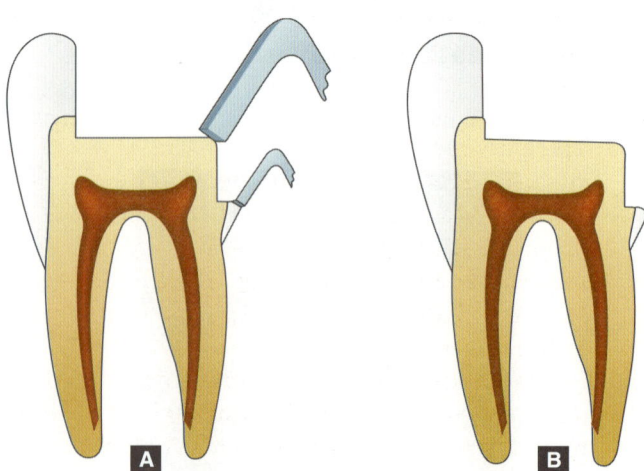

Figs 12.14A and B: (A) Finishing of axiopulpal line angle and gingival cavosurface margin; (B) Finished axiopulpal line angle and gingival cavosurface margin

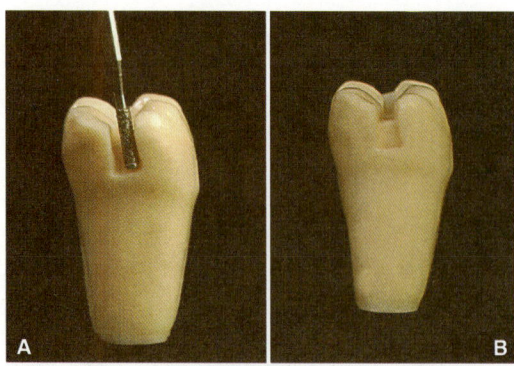

Figs 12.12A and B: Preparation of the buccal and lingual proximal walls of Class II cavity in mandibular first molar

Care is taken to place the gingival wall in enamel involving both enamel and dentin. The approximate width of the gingival wall is 1.0 mm or 1.5 mm, out of which 70% should be in dentin and the rest may be in enamel. The proximal box walls should have sufficient dentin (not less than 0.6 mm) so as to enable the operator to make retentive grooves or locks, if need arises.

In case where the extension of gingival wall is in the cementum, the width of the gingival wall should always be less than 1.0 mm (approximately 0.7-0.8 mm).

The proximal box so formed is wider at the gingival area as compared to the occlusal, i.e. the buccal and lingual walls are converging at the occlusal surfaces. The bucco-lingual width of gingival wall is more than the bucco-lingual width of occlusal area. This type of occlusal convergence contributes to the retention form and the desirable extension of buccal and lingual proximal walls into the embrasure areas facilitates the restoration to be self-cleansing. The marginal ridge is also conserved by keeping the proximal walls convergent occlusally (Figs 12.15A and B).

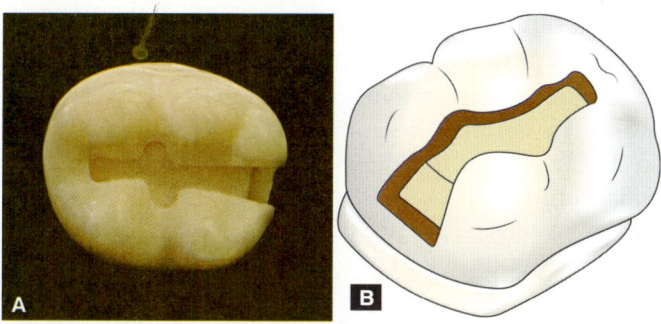

Figs 12.15A and B: Convergent proximal walls conserve marginal ridge

Primary resistance and retention form is achieved by the following features:
- The gingival and pulpal floor is flat and perpendicular to the long axis of the tooth.
- All walls create 90° cavosurface angle for the amalgam.
- The extension of walls is in such a way that the cusps and ridges have sufficient dentin support.
- The internal line angles are rounded off especially the axio pulpal line angle so as to have maximum bulk of silver amalgam at the axiopulpal area and to avoid stress concentration in the tooth.
- Pulpal floor is prepared adequately into the dentin so as to provide sufficient bulk of restorative material. This provides both resistance and retention form.
- Occlusal convergence of the walls provides primary retention form.

Removal of residual caries at the pulpal floor is accomplished in the same way as described for class I cavities.

Similarly, caries in the axial wall does not dictate cutting the entire axial wall towards the pulp. A small round bur is utilized for this purpose. The particular area is filled with calcium hydroxide or zinc oxide eugenol cement.

If remnant of caries is left in the gingival wall, the small portion can be extended cervically with small round burs leaving the other portion intact.

In case residual caries are left in one or both the side walls of the proximal box, i.e. buccal and lingual/proximal walls, then the extension of the walls is permissible keeping in mind the following points:

 i. The extension does not cross the line angle of the tooth.
 ii. The wall is not weakened from inside.
 iii. It does not hinder the support of the amalgam on the gingival wall.
 iv. The extended area remains accessible.

In case all these features are not satisfied and the caries still present, the cuspal coverage can be considered.

Secondary Retentive Devices

Many a times, after the cavity preparation, the final shape lacks the required retention form. The extra retention can be achieved by utilizing one or two extra retentive devices. These devices should be used only in cases where the retention form is not appropriate otherwise. This type of retention form is independent in the occlusal and the proximal areas of the cavity preparation.

The devices used for silver amalgam restorations are:
1. Slots or horizontal grooves
2. Locks or partial vertical grooves

1. Slots or Horizontal Grooves

This is a minor but definite depression in the pulpal and/or gingival wall. Slots are prepared with ¼ or ½ round bur depending upon the width required or available. These are made 0.5 to 1.0 mm deep and 0.2-0.5 mm wide. The slots are always given in dentin. In case of gingival wall the slots are given 0.2 to 0.5 mm inside the dentino-enamel junction depending upon the amount of dentin available. The bucco-lingual width of the slots is generally the bucco-lingual width of the gingival floor or the respective pulpal wall.

2. Locks or Partial Vertical Grooves

The locks are generally prepared in proximal box only. However, in occlusal areas, minor undercuts given by inverted cone bur serve the same purpose.

Locks can be prepared with round bur, inverted cone bur or tapering fissure burs (Figs 12.16A and B). The selection of the diameter of the bur depends upon the required depth of the lock. The greater the width of the proximal box, greater would be the width of the lock.

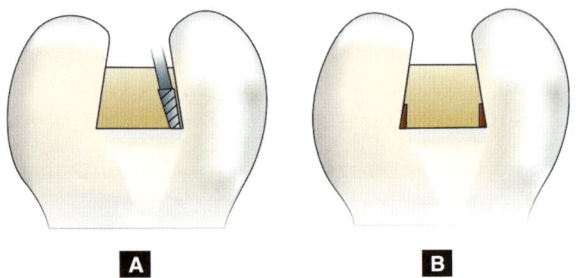

Figs 12.16A and B: Convergent proximal walls conserve marginal ridge

After the selection of the bur, the bur is moved in axio-lingual line angle 0.2-0.5 mm inside the dentino-enamel junction and keeping the pressure both on the lingual and axial side. Remember the pressure should be on both the walls. The pressure only on axial wall can lead to exposure and such a cutting might not aid in retention. This type of deepening usually finishes at axio-pulpal line angle. In case this height is less, the lock can be prepared at the expense of lingual dentin terminating below the dentino-enamel junction occlusally.

Similarly a lock is prepared on the axio-buccal line angle of the opposite side.

Position of axio-buccal and axio-lingual line angle is important prior to placement of locks. In shallow line angles proper amount of dentin is not available and in case of deep line angles, further cutting has the risk of exposure.

Different authors have conflicting studies regarding the use of these proximal locks. Latest studies suggest that with the use of amalgam with a creep value less than 1% the locks are of no use. Most of the high copper alloys available these days have this specified creep value. It has also been established that the marginal extension of amalgams are related to the creep values. Amalgams with higher creep values usually overextend at the margins.

Finally, the enamel margins are finished, making them straight and smooth. The cavosurface angle for silver amalgam should be 90° ± 5°. This type of butt joint between silver and enamel is necessary since silver being brittle, gives way under occlusal stresses at the thinner margins.

The gingival wall is beveled 20° towards the cavosurface margin to ensure full-length enamel rods. This is achieved by using gingival marginal trimmers. Such an angulation or bevel is only given in enamel and if the gingival wall is in cementum, such an angulation or the bevel is not required (*see* Fig. 10.27).

Modification of Class II Cavity (caries involving both proximal sides of posterior teeth)

In case the caries involves both the proximal surfaces; the preparation design is as good as two class II preparations. These two preparations vary only in the proximal box, where the buccal and lingual proximal walls are to include the contact areas. The disto-occlusal area and the distal-proximal box would be little wider than the mesial occlusal area and the mesial proximal box. The union between these two proximal boxes at the occlusal level depends upon following factors:

i. Whether the connecting fissures are carious or not.
ii. The remaining thickness of the oblique ridge should not be less than 1.0 mm in maxillary molars.
iii. The oblique ridge or the transverse ridge is not undermined by caries.

Remember, the occlusal cutting should be precise without involving the cuspal planes. In case, the caries so dictates, the capping of the particular cusp can be considered.

In a few cases, the proximal lesions, whether on one surface or both, may have lesions on the buccal and/ or lingual surfaces. These lesions can be treated separately, if the carious lesions are separate and the marginal ridge areas are not involved. However, if the caries is undermining the marginal ridges or after individual preparation of buccal/lingual lesion, the remaining width is less, the lesions can be joined as described in class I cavities (Figs 12.17 A and B). The position of the pulpal floor, axial wall and the gingival wall is maintained as instructed for such modifications in class I cavities (Fig. 12.18).

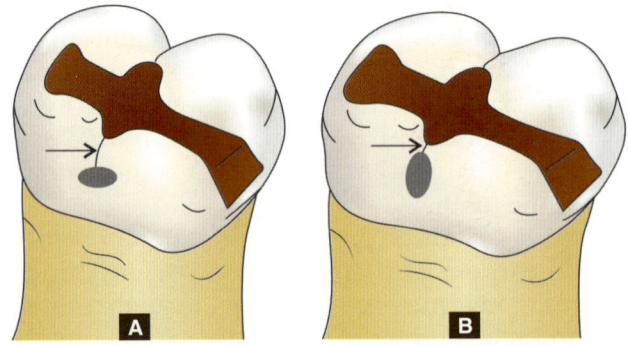

Figs 12.17A and B: Extension of cavity margins towards marginal ridge: **(A)** Adequate marginal ridge; **(B)** Thin marginal ridge – candidate for proximal preparation(→)

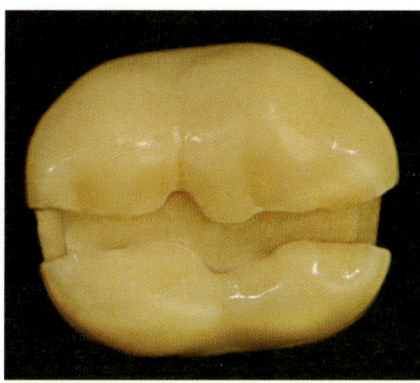

Fig. 12.18: Mesioocclusodistal cavity on mandibular first molar

Occasionally, the proximal lesions are joined or connected to the cervical carious lesions through proximal line angles or from the occlusal portion through buccal and lingual grooves.

In such cases cervical cavity is prepared separately (described later) and proximal lesion is prepared separately. These two are joined cutting the tooth structure in between. Such unions are mostly apical to the contact areas (Fig. 12.19). As regards restoration of such lesions, the cervical portion or the Class V preparation is filled and overfilled proximally with glass-ionomer cements, glass cermets and/or composites depending upon the occluso-cervical height of the lesion. After complete setting, the proximal box of the lesion is reshaped having restorative material at one end. In case both the lesions are to be filled with silver amalgam, first fill cervical lesion as mentioned earlier, over-fill, wait for 24 hours, reshape the proximal box and finally fill silver amalgam in proximal lesion as in routine.

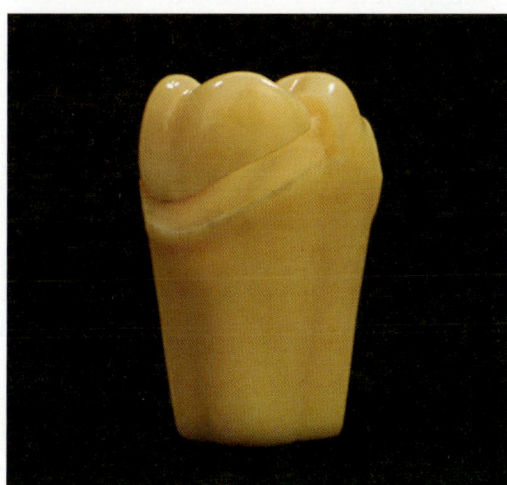

Fig. 12.19: Class II + Class V joined cavity

The extension of proximal box on the buccal and lingual surfaces cervically can be on one side or both sides depending upon the dictates of the caries. The operator has to decide whether to sacrifice the related cusps depending upon the extent of caries undermining these areas. Usually, if the union of proximal box and the buccal/lingual cervical lesion is well above the contact areas, the capping of cusps is considered.

Using enamel hatchets, the cavosurface margins are finished to achieve butt joint between the tooth and the silver amalgam.

Class III (Cavities involving the proximal surface of anterior teeth without involving the incisal edges or the contact points)

Mostly the distal surfaces of canines are the only lesions among anterior teeth which are filled with silver amalgam. The incisors and the mesial surfaces of canines are not restored with silver amalgam because of esthetic reasons.

Resins are usually avoided in the canines because the teeth are subjected to all three types of forces, i.e. compressive, tensile and shear. These teeth are also subjected to forces during protrusive, and lateral movements. The anterior component of forces is resisted by the distal surfaces of canines. Because of its position in the arch, all these forces, lead to continuous rubbing action of the distal side of the tooth. That is why the resin restorations because of their poor wear resistance may wear off easily. However, in certain conditions resin restorations become necessary such as:

i. Caries involving the labial side or the incisal edges of the canines.
ii. The removal of caries will leave very thin enamel covering labially and the amalgam will shine from within.
iii. Esthetically over conscious patients.

The outline of cavity is planned in such a way so that minimal cavity cutting may be performed. A small round bur, No. ½ or 1 is used to enter the carious lesion from the marginal ridge lingually. The direction of the bur is maintained perpendicular to the lingual surface of the tooth. The bur is moved 0.5 mm inside the dentino-enamel junction. The labial wall should have intact enamel as far as possible. With an inverted cone bur, the incisal and gingival walls are smoothened (Fig. 12.20). The lingual outline in such cavity preparation blends with the incisal and gingival margins, creating a cavity preparation without lingual proximal wall (Fig. 12.21).

In many cases, this much outline does not suffice for proper retention form and the preparation is extended lingually to create a lingual lock. With the same inverted cone bur or small flat fissure bur, the lingual portion is extended incisally as well gingivally. The lingual extension in no case is extended beyond

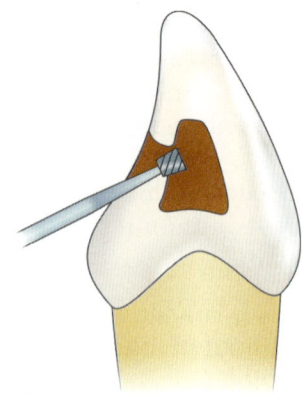

Fig. 12.20: Smoothening of cavity walls

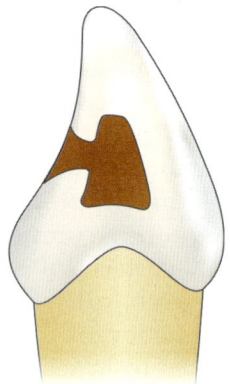

Fig. 12.21: Class III cavity without lingual proximal wall

the imaginary half of the lingual surface. The isthmus between the lingual and proximal preparation is kept approximately 1.5 mm.

All cavosurface angles are at 90° to the margins. The labial, incisal and gingival walls should meet the axial wall at right angle. The lingual wall, if present, may be making an obtuse angle with the axial wall (Figs 12.22A and B).

Preferably the contact point is not disturbed, until and unless dictated by caries. The drifting of canines

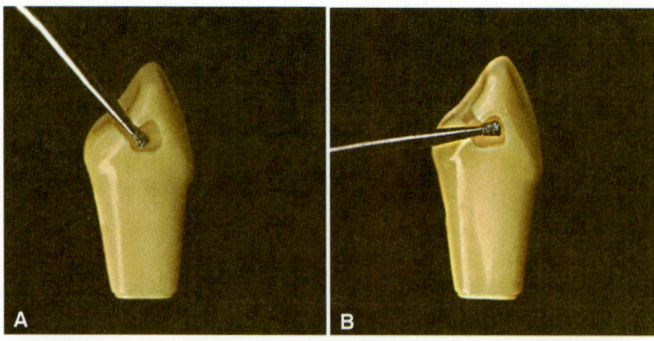

Figs 12.22A and B: (A) Gingival preparation for amalgam in Class III cavity on distal side of maxillary canine; (B) Labial wall preparation for amalgam in class III cavity on distal side of maxillary canine

distally is very common; therefore, proper contact will prevent or minimize the movement of the tooth.

Resistance form is provided by:
  i. Cavosurface angles of 90°
  ii. Definite internal line angles
  iii. Sufficient bulk of the material, i.e. adequate depth

Retention form is provided by preparing a gingival and incisal groove or undercut (Figs 12.23A and B). The gingival groove is placed at the axio-gingival line angle using small round or inverted cone bur. The bur is directed gingivally and pulpally. The groove is usually 0.2 mm wide and in dentin only.

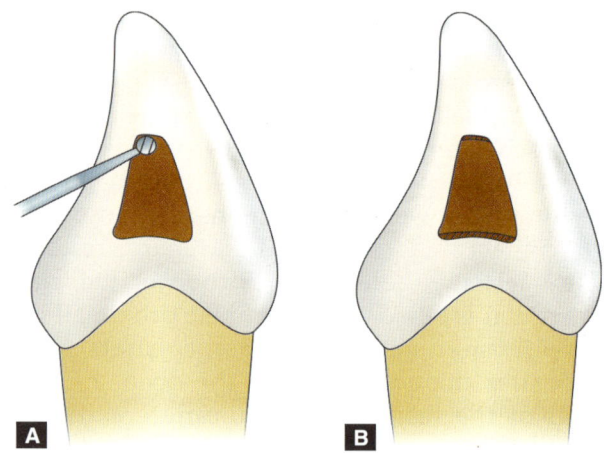

Figs 12.23A and B: Incisal and gingival undercut/groove

Care is taken not to place the groove entirely in the axial wall as it may lead to pulp exposure and also such grooves are less retentive.

Similarly the incisal groove is prepared in the inciso-axial line angle or inciso-axio-labial point angle as the shape of cavity dictates. A small round bur or inverted cone bur is utilized for the purpose as described for gingival groove.

If the incisal wall is not bulky enough to accommodate a retentive groove without undermining the distal slope it may be replaced mainly by a labial and to a lesser extent lingual groove. In case sufficient labial and lingual walls are not present, it is essential to create short walls by deepening the axial walls and pronouncing the axio-labial and axio-lingual line angles.

Such grooves can also be placed on the lingual extensions (lingual dove tail) of the preparation for added retention (Fig. 12.24). Finally the cavity margins are smoothened to have 90° cavosurface margin.

Modification of Class III (Caries involving both the proximal surfaces of anterior teeth)

If the caries are present on both the proximal walls of anterior teeth, the restoration with silver amalgam is

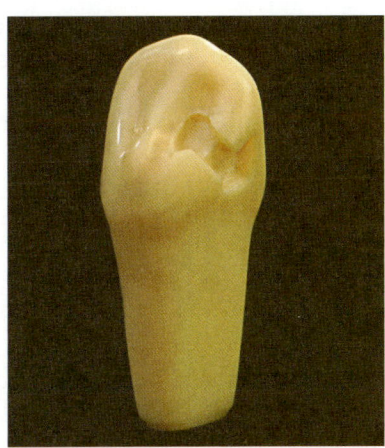

Fig. 12.24: Lingual dove-tail preparation for class III cavity preparation

not indicated mainly because of esthetics. However, the cavity preparation is same as described for Class III, i.e. two proximal cavities will be prepared. Such cavities are generally united on the lingual side. The two lingual dovetails of individual cavities can be made separately if width of the intervening ridge is at least 1.0 mm.

Rest all other features viz. angulation of walls, line angles, grooves, etc. are as described earlier.

Class IV (cavities involving proximal surfaces of anterior teeth with involving the incisal edges or contact points)

Silver amalgam is not indicated in class IV cavities because of its poor edge strength and also poor esthetics.

Class V (Caries on the cervical one third of labial/lingual surfaces of all the teeth)

Caries or defects on the cervical areas of teeth are more cumbersome to prepare and restore. The incipient lesions are often overlooked and difficult to diagnose since the lesion might be under the gingival tissues. Abrasion and erosion lesions are also very common in these areas. These lesions can be entirely in cementum or partially in enamel and cementum.
The selection of the material in these areas depends upon the esthetics as well as the caries index of the patient. These lesions need immediate care since these areas become sensitive very soon and also the deeper lesions would weaken the tooth. By and large, the labial and lingual surfaces of posterior teeth can be restored with silver amalgam while the labial surfaces of anterior teeth can be restored with composite resins.

These restorations, though thought to be free of physical stresses, are subjected to these stresses during protrusive and lateral movement of the mandible. These types of forces tend to dislodge the restoration buccally and create a minor gap at the occlusal/cervical surface of the restoration.

This gap is very mild and usually creates no problem. However, with repeated movements the restoration may get dislodged. These factors should be kept in mind while preparing the cavity.

Cavity Preparation

A flat fissure bur of appropriate size is used to enter the centre of the lesion at the depth of 0.5 mm inside the dentino-enamel junction. By keeping the bur perpendicular to the long axis of the tooth, the bur is directed mesially and distally and then occlusally and gingivally (Fig. 12.25). The mesial and distal extension of the preparation should be upto the line angles of the tooth until and unless the extension beyond the line angles is dictated by caries. The gingival wall is contoured according to the cemento-enamel junction and the occlusal wall is, by and large, straight. The axial wall is also contoured mesio-distally following the outer contour of the tooth. The depth of the gingival wall is usually 0.75 mm and the occlusal wall is 1.25 mm.

All the four walls of cavity preparation, i.e. mesial, distal, occlusal and gingival diverge outward. The gingival wall, if placed in cementum is kept straight. A small round bur (No. ¼ or ½) or inverted cone bur is used to prepare the retention grooves, one in axio-occlusal line angle directing occlusally and the other in axio-gingival line angle directing gingivally (Figs 12.26A and B).

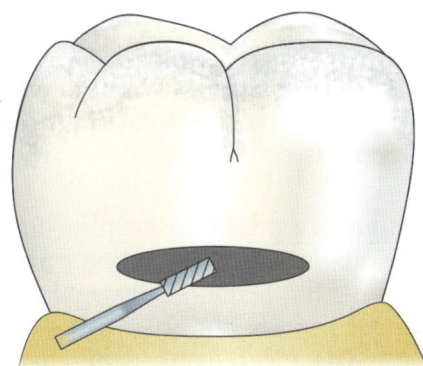

Fig. 12.25: Entry into the lesion with fissure bur

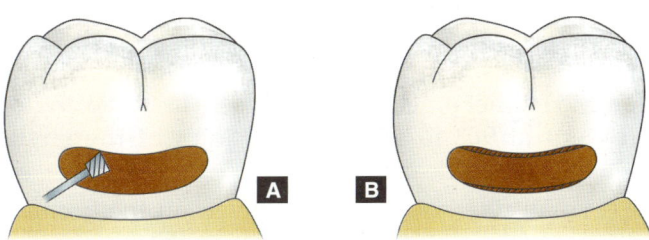

Figs 12.26A and B: (A) Bur directed occlusally; (B) Completed

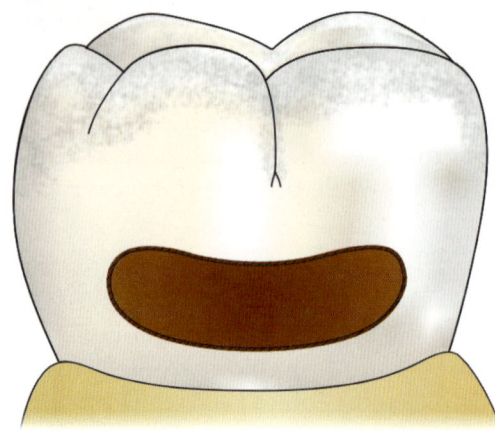

Fig. 12.27: Groove given all around the four walls of the cavity

In rare cases, if the cavity is extensive, the groove can be given all around the four walls of the cavity (Fig. 12.27).

The axial wall and the outer walls are finished with the help of the sharp chisel. The cavosurface margins are kept at 90° for the proper resistance form.

In rare instances the cervical lesions are extended occlusally on the side walls. This extension can be on one side or both the sides depending upon the extent of caries. The cavity preparation remains the same, with the extension of the occlusal wall on that particular side occlusally crossing the height of contour of that side of the tooth. The finishing of enamel margins is carried out as described earlier.

Modification of Class V (Cavities on the line angles of the posterior teeth, both lingual and buccal surfaces)

This type of lesion or cavity preparation was not included in Black's classification, though the operative dentist is confronted with such lesions in routine.

These lesions are prepared keeping in mind the extent of carious lesion. The outline form depends upon the size of the lesion. The usual form of the cavity outline is rounded or oblong and is prepared as described in Class V, the only difference being the location.

A tapering fissure bur can be utilized for gaining access into the centre of the lesion and extended all along to create a round or oblong shape as dictated by the caries. The depth is kept 0.5 mm into the dentinoenamel junction. The cavosurface line angles are kept at 90° to achieve butt joint of the silver amalgam with the cavity walls.

A small retentive groove is given on the occlusal and gingival wall of the preparation with ¼ or ½ round bur to achieve retention form wherever necessary.

A small chisel is used to finish the enamel and the axial wall.

Class VI (Cavities on the incisal edges and cusp tips)

The lesions on the incisal edges are usually not restored with silver amalgam, hence not discussed here.

The cusp tip may be carious or hypoplastic and can be restored with silver amalgam.

The centre of lesions is penetrated with small tapering fissure bur and extended all around to involve the caries. The depth is usually inside the dentin and the walls should have definite dentin support. A 90° cavosurface angle is usually given and if the cuspal planes are steeper, the cavosurface angle can be modified accordingly. A small retentive groove using ¼ round bur or inverted cone bur can be given all around the internal line angle. The shape of the cavity is usually round.

CONSERVATIVE CAVITY PREPARATION

For a long time, Black's principles of cavity preparation, by and large, were accepted by everyone in the profession. Summarily Black's cavity preparation includes:

i. Concept of extension for prevention, i.e. to involve even the non-carious pits and fissures.
ii. Wide occlusal isthmus, i.e. 1/3rd of the intercuspal distance.
iii. Extension of buccal and lingual proximal walls to self-cleansing areas.
iv. Sharp internal line angles.
v. Placement of gingival wall below the free margins of gingiva.

It was as early as in 1920, Prime reported that *the time has come to adapt the filling materials to the requirement of the tooth rather than force the tooth to meet the requirements of the filling material.*

As the cavities generally increase in size when the restorations are replaced, consequently weakening the tooth; therefore, it is emphasized to keep the cavity cutting as minimal as possible. The researchers favouring conservative cavity preparation, in no way defy Black's principles; they only favour modifications, keeping in mind:

- Advancements in understanding of dynamism of caries.
- Potential of preventive measures being effective.
- Advancements in restorative materials and techniques.

The area, which requires immediate attention, is the *'Outline form'* of Black's cavity preparation, which includes the concept of *'Extension for prevention'*. With the advent of adhesive restorative materials, the overzealous removal of tooth structure can be avoided.

Another feature, which is also controversial, is the extension of cavity into the dentino-enamel junction. Various authors are of the view that until and unless dictated by caries, the cutting into dentin is not required.

Preparation of cavities only in enamel: One school of thought regarding conservative cavity preparation is to prepare the cavity only in enamel when the caries has not reached dentin. The usual thickness of enamel at the occlusal areas is 1.5 mm and the depth of the cavity can be kept 1.0 mm. The width of the cavity is approximately that of width of number one flat fissure bur, i.e. less than 1.0 mm. The direction of the enamel rods is such that the depth of cavity only in enamel can withstand the forces of mastication.

An ultra small undercut is given at the base of the cavity for retention (Figs 12.28A and B). The usual sites for undercuts are where the enamel rods are mostly inclined inwards. A mini condenser (0.7 mm diameter) is used to condense the silver amalgam into the cavity. The carving mostly is not required, however the excess of amalgam is removed from the cavosurface margins. The restoration is finished and polished in routine.

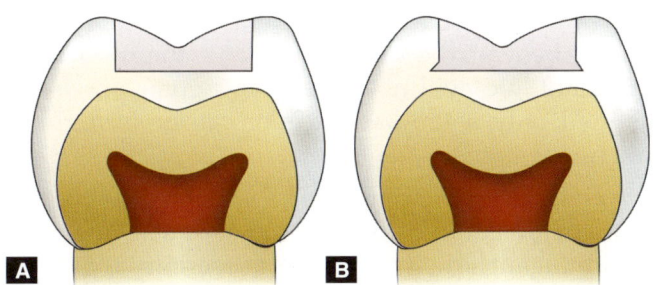

Figs 12.28A and B: Cavity preparation only in enamel: **(A)** No undercut; **(B)** Undercut

The proposed cavity has the following advantages:
  i. Painless cavity preparation
  ii. Since minimum tooth substance is sacrificed, the strength of the tooth is maintained
  iii. Since the width of the cavity is small, the chances of marginal breakdown are less
  iv. Less time consuming
  v. Economical

The feature *'extension of proximal walls into self cleansing areas'* is also questionable. The gingival sulcus is not bacteria free as established earlier. Any restoration, which can be polished, is self-cleansable; therefore, extension of these walls into the embrasure is not required.

The width of occlusal outline is narrowed to 1.0 mm or even less. A wider occlusal cavity preparation as advocated by Black may weaken the tooth and lead to cuspal fracture. *Vale* concluded that reduction of intercuspal distance from 1/3rd to 1/4th resulted in greater strength in the prepared tooth.

Another principle of conservative amalgam restoration is that each half of the restoration, i.e. proximal half and the occlusal half should be self retentive. The proximal part can be retained by buccal and lingual retention locks, while the occlusal part by converging walls occlusally. With the exception of the gingivo axial line angle, none of the internal line angles in the conservative amalgam need be sharp. The rounded line angles help in dissipation of the forces equally and smoothly. Access in the proximal area without involvement of the occlusal area should be through the marginal ridge and a box type preparation is made along with retentive locks. The authors who are not in favour of placing locks explain that in case of locks and undercuts, the silver cannot expand uniformly. The expanding amalgam is forced against the elastic dentin resulting in pressure on the dental pulp causing pain. Moist amalgams can expand up to 300–400 µ/cm, although 3–13 µ/cm is the acceptable expansion limit for amalgam. They are of the view that extra retention is not required in silver amalgam restorations.

Another conservative cavity preparation, which was designed with an idea to preserve the marginal ridge, is the *'tunnel restoration'*. Though mainly used with glass-ionomer cement, it has also been tried with silver amalgam restoration (Refer chapter No. 19). It may be used on a tooth with a carious lesion only on the proximal side and not involving the occlusal side. The access is gained through the mesial or distal pit depending upon the side involved. Prior to cavity preparation, the adjacent tooth is protected using the matrix bands. Starting at the concerned pit and by moving the small round bur directing approximately at 45°, pierce under the marginal ridge towards the proximal carious lesion. Once the lesion is approached, the access can be slightly widened using tapering fissure burs. The carious lesion is thoroughly excavated with round burs, moving the bur in occlusal and gingival directions. Till the completion of the cavity preparation, the band is to be kept intact so as not to injure the adjacent tooth.

The *advantages* of the tunnel restorations are:
- Marginal ridge is retained and maintains the strength of the tooth
- A normal contact area is maintained
- Risk of overhangs is minimum

The clinical durability and success of tunnel restorations has not been documented properly. On an average 10–20% failure rates have been observed.

Many authors have reported no improvement in maintenance of strength of the tooth and also the complete excavation of caries is difficult with these restorations.

MINIMAL INTERVENTION DENTISTRY

It has been established that extra tooth structure is lost with replacement of restoration each time. The so called *'replacement dentistry'* leads to weakening of tooth structure and eventually total loss of tooth. With the advent of adhesive restorative materials coupled with increased knowledge of dynamism of caries activity, the concept of *'minimal intervention'* cavity preparation has evolved. The treatment of caries is preferably done by biological approach, rather than surgical means. The recent adhesive restorative materials prevent microleakage and also, to some extent, reinforce the remaining tooth crown. Traditionally, failed restorations have been totally replaced but recent thrust is to adopt *'repair'* approach, consequently preserving the tooth structure. Ever since Levine proposed the theory of *'ionic see-saw'* mechanism in caries etiology, it is now well recognized that the enamel/dentin demineralization is not a continuous irreversible process. Depending upon the environment there is demineralization/ remineralization cycle in which the tooth structure alternatively loses and gains calcium and phosphorous ions. Because of lower pH, demineralization occurs and as the pH rises, remineralization starts.

Generally the rate of caries progression is slow except in few individuals. This progression is much slower in individuals drinking fluoridated water. This time lapse is crucial for the *'biological'* management of caries. There are two basic elements of biological approach; alternation of oral environment in order to minimize demineralization and application of external agents to stimulate remineralization. The operative intervention is delayed as far as possible; however, the individual is kept under observation regarding progress of caries.

The application of all these concepts is the basic principles of *'minimal intervention dentistry'*. Summarily, the principles are:
- Remineralization of early lesions
- Arresting active lesions
- Minimum surgical intervention
- Repair rather than replacement
- Changing the oral environment

REPAIR OF DEFECTIVE RESTORATION

Replacement of existing restoration after few years of service is a common practice, may be because of secondary caries, fracture, marginal ditching and, etc. It has been reported that on an average 50–75% restorations are replaced within five years. Replacement of old restorations, as said earlier, always leads to increase in surface area of the cavity. This increase is much more pronounced in resin restorations. The increased surface area every time tends to make more complex form of restoration. To avoid this, *'repair'* of the existing restorations are being tried. The repair should maintain the strength of the tooth and also does not compromise with the retention of both new and old restorations.

The success of repair mainly depends upon isolating the low caries risk patients from high-risk patients. Proper diagnosis of secondary caries and its extension to pulpal wall is important before repair process is started. The decision is quite complicated and depends upon various factors such as patients risk for caries, professional judgement of the extent of damage and the conservative approach of the repair.

For a small localized marginal defect, recontouring and repolishing should be the first choice. This is more favourably indicated in amalgam restorations. Application of sealant around the defective margins can also improve the life span of the old restorations. However in high caries risk patients the caries usually extends beneath the restoration, hence the application of sealant, etc. will not be useful. Repair process is justified only if the patient is or can be brought to low caries status.

Amalgam restorations are repaired by cutting the required defect and making the area self-retentive. The amalgam side is wetted with mercury rich layer and the rest is condensed with conventional amalgam. Many authors do not advocate wetting the restoration because of mercury vapours. It has also been reported that the total strength is decreased by 50% in such restorations. Recently *'bonded amalgam restorations'* are showing promising results. Bonding agent is applied on all the surfaces and the defect is restored with amalgam.

Repair with composite resin restorations are little difficult. The surface of the composite layer left is micro etched and a layer of bonding agent is applied and restored in routine. The process of micro etching requires an instrument specially designed for the purpose. Recently the defect is restored with glass-ionomer cements taking advantage of reliable adhesion and the fluoride release.

The repair process can be beneficial; however, the long-term success of the repair may depend upon the patient being shifted to low caries risk status.

MANIPULATION OF SILVER AMALGAM

The manipulation of amalgam involves many variables. A successful amalgam restoration should be based on following sequence of events.

Selection of Material

The selection criteria for an alloy for amalgam restoration are extensive. The operator has plenty of options to choose from. The following features are considered:

a. *Type of alloy*: Among the various types of alloys available, the choice depends on the properties and their composition like:
   - Size and shape of particles: these dictate the amount of mercury required.
   - Alloys containing zinc or without zinc
   - Percentage of copper in given alloy, i.e. high copper (>13%) and low copper (<6%)
b. *Anatomic position of restoration*: For restoration subjected to heavy occlusal forces, an amalgam with high resistance to marginal fracture is desirable.
c. *Operator's skill and armamentarium*: The operator's ability to isolate the tooth completely shall determine the choice between zinc containing or zinc free alloys. And also whether the operator has mechanical condenser and triturator or not.
d. *Early disposal of patient*: The mentally retarded patients and patients with heart diseases should be disposed off early and in such cases quickly setting type of alloy is required.
e. *Extent of the cavity*: Wider cavities have more chances of deterioration, so alloys with very low creep values are required for such cases.

Proportioning of Alloy and Mercury

Alloy/mercury ratio is an important variable for successful manipulation. Mercury must wet the alloy particles before two components can react. The wetting, however, is dependent on a number of factors like alloy composition, surface condition, particle size and shape. As these properties are different for different alloys, so manufacturer's recommendation of mercury and alloy ratio should be followed. The more quantity of mercury is generally required with hand mixing while low quantity of mercury is required for mechanical mixing. The spherical particles require less mercury (40%) as compared to lathe cut particles (45%). For optimum properties the final mass should contain less than 50% mercury. In routine, alloy/ mercury ratio is kept as 5:8 or 5:7, although *Eames* has preferred 1:1 ratio. If extra mercury is taken, there will be more chances of formation of weaker γ_2 phase and if less mercury is taken, it might not sufficiently wet the alloy particles leading to porous amalgam.

Dispensing of Alloy and Mercury

The alloy can be dispensed either by weight or by volume. Volumetric dispensing is accurate if manufacturer's instructions are followed properly.

Mercury is commonly dispensed by volume. Bottle should be held vertically and kept at least half full to ensure uniform spills.

Semi automatic dispensers are commonly employed which also carry out trituration. These dispensers have two containers containing alloy and mercury. The ratio is set by the operator. On pressing the button given amount of mercury and alloy is released. In case of large cavities, button can be pressed twice.

Another method used these days is the use of encapsulated alloy/mercury material. The required proportion of alloy and mercury is separated by a thin membrane. In a mechanical mixer, the membrane is broken as the mixer starts vibrating.

Trituration

The process of mixing of alloy with mercury is called trituration. Trituration can be carried out by hand or by mechanical amalgamators. Hand trituration is performed in glass mortar and pestle, preferably with a roughened surface. Mechanical mixing is carried out in semi automatic or fully automatic amalgamator.

The following factors control the quality of trituration:

a. Time
b. Speed
c. Force

a. *The time* of trituration varies from 6 to 20 seconds and even it can be 40 seconds. The time varies corresponding the following features:
   - It is higher for spherical low copper alloys and less for spherical high copper alloys.
   - Types of amalgamators.
   - Pestles of different weight and size.
   - Various sizes of mix viz. increasing the size of the mix increases the mixing time.
b. *The speed* mostly depends upon the unit. In case of mechanical amalgamators, the speed is set by the manufacturer. With time and use, the amalgamator becomes worn, thus speed is altered and leads to altered degree of trituration. In hand mixing the speed varies from operator to operator.

c. **The force** applied during mechanical amalgamation is a function of:
- Weight of pestle (more weight more is force)
- Size of capsule (bigger size of capsule so longer pestle required).
- The design of the pestle.

In hand trituration, forces are variable. Even the two mixes produced by the same operator vary considerably. Excessive force during trituration may lead to splintering of alloy particles leading to weak matrix. During trituration, the operator should take the following precautions:
- The mortar should be rested on a firm base
- Uniform pressure should be applied.
- Time should be well controlled.
- The surface texture of pestle and mortar should be rough.

This is done to produce enough friction so as to remove oxide layer of alloy particles and to ensure proper coating of alloy particles with mercury.

When more mass of amalgam is required for a given restoration, then a double mix should be used (about 800 mg of alloy mixed with mercury at one time).

When less mass of amalgam is required, then a single mix should be used (about 600 mg of alloy mixed with mercury) and unused sacrificed. But if mixes are oversized/undersized as compared to the containers in which they are mixed, proper amalgamation may not take place leading to inferior mix.

Following trituration, the consistency of the mix can be normal or it can be under mix or over mix.

The *normal mix* consistency is convenient to handle, shiny in appearance, warm, homogenous and has good strength.

The *over mix* consistency is soupy, can't be held in a form, difficult to remove from the capsule and pestle and has low strength.

The *under mix* consistency is dry and crumbly, dull in appearance and inconvenient to manipulate during insertion.

The **mechanical amalgamator** offers following advantages:
i. Mix is uniform.
ii. Trituration time is less.
iii. No need to squeeze excess of mercury, since the alloy/mercury ratio is proportioned by the manufacturer.
iv. Reduces the risk of environmental mercury contamination.

Mulling

It is the process by which the mix is given a cohesive form. After hand trituration mulling is carried out by taking mix in hand and rubbing between fingers.

After mechanical trituration, mulling is done by rotating the mix in a pestle free capsule. It gives mix a cohesive form.

After mulling, the mass is taken in a muslin cloth and squeezed properly to remove excess mercury especially in hand trituration. This squeezing should not be performed in an open environment of clinic as it can lead to increased mercury vapour content in the atmosphere.

It has been seen that even non γ_2 amalgams are not completely free of γ_2 phase. The reason behind this is the presence of residual mercury content.

The residual mercury content affects the various properties as:

a. Strength: 1.0% increase of residual mercury content corresponds to 1.0% decrease in compressive strength.
b. Dimensional Change: If residual mercury contents increase more than 55 wt%, then hardening expansion dramatically increases.
c. Increased creep rate.

Condensation

Condensation is a process by which the mix is compacted into the prepared cavity to attain a dense mass.

Aims

a. Helps in development of a continuous matrix.
b. Helps in removal of excess of mercury, minimizing porosity.
c. Proper adaptation of the material to all parts of the cavity walls.
d. Better adaptation of the incremental layers of amalgam.

Operator should condense the mass as early as possible after tritutration. If the time lapse between trituration and condensation is more than 3 to 4 minutes, then the mix should be discarded. Within this time the setting reaction partially hardens the mass and it will not be condensed properly.

Types of Condensation: There are three types of condensation:
a. Hand condensation
b. Mechanical condensation
c. Ultrasonic condensation

A. Hand Condensation

Hand condensation is carried out by hand instruments (Figs 12.29 and 12.30). Various types of condensers are available to suit the operator and cavity configuration. Factors regulating it are pressure, direction of condensation and the size of increment used.

$$\text{Pressure 'P'} = \frac{\text{Force}}{\text{Area of cross-section}}$$

Thus, increasing the area of condensation decreases the amount of pressure acting at the bottom of the condenser. The condensation should preferably start from center to periphery.

The increments should be small at one time. Large bulk of increments leads to air entrapment and leads to a porous and a weak restoration (Figs 12.31A and B). The cavity is overfilled slightly, which help in burnishing and carving (Fig. 12.31C).

Condensation pressure in the range of 4 to 8 lb is regarded as most appropriate. If the forces of condensation are unduly increased, then the mass of amalgam under condenser goes along with the packing instrument rather than being adequately condensed.

Various studies have indicated that use of extremely high condensation pressure substantially

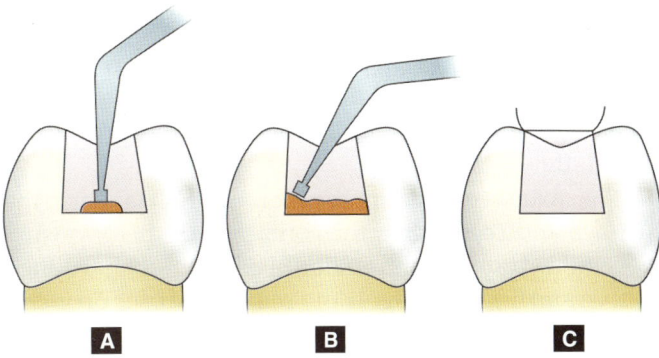

Figs 12.31A to C: (A) Condensation of silver amalgam at the centre; (B) Condensation of silver amalgam at the periphery; (C) Overfilled cavity

reduces the residual mercury content but there seemed to be no correlation between strength and residual mercury content when it was within the range of 45 to 53%. However, once the concentration level reaches more than 53%, the compressive strength is impaired.

Higher condensation pressure leads to close packing of the mass, so the residual mercury rises on the surface, which can be removed during burnishing and carving.

After proper condensation the surface of restoration becomes shiny. This is due to accumulation of residual mercury at the surface of restoration.

Should condensers be smooth or serrated, remained controversial. Authors favouring serrated condensers are of the view that serrations make the surface of increment rough so that when next increment is added, mechanical bonding would take place. Authors favouring smooth condensers are of the view that mechanical retention is of least importance in packing various increments of amalgam mix because bonding occurs due to residual mercury which occurs at the surface of each increment.

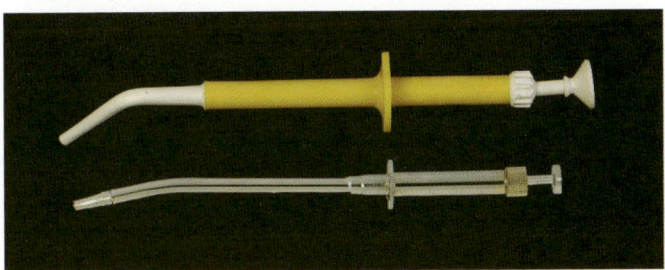

Fig. 12.29: Various types of amalgam carrier

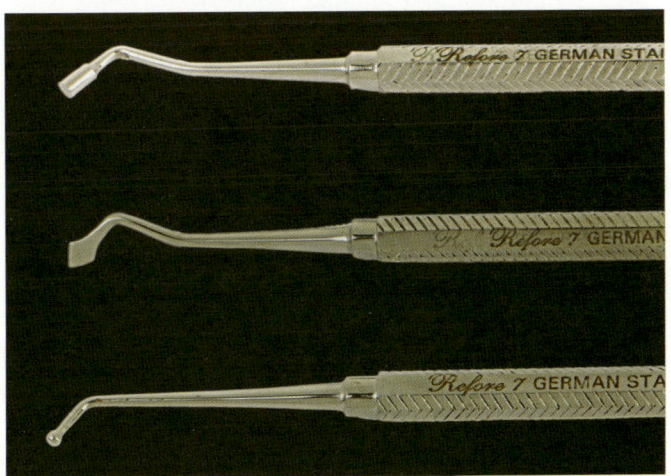

Fig. 12.30: Amalgam condenser, carver and burnisher

B. Mechanical Condensation

Mechanical condensing instrument or tools of various shapes and sizes are available. Usually the mechanical tools apply high loads, which may damage the tooth and even lead to cuspal fracture.

C. Ultrasonic Condensation

Ultrasonic condensers are usually not recommended because these produce local heating of amalgam leading to release of mercury.

Proper isolation measures should be taken during condensation as moisture contamination may lead to:

    i. Delayed expansion of zinc alloys
    ii. Improper adhesion between various increments.

Finishing and Carving

Initial finishing and carving is carried out to produce/simulate functional anatomy of the restoration. After establishing proper anatomy, the carving procedure is initiated.

The objective is to remove mercury rich layer on the surface and reestablish the contact with the opposing dentition. The alloy mass should be properly hardened before starting carving. If the mass is not set properly or is still plastic, then initiation of carving leads to pulling out of amalgam from the margins.

In case the mass is hardened completely, the carving will be very difficult.

When scraping silver amalgam with carver, a "ringing sound" appears or heard that is taken as a guide for appropriate time of carving.

Carving should be carried out by keeping half of the blade of carver on tooth structure and half on restoration following the incline plane of each cusp.

Burnishing is a process in which a smooth, rigid instrument is used for smoothening restoration surface which has become rough by carving. There are conflicting views as to what should be carried out first, carving or burnishing.

If carving is done before burnishing, the effect of carving is lost. If burnishing is done before carving, then the carving leads to production of rough surfaces.

This has led to the concept of pre-carve and post-carve burnishing.

Pre-carve burnishing is carried out before carving, which provide smooth margins and shapes the contours and curvatures (Fig. 12.32).

Post-carve burnishing: After carving, the rough surface so produced is smoothened by final burnishing. At this stage, the mass is hard/set enough to prevent any disturbance of anatomy formed by carving.

Final smoothening can be done by rubbing the surface with moist cotton pellet.

Final polishing is delayed until 24 hours so that the setting reaction has completed.

FAILURES OF DENTAL AMALGAM

A wise man once said – *"In the wide arena of the world, failure and success are not accidents as we so frequently suppose, but the strict justice of nature. If you sincerely do your work, you are certain to get reward – in praise or padding, whichever happens to suit your taste."*

Dental amalgam is one of the most frequently used restorative materials for restoration of posterior teeth. In routine properly restored silver amalgam may not last for more than ten years. Early restored teeth appear excellent but gradually peculiar things begin to happen altering the technical details of the restoration. These may lead to fracture of restoration, tooth fracture, recurrent caries, corrosion, loss of restoration, etc.

On the basis of specifications that have been established by the *National Bureau of Standards*, there are little chances of the manufacturers selling inferior dental alloys; hence the observed amalgam failures are most likely because of factors other than the material itself. The success of the amalgam restoration depends upon the control and attention to many variables. Everything that is done, from the time of cavity preparation until the restoration is polished, has a definite effect upon the success and failure of the restoration.

The different types of failure (Figs 12.33A to D) in an amalgam restoration are:

- At visual level
  - Secondary caries
  - Marginal fracture
  - Bulk fracture
  - Tooth fracture
  - Dimensional change
- At the microstructural level
  - Corrosion and tarnish
  - Stresses associated with masticatory forces
- Pain following amalgam restoration
- Pulp and/or periodontal involvement

Failures in an amalgam restoration can be studied in detail under three main headings:

  I. Failures due to faulty cavity preparation
  II. Failures due to poor matrix adaptation
  III. Failures due to faulty amalgam manipulation

Faulty Cavity Preparation

Most clinical studies that have evaluated causes of failure in amalgam restorations have concluded that

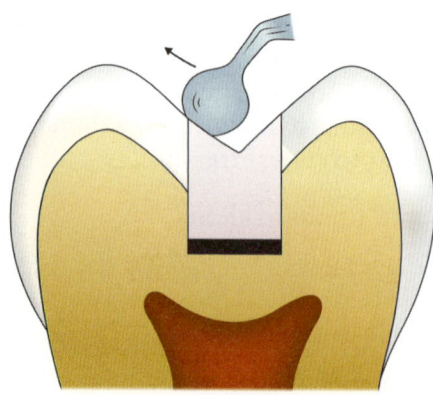

Fig. 12.32: Precarve burnishing helps in removing excessive mercury from overpacked amalgam. Always move ball burnisher from central groove to the margin using firm pressure

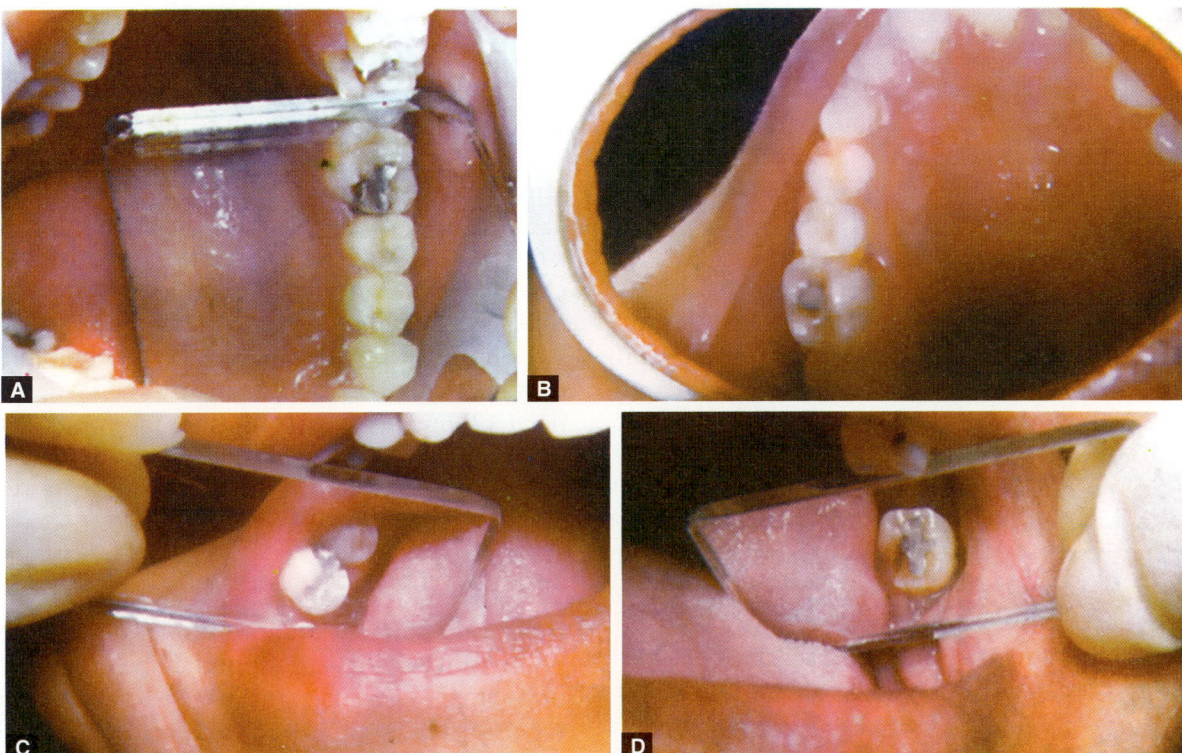

Figs 12.33A to D: Failures of amalgam restoration: **(A)** Ditching; **(B)** Secondary caries; **(C)** Fractured amalgam and **(D)** Fractured tooth

improper cavity preparation leading to recurrence of caries and fracture is the greatest single factor responsible for failure.

Earlier studies evaluating defective amalgam restorations have reported that 56% of the failures were because of improper cavity preparation and 42% of the failures were because of faulty manipulation of amalgam.

The different causes of failure that can occur at various steps while preparing a cavity for amalgam are as follows:

a. *Inadequate occlusal extension:* Inadequate extension to include pits and fissures increases the chances of caries recurrence particularly in oral cavities with high dental caries index. On the occlusal surface the preparation should be extended to include all the susceptible pits and fissures while terminating the margins in areas that can be finished.

b. *Inadequate extension of the proximal box:* If the proximal box walls are not adequately extended into the embrasures they are not amenable to brushing and cleaning by mastication, which predisposes to secondary caries. However, radical extension of the proximal box margins can result in the weakened tooth. Special attention should be directed towards lower bicuspids and the distal regions of the maxillary and mandibular first molars where frail walls can be formed easily.

c. *Overextension of the cavity preparation walls:* The ideal facio-lingual width of the cavity preparation for amalgam should be 1/4th the intercuspal distance. If the cavity preparation extends to half of the intercuspal distance, consideration should be given to capping of the cusps. If the cavity preparation extends to 2/3rds of the intercuspal distance, cusp capping becomes mandatory. If the remaining cusps are not capped in large amalgam restorations, there are chances that the cusps can fracture. This is because amalgam restoration acts as a wedge and tends to split the opposing cusps apart. During cusp capping amalgam should be present in a minimum thickness of 2.0 mm over functional cusps and a minimum thickness of 1.5 mm over non-functional cusps to give it adequate strength. If the required thickness of restorative material is not present, there are chances of fracture of the restoration.

d. *Inadequate depth:* Amalgam cavity preparations should have a minimum depth of 1.5 mm to provide the bulk and hence resistance to fracture.

e. *Curved pulpal floor:* If the pulpal floor of the cavity preparation is not flat but curved, the restoration produces a wedging effect thus increasing the chances of the fracture of tooth. Flat pulpal floor should be provided around the excavation site of caries. If this is not possible at least three flat seats should be provided to resist the forces directed along long axis of the tooth. Appropriate amount of dentin must be present around each excavated site.

f. *Acute/obtuse cavosurface area:* To assure strong junctions between amalgam and tooth regardless of its location, butt joints should be created particularly in those regions where occlusal stresses are to be encountered. If the cavosurface angle is acute, there are chances of fracture of the tooth margins; whereas if the cavosurface angle is obtuse, the acute marginal amalgam is likely to collapse under occlusal stress. The cavity margins should be adequately finished to remove any unsupported enamel rods, which are susceptible to fracture leading to gap formation and subsequently secondary caries.

g. *Sharp axio-pulpal line angle:* Failure to round off the axio-pulpal line angle as well as internal line angles and point angles can lead to concentration of stresses and fracture of the tooth or restorative material. The rounding off of the axio-pulpal line angle also provides bulk of the silver which is required for its strength

h. *Inadequate isthmus width:* Occasionally, fracture may be seen at the isthmus portion of the proximo-occlusal restoration, which may be because of a very narrow isthmus relative to the rest of the cavity preparation or inadequate proximal retention form

i. *Undermined marginal ridge enamel:* Failure to diverge the mesial and distal walls of the occlusal cavity preparation. When the mesiodistal extention of the cavity is extensive it can cause fracture because of the undermining of the mesial and distal marginal ridge enamel.

j. *Improper retentive devices:* Retentive devices should be prepared entirely in dentin without undermining the enamel.

k. *Use of low speed for cutting:* Post operative pain can also be a routine failure. The dentist should use high speed rotary instruments, with intermittent cutting and adequate cooling of tooth structure thereby minimizing the post operative pain.

Poor Matrix Adaptation

The areas and relationship of contacts, the anatomical design of the marginal ridges, the marginal continuity of the restoration all play important roles in assuring that the tissues of the periodontium will maintain a state of health. The proper contacts and contours in a restoration can be obtained by a properly contoured and applied matrix. The matrix should be very stable after it has been applied. Instability of a matrix results in a distorted restoration, gross marginal excesses and an uncondensed soft amalgam. The cervical excesses can irritate the periodontium, gradually and progressively destroying the periodontium. A complete and effective condensation cannot be attempted against a poorly stabilized matrix, which will result in a soft amalgam filled with voids. Hence, establishing proper contacts and contours with the help of matrices is fundamental for a successful amalgam restoration.

Premature removal of matrix band may lead to restoration fracture.

Faulty Amalgam Manipulation

It has been stated that more amalgam restorations fail because of poor manipulation than because of the use of poor alloys. Successful restoration can be achieved when variables are kept under strict control. The basic principle of all these manipulative procedures is to produce a well-prepared amalgam with the mercury content in the amalgam under control.

A. Mercury Alloy Ratio

A considerable loss of strength occurs when the residual mercury is in excess of 55% in the restoration. The clinical result of excess residual mercury includes reduced crushing strength, increased flow and increased susceptibility to tarnish and corrosion. Unfortunately, higher the mercury content used in mixing higher is the residual mercury, which cannot be effectively removed by squeezing and condensation. It is preferable to use a minimal mercury technique with dispensers used for the correct proportioning.

Mulling is a continuation of the trituration process and is carried out to ensure that all alloy particles are duly coated with mercury. It can be done manually or mechanically. While doing it manually, moisture can be incorporated into the material if bare hands are used. Mechanically, mulling is done in the amalgamator. The pestle is removed from the capsule and trituration repeated for 1-2 seconds. This procedure helps in cleaning the capsule of amalgam remnants. Amalgam, which hardens in the capsule if not removed will contaminate future mixes and is frequently a cause of hard amalgam islands that pull out of the plastic mass while the filling is being carved. Hence the capsules should be checked carefully for cleanliness after each use.

Both under trituration and over trituration can lead to failures of amalgam restoration. Under trituration leads to soft powdery non-coherent mix; whereas, overtrituration may break the already forming matrix.

B. Condensation

The rationale of condensation is to reduce residual mercury content, to ensure amalgam reaches all parts of the preparation and to obtain a homogenous restoration devoid of voids.

Freshly prepared amalgam has more desirable working properties. The effectiveness of removing residual mercury from the restoration is possible only if the amalgam is used within four minutes of trituration. Delayed use of triturated amalgam does not allow proper condensation of the material and also does not remove mercury from the restoration. Replasticizing the mix by adding mercury will seriously reduce its strength.

If a larger cavity demands that the working time of the amalgam exceeds 3-4 minutes, the use of multiple mixes will allow the operator to handle plastic amalgam throughout the condensation procedure and ensure building a homogenous restoration.

There are limits to the removal of mercury also. Certain amount of mercury is necessary to bind the mass together in a homogenous form. Elimination of mercury by excessive squeezing may induce a laminated effect and seriously reduces the strength of the restoration. The end result is similar to working with a partially crystallized or set amalgam. The critical reduction of mercury levels below 55% is however obtained during packing.

Condensation can be carried out either manually or mechanically. Condensation should be done using the stepping process to drive away any voids from the restoration. Small increments should be used rather than large increments to ensure proper condensation. Very small plugger sizes may punch holes in the amalgam whereas very large plugger size may not condense the amalgam in all corners. Condensation pressure used should be adequate. The packing motion is most effective if the condenser is rocked under a heavy steady thrust. Light tapping, will remove very little mercury to the surface. Mechanical methods of condensation have shown to provide restorations that harden sooner and have a slightly higher ultimate compressive strength. The mechanical condenser, however, should be used with caution to avoid fracturing of enamel margins.

C. Contamination

Contamination of the amalgam mix with moisture during trituration, mulling and condensation weaken amalgam restoration especially with zinc containing alloys. There occurs delayed expansion, which could possibly result in marginal flaws, tarnish, pitting, corrosion and blistering, etc. Expansion may also lead to pain.

D. Finishing and Polishing

The amalgam should be finished gently. Occasionally, during finishing, excess amalgam at the margins is dressed down to thin flakes or spur like overhangs, which can fracture from the restoration sooner or later, thus leaving susceptible crevices in vulnerable areas of the tooth surface.

Over carving the restoration to create normal, deep anatomic features should be avoided. An over carved restoration will reduce the thickness of amalgam and increase chances of fracture.

Amalgams that have a greater tendency for tarnish and corrosion do not retain surface polish for a long time. They may also offer resistance to polishing. A rough pitted and corroded surface only predisposes to failure.

Failure to polish may accelerate corrosion because of surface irregularities. Also the restoration surface is rough promoting plaque accumulation and gingival irritation.

Polishing should be done judiciously. When temperatures above 65°C are generated, mercury is released from the amalgam leading to defective restorations.

E. Post-operative Pain

This may occur following an amalgam restoration because of:
- *Hyper occlusion*: leads to inflammation of the apical periodontium.
- *Cracks in tooth*: such cracks cause pain during chewing because of expansion/contraction of tooth structure with every bite.
- *Galvanism*: not only the adjacent/antagonist dissimilar metal restorations lead to galvanism, but in poorly condensed silver amalgam, variation in silver concentration at different areas of the same restoration, also leads to galvanism.
- *Delayed expansion*: is peculiar to zinc containing alloys
- *Inadequate pulp protection*: Failure in the form of pain may occur if inadequate pulp protection is present. Amalgam is a good conductor of heat. If a base is not given, heat may be conducted to the pulp resulting in its damage.

Varnish should be routinely applied under amalgam restorations. Failure to apply proper varnish layer can lead to continuous leakage around the restoration. This leakage may cause postoperative sensitivity and *amalgam blues* due to penetration of corrosion products into dentinal tubules.

The restoration fracture may occur if the patient does not follow the instructions properly and bites on restoration before it sets.

GALLIUM ALLOYS

Silver amalgam, though an accepted restorative material, yet the mercury controversy limits its use. The toxic effects of mercury coupled with problems of mercury hygiene, led the researchers think of mercury-free alloys. Gallium alloy is the first of its kind which came into being in early 80s.

Properties

The melting point of gallium is 24.78°C and the boiling point is 1983°C. The density of the gallium is 5.90 gm/cm^3. It has the property of wetting many materials including tooth structure. The alloys of gallium are mixed and condensed as silver amalgam using almost the same instruments. It sets in reasonable time and possesses strength, diametrical stability and corrosion resistance equal to or even greater than silver amalgam.
- The compressive and tensile strength increases with time comparable with silver amalgam.
- Creep values are as low as 0.09%.
- It sets early so polishing can be carried out the same day.
- They expand after mixing, therefore provide better marginal seal.

The physical properties of high copper silver alloys and gallium alloys are depicted in Table 12.2.

Table 12.2: Comparative properties between (High copper) Silver alloys and Gallium alloys

Alloy	Creep %	Compressive strength (after 6 hours)	Setting contraction/ expansion (%)
Silver alloy (High copper)	1.04 ± 0.06	370 MPa	− 0.05
Gallium alloy	0.09 ± 0.03	350 MPa	+ 0.39

Composition

The earlier composition of gallium alloy was:

Powder	
Silver (Ag)	50%
Tin (Sn)	25%
Copper (Cu)	15%
Palladium (Pd)	10%
Liquid	
Gallium (Ga)	65%
Indium (In)	19%
Tin (Sn)	16%
Silver	Traces

The recent gallium alloy has the following composition:

Powder	
Silver (Ag)	60%
Tin (Sn)	25%
Copper (Cu)	13%
Palladium (Pd)	2.0%
Liquid	
Gallium (Ga)	62%
Indium (In)	25%
Tin (Sn)	13%
Bismuth	Traces

The early alloy contained 10% or even more of palladium; however, the corrosion problem increased and the researchers reduced the concentration to 1.0-2.0%.

Reaction

The alloy and the liquid are mixed as usual. The structure of the gallium alloy resembles that of silver amalgam. The reaction between AgSn particles and liquid gallium involves the formation of AgGa phase and a pure tin phase

$$AgSn + Ga \longrightarrow AgGa + Sn$$

The basic reaction remains the same, however, the composition of the alloy gallium varies considerably.

After mixing, the alloy tends to adhere to the walls of the capsule and thus reported to be more difficult to handle. However, as per manufacturer's instructions, by adding a few drops of alcohol, the problem of sticking can be minimized.

Biological Considerations

Biologically, the results are not promising. In early gallium alloys, surface roughness, marginal discoloration and fracture were reported. With the improvement in composition these defects were significantly reduced but not totally eliminated.

The problem of setting expansion though considered good initially later proved to be deleterious. The gallium alloys could not be used in larger restorations as the expansion led to fracture of the weakened cusps. The expansion may lead to postoperative sensitivity.

The creep values are best suited for gallium alloys. Even high copper alloys which are γ_2-free still exhibit significant creep value. Gallium alloys exhibit negligible creep value, which is beneficial for the life of the restoration.

The compressive strength is adequate; therefore, it can be given in stress-bearing areas. However, its manipulation is difficult. Since these alloys are sticky, their condensation into the cavity is time consuming. This also creates problem with removal of matrix bands. The cleaning of instrument tips and carriers is also difficult and time-consuming.

It is also less popular because of its cost, which is approximately 16 times that of silver alloys.

BONDED AMALGAM RESTORATIONS

To overcome one of the major disadvantage of silver, i.e. it does not adhere properly to cavity walls, adhesive systems designed to bond amalgam to enamel and dentin have been introduced. It also improves its adhesion, inability to strengthen remaining tooth structure and the need for removal of healthy tooth structure for gaining retention.

One of the earliest methods to bond and hence improve retention of amalgam restorations to the cavity surface relied on painting the walls of the cavity with a layer of zinc phosphate cement and then condensing amalgam over the wet surface.

Later, the *'selective interfacial amalgamation liner'* was tried. This liner was developed by combining the components of polycarboxylate cement and amalgam alloy particles. Though these techniques improve bond strength by 2.3 MPa but were not sufficient and desirable.

Further improvement in amalgam bonding became possible with the introduction of adhesive resins meant for the *'Maryland bridge'* technique. Two Japanese manufacturers marketed special adhesive resin systems, Superbond (Sun Medical) and Panavia (Kuraray) which contained monomers and enhanced bonding to metal surfaces after air abrading or tin plating these surfaces. Superbond was based on 4-META/Methyl methacrylate—Tri-n-butyl borane (MMA-TBB) resins while Panavia was based on a BisGMA phosphonated ester.

The use of Panavia Ex to reduce microleakage of amalgam restorations with or without a glass-ionomer base has not been documented well in literature. Shear bond strengths for Panavia Ex to etched enamel and dentin were reported to be 10MPa and 6.4MPa respectively. Panavia used in combination with glass-ionomer cement was more effective then Panavia used alone and Panavia in combination with both fluoride and glass-ionomer cement was even more effective.

Since then not only resin cements but dentin bonding agents have also been a subject of bonding amalgam to dentin in a number of studies. Various agents that have been tried are amalgam bond, amalgam bond with HPA (Parkell), All Bond 2 (Bisco), Optibond 2 (Kerr), Panavia 21 (Kuraray) (Fig. 12.34), Clearfil Linerbond 2 (Kuraray), Scotchbond MP (3M), etc.

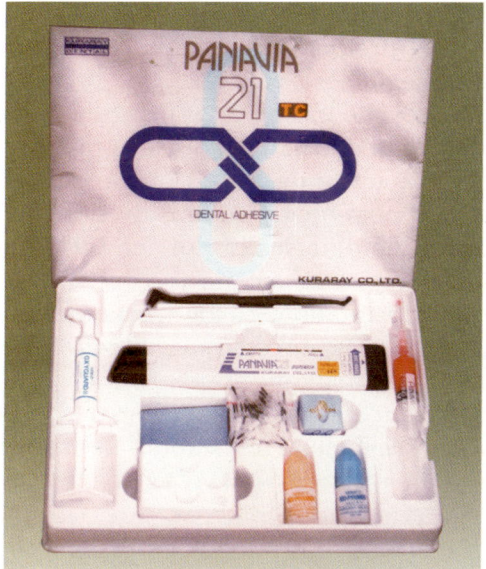

Fig. 12.34: Panavia 21

Indications

In the light of present knowledge, *'bonded amalgam restorations'* are referred to as amalgam restorations, which adhere to the underlying tooth structure through a resin mediated attachment.

- These are indicated in situations that warrant auxiliary retention, reinforcement of remaining tooth structure, conservative preparations and improvement of marginal seal.
- Bonded amalgam restorations are specially indicated for extensively carious posterior teeth where the more expensive cast metal restorations and metal ceramic crowns cannot be afforded by the patient.
- It also allows use of amalgam in teeth with low gingivo-occlusal height where conventional amalgam, pin retained amalgam, inlays, onlays and complete cast crown restorations are difficult to place.
- Bonded amalgam restorations may be used as a temporary restoration, which later can be reduced to a core under a cast crown.
- Can be used as amalgam sealants.

Advantages

Following advantages are provided by a bonded amalgam restoration:
- It permits more conservative cavity preparations because it does not require extensive undercuts and additional mechanical retention unlike conventional amalgam, pin retained amalgam, inlays, onlays and complete cast crown restorations.
- It reinforces tooth structure weakened by caries and cavity preparation.

- It eliminates the use of retention pins and their associated problems like periodontal perforation and pulp exposure, etc.
- It decreases the incidence of marginal fracture.
- It provides a bond at the tooth restoration interface and hence minimizes microleakage, recurrent caries and post-operative sensitivity.
- It allows biologic sealing of the pulpo-dentinal complex.
- It permits restoration of a tooth in one appointment compared to cast or ceramic restorations that may require more than one appointment.
- It is a cost effective treatment compared to the more expensive cast metal restorations or metal ceramic crowns.

Limitations and Disadvantages

- It is technique sensitive, as it requires the amalgam to be introduced into the cavity while the adhesive resin is still wet.
- It requires time to adapt to the new technique.
- Long term results of its clinical performance are not yet documented to prove its success.
- Experiments have shown no sustained effects of amalgam bonding when subjected to thermocycling.
- Hydrolytic stability of the bond is questionable over a prolonged time period.
- It increases the cost of an amalgam restoration.

Manipulation

The design of cavity for bonded amalgam restorations does not require the traditional form of cavity preparation. The unnecessary removal of healthy tooth structure is avoided as bonded amalgam technique preserves the remaining tooth structure. The cavity form is conservative yet an adequate form of resistance should be provided, as the bonding agent does not remove the need for parallel walls, grooves and box forms.

A high copper single composition alloy is selected as it offers excellent strength and immediate mechanical qualities that permit early polishability.

The bonding agent to be chosen under amalgam should preferably be chemically cured or dual cured. The most commonly used amalgam adhesives are based on the 4-META system or 10 MDP (Methacryloyloxy decyl dihydrogen phosphate) system. Amalgam bond, which utilizes the 4-META system, uses a solution of 10% citric acid and 3% ferric chloride to remove the smear layer and demineralize the dentin surface. A primer is subsequently applied on the conditioned dentin followed by a self curing 4-META system. High performance additive powder (HPA) in Amalgam bond plus, contains polymethyl methacrylate fibers, which may cross the interface between the amalgam and the bonding resin producing a reinforced connection between the two materials.

Panavia resin is a chemically activated, Bisphenol glycidyl methacrylate based resin cement. The addition of 10 MDP in the formulation contributes to the adhesive properties. Panavia Ex is a powder liquid system while Panavia 21 is a paste system. Both products are chemically cured and will not polymerize when oxygen is present, i.e. are anaerobic in nature. Panavia 21 includes application of a self etching primer followed by the application of the resin.

The procedure for a bonded amalgam restoration is illustrated using All Bond 2 (Bisco) resin (Figs 12.35 A to C).

A rubber dam is applied to isolate the concerned tooth.

- The carious lesion is removed with a slow speed round carbide bur. The unsupported enamel is removed and finished.
- The cavity preparation is gently rinsed with water and dried. If the depth of the cavity so dictates, a protective base of chemically cured or light cured glass-ionomer cement can be placed.
- Remember fragile cusps need not be sacrificed.
- Properly fitted auto matrices and wedges are applied. Automatrix is preferred as it is convenient to place and does not hinder manipulation. Wedges may have been inserted earlier prior to cavity preparation if there are chances of damaging the rubber dam during cavity cutting.
- Enamel and dentin are etched with a 10% phosphoric acid gel for 15 seconds after which the acid gel is removed with an air water spray.
- The vital dentin and enamel are dried with absorbent paper or gently with air through chip syringe. Properly etched enamel will have a dull white frosted appearance.
- Adhesive primer (Primer A + Primer B, All Bond 2 System) is applied thoroughly throughout the cavity surface.
- The enamel dentin bonding agent (All Bond Liner F) is applied with a disposable brush.
- Freshly initiated amalgam which has been triturated by an assistant is condensed immediately into the cavity while the resin is still wet, i.e. has not polymerized.
- The restoration is carved, finished and polished.

The Bonding Interface

The tooth restoration interface in a bonded amalgam restoration is characteristically composed of the tooth,

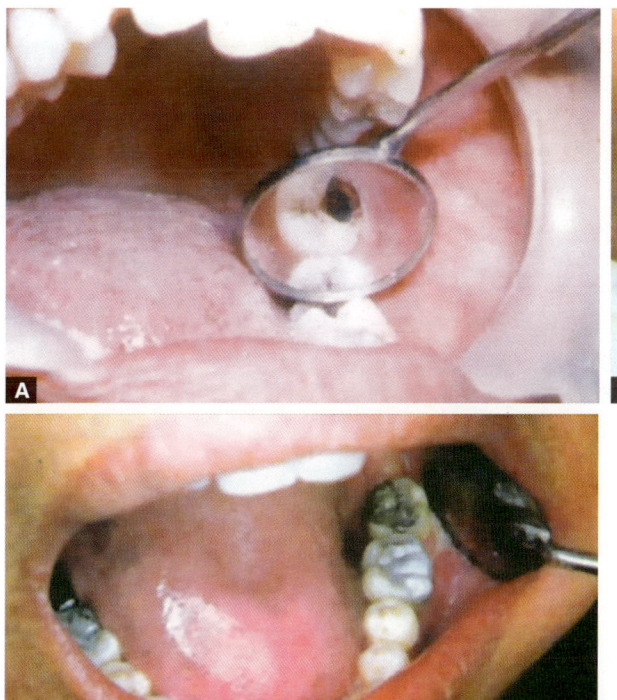

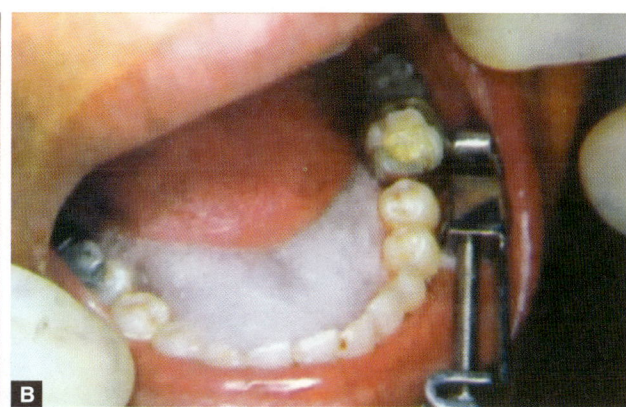

Figs 12.35A to C: (A) Carious lesion on mandibular left first molar; (B) Bonding resin applied on cavity preparation; (C) Completed bonded amalgam restoration

intervening adhesive resin and the amalgam. The tooth-resin bond is similar to the tooth-resin bond in any other composite restoration, i.e.

a. It may include tag formation,
b. Formation of precipitates on pretreated dentin surfaces to which an adhesive resin mechanically or chemically binds,
c. Chemical binding to the inorganic and/or organic components of dentin, or
d. Diffusion and impregnation of monomers into the substrate of pretreated dentin and subsequent polymerization resulting in a hybrid layer of reinforced dentin.

The scanning electron microscopic picture of fresh amalgam - tooth interface, amalgam-resin-tooth interface is shown in Figs 12.36A to C and old amalgam-tooth interface is shown in Fig. 12.37.

The bond formed between the resin and amalgam on the other hand is primarily micromechanical. The alloy is condensed against the adhesive resin before polymerization allowing the resin to surround the amalgam particles and lock into it as both the alloy and the resin set. Additionally, with the use of 10 MDP systems, the phosphate monomer may interact with the metallic (tin) ions in amalgam to provide chemical adhesion.

The attachment between the adhesive resin and the tooth structure is generally stronger than that between the adhesive resin and amalgam hence the weak link still appears to be the amalgam resin interface, i.e. an adhesive failure rather than cohesive failure in the resin is more likely at the interface. However, studies have also shown cohesive failure in the amalgam thereby indicating that the adhesive bond transfers sufficient stress across the interface to result in its cohesive failure. Also, cohesive failure in the tooth has been reported leaving a portion of the tooth material attached to the amalgam restoration.

Future of the Bonded Amalgam Restoration

A restoration technique that combines the best properties of amalgam and the principles of conservative preparation and marginal seal provides an attractive restoration for the posterior teeth. The technique however is lacking long-term clinical evaluation though comparative studies establish its advantages over the conventional technique. The success and failure of these restorations cannot be based solely on the adhesives but other factors like cavity preparation, type of alloy used, amalgam condensation, occlusion and the patient's dietary and hygienic habits, etc. also play a significant role.

It has been established that the bonded restorations are functioning properly, especially in case of smaller occlusal heights. Bonded amalgam restoration could be an asset in such special situations where minimal retention form is available in the cavity.

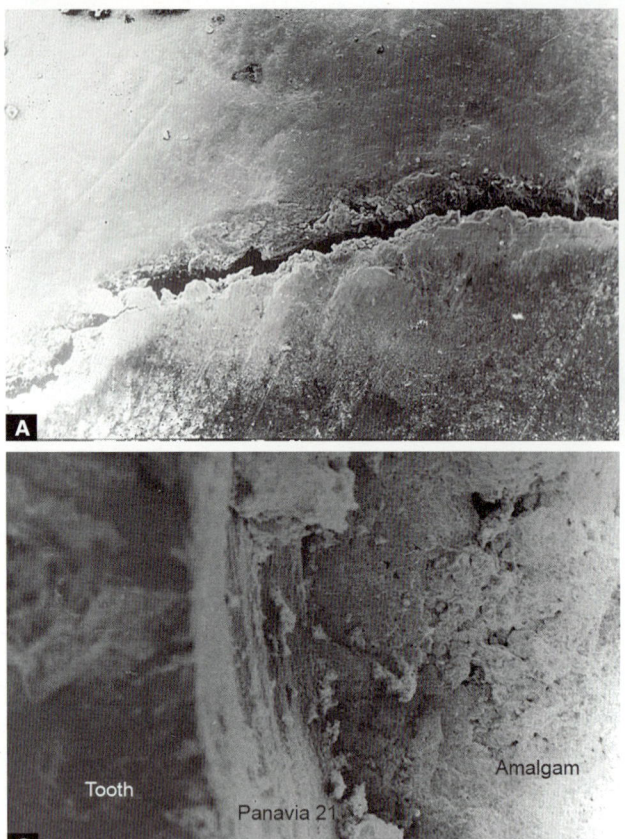
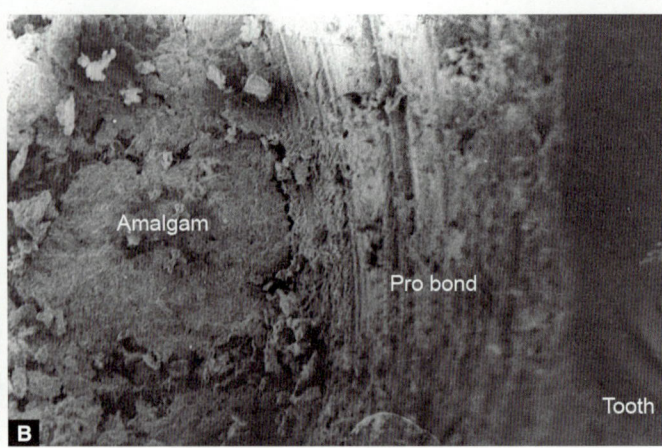

Figs 12.36A to C: Scanning electron microscopic picture of: **(A)** Fresh amalgam-tooth interface; **(A & B)** Amalgam-resin-tooth interface

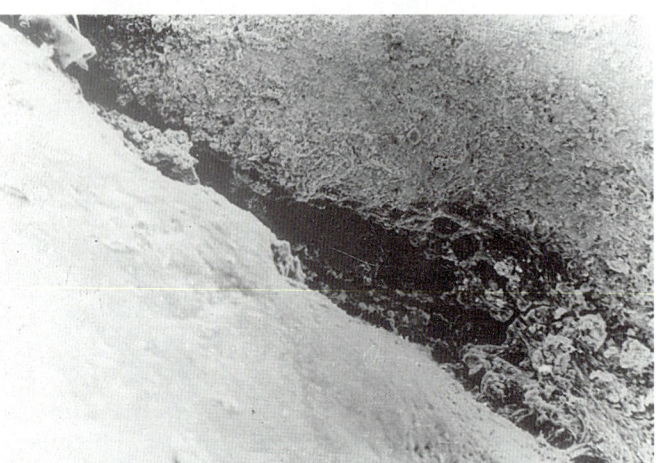

Fig. 12.37: Scanning electron microscopic picture of old amalgam-tooth interface

Ability to maintain adhesive bond over a long period of time under hydrolytic environment still remains questionable. Laboratory experiments have failed to show any added advantages with bonded amalgam restorations when the latter were subjected to cyclic loading and thermocycling tests.

In the future, amalgam adhesives will have a significant and increasing role to play in the daily restorations provided that the restorations are subjected to adequate clinical testing. Preservation of tooth structure, low placement costs and reduced chair time will continue to make amalgam the material of choice for many patients and it is not far that bonded amalgam restorations will become a routine.

FLUORIDATED AMALGAM

Fluoride, being cariostatic, has been included in amalgam to deal with the problem of recurrent caries associated with amalgam restorations. The problem with method is that the fluoride is not delivered long enough to provide maximum benefit. Several studies investigated fluoride levels released from amalgam. These studies concluded that a fluoride containing amalgam may release fluoride for several weeks after insertion of the material in mouth. As an increase upto 10-20 fold in the fluoride content of whole saliva could be measured, the fluoride release from this amalgam seems to be considerable during first week. An anticariogenic action of fluoride amalgam could be explained by its ability to deposit fluoride in the hard tissues around the fillings and to increase the fluoride content of plaque and saliva, subsequently affecting remineralization. In this way, fluoride from amalgam could have a favourable effect not only on caries around the filling but on any initial enamel demineralisation. The fluoride amalgam thus serves as a "slow release device".

CONSOLIDATED SILVER ALLOY SYSTEM

One amalgam substitute being tested is a consolidated silver alloy system developed at the National Institute of Standards and Technology. It uses fluoroboric acid to keep surface of silver alloy particles clean. The alloy, in a spherical form is condensed into a prepared cavity in a manner similar to that for placing compacted gold. The problem associated with the insertion of this material is that alloy strain hardens, so it is difficult to compact it adequately to eliminate internal voids and to achieve good adaptation to the cavity without using excessive force.

AMALGAM RESTORATIONS AND ORAL ENVIRONMENT

Amalgam restorations interact with oral environment as they are subjected to chemical, biological, mechanical and thermal forces. The environment include biochemistry of the adjacent tissues, formation of biofilm on the amalgam surfaces, galvanism, abrasion and other synergistic effects. The metal ions and the mercury are released into the oral cavity from the amalgam restoration.

Usually, for most of the time the environment for external surface of amalgam fillings is saliva. The chemistry of saliva varies with time, food intake, medical/psychological conditions and other related factors. At the interface between a filling and tooth structure, the environment is provided mainly by leakage of fluids from the oral cavity; however, the chemistry is different as a result of electrochemical reactions taking place at this junction. The fillings are covered initially with acquired pellicle, formed by salivary glycoproteins. This film affects the transport of ions to and from the surface. These modified metal organic complexes along with production of metabolites of microorganism are potentially significant factors in the corrosion processes (Fig. 12.38).

Biodegradation of Amalgam Restorations

The amalgam restorations are subjected to various forces, which lead to their degradation in the oral cavity. The electrochemical reactions constitute one of the major interactions between dental amalgam and the oral fluids. The other cause of degradation is the mechanical forces to which the fillings are subjected. There can be formation of biofilm, release of mercury from the amalgam or even wear and fracture of the restoration.

Corrosion

Corrosion processes are those electrochemical reactions that result in degradation of the structure

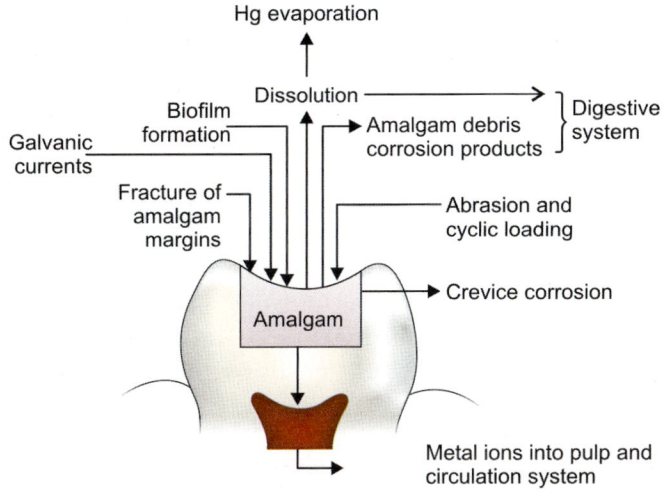

Fig. 12.38: Interactions between amalgam restoration and the oral environment

and mechanical properties. The phenomenon is related to presence of tin and copper in the amalgam along with chlorides in saliva. Low copper amalgams are susceptible to corrosion because of γ_2 (SnHg) phase. In high copper amalgams in which the amount of tin mercury phase is reduced or absent, the copper-tin phase η (CuSn) is resistant to corrosion.

The most severe corrosion of amalgam filling takes place in localized corrosion cells, such as pit and crevices. Because of the localized chemical changes within these occluded cells, such as depletion of dissolved oxygen and an increase in acidity and concentration of chloride ions, the protective film is not stable and fast corrosion results. If the amalgam restoration comes into contact with another metallic restoration its electrode potential and the corrosion rate changes. The corrosion is accelerated. This is severe for low copper alloys because γ_2 phase suffers a potential dependent breakdown of positivity followed by rapid dissolution.

A restoration is a very complex electrode with different parts of the surface corroding under different conditions. The rate at which corrosion occurs varies with different locations and patients. Corrosion degrades the strength of the dental amalgam. Loss of compressive strength and related implications have been reported as high as 50% for low copper alloys and much less for high copper alloys.

Tarnish

The discoloration of the amalgam restorations with the formation of silver and copper sulphides is known as tarnishing. The degradation is mainly concerned with the esthetics. The chemical reaction may cause formation of visible surface films. Thicker tarnish layer may result from an accumulation of complex deposits of both corrosion products and substances from the environment. Tarnish doesn't lead to loss of strength of the tooth.

Wear and Fracture

With the functional occlusal load, the surface of the filling is abraded, known as wear. In case the load is abnormal, it may lead to fracture of the restoration. A phenomenon known as *'ditching'* is common with these types of the abnormal loads. The causes of these types of problems include tensile overload, creep and metal fatigue.

Release of Amalgam Components

The process of corrosion results in conversion of metallic solid into dissolved metal ions and nonmetallic corrosion products. Most of the soluble metal ions are released into the oral fluids, while a substantial part of solid corrosion products remain within the amalgam structure. Some of these products are continuously removed by abrasion. Some metallic ions may interact with soft tissues in the oral cavity, most of the wear and dissolution products are carried into the gastrointestinal tract. Some of the components are absorbed into the tract by acidic juices of the system. The ions can also travel from restoration to pulp, tooth structure and transport to the circulation. Amalgam debris occasionally get embedded into the gingiva in the form of amalgam tattoo, releasing the element into the tissue fluids.

Solid corrosion products detected in retrieved amalgam restoration include tin and copper oxides, copper chloride and mercury sulphides. The rate of their release has not been documented well.

Release of Mercury

The release of mercury from dental amalgam restoration by dissolution and evaporation differ in some important aspects from corrosion and other forms of degradation. The dissolution and evaporation of mercury do not seem to cause substantial degradation of either appearance or function of restorations. Mercury can evaporate from Ag-Hg matrix phase of dental amalgam directly into the atmosphere. In the oral cavity this form of release is insignificant. Usually the mercury release is prevented or minimized by a protective film of oxide on the surface. The mechanical removal of the film by abrasion causes substantial increase in the evaporation rate. In the oral cavity, during partial removal of the film by chewing or brushing, the atomic mercury does not evaporate but dissolve in fluids. The dissolved mercury then either evaporates from the liquid solution or is oxidized to an ionic form (Fig. 12.39).

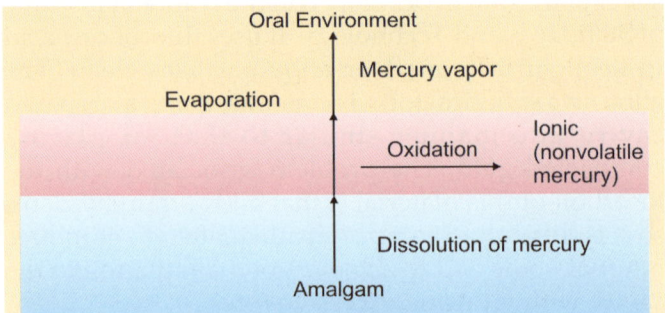

Fig. 12.39: Dissolution of mercury in oral environment

The analysis of retrieved amalgams has not shown a loss of mercury below the corroded layer. The average loss of mercury per day has not been documented properly. During the transport from the oral cavity throughout the gastrointestinal tract, the chemical transformation of mercury is even more complex than for other elements. The possibility of the formation of highly toxic organic form of mercury due to action of bacteria has also been reported. The average intake of mercury vapour has been varied between 0.4 to 4.4 µg per day depending upon the number of amalgam fillings.

The mercury release is a complex phenomenon, which is inadequately understood. There is paucity of clinical data as regards the effects of biodegradation. There is need for development of amalgam with improved corrosion resistance and minimum mercury release.

MERCURY AND ITS MANAGEMENT

Mercury has been used for more than 2000 years in preparations such as diuretics, antibacterial ointments, laxatives and skin ointments. It has also been used as a component of dental amalgam since long. Mercury vapours in atmosphere are considered to be toxic, therefore management of free mercury in dental operatory is of paramount importance.

Chemical forms and Source of Mercury

Mercury exists in three chemical forms:
a. Elemental mercury
b. Inorganic mercury (salts of mercury)
c. Organic mercury (organomercurials)

Elemental mercury is most volatile out of three forms. The exposure to this form can result from accidental spills, improper handling and poorly ventilated laboratories. Inorganic mercury exists as a mercurous or divalent mercuric salts. Salts of mercury can be acutely toxic and irritating. Organomercurials are not a hazard in dentistry but can be an environmental hazard. The alkyl mercury salts are most toxic and methyl mercury is the most common out of all.

Mercury Exposure Related to Dentistry

Mercury from dental amalgam is released in two forms, i.e. mercury vapours and mercuric ions.

Mercuric ions (Hg^{++}) are released due to corrosion. The absorption of mercuric ions from gastrointestinal tract is minute therefore this form has very little toxic effect. However, Hg^{++} play a role in allergic reactions.

Mercury vapours are carried to lungs from intraoral air where it is rapidly absorbed into blood stream. This form is rapidly oxidized from body.

Mercury exposure in dental office can result from:
a. Incorrect storage of mercury or waste amalgam.
b. Spillage of mercury or waste amalgam.
c. Mixed but unhardened dental amalgam during trituration, insertion and intraoral setting.
d. During finishing and polishing of amalgam.
e. Removal of amalgam.

Mercury Concentration in Urine and Blood

There exists a good correlation between mercury level in air and mercury level in urine and blood.

$1 \mu g/m^3$ is considered as the lowest threshold of mercury vapour in air. The $15 \mu g/l$ of mercury in urine and $4 ng/ml$ of mercury in blood is acceptable normal value for public surviving in such air.

Monitoring Mercury Levels

There are number of methods which can determine concentration of mercury in dental surgery atmosphere.

- Mercury vapour may be determined by using a mercury detection meter such as mercury sniffer. Such meters are very costly.
- Paper discs impregnated with palladium chloride can be used. The major disadvantage is lack of reaction specificity for mercury.
- A badge system may be used in which mercury is adsorbed on gold foil.
- Mercury in vapour and dust form may be determined by passing the known volume of air through an absorbing system and then quantifying the absorbed mercury.

Mercury Allergy

Allergy to mercury is very rare. Mercury can act as incomplete antigen. Mercury hypersensitivity is an allergic response mediated by immune system. It is a type IV or cell mediated response. Delayed hypersensitivity to mercury results in contact eczematous reactions on skin and mucosa. Mercury allergy can be confirmed by patch test.

Occupational contact dermatitis can also occur due to contact with mercury. This can be easily avoided by use of latex gloves and no touch technique.

Allergic Reaction to Amalgam Restorations

Allergic reaction to amalgam restorations usually occur 24–48 hours after insertion of amalgam fillings. Women are seen to be more affected than men. Usually cutaneous signs and symptoms are predominant. Symptoms include dermatitis, urticaria, eczema, erythema, odema and itching occurring in face, neck and limbs. Oral manifestations include gingivostomatitis, hypersalivation and erosive lesion. Symptoms usually resolve within few days to two weeks after removal of amalgam restorations.

Mercury Toxicity

In recent years there has been increased concerned related to mercury toxicity from amalgam fillings. Mercury from amalgam fillings have been evaluated for its toxicity related to nervous tissue, kidney, immune system and general health of patient but no cause and effect relationship have been found.

Hygiene Recommendations for Mercury in Dentistry

- Mercury containing products should not be stored in open but in closets or cabinets to minimize local concentration in rest of the office. Storage locations should be near a vent that exhausts air out of building.
- Local spill or spatters of triturated materials should not be collected with a vacuum aspiration. Spilled mercury can be made harmless by dusting with sulphur powder or spraying with a solution of sodium thiosulphate.
- Mercury droplets are very difficult to remove from artificial floor coverings so such coverings should either be avoided or intermittently replaced.
- To control the vapours of mercury during placement and condensation procedures, rubber dam should be used to isolate the patient and high volume evacuation should be used to prevent intraoral vapour from diffusing.
- Scrap dental amalgam from condensation procedures should be collected and stored under water, glycerine or spent x-ray fixer in a tightly capped jar.

- Silver mercury has a very low melting point and easily melts during finishing producing mercury rich liquid phase, so amalgam should be polished at slow speed using water spray.
- Instruments used for inserting, finishing, polishing or removing dental amalgam may contain some amalgam material on their surface. During instruments sterilization this material may be heated and release mercury vapour. Therefore, it is advisable to properly isolate or vent air from sterilization areas.
- Provide proper ventilation in work place by having fresh air exchanger and proper replacement of filters, which may act as trap of mercury.
- Mercury vapour level in office should be periodically monitored.
- Office personnel should also be periodically monitored.
- Precapsulated alloys should be used to eliminate the possibility of bulk mercury spill.
- Amalgamators should be covered.
- Skin contact with mercury or freshly prepared amalgam should be avoided.
- Change masks after removing amalgam restorations.
- Mercury contaminated items should be deposited in sealed bags.
- Spilled mercury should be cleaned with trap bottles, tapes or fresh mixes of amalgam.
- In dental operatory, professional clothing should be worn.

Amalgam is being used for the last hundred years or more. The present evidence does not demonstrate that amalgam restorations are a hazard to health of general public. However, occupational hazard to mercury is a potential hazard for dental personnel. In continuing to use amalgam, dentists should observe strict mercury and amalgam hygiene procedures.

BIBLIOGRAPHY

1. Akerboom H.B., Advokaat J.G., Van Amerongen W.E. and Borgmeijer P.J.: Long-term evaluation and restorations of amalgam restorations. Comm. Dent. Oral Epid.: 21, 45, 1993.
2. Allander, L., Birhed, D. and Bratthall, D.: Reasons for replacement of class II amalgam restorations in private practice. Swed. Dent. J.: 14, 179, 1990.
3. Almquist, T.C., Cowan, R.D. and Lambert, R.C.: Conservative amalgam restorations. J.P.D.: 29, 524, 1973.
4. Aminzadeh, K.K. and Etminan, M.: Dental amalgam and multiple sclerosis: A systematic review and meta-analysis. J. Public Health Dentistry: 67, 2007.
5. Berglund, A., Pohl, S., Olsson, S. and Bergman, M.: Determination of the rate of release of intraoral mercury vapour from amalgam. J.Dent.Res.: 67, 1235, 1988.
6. Blair, F.M., J.M. and McCabe, J.F.: The physical properties of a gallium alloy restorative material. Dent. Mater.: 11, 277, 1995.
7. Bona A.D. and Summitt J.B.: The effect of amalgam bonding on resistance form of class II amalgam restorations. Quint. Int.: 29, 95, 1998.
8. Browning, W.D.: Incidence and severity of post-operative pain following routine placement of amalgam restorations. Quint. Int.: 30, 484, 1999.
9. Browning W.D., Johnson W.W. and Gregory P.N.: Clinical performance of bonded amalgam restorations at 42 months. J.A.D.A.: 131, 607, 2000.
10. Calamia J.R., Styner D.L. and Rattet A.H.: Effect of amalgam bond on cervical sensitivity. Am. J. Dent.: 8, 283, 1996.
11. Chandler J.E., Messer H.H. and Ellender G.: Cytotoxicity of gallium and indium ions compared with mercuric ion. J.D.R.: 73, 1554, 1994.
12. Chin G. Chong J., Kluczewska A.L. Gorjy S and Tennant, M.: The environmental effects of dental amalgam. Aust. Dent.J. 45, 246, 2000.
13. Covey D.A., Kent D.K., Dunning D.G. and Koka, S.: Qualitative and quantitative determination of dental amalgam restoration volume. J.P.D.: 82, 8, 1999.
14. DoAmaral Zenkner, J.E., Baratieri, L.N., Monteiro, S., Caldeira De Andrada, M.A. and Vieira, L.C.C.: Clinical and radiographic evaluation of a cermet tunnel restorations on primary molars. Quint. Int.: 24, 783, 1993.
15. Duncalf W.V. and Wilson N.H.F.: Adaptation & condensation of amalgam restoration in class II preparation of conventional & conservative design. Quint. Int.: 23, 499, 1992.
16. Dunne S.M. Wilson N.H.F. and Gainsford, I.D.: Current materials and techniques for direct restoration in posterior teeth. Part I - silver amalgam. Int. Dent. J.: 47, 123, 1997.
17. Elderton R.J.: The prevalence of failure of restorations: a literature review. J. Dent.: 4, 207, 1976.
18. Elderton R.J.: Assessment of the quality of restorations: a literature review. J. Oral Rehab.: 4, 217, 1977.
19. Engle, J.H., Ferracance, J.L., Wichmann, J. and Okabe, T.: Quantification of total mercury vapour released during dental procedures. Dent. Mater.: 8, 176, 1992.
20. Hunter A.R., Treasure E.T. and Hunter, A.J.: Increase in cavity volume associated with the removal of class II amalgam and composite restorations. Oper. Dent.: 20, 2, 1995.
21. Holmstrup P.: Oral mucosa and skin reactions related to amalgam. Adv. Dent. Res.: 6, 120, 1992.
22. Jordon R.E., Suzuki, M. and Boksman, L.: The new generation amalgam alloys: clinical considerations. Dent. Cl. NorthAm.: 29, 341, 1985.
23. Knight G.T. and Berry T.G.: Clinical application of a direct placement mercury - free alloy. Am. J. Dent.: 10, 52, 1997.
24. Letzel H., van'tHof, M.A., Marshall, G.W. and Marshall, S.J.: The influence of the amalgam alloy on the survival of amalgam restorations: a secondary analysis of multiple controlled clinical trials. J. Dent. Res.: 76, 1787, 1997.
25. Letzel H., Van't Hof M.A., Vrijhoef, M.M., Marshall, G.W. Jr. and Marshall, S.J.A.: A controlled clinical study of amalgam restorations: survival, failures, and causes of failures. Dent. Mater.: 5, 115, 1989.

26. Mahler D.B., Adey J.D. and Marek M.: Creep and corrosion of amalgam. J.Dent.Res.: 61, 33, 1982.
27. Mamoun J.S. and Ahmed M. : Amalgam matrix for class II and class V preparations connected at the proximal box. J.A.D.A. : 137, 186, 2006.
28. Martin J.A. and Bader J.D.: Five year treatment outcomes for teeth with large amalgams and crowns. Oper. Dent.: 22, 72, 1997.
29. Mash L.K. Miller B.H. Nakajima H. Guo, I.Y. and Okabe, T.: Handling characteristics of a gallium alloy triturated with alcohol. Am. J. Dent.: 10, 199, 1997.
30. Mclean J.W.: The failed restoration: Causes of failure and how to prevent them. Int. Dent. J.: 40, 354, 1990.
31. Miller B.H. Woldu M. Nakajima H. and Okabe T.: Strength and micro-structure of gallium alloys. Dent. Mater. : 18, 96, 1999.
32. Navarro M.F.L. Franco E.B. and Bastos P.A.M. *et al*: Clinical evaluation of gallium alloy as a posterior restorative material. Quint. Int.: 27, 315, 1996.
33. Oddera M.: Conservative amalgam restoration of class II lesions - The 'Slot restoration' - A case report. Quint. Int.: 25, 493, 1994.
34. Papa, J., Cain, C., Masser, H.H. and Wilson, P.R.: Tunnel restorations versus class II restorations for small approximal lesions: a comparison of tooth strengths. Quint. Int.: 24, 93, 1993.
35. Plasmans P.J.J.M. Crengers, N.H.J. and Mulder J.: Long term survival of extensive amalgam restorations. J.D.R.: 77, 453, 1998.
36. Rasheed A.A.: Effect of bonding amalgam on the reinforcement of teeth. J.P.D.: 93, 51, 2005.
37. Roberts H.W. Charlton, D.G. and Murchison D.F.: Repair of non carious amalgam margin defects. Oper. Dent. 26, 273, 2001.
38. Shaini F.J. Fleming G.J.P. Shortall A.C.C. and Marquis P.M.: A comparison of the mechanical properties of a gallium-based alloy with a spherical high copper amalgam. Dent. Mater. : 17, 142, 2001.
39. Smart E.R. McLeod R.I. and Lawrence C.M. : Resolution of lichen planus following removal of amalgam restorations in patients with proven allergy to mercury salts : a pilot study. B.D.J. : 178, 108, 1995.
40. Spencer A.J.: Dental amalgam and mercury in dentistry. Aust. Dent.J. 45, 224, 2000.
41. Summitt J.B. Osborne J.W., Burgess J.O. and Howell M.L.: Effect of grooves on resistance form of class II amalgams with wide occlusal preparations. Oper. Dent.: 18, 42, 1993.
42. Svanberg M.: Class II amalgam restorations, glass-ionomer tunnel restorations and caries development on adjacent tooth surfaces. Caries Res.: 26, 315, 1992.
43. Terkla L.G. and Mahler D.B.: Clinical evaluation of interproximal retention grooves in class II amalgam cavity design. J.P.D.: 17, 576, 1967.
44. Tyas M.J.: Dental Amalgam - what are the alternatives? Int. Dent. J.: 44, 303, 1994.
45. Walls A, W., Murray J.J. McCabe J.F.: The management of occlusal caries in permanent molars. A clinical trial comparing a minimal composite restoration with an occlusal amalgam restoration. B.D.J.: 164, 288, 1988.
46. Williams, P.: Goodbye Amalgam, Hello Alternatives? Dent. Mater.: 62, 139, 1996.
47. Winkler M. M. Moore B.K. Allen J. Rhodes B.: Comparision of retentiveness of amalgam bonding types. Oper. Dent. 22, 200, 1997.
48. Zidan O. and Abdel K.U.: The effect of amalgam bonding on the stiffness of teeth weakened by cavity preparations. Dent. Mater. : 19, 680, 2003.
49. Zyman P.: Adhesive amalgam restoration technique: Clinical tips. J. Esthet. Dent.: 9, 131, 1997.

13

Cast Restorations

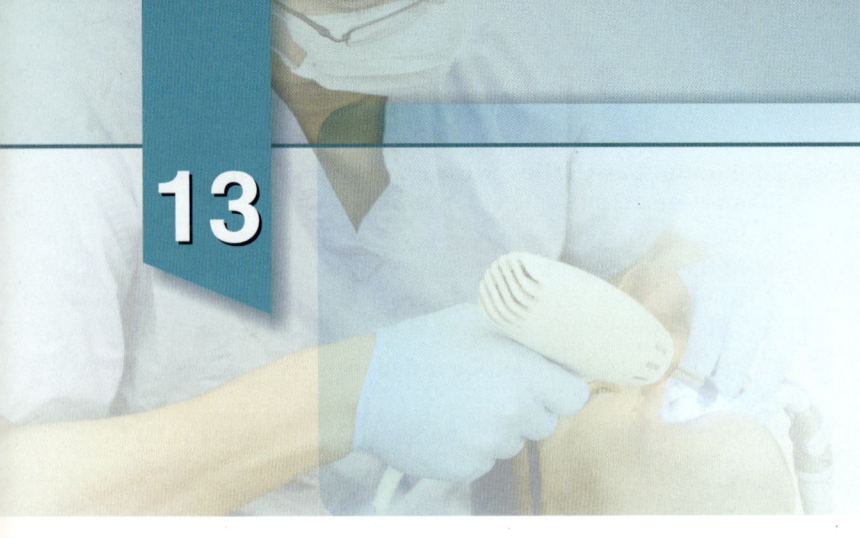

Many instances and clinical situations warrant the clinician to opt for cast restoration. These provide long lasting restorations and maintain the proximal contact for a considerable period of time. The configuration of contacts and contours can also be modified with the help of these restorations. Basically, the cast restorations are fabricated from either noble metals or base metals. *'Noble'* refers to metals with marked resistance to oxidation and chemical reaction. Sometimes, the term *'precious'* is also used. Precious usually refers to economic value. *'Base metal'* refers to the metal elements that are chemically reactive to their environment. Recently, titanium has also been used for casting. These restorations require meticulous approach towards cavity preparation and its fabrication.

History of casting of objects in gold by the wax elimination process dates back to four or five thousand years ago by Chinese. Italian artisan Benvenuto Cellini described the use of this techniques to make statutes and artistic pieces. In 1884 Aquilhon de Saran of Paris melted 24 Carat gold in an investment mould to form inlays.

Dr. D. Philbrook in 1897 was credited with casting the first restoration, which was without any evidence. *Taggart* in 1907 was credited for improving cast restoration with lost wax procedure giving details of the casting procedures.

The chemical composition of noble and base metal alloys is given in the Table 13.1, and the properties of individual constituents are given in Table 13.2.

Gold alloy is most commonly used for cast restoration because it has noble metal properties such as resistance to tarnish and corrosion and ductility and malleability. The gold alloy is divided into four types. In all these types, gold should be above 65–75%. The rest of the percentage contains silver, copper, palladium, platinum and zinc, which comprises of a smaller percentage of the alloy.

Type I } Gold percentage between 75–80% to
Type II } preserve the noble metal properties

Type III } Gold percentage between 65–75%
Type IV }

Previously 0.5% platinum was added to increase strength and corrosion resistance. Since platinum is

Table 13.1: Chemical composition of noble and base metal alloys

	Noble metal		Base metal	
	(Gold based)	(Palladium based)	(Cobalt based)	(Nickel based)
Major constituents	Gold	Palladium	Cobalt	Nickel
	Silver	Silver	Chromium	Chromium
	Copper	Copper	Tungsten	Iron
		Gold	Molybdenum	
Minor constituents	Palladium	Zinc	Copper	Molybdenum
	Platinum	Indium	Silicon	Manganese
	Zinc	Iridium	Gallium	Boron
	Iridium	Gallium	Aluminium	Copper
	Germanium	Tin	Nickel	Beryllium
	Tin	Ruthenium	Tantalum	
	Iron		Ruthenium	

Cast Restorations

Table 13.2: Properties of individual constituents

Constituent	Property
Gold	Adds high corrosion resistance, ductility and good castability
Silver	Reduces density, whitens the alloy counteracting redness of copper
Copper	Strengthens gold based alloys
Platinum/Palladium	Increases casting temperature, strength and corrosion resistance. Palladium lowers the cost and increases rigidity
Zinc	Increases castability
Iron	Improves mechanical properties and also bonding in metal ceramics
Tin	Acts as bonding element in metal ceramics, also increases strength
Iridium	Acts as grain refiner
Indium	Serves as bonding agent in metal ceramics
Germanium	Increases the castability of gold copper alloys
Gallium	Contributes the homogenous structure, improves castability
Ruthenium	Used as grain refiner
Cobalt	Provides strength, hardness and corrosion resistance
Chromium	Provides hardness and resilience and increases corrosion resistance to some extent
Nickel	Increases ductility and lowers melting temperature
Molybdenum	Increases the strength and hardness of alloy
Manganese	Acts as de-oxidizer
Tungsten	Helps reduce formation of chromium depleted areas
Aluminium	Increases strength and hardness
Boron	Decreases alloy melting temperature
Beryllium	Decreases melting temperature and corrosion resistance

very costly so it was replaced by palladium for achieving the same properties.

Type I and II are most commonly used for inlays where stress-bearing area is less. Type III and IV can be used where more stress bearing areas are involved in cavity preparations such as large inlays, crowns, long span fixed partial dentures, etc. As the gold alloy is very expensive, alternative materials such as base metal alloys and titanium are also being used.

The common disadvantages of base metal alloy are microleakage, difficult finishing and polishing, and difficulty in obtaining finer details.

Recently, titanium alloys are being used for cast restorations, though still in experimental stage. It is more biocompatible compared to base metal alloys. These also have certain disadvantages such as microleakage and difficulty in finishing and polishing.

This chapter deals mainly with cast gold restorations.

DEFINITION

An *inlay* is primarily an intracoronal cast restoration that is designed mainly to restore occlusal and proximal surface(s) of posterior teeth without involving the cusps and rarely the proximal surface of anterior teeth. An *onlay* is a combination of intracoronal and extracoronal cast restoration when one or more cusps are covered, and a *full veneer crown* is an extracoronal cast restoration where all cusps are covered.

INDICATIONS OF CAST RESTORATION

1. *Extensive tooth involvement*: Amalgam is limited in its ability to replace extensive loss of tooth structure, beyond this limit it can only act as a foundation. Cast restorations are efficient in replacing lost tooth structure and also for supporting remaining tooth structure (Fig. 13.1).

   Repeated removal of amalgam restorations also lead to extensive loss of tooth structure. Fractured teeth or fractured marginal ridges are also indications for cast restorations.
2. *Adjunct to periodontal therapy to correct tooth anomalies, which predispose to periodontal problems.*

   Cast restorations are indicated in physiologically restoring and maintaining the dimensions of the contact, contour, marginal ridges and embrasure areas, which are vital for the health of the periodontium (Fig. 13.2).
3. Superior control over contacts and contours.
4. *Correction of occlusion*: If any change for occlusal table is planned, cast restorations are ideal (Fig. 13.20A).

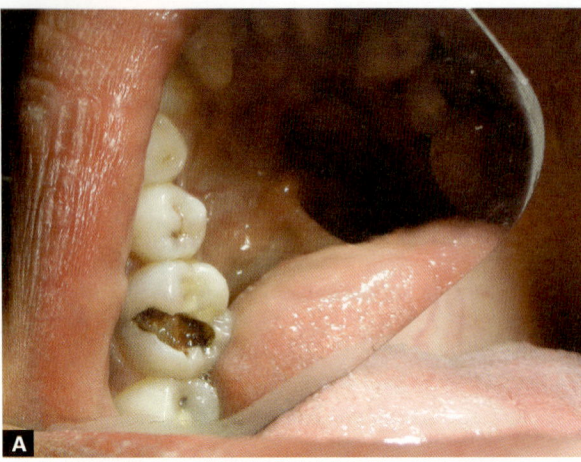

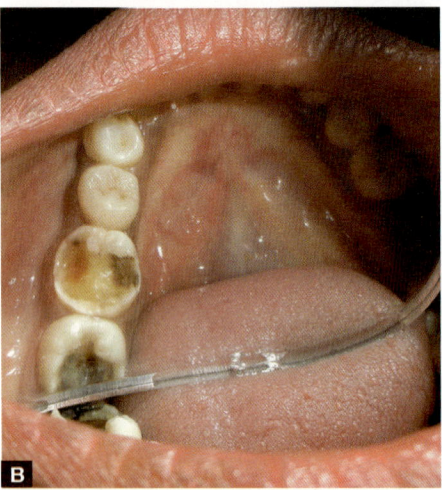

Figs 13.1A and B: Extensive tooth loss in mandibular right molar, indicated for a cast restoration

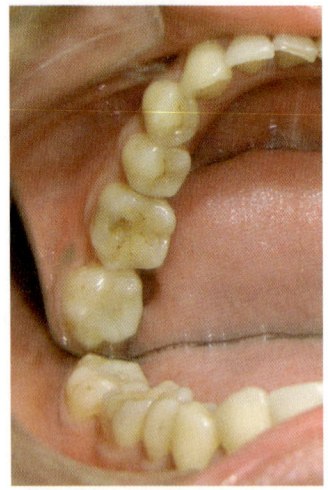

Fig. 13.2: Cast restoration indicated to modify the embrasure and contact

moisture is impossible, properly finished and polished gold alloys are the restorative materials most compatible with the periodontium. Therefore, these restorations are considered the most practical for subgingival lesions (Fig. 13.3).

8. *Patients with low incidence of plaque accumulation*: Patients to receive a cast restoration should have their plaque accumulation under rigid control to avoid problems due to the weak link of the tooth-cement-cast interphase.

9. *Fracture lines*: Fracture lines in the enamel, especially in teeth having extensive restorations, should be recognized as cleavage planes for possible future fracture of the tooth. Restoring these teeth with a restoration that braces the tooth against future injury is a highly valued preventive service.

10. *Esthetics*: Of all metallic restorations (with the exception of direct gold restorations), properly fitted cast restorations are most pleasant esthetically.

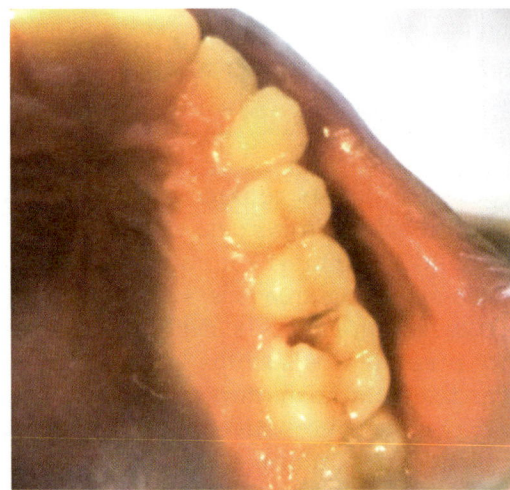

Fig. 13.3: Subgingival lesion on maxillary first molar

CONTRAINDICATIONS

Physiologically, young dentition with large pulp chambers and incompletely mineralized dentin are poor candidates for cast restorations.

1. *Developing and deciduous teeth*: Growth or resorption may be affected by the traumatic nature of the procedures for cast restorations.
2. *High plaque/caries indices*: Patients with rampant caries and poor oral hygiene should not be given cast restoration.
3. *Occlusal disharmony*: Cast restorations should not be used in patients with severe occlusal interference or other defects in the stomatognathic system.

5. *Restoration of endodontically treated teeth (on lays, full crown)*
6. *Retainers for fixed prostheses*
7. *Subgingival lesions*: In cavities with subgingival margins and where the prolonged exclusion of

4. *Dissimilar metals*: Gold-based castings are avoided in patients already having silver restorations.
5. Where esthetics is prime consideration because metallic restorations display metal color.
6. In case of extensive occlusal wear facets involving the remaining ridge of the tooth, inlays and onlays are generally contraindicated.

Advantages

- Yield strength, compressive strength, tensile strength and shear strength of alloys used for cast restorations are far greater than those of any materials used intra orally (some cast alloys have five times the ultimate strength of amalgam). One of the main uses of cast inlay in operative dentistry is in situations when a restorative material is needed to impart resistance to the tooth rather than depending on tooth structure to provide resistance form to the restoration.
- Cast techniques and materials are capable of reproducing precise form and minute detail. Additionally, these materials will maintain this detail under functional stresses.
- As the cast inlay contains one or more noble metals, they are not significantly affected by tarnish and corrosion processes in the oral environment. This major advantage improves longevity, esthetics and biologic qualities of inlays.
- The nature of building a metallic restoration instantaneously with a casting procedure as opposed to an incremental build-up in amalgam imparts advantages to the final restoration, e.g. fewer voids, no layering effect, less internal stresses, fairly even stress patterns of the entire structure and maximum bonding between the component phases.
- Cast restorations can be finished and polished outside the oral cavity, thereby producing surface with maximum biological acceptance.
- Freedom from volume change after placement.
- Gold castings have a coefficient of thermal expansion ($12 \times 10^{-6}/°C$) similar to that of tooth structure.

Disadvantages

- Being a cemented restoration, several interphases will be created at the tooth cement casting junction. These inter phases and the leakage accompanying them will become more significant due to the fact that cast fabrications involve a number of channels using different materials like impressions, models, etc. each of which possesses inherent discrepancies. This produces a restoration, which is microscopically ill fitting. Leakage around and under a cast restoration is the most complicated and has the highest dimension among all restorative materials. This leakage is pronounced gingivally than at other parts of the restorations.
- Cast inlay restorations necessitate extensive tooth involvement in the preparation, which creates possible hazards for the vital dental tissues.
- The cathode nature of cast gold dental alloys towards amalgam may lead to galvanic deterioration of amalgam if these two restorations are placed adjacent to or opposite to each other. As a byproduct of this dissimilar metal cell corrosion, the freed mercury will contaminate the cast alloy itself.
- The procedure for cast inlay restoration fabrication is lengthy, requiring more than one visit. It may require temporary coverage during inter-appointments. Cast alloys are much more expensive than other restorative materials, due to the inherent expense of the alloy.
- Some cast alloys and ceramics have a very high abrasive resistance, much more than that of tooth enamel. So, if a restoration is made for a patient replacing occluding surfaces and opposing natural teeth during functional mandibular relations, there may be abrasive differences between natural dentition and cast restoration, with the teeth being abraded much more easily. Such an abrasive difference will lead to an imbalance in occlusion resulting in tooth shifting, tilting or rotating and leading to occlusal interferences during mandibular movements.
- They are more technique sensitive.

BASIC CONCEPTS OF CAVITY DESIGN

The cast restoration is fabricated in noble metal by the replacement of a wax pattern formed directly in the prepared tooth or indirectly on a die. Therefore, removal of this wax pattern from the tooth or die without distortion is essential. Removal of the pattern and subsequent insertion of the casting can be accomplished only when the prepared cavity exhibits a fundamentally different form compared to the form with slight undercuts, which is used for the direct filling materials.

Three basic systems of preparation have been developed for the cast gold restorations:

a. *The first system* is based almost entirely upon the principles of cavity preparation as outlined by Black. The cavity is prepared with parallel axial walls, which are at right angles or nearly so, to the pulpal and gingival walls. To allow for the withdrawal of the wax pattern a flare of 2° to 5° from parallelism is incorporated in the vertical walls.

However, because of the inherent contraction of metal castings, there was some difficulty in fitting the larger and more complicated types of inlays. To overcome this difficulty, *Ward* suggested a preparation wherein the flare of the wall was increased from 8 to 20 percent per inch. This modification helped to seat the castings more easily within the cavities. However, such restorations were poor in retention.

A slice type of cavity preparation in which the convexity of a tooth was removed from the proximal surface and the margin extended gingivally so that it finished below the crest of the gingival tissue, was suggested almost a century ago.

b. *The second system* is based on the application of the groove principles of retention.
c. *The third system* is the use of the casting process to construct complete veneer metal crowns and their modifications.

Prior to the removal of any calcified tissue, the tooth must be studied carefully for the factors that influence the design of the cavity to be prepared. They are:

- The length of the clinical crown.
- The anatomic characteristics of the occlusal, proximal, buccal and lingual surfaces.
- The position of the tooth in the arch.
- The occlusal and proximal relationships.
- Unusual esthetic problems.
- The relationship and condition of the soft tissues.
- The extent and the location of the carious lesions.

PRINCIPLES OF CAVITY PREPARATION

Outline Form

I. External Outline Form

The external outline form of the cavity preparation with No.271 and No.169L burs for inlay should consist of straight lines and smooth flowing curves, avoiding any short angles. The finishing line should be extended on the occlusal surface to include retentive fissures or other faults and on to the proximal and cervical areas until the carious lesion is removed and the margins are convenient for finishing of the preparation as well as for casting. Enamel rods at the cavosurface margin should be supported by dentin and supported laterally by rods that lie within the preparation. Enamel that has been undermined by caries is removed. In order to obtain a well-fitted casting, the cavosurface margin is placed in sound, unbroken tooth tissue.

The external outline form for the gold inlay follows a similar external form as that for the amalgam cavity. Application of the concept of taper will necessitate a change in the proximal outline form from that used in the amalgam cavity (Figs 13.4A and B). The placement of bevels makes the outline form slightly wider for cast restorations.

II. Internal Outline Form

The pulpal floor and the axial wall of the gold inlay preparation must be placed in dentin. Care must be taken to protect the pulp. When the preparation has to be taken beyond its usual internal limits because of the extent of the lesion or injury, the additional loss of dentin is replaced with an appropriate cement base. The amount of taper required varies with the depth or length of the preparation from the occlusal to cervical aspect. The taper should not be visible to the eye. In shallow preparations, parallelism enhances the resistance and retention form of the preparation. Deep cavities require taper to facilitate seating of the restoration.

While it is difficult to establish an exact measurement for the length of the occlusal walls, owing to the anatomic variations of teeth, the pulpal floor will usually be positioned 0.5 mm or 1.75 to 2.0 mm into dentin below the central groove (Fig. 13.5).

The cervical floor should be in sound tooth tissue. When a cement base is placed to form a portion of this floor, it is necessary to maintain at least one half

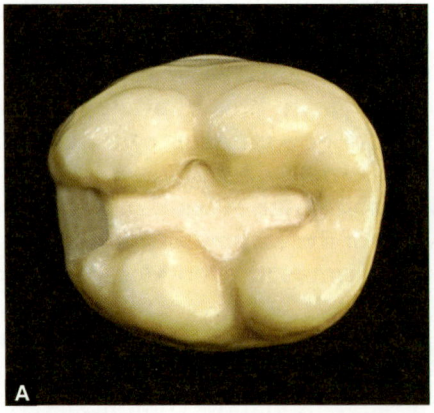 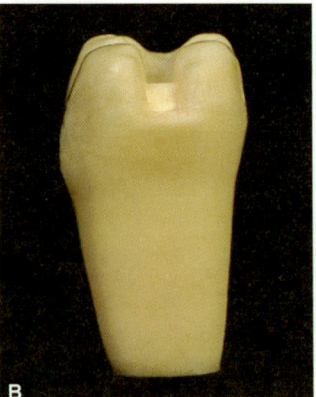 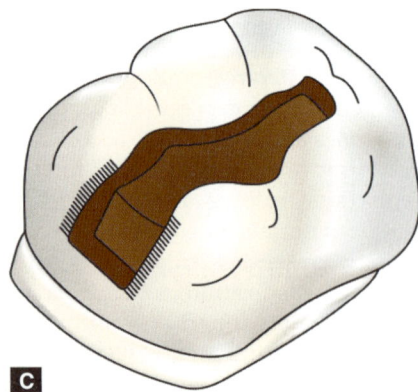

Figs 13.4A, B and C: Class II cavity preparation for cast gold: **(A)** Occlusal view; **(B)** Proximal view; **(C)** Diagrammatic representation (lines indicate secondary flare)

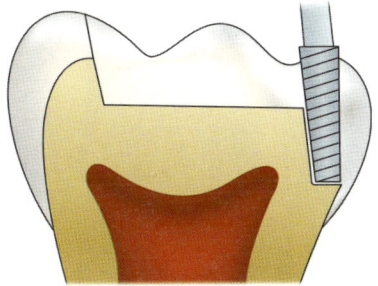

Fig. 13.5: Occlusal and axial walls are in dentin with slight taper of the axial wall

of the area in sound tooth tissue to support the restoration. The cervical floor is positioned after caries removal. The bevel is placed to establish the finishing line.

Line angles in both the occlusal and proximal portions of the preparation should be well defined. The axio-pulpal line angle is slightly rounded (Fig. 13.6). The flare of the proximal walls should form axioproximal angles of 100 to 110 degrees.

Providing sufficient taper to these walls, which will maintain adequate dentin support for the enamel, should enhance the integrity of mesial or distal marginal ridges. All questionable grooves or fissures should be included and cavosurface margin established on sound enamel. Fissures terminating near or in marginal ridge areas pose a special problem. It is sometimes desirable to incline the cutting instrument so that it forms either an exaggerated taper from cavosurface to pulpal floor or a long bevel on that area of the wall. This procedure protects the thin wall of enamel that remains at the cavosurface by maintaining a supporting edge of dentin (Fig. 13.6).

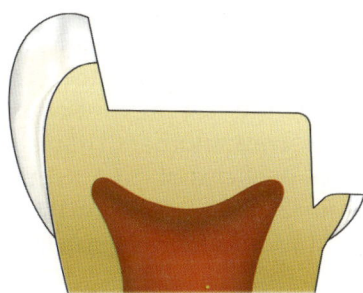

Fig. 13.6: Rounded axiopulpal line angle and reverse bevel at the gingival wall

Resistance and Retention Forms

The preparation of the tooth for a cast gold restoration must be so designed that it will resist the dislodging forces of compression and tension. The design must take into consideration occlusal forces that may cause fracture of the tooth.

Lateral or tangential forces may cause displacement of the restoration unless adequate resistance and retention have been incorporated in the preparation. Frictional retention can be achieved by the action of dentin and enamel walls grasping the restoration (intra coronal retention). Most dental cements are not adhesive. The strength of the cement bond alone will not provide retention for the casting. Cement provides only a moderate mechanical lock between the minute irregularities of the cavity walls and the casting surface.

Inlay Taper

A basic requirement of all cavity preparations for the intracoronal cast gold restoration is that the cavity walls must diverge from the floor of the preparation externally. A similar requirement for all extracoronal preparations is that walls must converge from the cervical to the occlusal surface. This is the concept of taper. Removal of wax pattern and insertion of casting is facilitated by the taper.

Each intracoronal and extracoronal preparation has a line of draw that describes the path of insertion and removal of the casting, which determines the axis of taper (Figs 13.7A to C and 13.8A and B). The axis of

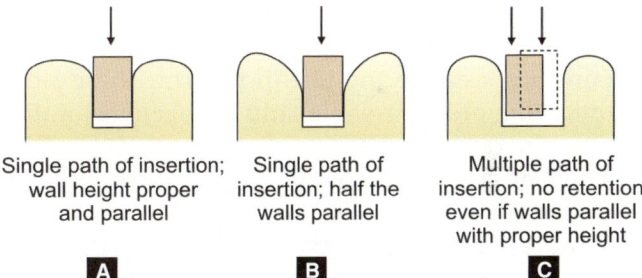

Figs 13.7A to C: Inlay taper: **(A)** Single path of insertion; wall height proper and parallel; **(B)** Single path of insertion; half of the wall height parellel; **(C)** Multiple paths of insertion; no retention even if parallel walls with proper height

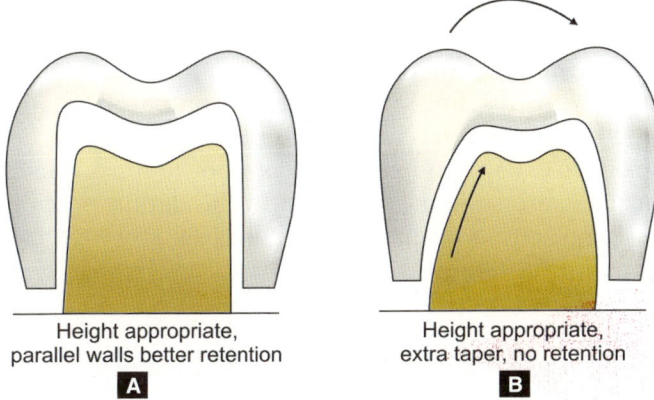

Figs 13.8A and B: Extra-coronal taper: **(A)** Appropriate height and parallel walls give better retention; **(B)** Appropriate height but extra taper give no retention

taper for a Class I and II preparation generally parallels the long axis of the tooth, for a Class V, axis of taper generally is perpendicular to the long axis of the tooth. Line of draw bisects the angle formed by the convergence of the tapered cavity walls to a point of their intersection. The amount of taper upon opposing cavity walls is described by this convergent angle. No single degree of convergent angle taper is considered ideal. A range between 8 to 12 degrees is used because empirically it has provided for adequate retention of the cemented casting, and one is able to clinically make a reliable visual assessment of this amount of taper upon opposing cavity walls. The axial length of the preparation will influence the amount of taper. Longer preparations require taper in the higher range, short preparations in the lower range. The correct taper of the cavity walls of a preparation is an important factor in providing satisfactory resistance and retention form. The degree of taper cannot be so great so as to lose the frictional grasp between tooth and the restoration. It must however be sufficient to allow the complete seating of the restoration in the cavity. Pulpal and cervical floors ideally should be perpendicular to the lines of force that will influence the restoration. Floors positioned perpendicular to these lines of force absorbs the stress over a broad area of tooth (Fig. 13.5).

Well-defined line angles are also important in obtaining resistance and retention form. These aid in maintaining precise relationship between restoration and tooth tissue.

The axiopulpal line angle is slightly rounded to dissipate the stresses (Fig. 13.6).

The slice is frequently used to increase the resistance and retention form by exposing a larger amount of tooth surface to the frictional grasp of the restoration.

The occlusal interlock or dovetail is a major factor in resistance and retention form.

Specially designed features are frequently incorporated to increase the resistance and retention form. Pinholes or postholes are sometimes placed parallel to the line of draw of the preparation and with appropriate concern for the pulp. Tapered grooves extending form cervical floor to the occlusal surface, are sometimes placed in the dentin portion of the proximal walls to form a locking key to aid in preventing lateral dislodgement of the restoration (Figs 13.9A and B).

Factors Affecting Retention of Cast Restorations

Certain forces collectively act on a cemented restoration mainly in the same direction as the path of withdrawal. The quality of preparation that

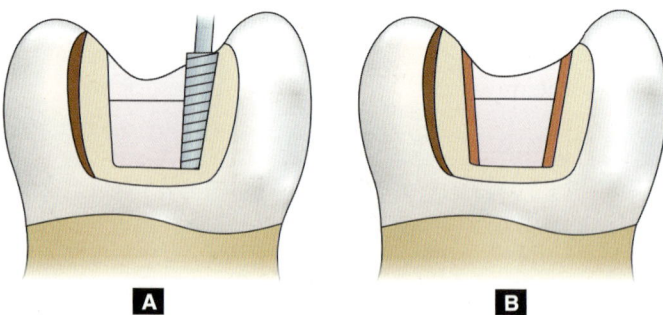

Figs 13.9A and B: Proximal grooves are incorporated to improve retention form: **(A)** Preparing grooves with tapering fissure bur; **(B)** Prepared grooves

prevents the restoration from becoming dislodged by such forces is known as retention.

The following factors affect the overall retention of the cast restorations:

1. *Magnitude of the dislodging forces*: Forces that tend to remove a cemented restoration along its path of withdrawal are small compared to those that tend to tilt it. Generally exceptionally sticky foodstuffs act as a pulling force. The quantum of vertical and oblique forces also tends to dislodge the restoration. The magnitude of the dislodging forces depends on the stickiness of food, occluding and lateral movement forces of the jaws and the surface area and texture of restoration being pulled.
2. *Geometry of the tooth preparation*: Retention of cast restorations depends on the geometric form of the preparation rather than on the intervening cements. This is because most of the traditional cements (e.g. zinc phosphate) are non-adhesive, i.e. they act by increasing the frictional resistance between tooth and restorations. The grains of cement prevent two surfaces from sliding, although they do not prevent one surface from being lifted from another. This is analogous to the effect of particles of dust within machinery. They do not have a specific adhesion to metal, but they do increase the friction between sliding metal parts.

   Cement is effective only if the restoration has a single path of withdrawal, i.e. the tooth is prepared to restrain the free movement of the restoration. The geometrical forms generally responsible for retention are:
   a. *Taper*: Theoretically, maximum retention is obtained if a tooth preparation has parallel walls. However, it is impossible to prepare a tooth this way using current techniques and instrumentation.

A slight taper is necessary for the fabrication of wax pattern. As long as this taper is small, the movement of the cemented restoration will be effectively restrained by limited path of withdrawal. As the taper increases, there will be free movement of the restoration along the path of withdrawal.

The maximum convergence between opposing walls should not be more than 6 degrees. The rotary instrument should be moved over the tooth in such a way that the taper of the instrument should produce the designed axial wall taper on the completed preparation. At least two opposite surfaces must always be parallel in a cast restoration.

b. *Surface area:* Provided the restoration has a limited path of withdrawal, its retention is dependent on the length of this path or more precisely on the surface area in sliding contact. Therefore, restorations with long axial walls are more retentive than those with short axial walls, e.g. restorations for molars are more retentive than for premolars. Surfaces where the restoration is essentially being pulled away rather than sliding, e.g. occlusal surface, do not add much to total retention.

c. *Stress concentration:* Various studies have shown that when a retentive failure occurs, it occurs due to cohesive failure in the cement layer because the strength of the cement was less than the induced stresses. These stresses are not uniform throughout the cement but are concentrated around the junction of the axial and occlusal surfaces.

d. *Type of preparation:* Different type of restorations have different retentive values and these correspond fairly close to the surface area of the axial wall, provided other factors are kept constant. Thus, the retention of a complete crown is about double than that of partial coverage restoration.

Adding grooves to a preparation with a limited path of withdrawal does not markedly affect its retention because the surface area is not increased significantly. However, where the addition of a groove limits the path of withdrawal, retention is increased.

3. *Roughness of the surfaces being cemented*: When the internal surface of a restoration is very smooth, retentive failure occurs through the cement restoration interface. Under these circumstances, retention will be increased if the restoration is roughened or grooved. This can be done by air abrading the inner surface with 50 μm alumina.

4. *Materials being cemented:* The more reactive the alloy is, the more will be adhesion with the luting cement. Therefore, base metal alloys are better retained than less reactive high gold content metals.

5. *Type of luting agent:* The data suggests that adhesive resin cements are the most retentive, although long term studies regarding the durability of the bond are not available.

Removing Carious Dentin

Removal of deeper carious lesion frequently precedes the establishment of resistance and retention form.

Convenience Form

Convenience form provides the accessibility and visibility required to complete operative procedures thoroughly and accurately. Opening the preparation to its approximate final outline form to establish an intact dentinoenamel junction enhances access and visibility for removal of carious dentin or old restorative materials. Extension, taper and flare of proximal walls to permit access for disking and bevel placement, and extension to allow proper finishing and adaptation of the margins of the restorative material are all examples of convenience form.

Finishing Enamel Walls and Margins

Excellent adaptation of the gold restoration to the walls and margins of the cavity preparation can occur only if the surface of the calcified tooth tissue has been finished properly. Regular grit diamond instruments and cross cut fissure burs leave roughened surfaces. Even hand instruments may leave notched irregularities on walls and margins. The marginal fit of a gold restoration depends upon the approximation of cast metal to tooth tissue and this cannot be accomplished accurately unless the surfaces recorded in the wax pattern or impression material are smooth.

If coarse or medium grit diamond instruments have been used during cavity preparation the walls and margins should be finished with carbide finishing burs or fine abrasive disks. Unlike cross cut fissure burs, plain fissure burs impart a relatively smooth surface to tooth tissue.

The cervical bevel of the indirect preparation is most frequently placed with the flame shaped extra fine finishing bur or flame shaped extra fine grit finishing diamond point or gingival marginal trimmers (Figs 13.10A and B). These instruments are used primarily because of their convenience. They provide a steeper bevel to prepare for an effective

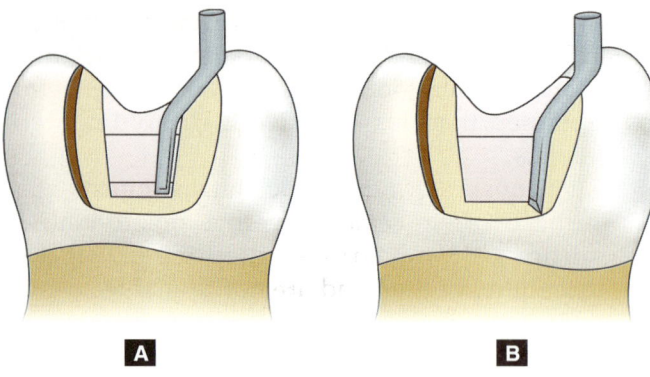

Figs 13.10A and B: **(A)** Gingival marginal trimmer used for finishing cervical wall; **(B)** Gingival marginal trimmer used for making cervical carvosurface bevel

adaptation of the metal margin. A bevel placed with a flame shaped rotary instrument will establish excellent cervical margin and will further blend together with the buccal and lingual proximal finish lines.

The greater bulkiness of the cervical margin produced by the flame shaped instrument, compared to that formed when the disk slices the cervical area is of advantage in gaining the impression and finishing the casting.

Whenever a direct wax pattern is to be formed, the bevel used is of greater bulk and extends a greater width across the cervical floor. Thus a bevel on the cervical margin of a box preparation for the direct technique should be uniformly about ¼ to ½ of mesiodistal width of the cervical floor and must include the proximal cervical cavosurface angles. Such a bevel is placed with a gingival marginal trimmer prior to finishing the proximal enamel walls.

The sharp point angle formed at the occlusal outline by the junction of the proximal wall and the slice is a hazard to good cavosurface margin adaptation of the casting. These angles should also be bevelled (Figs 13.11A to D).

Cleaning and Critical Appraisal of the Cavity

Upon completing the cavity preparation, the walls, floors and margins should be cleaned with water. After drying with cotton pledgets and a gentle stream of warmed air, the cavity should be scrutinized carefully for any imperfections. A trial impression with gutta-percha or impression compound is always a helpful procedure to evaluate taper and the line of draw of the preparation (Fig. 13.12). Even relatively minute under cuts are readily apparent in a compound impression, as is any discrepancy between the line of draw of the occlusal and proximal portions of a cavity preparation. A compound impression will also give

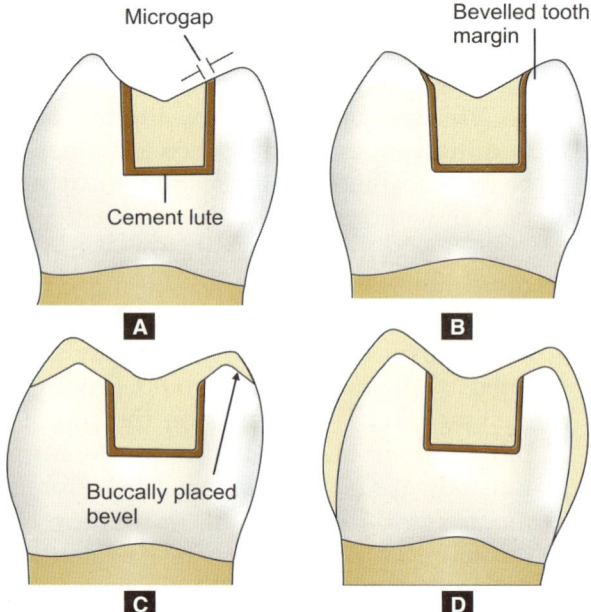

Figs 13.11A to D: **(A)** Significant microgap is seen with a non-bevelled intra-coronal inlay; **(B)** Microgap is reduced with bevelled intra-coronal inlay; **(C)** Microgap is reduced when intra-coronal inlay has buccal and lingual bevels; **(D)** A bevel parallel to the path of insertion reduces the cement thickness to almost nil at the margins

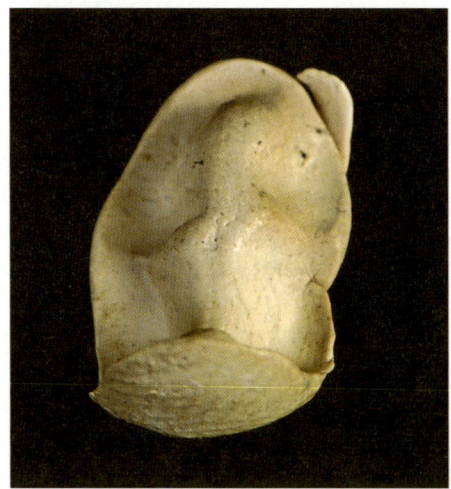

Fig. 13.12: Trial impression with gutta-percha

details regarding bevels, line angles, and the definition of finishing lines.

Types of Margins in a Cast Restoration

The various types of margins, which can be employed in a cast restoration, are depicted in the Fig. 13.13A to G). The relevant indications, advantages and disadvantages are tabulated in the Table 13.3. However, the bevel, chamfer and the shoulder are commonly used margins. The difference between chamfer and shoulder is that chamfer is less than 0.5 mm wide and is rounded while shoulder is 0.75 mm

Cast Restorations

Table 13.3: Margin designs

	Advantage	Disadvantage	Indications
1. Feather edge	Conservative	Does not provide sufficient bulk	Not recommended
2. Chisel edge	Conservative	Location of margin is difficult to control	Occasionally on tilted teeth
3. Bevel	Removes unsupported enamel, allows finishing of metal	Extends preparation into sulcus if used on apical margin	Facial margin of maxillary partial coverage restorations
4. Chamfer	Distinct margin, adequate bulk, easier to control	Care needed to avoid unsupported lip of enamel	Lingual margin of cast metal restorations and metal ceramic crowns
5. Shoulder	Bulk of restorative material	Less conservative	Labial margins of complete ceramic crown and metal ceramic crowns
6. Sloped shoulder	Bulk of material, advantages of bevel	Less conservative	Facial margin of metal ceramic crown
7. Shoulder with bevel	Bulk of material, advantages of bevel	Less conservative, extends preparation apically gingival margins	Facial margin of posterior metal ceramic crowns with supra-gingival margin

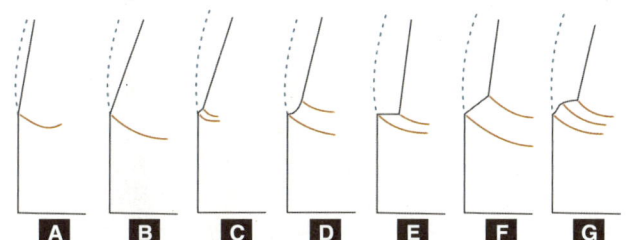

Figs 13.13A to G: Different margin designs: **(A)** Feather edge; **(B)** Chisel; **(C)** Bevel; **(D)** Chamfer; **(E)** Shoulder; **(F)** Sloped shoulder; **(G)** Shoulder with bevel

to 1.0 mm wide and sharp. Chamfer is mostly given on the lingual sides while shoulder is given on the labial sides. Alternatively the chamfer is given where less bulk is required and the metal is malleable whereas the shoulder is given where more bulk is required and the metal is not malleable.

Bevels

The weakest link in any cast restoration is the tooth cement cast joint complex. An accurate wax pattern and reproduction in gold does not assure a casting margin well adapted to the tooth surface. Special attention should be paid to the marginal peripheries of the preparation, and every effort, should be made to design and prepare these marginal peripheries to create the most favourable relationship with the restoring casting and luting cement. This peripheral marginal anatomy of the preparation is called "*circumferential tie*" and it should have the following features. Enamel must be supported by sound dentin, enamel rods forming the cavosurface margin should be continuous with sound dentin, enamel rods forming the restorative material and angular cavosurface angles should be trimmed.

Function of Occlusal and Gingival Bevels

Bevels satisfy the requirements for ideal cavity walls, create obtuse-angled marginal tooth structure, which is the bulkiest and the strongest configuration of any marginal tooth anatomy and produce an acute angled marginal cast alloy substance, which in such configuration is most amenable for burnishing. Marginal bevels reduce the error factors by (space between cast and tooth substances) three or more folds at the margins compared to their internal dimensions, depending on the bevel's angulation. Bevels indirectly improve retention forms for a cast restoration since bevels decrease the direct frictional component between the tooth and the casting. The circumferential tie of tooth-casting interphase is a susceptible friction zone and if left to direct contact will lead to less retention of the restoration. The bevels available for cast restorations are (Figs 13.14A to D):

a. *Partial bevel:* It involves part of the enamel wall. Such type of preparation is indicated in direct filling gold restorations. A few authors advise giving partial bevel in composite restorations to have more surface area.
b. *Short bevel:* It involves the entire enamel wall. This type of bevel is best suited in cast gold restorations.

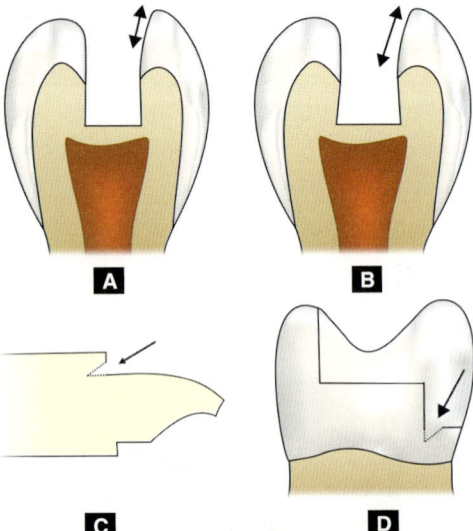

Figs 13.14A to D: Types of bevels: **(A)** Partial bevel; **(B)** Short bevel; **(C)** Inverted bevel; **(D)** Reverse bevel

c. *Inverted bevel:* It is given on the labial shoulder of metal ceramic crowns to effectively improve the esthetics at the margins.
d. *Reverse bevel:* A reverse bevel is placed at the dentinal portion of the cervical wall towards the axiogingival line angle. The hydrostatic pressure during cementing a cast restoration can produce a rotational displacement of the casting with flat gingival walls. This effect is resisted by the reverse bevel resulting in even seating of the cast restoration.

Types and Design Features of Facial and Lingual Flares

a. *The primary flare*: This is the conventional and basic part of the circumferential tie facially and lingually of the proximal box for an intracoronal preparation. It is very similar to a long bevel formed of an enamel and part of the dentin on the facial or lingual proximal wall. Primary flares have 45° angulation to the inner dentinal wall proper (Figs 13.4A and B).

  Functions and indications: These design features bring the proximal facial and lingual margins of the cavity preparation to cleansable finishable areas. They are indicated for any facial or lingual proximal wall of an intra-coronal cavity preparation, when the normal contacts are present and there is minimal extension of caries in buccolingual direction. It is prepared on enamel and dentin.

b. *The secondary flare:* The secondary flare is a flat plane superimposed peripherally to a primary flare. Usually it is prepared solely in enamel, but sometimes it may involve some dentin in all or parts of its surfaces. Unlike primary flares secondary flares may have different angulations, involvement and extent depending on their function (Figs 13.4A and B). Secondary flare is not given in the areas where aesthetic is more important.

  Functions and indications: In very widely extended lesions buccolingually, the buccal and lingual tooth structure will be badly thinned; the primary flare will end in an acute-angled marginal tooth structure, occasionally with unsupported enamel. A secondary flare at the correct angulation can create the needed obtuse angulation of the marginal tooth structure. In very broad contact areas or malposed contact areas, the primary flare will not bring the facial and lingual margins to finishable cleansable areas. A secondary flare placed peripheral to the primary flare will accommodate this without changing the fixed 45° angulation of the primary flare necessary for resistance and retention.

  In ovoid teeth, marginal undercuts can be present occluso-gingivally on the facial and/or lingual peripheries of the cavity preparation. Elimination of these undercuts with primary flare extension will unnecessarily involve more tooth structure subsequently weakening the same. However, a secondary flare superimposed on a primary flare in the correct angulation and extent can eliminate these undercuts with minimal sacrifice of tooth structure. Surface defects or decalcifications can be involved in the preparation with a secondary flare.

Variations in Proximal Marginal Design

The design of the proximal margins will vary depending upon the following factors:
- The extent of tooth tissue loss
- The location of that loss
- Tooth form, i.e. curvatures and embrasures
- The positional relationship with adjacent teeth
- The need for retention form
- Convenience

The modified preparation, following the guidelines of the above said factors, can be:

I. Box Preparation

This is basically the conventional technique. The direct wax technique requires the proximal margin to be so designed, such that it can be manipulated in the mouth. Margins are prepared to permit a great bulk of wax, which is consistent for the subsequent finishing and adaptation. The buccal and lingual proximal walls are finished in such a way so that the cavosurface angle formed by the proximal flare and the tooth surface will be at right angle or slightly obtuse angles. A cervical bevel is required.

The box design is preferred with the proximoocclusal preparation for the direct method of wax pattern formation.

II. Slice Preparation

Historically, *a slice referred to the placement of extracoronal taper using a disk of adequate diameter to contact nearly the entire proximal surface.* Slice established a cervical finish line for the preparation, but it also eliminated much of the proximal anatomic under cut which facilitated taking an impression with a non-elastic impression material. With introduction of the elastic impression materials such gross reduction of the proximal contour was unnecessary. Present slice preparation involves conservative disking of the proximal surface to establish the buccal and lingual extent of the finish lines and provide a lap joint for finishing. These slices are placed on the buccal and lingual proximal surfaces independently. The slice is extended to the cervical floor or slightly occlusal to cervical floor by keeping the factor in mind that the tooth tissue should be preserved (Fig.13.15A and B). Radiographic and intraoral examination of the tooth form will decide as to how much cervical extension is necessary. Teeth with proximal contours of the square tooth form require slice preparation extending upto cervical floor and for teeth with tapering or ovoid tooth form slice formation extending short of the cervical floor. Placement of a proximal slice for the indirect inlay produces excellent definition for the finishing line.

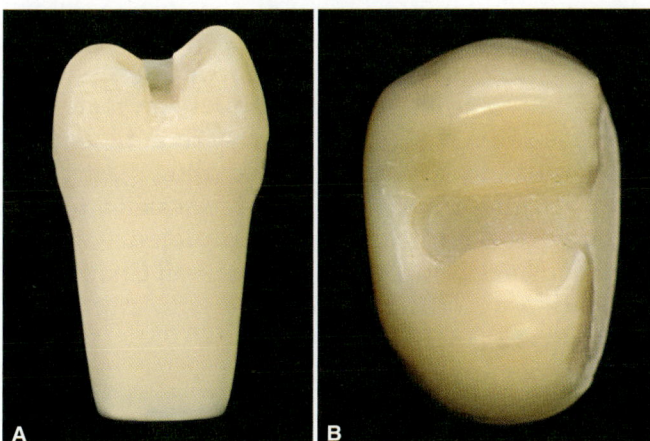

Figs 13.15A and B: Slice preparation: **(A)** Proximal view; **(B)** Occlusal view

III. Auxiliary Slice

Slice preparation provides external support of weakened tooth or areas subjected to high stresses during function. The auxiliary slice partially wraps around the proximal line angles thus providing additional support (Fig. 13.16). Minimal bulk of tooth tissue is lost but greatly enhances the resistance form, reducing the possibility of tooth fracture. The auxiliary slice can be employed to provide retention form. An auxiliary slice around the lingual proximal line angle of a tooth will aid in preventing a buccal displacement of the casting. When a buccal proximal wall is impossible to establish because of the loss of tooth tissue due to dental caries or trauma, an auxillary slice can also be conservatively included within the inlay preparation.

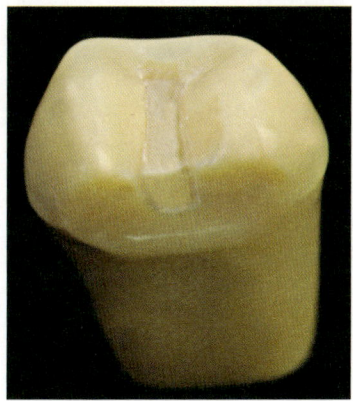

Fig. 13.16: Auxiliary slice preparation

IV. Modified flare Preparation

The modified flare is hybrid of the box and slice preparation. Buccal and lingual proximal walls are initially formed with minimal extension, and then disked in a plane that only slightly reduces the proximal wall dimension. Extensive disking will reduce the retention of these walls. The obtuseness of the cavosurface angle is enhanced.

The box, the slice preparation or the modified flare preparation may be selected as most suitable as per the mechanical and biological considerations or for esthetic reasons.

CUSP CAPPING/ONLAY

Cusp capping or onlays are usually indicated where one or more cusps, which are weakened by caries or trauma, are to be covered occlusally with the restorative material. The most suitable restoration is the cast restoration especially when functional cusps are to be capped. It is partly an intracoronal and partly extracoronal type of restoration. As already described, if the cavity involves more than half of the cusp inclines, cuspal coverage is mandatory.

A tapering fissure bur of appropriate size is taken and the cusp is reduced occlusally by 1.0-1.5 mm. The different sizes and shapes of burs for cast preparation are shown in Fig. 13.17. The total height of the wall in the cavity is not included (Figs 13.18A and B). The extracoronal margins are placed at the enamel and the design of the margin can be selected depending upon the restorative material. Usually chamfer is indicated with cast gold restoration. Because of the ductility and malleability of the material, the margins can be burnished and adapted to the tooth surface (Fig. 13.19).

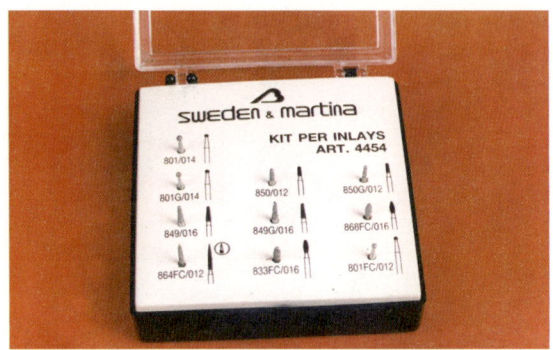

Fig. 13.17: Different sizes and shapes of burs for cast preparation

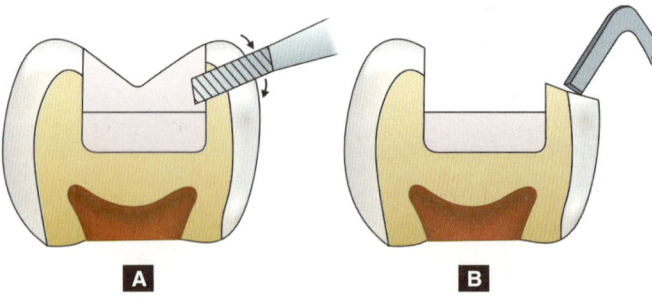

Figs 13.18A and B: **(A)** Cusp being reduced with a bur; **(B)** Margin being refined with a hand instrument

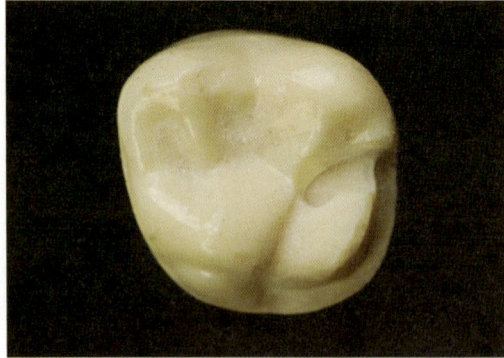

Fig. 13.19: Class II cavity preparation with distolingual cusp reduction - indicated for cast restoration

In case, functional cusps are capped, it is advisable to make contra retention on the opposing tooth surface. For example, if both the buccal cusps of mandibular molars are capped, lingual extension of the cavity is mandatory as is done in lingual complex of class I cavities.

PIN-RETAINED CAST RESTORATIONS

Indications

1. When one wall of a proximal box is shorter than opposing proximal wall.
2. When a proximal preparation is unusually long.
3. In case of over tapered full crown preparations.
4. Full crown preparations with one wall very short and opposite wall very long.
5. Attritioned or abraded teeth where occlusogingival height is excessively reduced.
6. Large occlusal inlays and cuspal fractures.

Methods

The pin channels are slightly wider in cast pin restorations and a depth of 3.0 mm is required with such pins. In case, two or more pins are required to be inserted, the parallelism between the pins is to be maintained.

The wax pattern can be drawn by two methods:
1. *Direct:* In direct method, the wax pattern is made in the oral cavity itself. After making necessary pinholes, nylon bristle of the size of the pinhole is seated in each pinhole and wax pattern is made, incorporating the external part of the bristle. The outer end of the bristle is flattened so as to enable the end to be incorporated into the pattern. This wax pattern along with the incorporated bristle is invested, and casting is completed.
2. *Indirect:* In indirect method, a stainless steel pin ground to the size of pin channel, is inserted and stabilized using inlay wax. An impression is taken using rubber base impression materials. This impression is used to make a die and on this die, wax pattern is made using plastic pins as in the direct method. This wax pattern is invested and casting is completed with the requisite alloy. Details are given in Chapter 16.

A case of occlusal rehabilitation with cast pins is shown in Figs 13.20A to I.

TUCKER'S TECHNIQUE

Dr. Richard Tucker developed a conservative cast gold inlay preparation technique. The cavity preparation sequence is as follows:

After placement of rubber dam, the existing restoration, if any, and carious tooth structure is removed. Then, a thin film of calcium hydroxide (Dycal, Dentsply) is placed on the internal surface of the preparation with a small cotton pellet. It acts a separator

Cast Restorations

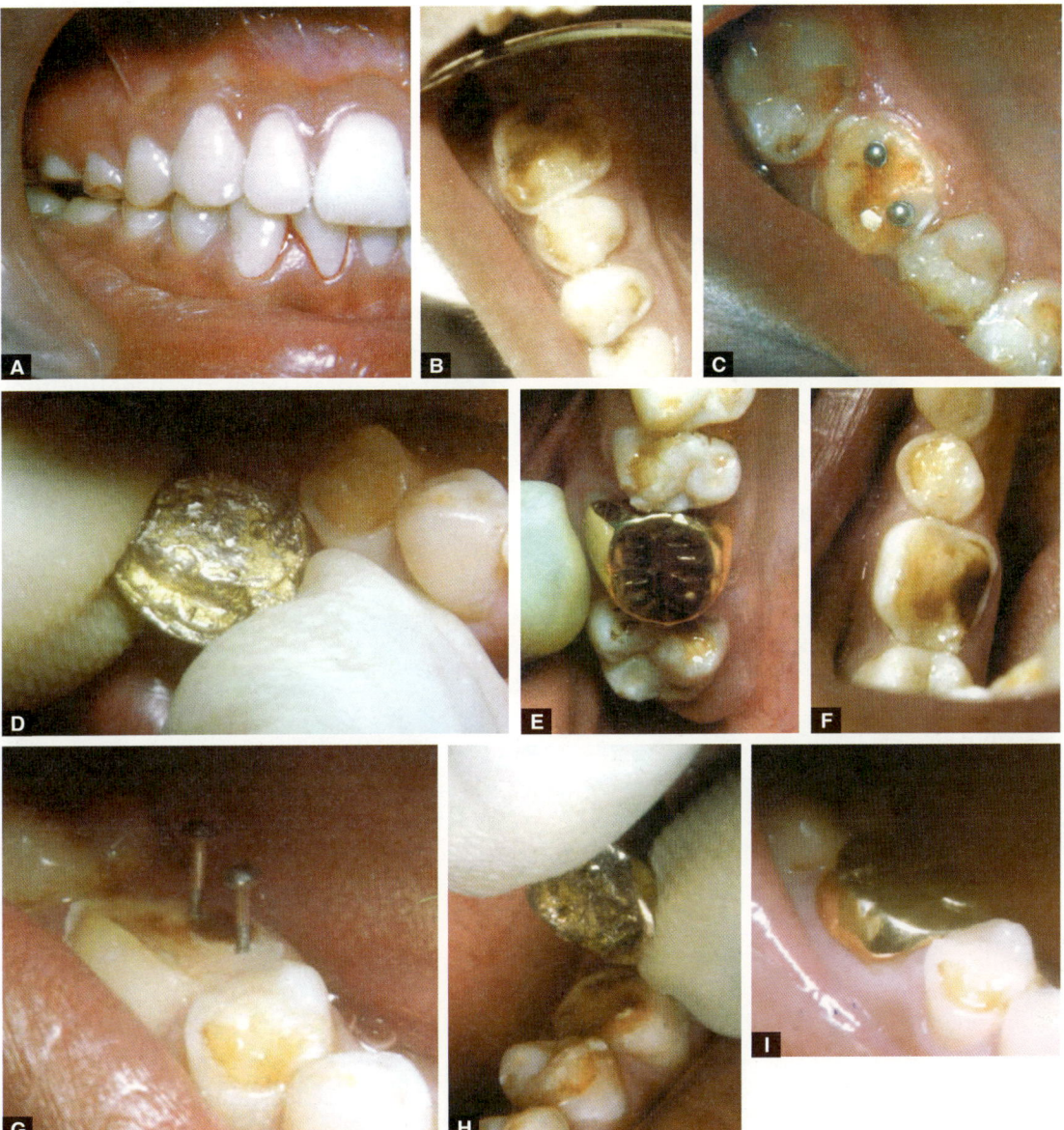

Figs 13.20A to I: Occlusal rehabilitation using cast pins on maxillary right first molar: **(A)** Pre-operative photograph (facial view); **(B)** Pre-operative photograph (occlusal view); **(C)** Pins placed in pin-channel preparation; **(D)** Casting obtained; **(E)** Casting in place. Occlusal rehabilitation using cast pins mandibular right first molar; **(F)** Pre-operative photograph; **(G)** Pins placed in pin channels; **(H)** Casting obtained; **(I)** Casting in place

for easy removal of composite build up prior to cementation. The use of resin composite build up conserves tooth structure. The resin composite build up allows the operator to cut a precise cavity preparation that has an ideal taper, smoothness and proportions. An autocure resin composite can be placed with a packing instrument or a syringe. The build up is usually entirely removed prior to cementation. The casting often seats more completely because of the absence of the composite pulpal wall and the area of the previous build up is filled with luting cement.

The occlusal box is prepared with straight fissure bur and pulpal floor are placed to a depth of 1.5 to 2.0 mm and a uniform inclination of the walls of 3 to 5 degrees. The proximal box form is established next and is blended with the occlusal preparation. The buccal and lingual walls must be extended sufficiently (1 mm) beyond the adjacent tooth. The proximal walls have slight flare (45°) that eliminate unsupported enamel rods. Occlusal and gingival bevels are placed and cavity walls are finished. The gingival bevel is a small bevel 0.5 to 0.75 mm wide. The bevel should be definitive and smooth but not too wide. Tucker's gingival margin trimmer are used in this technique. The No.232 Tucker (10-98-10-16) GMT is used on distal aspect and the No.233 Tucker (10-78-10-16) GMT is used on the mesial aspect. The bevels on non-Tucker GMT instruments are less acute 45 degree) than the ones marked Tucker (30 degree). The occlusal bevel is placed with the straight fissure bur inclined only a few degree more than that of the occlusal wall. The finishing of the proximal walls is completed with a 0.5 inch garnet disk. The technique is illustrated in Fig. 13.21.

Differences in cavity preparation for silver amalgam and cast restorations: The differences in cavity preparation for silver amalgam and cast restoration is given in Table 13.4.

FABRICATION OF CAST RESTORATIONS

Fabrication of cast restoration involves various procedures. Many of these procedures are to be carried out in laboratory. These procedures are equally important as that of cavity preparation for the success of the treatment. The procedures are:

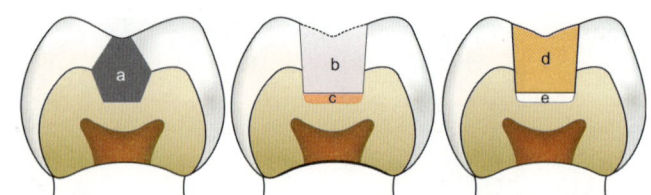

Fig. 13.21: Tucker's Technique: **(a)** Carious Lesion; **(b)** Cavity Preparation for Inlay; **(c)** Composite Build-Up; **(d)** Inlay; **(e)** Luting Cement

A. Impression Technique

An impression is a negative replica of any object. In dentistry impression is the negative replica of teeth and surrounding tissues. From this negative form of the teeth and the surrounding structures, a positive reproduction, or cast, is made. The cast must exactly duplicate the prepared tooth and the preparation in order to have the precision fitting castings.

Table 13.4: Differences in cavity preparation for silver amalgam and cast restorations

Silver amalgam	Cast restorations
i. Intercuspal width is 1/4th intercuspal distance (outline form is narrow).	Intercuspal width is 1/3rd intercuspal distance (outline form is wide).
ii. Cavity depth is more.	Comparatively less depth.
iii. Cavity walls are kept convergent occlusally (minor undercuts).	Cavity walls are kept parallel (no undercuts).
iv. Buccal and lingual proximal walls are convergent occlusally.	Buccal and lingual proximal walls are parallel.
v. Cavosurface bevel is contraindicated (butt joint is preferred).	Cavosurface bevel is given.
vi. All line angles and point angles are rounded and axio pulpal line angle is bevelled.	All line angles and point angles are well defined and axiopulpal line angle is slightly rounded.
vii. No reverse bevel is given.	Reverse bevel is indicated.
viii. Grooves are not given, only locks are given.	Grooves are given, locks are not given.

Cast Restorations

Several types of impression materials are available and considered accurate enough for use in the fabrication of cast restorations. The choice is based on ease of manipulation, dimensional stability and to some extent the cost of material. Most of newly available materials have excellent accuracy and can be used without doubt.

The impression can be taken on prefabricated tray or the tray can be fabricated outside the oral cavity.

Selection of Impression Tray

For reversible hydrocolloid, a water-cooled stock metal tray is used. For polysulfide and polyether material, a custom tray is used. Condensation and addition silicones can be used with stock or custom trays.

Custom trays are usually preferred because they allow a more uniform, thin layer of 2.0-3.0 mm of the impression material. A uniform thickness of impression material will lead to less distortion. Elastomeric impression materials in thicknesses greater than 3.0 mm show greater shrinkage and distortion. Thickness of less than 2.0 mm would either tear or distort easily.

It has been reported that the mean difference in material thickness between custom and stock trays is less than 1.0 mm and that variations from uniform thickness of impression material exist in both custom and stock trays. It has been established that there is no significant difference in the marginal fit of single tooth restorations on casts made from polyvinyl siloxane impressions in custom and stock trays. Thus, for single tooth restorations, stock trays serve the purpose adequately (Fig. 13.22). However, for long span fixed partial dentures inter-preparation and cross-arch discrepancies may occur with these trays. Some authors have described a technique of making a custom tray by lining a stock-tray with modeling compound. But this is not an effective method because plasticizer in the elastomeric material can soften the compound and distort the impression.

Fabrication of Custom Tray

Acrylic resin is used to form a custom tray. A study model provides the basis for forming the tray. To provide space within the completed tray for the impression material, the study model is covered with base plate wax. A sheet of base plate wax is heated over a flame to soften it. It is then folded in half and placed on the diagnostic cast. It is trimmed so that it extends 2.0-3.0 mm beyond the necks of the teeth. A horseshoe shaped form is used for both arches, palatal coverage is not required for the maxillary arch. The diagnostic cast must be covered with tin foil before the wax is adapted. A 3.0 × 3.0 mm hole is cut through the wax over the posterior teeth on both sides and in the incisor area. The tray resin will touch the teeth in these areas to form tray stops. This will prevent the tray from being seated inaccurately. On the side of the prepared tooth, the stop is placed distal to the prepared tooth.

Before the resin tray is made, the wax is covered by a layer of tin foil to prevent the wax from impregnating the surface of the tray during the exothermic polymerization of the resin. The waxy layer on the tray will diminish bonding action to the tray adhesive.

The cold cure acrylic resin is mixed and allowed to stand till the dough stage is reached. It is then rolled to form a horseshoe shape and flattened. Some extra bulk is left in the middle. The acrylic is adapted over the wax. The bulk in the middle is used to make a handle. Two lateral extensions in the posterior region may be placed to aid in removal of the tray from the mouth (Fig. 13.23).

When the tray is hard, but still warm to touch, it is removed from the cast and the tin foil is peeled off. The tray undergoes polymerization shrinkage for at least 40 minutes after fabrication and minor changes continue to occur for upto six hours. Thus, it should be prepared at least six hours prior to making the final

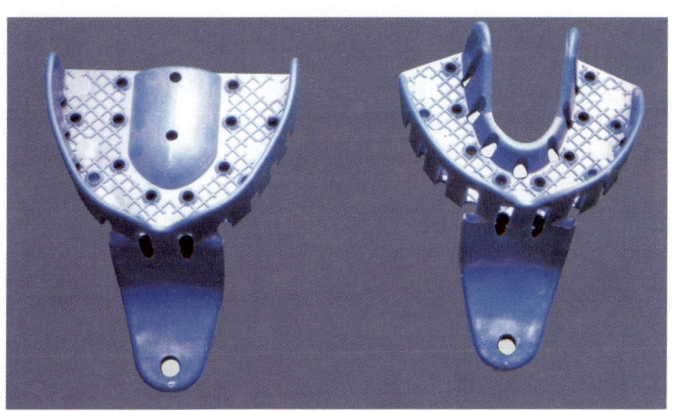

Fig. 13.22: Stock impression trays

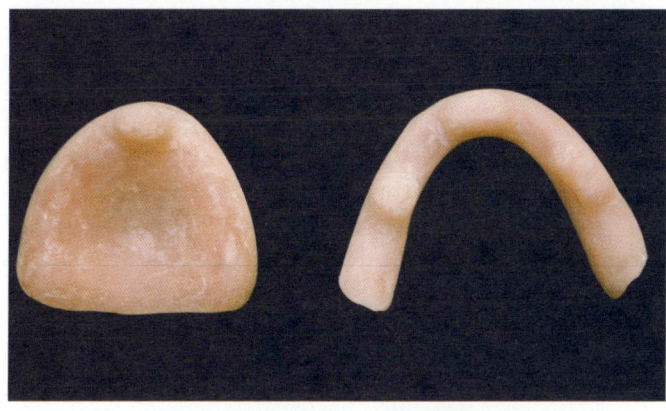

Fig. 13.23: Custom impression trays

impression. The tray is then coated with the tray adhesive. Different tray adhesives are available. The adhesive must be painted and allowed to dry for at least 15 minutes before the material is loaded. The bonding strength of the adhesives used with polyvinyl siloxane can be improved nearly 50% by adding perforations to the tray and approximately 40% by roughening the inner surface of the tray.

When plastic perforated impression trays are used with polyvinyl siloxane impression material the adhesion is usually adequate but can be improved when a tray adhesive is used.

Technique for Making Impression with an Elastomeric Material

The various elastomeric impression materials can be used with minor variations in technique. Mostly, the polyvinyl siloxane (addition silicones) is used.

Local anaesthesia is administered. Gingival retraction procedures are carried out. The retraction cord is packed into the sulcus for displacement of the gingival sulcus to provide access to subgingival margins of the preparation. The retraction cord is left in place for 3–5 minutes depending upon the retraction needed.

Most silicones are available in the form of two pastes (base and catalyst) that are mixed prior to application on the tooth. For still more convenience, materials are also available in disposable auto-mix cartridge dispensing systems.

The armamentarium required for mixing is – two mixing pads, two spatulas, a syringe, a tray, heavy body and light body material.

A funnel is prepared using a sheet from the mixing pad. First the sheet is folded in half, then a second fold is made by folding on an angle so than one end is slightly wider than the other. A third fold is then made similarly. This now forms a paper funnel, which is used to load the light body material in the syringe.

The dentist and his assistant simultaneously mix the two consistencies. The heavy body material is loaded into the impression tray, which is already coated with tray adhesive. The paper funnel can be used to introduce the light body material in the syringe.

The retraction cord is now removed. The cord must be slightly damp before removing so that it does not tear the sulcular epithelium. The impression material is immediately injected into the sulcus. The tip of the syringe is held just above the opening of the sulcus and moved carefully along the entire circumference of the prepared tooth. An air syringe can be used to direct a stream of air against the material to spread it evenly. The tray is then seated with the help of stops holding the tray firmly in one position. The impression tray is held for 6–8 minutes in place. The set of the heavy body material is tested wherever it is accessible at the periphery of the tray.

The impression is removed as quickly as possible and in vertical direction. It is rinsed, dried and disinfected using 2% gluteraldehyde for ten minutes and is then ready for pouring (Fig. 13.24).

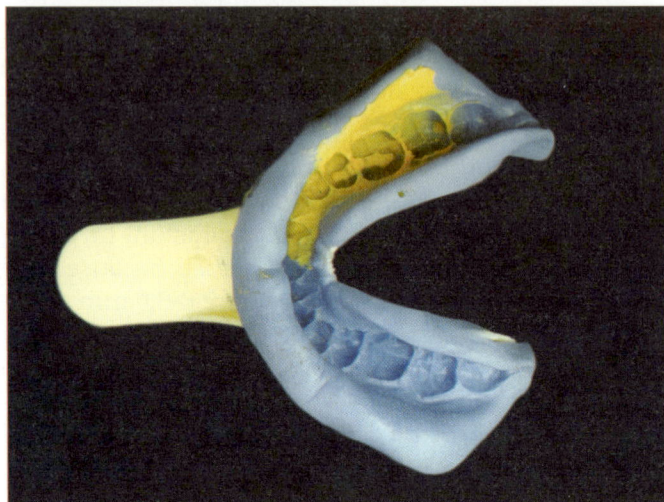

Fig. 13.24: Elastomeric impression ready for pouring

Mixing of the impression material can also be carried out by the auto-mix technique. The armamentarium required for this technique is two dispensing guns and cartridges of light and heavy body material. A disposable auto-mixing tip is provided that fits onto the end of each cartridge. The light body mixing tip may have an accessory tip to gain access to the remote areas of the cavity.

When the trigger of the dispenser is pulled the plunger is driven forward so that the base and accelerator pastes are forced from the two cartridges into the mixing tip containing the spiral mixer. The pastes pass down the bore and over and through the spiral, which has sections which rotate at 180° to one another. It then exits at the reservoir as a uniformly mixed paste.

The advantages of the auto-mixing technique are:
- Greater speed
- More consistent mixing
- Fewer voids and bubbles
- Lesser armamentarium required
- Lesser possibility of contamination of material

Putty Silicon Technique

The putty silicone is dispensed with a scoop and the recommended number of drops of the liquid catalyst is added to it by use of a spatula until no streaks are present. Kneading the material in moist hands completes mixing. It is loaded into the impression tray as if it were softened impression compound. The tray is filled and seated and then moved in all directions in order to enlarge the space occupied by the teeth. This completed impression serves as a custom tray. The syringe material is injected into the preparation and the tray is held there till the material sets.

Technique for Making Impression with Reversible Hydrocolloid Material

Reversible hydrocolloid has been used extensively as an impression material for cast gold restorations. It is packaged as a semi-solid gel in polyethylene tubes. It is liquefied by placing in boiling water. It is then tempered to reduce the temperature and increase the viscosity of the material in the tray. After the material is tempered, it is placed in the mouth, cool tap water is circulated through the tray tubing, the impression is removed from the mouth and is ready to be poured.

The ideal hydrocolloid conditioner has three baths:
- *Liquefying bath*: Tubes of the impression material are boiled for ten minutes. Propylene glycol can be used in the bath.
- *Storage bath*: The tubes filled with liquefied material can be stored for five days at temperature of 150°F. If the material is not used within five days, then it should be re-liquefied by boiling it for 12 minutes.
- *Tempering bath:* Loaded impression trays are tempered in this bath at 110°F to 115°F for five to ten minutes before placing them in the mouth.

A metal stock tray with tubing is taken. Adhesive plastic stops are placed in the front of the tray and at the back of each side. The impression, which was liquefied and kept in the storage bath, is loaded in the impression tray. The tray is placed in the tempering bath for ten minutes. A cartridge of agar-agar is removed from the conditioner bath. The retraction cord is removed and using the tip of the syringe, reversible hydrocolloid is injected into and around the prepared tooth.

An alternative way of applying the syringe material is called *Wet Field Technique*. The prepared teeth are bathed in warm water and syringe material is deposited in generous quantities only on the occlusal surfaces of the teeth. The tray material is seated. The hydraulic pressure of the viscous tray material forces the fluid syringe hydrocolloid down into the areas to be restored. This motion displaces the syringe material, blood, and debris with the stronger tray material throughout the sulcus.

The impression is removed with a sudden snapping motion rather than teasing it out to avoid distortion.

B. Construction of the Die and the Working Model

A *'Die'* is the positive replica of one tooth. Usually the prepared tooth is separated from the cast (die making) and the rest of the procedures are carried out on the die.

The *'dies'* can be constructed in two ways.
 I. Techniques utilizing two sets of pours
 II. Techniques utilizing one set of pour.

Techniques Utilizing two Sets of Pours

- Two pours can be had if elastomeric impression materials are used
- Two separate impressions are required if reversible hydrocolloid is used.

Dies are prepared from the first pour. These dies are not incorporated into the working model. Working models are poured from the second impression or are obtained from second pour of the same impression depending upon the impression material.

Advantages
- The mounted casts are not subjected to distortion since mechanical removal and insertion of the die may induce stresses and may interfere with its relationship with the master cast.
- There is complete immobilization of the prepared tooth replica, during building the anatomy, contact and contour of the wax pattern.

Disadvantages
- Moving the wax pattern from the working model to the die and vice-versa can induce stresses in the wax.
- The two replicas of the tooth may not have the same exact dimension and shape, thus inducing stresses in the wax pattern.

A pre-measured amount of water is placed in a plastic bowl and a measured amount of die stone is added to the water. Die can be poured with approximately 50–70 gms. of stone. Full arch impressions require approximately 200 gms.

The water and powder is vacuum mixed. Excessive water is blown from the surface of the hydrocolloid impression material without actually dessicating it. In case of elastomeric impression material, a surface wetting agent may be sprayed on it. A small amount of stone is then carried on the side of the impression above the preparation and then vibrated until stone reaches the 'bottom' of the preparation. Small increments are continually added till the impression is filled completely. After the preparation is filled, stone is poured into the tooth on either side of the impression. Stone is built to approximately one-inch height to allow adequate bulk for preparation of a handle on the die. After this pour is hardened, the impression is poured again (for elastomers); second impression can be used for hydrocolloids to obtain full arch working models. Hydrocolloid impressions are placed in a humidor while the stone hardens, while elastomeric impressions are kept open.

The cast from which die is poured is trimmed. Wet it slightly prior to trimming. All excess stone around the prepared tooth is removed. A handle is cut for the die. The handle should be slightly larger in diameter than the preparation and octagonal in cross-section. Its sides ought to be parallel or slightly tapered toward the base. The handle should be parallel to the long axis of the tooth preparation. It should be approximately 1 inch long. The die is trimmed 'apical' to the finish line. There should be adequate access to rest a burnisher on this part of the stone die when the margins are finished. The contour of the die apical to the finish line should approximate that of the root to facilitate good axial contours in the finished restoration. The full arch models are articulated.

The wax pattern contacts, contours and occlusal morphology is build on the working casts. The dies are reserved for final margination, detail adjustments, surface treatment and spruing of the wax pattern.

Techniques Utilizing one set of Pour (Cast)

In these techniques, the die will be part of the working cast, where it can be used to build occlusion, contact and contour of the wax pattern. The die can be removed from the working cast to marginate, adjust and treat the wax pattern.

Advantages
- It saves time and effort by using only one cast.
- It eliminates dimensional discrepancies between dies.
- There is less distortion of the wax pattern since it is not moved from one die to another.

Disadvantages
- Mobility in one or more directions is not completely prohibited, especially with the loss of interproximal gypsum of adjacent teeth.
- Necessity for additional tools and equipment.

Dowel Pin System

In this system, a dowel pin is positioned over the prepared tooth in the impression after partially pouring the cast. The accurate positioning of the dowel pin is a must. Inaccurate placement might cause them to interfere with the margins, weaken the die or prevent the die from being easily removed from the cast. After initial setting, the pin, which is visible, is coated with some lubricant and then the final pouring is done.

Alternatively, it is advised to preposition and stabilize the dowel pin before stone is poured into the impression. There are devices made specifically for precise positioning of dowels before the pouring of an impression. One such device uses a moveable base to hold an impression in an exact, repeatable position, while pins are suspended above the impression from magnets on a larger immoveable base. Anaesthetic needles, bobby pins, paper clips and paper matches have been used to orient dowel pins.

A technique using bobby pins is common. A straight pin is pushed between the arms of the bobby pin and into the impression material on both the buccal and lingual surfaces of the impression of the prepared tooth. Dowel pin is stabilized in the bobby pin, the round side of the dowel in one of the corrugations and the flat side of the dowel against the flat arm of the bobby pin. The bobby pin is then stabilized against the straight pins with sticky wax. The dowel pin should be parallel to the long axis of the preparation and must not touch the impression.

Die stone is poured into the impression. Paper clips can be set in the partially set stone to provide retention for the base that will be added later. When the stone has set, the straight pins and bobby pins are removed from the impression. A small ball of soft utility wax is applied to the tip of each dowel. A U-shaped buccolingually orientation groove or a round dimple on each die is cut to aid in reseating the die completely and accurately during use. Then the stone around each die is lubricated with a separating medium. Stone is then poured to form the base of the cast.

When the stone is hard and dry, use a saw frame with a thin blade to cut through the layer of die stone. Mechanical die cutters are also available (Fig. 13.25). A cut is made on the mesial and distal side of each die. The cuts should taper slightly toward each other from occlusal to gingival. The end of the dowel is tapped lightly to loosen the die. The die is then trimmed (Figs 13.26A and B).

Strip Technique

Stainless steel strips are cut from ribbon material that is 8 mm wide and 0.05 mm thick. Two strips for each tooth are required. The gingival end is trimmed to follow the proximal gingival outline. The strips are trimmed so that they follow but do not touch the

Cast Restorations

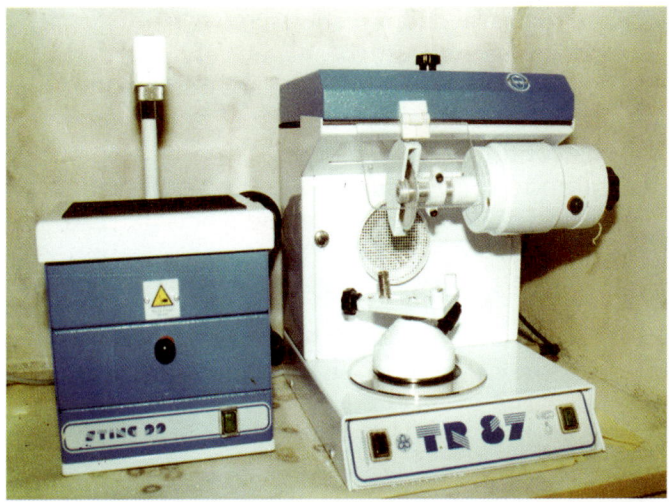

Fig. 13.25: Die cutter

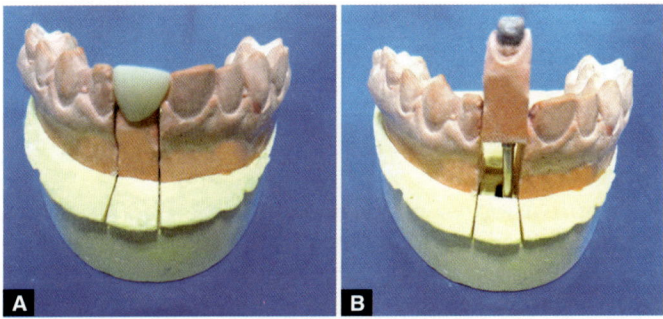

Figs 13.26A and B: (A) Trimmed die; (B) Removal of die from the cast

facial, lingual and gingival contours of the impression. The strips are positioned so that they converge slightly away from the impression. However, they must not converge so much that they interfere with head of the dowel placed subsequently. When the gingival margin is adjacent to an edentulous region, the strip is positioned 1.0-2.0 mm away from the impression of the gingival margin. After the strips have been adequately trimmed, they are placed aside. Utility wax 1.0-2.0 mm is poured on the facial and lingual flange area of the impression.

Now each strip is heated in an open flame, held in a tweezers. The strips are heated so that they will readily enter and move into the wax. The strips are positioned adequately in the wax and sealed with the help of a heated spatula.

Now dowel pins are checked for correct positioning in the impression and placed aside. A mix of high strength die stone is made using vacuum mixing and poured with the help of a vibrator. The die stone is poured so that 1.0 mm of the strips is left exposed. Gently the head positions of the tapered brass dowel pins are inserted into the stone. The dowel pins are aligned vertically so that they are parallel to one another and to the long axis of the tooth. After the die stone has set, a separating medium is poured on the stone and the boxed impression is poured. The base of the cast must be at least 10 mm for adequate strength with 2.0 mm of the dowel pins are left exposed. After the stone has hardened the boxing wax is removed and the ends of the dowel pins are tapped lightly with the end of an instrument handle until a different 'ring' is heard. This indicates that the die has moved slightly from its seating. The dies are then gently pushed out. The metal strips and the v-shaped wedges that are between the adjacent dies are removed.

Advantages

- Offers more control resulting in fewer difficulties, especially in the separation of those dies, which are extremely close to each other.
- It provides landmarks so that dowel pins are positioned precisely in the centre of the die base.
- It provides a concave die base that helps index the die on the cast.
- Allows speedy separation of dies without the use of rotary instruments or saws.

Materials for Die Construction

Various materials have been used for construction of dies. Some of the *basic requirements* for such materials are:

- It should be compatible with the impression material.
- It should be dimensionally stable.
- It should have a smooth, non-abradable surface.
- It should be able to accommodate auxiliary restoration retention (e.g. pins).
- It should be able to receive a spacer in selected areas to create space for the luting agent of the casting.

The materials used for construction of dies are:

Gypsum

The most commonly used die materials are type IV and type V dental stone, the properties of which are tabulated in Table 13.5.

Strength of these materials is greatly increased by decreasing the porosity, thus pouring under vacuum is helpful. Decreasing the water/powder ratio increases the strength. In limits, increase in the mixing time will increase the strength.

Some investigators have tried incorporation of amalgam powder to increase strength. Incorporation of accelerators and retarders cause a loss of strength.

Certain water substitutes can dramatically increase the strength and hardness of gypsum, e.g. aqueous

Table 13.5: Physical properties of gypsum

Properties	Water/Powder ratio	Setting time (min.)	Setting expansion (%)	Compressive strength (psi)
Type IV	0.22-0.24	12 ± 4	00.0-0.10	5000
Type V	0.18-0.22	12 ± 4	0.10-0.30	7000

solution of colloidal silica or soluble resin solutions by increasing the friction between the dehydrate crystals.

Setting time can be accelerated by the operator by use of fine particle gypsum, low water/powder ratio, long and fast mixing, use of 3% potassium sulphate solution or the use of slurry water. The use of slurry water is the safest method.

Gypsum products are sometimes modified to:
- Make the material more abrasion resistant. This can be done by using die-hardening agents such as cyanoacrylate and acrylic resin lacquer. These hardening agents must be used in very thin coats to avoid any unacceptably thick relief at the margins of the preparation. The thickness of cyano-acrylates at the margin can range from 1.0 to 2.5 μm while acrylic lacquers can add 4 to 10 μm thickness.
- Change the dimensions of the die. This is most commonly done by using a die spacer. The most common die spacers are resins. Models paint, colored nail polish or thermoplastic polymers dissolved in volatile solvents may also be used. The thickness varies with the number of coats applied. Usually a relief of 20 to 40 μm is desired. The tooth preparation on the die is painted to within 0.5 mm of the finish line. The longer the surrounding walls thicker the spacer required.
- Increase the refractoriness of the die. In this technique the die material and the investment have a comparable composition. The die is made of this material and the wax pattern is constructed on it. Then the entire assembly (die and pattern) is invested in the same material, thereby eliminating the possibility of distortion of the wax pattern upon removal from the die or during the setting of the investment.

Electroformed Dies

Certain metals having high strength, hardness and abrasion resistance can be electroplated on the impression forming electroformed dies.

Electroplating is the result of electrolysis. When electric field is superimposed on the electrolytic solution, the ions in this solution are attracted and begin to move to oppositely charged electrodes. The positively charged ions (cations) move to the negative electrodes (cathodes), the negatively charged ions (anions) move to the positive electrode (anode).

The anode is a bar of pure metal, supplying metal cations continuously. The deposition takes place on the cathode (impression). The impression must be made electrically conducting and it acts like cathode.

A. Copper Plating

This method is usually used with impressions of impression compound or addition silicone rubber base material.

Technique

The two methods frequently used are:
- The cavity surface may be lightly oiled and coated with a thin film of colloidal metal.
- The cavity surface may be coated with a film of graphite.

The graphite is mixed with water to a fairly concentrated consistency, painted onto the cavity surface of the impression and dried under the blast of a chip blower.

Application of graphite is the method of choice because it is more readily wetted by the copper sulphate solution.

A thin copper wire, 28-gauge, is wrapped around the copper tube and twisted. A sheet of tacky casting wax is cut into strips. One of the strips is open for a short distance at its midpoint. The strip is passed through the flame of a Bunsen burner, the slit of the wax accommodates the circuit wire, while the wax is wrapped around the copper tube and tucked over its bottom edges. A second strip of wire is wrapped around the circuit wire. Wax is melted and used to seal all joints and to cover any remaining exposed metallic surfaces. The wax wrapping the circuit wire is bent and acts as a handle and permits ready visibility during the electrodeposition.

The manufacturer provides a 'holder' for the impression. The impression is wrapped in wax and then held in a stream of cold water. The force of stream will flush out the pattern and force any pocket of air before it. Any pocket of air will result in a failure of electrodeposition in the area.

The water-filled impression is then submerged in the electronic bath, and the circuit wire is twisted about the contact bar of the impression holder. A cathode 'tapping' wire is placed in the bath. This taps some of current so as to reduce the rate of deposition.

The electroformer apparatus are merely devices, which step down the line voltage, rectify the alternating current, and provide rheostatic control to regulate the rate of electrodeposition.

Electroforming must begin at a very low amperage, otherwise the initial deposit of copper is granulated and since this deposit will be along the margins of the preparation such dies are worthless. When copper deposition has begun satisfactorily, the tapping wire may be removed. After the entire cavity surface is coated with copper, the amperage may be stepped up to accelerate the electroforming.

The composition of the solution for copper plating is:

Copper sulphate	200 gm
Sulphuric acid	30 ml
Phenol Sulphuric acid	2 ml
Distilled water	100 ml

Plating is allowed to proceed for 12-15 hours. After electroforming, the impressions are washed off the elctroforming solution. Acrylic resin or dental stone can be poured.

B. Silver Plating

These dies are restricted to polysulfide, polyether and silicone rubber base materials, however some silicone rubber impression materials might not produce acceptable silver plated dies.

Same apparatus as copper plating is used, but small current is required. The surface of the impression is metallized with a fine silver powder. A silver cyanide bath is preferred over an acid copper bath. The reliability of silver cyanide bath is better and also polysulfide is more dimensionally stable in the alkaline cyanide bath than in the acid copper bath.

An anode of pure silver at least twice the area to be plated is used.

Electroplating is carried out for approximately 10 hours.

The composition of the silver-plating bath solution is

Silver cyanide	36 gm
Potassium cyanide	60 gm
Potassium carbonate	45 gm
Distilled water	100 ml

Precautions

- The silver-plating solution is poisonous so care should be taken that hands, workbench area or clothes are not contaminated.
- Silver-plating solution should be kept as a basic solution. Addition of acid will cause formation of hydrogen cyanide gas, which is poisonous.
- Copper plating shouldn't be done in the same area where silver plating is done because of risk of contaminating the basic silver solution with acidic copper solution.
- The silver-plating solution should be covered at all times to control evaporation and dissipation of fumes.

C. Low Fusing Alloy Such as Bismuth, Lead, tin and Cadmium

Low fusing alloy such as bismuth, lead, tin and cadmium have also been used. They are usually used to form extensions on electroformed dies.

Amalgam Dies

Conventional amalgam is also used to make dies similar to the silver amalgam which is used to restore teeth.

Technique

An impression is made in a copper band with modelling compound. A thin piece of boxing wax, 28 to 30 gauge, is wrapped around the impression and band matrix and extended about 3/8 inch beyond and along the gingival margins of the band and its contained impression. The boxed impression is embedded with the open end showing the cavity facing up, in a mix of plaster, which has been previously placed in a small rubber ring to hold it steady and prevent it from spreading during setting.

After the plaster base has hardened, a plastic mass of amalgam alloy is mixed. The amalgam is condensed into the impression as is done in making a good restoration.

After it has thoroughly set, the rubber ring and plaster is removed and the die is immersed in warm water to remove the impression compound and wax.

The die is then trimmed and tapered so that it simulates the shape of a tooth root.

An impression of the upper and lower arches is made. The amalgam die is placed in the impression of the prepared tooth and the cast is poured.

Amalgam dies and all metal dies are good conductors of heat and so softened wax applied to them cools rapidly. This rapid cooling of the wax may produce internal stresses, which can cause distortion of the wax pattern. The sudden cooling of the liquid wax when applied to a metal die may also result in the contraction of wax away from the die and discrepancies may arise because of imperfect adaptation of the wax pattern to the die.

These problems can be avoided by:

- Warming the metal die to mouth temperature or slightly below.
- Some operators prefer to place an electric heating pad on the bench which serves to keep the die

and all carving instruments at a suitable temperature to avoid sudden cooling of the inlay wax.

In case of amalgam dies, the die should be lubricated with oil prior to fabrication of the wax pattern. After the inlay is tried on the amalgam die it must be pickled to remove any traces of amalgam.

Silicophosphate Cement Dies

These are sometimes used to make dies in compound impressions. They give harder dies than dental stone.

One disadvantage of these materials is that they shrink on setting and the surface of the cement has a tendency to loose water upon standing making it friable. Therefore, the cement dies are stored in water or glycerine.

Epoxy Resin Dies

Epoxy resins are supplied in two or three parts that are mixed before insertion into the impression. The first part contains 50–60% epoxy polymer, 30–40% vinyl cyclo-hexene diepoxide and the rest are copolymers. The second part consists of partially hydrolyzed benzophene tetra-carboxylic acid dianhydride. The third part is a tertiary amine catalyst.

The material is mixed in vacuum and then poured into the impression. It is compatible with all impression materials except hydrocolloids. The resin cures in about half an hour at room temperature.

During this curing it shrinks about 0.02 to 0.6% depending on configuration and bulk of the die.

This shrinkage can be compensated for by thermal treatment of the die. It is heated in steps of 10° per minute to 160°C and then held at 160°C for one hour. The temperature should not exceed 200°C. It is then rapidly cooled to room temperature. The exact mechanism of this expansion of the material is not known. One hypothesis is that further cross-linking of the polymer occurs which generates water causing expansion.

Epoxy dies are stronger and more abrasion resistant than gypsum dies and also the reproduction of detail is much better than with gypsum dies.

C. Preparing the Wax Pattern

There are two methods of making a wax pattern for an inlay; the direct method (fashioned on the tooth) and the indirect method (fashioned on a die).

Direct Method

Indications
- A tooth is in an area of easy accessibility, i.e. the tooth should be clearly visible and easy to work on. The second and third molars are usually not suitable.
- Cavity preparations with minimal proximal extensions, i.e. relatively small cavity preparations which leave a good deal of supporting tooth structure to help stabilize the pattern during carving.
- Cavity preparation where the walls are flat, internal line angles are sharp and gingival bevel is definite.

Advantages
- The pattern is carved on the tooth and not on a model which may not be a perfect replica of the tooth because of possible inaccuracies during each stage of preparation of the model.
- Little laboratory work has to be done compared with the indirect method.
- *Time saving:* Although chairside time is increased but the overall time required for fabrication is decreased.

Disadvantages
- Great skill and patience is required to carve patterns in the mouth.
- When wax is carved by indirect vision in a mirror, manipulation becomes difficult and fatiguing.
- Discrepancies of the pattern at the gingival margin are difficult to detect until the pattern has been carved and withdrawn.
- As most of the adjusting and polishing has to be done on the tooth, valuable chairside time is lost.
- If the casting fails, the patient has to be recalled thereby wasting time and energy.

Manipulation of the Inlay Wax

The stick of inlay wax can be softened in hot water or using dry heat. Softening in a water bath can result in inclusion of droplets of water that could splatter on flaming, smear the wax surface during polishing and distortion of the pattern due to thermal changes.

When wax is softened directly over a flame, care must be exercised to ensure thorough heating of the wax stick. The wax should be kept moving till it becomes shiny and then removed from the flame. It should then be compressed between the fingers and again warmed. The process is repeated until the wax is warm throughout. It is kneaded using the thumb and first finger which are lubricated with vaseline to avoid sticking of the wax. The wax stick can be flattened to expose more wax surface to the flame and thereby obtain a uniform softened texture.

A wax annealer, which maintains a constant temperature of 65°C can also been employed.

It has been observed that higher the temperature of the wax during manipulation, the lesser the internal strain and distortion upon storage. Plastic mass should be inserted into the prepared cavity at as high a temperature as can be tolerated and held under pressure. The surface is cooled in running water.

The pattern should be prepared in such a manner that no addition of wax would be required, as wax, which is added after the initial cooling introduces stresses which will distort the pattern.

The wax pattern by direct method can be prepared with and without the application of matrix band.

Wax Pattern Prepared with a Matrix Band

The retainer and band are tried loosely on the tooth, making certain that the gingival margins are covered by the band before fitting and applying a wedge. The internal surfaces of the band are lightly lubricated with a separating medium such as castor oil. With the finger used as a plunger to confine the occlusal portion of the wax, the band is tightened until a snug fit is obtained.

Finger pressure is maintained while the wax is cooled and hardened. The bulk of excess wax is then trimmed (Fig. 13.27). The matrix retainer is loosened and removed. The wax is held firmly in place and the band is removed. Excess wax is trimmed from the cavosurface margins. Trial removal of the pattern is attempted at this stage.

A narrow strip of copper ribbon is bent into a 'V' or 'U' shape, heated over the flame and quickly inserted as a staple into the marginal ridge areas of the wax pattern. The staple is kept stable for 2-3 minutes so as to let it cool down. An instrument is inserted under the staple to lift the pattern out of the cavity in an occlusal direction.

The pattern is carefully inspected for:
- Sharp internal details.
- Good reproduction of the cavosurface and gingival margins.

If either is lacking it is better to start again rather than attempt to repair the same.

The gingival flash, if any, is removed with a sharp scalpel.

The pattern is again seated in the cavity. A heated instrument is held lightly against the copper staple, thus facilitating its removal. The pattern is then carved with the help of plastic instruments. To test the occlusion, the tooth is carefully isolated and dried with cotton rolls. The opposing tooth is also dried. With a camel hair brush, talcum powder is dusted on the occlusal surface of the wax and the patient is instructed to close the teeth lightly. Cuspal contact with the wax pattern is indicated by a shiny burnished spot on the pattern. The spots of hyperocclusion are carved away using warm carvers.

The occlusal surface may be polished by rubbing a wet pledget of cotton over the area. The pledget of cotton can be warmed over a flame for better results. Proximal surfaces are polished by wrapping a smooth linen strip tightly around the tooth and clinching it upon the buccal side.

Copper bands can also be used instead of matrix bands.

Wax Pattern Prepared Without a Matrix Band

Attempts have been made to prepare wax patterns without the use of a matrix band. Here the inlay wax stick is softened to form a pointed end. The softened pointed end is forced into the cavity, the harder end acting as a plunger so as to confine the wax to the approximal part of the cavity; the thumb and forefinger of the free hand are pressed into the buccal and lingual embrasures. Excess wax is cut off occlusally and an egg shaped burnisher is used to press the wax further into the cavity until it ceases to move under pressure.

It is now bathed with several syringes of water at 110–115°F. The patient is asked to close his teeth to force the wax further into the cavity and to locate the occluding cusps. The wax is again bathed in warm water. The occlusal surface is carved with a wax carver. Wax in the embrasures is rimmed. The remaining wax in the approximal space is removed with curved probes. At this stage a piece of silk thread is passed through the contact point to make sure all the wax has been removed. The thread is held just

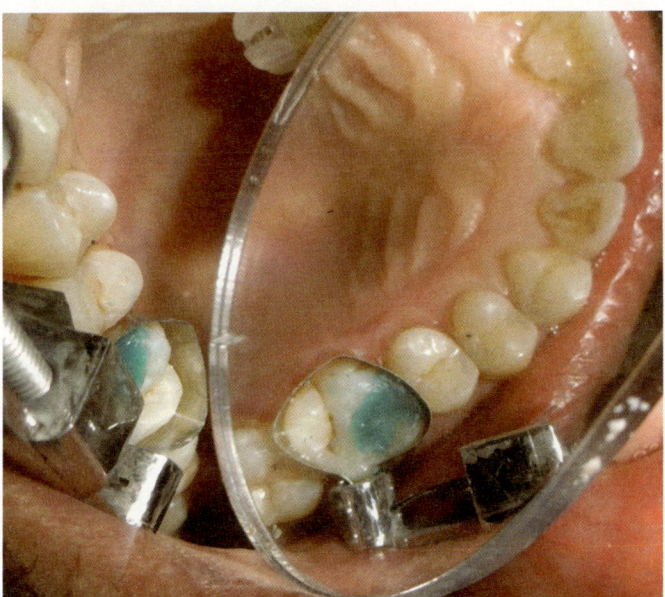

Fig. 13.27: Wax pattern fabricated with band applied

below where the contact point will be and then moved gingivally under pressure against the approximal surface of the wax pattern. In this way the thread cuts the approximal excess leaving a triangular section of wax in the approximal space which can be removed with plastic instruments. Finally the approximal surface is burnished with a smooth linen strip. Care should be exercised to hold the strip so that it does not burnish the wax away from the cavity margin. Hence when it is being withdrawn against the buccal part of the pattern it must be held away from the lingual margin (Fig. 13.28).

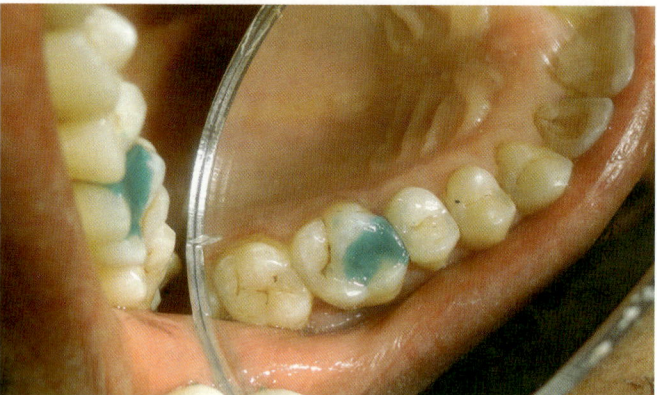

Fig. 13.28: Wax pattern fabrication without band applied on tooth

The proximal contour and contact of the pattern deserves special attention. It is important that contacts be of proper form as in the right position. In order to evaluate the contact form the ligature (dental floss) is first passed to the gingival of the contact; the two ends are then held parallel in the occlusal direction as shown for the contact between the premolars (Fig. 13.29). This measures the faciolingual width of the contact or very near approach of the two surfaces.

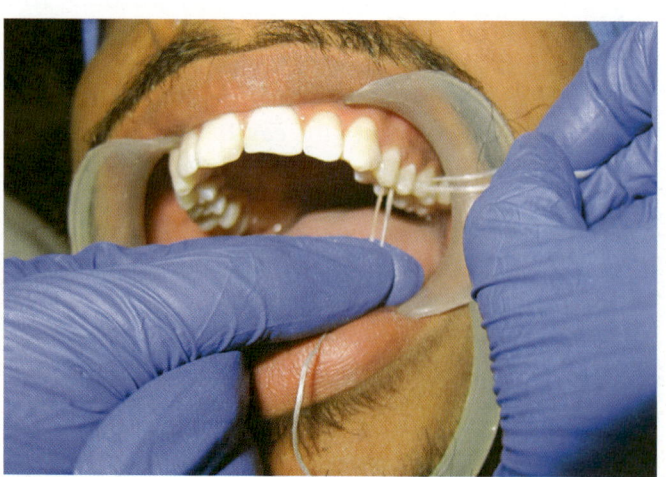

Fig. 13.29: Method to measure contact

Without removing the ligature, the two ends should be held parallel in the facial direction as shown for the contact between the two premolars. This measures the occlusogingival width of the contact. In either position of the parallel strands are more than 1½ or 2 mm apart the contact is too broad.

Indirect Method

After the preparation of the die, a lubricant is applied to facilitate the withdrawl of the pattern from the die. Various lubricants used are castor oil, machine oil, petroleum jelly, cocoa butter, etc. The time for the application of the lubricant depends upon the wetness of the die, the humid die will take less time and vice versa. Few authors are however, not in favour of using lubricants since, these may lead to change characteristics of the inner side of the wax pattern.

In case of large patterns, mostly with full crowns and fixed partial dentures, die spacer is used to compensate the solidification shrinkage of the casting alloy (Fig. 13.30).

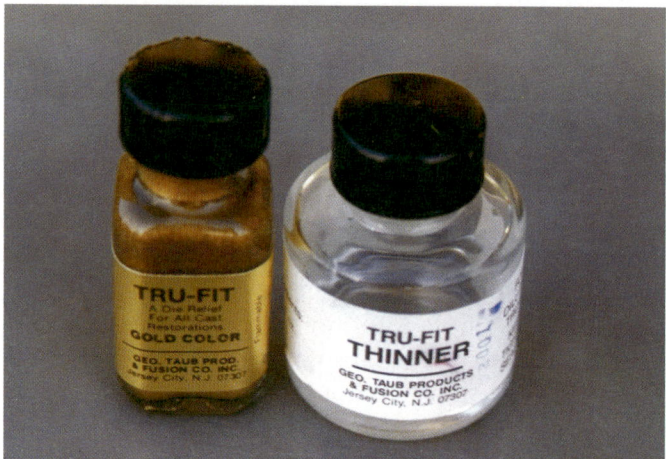

Fig. 13.30: Die spacer and thinner

The blue inlay wax is softened, molded and pushed into the cavity as in direct pattern technique. The rest of the finishing and carving is carried out as in direct pattern.

D. Removing the Pattern from the Cavity

The pattern must be removed without distortion and maintaining the path of removal parallel with the direction of the cavity walls. The sprue former should be attached to the pattern while it is still on the tooth to minimise distortion of pattern due to heat and mechanical induction of stresses. The sprue former of exact size and shape is selected, keeping in mind the size of wax pattern, casting machine to be used and the metal to be cast. Sticky wax is applied to one end of the sprue and attached to the pattern site. A little wax can be added, if need be, at the joining of the sprue and the pattern. After keeping the sprue for 2-3 minutes, trial removal can be carried out. If the pattern cannot be freely sprued on the tooth, indirect procedure can be used (the same procedure as used for trial removal of the pattern). A copper staple or a 24 gauge twisted brass wire is inserted into the occlusal part of the pattern. For MOD patterns, the prongs of the wire are placed near the marginal ridges (Fig. 13.31) and for disto-occlusal or mesio-occlusal patterns, the prongs are inserted at an angle of 45° near the marginal ridge (Fig. 13.32). Using the staple, the pattern is lifted out of the cavity with a direct pull parallel to the cavity walls. The sprue is then inserted into the wax pattern and the staple removed by holding it with warm pliers to melt the wax holding the staple (Fig. 13.33). A heated blunt explorer is used to fill in the holes left from the staple. If the staple is made of the same alloy or one of the component metals of the alloy used for casting then it can be left in the pattern and cut off after casting.

The purpose of the sprue former is to provide a channel through which molten alloy can reach the mold in an invested ring after the wax has been

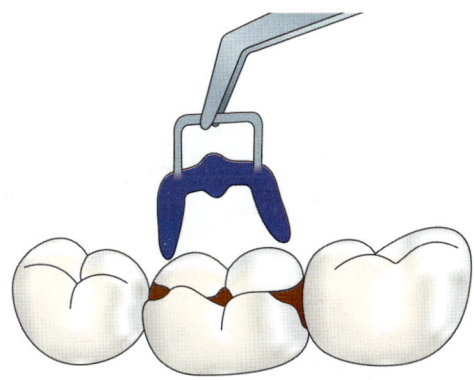

Fig. 13.33: Removal of pattern from the tooth

eliminated. Low fusing inlay wax is flown over the contact area and flushed with the proximal surface to build the contact (Fig. 13.34).

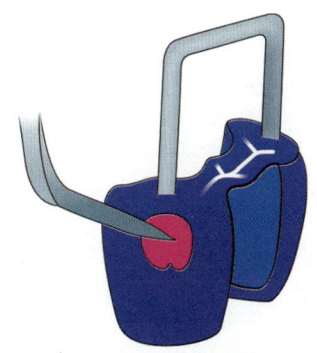

Fig. 13.34: Building of the contact area

E. Sprue Former

Sprue Former Material

The sprue former can be made of wax, resin or metal. Wax and resin sprue formers have the advantage of being burnable and so do not need to be mechanically removed (Fig. 13.35). Further, the wax or resin have a fusion temperature lower or almost same as that of the pattern wax. However, disadvantage of wax sprue formers is that they lack rigidity.

Metal sprue formers can be solid or hollow. Hollow sprue formers are preferred since they hold less heat than a solid sprue former and so will cause less heat transfer to wax pattern resulting in less distortion. Also their retention to the wax pattern is better. To further improve retention and reduce thermal conductivity, the sprue former can be filled with sticky wax.

The metal sprue former must be mechanically removed prior to burnout. This could cause investment to loosen from the walls. To avoid this, metal sprue formers are uniformly coated with wax before investing so that at the time of burn out, the sprue former comes out on its own because of melting of wax. This way the loosening or breaking of investment can be avoided.

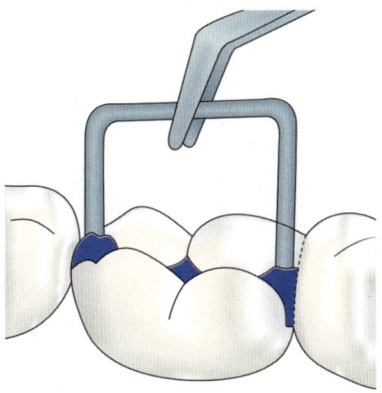

Fig. 13.31: Copper staple for removing wax impression of MOD cavity

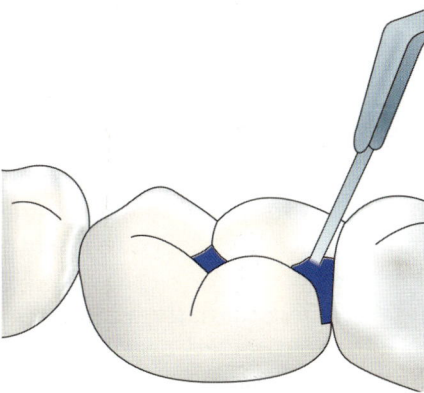

Fig. 13.32: Staple inserted at 45° for mesiocclusal or distoocclusal preparation

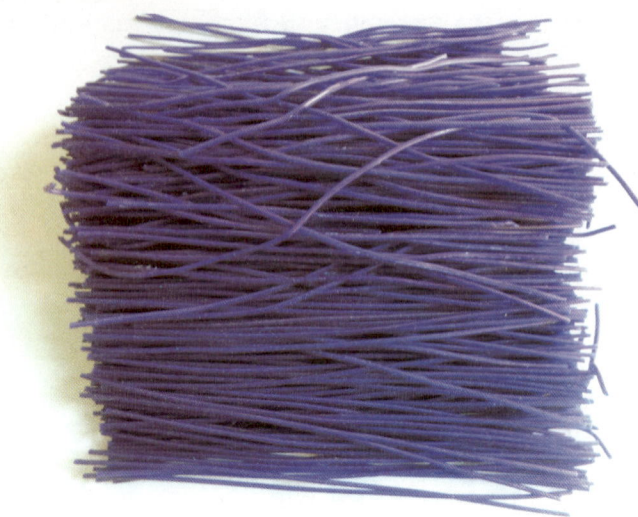

Fig. 13.35: Inlay wax for making sprue former

Sprue Former Diameter

The diameter of the sprue former will depend on the size of the wax pattern, the quality of casting machine, and the ring, which is used to form the mold.

In general, a sprue former with a larger diameter is preferred to one with a smaller diameter, because the greater the diameter the less likely is the molten alloy to solidify before the mold is filled. On the other hand, since the sprue former is attached to the wax pattern by heat, the heat from a large sprue former might cause distortion or actual melting of the pattern if a very small wax pattern is involved. Preferably the diameter of the sprue former should not be more than 1/4th of the total area of the wax pattern.

Suggested Sprue Former Diameters

Gauge no.	Diameter (cm)
06	0.4115
08	0.3264
10	0.2588
12	0.2053
14	0.1628
16	0.1291
18	0.1024

Tabulation of sprue sizes and their application		
Sprue size	Approximate diameter (mm)	Comments
16	1.3	Thin inlay onlay; may need reservoir
14	1.7	Largest size for air pressure casting
12	2.1	Best for most inlays
10	2.6	Use on heavy crown only

The diameter of the sprue is the most important factor in determining the speed with which the molten metal enters and fills the mold. Melt velocity is directly proportional to sprue diameter.

If gold is to be melted immediately above the entrance (air pressure technique) the sprue former must be small in diameter so that the molten gold will not be able to flow into the sprue hole before the pressure of the casting is applied.

Sprue Former Length

The length of the sprue former depends upon the length of the casting ring. The length should be adjusted so that the wax pattern is within 6.5 mm (1/4 inch) of the open end of the ring for gypsum-bonded investments and 3.25 mm (1/8 inch) for phosphate bonded investments. If the pattern is too close to the end of the ring, the molten alloy may blast through the investment during casting; if it is too far away, gases may not escape rapidly enough to allow metal to fill the mold space.

The sprue former should not be too long so that the gold will begin to solidify in the sprue and cause porosity in the casting.

Location of Sprue Former

The sprue former should be attached to the bulkiest part of the wax pattern because of the following reasons.

- This will minimise the effect of released residual stresses by the heat of attaching the sprue.
- It will ensure that the thinner cross-section of the mold will be filled completely.
- The melt will always be fluid enough and available until all lesser dimension sections are adequately filled.

The general rule is to attach the sprue former in a position so that the molten metal will reach the mold areas farthest from the attachment of the sprue former at the same time.

Sprue formers should be attached to the least anatomical area of the wax pattern.

Angulation of the Sprue Former

It should not be attached at right angle to a broad surface because the melt may impinge the mold surface and produce a so-called *'hot spot'* producing suck back porosity.

An angle of 45° is usually adequate. The sprue former should be directed away from any thin or delicate parts of the pattern, since molten metal may abrade or fracture investment in this area and result in casting failure.

Number of Sprues

If the wax pattern is designed such that attachment of the sprue former at the bulkiest portion allows the metal to flow uninterrupted from the sprue to the farthest end of the mold then a single sprue is adequate.

However, should the wax pattern have a thin area between the sprue and the periphery of the pattern, the melt will solidify at the reduced cross-sectional area preventing complete filling of the mold. Here two sprues can be used.

If multiple sprues are used, they should join together at the crucible former level in a reservoir larger in diameter than all the sprues combined.

Sprue Former Attachment

The sprue pattern joint must be smooth and uninterrupted. If high velocity ingress of the melt into the mold is required, the junction should be flared. If low velocity ingress is required, a constricted junction is made.

To minimise stress release while joining a sprue former to a wax pattern, a drop of sticky wax should be applied to the wax pattern. Then the sprue also, with a bead of sticky wax is brought in contact with the sticky wax on the wax pattern and held immobile until the sticky wax is solidified.

Patterns can be sprued directly or indirectly. In direct spruing, the sprue former provides direct connection between the pattern area and the crucible former.

Reservoir

In case, the diameter of the sprue is smaller than the average cross sctional area of the pattern, a reservoir is attached with the sprue as near as possible to the pattern sprue junction. The diameter of the reservoir should be more than the average cross sectional area of the pattern. The rationale of adding reservoir to sprue is to provide molten metal to prevent localized shrinkage porosity.

When molten metal strikes against the mold wall at 90 degree angle and if the mold-metal temperature differential is more, it creates a hot-spot, the molten metal in this area will solidify last, leading to localized shrinkage porosity, if there is no continuous supply of molten metal. The reservoir provides the molten metal to compensate for this localized shrinkage porosity at the casting sprue junction.

If we use a sprue former, the diameter of which is greater than the diameter of the cross-sectional area of the pattern, there is no need for providing reservoir. The sprue will itself provide the molten metal.

F. Forming the Crucible and Attaching the Pattern

The crucible part of the investment assembly is cone shaped. The sprue is attached to the crucible in the same way as the sprue is attached to the mold, i.e. it should be bulkiest in cross-section, flared and smooth.

The depth of the crucible and the inclination of its walls towards the sprue are dictated by factors similar to those governing the diameter of sprue, i.e. alloy density, casting machine energy, melt viscosity, size of a pattern, porosity of investment, etc. The deeper the crucible is and the more inclined its walls are, more velocity will be imparted to the melt on its way to the mold.

Venting

In some situations, there is some doubt about the speed with which the mold gases will escape relative to the speed at which the molten metal is entering. A wax rod is added to the farthest, or close to the farthest part of the pattern, which will stop short of the ring (investment) surface. In most cases, they are curved towards the sprue. Gases that will not escape fast enough ahead of the ingressing melt will be compressed and trapped in these vents.

G. Preparation of the Ring for Casting

In the past, several metals have been used for making casting rings. The metal used in the construction of a ring should be non-corrodible, hard and with a thermal expansion similar to the investment used. Stainless steel has been found to produce the most acceptable rings. The thermal expansion of stainless steel is 12% at 700°C, which is compatible with the expansion of investments, provided a liner is used.

The dimensions of the ring may vary according to the desire of the operator, but the average dimensions are approximately 29 mm (1 1/8 inch) in diameter and 38 mm (1½ inches) in height.

Need for Liner

A resilient liner is placed inside the ring to provide a buffer of pliable material against which the investment can expand to enlarge the mold. If there is no liner present, the investment is in direct contact with the walls of the mold and will not be able to expand outward (because of the resisting action of the walls of the ring) and so will expand in the direction providing less restriction, i.e. towards the centre of the mold thus resulting in distortion of the casting. The liner if wetted allows for semi-hygroscopic expansion of the investment. It becomes easier to remove the investment and casting from the ring, if a liner is used.

Liner Material

For many years, asbestos was used to line casting rings, but now its use has decreased because of concern over its carcinogenic properties. It has been proved that asbestos fibres can cause asbestosis, bronchogenic lung cancer, mesothelioma, etc. The currently accepted threshold limit value for asbestos fibres ranges from 2×10^5–20×10^5 fibres/m^3. This limit is considerably exceeded when dental castings are recovered from asbestos lined rings.

Alternatives to asbestos liners have been introduced, these include absorbent cellulose and nonabsorbent ceramic materials. Cellulose liners readily absorb water when immersed and therefore must be wetted before use. Ceramic liners are virtually nonabsorbent and can be used dry.

It has recently been suggested that fibres from ceramic lining material can be of similar dimensions to those from asbestos liners, and so may also be a potential health risk. But other studies claim that these fibres dissolve quickly in lung tissues and so have little harmful effect.

Most studies carried out to determine suitability of these alternative liners have concluded that both cellulose and ceramic liners could produce satisfactory castings provided some alterations were made to the investing technique, which is routinely used with asbestos. When using ceramic liners one should not use vacuum investing technique. A dry ceramic liner produces very inconsistent castings, which are clinically unacceptable. So one can saturate the liner with a dilute wetting agent prior to investing. An investment with an increased potential expansion should be used.

The relative incompressibility and the high water sorption of cellulose liners must be considered and also the fact that they burn out of the ring at temperatures over 600°C.

A study comparing asbestos and ceramic liners showed that asbestos could be compressed 10 percent of its original thickness when dry and 30 percent when wet. Ceramic liner could be compressed 50% of its original thickness when dry or wet. Thus on the whole, ceramic material is not only an adequate substitute for the traditional asbestos liner, but an improvement as regard the requisites of the liner.

How to use a Liner?

A liner can be used dry or wet. A dry liner will allow greater normal setting expansion in the investment.

Theoretically, a wet liner will allow greater normal setting expansion and semi-hygroscopic expansion, but it also reduces the powder-water ratio, which in turn will reduce the thermal expansion of the investment. As a result, the net expansion with a dry liner will be slightly greater than with a wet liner. However, because the effect of a dry liner depends on its volume relative to that of the investment, which varies with the diameter of the ring, a damp liner is preferred for the sake of consistency.

The maximum thickness of a liner is 1.0 mm. A thicker liner or two layers of liner can also be used.

The liner is cut to fit the inside diameter of the ring with no overlap. The length of the liner is a controversy.

Few authors are of the view that when a liner is placed 1/8th to 1/4th inch short at each end of the ring, the investment cannot expand laterally at the ends of the ring. In the central portion of the ring it does expand laterally to a limited extent. Thus the mold cavity is distorted.

Many others feel that expansion of the investment is always greater in the unrestricted direction (longitudinal) rather than in the lateral direction (towards the ring itself). Thus it is important to reduce expansion in the longitudinal direction. Liner should be placed 1/8 inch short at the ends to get less distortion of the mold.

Others believe that placing the liner flush with the open end of the ring gives maximum expansion.

When cellulose liners are used, they burn out before the casting is made. This deprives the investment of support by the ring, and may result in cracking of the investment. Thus 3.0 mm of the ring is left unlined at each end to support the investment.

After the liner has been placed in the ring, the ring is dipped in water for 10 seconds (in case of asbestos or cellulose liners) and then gently shaken to remove excess. Squeezing the liner would result in removal of excess and variable amounts of water. The diagrammatic representation of the ring, crucible former, sprue former, and wax pattern is shown in Fig.13.36.

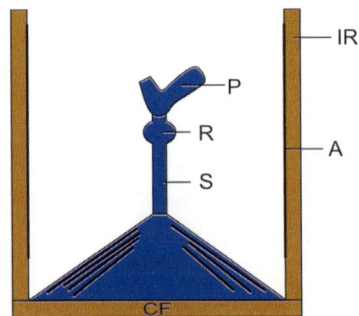

Fig. 13.36: The length of the sprue is so adjusted to bring the wax pattern(P) to 6 mm from the top of the ring. Crucible former (CF), investment ring (IR) lined with wet asbestos (A) kept short of the ring on both sides and reservoir (R) added to the sprue (S).

Preparing the Wax Pattern for Investment

The wax pattern should be cleaned of any debris, grease or oils before it is positioned in the ring. This will decrease the surface tension and improve the wettability of the wax pattern.

Gentle washing with liquid soap using no. 2 paint brush is effective. The soap should be thoroughly rinsed off with water at room temperature and the pattern dried with a stream of clean air. A debubblizing solution provided by the manufacturer may also be painted on the surface of the pattern, taking care to avoid pooling around the internal line angles.

INVESTMENT OF THE PATTERN

Investment Materials

An investment can be described as a ceramic material which is suitable for forming a mould into which molten metal or alloy is cast. The procedure for forming the mould is described as investing. These materials can withstand high temperatures. Therefore, also known as refractory materials.

There are three types of investment materials:
- Gypsum bonded investments
- Phosphate bonded investments
- Silica bonded investments

General composition

All investment materials contain:
- Refractory
- Binder
- Modifiers

Gypsum Bonded Investment

Composition

Refractory – silica (Quartz or cristobalite)	60–65%
Binder – Alpha-hemihydrate	30–35%
Modifers – Carbon, Boric acid or sodium chloride	5%

Silica is a refractory material which withstand high temperature, it regulates thermal expansion and increases setting expansion.

Alpha-hemihydrate binds and holds the silica particles together, contributes to mould expansion.

Carbon provides reducing atmosphere in the mould, it reduces any oxide formed on the metal.

Boric acid or sodium chloride regulate setting expansion and setting time.

Setting Reaction

$CaSO_4 \cdot \frac{1}{2}H_2O + 1\frac{1}{2} H_2O \longrightarrow CaSO_4 \cdot 2H_2O$

Properties

1. Thermal behavior of gypsum – When gypsum is heated to high temperature, it shrinks and fractures. At 700°C it shows slight expansion and then great amount of contraction.
2. Thermal behavior of silica – when heated quartz and crystoballite changes its crystalline form. The α (alpha) form converted into β (beta) form, which is table only above transition temperature. Density decreases as a changes to β (beta) form, with resulting increase in volume and rapid increase in linear expansion.
3. Normal setting expansion – A mixture of silica and dental stone results in greater setting expansion than gypsum product alone. Silica particles interfere with the intermeshing of the crystals as they form.
4. Hygrosopic setting expansion – When gypsum products are allowed to set in contact with water, the amount of expansion exhibited is much greater than normal setting expansion. The increased amount of expansion is because, water helps in the outward growth of crystals.

Phosphate Bonded Investment

The metal ceramic alloys and cobalt chromium alloys have high melting temperatures. They are cast in moulds at 850 to 1100°C. At high temperatures, gypsum bonded investment disintegrates. Hence investment which can withstand higher temperature are required. The investment used for this purpose are phosphate bonded and silica bonded.

Composition

- Powder
- Refractory – Silica
- Binder – Ammonium diacid phosphate
- Magnesium oxide – reacts with phosphate ions, liberated by ammonium diacid phosphate
- Liquid – Silica solution in water

Setting Reaction

$NH_4H_2PO_4 + MgO + H_2O \longrightarrow NH_4MgPO_4 + H_2O$

At room temperature, ammonium diacid phosphate reacts with magnesium oxide to give the investment green strength. At high temperature, a superficial reaction between P_2O_5 and SiO_2 to form silicophosphate, which increases the strength of investment at higher temperature.

Silica Bonded Investment

In silica bonded investment, the silica is used as binder. It is derived from ethyl silicate or aqueous dispersion of colloidal silica or sodium silicate.

Ethyl silicate as a binder – Silica bonded investment bonded by hydrolysis of ethyl silicate in the presence of hydrochloric acid. The product of hydrolysis in the colloidal solution of silicic acid and ethyl alcohol.

$$Si(OC_2H_5)_4 + 4H_2O \xrightarrow{HCl} Si(OH)_4 + 4C_2H_5OH$$

Ethyl silicate has the disadvantage of containing inflammable components which are required for manufacture.

Sodium silicate and colloidal silica are more commonly used as binders.

Methods of Investment

Two methods of investing may be used.
- Manual investing
- Vacuum investing

Manual Investing

Water and powder may be incorporated in the appropriate ratio (indicated by manufacturer) in a rubber bowl with a hand spatula using a rubbing motion and slowly rotating the bowl during the mixing period. Mixing is carried for one minute. The mix is placed on a vibrating table and stirred very slowly for 30 seconds to remove any entrapped air. The investment is then carefully applied to the pattern, using a small sable brush, starting in one place and carrying the investment forward until the pattern is completely covered. The investment is allowed to set partially. The rest of the lined ring is then filled with investment.

Vacuum Investing

In this technique, the investment is mixed and the pattern is invested under vacuum. Several types of vacuum investing equipment are available in the market (Fig. 13.37). The basic method used is as follows:

The investment and water are measured as usual. The mix is placed in a specially constructed mixing unit. The unit is motor driven, and the air evacuated by means of a tube attached to the mixing unit from a vacuum pump. During mixing, air is evacuated and the possibility of bubble formation is thereby reduced. Also while under vacuum, the investment is vibrated into the casting ring and over the wax pattern.

Although good results can be obtained both with hand and vacuum investing, the latter technique is preferred because it is more likely that the casting will be smooth and free of nodules with this technique.

CASTING OF THE PATTERN

Time Allowable for Casting

The investment contracts as it cools because of the liner and the low thermal conductivity of the investment. A short period can elapse before the temperature of the mold is appreciably affected.

Approximately one minute can pass without a noticeable change in dimension.

Casting Machines

Casting machines are divided into three groups depending upon the technique by which gold is pushed into the mold.
- Those which exert pressure on the gold, as by air, nitrous oxide gas or steam.
- Machines which draw the gold into the mold by a vacuum.
- Machines which revolve and gold is carried into the mold by centrifugal force.

Air Pressure Casting Machine

The alloy is melted in the hollow left by crucible former and then air pressure is applied through a piston, which is pushed downward into contact with the top of the ring, enclosing the molten gold alloy. A pressure of 10-15 psi is usually applied (Fig. 13.38).

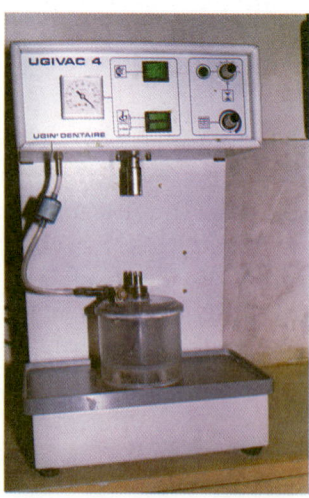

Fig. 13.37: Vacuum mixer

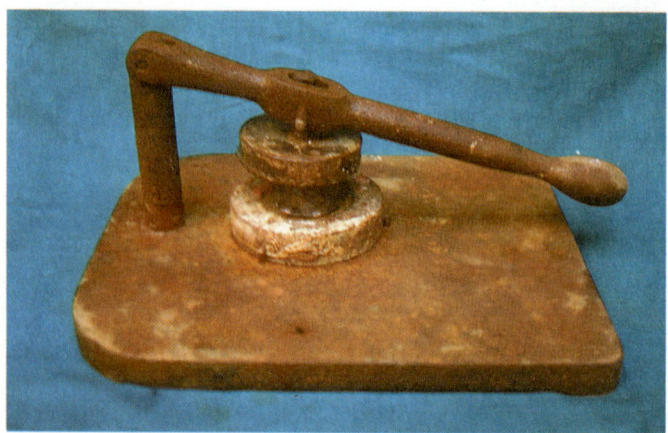

Fig. 13.38: Air pressure casting machine

The pressure gradient along the sprue axis and casting is nil, the thinner the section the faster it solidifies. The button is the thickest portion and so it solidifies last.

Carbon dioxide, carbon monoxide or nitrogen gas can be used.

Vacuum Casting Machine

Here a vacuum is applied through the base beneath the casting ring and the molten alloy can be drawn into the mold by suction. It cannot work alone in filling the mold, even if gravitational forces are used in driving the melt. Therefore, machines are employed that use a combination of centrifugal pressure and a vacuum, gas pressure and a vacuum or centrifugal and gas pressure with the vacuum to create the driving force.

Centrifugal Casting Machine

Various designs of the centrifugal casting machines are now available (Fig. 13.39). The most commonly used design of casting machine is shown in the Fig. 13.40. The machine basically has a strong spring encased in the base of the casting machine, which can be wound into tension by rotating the arms with the weights at one end and the casting ring at the other. In front of the ring is a separate crucible in which the gold alloy is melted. When the spring is released the two arms rotate rapidly, and the molten metal is forced into the mold by centrifugal force. If a '*broken arm*' principle is incorporated in the machine it further accelerates the effective initial rotational speed of the crucible and casting ring, thus increasing the linear speed of the liquid casting alloy as it moves into the mold. A pressure gradient, which is parabolic in shape is created so that a pressure of 30-40 psi (highest) is

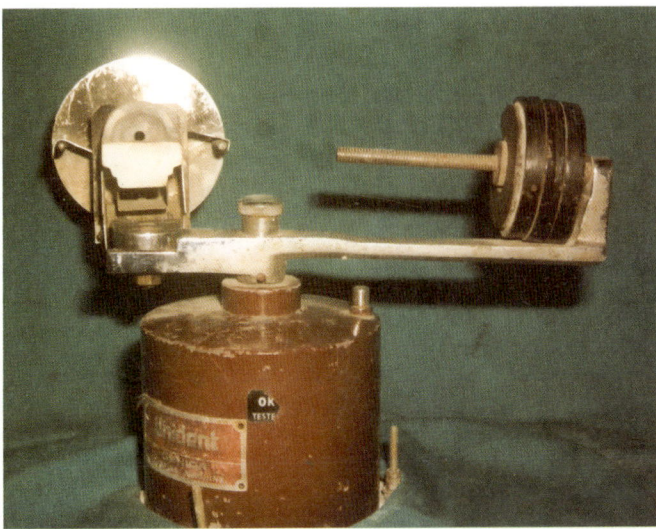

Fig. 13.40: Centrifugal casting machine

created at the tip of the casting and zero at the button surface. The gradient of heat transfer is such that heat transfer is maximum at higher pressure end thus this further ensures that the tip solidifies first.

Time required to cast gold alloy by centrifugal force depends on the cross-sectional area of the sprue and the number of winds of the machine.

When the size of the sprue is increased, the casting time is reduced. When the number of winds is increased and therefore the force is increased, the casting time is reduced. It is observed that the crosssectional area has a greater influence on casting time than does the number of winds of the machine.

Time required to cast gold through 11 gauge, 14 gauge and 17 gauge sprues by centrifugal force produced with 5, 4 and 3 winds of the machine is given in Table 13.6.

Table 13.6: Time taken to cast gold with different gauge of the sprue and winds of the centrifugal machine			
	5 wind	4 wind	3 wind
11 gauge sprue	0.38 min.	0.39 min.	0.46 min.
14 gauge sprue	0.42 min.	0.44 min.	0.54 min.
17 gauge sprue	0.51 min.	0.54 min.	0.67 min.

It is concluded that:
- Centrifugal force is directly proportional to the square of the speed of the machine in revolutions per second.
- Centrifugal force varies directly with the radius of the circular path. Doubling the length of the arm of machine doubles the force.
- Centrifugal force is directly proportional to the weight of the metal directly over the sprue.

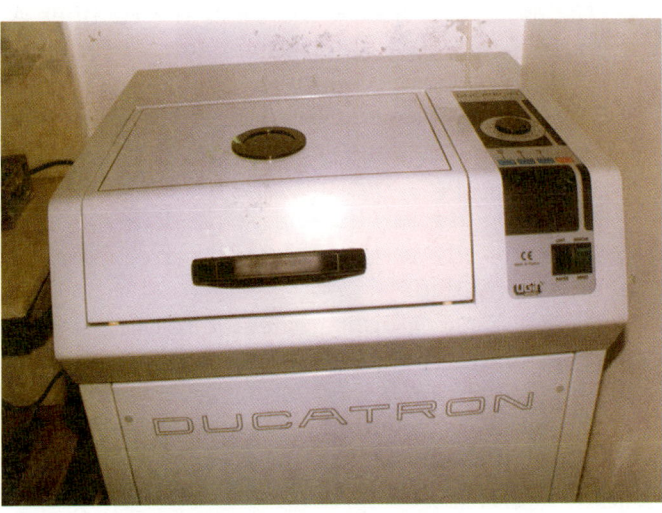

Fig. 13.39: Induction casting machine

When a larger sprue is used the weight of the effective mass of metal is increased thus large sprues are used. More speed of the machine is required to cast small designs since the weight of effective mass of metal is reduced.

Casting Procedure Using Centrifugal Casting Machine

The counter weight of the casting machine is grabbed in the right hand and wound clockwise 2-5 times. The pin is raised from the base so that it rests in front of the crucible assembly, preventing the spring from unwinding.

Casting alloy is placed in the crucible. Enough bulk of the metal must be used in casting to fill the mold, the sprue and part of the crucible former. This metal is melted using one of the methods described earlier. The oxygen gas along with blow-pipe is commonly used. A small multiorifice tip is ideal. Single orifice tips may be used if they are large enough. The small soldering tips should not be used for melting the alloy. Before any torch is lit each knob must be checked. The oxygen valve should be opened slowly to prevent sudden high pressure from hitting the regulator and producing high recompression heat. Gas is ignited first and extinguished last.

A conical flame about 40 mm long is obtained by adjusting the torch. The parts of the flame are identified (Fig. 13.41). The first long cone emanating directly from the nozzle is the zone in which the gas and oxygen are mixed before combustion. No heat is present in this zone. The next cone, which is green in color is the combustion zone. Here the gas and air are partially burned. This is an oxidizing zone. The next zone, dimly blue is the reducing zone. It is the hottest part of the flame and is just beyond the tip of the green combustion zone. This area of the flame should be used to melt the metal. Beyond this is an outer oxidising zone where combustion occurs with oxygen in the air. Contact with the oxidising zone will cause copper and other metals in the alloy to form oxides and thus alter the properties of the alloy.

A small amount of *flux* should be sprinkled onto the warm metal. *Borax* when used as a flux will help to exclude oxygen from the surface of the alloy and dissolve any oxides that are formed.

Reducing flux, which contains carbon in addition to borax, will also reduce any oxides that happen to form. When the reducing zone of the flame is in contact with the metal the surface will be bright and mirror like. As the alloy melts it first appears spongy, and finally it assumes a spheroidal shape and moves with the flame.

Keeping the flame on the gold, the casting ring is removed from the oven and carefully placed in the cradle of the casting machine.

When the metal is a light orange in color and tends to spin or follow the flame when moved, it is ready to be cast. At this juncture it is approximately 38° to 66°C above the liquidus temperature.

Gentle clockwise pressure is applied on the counterweight so that the pin drops. The weight is released allowing the machine to spin. The metal will be thrust into the mold space.

The amount of driving energy used is a matter of judgement but is dictated by the following factors.

a. *The density of the cast metal*: the lower the density, the higher the energy needed.
b. *The porosity of the investment*: the more the porosity, the less the energy needed.
c. *The number of sprues*: the more the number of sprues, the more the driving energy needed to force the melt into them.
d. *The length of the sprue*: the longer the sprue, the more the energy needed.
e. *The size of the sprue*: the larger the diameter of the sprue, the less the energy needed.
f. *The size of the pattern*: larger the size, more the energy needed.
g. *The amount of the melt*: greater the amount of melt, relative to mold size, less the energy used.
h. *The angulation and funnelling of the sprue*: the more the sprue is oriented for immediate and fast filling of the mold, less the energy used.
i. *The differential temperature between the melt and mold*: the more the lag between the two

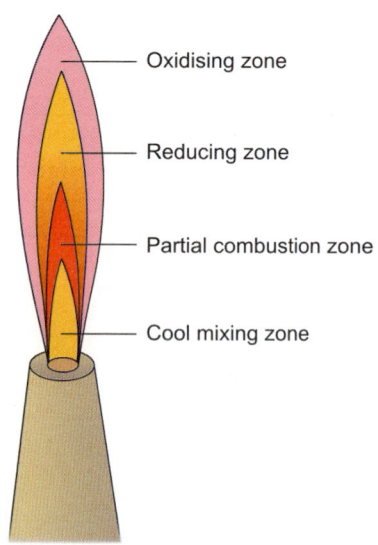

Fig. 13.41: Different zones of the flame

temperatures, the less the energy required within a limit.

j. *The configuration and details of the pattern*: the more the details, the more the energy required.

Casting Techniques

There are two casting techniques usually being used.
- Thermal expansion technique (high heat technique)
- Hygroscopic expansion technique (low heat technique).

Thermal Expansion Casting Technique

The investment is allowed to harden for a minimum of 45 minutes. The excess investment is levelled off the surface of the ring before it sets. Scraping of the investment at a later stage will fill in the pores, decreasing the porosity of the investment.

After the investment has thoroughly set, the crucible former is removed. At this stage any loose particles of investment should be removed and prevented from blocking the ingate formed by the sprue former. The metal sprue former is warmed slightly over a gas flame and carefully removed with pliers. With the ring inverted, a dry brush is used to remove any loose particles of investment remaining around the edges of the sprue hole. The inverted ring is then tapped lightly on the laboratory bench to remove any loose particles, which may have fallen into the mold space.

If the burnout and casting procedure are to be delayed for several hours or overnight, it is advisable to place the invested pattern in humid environment to prevent excessive drying. Excessive drying of the investment prior to burnout will cause the molten wax produced during burnout to be absorbed into the investment.

Burnout Procedure

The casting ring should be placed in an oven preheated to approximately 900°F (480°C), held at that temperature for 20 minutes, and then the temperature is slowly raised to 1290°F (700°C) and held for 30 minutes.

A cold furnace may be used to start the burnout and the temperature is raised slowly and uniformly till 1290°F. The ring is held at this temperature for an adequate period of time to assure complete wax elimination.

Care should be taken to avoid heating gypsum bonded investment above 1290°F. This is because above 1290°F (700°C) calcium sulphate is reduced by carbon molecules releasing sulphur dioxide gas. The sulphur dioxide gas, thus released may contaminate the gold alloy as it enters the mold.

It is advisable to burnout with the sprue hole facing downward, since this will allow the wax to run from the mold and carry investment inclusions out of the mold cavity.

The mold should be protected from variations in temperature by placing it in the centre of the furnace away from the heating coils and the door of the furnace.

Melting Gold Inlays

The gold alloy is melted in one of the following ways.

A. Using a torch flame

a. *Natural gas (mainly propane) and air*: This supplies the lowest temperature of all sources, and is very efficient for small inlays and Type I and Type II alloys.

b. *Natural gas and oxygen*: This supplies a higher temperature and can be used for extensive alloys.

c. *Acetylene and oxygen mixture*: This is the hottest of all gas fuels. It may be too hot for cast gold alloys. It is used for melting base metal alloys.

B. Using electric energy

Induction heat is the most efficient and popular method of melting an alloy. The metal is melted by an induction field that develops within a crucible surrounded by water-cooled metal tubing.

The metal can be melted in a separate crucible and then pushed into the mold space or in the same crucible.

Generally, three types of casting crucibles are available- *clay (ceramic), carbon and quartz*. For gold alloy, clay or carbon crucibles are used. Clay crucibles are more popular. They are lined with asbestos or kaolin, which after casting insures non-contamination of the crucibles, hence may be re-used.

Hygroscopic Expansion Technique

This technique involves the immersion of the metal ring with investment into a warm water bath set at 37°C or 100°F. The technique *compensates shrinkage* by three mechanisms.

- 37°C water bath expands the wax pattern.
- Water entering the investment provides greater volume into which gypsum crystals can grow and hence provides some hygroscopic expansion.
- Thermal expansion at 468°C (burn out temperature for hygroscopic setting expansion).

The amount of hygroscopic expansion can be controlled by:
- *Water/Powder ratio:* The higher the water/powder ratio, the lower the amount of expansion.
- *Time of immersion in the water bath:* The longer the delay before the investment is immersed in the water bath, the less is the hygroscopic expansion.
- *Controlling the amount of water* added during the setting.

Hygroscopic expansion can be achieved by two ways:
- Immersing the filled casting ring in a water bath.
- By addition of a known quantity of water to the exposed surface of unset investment in the casting ring (controlled water technique).

I. Water Bath Technique

The essential features of water bath technique are:
- The pattern is washed with soap and water.
- Definite proportions of water and investment are used.
- Investment must be slow setting (from twenty to thirty minutes) to allow sufficient time to expand.
- The wax pattern is invested.
- Both ends of the ring are sealed and it is placed in the water bath at 43°C for inlays and at 44°C to 45°C for crowns until the investment has completely set. In actual practice, these temperatures are governed by prevailing conditions and the exact temperature to be used must be worked out by the practitioner.
- The wax is then burned out and the metal is casted.

II. Controlled Water Technique

It has been shown that the amount of hygroscopic expansion is directly related to the amount of water available to the setting investment and that by adding a specific amount of water to the setting investment, a specific amount of expansion results. The controlled water added technique is based on this principle.

Equipment Required

The equipment consists of a rubber sprue former, around which a rubber ring is placed. A thin metal ring is placed around the rubber ring, to prevent its collapse during vacuum investing or for convenience during hand investing. It is removed after the rubber ring is filled. A syringe of 200 ml capacity is used to add controlled amounts of water with an accuracy of 0.1 ml.

Procedure

In all techniques involving setting expansion of the investment, the expansion takes place in the presence of the wax pattern. The wax pattern can restrict expansion of the investment. In order to soften the wax the ring can be immersed in water held at a temperature of 37°C. But care is taken to see that the level of water is below the top of the rubber ring and no water is allowed to come in contact with the investment.

The investment used for this technique is an investment especially compounded to provide high hygroscopic expansion.

The investment is mixed and poured into the rubber ring with supporting metal ring in place. Immediately after investing, the metal ring is removed so as to avoid restriction of the expansion of investment. The investment is flushed with the top of the rubber ring and the reservoir collar inserted. The syringe is filled with water and the water is carefully dispersed into the reservoir collar. For an inlay, generally 1.1 ml of water is added. If a warm water bath is used then some expansion of wax has already occured so about 0.6 ml water is added.

Before burn out, the investment is allowed to set for a minimum of 45 minutes. After the investment has set, the rubber ring is removed and the investment mold without the support of a metal ring is subjected to burn out and the alloy is cast into the mold. The purpose of the rubber ring is to eliminate the asbestos liner, which would absorb the added water, thereby mitigating the accuracy of the water addition.

In the hygroscopic technique the ring is heated not higher than 468°C because thermal expansion of the investment is not desired. The mold should be held at this temperature for 60 to 90 minutes because the chances of a carbonaceous residue are very high.

Cleaning the Casting

After the casting has been completed, the ring is removed and quenched in water as soon as the button emits a dull red glow.

Advantages of quenching are:
- The noble metal alloy is left in an annealed condition for burnishing, polishing, etc.
- When water contacts the investment, it is absorbed into the investment pores. It undergoes immediate vapourizing within the hot mass. Steam in large amounts produces cracking of the investment into small pieces. This simplifies cleaning the casting.

Sandblast technique is also used to remove the remaining investment material on the casting.

FINISHING AND POLISHING OF CAST RESTORATIONS

Finishing and polishing of restorative dental materials are important steps in the fabrication of clinically successful restorations. The techniques employed for these procedures are meant not only for the removal of excess material but also to smoothen the rough surfaces.

Chemical

After casting the gold alloys become discolored or dark due to contamination and due to the presence of sulphide in the investment material. To remove these discolorations, pickling procedure is done. The solutions used for pickling are 50% hydrochloric acid or 50% sulphuric acid. The best pickling solution for gypsum bonded investment is 50% HCl acid solution. The disadvantage of hydrochloric acid is that fumes from acids are likely to corrode laboratory equipments and can cause health hazards. A similar solution of sulphuric acid is more advantageous in this respect. Its action is enhanced by addition of potassium dichromate. However, sulphuric acid solution also proves dangerous. The best method of pickling is to place the casting in a test tube or dish and pour the acid over it. It may be necessary to heat the acid but boiling should be avoided. After pickling, the acid is poured off and the casting is removed. The pickling solution should be renewed frequently because it is likely to become contaminated. Casting should not be held with steel instruments as this may contaminate the pickling solution and casting. This is because the pickling solution usually contains small amounts of copper dissolved from previous castings. When the steel tongs contact this electrolyte, a galvanic cell is created and copper is deposited on the casting at the point where tongs grip it.

Another procedure to be avoided is heating the casting and then dropping it in the pickling solution. This may cause delicate margins of the casting to melt or the casting may be distorted by sudden thermal shock when plunged into the acid. After pickling, the casting should be washed in running water to remove the acid.

Mechanical

The casting that is retrieved from the investment possesses a surface that is too rough to be used in the mouth. To remove the roughness of the casting surface, different abrasives are used. There are coarse materials, which help in removing the surface irregularities and impregnation. Different abrasives used are diamond, silicon carbide, emery, aluminium oxide, garnet, sand, tripoli, rouge, etc. The outer surface of the casting is smoothened with these abrasives using consecutive and progressive small particle sizes. The finishing process not only removes the surface blemishes and imperfections but also it gives the casting a shape to an ideal form or a desired state.

Polishing

Finishing procedures tend to leave microscopic scratches on the casting. During the final polishing stage these scratches are eliminated or reduced to a microscopic size which results in a microcrystalline surface layer known as Bielby layer.

Polishing can be accomplished with the help of rubber abrasive points, fine particle disks, strips, flexible paper backed disks finishing burs and polishing paste used with rotary instrument. Polishing paste is applied with soft felt points, muslin wheels, prophy cups or buffy wheels. Therefore, polishing is one of the more refined finishing processes which should be done to keep the casting restoration clean as it also aids in corrosion resistance. The details of finishing and polishing are given in Chapter 27.

Try in

Remove the temporary restoration, making sure that all the temporary cement has been dislodged from the preparation walls and cleared away. Now confirm the fit of the casting. A gauze sponge should be placed as a 'throat screen' to catch the casting, if it is accidently dropped. Try the casting on the tooth using light pressure. Do not force the casting on the tooth. If the casting does not seat properly, most likely cause is an overcontoured proximal surface. Using the mouth mirror, judge where the proximal contour needs adjustment to allow final seating of the casting, producing the correct position and form to the contact. Passing the dental floss through the contact will indicate tightness and position of the contact. If the floss will not enter or tears on entering the contact is excessive. To adjust the proximal contour and to correct contact relationship several trials on the tooth are required but it is best not to remove too much at a time. This contact should be passive. If contact is open, a new contact area must be soldered to the casting. An open contact is best detected by visual inspection with the aid of the mouth mirror. The soldering can be done by cleaning the contact area using a mild acid. Cut a small piece about 2.0 to 3.0 mm of solder out of solder strip. Apply borax type flux on the contact area of the casting and on the both surfaces of the piece of solder. Place the solder on contact area requiring build-up and direct the pinpoint flame of Bunsen burner to the solder with the help of blow pipe so that the solder melts and flows.

When the proximal contacts have been adjusted and the casting is satisfactorily seated on the tooth occlusion is verified. Occlusion is verified both in centric occlusion and during lateral excursive movements. Any high points and areas of heavy occlusal contacts are reduced with suitable abrasive stones.

CEMENTATION

Before cementation, the tooth is isolated with the air syringe, dry the preparation walls but do not dessicate them. Now mix the cement following manufacturer's instructions. Cement mix is generously applied to the preparation side of the casting, start the casting to place with fingers. Place the ball burnisher in the pit area to exert firm pressure to seat the casting. Ask the patient to close and exert biting force, several seconds of this pressure is sufficient. Complete seating of the casting is verified by inspection after wiping the excess cement away from the margins.

After the cement has hardened, excess is cleared off with an explorer and air waterspray. Dental floss should be passed through the contact and clean the gingival embrasure.

Burnishing of the margins depends on the cement used. Burnishing of the margins was done after 24 hours, if zinc phosphate cement was used, as zinc phosphate cement is soluble in oral fluids whereas burnishing can be done after 15–20 minutes if resin cements were used because they are very less soluble in the oral cavity.

CASTING DEFECTS

Various casting defects, their probable causes and solutions are given in Table 13.7.

Porosity is a major defect in casting, so is discussed separately here.

Porosities in noble metal alloy castings can be classified as:

Those Caused by Solidification Shrinkage

a. *Localized shrinkage porosity*: When the alloy solidifies from liquid state, a shrinkage of at least 1.25% occurs. Thus during solidification of metal in mold, if additional molten metal is not available to compensate for shrinkage then porosity occurs.

It can occur if the metal freezes in the sprue before it does in the mold. It generally occurs at the sprue casting junction.

It could also be the result of formation of a *hot spot* when metal impinges on a mold surface so that here the metal remains molten whilst it solidifies everywhere else.

This kind of porosity is avoided by:
- Flaring the point of sprue attachment.
- Placing sprue in such a way so that a hot spot formation is avoided.
- Not using an excessively long sprue.
- Using a reservoir.
- Reducing the mold-melt temperature differential (i.e. lowering the casting temperature by about 30°C).

b. *Micro porosity*: It occurs due to premature solidification of the metal and is the result of solidification shrinkage. The voids produced are irregular in shape. This defect is discovered only if the casting is sectioned.

It occurs due to unduly rapid solidification of the metal or casting temperature is too low.

Porosities Caused by Gas

a. *Pinhole porosity*.
b. *Gas inclusion porosity*.

Both produce spherical defects; the defects in case of gas inclusion porosity are larger.

The metal absorbs gases when it is in molten state. Upon solidification, the absorbed gases are expelled and pinhole porosity results.

Larger spherical porosities are caused by gas occluded from a poorly adjusted blowpipe flame or if the reducing zone of the flame is not used.

Subsurface Porosity

The exact reason for this has not been established. It may be due to the simultaneous nucleation of solid grains and gas bubbles at the first moment that the metal freezes at the mold walls. This can be diminished by controlling the rate at which the molten metal enters the mold.

Back Pressure Porosity

Porosity produced due to air entrapped on the inner surface of the casting. Usually occurs if for some reason gas is not vented from the mold.

To prevent this the burnout should be adequate so that carbonaceous residues do not decrease porosity of investment. Mold and casting temperature should not be too low so as to allow metal to solidify rapidly.

The water/powder ratio of the investment should be correct.

The casting pressure should be adequate.

The rest of the defects are tabulated in Table 13.7.

Cast Restorations

Table 13.7: Various casting defects, their causes and solutions

Casting defect	Causes	Solutions
Incomplete castings	• Inadequate spruing (sprue former too small)	• Use larger size of sprue former. Place sprue former in such a way so that all areas of the mold are fed by molten alloy.
	• Alloy not hot enough	• Have casting temperature at least 150°F (57°C) above fusion temperature of alloy.
	• Mold too cold	• Mold should soak heat for approximately one hour at burnout temperature. The temperature of the oven should be checked regularly with a pyrometer. Mold should be removed from burnout oven and casting completed within one minute.
	• Ingate obstructed	• Ensure that no debris blocks the ingate. The ring should be held with sprue hole down when removing crucible former and sprue former (metal).
	• Insufficient casting force	• Use the adequate amount of force for casting.
	• Insufficient gold	• Cast enough gold to allow for a good button in the crucible of the ring.
Rounded margins	• Incomplete burnout of wax pattern	• Carbon residues in the mold can produce shiny rounded margins. Ensure adequate burnout time and temperature to cause the carbon to get converted to carbon monoxide or carbon dioxide.
	• Insufficient heating of alloy before casting	• Heat alloy to 150°F (57°C) above fusion temperature.
	• Improper diameter/length of sprue restricts flow of alloy into the mold. The metal freezes before margins are complete.	• Average casting should have 10 gauge sprue and approximately 6.0 mm long.
Pits in casting	• Debris in mold	• Join the sprue former, crucible former and pattern with continuous smooth surface with no jagged areas of investment, which can break off and enter mold.
	• Dirty wax	• Use clean, new wax for patterns and sprues.
	• Loose debris in crucible	• Use clean crucible for each casting
	• Mold temperature too hot	• At very high temperature the investment can break. Avoid overheating.
Distortion	• Distortion of wax pattern	• Proper handling and manipulation of the wax pattern.
	• Due to uneven movement of the walls of the pattern when the investment is setting. The gingival margins are forced apart by the mold expansion, whereas the solid occlusal bar of wax resists expansion during the early stage of setting.	• Not much can be done to avoid this.
Surface roughness, irregularities	• Air bubbles on the pattern	• Use vacuum investing technique. • Vibrate before and after mixing. • Use a wetting agent to reduce surface tension of wax pattern. • Air dry the wetting agent as excess water will dilute investment, causing irregularities.
	• Water films causing ridges and veins on the surface	• Avoiding movement, vibration of pattern after investment. Painting investment properly on the pattern to ensure intimate contact. • Using a wetting agent.

(Contd.)

Table 13.7: Various casting defects, their causes and solutions (*Contd.*)

Casting defect	Causes	Solutions
	• Too rapid heating resulting in fins or spines	• The mold should be heated gradually, 60 minutes taken to heat the ring from room temperature to 700°C. • Rapid heating will cause flaking of investment when steam forms. Also a surge of steam may carry salts used as modifiers into the mold.
	• Underheating causing incomplete elimination of wax	• Heat the ring for adequate period of time so that the carbonaceous residue is removed.
	• Inappropriate W/P ratio	• Both excess W/P and low W/P ratio causes rough castings. Thus W:P should be accurate Low W:P ratio causes roughness because it cannot be painted on properly and during vacuum investing air might not be removed completely.
	• Prolonged heating	• Gypsum bonded investment should never be heated above 700°C because sulphur compounds are formed and investment starts disintegrating.
	• Temperature of alloy too high	• The color of the molten alloy just prior to casting should be no lighter than light orange. Very hot alloy will attack surface of investment causing roughness.
	• Casting pressure too high	• Pressure required for casting should be adjusted.
	• Foreign bodies	• Avoid carrying pieces of investment loosened during removal of sprue former and crucible former. • A piece of carbon from the flux could be carried into the mold to cause a bright appearing concavity.
	• Impact of molten alloy	• The direction of sprue former should be adjusted so that it does not strike a weak part of the mold surface at an angle of 90°.
	• Pattern position	• Several patterns when placed in the same ring should not be placed too close together because expansion of wax can cause break down of investment if a thickness of several mm is not present.
Discoloration	• Sulphur contamination of casting causing black castings	• This could be due to (a) heating the investment above 700°C causing its breakdown and formation of sulphur compounds. It can be avoided by avoiding overheating of investment. (b) sulphur content of the torch flame. The problem can be solved by changing the source of heat.
	• Contamination with copper during pickling	• Avoiding the use of steel tongs to hold casting during pickling. If they must be used then the tips of the tongs should be covered with rubber.
	• Contamination with mercury	• Castings should never be placed with amalgam dies or kept on a table where amalgam scrap is present.

BIBLIOGRAPHY

1. Allan, F.C. and Asgar, K.: Reaction of cobalt-chromium casting alloy with investment. J.D.R.: 45, 1516, 1966.
2. Barreto, M.T., JonGoldberg, A., Nitkin, D.A. and Mumford, G.: Effect of investment on casting high fusing alloys. J.P.D.: 44, 504, 1980.
3. Bessing, C.: Evaluation of the castability of four different alternative alloys by measuring the marginal sharpness. Acta. Odontol. Scand.: 44, 165, 1986.
4. Blockhurst, P.J., McLaverty, V.G. and Kasloff, Z.: A castability standard for alloys used in restorative dentistry. Oper. Dent.: 8, 130, 1983.
5. Chan, D.C.N., Brackman, R., Kaiser, D.A. and Chung, K.: The effect of sprue design on the marginal accuracy of titanium castings. J. Oral Rehabil.: 25, 424, 1998.
6. Chew, C.L., Land, M.F., Thomas, C.C. and Norman R.D.: Investment strength as a function of time and temperature. J. Dent. 27, 297, 1999.
7. Christensen, G.J.: Marginal fit of gold inlay castings. J.P.D.: 16, 297, 1966.

8. Corso, P.P. Jr., German, R.M. and Simmons, H.D.: Corrosion evaluation of gold based dental alloys. J.D.R.: 64, 854, 1985.
9. Corso, P.P. Jr., German, R.M. and Simmons, H.D.: Tarnish evaluation of gold based dental alloys. J.D.R.: 64, 848, 1985.
10. Dewald, E.: The relationship of pattern position to the flow of gold and casting completeness. J.P.D.: 41, 531, 1979.
11. Eames, W.B. and MacNamara, J.F.: Evaluation of casting machines for ability to cast sharp margins. Oper. Dent.: 3, 137, 1978.
12. Earnshaw, R.: The compressive strength of gypsum-bonded investments at high temperatures. Aust. Dent. J.: 14, 264, 1969.
13. Eichner, K.: Applications of metal alloys in dentistry: A review. Int. Dent. J.: 33, 1, 1983.
14. Farah, J.W., Dennison, J.B. and Powers, J.M.: Effects of design on stress distribution of intracoronal gold restorations. J.A.D.A.: 94, 1151, 1977.
15. Frates, F.E.: Inlays. D.C.N.A.: 11, 163, 1967.
16. Fusayama, T. and Yamane, M.: Surface roughness of castings made by various casting techniques. J.P.D.: 29, 529, 1973.
17. Gable, A.B.: Mechanical principles of operative dentistry. J.A.D.A.: 43, 153, 1951.
18. Geurtsen, W.: Biocompatibility of dental casting alloys. Crit. Rev. Oral Biol. Med.: 13, 71, 2002.
19. Hess, TA. and Wadhwani, CPK.: The Tucker Technique: Conservative molar inlays preserving the transverse ridge. Oper Dent.: 37, 93, 2012.
20. Hirano, S., Tesk, J.A., Hinman, R.W., Argentar, H. and Gregory, T.M.: Casting of dental alloys: Mold and alloy temperature effects. Dent. Mater.: 3, 307, 1987.
21. Ho, E K-H and Darvell, B.W.: A new method for casting discrepancy: some results for a phosphate-bonded investment. J. Dent.: 26, 59, 1998.
22. Kelly, G.P.: Study of porosity and voids in dental gold castings. J.D.R.: 49, 986, 1970.
23. Lacy, A.M., Fukui, H. and Jenderesen, M.D.: Three factors affecting investment setting expansion and casting size. J.P.D.: 49, 52, 1983.
24. Leinfelder, K.F.: An evaluation of casting alloys used for restorative procedures. J.A.D.A.: 128, 37, 1997.
25. Leinfelder, K.F.: Low gold alloys: A laboratory and clinical evaluation. Quint. Int.: 5, 483, 1981.
26. Luk, H.W.K. and Darvell, B.W.: Casting system effectiveness measurement and theory. Dent. Mater.: 8, 89, 1992.
27. Luk, H.W.K. and Darvell, B.W.: Effect of burnout temperature on strength of phosphate-bonded investments. J. Dent.: 25, 153, 1997.
28. Luk, HW-K and Darvell, B.W.: The effect of burnout temperature on the strength of phosphate bonded investments: Part II: effect of metal temperature. J. Dent.: 25, 423, 1997.
29. Mahler, D.B. and Ady, A.B.: The influence of various features on the effective setting expansion of casting investments. J.D.R.: 13, 365, 1963.
30. Manhart, J., Chen, H.Y., Hamm, G. and Hickel, R.: Review of the clinical survival of direct and indirect restorations in posterior teeth of the permanent dentition. Oper. Dent.: 29, 481, 2004.
31. Marsaw, F.A., Rijk, W.G., Hesby, R.A., Hinman, R.W. and Peller, G.B.: Internal volumetric expansion of casting investments. J.P.D.: 52, 361, 1984.
32. Moon, P.C. and Mdjeski, P.J.: The burnishability of dental casting alloys. J.P.D. ; 36, 404, 1976.
33. Morey, E.F. and Earnshaw, R.: The fit of gold alloy full crown castings made with ceramic casting ring liners. J.D.R.: 71, 1865, 1992.
34. Morey, E.F. and Earnshaw, R.: The fit of gold alloy fullcrown castings made with pre-wetted casting ring liners. J.D.R.: 71, 1858, 1992.
35. Morey, E.F.: Dimensional accuracy of small gold alloy castings. Part I: A brief history and the behaviour of inlay waxes. Part II: Gold alloy shrinkage. Part III: Gypsumbonded investment expansion. Part IV: The casting ring and ring liners. Aust. Dent. J. 36, 302 and 391, 1991 and 37, 43 and 91, 1992.
36. Mori, T. Study of gypsum-bonded casting investment. Part I & Part II. 38, 220-306, 1993.
37. Myers, R.E.: Time required to cast gold by centrifugal force. J.A.D.A.: 28, 2001, 1941.
38. Olivera, A.B. and Saito, T.: The effect of die spacer on retention and fitting of complete cast crowns. J. Prosthodont.: 15, 243, 2006.
39. Pretson, J.D.: Metal mold equilibrium with vacuum pressure induction casting. J.D.R.: 64 (Abst. 1590), 1985.
40. Rawson, R.D., Gregory, G.G. and Lund, M.R.: Photographic study of gold flow. J.D.R.: 51, 1331, 1972.
41. Rosenstiel, E.: To bevel or not to bevel? B.D.J.: 138, 389, 1975.
42. Santos, J.F. and Ballester, R.Y.: Delayed hygroscopic expansion of phosphate bonded investments. Dent. Mater.: 3, 165, 1987.
43. Schmaltz, G. and Garhammer, P.: Biological interactions of dental cast alloys with oral tissues. Dent. Mater.: 18, 396, 2002.
44. Smales, R.J. and Etemadi, S.: Survival of ceramic onlays placed with and without metal reinforcement. J.P.D.: 91, 548, 2004.
45. Stevens, L.: The effect of time between mixing and heating on the expansion of phosphate-bonded investment. A.D.J.: 31, 207, 1986.
46. Stoll, R., Siewek, M., Pieper, K., Stachniss, V. and Schulte, A.: Longevity of cast gold inlays and partial crowns – a retrospective study at a dental school clinic. Clinical Oral Investigations: 3, 100, 1999.
47. Sturdvent, J.R., Sturdvent, C.M., Taylor, D.F. and Bayne, S.C.: The 8-year clinical performance of 15 low gold casting alloys. Dent. Mater.: 3, 347, 1987.
48. Tschernitschek, H. and Borchers, L.: Non-alloyed titanium as a bioinert metal – a review. Quint. Int.: 36, 523, 2005.
48. Tucker, R.V.: Variation in inlay cavity design. J.A.D.A.: 84, 616, 1972.
50. Werrin, S.R., Jubach, T.S. and Johnson, B.W.: Inlays and onlays: Making the right decision. Quint. Int.: 11, 13, 1980.
51. Whitlock, R.P., Hinman, R.W., Eden, G.T., Tesk, J.A., Dickson, G. and Parry, E.E.: A practical test to evaluate the castability of dental alloys. J.D.R.: 60 (Abst. 374), 1981.
52. Zidan, O. and Ferguson, G.C.: The retention of complete crowns prepared with three different tapers and luted with four different cements. J.P.D.: 89, 565, 2003.

14

Complex Restorations

The operative dentist is confronted with restoration of extensively damaged teeth in routine. Many a times, the damage, which may be because of caries, trauma or previous restorations, involves half or more than half of the tooth structure. The remaining tooth structure is not sufficient to retain the restoration and require modification of classic preparation design by incorporation of various retentive means. The earlier authors defined complex restorations as the restorations involving more than two tooth surfaces. However, many lesions warrant the use of extra retentive devices involving single tooth surface also. Such restorations, which require extra retentive device for their retention, are labeled as '*complex restorations*'.

CLASSIFICATION OF CORONAL TOOTH DESTRUCTION

Location, as well as extent of coronal destruction, plays an important role in selection of material and design of cavity preparation employed in restoration of tooth. Location of destruction can be categorized as peripheral, which occurs on the axial surfaces of the teeth (Fig. 14.1); central, which occurs in the central portion of the tooth (Fig. 14.2); and combined, which incorporates destruction in both areas (Fig. 14.3).

Minimal destruction of tooth structure in central, peripheral and combined locations usually can be restored with an amalgam or composite resin restoration. An amalgam or composite resin restoration can also be employed on mostly moderately damaged teeth. However, combined destruction may require onlay, if the potential for fracture of unsupported cusp becomes too great (Table 14.1).

Peripheral destruction, even when not pulp threatening, can require extra retentive devices. Extensive central destruction that undermines much of the enamel will require the placement of amalgam core followed by a crown.

Severe destruction of the crown of the molar can be treated by placement of pin-retained amalgam or composite resin core, followed by placement of crown.

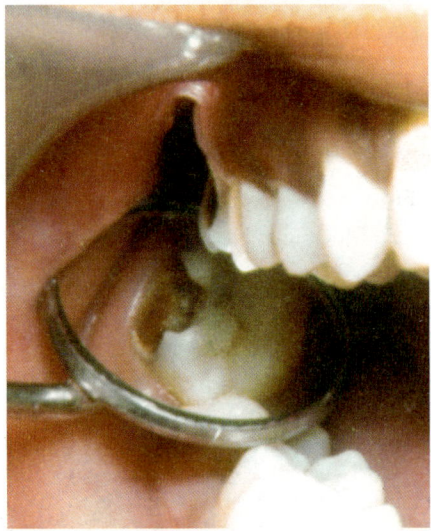

Fig. 14.1: Peripheral tooth destruction

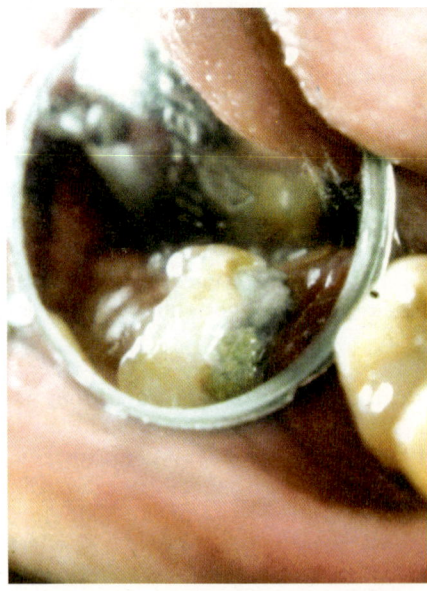

Fig. 14.2: Central tooth destruction

Restoration of a premolar in similar circumstances may require elective devitalization of tooth followed by dowel-core.

Complex Restorations

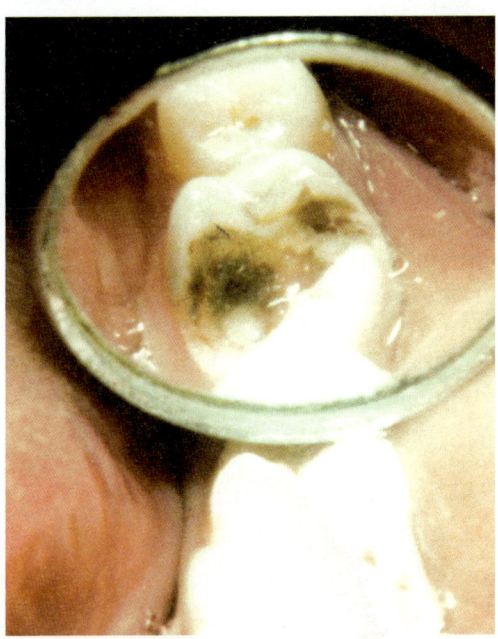

Fig. 14.3: Combined tooth destruction

EXTRA RETENTIVE DEVICES

Certain rules should be followed to avoid excessive tooth destruction while creating retention in already weakened tooth

- Central core (the pulp and the 1.0 mm thick surrounding layer of dentin) must not be invaded in vital teeth: No retentive feature should extend more than 1.5 mm into the dentin from the cervical line and/or central fossa. If caries removal results in deeper cavity, any part lying within vital core should be filled with glass-ionomer cement.
- No dentin wall be reduced to thickness less than 1.0 mm for the sake of retention as it is required for the placement of the foundation restorations.

To compensate the lost tooth structure, may be moderate, severe or total, one or more than one retentive device is utilized (Table 14.2). The routinely used retentive devices are:

i. Slots
ii. Grooves/Locks
iii. Crown lengthening
iv. Pins

i. *Slots:* Slots are given to increase the surface area for the restoration. A 0.75-1.0 mm deep and 1.0-3.0 mm wide cut is given on the pulpal and/or cervical wall. This rectangular depression in these walls increases the bulk for the restoration, and also increases the area for bonding (Fig. 14.4).

ii. *Grooves/Locks:* The locks are given in direct restorations while the grooves are given in indirect restorations. The major difference between the groove and the lock is, that the lock extends upto the pulpal wall (from cervical to pulpal) and the groove extends upto the cavosurface margin (from cervical to cavosurface). The groove maintain the parallelism of walls while the lock converge occlusally. The grooves/locks are given at

Table 14.1: Treatment options

	Minimal	Moderate	Severe
Central	• Amalgam • Composite	• Bonded amalgam • Sandwich technique	Amalgam core + crown
Peripheral	• Amalgam • Composite	• Pin amalgam • Pin composite • Cast restoration • Crown	Full crown
Combined	Amalgam	• Pin amalgam • Onlay	• Amalgam core + crown • Cast pin restoration

Table 14.2: Compensation for lost tooth structure

Loss of tooth structure	Explanation	Compensating procedures	Final restoration

Moderate	One or two cusps missing but more than 50% of coronal tooth structure remaining. Thickness of remaining walls : at least 1.0 mm thick	• Modify existing preparation features:
		  – Grooves
		  – Pin
		• Remove questionable tooth structure
			Full or partial veneer crown

Severe	Loss of 50% or more of crown. Thin walls (less than 1.0 mm)	• Apply • Lengthen the crown surgically, if need be	Full veneer crown
Total	All cusps destroyed, Supra-gingival height 1.0 mm or less	• Place amalgam or composite resin core with pins • Elective devitalization and dowel core for premolars • Lengthen crown surgically if need be	Full veneer crown

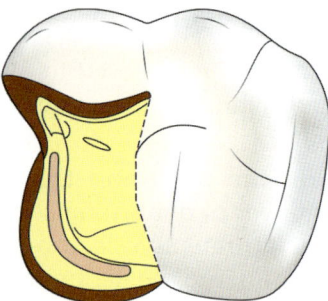

Fig. 14.4: Slot placement

axiobuccal and axio-lingual line angle, inside dentino-enamel junction, putting more pressure on buccal and lingual walls rather than at the axial walls.

Multiple grooves can also be given for enhanced resistance. They may also be added to the angles of oversized box forms to augment the resistance provided by the box walls. Care should be taken to place the grooves in one plane. More than one groove per wall is rarely indicated and if necessary, can be given keeping proper parallelism and dentin around each groove.

iii. *Crown lengthening*: In moderate to severe loss of tooth structure, one of the compensating procedures is to lengthen the crown surgically (Fig. 14.5). The clinical crown can sometimes be lengthened surgically by electrosurgery, but this is limited by the width of the attached gingiva. Any exaggerated apical placement of finish line, whether accompanied by surgical crown lengthening or not, will result in apical migration of epithelial attachment and alveolar crest of bone. Eventually the alveolar crest will migrate to a level of approximately 3.0 mm apical to the margin of the restoration. In addition to periodontal pocket that will be created, the crown root ratio may also be compromised.

iv. *Pins*: Restorations using pins have been and are still being tried to achieve the required retention.

Pins have long been utilized for retention purposes in dentistry, but were not popular earlier because of the lack of expertise, efficient tools and materials. Extensive research has eased pin placement and fabrication of pin retained restorations. With their introduction, it became possible to salvage extensively decayed teeth; may be as individual restorations or as abutments for fixed and removable partial dentures. Though recently, alternative techniques to some extent have overcome the dangers associated with pin placement, the use of pins cannot be totally eliminated. A complete knowledge about their characteristics and use is desirable for better results.

RATIONALE FOR USE OF PINS

Pins help to support the restorative materials and resist their dislodgement in teeth that have been severely damaged and weakened. Conventional cavity preparation in badly mutilated cases require removal of large amounts of tooth structure for obtaining retention and resistance forms. Pins provide efficient and adequate retention to the restorations with the least possible sacrifice of healthy tooth structure. With the use of pins, cavity preparation can also be limited to only damaged surfaces thereby preserving esthetics and contours.

Markley had referred to the pin retained restorations as analogous to reinforced concrete architecture. The simple inference was that pins strengthened restorative material. However, no concrete evidence was presented by Markley concerning the additional strength of pin retained restorations. On the contrary, various studies concluded that stainless steel pins in amalgam did not actually strengthen it. Hence, the use of pins is restricted for extra retentive purposes. It is emphasized that pins are auxiliary aids of retention and should be used only after primary retentive features like establishment of parallel walls, boxes and grooves are not sufficient to provide the desired amount of retention.

INDICATIONS

1. Pins are indicated as auxiliary aids of retention in badly broken down or mutilated teeth, large class II, class III, class IV and class V cavity preparations.
2. In teeth with guarded prognosis, i.e. in endodontically and periodontically involved teeth, pin retained restorations are more useful than comparatively expensive treatments.
3. Pins may be used in foundations for full or partial metal or metal ceramic restorations.
4. Pin retained restorations may facilitate rubber dam application and subsequent procedures on the concerned tooth.

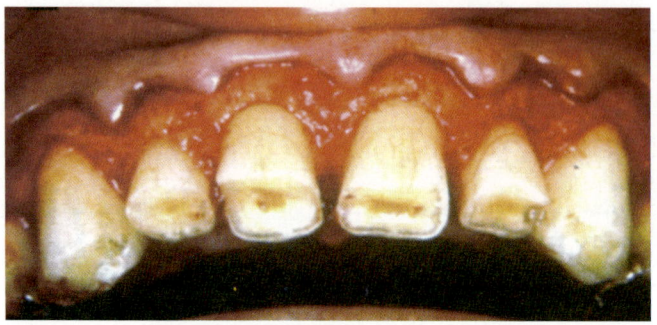

Fig. 14.5: Crown lengthening

Advantages

- Offer retention without the need for extensive preparation of tooth structure.
- May increase resistance form of the preparation to some extent.
- Relatively less time consuming than cast restorations, which require multiple appointments.
- Comparatively less expensive than cast restorations for salvaging badly broken down teeth.

Disadvantages

- Do not increase the compressive strength of the overlying restorative material, and may reduce the transverse and tensile strengths significantly.
- Induce stresses in dentin in the form of cracks or craze lines, which may increase the potential for fracture of tooth, microleakage, pulpal damage, etc.
- Increase the chances of perforations into pulp or on external tooth surface.
- Chances of microleakage exist at the pin dentin interface if the overlying restoration leaks.

CLASSIFICATION OF PINS

Pins can be classified as:
- Direct pins/non-parallel pins
- Indirect pins/parallel pins

1. *Direct pins* are usually made of stainless steel, and inserted into dentin followed by the placement of a restorative material like silver amalgam, resin or cement directly over them. Other materials of which the pins can be made of are silver, titanium, stainless steel with gold plating, etc. These have also been referred to as the *non-parallel pins* since they can be inserted directly into the tooth structure and hence need not be parallel. Further, this category of pins includes cemented, friction locked and threaded pins of which the last category of pins is the most popular.
2. *Indirect pins* are slightly undersized compared to their pinholes and are an integral part of a cast restoration. These are also known as the *parallel pins* as the method necessitates placement of pins parallel to each other as well as parallel to the path of insertion of the restoration. The pins are held in the pinholes by means of a cement. Retention offered by the parallel pins is definitely less than that offered by the non-parallel pins. There are basically two types of pins used in the parallel pin technique.
   a. *Cast gold pins*, which have a relatively smooth surface. Restorations using these pins are fabricated by placing nylon bristles or plastic pins in the pinholes over which the rest of the restoration is built in the conventional form with a blue inlay wax. The whole assembly is invested and cast, with pins forming an inherent part of the cast restoration.
   b. *Wrought precious metal pins* have surfaces that have been deformed or roughened by means of threaded or knurled patterns. These pins are alloys of gold, platinum, palladium or platinum-iridium. The pins are placed in the pinholes and included in the wax pattern. Their high melting point and tarnish resistance enable them to be incorporated into the final gold casting. Threaded wrought pins have shown to be 20–30 percent more retentive than the smooth cast pins.

DIRECT PINS

The three major categories of direct pins are cemented, friction locked and threaded pins.

a. Cemented Pins

Markley introduced this type of pin in early 1950s to achieve greater retention in a large silver amalgam restoration. In this technique, the pins are 0.0013"-0.0023" smaller than their pin channels and the difference in diameter provides space for the cementing medium. The pins can be of varying sizes – 0.0183" to 0.0303" and the corresponding pin channel sizes are then 0.0203" to 0.0323" respectively. Cemented pins are generally indicated in cases where least crazing and stresses are desired in the remaining tooth structure, e.g. endodontically treated teeth, where bulk of dentin to accommodate the pin is limited, where there is no other choice but to place the pin near the dentino-enamel junction and when dentin has lost its elasticity because of sclerosis or dehydration. It is the preferred technique for class IV preparations where the pins need to be bent in the form of U or L, or when crosslinking two parts of the same tooth is required.

Technique

The technique for placement of cemented pins is as follows (The basic instruments required are given in Table 14.3):

The method commonly utilizes pins in the form of stainless steel wires, which are serrated or threaded and cut to the required length. Pinholes extending 2.0–4.0 mm into dentin are prepared using twist drills. If the pin channel is directly accessible and visible and the operator has full control on the manipulation of the pin, the wire can be cut extraorally to the desired length with a wire cutter or a Dial-A-Pin cutter. The length should be such that after seating the pin into the pin channel completely, the pin extends not more

Table 14.3: Basic instruments required for cemented, friction locked and threaded pin techniques		
Cemented pin	*Friction locked pin*	*Threaded pin*
Threaded stainless steel wire	Threaded stainless steel wire	Pins
Twist drill	Twist drill	Twist drill
Machinist's wire cutter or Dial-A-Pin cutter	Machinist's wire cutter or Dial-A-Pin cutter	Hand wrench
		Auto clutch slow speed contra-angle handpiece
Locking tweezers or grooved hemostats	Locking tweezers or grooved hemostats	High speed handpiece and bur
Contouring pliers	Contouring pliers	Contouring pliers
Carborundum disc	Carborundum disc	
Paper points	Anterior and posterior pinsetters	Wire cutter
Zinc phosphate cement or any other luting cement	Mallet/tapper	Carborundum disc
	High low speed handpiece and bur	
Glass slab		
Cement spatula		
Lentulospiral		
Root canal file		
Perioexplorer		

than 2.0-3.0 mm above the base. Dial-A-Pin cutter produces a square smooth end on the pin without deformation where as a wire cutter produces a deformed end which needs to be rounded with a carborundum disc to facilitate insertion to the full depth of the pinhole. The pin is held in the locking tweezers or grooved haemostats and placed in the pinhole for checking its fit and length. If necessary, the pins can be bent with contouring pliers to keep them within the contours of the restoration. When access to the pin channel is difficult and there exists a possibility of losing or mislocating the pin during its try-in, the wire should not be cut completely but a groove made at the desired length. The rest of the wire serves as a handle during the try in and seating of the pin, which can be separated from the pin after cementation by simply bending it. Any roughness on the protruding end of the pin is smoothened using a carborundum disc.

In teeth where more than one pin is to be inserted, each pin is selected and kept aside, until cementation. The pins are so kept that they allow easy identification of the pinholes for which they are intended. For this, the pins are placed on corresponding circles on a map of the prepared tooth. To facilitate location of the pin channel at a later stage, it is advisable to mark the pin channel end as well as the cavity end of the pin with a permanent marker.

The pin channels are dried with precut endodontic paper points. For cementation purposes, zinc-oxyphosphate cement is mixed to a luting consistency on a cool glass slab. Other agents that can be used for cementation are polycarboxylates and light cure glass-ionomer cements. When Zinc phosphate cement is selected, the operator should consider applying a thin layer of copal varnish to the walls of the pin channel with endodontic paper points. The cement mix is introduced into the pin channel with a root canal file or an explorer or a lentulo-spiral running at slow speeds of 1000 rpm or less. The pin held in the forceps is also coated with the cement and inserted into the hole. An amalgam condenser is used to assure full seating of the pin. The pin is held in its position till it sets. The excess cement is flicked off with an explorer point. Any bending of the pin should be done prior to cementation to avoid loosening of the cement joint and introduction of stresses into dentin. All other pins are similarly placed in their channels, one by one.

This technique was later modified using threaded stainless steel pins of the same size as the twist drill. Most commonly used size is the 0.027". The advantages offered by this technique are: close contact between the pin and channel and increased lateral stability. The pin is cut and modified by creating a longitudinal facet with a carborundum disc. This facet serves as a vent and is necessary to allow escape of excess cement especially when the pin and the channel diameters closely match.

Advantages

1. Cemented pins are approximately 0.001"-0.002" (0.025 mm-0.050 mm) smaller than their pinholes and hence are more likely to be seated to the full depth of the hole.
2. Since they are passively retained in the dentin, they virtually place no stress on the surrounding dentin during or after placement.
3. Because the cement seals the interface between the pin and the tooth, chances of microleakage are reduced.
4. These can be cut or bent to their final configuration before fixing them in the pin holes.

Disadvantages

1. They offer less retention compared to the friction locked and threaded pins.
2. It is often difficult to insert cement into the pinhole and later locate the hole after cement has been introduced.
3. At times, a poorly cemented pin is easily dislodged when the filling material is being inserted.
4. Greater time is required for the mixing and hardening of the cement.

b. Friction Locked Pins

With the idea to improve upon the disadvantages of cemented pins, *Goldstein* introduced the friction locked pins. These pins are 0.001" larger than their pin channels and hence utilize the elasticity of dentin for retaining the tapped pins in a vise like grip, e.g. a pin of size 0.022" is inserted into a pin hole of size 0.021". These pins are indicated in teeth that are vital and periodontally sound, and where direct access is possible so that the tapping force can be applied parallel to the long axis of the pin. These pins are indicated only when sufficient amount of dentin is available to surround the pin and in no way should they be placed closer than 1.5 mm to the dentino enamel junction.

Technique

The minimum instruments required for the technique are given in the Table 14.3. A self-centering spiral drill mounted in a low speed handpiece is used to prepare the pin channel in dentin to a depth of 2.0-3.0 mm, 1.5 mm inside the dentino-enamel junction. The channel must be kept dry until the pin is inserted. Friction locked retention pins are smooth surfaced and may be prefabricated from stainless steel wires with a cutting plier or carborundum disc. It is advisable to cut as close as possible to the desired length extraorally itself as the pin cannot be inserted into the pinhole for try-in and adjustment, and also to minimize inducing further stresses in dentin because of cutting. Both ends of the pin are smoothened with a carborundum disc or a abrasive wheel. Roundening off of the trimmed end of the pin facilitates insertion. The depth to which the pin channel has been drilled is marked on the pin with a permanent marker. The pin is inserted into a pin setter and carried to the pinhole. A mallet is used to apply force parallel to the axis of the pin. Only moderate force similar to that used for condensing gold foil is applied to avoid any damage or discomfort. Forces are applied until the established mark on the pin reaches the cavity floor. Additionally, the pin is felt to reach the bottom of the pinhole by sense of touch and sound. Do not use cement under any circumstances. Any excess length is then removed with a small round bur in an air rotor handpiece with adequate air water coolant. If required, the pin is bent at a desirable angle with a contouring plier.

Advantages

1. Cement is not required so one does not have to wait for the cement to set and other related problems.
2. Pins acquire stability from the moment they are inserted.
3. Better retention than the cemented pins.

Disadvantages

1. The length of the pin is judged by trial and error. It cannot be removed from dentin for cutting to the desired length once inserted.
2. Bending or contouring of the pin after it has been inserted into the pinhole leads to further stresses.
3. Driving pins into their respective pinholes generates stresses in dentin in the form of cracks or craze lines.
4. Many a times, the pins do not reach the full depth of the channel because of gouging, and hence may lose some of their retentive capacity.
5. Microleakage is higher than for cemented pins, if the overlying restoration leaks.

c. Threaded Pins

The use of threaded pins was first described by *Going*. In this technique, the pins are 0.0015"-0.002" larger than their pin channels and like the friction locked pins they are also retained by the elasticity of dentin. Additionally, they actively engage the tooth structure through their threads similar to a screw inserted into a wooden block. Currently, threaded pins are most popular amongst the three pin systems. The reasons for their rising popularity are ease and rapidity of insertion, and maximum retention offered. However, the amount of stresses induced in dentin in the form of cracks and craze lines is also maximum with the threaded pins. These pins are indicated in vital teeth and where maximum retention is desired. These pins should be given only when sufficient amount of dentin is available to surround the pin.

Four varieties of threaded pins are available depending on their sizes (in decreasing order of sizes) as:

Regular - 0.030", 0.031"
Minim   - 0.024", 0.025"
Minikin - 0.019", 0.020"
Minuta   - 0.014", 0.015"

The four basic designs of threaded pins are:
- Standard design
- Self shearing single pin design
- Two-in-one design and
- Disposable latch head design

The *standard pin* is a full length pin, i.e. 7.0 mm long which can be cut to the required length after placement. It provides a flattened head for engagement with the hand wrench or the handpiece chuck.

The *self shearing single pin design* is available in varying lengths depending upon the diameters (Fig.14.6). The pin is designed so that when it reaches the bottom of the pinhole, the head separates automatically at the shear line, leaving a portion of it to project from the dentin. Shearing occurs when there

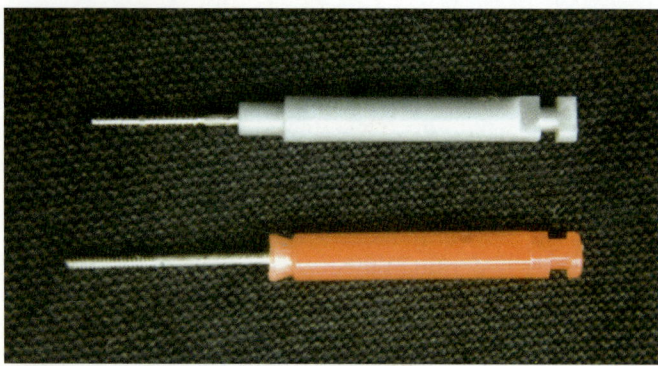

Fig. 14.6: Pins. Two types; Link series (Red), Link plus series (White)

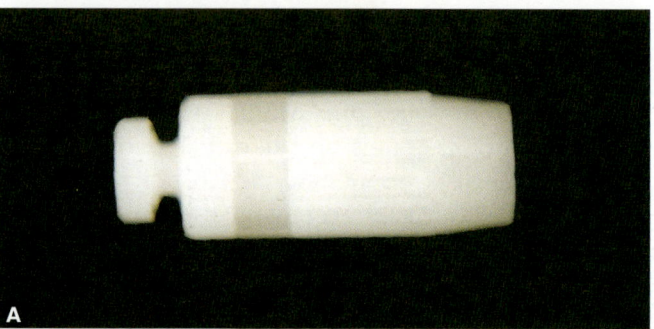

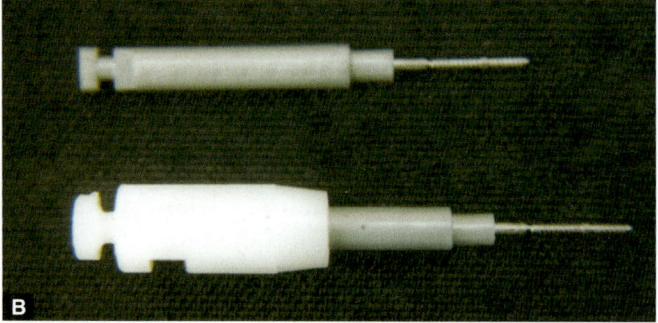

Figs 14.7A and B: (A) Hand wrench; (B) Pin; and pin in the hand wrench

is marked resistance to turning, i.e. pin insertion is torque limited. A flattened head on one end of the pin is shaped to engage the slot in the hand wrench or the handpiece chuck (Figs 14.7A and B) Studies have shown that self shearing pins may not reach the full depth of the pin channel.

The *two-in-one design* is one in which two pins are connected to each other at a joint. This joint serves as a shear line for the peripheral pin. The two-in-one pin is approximately 8.0–9.0 mm in length and provides two pins of equal lengths. It has a flattened head to engage the slot of the hand wrench or the handpiece chuck. Out of the two pins, one which is released first is known as the pin A or the peripheral pin, where as the one which is released second is known as the pin B or the wrench attachment pin. As the name indicates, it is pin B which provides a head for attachment to chuck or wrench. After the first pin has been threaded to the floor of the pin channel, it shears off at the connecting joint leaving behind the second pin alongwith its attachment to be used in another pin channel. A variation in this design is the presence of a shear line a few mm from the tip of the wrench attachment pin, but this shear line is more resistant (less grooved) than the shear line between the two pins to avoid shearing off first at this groove. One major advantage with the two-in-one pin is that the handpiece need not be reloaded during two pin insertions. All of the above three designs may be manufactured with pre-attached wrenches, meant to be disposed off after the pins have been inserted.

The *disposable latch head design* has a plastic sleeve/head designed to fit in a slow speed contrangle handpiece. The pin appears to float freely in the plastic sleeve. This aids in self alignment as the pin is driven into the pinhole. After the pin reaches the bottom of the pinhole, the resistance offered causes the head to separate from the pin at the shear line. The plastic sleeve is then discarded. To facilitate identification of different sizes of pins, the plastic sleeves are color coded. In the commercially available TMS system of pins, this design is known as the '*Link Series*'.

A slight variation to the above design is the incorporation of sharper threads, a shoulder stop and a tapered tip to more readily fit the bottom of the pinhole. This design in the TMS system is known as the '*Link Plus Series*'. It is believed that stresses induced in the surrounding dentin (especially the apical stresses) during pin insertion are greatly reduced because of these modifications.

Examples of threaded pin system are given in Table 14.4.

Technique

The minimum instruments required for the technique are given in the Table 14.3. The technique for threaded pins is easily understood, if one is familiar with the different designs of pins.

Prepare the pin channel in dentin to a depth as required or instructed by the manufacturer depending upon the length of the pin. Pins are inserted either manually or mechanically.

For manual insertion, pins are attached to the hand wrench and threaded slowly into position. Tactile sense is a major factor in determining whether the pin has reached the bottom of the pin channel. For mechanical insertion, pins are engaged in the appropriate handpiece chuck or may have an attached latch head to be inserted into the handpiece. With the handpiece operating at slow speed, the pin is inserted

Complex Restorations

Table 14.4: Examples of threaded pin systems

Source	Pin name	Metal	Size	Pin diameter mm (inches)	Drill diameter mm (inches)	Features
Brasseler USA, Savannah, GA	FO Pins PCR Pins	Titanium Titanium	2 4	0.52 (0.020) 0.70 (0.028)	0.43 (0.017) 0.54 (0.021)	FO for amalgam PCR for composite
Fairflax Dental Inc., Miami, FL	Stabilok	Stainless steel or titanium	Large Small	0.76 (0.030) 0.61 (0.024)	0.69 (0.027) 0.53 (0.021)	Single-shear hand-piece shank
Union Broach Corp., New York, NY	Retention Pins	Stainless steel	Large Medium Small	0.76 (0.030) 0.61 (0.024) 0.51 (0.020)	0.59 (0.027) 0.53 (0.021) 0.43 (0.017)	Single-shear hand-piece shank
Union Broach	Dolphin Retention Pins	Stainless steel		0.76 (0.030) 0.61 (0.024)	0.69 (0.027) 0.53 (0.021)	Single-shear pin attached to finger wrench
Vivadent USA, Amherst, NY	Filpin	Titanium	Large Universal	0.76 (0.030) 0.63 (0.025)	0.69 (0.027) 0.53 (0.021)	Single-shear hand-piece shank
Coltene/Whaledent Inc., New York, NY	Threadmate System (TMS)	Gold-plated, Stainless steel or titanium	Regular Minim Minikin Minuta	0.76 (0.030) 0.635 (0.025) 0.51 (0.020) 0.37 (0.015)	0.69 (0.027) 0.53 (0.021) 0.43 (0.017) 0.34 (0.0135)	Separate wrench; single-shear and double-shear with separate finger wrench
Coltene/Whaledent Inc.	TMS link	Gold-plated stainless steel or titanium	Regular Minim Minikin Minuta	0.76 (0.030) 0.635 (0.025) 0.51 (0.020) 0.37 (0.015)	0.69 (0.027) 0.53 (0.021) 0.43 (0.017) 0.34 (0.0135)	Single-shear and double-shear hand piece shank
Coltene/Whaledent Inc.	TMS link plus	Gold-plated stainless steel or titanium	Regular Minim Minikin Minuta	0.76 (0.030) 0.635 (0.025) 0.51 (0.020) 0.37 (0.015)	0.69 (0.027) 0.53 (0.021) 0.43 (0.017) 0.34 (0.0135)	Single-shear and double-shear hand piece shank plus shoulder stop
Coltene/Whaledent Inc.	Bondent	Stainless steel or titanium		0.48 (0.019)	0.425 (0.017)	Nail head for composite; 2 lengths : 2.0 and 2.5 mm

with light pressure. On reaching the full depth, resistance is increased and the pin shears off at the shear line or disengages from the handpiece drive. If there is no provision for shearing, the pin can be separated from the head with a rotating bur.

After the pin has been placed into dentin, it is checked from all sides for length and angulation. The ideal pin length extending out of dentin should be 2.0 mm while providing space for 1.0 mm of restorative material peripheral to the pin and 2.0 mm occlusal to the pin. Any excess length is removed with a rotating bur or cutting pliers. If required, the pin is bent slightly with a contouring plier. Any sharp ends are smoothened with a round bur or carborundum disc.

Advantages
1. Ease of insertion.
2. Maximum retention is offered.

Disadvantages
1. Excessive stresses in the form of cracks and craze lines are generated in the surrounding enamel and dentin, especially with the large sized pins.
2. Pins may need to be bent, cut or contoured after insertion, which places extra stress on the tooth or may loosen the pin.
3. When the pin is forced into the channel, it may strip the sides of the dentin resulting in a loose fit.
4. Pins may fail to seat completely.
5. Microleakage is higher than the cemented pins if the overlying restoration leaks.

L or T shaped threaded pins – Mattos (1973) introduced these pins to overcome the need for bending pins after their placement. The L or T shaped pins are well suited for class IV preparations as it devoids the need for a second pin at the incisal third.

The transverse portion of the L is allowed to rest in a depression specially prepared in the dentin. These pins have either a square head or a flat extended head for attachment to the hand wrench. The extended head has a shallow groove at its junction with the pin at which it separates once the pin reaches the bottom of the pinhole.

PIN MATERIALS

Materials used for the construction of pins include stainless steel, titanium, silver, cast gold alloys, platinum-palladium, platinum-iridium, plastic, aluminium, acrylic, etc. (Fig. 14.8).

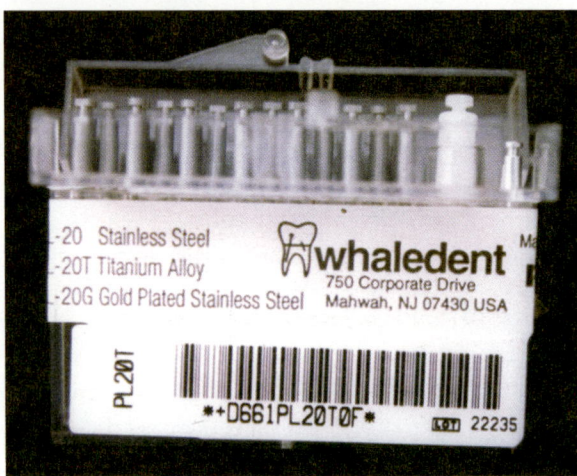

Fig. 14.8: Whaledent pins

Stainless steel, titanium and silver pins are commonly used for the direct/non-parallel pin technique, of which the stainless steel pins are used most frequently. Stainless steel pin is stronger than its gold and titanium counterparts but has the disadvantages of getting corroded and non-adherence to silver amalgam and composite restorative materials. Titanium pins have the advantages of being the least corrosive and most biocompatible of the metals but their strength and modulus of elasticity is less compared to that of stainless steel and high gold content alloys. Titanium pins also do not show any adherence to silver amalgam or composite restorative materials. Silver pins were introduced with the idea of achieving a true adhesive bond between the pin and silver amalgam material so as to render them an integral part of the restoration. An excellent bond does exist between silver pins and silver amalgam as shown by Moffa *et al.* (1972), but solid silver pins are soft and easily deformed.

Pins constructed in cast gold, platinum-palladium or platinum-iridium are used with the indirect/parallel pin technique. These pins are relatively corrosion resistant. Pins in cast gold are formed when impression of the pinholes is taken with nylon/plastic pins that are incorporated into the wax pattern, which is subsequently burnt out and cast in gold. Platinum-palladium or irido-platinum pins are available as prefabricated pins and are cast directly to the overlying gold restoration.

Plastic pins are used in the indirect parallel pin technique but do not serve as a part of the final restoration. They are meant for taking impressions of the pinholes for fabricating a cast gold alloy restoration.

Aluminium pins are used for retaining a temporary restoration until the final restoration is fabricated and inserted.

Acrylic pins have been tried for use with composite resins, but are not very popular. Silver plated and gold plated stainless steel pins have also been tried to achieve a true adhesive bond between steel and silver amalgam. However, these pins did not prove to be very successful. Microscopic observation revealed no difference in the interphase of silver plated pins and amalgam with that of the non-plated pins and amalgam (Moffa et al, 1972). It was speculated that there occurred a complete dissolution of the silver plate in the amalgam matrix resulting in voids and an irregular interphase. Bonding of amalgam to gold plated pins is also difficult to achieve because of the inability to maintain a gold surface free of contaminants especially under oral conditions.

Gold plated pins are usually preferred under composite resins to reduce the 'shine through' of stainless steel pins.

PRINCIPLES OF PIN PLACEMENT

The placement of pins, whether any size and shape, utilizing any technique should follow certain principles for the success of the restoration. The principles are as follows:

1. *Number of pins*: The number of pins that should be given in a tooth are based upon the simple rule of one pin per missing cusp or one pin per missing axial line angle (Figs 14.9 and 14.10). The operator occasionally may need to modify this rule depending upon the amount of tooth structure missing, the amount of retention desired, the amount of dentin available and the size of pins. Increasing the number of pins increases the chances of increased stresses, pulpal damage and/or perforation, hence the aim should be to achieve adequate retention with minimum possible number of pins.

2. *Pin site*: Deciding on the location for a pin requires adequate knowledge about the pulpal anatomy and external contours of the concerned tooth, the

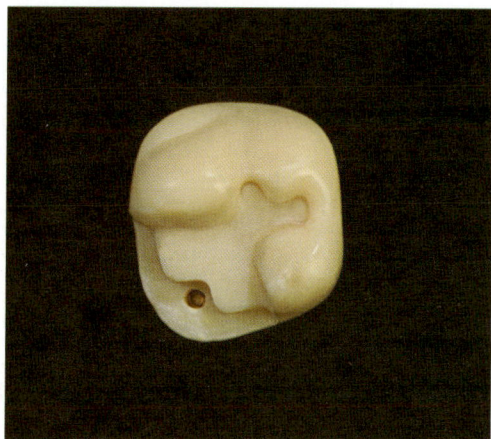

Fig. 14.9: Pin channel preparation

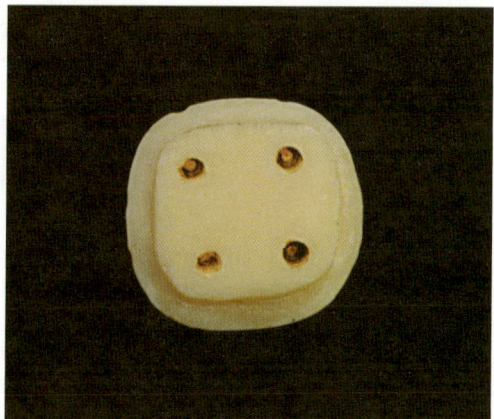

Fig. 14.10: Multiple pin channels prepared

patient's age, a recent radiograph of the tooth, and a periodontal probe. The radiograph though is a two dimensional image of the tooth, it gives an indication of the pulpal anatomy, external contours of the tooth, and the distance between the pulp space and the external outline of tooth on mesial and distal sides. Patient's age is important as young patients have higher pulp horns and this needs to be considered when placing a pin. The operator should be aware of sites safe for the placement of pins. Noting the inclination of a periodontal probe placed along the adjacent external surface of a tooth gives an indication of the presence of any abnormal contours in the tooth outline. The most desirable locations for pinholes are the facio/linguo-proximal line angles (Figs 14.11A to D) or corners of the tooth and the least desirable locations are in the middle of the facial, lingual, mesial and distal surfaces of a tooth. Placing pinholes in locations overlying furcations (i.e. middle of the facial, mesial and distal surfaces for maxillary molars) and concavities (e.g. mesial concavity of a maxillary first premolar) are particularly hazardous. The operator should try and place pins in locations where they will be surrounded by optimum bulk of dentin and restorative material. Based on these considerations, several authors have explained differently the ideal location for pinholes such as:

a. The site should be half way between the pulp and the dentino-enamel junction/external surface of the tooth. The problem with this view is that it is difficult to visualize the outline of the pulp chamber externally, so one has to again depend upon radiographs which do not provide accurate assessment because of their two dimensional nature.
b. There should be atleast 1.0 mm of sound dentin aorund the whole circumference of the pin.
c. Pins should be located no closer than 0.5 mm to the dentino-enamel junction to avoid crazing of enamel.

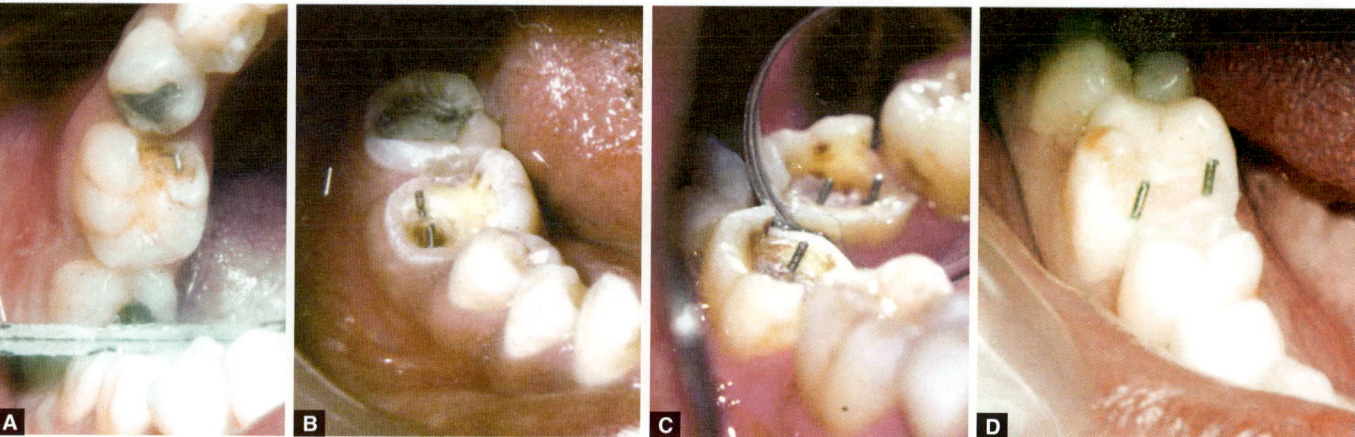

Figs 14.11A to D: (A) Pin placed at the mesiolingual line angle of the tooth; (B) Pins placed at the mesiobuccal and distobuccal line angles of the tooth; (C) Pins placed at the mesiolingual and distolingual line angles of the tooth; (D) Pins placed at the mesiobuccal and mesiolingual line angles of the tooth

d. Dentin thickness around each pin should be at least 2.5 times the diameter of the pinhole.
e. Pin placement should allow at least 1.0 mm of dentinal thickness between the pulp and the pin to prevent any severe inflammatory response.

To best conclude, pinholes should be located such that 1.5-2.0 mm of sound dentin surrounds them along the entire periphery. If at all this is not possible, the clinician should compromise by placing pins more in the pulpal direction because crazing towards the pulp is better tolerated. Placing pins more towards the external surface will produce craze lines in communication with the external environment that could prove to be more harmful because of continuous microleakage and chances for increased fracture of the remaining thin portions of the tooth.

In anticipation of pinhole preparation, if one realizes that pin placement would present the pin being very close to the longitudinal wall of the cavity preparation such that condensation of restorative material between the pin and wall becomes difficult, it is advisable to cut a cove in the adjacent vertical wall. A cove is prepared using appropriate bur which creates space for pinhole preparation as well as allows a clearance of 0.5 mm around the pin for proper condensation of material (Figs 14.9, 14.12, 14.13A to C).

Pin holes should be located on flat surfaces. It is difficult to stabilize a pin drill on an inclined surface and moreover an inclined plane interferes with the shoulder stop of a drill preventing its penetration to full depth. Thin portions of dentin left after drilling are also more susceptible to fracture.

When three or more pins are to be placed in the same tooth, they should preferably be located in different planes/levels to preclude interaction of stresses in the same plane.

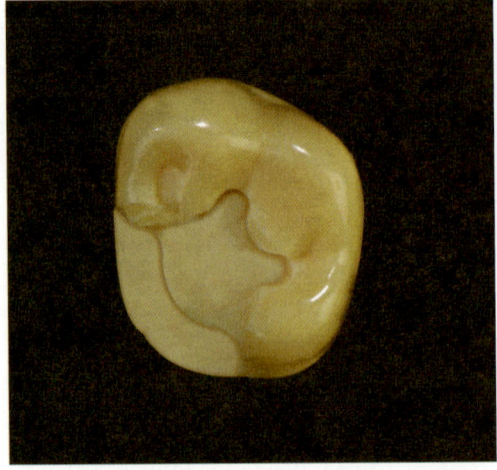

Fig. 14.12: Cavity preparation in which pin placement would present the pin being very close to the longitudinal wall the cavity

3. *Pin orientation*: Pins should be oriented parallel to the long axis of the tooth. However in excessively cervically placed areas towards the cemento-enamel junction where sharp constrictions are likely to be present and dentin thickness is reduced, it is mandatory to direct the pin parallel to the closest external surface of the tooth and then bend it slightly as needed. This would mean compromising on factors like increasing stresses in the tooth but would save the clinician of the trauma of perforation. The best possible way to determine presence of any abnormal contours is to place a probe adjacent to the surface close to the intended location and examine its direction. Radiographs can also be helpful.

4. *Pin diameter*: The selection for the diameter of the pin depends upon (a) the amount of dentin available (b) the size of the concerned tooth and (c) the amount of retention required. Generally, increasing the diameter of the pin offers increased retention, but large sized pins are also associated

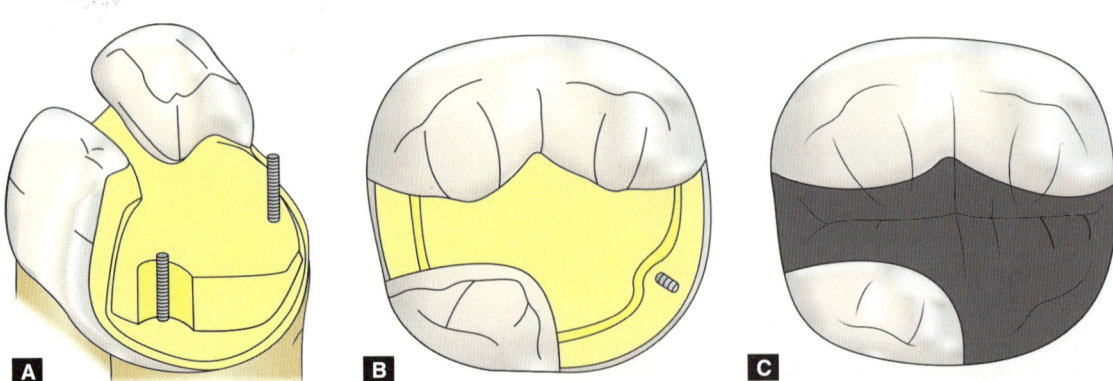

Figs 14.13A to C: (A) When pin placement would be close to the longitudinal wall of the cavity, a cove is prepared in the adjacent vertical wall to create space for pin placement (proximo-occlusal view); (B) Mesioocclusodistal cavity in mandibular second molar with one pin replacing the disto-lingual cusp (occlusal view); (C) Completed pin-retained restoration

with a heavy concentration of stresses in dentin. Preferably, the depth should be more than the diameter.

5. *Pin length*: The optimum ratio of pin length in dentin to pin length in restorative material varies with the different types of pins, i.e. for cemented pins it is 3.0 mm and 2.0 mm; for friction locked pins it is 3.0 mm and 3.0 mm; and for threaded pins it is 2.0 mm and 2.0 mm respectively. Preferably the length of the pin inside the dentin and the length of the pin in restorative material should be equal. These optimum lengths may not be achievable under all circumstances, and minor adjustments should be acceptable.

6. *Interpin distance*: When greater than two pins are to be placed in the same tooth, interpin distance should be considered to allow space for insertion of restorative material between the pins and prevent excessive concentration of residual stresses in dentin. The optimum interpin distance depends upon the type and size of pins. The minimal interpin distance is 2.0 mm for cemented pins, 4.0 mm for friction locked pins, 3.0 mm for Minikin threaded pins and 5.0 mm for Minim threaded pins. The accepted principle is to have 2.0 mm of dentin around each pin.

PINHOLE PREPARATION

Pinholes are prepared using a device called *'twist drill'* (Fig.14.14). This is an end cutting instrument that performs cutting when rotated clockwise at low speeds. The drill has two blades which revolve at precisely equidistant points from the centre, and is helix fluted to allow escape of the cutting debris. Twist drills may be either made in one piece or two piece. One piece twist drill is made of steel, is less expensive and more likely to fracture. Two piece drill is made of steel that is swaged onto an aluminium shank, is more expensive, stronger and less likely to fracture. Carbide is not used for construction of twist drills as it is brittle. The recommended speed for drilling channels is 300–500 rpm (ultralow speed) or 1000 rpm (low speed). Very little heat is generated at these speeds and hence water or air cooling is not required.

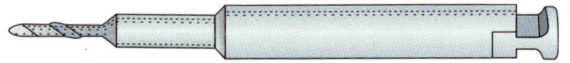

Fig. 14.14: Common type of twist drill for making pin holes

There are four basic designs of twist drills (a) *Regular twist drills* which have their cutting parts 4.0 mm or more in length without a limiting shoulder/stop. (b) *Limited depth twist drills* which have a stop or shoulder to limit the depth of cutting. These stops are either prefixed or adjustable. When fixed, they are generally located at 2.0 mm lengths from the cutting end of the drill. (c) *Miniature twist drills* which are regular or limited depth type but their overall length is shorter (17.0 mm) and (d) *Twist drills with parallelometer attachment*. These again are regular or limited depth type drills designed to function with paralleling instruments. They have narrowed shanks that pendulate freely in the bur sleeve of the handpiece and a sleeve to fit in the parallelometer. Their use becomes necessary when parallel pins are required under cast restorations.

For easy identification of diameters, the manufacturer may also color the shank of twist drill differently. Occasionally in areas of difficult access, the neck thickness may interfere with drill penetration. To overcome this hindrance, the neck is ground back with an abrasive wheel and the diameter checked with a micrometer. For two piece drills, the dimensions of the reduced neck should be a minimum of 0.004" larger than the diameter of the drill to retain the drill to the neck. The necks of one piece drills can however be trimmed to sizes similar to or even less than the diameter of the drill. This process is referred to as the *'slimming of a drill'*. When necks are trimmed 0.003"-0.004" smaller than the drill diameter, a reverse taper is said to have been given. Reverse taper aids in removal of the cutting debris, reduces lateral friction and consequently heat generation, and also reduces the chances of jamming within the channel.

The proposed pinhole locations are marked with a marker before the pin channels are prepared with the twist drill. A No.1/4 round bur at low speed is dipped to about half the diameter at these marks to create starting points known as *lead holes* or *pilot holes*. The purpose of these holes is to permit more accurate positioning of the twist drill and to prevent its skidding out laterally into unfavourable locations. For making lead holes in metal alloys, a No. ½ round carbide bur should be used at high speeds under sufficient air water coolant. Pinholes should be located only in areas that provide adequate access to the site. Any difficulty in proper access increases the incidence of associated complications like pin or drill breakage, perforation, pulp exposure, etc.

The pin channels are cut with drills held in 10 to 1 gear reduction handpiece running at speeds of 300-1000 rpm. Conventional slow speed contrangle handpieces have also been recommended. Slight pressure is applied in an apical direction when the drill starts cutting into dentin until it penetrates to its marked length or the shoulder stop is reached. The drill should be dipped only once in dentin and quickly removed allowing only a very brief period of rotation at the bottom of the pinhole. It should be rotating when it enters and leaves the dentin and at no time stopping in between. The following points need to be kept in mind when drilling a pin channel:

- Repeated insertion and removal of a drill in the same channel can result in enlarged channels and/or conical or eccentric shapes of the channel.
- Lateral stresses applied while drilling can induce additional stresses in dentin and increase the chances of drill breakage.
- Rotating pin drills for longer period after they have reached the bottom of the pin channel can result in large sized holes.
- Stopping the pin drill during the drilling procedure increases the chances of drill breakage.

After the pin channels have been completed, radiographs taken, their depths are read and confirmed with depth gauges that read in millimeters. The pins are inserted following the techniques described earlier for cemented, friction locked and threaded pins.

PIN BENDING AND PIN TRIMMING

Following pin insertion, conditions may necessitate bending or trimming of pins. Ideally, the maximum amount of bending and trimming should be performed prior to placement of pins but often this is not possible in friction locked and threaded pins. Cemented pins on the contrary can be contoured and bent to the desired angulation prior to being cemented.

After having inserted the pins, evaluate the length and position of the exposed pin from all aspects especially the occlusal aspect. This gives an indication of whether the free ends of the pin need to be included within the contours of the restoration or if the length of the pin needs to be adjusted. Preferably, at least 1.5 mm of the pin should be exposed, at least 1.0 mm of the space for restorative material around the periphery of the pin and at least 2.0 mm of space occlusal to the pin should be available. Pins should not be bent with the aim of increasing retention. Often bending is required to facilitate condensation of restorative material in an occluso-gingival direction.

Proper bending tools or contouring pliers should be used to bend the pin smoothly at a distance from the pin dentin interface. Use of hand instruments or spoon excavators are contraindicated as they are more likely to produce a sharp bend at the pin dentin interface and increase the chances of fracture. Bending a pin after it has been seated may cause stress development and fracture of the dentin or the pin.

If the operator decides to trim the pin, it should be cut short with a sharp fissure bur running in a high speed handpiece. Adequate coolants should be used to prevent heat generation and proper measures taken to retrieve the sheared fragment. The bur is oriented perpendicular to the pin and to the left. If placed on the right side, the clockwise rotation of the high speed handpiece may unseat the pin by moving it counterclockwise. At times, the access necessitates holding the bur parallel to the long axis of the pin. In such circumstances, a small inverted cone bur or wheel shaped bur can be used in a slow speed handpiece that rotates in a reverse/anticlockwise manner. To avoid the pin from getting loosened in its channel, stabilize the pin with a haemostat or plier while lateral pressure is applied, and if possible use light intermittent high speed cutting only.

PIN REMOVAL

Occasionally, replacement of a pin retained restoration may necessitate removal of pins. Reusing the same pin around which the restorative material has been removed is associated with the danger that in function or in restoration removal, the pin may have been loosened. Moreover, it is difficult to place pins at new sites because of the limited availability of dentin and the chances of pulpal exposure and external tooth perforation. Removing pins is advantageous, as the same pin sites could then be reused without much loss of tooth tissue. Several methods have been advocated for pin removal.

- Pin can be grasped directly with an artery forceps and unwound. The procedure is however possible only when sufficient length of the pin is available for engagement by the ends of the forceps, and access allows forceps to be held in line with the pin. Difficult access prevents proper alignment of the forceps and hence large leverage on the pin. An alternative approach is to bond a tube to the pin with a cyano-acrylate adhesive, which may facilitate unscrewing the pins with forceps especially for those pins, which are short in length. Both these methods can be used only for removing threaded pins.
- A pin can be removed with a rotating bur that produces anticlockwise rotation in the pin. The latter is possible when a bur rotating at high speeds is placed perpendicular to the pin and to its right or parallel to the pin. Only a fleeting contact should be made between the pin and the bur with the aim of unscrewing it rather than cutting it. The hazards include cutting the pin if excessive pressure is applied or cutting of tooth substance lateral to the pin. This method also can be used only for removing threaded pins.
- A pin can be removed with ultrasonic tip also. The vibrating tip is held in contact with the pin and

rotated anticlockwise in an unscrewing motion. It is believed that the torque applied by the mechanical vibration of the ultrasonic tip in contact with the pin is responsible for its unscrewing. The lateral contact between the tip and the pin may be ineffective in removing pins as oscillations of the sonic tip in the lateral direction are easily stopped. The prescribed method is used for removal of threaded pins. Ultrasonics can also be used for removal of cemented pins. Under ultrasonic vibrations, the cement is broken down and the dislodged pin easily removed. Frequently, pins may be fractured at the level of dentin. Removal of such pins is quite difficult though not impossible. The first two methods cannot be employed, as the procedures require some amount of exposed pin for pin removal. Ultrasonics may be used with some degree of success.

CLASS II PIN RETAINED RESTORATIONS

Pins are indicated in class II cavities when the cavity is shallow and wide with little or no axial wall height remaining, when one or more cusps of posterior teeth are missing, when the tooth presents a flat occlusal surface or when to retain foundation for a future cast restoration.

Cavity Design and Pin Placement

Prepare the initial cavity following basic principles of cavity preparation. Cusps that have been severely weakened should be reduced to restore the resistance form of the tooth. Maximum retention should be gained with primary retentive features like opposing walls, boxes and dovetails (Figs 14.13A and B). After the initial cavity has been prepared, any remaining infected dentin is removed. A radiograph of the concerned tooth is taken to aid in determining the pulpal anatomy and external contours of the tooth. The angulation of a probe positioned alongside the external surface gives an indication of the presence of any abnormal contours. Pin channel locations are selected and marked following the principles of pin placements. Pinholes are drilled and pins inserted as described earlier.

Following the establishment of secondary retentive features, finishing of the cavity is done. The cavosurface margins are refined to 90° for silver amalgam restorations. The preparation is debrided and cavity varnish is applied. If required, a cavity liner/base is also given. When adequate tooth structure is present for retaining a band, the tofflemire retainer and band can be used successfully. However, if quite a lot of tooth structure has been lost, the compound supported copper matrix band is the best choice. An alternative is the use of automatrix. It is emphasized here that whatever be the matrix system used, it should be anatomically correct and perfectly stable. A poorly stabilized matrix results in a weak restoration.

A spherical or admixed high copper amalgam is preferred because of its high early compressive strength, good adaptation to the pins and adequate clinical performance. The amalgam alloy is triturated according to the manufacturer's instructions and inserted into the preparation using amalgam carrier. It is condensed thoroughly around the pins with 0.5–1.0 mm diameter round pluggers or small parallelogram shaped condensers. A large amalgam plugger can then be substituted only after the pins have been covered. Condensing amalgam well around the pins is quite time consuming but if done properly will definitely reduce the incorporation of voids into the final restoration. The preparation is slightly overfilled.

After the occlusal contours are partially carved, the matrix is removed. For this, the wedges are allowed to remain in place as they maintain a passive pressure on the band from the adjacent tooth. If a retainer has been used, it is separated from the matrix. The matrix band is opened out and pulled occlusally enough to snip the edge with crown scissors over each contact point. With pliers or hemostats, the band is gripped on either side of the scissor, cut and pulled apart for removal without damage to the proximal region of the amalgam. An another method for matrix removal is to loosen the matrix band around the tooth and move it obliquely towards the occlusal surface. The band should be removed in the direction of wedge placement to avoid dislodging it. The wedges are now removed and any interproximal excess amalgam sheared away with an explorer. Facial and lingual contours are established. The occlusal anatomy is also completed while checking for opposing occlusal contacts. The final restoration is checked for any discrepancies, finished and polished. Stepwise procedure for a pin retained amalgam restoration is shown in Figs 14.15A to E. Similarly pins can be given in composite restorations (Figs 14.16A to C).

CLASS III AND CLASS IV PIN RETAINED RESTORATIONS

With the introduction of improved esthetic restorative materials and better bonding mechanisms, pins in class III and class IV tooth colored restorations for improving retention have almost become obsolete. However, they may be indicated in certain situations like:

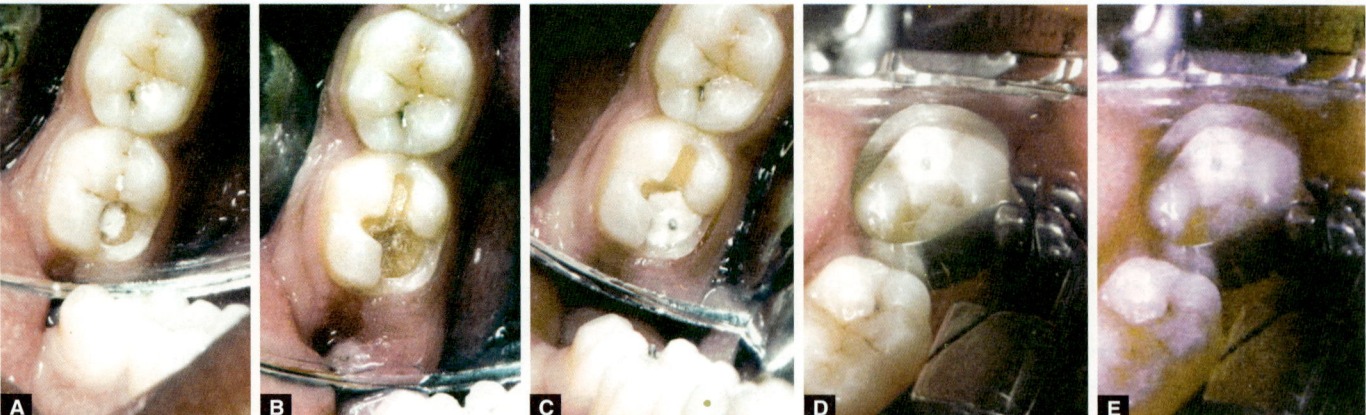

Figs 14.15A to E: (A) Distolingual cusp of mandibular right second molar is lost; **(B)** Cavity preparation on mandibular right second molar; **(C)** GIC base applied and pin inserted on the distolingual line angle of the tooth; **(D)** Tofflemire retainer and band applied; **(E)** Final restoration finished and polished

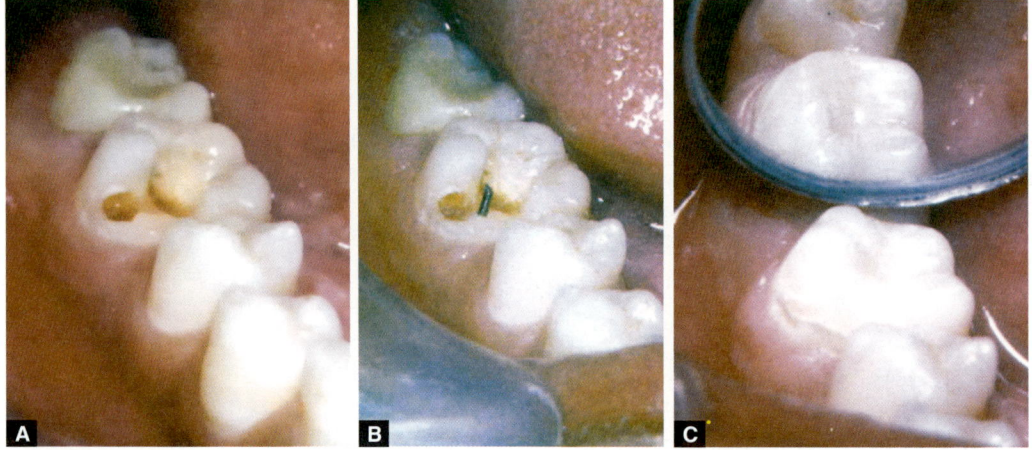

Figs 14.16A to C: (A) Carious lesion with mesiobuccal cusp lost on mandibular right first molar; **(B)** Cavity preparation with pin placed at mesio-buccal line angle; **(C)** Completed pin-retained composite restoration

- When adequate retention like grooves or boxes that will suit to the restoration size, cannot be offered without endangering the health of the pulp.
- If the final cavity is large and involves two thirds or more of the clinical crown length, or the incisal, labial and lingual walls are completely missing.
- When there is little or no remaining enamel on the tooth, e.g. in some structural disorders like enamel hypoplasia, or the restoration is to be subjected to forces in centric and excursive movements.
- When the restoration is to serve as a foundation or long term provisional restoration. Resin is contraindicated in these situations as the retaining enamel will be lost during tooth preparation for the final restoration.

Cavity Design and Pin Placement

Establish the gingival floor as pronounced as possible. The labial and lingual walls are created even if they have to be as little as 1mm long. At times this would mean extending the gingival floor apically and axial wall axially to produce these walls. In class III cavities, only one pin on the gingival floor will suffice. In class IV cavities, one pin site is located on the gingival floor and the second pin site is located on the incisal angle. Pin locations are selected so as to allow the two pins to form an approximate 90° angle near the incisal angle to be restored. Pins should be positioned entirely in dentin. Any contact of the pin with the enamel could result in cracking or fracture of the enamel and show the pin through the resin as a dark shadow. In unilateral class IV preparations, L shaped pins can also be used. The long arm of the 'L' is inserted into the pin channel prepared on the gingival floor where as the short arm fits incisally into a step or depression. In bilateral class IV preparations, U shaped pins are the most efficient. The two ends of the U pin are located gingivally. In both L shaped and U shaped cemented pin techniques, one should take care that adequate space is present between the vertical and horizontal arms of the material. The L and U shaped pins should be bent very gradually without inducing sharp corners so as to improve adaptability of the restorative material to the pin in these regions and avoid any possible fracture or stress accumulation.

Pin locations are marked and pilot holes made at the marked sites with a no. ¼ round bur. A pin drill of smaller size preferably 0.021″ is selected. Drill pinholes to depths of 2.0 mm using a labial or lingual approach depending upon the angulation or rotation of the tooth in the arch. When two pins have to be inserted, a two-in-one self threading pin is preferred. The peripheral pin is adjusted to the desired length and inserted in the incisal pinhole. The wrench attachment pin is released on the gingival floor. The pins are bent to proper alignment and the preselected restorative material inserted.

CLASS V PIN RETAINED AMALGAM

Pins are rarely used in class V cavity preparations but may be employed when cavities are large with little/no remaining mesial and distal walls, or when gingival floor cannot be established and also, when adequate retention suited to the restoration size cannot be offered without endangering the health of the pulp.

Cavity Design and Pin Placement

The cavity is prepared following the basic principles for routine class V amalgam restorations. It is emphasized that pin placement does not forbid the need for extension for prevention, adequate depth, sound mechanical retention, resistance features, convenience form, etc. After the basic cavity has been completed, the locations for pin channels are selected and marked. The ideal location for the pinholes is in the floor of the preparation, approximately 1.0-1.5 mm inside the lateral margins. Two pin channels directed mesially and distally provide adequate retention. Mesial and distal walls should be extended to proximal line angles in order to permit pin placement at the maximum distance from the pulp. If the cavity is large and additional retention is required, four pin channels can be prepared effectively (Fig. 14.10). A slight undercut in inciso/occluso axial and gingivo axial line angles will augment in the retention.

Pilot holes are prepared at the marked sites with a No. ¼ round bur. Since the thickness of dentin between the pulp and enamel at the cervical line is less, a small diameter pin is preferred. With a depth limiting twist drill of 0.021″ in a slow speed handpiece, drill pinholes to a depth of 2.0 mm. The drill is slanted about 5 to 10 degrees in the horizontal axis to preclude any possibility of pulp exposure and is directed parallel to the external surface of the tooth. However, care should be taken that the bottom of the pinhole does not touch the dentin side of the enamel. The pin drill is kept rotating as it enters or leaves the dentin, nowhere stopping in between. Clean the pin channels and coat with cavity varnish using endodontic paper points.

A 4.0 mm pin is generally too long and will protrude through the surface of the restoration. The pin extending approximately 1.0 mm above the floor of the preparation is considered adequate. Pins may be trimmed before or after penetration. A single or twoin-one self shearing pin is placed in the proper hand wrench or the chuck of the handpiece and carried to the pinhole. Light pressure is applied. The pin screws into dentin and shears off automatically at the shear line. Bending, if required, is done with a bending tool.

A rubber dam is applied, and one shortened matrix strip is secured on each proximal surface with a wedge and compound, if required, to facilitate condensation of amalgam. A base is placed when necessary and the rest of the cavity coated with cavity varnish. Silver amalgam alloy is mixed and inserted. Amalgam is then condensed around the pins and the cavity is filled. Careful hand condensation ensures proper adaptation of the alloy to the pin. The surface is contoured, finished and polished.

PIN AMALGAM FOUNDATION (PAF)

It is defined as a silver amalgam restoration using pin retention that is to be reduced to provide a core for subsequent cast restoration. Apart from silver amalgam, foundations can also be made of composite resins, glass cermets, compomers, etc.

Pin amalgam foundation differs from pin amalgam restoration in several aspects. The following discussion focuses on the differences while the similarities are not elaborated.

The principles of outline form dictate more conservative preparations for a pin amalgam foundation than for a pin amalgam restoration. All carious tooth structure and prior restoration is removed similar to a pin amalgam restoration. The margins need not be extended to self cleansing areas or to include susceptible pits, fissures or decalcified regions unless they are carious. Breaking contact is also not necessary. Weak or fragile enamel that is likely to fracture during matrix application, amalgam condensation or crown preparation shall be removed. However, if the undermined enamel appears strong enough to resist condensation forces and will not be extensively reduced during the final preparation, it is advantageous to retain that portion as it will ease matrix application and provide additional retention for the amalgam foundation.

The principles of convenience form remain the same, i.e. to provide adequate access to the preparation for placement of retentive pins, matrix band application and adequate condensation of amalgam. A cavosurface angle of 90° is recommended for a pin amalgam restoration to provide strength to enamel as well as amalgam. However, for a pin amalgam foundation, cavosurface angles can range from 45°–135° as they are not subjected to direct occlusal forces.

For placement of pins, the selection of areas is generally the same. Additionally, one needs to consider the extent of retention that will be lost after axial preparation, which will dictate the number and location of pins in the final preparation. The pins should be placed such that they accommodate the axial reduction as well as provide 0.5-1.0 mm of restorative material on the periphery of the pin. If restorative material equivalent to more than half the diameter of the pin is removed, the retentive effect provided by the pin is completely lost. Pins placed at the line angles of the tooth should be placed more towards the proximal surface. If the proximal surface presents a concavity, the pin is directed gingivo facially or gingivo lingually while paralleling the adjacent external surface. This allows not only for the occlusal reduction but also protects against perforation of the external concave surface. The pin length should be such that it allows 1.5-2.0 mm of occlusal reduction and some material covering the occlusal end of the pin. The extension of the pin close to or through the occlusal surface of the reduced foundation is however not very critical as the final cast restoration will distribute the occlusal load over the entire preparation. Minikin size of the pins should be used for the purpose of foundations as their smaller size fulfills most of the requirements.

The matrix band is applied and the amalgam condensed. A fast setting high copper alloy is the choice as it allows the foundation to be prepared at the same visit. Most single composition spherical alloys exhibit enough strength after 30 minutes of condensation to initiate crown preparation. High copper admixed alloys require longer setting times of about one hour before the preparation can begin. For slower setting alloys, preparation of the foundation should be delayed until the next appointment.

Carving and finishing of the amalgam foundation depends upon when the preparation is to be initiated.

a. If the foundation is to be reduced at the same appointment, most of the axial and occlusal reduction can be accomplished while carving the amalgam itself.

b. If the reduction is to be done at a subsequent appointment of less than 7 days, occlusal contacts need to be maintained to prevent supra eruption of teeth. Axial reduction can however be accomplished while carving amalgam.

c. If the foundation is expected to serve as an interim restoration for one week or greater, both axial contours and occlusal contacts should be ascer-tained similar to as in a pin amalgam restoration, for preserving tooth position and health of the periodontal and surrounding tissues. The final restoration is finished and polished.

When the operator is doubtful regarding the tooth's endodontic status, or if the periodontal treatment is to be completed, or because of financial limitations of the patient, a foundation could be needed to serve for periods longer than 6 months. It is, however, mandatory to maintain the restoration in a functioning state during this period.

Tooth colored restorative materials are preferred for foundations, when a matrix cannot be adapted properly in the gingival aspect of the tooth such as the furcation areas. Adequate isolation is however must when using these materials. The foundations should be of a shade or color that allows distinct differentiation from the natural tooth structure. This aids in reduction and prevents margin from being located on the foundation material. Amongst the direct restorative materials, amalgam is preferred because it is stronger and shows less microleakage. Cast post and cores, which serve as foundations are limited to root canal treated teeth with little or no remaining coronal tooth structure.

PINS, STRESSES AND TOOTH

Stresses are almost always associated with insertion of friction locked and threaded pins in dentin. It is quite obvious that stresses will be generated as pins are inserted into channels 0.001"-0.004" smaller than the diameter of the pins. Insertion of larger pins into smaller pin channels is possible because of the elastic properties of dentin. Once the elastic limit of dentin is exceeded, plastic deformation occurs. If the stresses sum up to a point where the dentin's plastic limit is exceeded, microscopic and/or macroscopic craze lines or cracks are generated. These fracture lines can lead to involvement of pulp or periodontium, cracked tooth syndrome, gross fractures, loose restorations, etc.

Cemented pins are known to induce the least stresses, threaded pins induce intermediate stresses and friction locked pins induce the maximum stresses. Friction-locked pins act as wedges and lateral stresses are the main type of stresses present around them, compared to threaded pins which are associated mainly with apical stresses. Impact forces introduced during insertion of friction locked pins are probably responsible for greatly magnifying the residual stresses in dentin. With the threaded pins some of the induced stresses are reduced by cutting and eliminating stressed dentin. Factors which *increase* the residual stresses in dentin are discussed below:

1. Pin morphology
   - Large diameter of the pin
   - Large difference between the pin and pin channel diameter especially in friction locked and threaded pins
   - Blunt threads
   - Narrow pitched threads, i.e. greater number of threads per unit distance
   - Excessively long threads extending outward from the core of the pin
   - Irregularities at pin ends induced during manufacturing or during adjustment
   - Inserting a flat ended pin into a chisel ended channel
   - Inserting pins into channels not prepared with matching drills
2. Placing pins close to each other causes interaction of the field of stresses of individual pins. This interaction is maximum when the interpin spacing is less than 2.0 mm.
3. Increasing the number of pins per tooth increases stresses.
4. Ratio of embedded pin and exposed pin length if not 1:1 induces harmful stresses.
5. Mismatch between the pin and pin channel circumference increases stresses by concentrating stresses at points of contact rather than being distributed evenly around the channel. This mismatch may be due to manufacturing defect, repeated insertion and removal of drill resulting in conical channels, because of drills with increased run out producing eccentric shaped channels.
6. A pin which is loose in its channel induces stresses on dentin when the overlying restoration is stressed. The magnitude of stress induced depends upon the amount and degree of pin movement in the channel.
7. An attempt to drive the pin further into its channel even after it has contacted the bottom, increases stresses.
8. Bending or shortening pins after they have been fully engaged in dentin can induce excessive stresses.
9. Incidence of cracks in enamel is higher with the friction locked and threaded pins and very negligible with the cemented pins. Friction locked pins are the most dangerous when placed at less than 1.0 mm from dentino-enamel junction. Threaded pins are relatively less damaging if placed 0.5 mm away from the dentino-enamel junction. The least damaging are cemented pins, which have not shown to induce stresses even when placed at dentino-enamel junction.
10. Cutting channels with drills that are dull, vibrating and with laterally applied forces, increase the stresses in dentin. Abnormal stress patterns are also induced.
11. Lesser the bulk of dentin surrounding the pin, greater are the stresses per unit volume of dentin. Regular primary dentin of young teeth because of its high elastic and plastic limits is least affected by the stresses produced during pin insertion. The ability of stress tolerance of different types of dentin in a decreasing order is: secondary dentin, sclerosed dentin, tertiary dentin and calcific barrier. Cemented pins are, therefore, the only preferred pins in endodontically treated teeth with non vital dentin.
12. Inserting pins in stress concentration areas like axial angles can complicate pre-existing stress patterns. Residual stress in dentin can be reduced if the above mentioned factors are prevented. Another method proposed for decreasing stresses around threaded pins is unthreading them by one fourth to one half turn after they have been fully seated to position. Unthreading does not adversely affect the retention values of pins in dentin.

PINS, STRESSES AND RESTORATIVE MATERIAL

Originally, when pins were introduced into dentistry, they were believed to reinforce amalgam in the same way as steel rods reinforced concrete. Subsequent studies, however showed that pins did not strengthen or reinforce a restoration but assisted in the retention forms only. Neither compressive strength nor transverse/tensile strength of amalgam was improved because of possibly stress concentrations around the pins and cleavage planes set up in the material by the arrangement of pins. It is indicated that stress concentration is more likely to be produced by pins as they are more rigid than amalgam.

Pins are likely to reduce the strength of amalgam and composite restorations because of the absence of any chemical union between the pin and restorative material at the interface. Voids and irregularities are present at the interface, or the pin in toto is believed to serve as a void in restorative material and hence act as a stress initiator. Fractures in the pin amalgam restorations are, therefore, commonly seen in planes involving pins. The adaptability of composite resins around the pins compared to silver amalgam is not very good. This may explain the higher number of failures associated with pin retained composite restorations.

Several attempts have been made to achieve a closely adapted interphase between the pin and restorative material by silver plating or gold plating stainless steel pins or using pins made of silver. As described earlier, these pins have not been proved to be very successful.

The formation of corrosion products at the interphase of pin and restorative material, either because of presence of two dissimilar metals or because of corrosion properties of the pin itself, reduces the fracture strength of pin retained restorations. The corrosion process requires the presence of an electrolyte like saliva or dentinal fluid for the corrosion to occur. The corrosion products act as stress concentration areas and their accumulation should therefore be prevented by all possible means. Reducing microleakage by varnish application is one method. Titanium pins are getting popular because they are corrosion resistant.

Factors relating to pins that *decrease* the compressive and tensile strength of a restoration are:

1. Pin ends in restoration may be wedge-shaped or irregular in shape, serving as areas of stress concentration.
2. Pins are close to or protrude through the outer surface of the restoration. This decreases the bulk of material between pin end and restoration surface, thereby not providing adequate strength to the material required for resisting mechanical loading, e.g. silver amalgam is weak if it is not present in thickness of 1.5-2.0 mm.
3. Pins are closer than 2.0 mm to each other. This increases the possibility of incorporation of voids because of the inability to properly insert and condense material between the pins and insufficient bulk of material is present around the pins.
4. An additional factor associated only with the tensile strength of restorative material is the relative direction of tensile stresses in relation to the direction of the pin. A 30–40% reduction in tensile strength of the restorative material is seen when the pins are at right angles to the direction of the tensile stresses during function. A 10% reduction is seen when the pins are at 45° to the direction of tensile stresses and no reduction in strength is seen when the pins are in line with the tensile stresses.

FACTORS AFFECTING RETENTION OF PINS IN TOOTH STRUCTURE

Several factors are known to control the retention of pins in tooth structure. These include:

a. *Pin type*: Among the three systems of pins, cemented pins are the least retentive. Friction locked pins show intermediate retention and threaded pins are the most retentive. Cemented pins are placed in channels which are 0.001 inch oversized than the pins, friction locked pins in channels which are 0.001 inch undersized than the pins, and threaded pins in channels which are 0.002-0.004 inches undersized than the pins. Friction locked and threaded pins are retained by the elasticity of dentin and this accounts for their higher retention. An oversized pin inserted into an excessively undersized channel however results in loss of retention. It was observed that when a 0.027" pin was seated in a channel, 0.021" in size, there was much crazing and crushing of the surrounding dentin, which actually decreased the ability to retain the pin. Enlarging the channel size from 0.021" to 0.026" for the same 0.027" pin decreased the amount of damage inflicted to the surrounding dentin but increased the retention by 250 percent. The difference between the pin and channel should therefore be limited to no more than 0.0043". Within the cemented pin technique, serrated or threaded pins offer more retention than smooth surface pins.

b. *Pin depth in dentin*: Increasing the depth of pin in dentin increases the retention values. The relationship is linear for the cemented pins, but non linear for the friction locked and threaded pins i.e. for these pins increase in retention is minimal at depths exceeding 2.0 mm. It is demonstrated that at depths greater than 2.0 mm, attempts to remove a smaller self threading pin (0.024") fractured the pin, where as a larger self threading pin (0.031") fractured the dentin. Similarly, for the friction locked pins, there is little danger of pin or dentin fracture as long as the depth is limited to 3.0 mm in dentin.

For attaining equal retention with the three types of pins, cemented pins should be 5.0-6.0 mm deep, friction locked pins 2.0-3.0 mm deep, and threaded pins only 1.0 mm deep.

c. *Pin diameter*: Within limits, as the diameter of the pin increases, the retention increases. It has been seen that the retention values almost double when the diameter of the pin increases from 0.0155" to 0.0190" and triples when the diameter of the pin increases from 0.0155" to 0.0230". However, the practical limitation of having appropriate amount of dentin around pin would warrant use of smaller diameter pins.

d. *Pin number*: Within limits, increasing the number of pins increases the retention in dentin. However, one should also take care of the potential problems associated with the increase in number of pins like increase in crazing of dentin and increased potential for fracture. At interpin distances of less than 2 mm, there is interaction of stresses in dentin resulting in loss of retention.

e. *Cementing agents:* The most commonly used agent for cementation of cemented pins is the zinc phosphate cement. It has been found to be more retentive than polycarboxylate and zincoxide eugenol cements. Glass ionomer cements may also prove to be more retentive.

Zinc phsophate cement is a potential pulpal irritant. To reduce the penetration of the constituents of the cement as well as to minimize leakage potential around the pins, varnish may be applied prior to placing the cement. However, varnish reduces the retentive ability of the cemented pins by almost 46 percent. This decrease in retention should be compensated by other measures like increasing the length, diameter or number of pins. Cavity varnish applied for the purpose of reducing leakage on the other hand has no significant effect on the retention of friction locked and threaded pins. When used with cavity varnish, threaded pins are eight times more retentive than the cemented pins.

f. *Association between pin channel and pin circumference:* Poor quality control in the manufacture of pins can induce discrepancies like mismatch between the pin and drill diameters, variations in the inside diameter and thread shapes of the pins, etc.

The pin channel circumference should closely match the pin circumference. A pin with circular cross section will show less retention when placed in elliptical pin channels. Similarly, a difference in the morphology between the pin shape and the conical shape of the channel results in incomplete thread engagement. Repeated insertion and removal of drill at slow speed produces conical channels. Eccentric shaped channels are produced when using drills with increased run out or when plunged into dentin more than once.

g. *Miscellaneous*: Young resilient primary dentin offers more retention than secondary dentin. Hypermineralization and dehydration greatly decrease the retaining potential because of the loss in elasticity of dentin.

Shortening the pins after they have been inserted into dentin affects retention. Cutting the excess pin with a plier is less disturbing than when cutting with a bur.

The type of contra-angle handpiece used for inserting pins, i.e. conventional slow speed or 10 is to 1 gear reduction has not shown to influence the retentive properties.

FACTORS AFFECTING RETENTION OF PINS IN RESTORATIVE MATERIAL

The following factors affect the retention of pins in restorative material:

a. *Pin length*: Within limits, increasing the length of the pin in restorative material increases retention. The relationship is linear for friction locked pins but non-linear for cemented and threaded pins. Friction locked pins can be safely used uptil depths of 3.0 mm without the danger of fracturing the pin or restorative material. In the case of cemented pins of sizes 0.018" and 0.025", and the smaller threaded pins of sizes 0.023", an embedment depth of greater than 2.0 mm increases the chances of restoration fracture. Hence the optimal length for these pins in the restorative material is considered to be 2.0 mm.

b. *Pin number, diameter and orientation*: Increasing the number of pins increases retention of the restoration to the tooth structure, but to a certain extent only. However, increasing the number of pins poses problem in condensation of restorative material and also decreases the overall strength.

Retention increases with the increase in diameter of the pin. Large sized threaded pins (0.031") offer maximum retention.

Pin orientation affects retention, i.e. pins placed in a non-parallel manner increase retention.

Bending pins may also improve retention but this should not be the sole aim as bending interferes with condensation of material around the pin, may loosen or weaken the pin as well as induce additional stresses in dentin.

Though increasing the number, depth and diameter of the pins increases retention of a pin restoration, a delicate balance between the three factors should be maintained to avoid pulpal involvement, tooth perforation or fracture of the tooth or restoration.

c. *Surface characteristics of the pin*: The number of surface deformations per inch influences the retention of pins in restorative material. Friction locked pins with 25 deformations per inch on their surface are the least retentive. The cemented pins are intermediate with 70 deformations per inch and threaded pins are the most retentive with 128 deformations per inch. Within the threaded variety, pins with threads placed closer together (narrow pitch) provide lesser retention because inadequate amount of material is contained between the threads. In contrast, wider pitched threads provide greater retention.

d. *Pin shape*: Retentive cleats (0.83 mm in diameter), and square or pear shaped heads on the pins improve retention to restorative material.

e. *Interpin distance*: Placing pins close to each other increases retention but is only limited to interpin distances of 2.0 mm. At distances lesser than this, there occurs a definite reduction in pin retention because of the less amount of material present in between the pins and increase in residual stresses in dentin.

f. *Type of restorative material*: Restorative material with a greater wetting ability provides closer adaptation to the pin surface and hence greater frictional retention. Spherical amalgam alloys and alloys with a combination of spherical and lathecut particles exhibit superior adaptation to all three types of pins – cemented, friction locked and threaded, whereas lathecut alloys exhibit good adaptation to only friction locked pins.

Retention of pins in composite resin is also influenced by the type of composite resin. Minuta and Minikin threaded pins are not very retentive in composite resins compared to Minim pins. For the minim pins, 2.0 mm length is considered optimal in Macro and intermediate filled composites, whereas the length needs to be increased to 2.25 mm for gaining equal retention in microfilled composite resins. If Minuta and Minikin pins are to be used, the strongest possible composite should be used with them.

g. *Pin restoration interphase*: An ideal interphase between the pin and material is one which is not interrupted. If the surface layer of the pin can chemically combine with the restorative material or one of its phases, a continuous interphase can be achieved. Unfortunately, this has not been possible as yet. Gold plated or silver plated stainless steel pins have been tried with the aim of reacting with silver amalgam but are not very effective. With the silver plated pins, voids have been observed at the inter-phase, possibly because of the mercury in amalgam reacting with the silver coating and dissolving it completely. If pins are gold plated, gold must be pure and free of any impurities for the mercury to react with it, but this condition is highly difficult to achieve especially in the oral cavity.

h. *Bulk of material surrounding the pin*: Pin retention decreases with the decrease in bulk of material surrounding the pin. Retention is almost completely lost when the material around the pin is less than half the diameter of the pin.

To summarize, any pin technique employed should permit optimal retention while inflicting minimal danger to the remaining tooth structure and restoration.

COMPLICATIONS DURING PIN PLACEMENT PROCEDURE

1. *Drill breakage*: The breakage of drill though not very common, can occur in following circumstances, when:
   - Lateral stresses are applied while drilling,
   - Dull drills are used,
   - The drill is allowed to stop rotating while entering or exiting from dentin or anywhere in between.

   'Precaution' is the only treatment. All factors that could lead to drill breakage should be avoided because removal of a broken drill is quite difficult. If removal is not possible, a new hole can be drilled 1.5 mm away from the first hole.

2. *Pin breakage*: The following factors lead to breakage of pins:
   - Excessive force is applied while driving the pin into its pin channel,
   - The pin is rotated despite being fully seated in the channel
   - The operator is not careful while bending the pin.

   All factors that could lead to pin breakage should be avoided because removal of a broken pin is quite difficult, however, it mainly depends upon the level of the pin breakage. When sufficient length of pin is available for holding, removal should be attempted. If unsuccessful in removing the pin or when the pin has broken at the level of dentin, a new hole can be drilled 1.5 mm away from the first hole.

3. *Loose pins*: Quite frequently the pins are loosely fitted in their channels. This may possibly be because of:
   - Repeated insertion and removal of the pin drill enlarging the pin channel,
   - Pin drill is rotated more than instructed, resulting in large sized channels,
   - Manufacturer's discrepancy, i.e. poor quality control between the pin drill and pin sizes
   - A self shearing pin fails to shear, resulting in stripped out dentin,

   Care should be taken that the pin drill rotates only for a brief moment. A single thrust without any lateral deflection of the twist drill avoids this complication. In case the pin is loosely fitted, then the channel should be enlarged with the next sized drill and a larger pin inserted. If the pin, which is loose in the channel is of the largest available size, or there exists a danger of encroachment into enamel on further enlargement, it is better to close the channel with appropriate materials and a new hole, 1.5 mm away from the first hole, is drilled.

A well fitted pin in the channel may also get loosened at a later stage. This often occurs while shortening the pin, when the rotating bur is held parallel to the pin or perpendicular to the pin on its right side, which causes the pin to rotate counter-clockwise. In this case, it is recommended to unwind the loosened pin completely. Since the pinhole has not been enlarged, a second pin of same size generally fits in well. If still loose, a hole larger in size is drilled and a larger pin inserted.

4. *The pin shears off before having reached its full depth*: In such cases, the treatment includes unthreading the pin, cleaning the channel and inserting a second pin of the same size.
5. *Twist drill dulling*: Cutting edges of a twist drill are dulled when the drill is repeatedly used. Dull drills have decreased cutting effectiveness, induce more stresses in dentin, and are more prone to breakage.

   Failure to remove clogged debris may also give the impression of dull drills. Coated drills show an increase in effective diameter and hence produce large sized channels.

   Treatment includes preventing repeated insertions and avoiding lateral forces on the twist drill. Twist drills should be thoroughly cleaned with hydrogen peroxide and should be discarded after preparing a maximum of 20 channels.
6. *The pin fails to bind and shear, but keeps rotating within its channel*: The best solution is to cement the pin or use one size larger.
7. *Heat generation*: Rise in temperature subsequent to the use of twist drills may be related to cutting deep channels, high rotational speeds used during channel preparations, large sized twist drills and repeated insertion of pin drills into dentin. Heat generation can be reduced by using 2.0 mm depth limiting drill and the smallest pin possible. Drills should be run at slow speeds. No injurious rise in intrapulpal temperature was seen by Ulusoy et al (1992)[53] when the twist drill use was limited to five times or below. Beginning with the sixth use, the rise in temperature was above 5.5°C which is sufficient to induce pulpal damage.

   Occasionally, while adjusting the height of the pin, excessive heat may be produced. This can be avoided by using burs at high speed with intermittent cutting and with adequate air water coolants. It has been seen that temperature rises only 1.7°C when air water coolant was used whereas temperature rises as high as 11.4°C when only air coolant was used.
8. *Microleakage*: Microleakage in dentin is evident under all types of pins and is related to the leakage potential of different restorative materials. With the use of amalgam, leakage generally diminishes in time due to accumulation of corrosion products. On the other hand, resin restorations show a gradual deterioration in the margin seal as a function of time. The use of pins conceivably aggravates the leakage problem by producing fine craze lines and cracks that behave as communication channels with the exterior and the pulp. The leakage of saliva at the pin/dentin and pin/restoration interface predisposes to formation of corrosion products. Leakage with cemented pins occurs around its whole circumference, whereas with friction locked and threaded pins occurs in a semilunar pattern. The characteristic leakage pattern is attributed to the round pin-ovoid hole combination. The dead space created by incomplete seating of pins may harbour bacteria and induce pulpal problems.

   Microleakage can almost be eradicated under amalgam restorations by applying cavity varnish on the entire cavity surface including the pin channels. However, when varnish is used under cemented pins their retention is drastically reduced. Retention of friction locked and threaded pins is not affected by use of cavity varnish. Pin channels prepared significantly inside the dentino enamel junction also reduce the possibility of cracks extending to the dentin defects or the external surface, hence reducing microleakage.
9. *Dentinal cracks*: Microcracks usually form subsequent to introduction of friction locked and threaded pins into dentin. Their details have already been covered under the section – *stressing effects of pins on dentin*.
10. *Perforation into the pulp space* (Fig. 14.17A): Pulp exposure under a pin is suspected if:
    - Bleeding occurs in the pin hole following removal of the drill from the pin channel.
    - Sudden lack of resistance is felt.
    - Sudden pain is experienced in a tooth while drilling, if the tooth is not anaesthetized.
    - The pin continues to thread greater than its intended depth.

    Radiographs may aid in detecting a pulp exposure if no dentin is visible between the pulp space and the pin, or the pin is seen to encroach

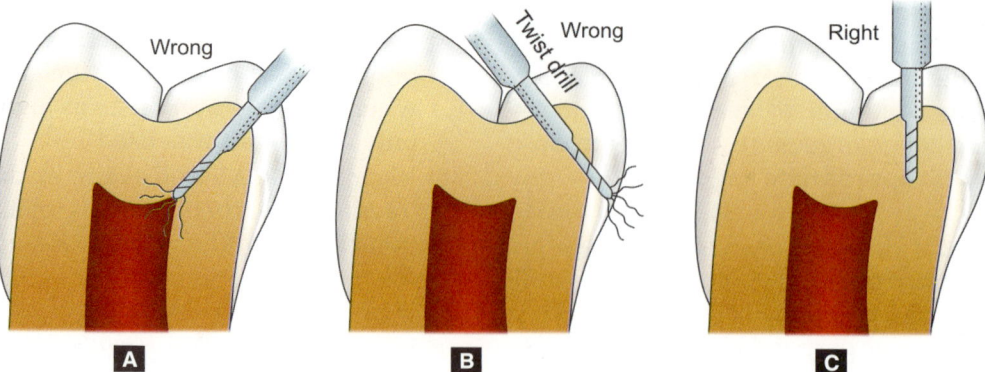

Figs 14.17A to C: Wrong angulation of the twist drill causes perforation; **(A)** In pulp chamber; **(B)** On external tooth; **(C)** Correct angulation of a twist drill

the outline of the pulp space. However, since radiographs are two dimensional images and superimposition can occur, this may not be a definite indication (Figs 14.18A and B).

Factors increasing the chances of pulpal penetration include inappropriate positioning and direction of the pin channels, use of large sized pins in small teeth, increased number and depth of pins in a single tooth, etc.

Pulpal perforation is not very disastrous provided that healthy dentin is penetrated prior to perforation, sterile conditions are present and can be maintained, and a hermetic seal can be provided. The treatment of pulp exposure by pin is similar to any other direct pulp cap procedure. If the perforation is discovered while drilling the pin channel, any resulting haemorrhage is first controlled and then the channel filled and sealed with calcium hydroxide. If the perforation is discovered after the pin has been inserted, it is wise to remove the pin, control any haemorhage and then place calcium hydroxide. The pin should be removed (a) for chances of post operative sensitivity being developed and (b) interference with subsequent root canal treatment. A new pin channel is then prepared 1.5-2.0 mm away from the first hole.

An alternative treatment is to control any haemorrhage and insert a sterile pin coated with calcium hydroxide just to the level of the pulp. Radiographs and pulp testing should be performed after every 3–6 months for confirming the vitality status of the pulp.

Generally, the teeth that are candidates for pin placement are extensively decayed and their pulpal status might be compromised. It is better to weigh between root canal treatment and pin placement especially when opting for cast restoration.

11. *Perforation onto the external tooth surface* (Fig. 14.17B): Perforation of the external tooth surface is suspected if:
    - Bleeding occurs in the pinhole following removal of pin drill.
    - Sudden lack of resistance is felt.
    - The pin continues to thread greater than its intended depth.

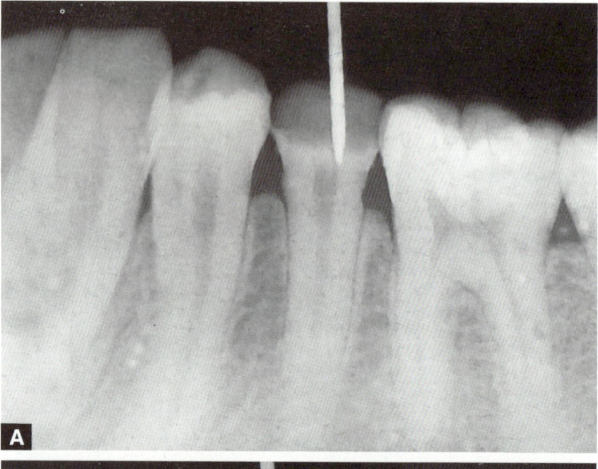
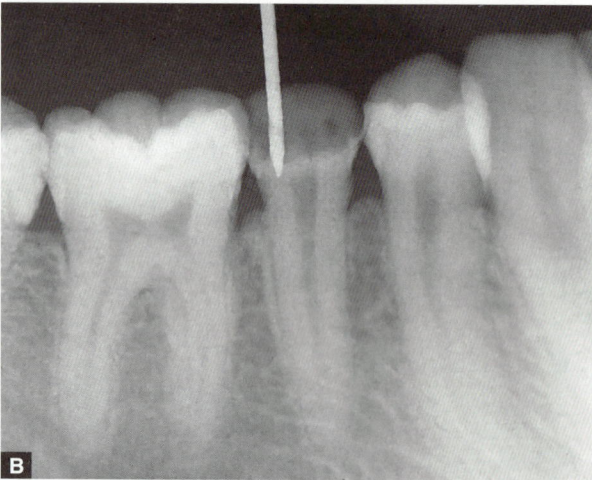

Figs 14.18A and B: Radiographs may not be a definite indication of perforation; **(A)** Pulp space does not seem to be exposed; **(B)** In same radiograph, pulp space seems to be exposed

Complex Restorations

- Pain is felt by the patient when the pin hole is being inserted in an unanaesthetized or root canal treated tooth.

Perforation should be confirmed with a probe and in a radiograph. Radiographs can verify an external perforation when the pin seems to project outside the tooth. However, since radiographs are two dimensional images, seeing a pin inside the tooth outline does not preclude the possibility of an external perforation. Additionally, observing the direction of a pin drill or pin indicates a possible lateral perforation.

Lateral perforations into the periodontal tissues are most often a result of careless pin placement and inadequate knowledge about the normal anatomy of a tooth.

The treatment of external perforations is determined by the site of perforation relative to the alveolar bone level. When the perforation is suprabony and the pin protrudes into the sulcus, there may occur plaque accumulation and bacterial colonization adjacent to the pin, followed by inflammation and periodontal problems. Three modes of treatment can be rendered in such situations when the perforation is coronal to the alveolar crest (a) Trim the protruding portion, flush the pin with the external surface, whether tooth or restoration and polish. No further treatment is deemed necessary (b) Trim the protruding pin, flush with external surface and polish. The perforation site is included beneath a cast restoration and (c) Back up the pin by about 0.5 mm, enlarge the external exit of the pin hole and seal in composite or amalgam with a fine condenser. One should not hesitate to raise the gingival tissue flap, if adequate treatment needs to be rendered.

When the perforation is infrabony, two modes of treatment can be rendered, insert the pin and observe periodically, uneventful healing might occur. In case periodontal problems arise, a flap is raised, the necessary bone removed, pin trimmed flushed with tooth surface and polished. In case the pin protrudes in an area with pre-existing pathology, no observation period is rendered but the surgical management performed as soon as possible.

The incidence of pulpal and periodontal perforations can be greatly reduced if the clinician is thorough with the pulpal and external anatomy of the tooth, observes radiographs carefully before the procedure, and follows the principle and techniques of pin placement carefully. Correct angulation of pin drill is shown in Fig. 14.17C.

FAILURES OF PIN RETAINED RESTORATIONS

Failures after pin placement and/or restoration may occur in five areas.

1. *In the dentin, i.e. fracture of tooth*: The solution is to reduce the area to a flat surface and re-drill a pinhole.
2. *At the dentin/pin interface, i.e. pin pulls out along with the restoration*: The treatment includes recementing if it is a cast pin restoration, or performing the whole procedure again if it is an amalgam restoration. It is generally difficult to determine the size of the pin that will suit the pinhole. Quite often, the patient brings along with him the lost restoration and in such cases the size of the pin can be measured with a micrometer and the next larger size chosen. If no pin is available for measurements, the operator should chose by using successive sizes of pin starting with the smallest size possible.
3. *In the pin itself, i.e. pin fractures*: Remove the remaining restorative material from the cavity preparation. Fractured pins are managed similar to as described earlier and the tooth is restored again.
4. *At the pin/restoration interface, i.e. restoration pulls away from the pins*: Formation of corrosion products at the interface is the most common cause for such type of failures. Titanium is the least corrosive pin. The treatment includes removal of any remaining restorative material. Pins are checked for loosening. There is every possible chance of having loosened the pins during restoration removal. Loose pins are managed as described earlier and the restoration done again.
5. *Failure of the restorative material itself, i.e. restoration fractures*: The most common cause for such type of failures is an improperly retained matrix. Any movement of the matrix during placement, condensation and setting of amalgam can severely weaken the restoration and result in a poorly adapted interface with the pin. For the same reasons, pre-mature removal of the matrix should be avoided, i.e. matrix should be allowed to stay in place for at least 10–15 minutes before removal. The occlusion should be checked thoroughly as any high point predisposes to restoration fracture.

The treatment includes repair of the restoration, if possible. When restoration cannot be repaired, the remaining restorative material is removed and the tooth restored again. Any pins loosened during restoration removal should be adequately managed. Adhesive failures are seen in cases 2 and 4 whereas cohesive failures are seen in cases 1, 3 and 5.

EFFECT OF PINS ON PULP

Quite often, pins are placed close to the pulp or there may be a minute pulp exposure while drilling into dentin. One wonders as to how the pulp will respond!

Haemorrhage into pin channel may not be present under all pulp exposures. The reasons may be attributed to the small size of the pinhole, dentin debris forced ahead of the drill into the pulp tissue acting as a hemostatic agent. Generally, the pulp responds positively to the pin and accepts its presence without any adverse effects. However, if the tooth is carious, symptomatic or a hermetic seal is not maintained under the restoration, the pulp may succumb to the injuries. Intentional insertion of pin in the pulp of vital tooth, which were later extracted and put to histological study revealed that after an initial inflammatory response, necrotic tissue was encapsulated and walled off. This was followed by fibrous tissue regeneration and coalescing of dentinal tubules by the formation of predentin by odontoblasts. Similar eventual healing occurs under direct pulp caps of zinc oxide eugenol, calcium hydroxide, etc.

The proximity of pin channels to the pulp tend to induce initial pulpal responses like destruction of odontoblastic nuclei, vascular dilation and inflammatory cell infilteration. Inflammatory reactions have been observed under all three types of pins, i.e. cemented, friction locked and threaded. The response under cemented pins is attributed to the type of cement used and its effect on pulp. Zinc phosphate cement without an underlying varnish layer induces a more severe inflammatory response compared to zinc oxide eugenol or glass-ionomer cement. Pulpal response under friction locked and threaded pins is probably because of the microcracks generated in communication with the pulp or disruption of the odontoblastic processes. Applying a varnish layer does not reduce the pulpal response of friction locked and threaded pins. The pulpal response is succeeded by normal defense reaction like formation of reparative dentin under all three pins.

Heat generation during pin placement procedure is also tolerated by the pulp as long as the twist drill is new and has not been used for drilling more than five channels, and adjustment of pin length is carried out under high speed burs, adequate air water coolant and intermittent cutting.

AMALGAPINS

Shavell (1980) introduced the concept of amalgapins as an alternative to the traditional stainless steel pins. *It is referred to as a vertical post of amalgam anchored in dentin* (Fig. 14.19). Amalgapins offer almost similar retention when compared to dentin retained pins yet seem to cause less internal stress in the dentin. They also do not reduce the compressive and transverse/tensile strengths of amalgam unlike pins. However, they are associated with a greater tooth substance

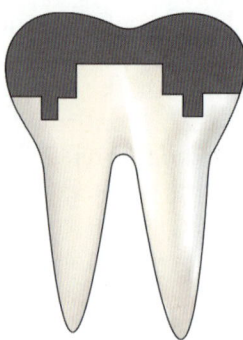

Fig. 14.19: Cavity preparation using amalgapins

removal. Gingival areas that are weak are areas ideal for their usage.

An inverted cone bur of appropriate size is used to create a ditch 1.0 to 2.0 mm deep and 0.5-1.0 mm wide, 0.5 mm inside the dentino-enamel junction. After making the channels, amalgam is condensed directly into them with fine pluggers or fine condensers (0.76 mm in diameter). One aspect which is very important in restorations with amalgapins is the stabilization of matrix. An attempt to remove the matrix before the amalgam has fully set may shear off the amalgapins quite easily. If the operator depends primarily on amalgapin rather than walls of dentin or enamel for stability, the matrix should be removed after 10 to 15 minutes.

PIN RETAINED CAST RESTORATIONS

Pins may be used for aiding retention in extensive cast gold preparations or short or excessively tapered preparations where adequate retention cannot be offered by other means. Pin placement also overcomes the need for extending preparations onto additional surfaces, limits extension of the preparation to areas not visible, and eliminates the need for subgingival extensions. Two basic casting designs that utilize pins are the '*pin ledge*' and '*pin lay*' castings. *A pin ledge casting is one in which the operator places pins in dentin as auxiliary aids for increasing retention.*

Ledges or seats for the pinholes are usually accompanied by a groove or box on at least one proximal surface. *A pin lay casting is one which has no grooves, boxes or flanges, but only a chamfered finish line which surrounds a flat area of missing tooth structure.* Pins here are not used as auxiliary aids for securing the casting in position but as primary means of retention. The use and advantages of pins in these restorations, however, does not preclude the principles of proper preparation and extension. In single restorations placement of one or two pins for retention may suffice whereas for abutment restorations under bridges three to four pins are required.

Pins used in a cast restoration are also referred to as parallel pins since it is necessary to place them parallel to each other as well as parallel to the path of insertion and removal of the restoration. This requires a cementing agent for retention. The retention values, therefore, vary depending upon the type of cement used. Stepwise procedure for a pin retained cast restoration is shown in Figs 14.20A to G.

Indications

1. One wall of a proximal box is shorter than the other proximal wall, may be in routine class II preparation or in a mesio occluso distal preparation.
2. The gingival floor of a proximal preparation is unusually deep.
3. One proximal wall of a mesio occluso distal preparation is exceptionally short.
4. Overtapered full crown preparations.
5. Attritioned or abraded teeth where the occlusogingival height of the tooth has been excessively reduced.
6. Full crown preparations where one wall is short and the other wall is long.
7. Can be given in cuspal fractures.

Restoration of a Single Tooth with Cast Restoration Utilizing Pins

The preparation of tooth for pin retained cast restoration follows the conventional principles of cavity preparation. The floor of the preparation, whether pulpal or gingival is kept flat and parallelism of the remaining walls is maintained. All remaining tooth structure is preserved as far as possible. The undermined caries is removed and the unsupported enamel finished. The features of cast gold restorations are achieved in the remaining tooth structure. Uneven areas or depressions at one or two particular areas can be filled with light cure glass-ionomer cements. The channel sites are marked and drilled as mentioned before, following the principles of pin placement and pinhole preparation. For the first channel to be drilled, the twist drill is carefully aligned with the angle of

Stepwise procedure for a pin-retained cast restoration

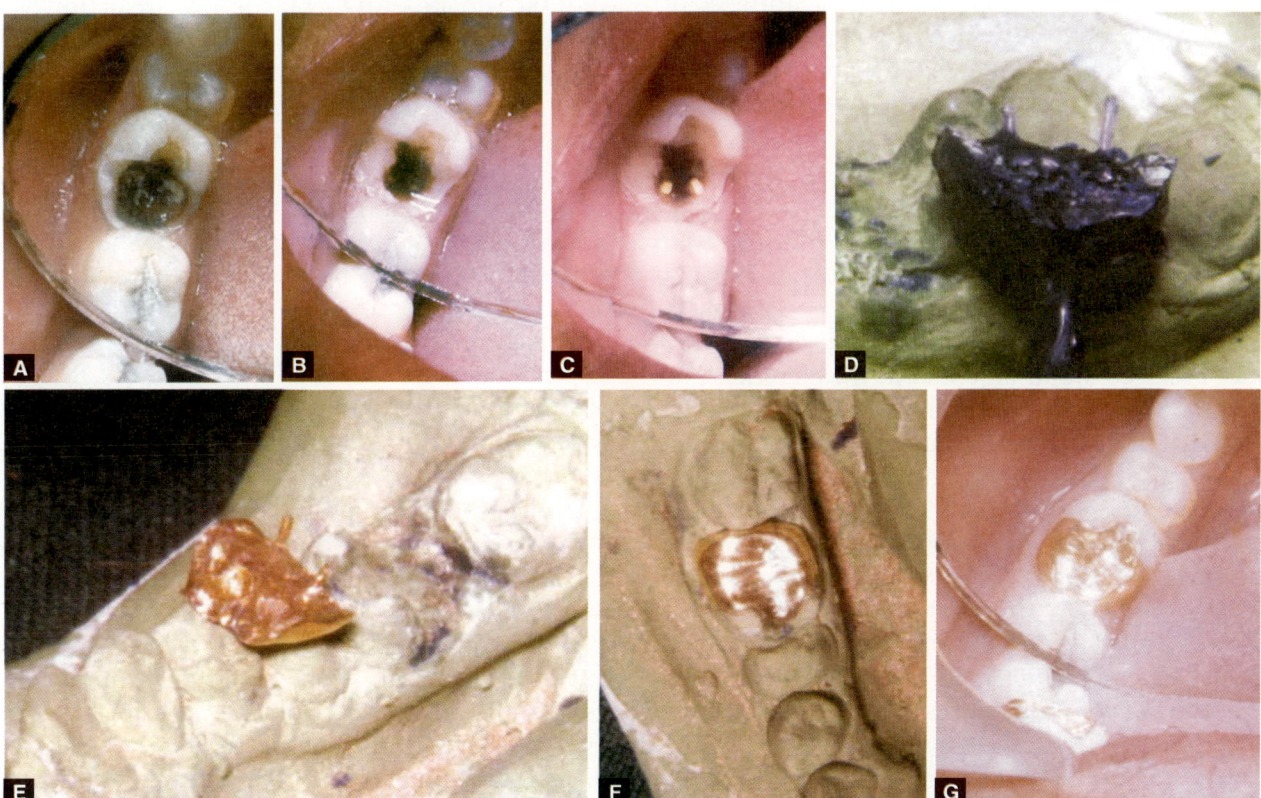

Figs 14.20A to G: **(A)** Carious mandibular right first molar, decided to be restored with a pin retained cast restoration; **(B)** Cavity prepared on mandibular right first molar; **(C)** Pins placed in cavity preparation following which an impression in rubber base is taken; **(D)** A cast is poured and a blue inlay wax pattern of the prepared tooth is made. Plastic pins are seen to be a part of the wax pattern; **(E)** Casting along with the cast pins; **(F)** Casting placed on the prepared tooth on the cast - finished and polished; **(G)** Casting placed on the prepared tooth in the oral cavity

the prepared wall and run to the described depth. The first pinhole is cut freehand and should be the distal most pinhole on the posterior abutment as it is utilized as a guide pin in preparing other pinholes parallel to this pilot hole. It is easier to move from posterior to anterior rather than anterior to posterior.

If only two pins are to be inserted, the second pinhole can be paralleled with the first pinhole visually without the need for more elaborate paralleling devices. A plastic or steel pin is inserted into the first pinhole to serve as a guide pin. For the second pinhole, the twist drill is positioned at the marked site and aligned in two planes with the guide pin. Once satisfied, the channel is drilled. Slight discrepancies of 5–8° are permissible as these can be tolerated by the flexibility of the metal pins and the 0.002" size gap between the pin and its channel. Moreover, a minimal adjustment of the deviating pin and beveling the pin end can ease insertion during tryin and cementation. A pin channel which deviates more than 8° can be corrected by using a large sized drill which includes the smaller channel and provides a channel which is in better alignment.

In teeth where more than two pins have to be inserted, a paralleling device is recommended for use. Paralleling devices are marketed in a number of designs. The use of these devices is not discussed here in detail. After the pin channels have been drilled, a wax pattern is made either by the direct method or the indirect method, invested and cast.

Direct Method

The channel and the tooth surface is thoroughly cleaned and dried. A thin layer of cavity varnish is applied inside the channel using small paper points. A plastic pin of slightly lesser diameter than the channel is selected and adjusted in the channel. The outer end of the pin is rounded off or coiled with the help of any hot instrument. Blue inlay wax is applied over the pin and seated in the channel. The final impression of the channel is checked by removing the pin from the channel and reinserting the same. The rest of the impression is taken by blue inlay wax as in routine for any cavity preparation.

In place of plastic pins, wrought pins can also be used. Precious metal pins have also been used which become the part of the final restoration. In case, two or more pins are used, these are stabilized by using pink wax or sticky wax.

The final pattern is removed and cast as in routine.

Indirect Method

The channel and the rest of the cavity is cleaned and dried. The channel is coated with thin layer of cavityvarnish. A stainless steel pin, cut according the need, or paper pin is inserted into the channel and stabilized. In case of loose pins, blue inlay wax can be applied over the pins. A rubber base impression is taken. The impression is withdrawn along with the pins and the model is poured.

To reproduce the pins in the preparation, plastic pins/nylon bristles, 0.002"–0.004" smaller than the pin channels are used. Several manufacturers supply plastic pins/nylon bristles in different sizes. Nylon bristles are egg shaped in cross-section and hence for the same pin channel, nylon bristles have to be used which are smaller than the plastic pins having a round cross section. If the dentist does not have special bristles, he can easily make one by cutting mono filament fishing line or plastic pins that are present in packed new shirts. Pin heads can be made by holding the end of the bristles close to the bunsen flame until a ball is formed. This ball is then pressed against a flat cold metal object resulting in knobbed pins/bristles that are easier to anchor in the elastic impression. Approximately, 5.0 mm of the pin should extend above the floor of the preparation. Because the pin is smaller in size it does not have a snug fit. To stabilize the pin in its channel, it may be rubbed against red beading wax before insertion which provides more adhesion.

The pins are placed in their respective channels. If these have not been stabilized earlier, they may be lightly stabilized by holding an index finger on their head while injecting light body hydrocolloid material around the pins. The finger should be removed sideways to avoid dislodging the pin. The tray loaded with heavy bodied hydrocolloid is then seated to position. Occlusal stops should be placed in the impression tray so that a sufficient thickness of impression material is provided without the danger of pins touching the tray. If a heavy bodied rubber base material is used for impression, knobbed bristles should be avoided, as separating the impression from the pins is difficult without the danger of fracturing the cast.

The impression material is allowed to set and then the tray carefully removed from the mouth. The impression is checked. Any pin, which has not come out with the impression is carefully removed from its channel and inserted in the appropriate location in the impression. Any fragments of impression material that have been forced around the bristles into the pin channel should be carefully trimmed with a blade.

The impression is poured immediately in die stone and allowed to set properly. If an electroplated die has to be constructed, steel pins should be used for impression instead of nylon/plastic pins. The cast is carefully separated from the impression. Pins are removed from the cast in line with the pin channels using pliers and discarded.

Wrought pins may be cast directly to the overlying cast gold restoration. For this, the model is coated with a film of separating medium. Threaded, serrated or knurled wrought pins that are 0.001"-0.002" smaller than the pin channel are selected and inserted into the pin channels. The pin length is adjusted to just short of occlusion. The pins are joined with molten pink wax, which after cooling provide stability. Blue inlay wax is added and the pattern completed.

The pattern is sprued, carefully removed from the die, invested and cast in Type I or Type II gold alloys. The casting so obtained is adjusted, finished, polished and seated following the procedures similar to that for any other restoration. Stepwise procedure for an indirect pin retained cast restoration is shown in Figs 14.21A to G.

Arbo M.A. (1970) described an alternative technique in which the wax pattern is not separated from the die but invested along with it. The procedure requires taking an impression in rubber base impression material using plastic/nylon bristles as mentioned before. The difference with this technique is that the model is poured in Die-investment rather than die stone as done in the previous technique. After the investment model has set, it is separated from the impression. Pins are not placed in the pin channels, rather blue inlay wax is melted adequately and directly luted to the die. The pattern is completed and contoured. Excess die material is removed with a model trimmer. The sprue is attached near the orifice of the pinholes and at an angle to permit the gold to flow directly into the pinholes before it crystallizes. The same investment material is used for investing the die and its pattern. The die then becomes a part of the investment after it has set. Rest of the procedure until seating of the casting is carried out conventionally.

Retention offered to the casting by the pins is determined by the type of cement used. Smooth cast pins are generally 20–30% less retentive than the threaded wrought pins. Examination of failed castings

Stepwise procedure for an indirect pin-retained cast restoration

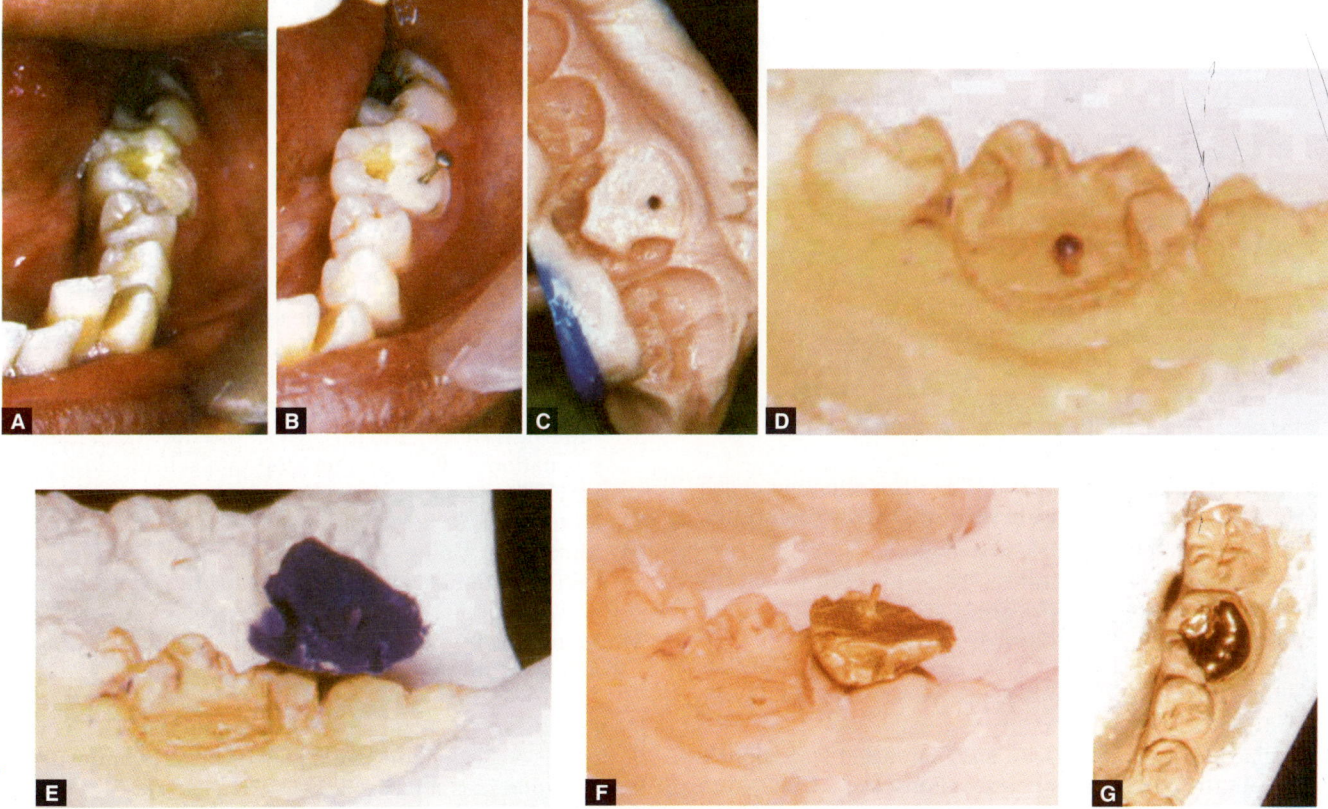

Figs 14.21A to G: **(A)** Cavity prepared on a mandibular left first molar, decided to be restored with a pin-retained cast restoration; **(B)** Pin placed in the cavity preparation to be later incorporated into the impression; **(C)** Full arch impression taken. Pin can be seen in the impression; **(D)** A cast is poured. Pin from the impression has been transferred onto the cast **(E)** Blue inlay wax pattern made on the prepared tooth. Pin on the cast has been incorporated into the wax pattern; **(F)** Casting along with the cast pin; **(G)** Casting placed on the prepared tooth on the cast—finished and polished

with smooth pins generally show no cement adhering to the cast pins, i.e. failure at the pin cement interface, whereas examination of castings with threaded wrought pins that have failed, usually show cement particles adhering to the pin, i.e. failure occurs at the cement-dentin interface or cohesively in the cement. The length, number and diameter of pins are also known to affect retention. Since these pins are cemented into their channels, increasing the length, number and diameter of pins increases the retention values without the danger of inducing harmful stresses.

Temporary protection of the prepared tooth is done by placing 1.0-2.0 mm of non-headed plastic pins or aluminium pins in the pin channels. Acrylic resin is applied with a brush to complete the temporary restoration. An aluminium or temporary crown filled with temporary cement may also be placed over the temporary pins.

BIBLIOGRAPHY

1. Arbo, M.A.: A simple technique for castings with pin retention. D.C.N.A. 14, 19, 1970.
2. Bailey, J.H.: Retention design for amalgam restorations: Pins versus slots. J.P.D.: 65, 71, 1991.
3. Barkmeier, W.W., Frost, D.E. and Cooley, R.L.: The two in one self threading self shearing pin. Efficacy of insertion techniques. JADA: 97, 51, 1978.
4. Bione, H.M., Wilson, P.R.: The effect of mismatch between the core diameter of self threading dentin pins and the pinhole diameter. Aust. Dent. J., 43, 181, 1998.
5. Brackett, W.W. and Johnston, W.M.: The retention of titanium pins in high copper amalgam and their influence on its fracture resistance. Oper. Dent.: 14, 136, 1984.
6. Burgess, J.O.: Horizontal pins: A Study of tooth reinforcement. J.P.D., 53, 317, 1985.
7. Butchart, D.G.M.: A new self threading dentin pin. Br. Dent. J.: 155, 83, 1983.
8. Butchart, D.G.M. and Llyord C.H.: The retention of self threading pin embedded in various restorative materials. Dent. Mater.: 2, 125, 1986.
9. Butchart, D.G.M. and Llyord, C.H.: The retention of self threading pins embedded in visible light cure composites. J. Dent.: 15, 253, 1987.
10. Certosimo, A.J., House, R.C. and Anderson, M.H.: The effect of cross-sectional area or transverse strength of amalga pin retained restorations. Oper. Dent.: 16, 70, 1991.
11. Chan, C.C. and Chan, K.C.: The retentive strength of slots with different width and depth versus pins. J.P.D.: 58, 552, 1987.
12. Collard E.W., Caputo, A.A. and Standlee, J.P.: Rationale for pin retained amalgam restorations. Dent. Clin. North Am.: 14, 43, 1970.
13. Collard, E.W., Caputa, A.A. and Standlee, J.P.: Invitro analysis of self-shearing retentive pins. J.P.D.: 45, 456, 1981.
14. Cookey, R.L. and Barkmeier, W.W.: Temperature rise in the pulp chamber caused by twist drills. J.P.D.: 44, 426, 1980.
15. Currens, W.E., Korostoff, E. and Von Fraunhofer, J.A.: Penetration of shearing and non-shearing pins into dentin. J.P.D.: 44, 430, 1980.
16. Davis, S.P., Summitt, J., Mayhew, R.B. and Hawley, R.J.: Self threading pins and amalgapins compared in resistance form for complex amalgam restorations. Oper. Dent.: 8, 88-93, 1983.
17. Dilts, W.E. and Coury, T.L.: A conservative approach to the placement of retentive pins. Dent. Clin. North Am.: 20, 397, 1976.
18. Dilts, W.E., Welk, D.A. and Laswell, H.R. et al: Crazing of tooth structure associated with placement of pins for amalgam restorations. J. Am. Dent. Assoc.: 81, 387, 1970.
19. Eberting, J.J.: A review of the amalgapin technique for complex amalgam restorations. Gen. Dent.: 48, 378, 2000.
20. Evans, J.R., Wetz. J.h.: The pin-amalgam restoration, Part 1-A Review. J.P.D., 37, 37, 1977.
21. Galindo, Y.: Stress induced effects of retentive pins– A review of the literature. J.P.D.: 44, 183, 1980.
22. Garman, T.A., Binon, P.P. and Averette, P. et al.: Self threading pin: Penetration into dentin, J.P.D.: 43, 298, 1980.
23. Going, R.E., Moffa, J.P. and Nostrant, G.W. et al: The strength of dental amalgam as influenced by pins. JADA: 77, 1331, 1968.
24. Ianzano, J.A., Mastrodomenico, J. and Gwinnett, J.A.: Strength of amalgam restorations bonded with amalgam bond. Am. J. Dent.: 6, 10, 1993.
25. Imbery, T.A., Burgess, J.O. and Batzer, R.C.: Comparing the resistance and pins in amalgam restorations. J.A.D.A.: 126, 753, 1995.
26. Jacobi.R., Shillinburg.H.T.:Pin dowels and other retentive devices in posterior teeth. D.C.N.A., 37, 367, 1993.
27. Lloyd, C.H. and Butchart, D.G.: Retention of core composite glass-ionomers, and cermets by a self-threading dentin pin: the influence of fracture toughness upon failure. Dent. Mater.: 6, 185, 1990.
28. Macpherson, L.C., Smith, B.G.N: Replacements of missing cusps: An in vitro study. J. Dent, 22, 118, 1994.
29. Mamoun, J.S. and Cervini, E.: A pin amalgam or composite core formation technique for teeth with minimal coronal structure. J.P.D.: 91, 599, 2004.
30. Marshall, T.D. and Cooley, R.L.: Evaluation of the Max titanium ally retentive pins. Am. J. Dent.: 2, 349, 1989.
31. Marshall, T.D., Porter, K.H. and Re, G.J.: Invitro evaluation of the shoulder stop in a self-threading pin. J.P.D.: 56, 428, 1986.
32. Mattos, F.M.: A new self-threading pin. J.P.D.: 29, 81, 1973.
33. Moffa, J.P., Going, R.E. and Gettleman, L.: Silver pins: their influence on the strength and adaptation of amalgam. J.P.D.: 28, 491, 1972.
34. Mondelli, J. and Vieira, D.F.: The strength of class II amalgam restorations with and without pins. J.P.D.: 28, 179, 1972.
35. Palaghias, G., Eliades, G., Vougiouklakis, G.: In vivo corrosion behaviour of gold plated versus titanium dental retention pins. J.P.D., 67, 194, 1992.
36. Pameijer, C.H. and Stallard, R.E.: Effect of self-threading pins. JADA: 85, 895, 1972.
37. Papa, J., Wilson, P.R. and Tyas, M.J.: Pins for direct restorations. J. Dent.: 21, 259, 1993.
38. Perez, E.R., Schoenech, G.A. and Yonahara, H.M.: The adaptation of non-cemented pins. J.P.D.: 26, 631, 1971.

39. Plasmans, P.J.J.M., Creugers, N.H.J. and Mulder, J. : Long term survival of extensive amalgam restorations. J.D.R. : 77, 453, 1998.
40. Podshadley, A.G., Storey, R.: Pinhole preparation of self threading pins. J.P.D., 65, 68, 1991.
41. Podshadley, A.G.: The retention of threaded pins in composite resin. J.P.D.: 61, 169, 1989.
42. Podshadley, A.G. and Storey, R.: Pin hole preparation for self-threading pins. J. Prosth. Dent.: 65, 68, 1991.
43. Roberts, H.W., Hermesch, C.B. and Charlton, D.G. : The use of resin composite pins to improve retention of class IV resin composite restorations. Oper. Dent. : 25, 270, 2000.
44. Roddy, W.C., Blank, L.W. and Rupp, N.W. et al.: Channel depth and diameter: Effects on transverse strength of amalgapin – Retained restorations. Oper. Dent.: 12, 2, 1987.
45. Shavell, H.M. The amalga pin technique for complex amalgam restorations. J. Calif. Dent. Assoc.: 8, 48, 1980.
46. Smales, Q.J. and Hawthorne, W.S. : Long term survival of extensive amalgam and posterior crowns. J. Dent. : 25, 225, 1997.
47. Smith, B.G. : Replacement of missing cusps : an in vitro study. J. Dent. : 22, 118, 1994.
48. Standlee, J.P., Collard, E.W. and Caputo, A.A.: Dentinal defects caused by some twist drills and retentive pins. J.P.D.: 24, 185, 1970.
49. Summitt, J.B., Burgess, J.O., Berry, T.G., Robbins, J.W., Osborne, J.W. and Haveman, C.W. : The performance of bonded vs. pin-retained complex amalgam restorations. A five year clinical evaluation. J.A.D.A. : 132, 923, 2001.
50. Summitt, J.B., Burgess, J.O., Berry, T.G., Robbins, J.W., Osborne, J.W. and Haveman, C.W. : Six year clinical evaluation of bonded and pin retained complex amlgam restorations. Oper. Dent. : 29, 261, 2004.
51. Tjan, A.H., Dunn, J.R. and Grant, B.E.: Fracture resistance of composite and amalgam cores retained by pins coated with new adhesive resins. J.P.D. : 67, 752, 1992.
52. Trengrone, H.G., Carter, G.M., Hood, J.A.A.: Stress relocation properties of human dentin. Dent. Mater., 11, 305, 1995.
53. Ulusoy, N., Denli, N., Atakul, F.: Thermal response to multiple use of a twist drill. J.P.D., 67, 450, 1992.
54. Van Nieuwenhuysen, J.P. and Vreven, J.: Maillefer and TMS pins compared for retention and penetration. Oper. Dent.: 10, 150, 1985.
55. Van Nieuwenhuysen, J.P., D'Hoore, W. and Carvallo, J. and Qvist, V. : Long term evaluation of extensive restorations in permanent teeth. J. Dent. : 31, 395, 2003.
56. Wacker, D.R. and Baum, L.: Retentive pins: Their use and misuse. Dent. Clin. North Am.: 29, 327, 1985.
57. Watson, P.A. and Gilmore, H.W.: Use of pins for retaining amalgam restorations: A synopsis. J. Canad. Dent. Assoc.: 1, 30, 1970.
58. Webb, L.E., Staka, W.F. and Phillips, C.L.: Tooth crazing associated with threaded pins: A three dimensional model. J.P.D.: 61, 624, 1989.
59. Wilson, P.R., Bione, H.M.: Ultrasonic removal of dentin pins. J. Dent, 21, 285, 1993.

15

Direct Filling Gold

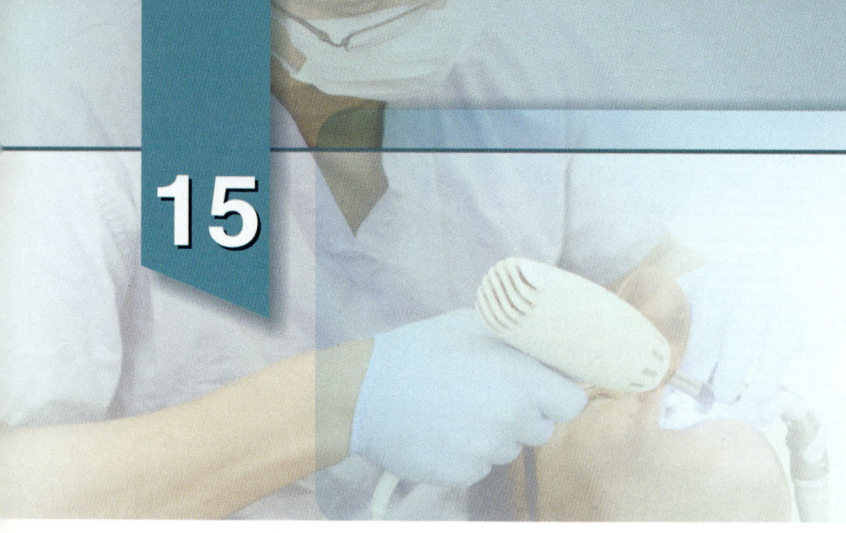

Gold foil was one of the earliest materials available for restoration of teeth. It is undeniably the most permanent restorative modality. Though the term 'gold foil' and 'direct filling gold' have been used interchangeably, gold foil is one form of pure gold used for direct restorations, and there are other forms also available.

In teeth with sound pulpal and periodontal health, this noble metal is a superior restorative material to fill small cavities. Even in persons with good oral hygiene measures, sometimes pit and fissure caries develop and when detected early, they can be prepared and restored conservatively with direct filling gold. When proper case selection is done and meticulous care is given to the cavity preparation and material manipulation, direct gold restorations can last for a life time, a claim that no other filling material can make to date.

Direct gold are those gold restorative materials that are manufactured for compaction directly into prepared cavities.

PROPERTIES OF PURE GOLD

1. Pure gold is soft, malleable, ductile and does not oxidize under the normal atmospheric conditions. It is the most ductile and malleable of all metals, second to it being silver. One grain of gold can be drawn into a wire of nearly 500 feet long. The percentage elongation seen is 12.8. Malleting produces a sheet as thin as 0.13 mms.
2. It is rich yellow in color with a strong metallic lustre.
3. Fuses at a temperature of 1063°C and boils at 2200°C.
4. The true density of pure gold is 19.0-19.3 g/cm^3. However, true density is difficult to achieve because of the voids, which are usually left behind in the restoration during condensation. Voids tend to decrease the final strength and density of the restoration. The measured or the apparent density is then found to be in the range of 14–15 g/cm^3, the higher values being for the gold foil.
5. Brinell's hardness number of pure gold is 25. This would seem to contraindicate its use as a restorative material. However, cold working while building the restoration increases its hardness to almost 58–82. This type of hardening is known as *'work hardening'* or *'strain hardening'*. Tensile strength after cold working increases from 19,000 psi to 32,000 psi while the yield strength raises from 0 to 30,000 psi.
6. Coefficient of thermal expansion (C.T.E.) is 14.4×10^{-6}/°C which is close to that of tooth structure, i.e. 11.4×10^{-6}/°C.
7. It has a high thermal conductivity of 0.710 cal/sec/cm^2 (°C/cm).
8. Gold is the noblest of all metals. Air or water at any temperature does not affect or tarnish gold. It is not soluble in sulphuric acid, nitric acid or hydrochloric acid, but readily dissolves in aqua regia (a combination of nitric acid and hydrochloric acid) to form trichlorides of gold ($AuCl_3$). It is also dissolved by a few other chemicals such as potassium cyanide and solutions of bromine and chlorine.
9. Small amounts of impurities have a pronounced effect on mechanical properties of gold, e.g. 0.2% lead makes gold very brittle. Bismuth and mercury have also shown to have adverse effects on gold. On the other hand, addition of small amounts of calcium, palladium and platinum are beneficial in improving its properties.
10. The most important property of pure gold which permits its use as a filling material is the ability to be cold worked and welded at room temperature. If two clean pieces of gold are pressed firmly together and a sufficient force applied, they unite at their point of contact and the gold is welded together without the application of heat. This

process is known as *'cold welding'*. Gold shows its maximum cohesiveness when it is 999 fine.
11. Direct gold restorations are the most efficiently sealing permanent fillings.

TYPES OF DIRECT FILLING GOLDS

There are several different forms of direct gold that can be employed in the restoration of a cavity. All of these forms are cohesive and 99.9% pure. It is necessary to understand the properties and indications of each material because the manipulation procedures vary with the choice of material. A combination of two different types of gold in a cavity is primarily indicated for convenience and conservation of time. The different forms of direct gold available are:

I. Foil
   - Sheets
   - Pellets (hand-rolled and commercially rolled)
   - Cylinders (preformed and hand-rolled)
   - Ropes
   - Corrugated foil
   - Laminated foil
   - Platinized foil
II. Electrolytic precipitated gold
   - Mat gold
   - Mat foil
   - Gold calcium alloy
III. Powdered gold
   - Goldent

All these forms of gold when properly condensed are of comparable strength, hardness and density as well as are equally resistant to wear and abrasion. The differences lie not in the end result but in their working characteristics.

Gold Foil

Gold Foil Sheets

Use of gold foil is the oldest amongst all forms of direct filling gold. Gold foil as a dental restorative material was first introduced in America by Robert Woffendale in 1795. The discovery of its property of cohesiveness is attributed to Robert Arthur in 1855. Sheets are manufactured by a process called *'gold beating'* or *'rolling'* (Fig. 15.1A). All light weight sheets are formed by beating and heavy weight sheets by rolling. The pure metal is first melted and formed into ingots of desired size. In the beating process, heavier mallets are used initially for beating gold ingots followed by the lighter ones when the gold gets thinner. In the rolling process, gold is passed continuously through the rolling mills until the desired

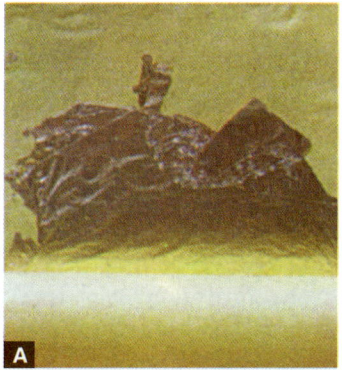

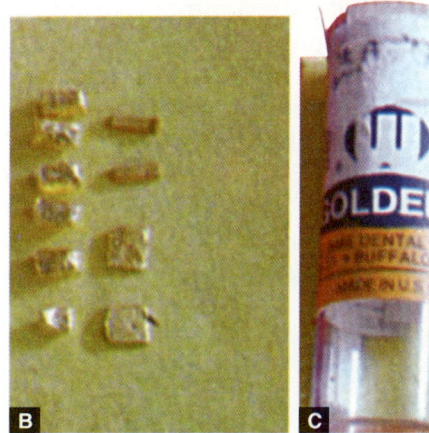

Figs 15.1A to C: Types of direct filling gold: **(A)** Gold foil between paper leaves; **(B)** Mat gold of different sizes; **(C)** Powdered gold (Goldent)

thickness is achieved. During the manufacturing process of gold foil, crystals of gold become elongated and assume a fibrous appearance (when viewed under a microscope). These fibres run in all directions interlacing with each other. Because of this property, fibrous forms of gold make a stronger restoration. Any of the processes mentioned above renders gold non-cohesive. In order to permit its use as a restorative material, gold should be first turned cohesive by annealing.

Gold foil sheets are bound in the form of books of 1/10 or 1/20 ounces. One book contains 12 sheets and each sheet commonly has the dimensions of 4" × 4". No. 4 gold foil is the standard size, which is usually used. It weighs 4 grains (0.259 gms/259 mgs) and is 0.51 mms thick. The numbering system refers to the weight of the sheet used, so it reflects the thickness as well i.e.:

No. 3 gold foil - weighs 3 grains (0.194 gms) - 0.38 mms thick

No. 2 gold foil - weighs 2 grains (0.130 gms) - 0.25 mms thick

Varying numbers of gold foil are available like No. 20, No. 40, No. 60, No. 90, etc.

Gold Foil Pellets

These may be hand rolled or commercially produced. An ideal pellet is produced from a No. 4 gold foil by the dentist or his assistant. Pellet sizes may vary from 1/2 -1/128 which represent the portion of the No. 4 gold foil used to form a pellet. The procedure for hand fabrication includes removing the No. 4 gold foil along with its tissue paper from the book. The foil is held on to the paper, marked (Fig. 15.2) and cut along with it. The paper supports the thin gold foil and prevents it from tearing and wrinkling during manipulation. Sizes, which are commonly used for rolling into pellets are 1/16 onwards. Larger sizes like 1/2, 1/4, 1/8 are used for forming cylinders. The desired piece of gold foil is then grasped from the centre and held between the thumb, index finger and middle finger of the left hand. Ends are tucked with tweezers towards the centre and rolled lightly into round balls of loosely packed mass of gold. Pellets are degassed and stored in separate compartments of a gold box.

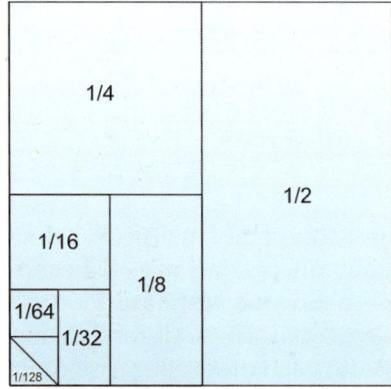

Fig. 15.2: Square showing various sections of gold foil sheet

Gold Foil Cylinders

This form can also be both hand rolled and commercially rolled. It is custom made by rolling cut segments of No. 4 gold foil usually 1/2, 1/4 and 1/8 into desired widths. Cylinders are degassed and stored in the gold foil box.

Corrugated Gold foil/Carbonized Gold Foil

Manufactured by placing thin sheets of paper in between the gold foil sheets, which are then ignited. The paper burns and gets charred. However, the gold foil remains unharmed, except that it becomes corrugated because of the shrivelling of paper. This was first observed by a dental dealer in the great Chicago fire of 1871.

Platinized Gold Foil

This is a sandwich of gold and platinum with the platinum content being 15%. It can be formed in two ways:

1. One sheet of pure platinum foil is sandwiched between two sheets of gold foil. These are then hammered until the thickness of one No. 4 gold foil is obtained.
2. Layers of platinum and gold are rolled over together so that there occurs fusion of the two even before the beating procedure has begun.

Platinum increases the hardness and wear resistance of the restoration. This form can therefore be applied in stress concentration areas like incisal edges and cusp tips.

Laminated Gold Foil

When a gold foil is beaten from an ingot, its crystals are elongated in a specific direction. A particular directional elongation allows forces to be better resisted in that direction. When two or three foils with crystals running in different directions are combined together, it results in a material that has fibres running in all directions. This makes it more resistant to the applied forces. Such a combination of 2-3 foils is known as *laminated gold foil*.

Cohesive and Non-cohesive Forms

Pure gold can be classified into *cohesive, semi cohesive* and *non-cohesive* forms. It should be emphasized here that two gold surfaces can cohere by welding at room temperature only if the surfaces are atomically clean. Hence, the manufacturer may supply gold foil to the dentist, which is essentially free of any surface contaminants and can be placed directly into the cavity preparation. Such a form of gold is called the *'cohesive gold'*. It is difficult to maintain the cohesive state as some adsorption of gases like carbonic acid gas, phosphoric acid gas, hydrogen sulfide gas, etc. are likely to occur during storage and transportation. Carbonic acid gas can get deposited from the exhalations of lung while both the sulphurous acid and phosphoric acid gases can emanate from the decaying matter like blood, pus, etc. and from burning matches. It is therefore recommended to degas even the cohesive forms before placing them in the cavity preparation.

The *'semicohesive gold form'* is one in which a protective gas film like ammonia is deliberately adsorbed on to the surface of gold by the manufacturer. This is beneficial as it minimizes the adsorption of other less volatile substances and also prevents premature cohesion of gold which may occur during storage and distribution. This volatile film is readily removed by heating and the foil is made cohesive.

'Non-cohesive form of gold' is one in which certain non-volatile contaminants like iron, sulphur or phosphorous are permanently deposited onto the surface. These cannot be driven away by heat and the gold therefore loses its cohesive property. Noncohesive forms are occasionally used as a starting material since they can be worked more easily than the cohesive forms. These however do not have sufficient strength and hardness compared to their counterparts.

With the introduction of newer instruments that provide better access, ease and convenience of manipulation, the non-cohesive forms are no longer used nowadays. The earlier category of semi-cohesive form is now retermed as the non-cohesive form and hence the classification is reduced to just two forms: *cohesive* and *non-cohesive* (ones in which there is a surface layer of adsorbed ammonia).

Electrolytic Precipitated Gold

This consists of the crystalline gold powder formed by electrolytic precipitation. The powder is formed into different shapes by heating at a temperature well below the melting point of gold. Diffusion of the particles occurs at the point of contact so that the particles coalesce and grow.

Mat Gold/Crystal Gold

In 1937, *Rule* first referred to crystal gold in his analysis of gold foil. This is electrolytic precipitated gold obtained by a process which is similar to electroplating but at an accelerated rate. The deposited material has a spongy structure with loosely arranged or fern like crystals. During subsequent heating process, branch ends of the crystals are rounded and tend to weld themselves together. These are available in the form of strips of medium widths (2.0 mm) and wide widths (3.0 mm) (Fig. 15.1B), which can be cut to the size that fits the cavity. Since mat gold is spongy in nature it can be easily compacted and adapted to the retentive portions of the prepared cavity. However its use is restricted to forming only the internal bulk of the restoration because of its large surface area, which does not permit easy welding into a solid mass. Also because mat gold is loosely packed, is friable and contains numerous voids between the particles, a gold foil is generally recommended for the external surface of the restoration.

Mat Foil

This is a sandwich of mat gold placed in sheets of No. 3/No. 4 gold foil. The sandwich is sintered by heating to just below the melting point of gold and cut into strips of different widths. The idea to use mat foil was to eliminate the need to veneer the restoration with a layer of gold foil. The gold foil cover holds the crystalline gold together while it is being condensed.

Electralloy

This is an alloy of electrolytic gold and calcium. The calcium content is usually 0.1-0.5% by weight. Its purpose is to produce stronger restorations by dispersion hardening. For convenience, the product is sandwiched between two layers of gold foil.

Powdered Gold

Powdered gold is in the form of minute particles. It can be obtained by atomization from a molten state or by chemical precipitation. In the latter process, gold is dissolved in aquaregia and precipitated by oxalic acid, sulphur dioxide or sodium nitrate. The average particle size is 15 µ. As a powder the material is impractical to manipulate, so is gathered into a conglomerate mass having a diameter of 1-3 mms. These masses are either sintered or lightly precondensed to facilitate slight adhesion between the particles and ease handling. However, even on mild provocation, these masses tend to fall apart. Because powdered gold produces a less porous surface compared to mat gold, veneering with a gold foil is not very much necessary.

Powdered Gold and Gold Foil Combination

This form was introduced in 1962 by *Baum and Lund*. Commercially available pellets of powdered gold wrapped in a gold foil are known as *'Goldent'*(Fig. 15.1C). The powdered particles are mixed with a soft wax and held in a No. 3 gold foil. Gold foil acts as a container for the powdered particles and facilitates their condensation. Each pellet contains approximately ten times more gold than a pellet of gold foil of comparable size. The ratio is 95% powder and 5% foil. Hand method of compaction is better than mechanical compaction for powdered gold.

ANNEALING/DEGASSING

'Annealing' a gold foil refers to the removal of surface contaminants. *'Degassing'* or *'desorption'* is the preferred term over *'annealing'* because at no stage is any recrystallization or stress relief intentional. The primary purpose is to produce an atomically clean

surface and render the material cohesive and workable. For non-cohesive gold, degassing is done to remove the protective ammonia film which had been deliberately placed on its surface by the manufacturer. In cohesive gold, various contaminants like sulphur and phosphorous compounds, oxides or water vapour may have been adsorbed on to the surface during storage and packaging. It is therefore highly desirable to anneal both the cohesive and non-cohesive forms to drive away all surface contaminants. Temperatures in the range of 600–1300°F must be produced on the surface of the gold to volatilize gases or other volatile contaminants. Following two methods can be used for degassing - the alcohol flame or the electric annealer.

i. *Alcohol flame:* This is the preferred method for degassing. Absolute or 90% ethyl/methyl alcohol without any additives is used in the lamp to produce a clean blue flame. It is important to use its middle zone for heating. Regular cohesive gold is held only momentarily for a few seconds in the flame until the color changes to dull cherry red. Powdered gold must be held in the flame until all the wax is burnt out and the pellet reaches a dull red glow. It may take 15–20 seconds for complete degassing of the powdered gold pellets.

Degassing may be done by piece method or bulk method. In the *piece method*, a single piece is annealed at one time, usually done by the dental assistant while the operator concentrates on the procedures for restoration. The gold is carried and held with a suitable instrument usually a nichrome wire (Fig. 15.3A) because it does not interfere with the cleaning process. Advantages of piece method are:

- Little waste
- Ability to select a piece of desired size
- Eliminates contamination amongst different pellets during their heating and use

'Bulk annealing' is the degassing of several gold pellets at the same time, usually takes five minutes for the process. Mica trays are used to hold the gold over the flame. Bulk annealing has the advantage of taking less time in the whole process compared to the piece method. However, gold pellets may stick together if the tray is accidentally moved during heating. Air currents may cause unequal heating of the tray and result in gold with poor welding properties.

Various precautions should be taken when using a flame for degassing.

1. The lamp should not run out of fuel during the procedure.
2. There should be no surface contaminants and waxes on the lamp and wick.
3. Wick should be properly trimmed and rounded to produce a tear drop flame.
4. Attention should be given during lighting as sulphur in the matches could adhere to the wick and contaminate the gold. Preferably ignite with the other end of the match stick.

ii. *Electric annealers:* These prove to be useful when one is working alone. The desired amount of gold is placed in the divided trays of the annealer and the lid closed. The gold is heated at a temperature of 850°F for 10 minutes and then allowed to cool before it is placed in the cavity. Disadvantages with an electric annealer are:

1. Inability to judge the correct requirements can lead to inadequate or excessive amounts being degassed.
2. Any remaining gold needs to be discarded because of possible irreversible contamination.
3. A temperature of 800°F may not be high enough to anneal the powdered gold. They require a temperature of 900°F-1200°F.

Care should be taken to avoid underheating or overheating during degassing. 'Underheating' does not adequately remove all surface impurities. This results in incomplete cohesion, because of remaining contaminants leading to overall inferior properties of the restoration. 'Overheating' leads to excessive sintering and possible contamination from the tray, instruments or flame. It may occur because of prolonged heating or use of too high temperatures. Following are its attendant consequences:

- Recrystallization and crystal growth
- The whole mass of particles adheres to each other instead of only the surfaces. This leads to a decrease in plasticity and poor compaction characteristics
- The heated portion becomes brittle

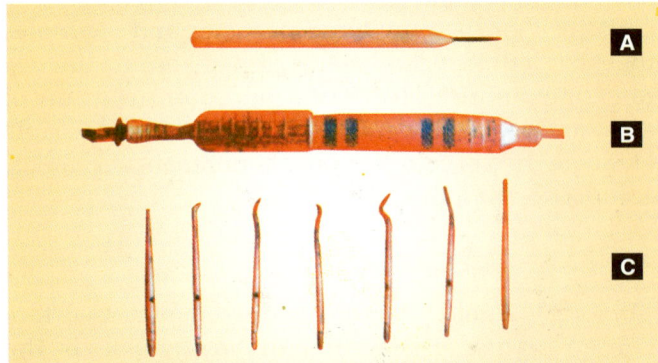

Figs 15.3A to C: Instruments used in a direct filling gold restoration; **(A)** Nichrome wire used for carrying gold; **(B)** Pneumatic condenser; **(C)** Detachable condensing tips

CONDENSATION/COMPACTION OF THE DIRECT FILLING GOLD

Condensation is the procedure used to condense and harden gold inside the cavity preparation. When performed thoroughly, it results in a dense non-porous gold restoration. Each pellet must be thoroughly condensed and hardened before the next is begun because once it has been covered by another pellet, it is not possible to reach the first one and remove the porosity. The objectives of compaction are:

1. Cohere two pieces of gold to each other. This process is known as welding.
2. Adapt the gold intimately to the walls and margins of the prepared cavity.
3. Cold work and thus harden the gold mass to increase its strength. When the gold is condensed, slip planes are developed and the resulting stress hardens the restoration.
4. To drive away air from in between the pieces of gold and gold-tooth interface.

Techniques for compaction vary with the different types of gold selected. Variables of compaction are: force of the blow, angulation and size of the condenser and the method of stepping the instrument.

i. *Force of the blow*: The average force required to condense gold with a condenser point of 1 mm diameter is 15 pounds. It has been found that this much amount of force can be obtained only when the operator applies maximum finger thrust. This would imply that the operator gets rapidly tired if hand pressure alone is used for condensation. Delivering forces from a mallet is hence recommended because it is rapid, easier and less strenuous. Blows from the mallet should neither be too strong nor too light. Stronger blows deliver heavier forces which could perforate the gold and damage pulp and supporting structures. With lighter blows, inadequate force is applied which could result in imperfect compaction, poor adaptation to cavity walls and a restoration full of voids. A force of 15 pounds is considered optimal and is well within the physiologic limits of the tooth. Factors which control the ultimate force delivered in a blow are (a) weight of the hammer and the velocity with which it is brought down on the condenser (b) resistance of the substance receiving the blow and (c) area of the condenser point in contact with the restoration. For the first two characteristics force is directly proportional to the weight and velocity of the mallet. Within limits, a thick periodontal ligament will sustain and dissipate forces better than thin ligaments. In such cases force of the blow should be increased slightly to attain the desired results. Size of the condenser nib, i.e. diameter and area also influence the amount of total force needed. Larger diameter condenser nibs require greater forces for compaction compared to smaller nibs. Forces of magnitude 3.75 pounds are recommended for condenser nibs of 0.5 mm diameter, 8.43 pounds for 0.75 mm diameter and 15 pounds for 1mm diameter nibs. It can be noted here that when the diameter of the instrument is doubled, forces required are increased four times. In other words, for a constant amount of force being applied on condensers of 1.0 mm and 2.0 mm diameter, the force per unit area in the latter is four times less compared to the former.

ii. *Direction of the applied force during condensation is called as the line of force.* Force applied with a condenser parallels the long axis of the instrument shaft regardless of the angle of the working point. While compacting in the centre of the cavity, forces are usually directed at 90° to the pulpal floor. Black advocated an angle of 45° to the cavity walls at the periphery such that the line of force bisects the line angles and trisects the point angles.

iii. Small condenser tips (0.5-1.0 mm) are usually considered adequate to achieve the desired compaction. Very small diameter nibs tend to perforate the gold. Very large diameter nibs on the other hand require very high forces for compaction and are less effective in forcing gold into the line and point angles.

iv. Uniform stepping of the condenser point is important to ensure hardening and welding of the entire restoration without leaving behind any voids. *Stepping is the overlapping of the previous area of the condenser's stroke by half or one fourth both in individual steps and in lines of steps* (Fig. 15.4). Stepping process can proceed in two ways (1) Moving parallel to the wall and wedging the final row between the already condensed mass of gold and cavity wall. (2) Moving prependicular to the wall. The final row wedges the gold between that wall and the already condensed gold.

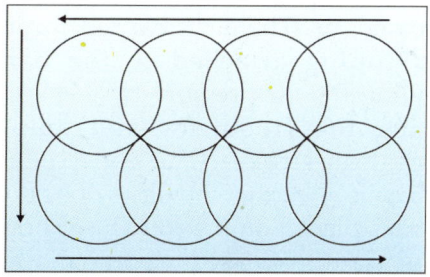

Fig. 15.4: "Stepping" pattern of the condenser

Condensers

Condensers/pluggers are instruments used to deliver the forces of compaction to the underlying restorative material. There are several methods for the application of these forces:

a. *Hand pressure*: As explained earlier, use of this method alone is contraindicated except in a few situations like adapting the first piece of gold to the convenience or point angles and where the line of force will not permit use of other methods. Powdered golds are also known to be better condensed with hand pressure. Small condenser points of 0.5 mm in diameter are generally recommended as they do not require very high forces for their manipulation.

b. *Hand malleting*: Condensation by hand malleting is a team work in which the operator directs the condenser and moves it over the surface, while the assistant provides rhythmic blows from the mallet. Long handled condensers and leather faced mallets (50 gms in weight) are used for this purpose. The technique allows greater control and the condensers can be changed rapidly when required. However, with the introduction of mechanical malleting, use of this method has decreased considerably.

c. *Automatic hand malleting*: This method utilizes a spring loaded instrument that delivers the desired force once the spiral spring is released. Disadvantage is that the blow descends very rapidly even before full pressure has been exerted on the condenser point.

d. *Electric malleting* (McShirley electromallet): This instrument accommodates various shapes of condenser points and has a mallet in the handle itself which remains dormant until wished by the operator to function. The intensity or amplitude generated can vary from 0.2 ounces to 15 pounds and the frequency can range from 360–3600 cycles/minute.

e. *Pneumatic malleting* (Hollenback condenser): This is the most recent and satisfactory method first developed by Dr. George M. Hollenback. Pneumatic mallets consist of vibrating condensers and detachable tips (Figs 15.3B and C) run by compressed air. The air is carried through a thin rubber tubing attached to the hand piece. Controlling the air pressure by a rheostat allows adjusting the frequency and amplitude of condensation strokes. The construction of the handpiece is such that the blow does not fall until pressure is placed on the condenser point. Then it continues until released. Pneumatic mallets are available with both straight and angled handpieces.

To obtain proper condensation and cause least discomfort to the patient, it is necessary that a small amount of hand pressure be combined with malleting. The condenser point is placed firmly in contact with the gold using slight pressure so as to condense it minimally and tense the periodontal fibres. It is only then that the blows from the mallet are applied. Forces applied when condensing gold are regulated by the capability of the periodontal ligament to resist pressure, by the density demanded in the restoration, etc. Teeth accustomed to heavy masticatory stresses would bear heavy malleting forces better than ones, which are used lightly. Multi rooted teeth because of their greater tooth support will stand greater condensation than single rooted teeth. Restorations placed on areas of heavy occlusal stresses such as the incisal edges and cusp tips require heavy condensation for obtaining a much harder bulk and surface. One should note that regardless of the type of condensation method used, the desired compaction should be achieved with forces that do not damage the tooth structure.

Hand condensers have a long handle, approximately six inch in length and a blunt end to receive blows from the mallet. On the other hand, ones which are to be inserted into the handpieces for mechanical malleting have short shanks of one inch in length. Condenser shanks may be straight, monoangle or offset. Nibs of the pluggers can be of various shapes like round, rectangular and parallelogram shaped. The latter two condensers compared to the former, require three times more force during compaction because of their large size. Pyramidal/wedge like serrations are present on the face of the condenser nibs to increase their surface area, exert lateral forces on their inclines, prevent slipping of the gold and to cut through the outer layers to allow entrapped air to escape. When using angled pluggers for condensation, the effective force is decreased because the force does not act at right angles to the nib surface. Since the force applied is oblique to the plugger end, resolution results in one component being perpendicular to the end and the other being in the plane of the end. The latter force tends to displace the nib from the surface of gold or to displace the gold itself.

Compaction Technique

The rules for compaction were originally established for the gold foil; though same principles also hold true for other forms of gold. The gold foil cut to the size and shape of the cavity is delicately manoeuvred and spread out in a smooth concave form by hand before the application of compacting forces. Gold is adapted lightly to the cavity walls, line angles and point angles by hand pressure. It is then held steady by a holding instrument, and a condenser of desirable size is used to begin malleting in the centre of the mass. Slowly, the condenser is moved to the periphery along straight lines using the stepping process. As it reaches the walls, the condenser is turned from 90° to 45° such that it bisects the line angles and trisects the point angles (Figs 15.5A and B). While building the restoration, forces of condensation must be directed at 90° to the previously condensed gold so as to prevent any shear components from displacing the already condensed pieces of gold.

The compaction of 1st layer produces a building shelf and thereafter a gold bank is developed onto it. The most important rule is to keep the gold banked against the walls ahead of the centre until the cavosurface margins are reached, thus creating a concave surface while building the restoration (Fig. 15.6). A concave surface permits comfortable access to the condenser point. The central concave area left in the restoration is filled last. When an improper building shelf is produced, gold bulges in the centre creating a convexity in the material. The hump prevents the condenser from reaching the cavity walls, thereby resulting in a porosity. It also prevents proper application of the force and hence poor adaptation results. Improper condensation could lead to 'bridging' of gold. Bridging is the covering up of small crevices and pits present in the deeper portions of the cavity especially adjacent to the cavity walls. It is essential that bridging be minimized to avoid deteriorating the properties of the restoration. Any voids at the surface of the restoration or cavosurface interface could serve as possible routes for microleakage to the interior of the restoration.

Crushing of the cavosurface enamel is a frequent mishap that occurs with the novice operator. To avoid this, some amount of gold should invariably be present between the condenser point and the enamel margins (Fig. 15.7). If such an injury is recognized early in the process, removal of the sheared components could reestablish a clean margin allowing condensation to continue to completion. Retention in a direct gold filling is best obtained by harnessing the elasticity of dentin. During condensation, forces tend to compress the dentin, so that when the filling is completed the dentin returns back to its original position thereby tightly holding the restoration. Hence measures should be directed to properly condense and wedge the gold between two opposing walls.

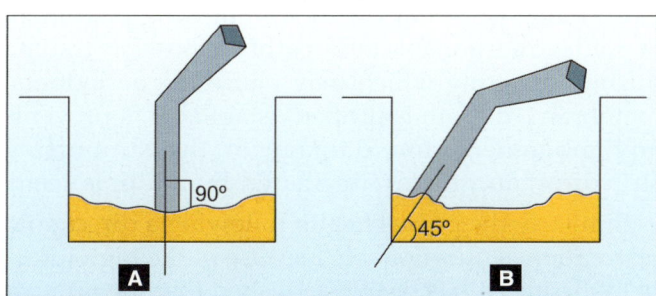

Figs 15.5A and B: (A) Condenser held at 90° to the pulpal floor in the centre of the cavity preparation; (B) Condenser held at 45° when it is moved towards the periphery of the cavity preparation such that it bisects the line angle and trisects the point angle

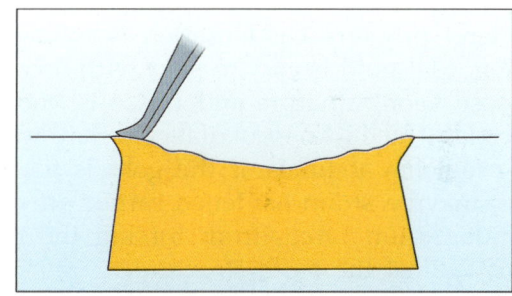

Fig. 15.7: Condensing gold in the cavosurface area

Condensation of Gold Foil

Gold foil has enough toughness even in thin sections and does not easily fragment under the pressure of a condenser. Because of the toughness and smaller mass per unit volume, gold foil can be easily manipulated in smaller cavity preparations and against preparation bevels. One difficulty encountered during its initial placement is the property of the material to roll out of the undercuts towards the condenser. This requires making sharp line and point angles in the cavity to serve as retentive locks and use of a holding instrument to secure the gold in position while it is being condensed. If pellets are used, the first gold pellet is condensed into a point angle (Fig. 15.8). A holding instrument is used to stabilize the previously condensed gold, while additional pellets are added one at a time slowly proceeding to the opposing undercut.

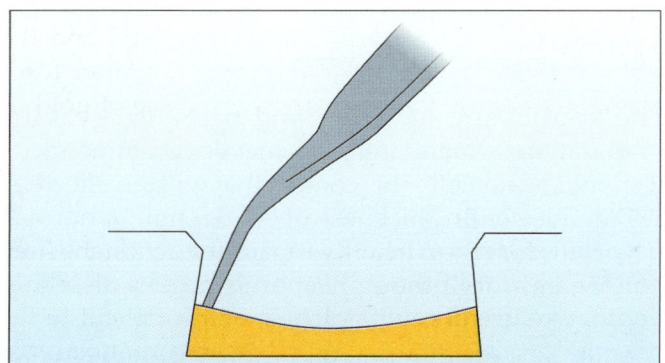

Fig. 15.6: Gold banked against the walls ahead of the centre thus creating a concave surface

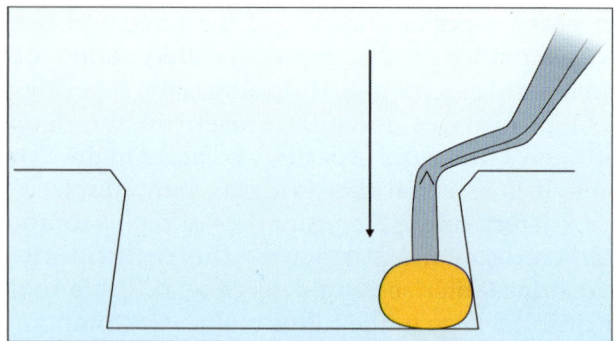

Fig. 15.8: First gold pellet being condensed into the point angle

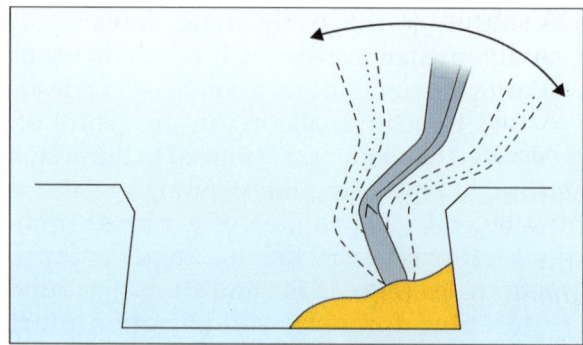

Fig. 15.9: Rocking motion of the instrument to condense the gold

Condensation of Mat Gold

The internal preparation of the cavity is similar to that for gold foil, i.e. sharp line angles and point angles to retain the gold and the bevelling of cavosurface margins. Mat gold is cut to the shape and size of the cavity and placed on the pulpal/axial walls of the preparation. It is condensed against the walls as a gold blanket using two condensers. One condenser stabilizes the gold while the other performs condensation. Two blankets of gold usually are a sufficient thickness to resist curling of the gold during subsequent condensation. Best results are obtained when hand pressure condensation is followed by malleting. Mat gold is easy to start with because of their loose spongy nature and hence is known as *starter gold*. The thickness of mat gold may however create problems at times. If the gold is too thick, surfaces may be strain hardened earlier preventing the condensation forces from forcing the deeper portions against the tooth structure.

Condensation of Powdered Gold

The cavity preparation for powdered gold differs slightly in two ways (1) It does not require sharp line angles and point angles (2) Flares and bevels in the cavity need to be minimized because powdered gold condenses more readily against butt cavosurface margins. These have a distinct clinical advantage during compaction because of their initial spreading quality. Upon contact with a condenser, the pellet of powdered gold tends to break apart and wedge itself into the opposing undercuts. It therefore does not require a holding instrument for stabilization and the indications include a proper box shaped cavity with sides, ends and a floor. Powdered gold should be firmly wedged between two opposing walls for condensation to be carried out properly. For this a pellet of larger size may be chosen or two or three pellets may be placed together to wedge the space. Pressure is then exerted with a rocking motion to adapt and harden gold initially in the retention forms and line angles (Fig. 15.9). Small faced condensers with a convex surface are considered ideal. After the periphery has been built by powdered gold, the centre of the ring is then filled.

BIOLOGICAL PROPERTIES OF PURE GOLD

A pure gold restoration is biologically sound; if proper techniques are used, cavity preparations are conservative and the teeth are properly stabilized with acrylic or compound before condensation. Pure gold is well tolerated by the gingival tissue. The periodontal health of the tooth following placement of gold is questionable because of the possible trauma during malleting which may injure the periodontal membrane. If tooth is properly stabilized, it prevents any movement and damage of the supporting structures, and forces are shared by multiple teeth.

Similarly the pulpal health following a direct gold restoration is questionable because of the high forces of malleting. It has been established that the number and intensity of pulpal reactions increase significantly after direct gold restorations. However, resolution occurs by the regeneration of odontoblastic layer and deposition of cementum after 35 days. Pulpal reaction includes displacement of odontoblasts, areas of internal haemorrhage and vesicle formation.

USE OF LINERS AND BASES

The application of liners and bases in a cavity preparation is mandatory whenever recommended. It should be noted in this context that with an effective remaining dentin thickness of 3.0-3.5 mm, a normal pulp will undergo a healthy reparative action. Hence, no intermediary base protection is necessary at this depth. The use of cavity varnish will suffice.

With an effective remaining dentin thickness of 1.0 mm, there will usually be an unhealthy reparative action. It is recommended to use:

- A subbase of zinc oxide eugenol followed by a cavity varnish and a base of zinc phosphate cement.
- A subbase of calcium hydroxide followed by a base of polycarboxylate cement.

With an effective remaining dentin thickness of less than 1mm, there will usually be destruction of pulp dentin organ. Hence a direct gold restoration is contraindicated in these situations.

INDICATIONS FOR DIRECT FILLING GOLD RESTORATIONS

1. *Incipient carious lesions*: Use of direct gold should be limited to only small conservative cavities. Because of its property to get easily deformed under forces, pure gold does not bear the onslaught of masticatory stresses very successfully. Hence, it is advisable not to expose the restoration to heavy stresses such as shear forces that occur during mastication. The indications include:
   - Class I lesions in premolar teeth and other accessible developmental pits (lingual pits on maxillary anteriors and facial pits on molars)
   - Class II lesions on premolar teeth. At times also indicated for small lesions on mesial proximal surfaces of molars.
   - Class III lesions in maxillary and mandibular anterior teeth.
   - Class V gingival lesions: Indicated for small lesions on the facial surfaces of premolars and canines and occasionally on the mandibular incisors. Maxillary incisors and molars are not good candidates, because of the limitations of esthetics in the former and poor accessibility in the latter.
2. *Erosion areas*: Indications are same as those mentioned above for gingival carious lesions.
3. *Atypical lesions*
   - Proximal lesions on teeth adjacent to crown preparations.
   - Vent holes in crowns and defective inlay/crown margins can be effectively repaired with direct gold.
   - Class VI lesions (cusps tips) and incisal edges (Figs 15.10A and B).
   - Retrograde root canal filling material.

CONTRAINDICATIONS

1. Teeth with very large pulp chambers because of their greater susceptibility to get damaged during condensation.
2. Severely periodontally weakened teeth as they will be unable to withstand the condensation forces.
3. Large carious lesions: These would increase the chances of the restoration being exposed to heavy masticatory stresses and would also require a greater expenditure of time and effort for its placement.
4. Handicapped, elderly or young patients who cannot give very long sittings.
5. Psychologically unsound patients who fear the malleting process.
6. When economics is a limiting factor.
7. Where esthetics is a prime requirement.
8. Inaccessible/poorly accessible areas.
9. Isolation unobtainable.
10. Areas of undesirable occlusal stresses.
11. Patients with a high caries index.
12. Hypoplastic areas, as forces required to condense gold against the enamel margins might fracture the latter.

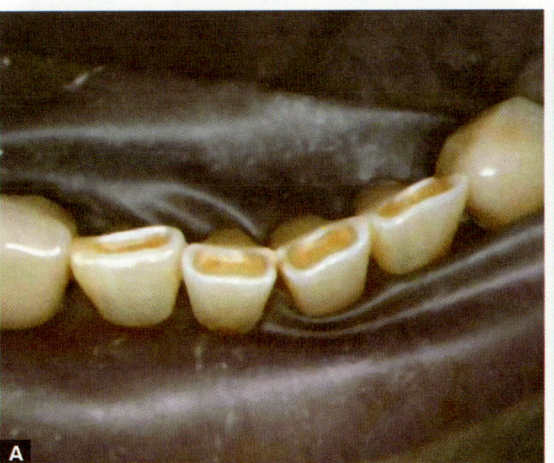
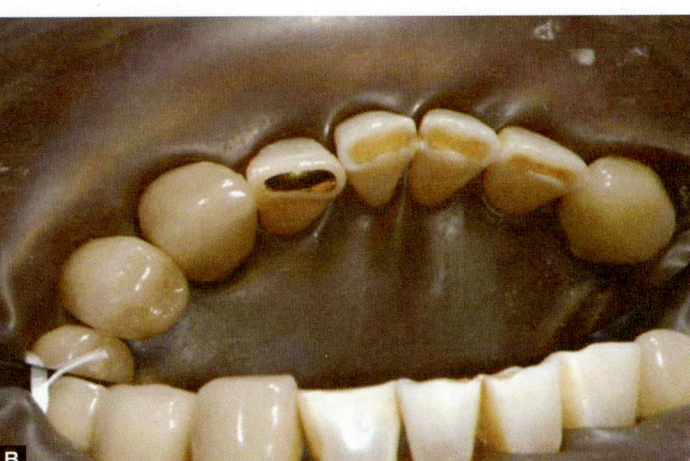

Figs 15.10A and B: (A) Attrition in mandibular incisor teeth; (B) Restored mandibular lateral incisor with gold foil

CAVITY PREPARATION AND RESTORATION

For the success of a direct gold restoration, adherence to Black's basic principles of cavity preparation is a must. Manipulation and placement also demands meticulous attention. If care is not exercised, the operator may be left frustrated in the end inspite of having put in his best efforts, time and energy for completing the restoration. Detailed description for the cavity preparation and restoration of class I, class V, class III and class II lesions is given in the following section. Before beginning any procedure for direct gold restorations it is mandatory to apply a rubber dam for proper isolation and access. It should be noted that even the breath of the patient could contaminate the surface of gold and render it non-cohesive.

Class I Cavity

Preparation

The external form of the cavity for direct filling gold is quite similar to that of silver amalgam. The marginal outline form is extended to include all the carious lesion and fissured enamel. Any defective pits and noncoalesced enamel are also included. The cavity is kept as small as possible consistent with suitable access for instrumentation and manipulation. In case of a pit defect, the outline may be simply triangular, oblong or circular (Figs 15.11 and 15.12). Margins are in the form of straight lines or smooth curves to make it more esthetic, and are terminated on sound and smooth areas so that they can be easily finished and polished. Internal outline form includes extending the pulpal floor to 0.5mm below the dentino-enamel junction. The carious lesion is entered with a No. 1 round bur and the outline form established with an appropriate pear shaped bur.

Opposing walls of the preparation are made parallel to each other. In wide cavities, mesial and distal walls need to be diverged slightly towards the occlusal surface so as to prevent any undermining and weakening of the marginal ridges. Pulpal floor is made flat and perpendicular to the occlusal forces. All enamel must be supported by sound dentine. All these features contribute to the resistance form of the cavity. Retention is provided by the parallelism of walls and sharp line angles and point angles. Accentuation of the angles is done with a No. 6½-2½-9 hoe. Additional retention if desired is given in the form of undercuts in dentin by a No. 33½ inverted cone bur or a No. 6½-2½-9 or 8-4-10 hoe. These retention grooves are placed facially and lingually in the occlusal preparation of posterior teeth at the facio pulpal and linguo-pulpal line angles respectively (Fig. 15.13). For the lingual surfaces of anterior teeth and facial surfaces of molars, these are given incisally and gingivally on inciso axial and gingivoaxial line angles respectively.

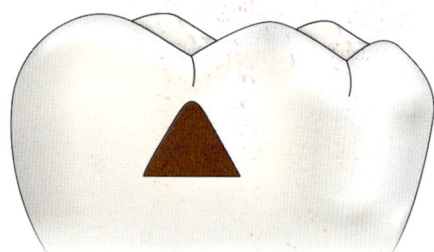

Fig. 15.11: Cavity preparation for direct gold restoration

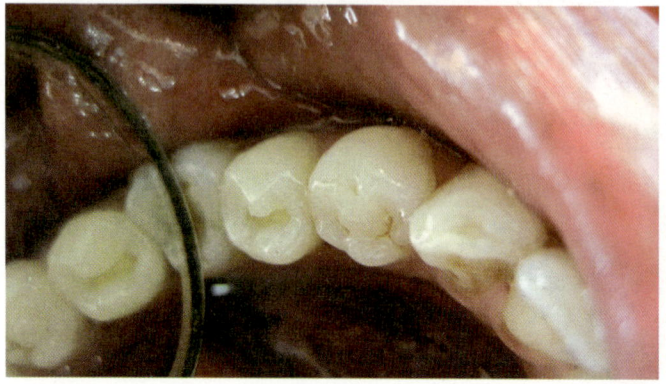

Fig. 15.12: Class I cavity prepared on mandibular premolar

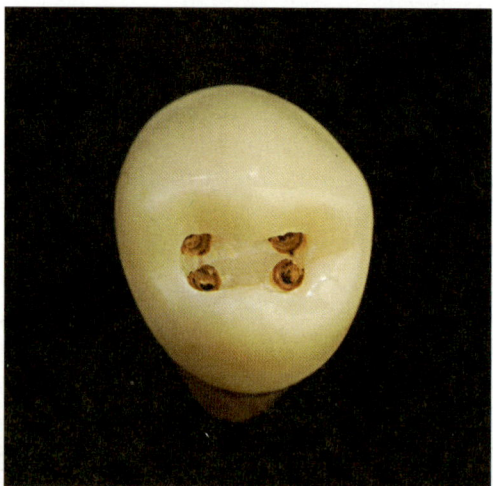

Fig. 15.13: Retention grooves placed facially and lingually in a class I cavity preparation for direct filling gold

Any remaining infected carious dentin is removed with a large No. 2 round bur and if needed a base is given. Planing of the walls is done with a No. 6½-2½-9/8-4-10 hoe. A very slight cavosurface bevel of 30-40° and 0.2 mm in width is placed on all the margins using a smooth finishing bur or a flame shaped white stone. Bevels aid in removing any rough enamel and create thin metals for ease of finishing.

This is the standard cavity preparation for restoration with gold foil or mat gold. Variations in design for powdered gold include rounding line angles and point angles and establishing butt cavosurface margins.

Restoration

The cavity is usually filled with mat gold and veneered with gold foil, although it may be entirely filled with gold foil or powdered gold also.

Procedure for Filling the Cavity with Combined Mat Gold and Goil Foil

Cavity varnish is applied on all the preparation surfaces and in case where the cavity is deep, a base is given. A piece of mat gold is cut to a size slightly larger than the cavity preparation, degassed and placed into position by a carrying instrument. Using two condensers, gold is spread out in the form of a blanket and intimately adapted to the preparation surfaces and retentive areas initially by hand pressure. For large cavities, parallelogram condensers are advocated. One condenser serves as the stabilizing instrument while the other is used for applying the forces. Malleting is not advised at this stage as the purpose of this step is to simply adapt the gold. It is only after the gold has been properly adapted, malleting is begun in the centre at 90° to the pulpal floor. A holding instrument is not necessary once a sufficient thickness of gold shelf (0.010″) that will resist buckling has been wedged into position. The condenser is moved by stepping process towards the periphery to complete the compaction into the pulpal line angles. On reaching the periphery, the line of force is changed to 45° to the cavity walls. Gold is condensed in such a manner that an excess is present towards the surrounding walls and a lesser amount in the centre (Fig. 15.6). Another increment is then added and condensed in a similar manner until the cavity is half to two thirds full. Building of the restoration should always proceed in a concave form to avoid humping in the centre or bridging of the restoration.

The remaining cavity is completed with a gold foil. For pit preparations, gold foil pellets of $1/64$ size are used where as for large preparations larger sizes of pellets such as 1/16 or 1/32 are advocated. The pellet is degassed and placed into the cavity along the wall restoration interface. It is first spread and secured against the already condensed mat gold with hand pressure and then mallet compacted. The rest of the portion is secured against the cavity wall. Similarly, additional pellets are placed and banked against all of the surrounding walls following the previously mentioned rules of compaction. Cavosurface margins are covered with gold as soon as possible. Gold should always be present between the condenser face and marginal enamel otherwise a direct blow from the plugger might injure the enamel. The central concave area is finally filled with gold to a slightly higher level. An excess on the surface allows for finishing and polishing procedures to be carried out. Finishing is necessary for contouring and conditioning the surface, increasing hardness of the restoration and providing closer adaptation of the metal to the tooth margins.

Burnishing begins the procedure of finishing. It is performed with a special spratley burnisher or a flat beaver tail burnisher or a ball burnisher that is run with considerable pressure from the restoration to the tooth surface (Fig. 15.14). Contouring is done with a green stone or garnet coated disks of small sizes or a gold file (Fig. 15.15). Gross excess at the margins is removed with a cleoid discoid carver or a gold foil carver (Fig. 15.16). Part of it should rest on enamel while it is pulled from the gold to the tooth surface so as to trim away any excess. After the excess has

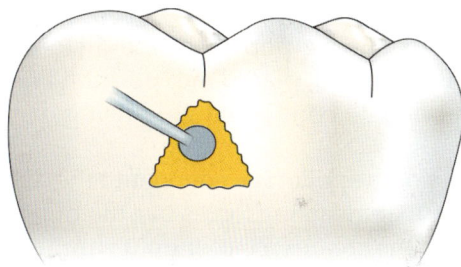

Fig. 15.14: Ball burnisher is used to rub the entire surface

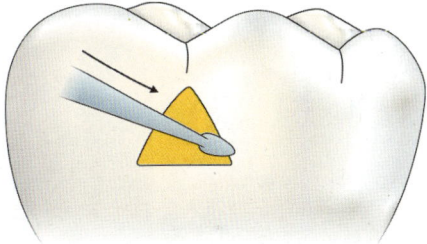

Fig. 15.15: Gold file is used with push-pull motion to develop the contour

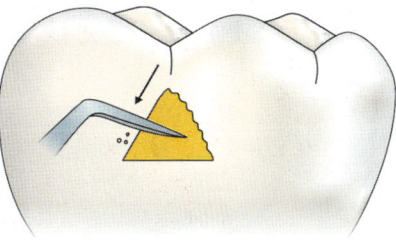

Fig. 15.16: Marginal excess or tags are clipped off with gold foil carver

been contoured and removed, burnishing is again performed. A high lustre is imparted to the restoration by using powdered abrasives like tin oxide, pumice or white rouge with a webless rubber cup at slow speeds.

Procedure for Filling the Entire Cavity with Gold Foil

When using gold foil pellets to completely fill the cavity preparation, the first pellet is placed in the most distal point angle say the disto-bucco-pulpal point angle. Using a holding instrument and a small round condenser of 0.5 mm diameter, the gold is firmly wedged with hand pressure between the three surrounding walls. The line of force is directed in the disto-bucco-pulpal direction. Malleting forces are then delivered to compact the gold. The second pellet is added on to the first one along the disto-pulpal line angle. This pellet is also first adapted by hand pressure followed by malleting in the disto-bucco-pulpal direction. Additional pellets are similarly condensed until two thirds or more of the line angle is covered. Next, a pellet size is chosen which will cover the remaining portion of the disto-pulpal line angle. It is degassed, placed into position and cohered to the previously condensed gold using disto-bucco-pulpal pressure.

The rest of the pellet is wedged into the distolinguo-pulpal point angle using forces in a distolinguopulpal direction. This creates a bar of gold running between two point angles. Similarly a gold tie is formed between disto-bucco-pulpal and mesiobucco-pulpal point angles; disto-linguo-pulpal and mesio-linguo-pulpal point angles; and mesio-bucco-pulpal and mesio-linguo-pulpal point angles. The concavity in the centre is then filled with medium to large sized pellets by directing forces in the four corners separately. Additional increments are similarly added in a concave form and the cavosurface margins covered with gold. The remaining depression in the central area is finally restored to a slight excess. The completed restoration is burnished, contoured and polished (Figs 15.17A to G).

Class V Cavity

As mentioned earlier, the use of rubber dam is necessary to provide adequate isolation. Access is facilitated by employing a No. 212 retainer or gingival retractor (developed by Dr. W.I. Ferrier). The hole for the tooth to be treated is punched 1mm facial to the actual position and an extra 1.0 mm of dam is left between this hole and the adjacent ones.

Preparation Design

The most commonly followed class V cavity design is the Ferrier's design. All fundamentals of cavity preparation should be adhered to when making the cavity. External outline is trapezoidal in form. Straight lines are preferred in the preparation as these are more

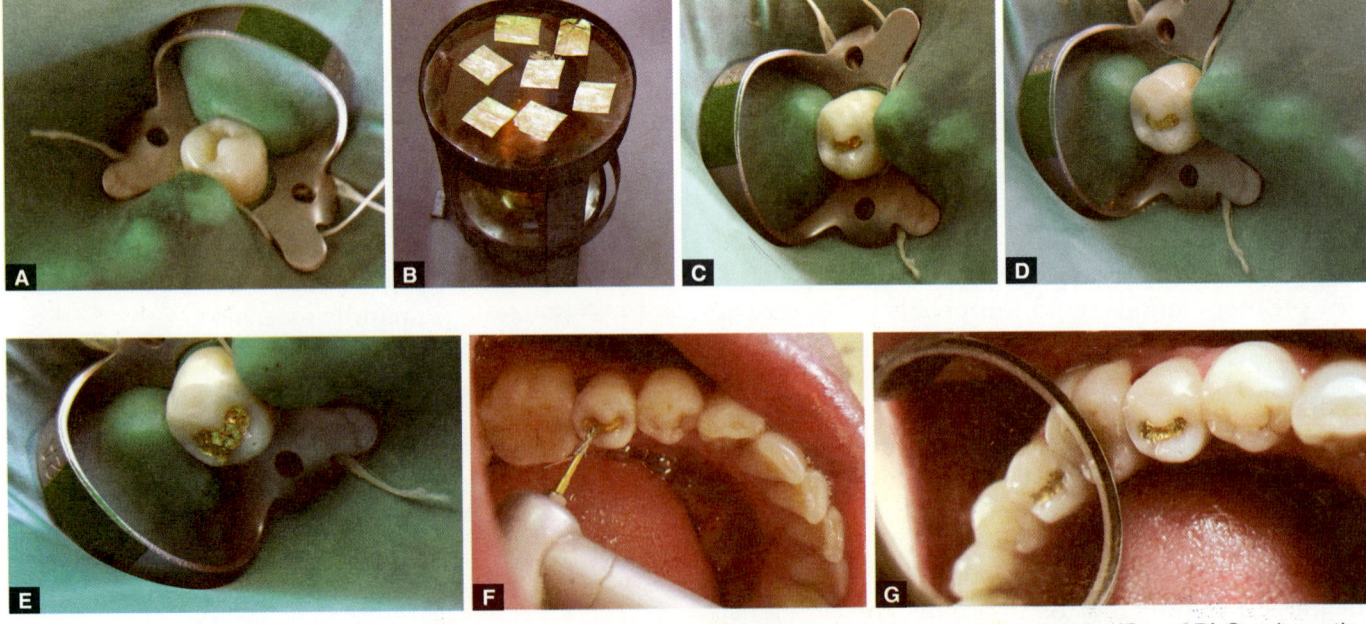

Figs 15.17A to G: **(A)** Class I cavity prepared on mandibular premolar; **(B)** Heat treatment of gold pellets; **(C and D)** Condensation of gold foils; **(E)** Condensation completed; **(F)** Burnishing and finishing; **(G)** Completed class I Restoration

esthetic and readily discernible when removing excess gold at the margins during finishing. Preparation is begun using a No. 33½ inverted cone bur and the cavity is extended to include all of the carious lesion. The same bur is used to establish the occlusal, gingival, mesial, distal and axial walls. The end of the bur forms the axial wall and the side forms the occlusal, mesial, distal and gingival walls.

Occlusally, the margin is straight and parallel to the occlusal plane of the treatment tooth. It extends beyond the carious lesion to sound tooth structure and is limited mesio-distally by the proximal line angles. Similarly the gingival margin is straight and parallel to the occlusal plane of the tooth but shorter than the occlusal margin. It extends gingivally beyond the carious lesion and mesio-distally is again limited to the line angles of the tooth. The gingival margin is placed well below the free margin of gingiva. Mesial and distal margins are extended sufficiently mesially and distally to be covered by the free gingiva. They are parallel to the proximal line angles of the tooth and meet the occlusal margin in a sharp acute angle and the gingival margin in a sharp obtuse angle.

End of the bur establishes the axial depth in dentin. The axial wall is straight occluso-gingivally and parallel to the facial surface of the tooth. Mesio-distally it has a slight curvature similar to the external contour of the tooth. This minimal curvature prevents encroachment on the pulp. The depth of the axial wall in occlusal half of the preparation is approximately 1.0 mm and in the gingival half is 0.75 mm. Axial wall forms a sharp right angle with the occlusal wall, an acute angle with the gingival wall and obtuse angles with the mesial and distal walls. The divergence of mesial and distal walls towards the surface prevents undermining the enamel.

Retention form is primarily provided by the gingival wall of the preparation. The acute axiogingival line angle is the key to retentive feature. It is prepared with a No. 6½-2½-9 hoe working from the cavosurface to the axial wall in a push stroke. The cut fragments are removed with an explorer or angle former. Sharp line angles and point angles also aid in retention. Starting points or convenience points in the form of coves or triangles are prepared incisally and gingivally at the point angles using a No. 33½ inverted cone bur. Any remaining caries is removed with a round bur. Planing the mesial, distal and gingival walls is done with a No. 6½-2½-9 hoe or 8-4-10 (larger hoe). The same hoe may also be used for establishing sharp line angles, retention grooves and finishing margins. Occlusal margin and the axial wall are planned using a wedelstedt chisel. A slight cavosurface bevel is given on all the margins using a wedelstedt chisel. A bevel on the gingival wall is not given when the latter extends to the cementum.

Variations in Design

a. When esthetics is the major demand, e.g. in anterior teeth, the occlusal outline may be curved to follow the gingival contour (Fig. 15.18A).

b. Thin strongly adherent gingival tissue may make it necessary to prepare a curved gingival wall (Fig. 15.18B).

c. At times because the height of contour is located very apically and when added esthetics is required, the gingival margin is curved in continuation with mesial and distal margins as if creating a circle. The occlusal outline is also made to follow the contour of the gingiva, so the general shape looks crescent shaped (Fig. 15.18C). This form of cavity is most commonly indicated for maxillary and mandibular canines and upper first premolars. Definite angles are however seen at the junction of the proximal and incisal/occlusal walls. Starting points in the form of coves are placed on the mesio-inciso-pulpal and disto-incisal-pulpal point angles.

d. Sometimes caries or decalcification extends from the gingival lesion towards the occlusal surface on the proximal line angles of the tooth. In such cases, extension/s may be added to the basic trapezoidal form in the form of a step or a moustache (Figs 15.18D to G), rather than carrying the whole of the occlusal wall occlusally. The angle where the occlusal wall meets the extension is rounded to remove unsupported enamel rods. Sharp angles in the extensions serve as excellent starting points for the condensation of gold. The cavosurface margins are bevelled as the rest of the cavity preparation.

e. Occasionally a carious lesion is seen to extend from the facial surface to the proximal surface/s of the tooth. In such situations, the basic class V cavity is prepared on the facial surface as mentioned before, with a parallelogram like extension on the mesial/distal surfaces (Fig. 15.18H). The proximal part known as the penhandle extension has only three walls: gingival, incisal/occlusal and facial/lingual. The internal form is similar to the basic trapezoidal form.

Restoration

Cavity varnish is applied thoroughly on all the preparation surfaces. Pieces of mat gold/mat foil/electralloy is used for forming the bulk followed by veneering with a gold foil. The cavity may be filled completely either with gold foil or powdered gold.

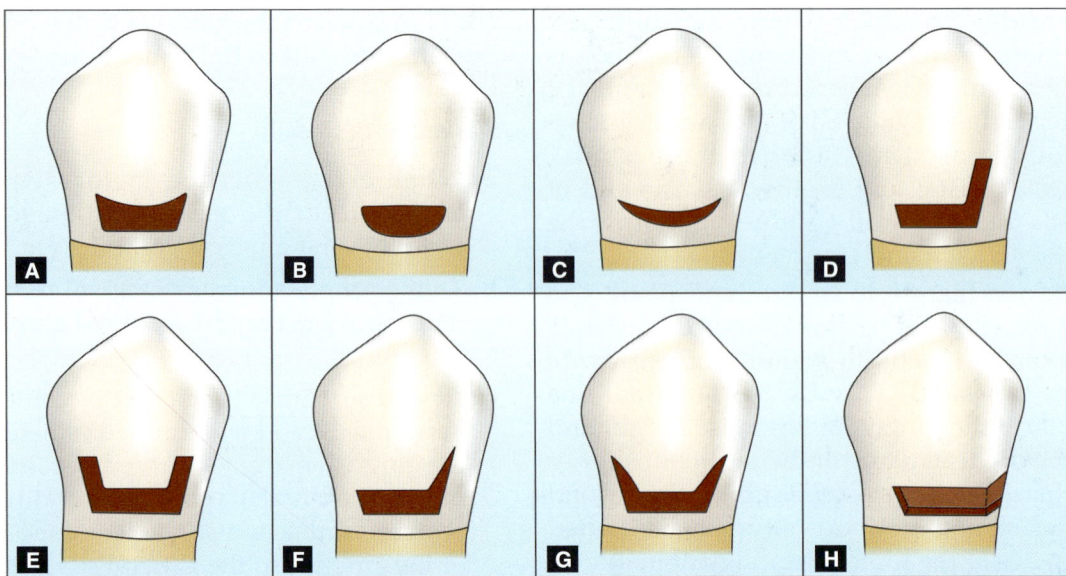

Figs 15.18A to H: Variations in class V cavity design for direct filling gold; **(A)** Curved occlusal outline to display less gold; **(B)** Curved gingival outline when gingival tissue is strong and adherent; **(C)** Partial moon-shaped cavity preparation; **(D)** Basic trapezoidal form with a unilateral step; **(E)** Basic trapezoidal form bilateral steps; **(F)** Basic trapezoidal form with a unilateral moustache extension; **(G)** Basic trapezoidal form with bilateral moustache extensions; **(H)** Class V cavity with penhandle extension

A piece of mat gold is cut to the shape of the cavity preparation but slightly larger. It is degassed and placed onto the axial wall with a carrying instrument. A pair of parallelogram condensers is used for the initial compaction of gold by hand pressure. One of the condensers serves in stabilizing the gold, while the other is used with rocking motion to adapt the gold against the axial wall and into the retentive line angles and point angles. The condenser should always be moved from the centre to the periphery and a concave surface maintained during compaction. After the gold has been secured, retaining one of the condensers as a stabilizing instrument; compaction is begun by delivering malleting forces with a 0.5 mm diameter round, serrated condenser nib. The holding instrument is removed once a building shelf of 0.013" is obtained. Additional increments of mat gold are added and compacted until the cavity is half to two thirds full using the previously mentioned principles of compaction. Remaining portion of the cavity is filled with gold foil pellets.

A medium sized gold foil pellet is chosen, degassed and placed in an area away from the operator, which is usually the disto-gingivo-axial area. The pellet is cohered to the already condensed mass of gold with a line of force directed disto-gingivo-axially. Additional pellets are added and condensed until half of the gingival and distal walls are banked. The same procedure is carried out on all the point angles and their adjoining walls. This results in a cavity that has been banked on all walls until the cavosurface margin, with a remaining concavity in the centre. Medium or large sized pellets (1/16 or 1/32) are used to fill the concavity to a slight excess. Any remaining defects can be sealed with small pellets of 1/128 size.

The excess which has been compacted is now contoured and finished. Burnishing is the first step and is performed with a spartley burnisher, ball burnisher or a flat beaver tail burnisher. Disks coated with garnet are used for contouring. These should be confined to the restoration, used along with a lubricant such as jelly and run at slow speeds. Morse scaler or Jones knife are also known to be good instruments for contouring and removing excess at the cavo-surface margins for class V restorations. Disks should be small enough which would allow them to be used within the No. 212 clamp and prevent any abrasion of the surrounding tooth structure. Their use should be avoided on the gingival margins for the fear of damaging cementum. Smoothening of the surface is done with cuttlefish disks used in an order of their descending abrasiveness. The final lustre is attained with tin oxide or white rouge applied with a soft webless rubber cup. The final restoration is shown in Figs 15.19A to C.

After the restoration has been completed, the No. 212 retainer and rubber dam are removed carefully. Avoid scratching of the restoration or the tooth during its removal. Any remaining abrasive is then thoroughly washed away. Gingiva is slightly massaged before sending the patient away so as to revive blood circulation which might have been hampered during the application of the retainer.

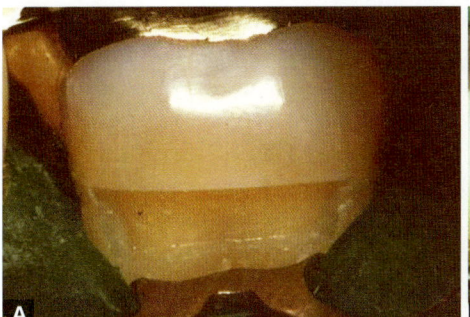
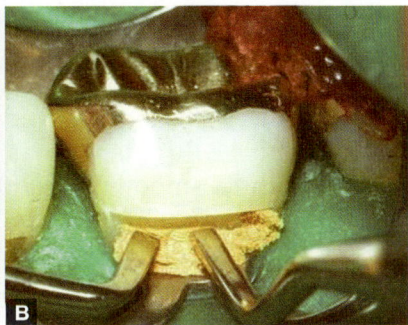
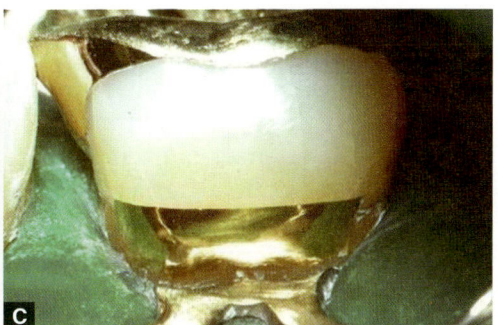

Figs 15.19A to C: **(A)** Preparation of class V cavity; **(B)** Condensation of gold foil; **(C)** Restored class V cavity

Class III Cavity

The class III preparation may be done either from the facial or lingual approach. Numerous designs such as the Ferrier design, Loma Linda design, Ingraham design, design by Lund and Baum and Woodbury design have been suggested. Preferably whenever any instrumentation or restoration of the cavity is performed, separation is done first with a Ferrier's separator. A minimal separation of 0.25 mm-0.50 mm is considered adequate. The separator should be removed as early as possible after having obtained the desired movement to prevent any damage to the supporting structures because of prolonged application.

Cavity Design by Ferrier

This design is indicated for small carious lesions when sufficient amount of thick labial, lingual and incisal walls shall remain. Access is obtained primarily from the facial approach, although lingual instrumentation may be needed in the maxillary teeth. Because of the entry being made from the facial surface, this design is indicated for those lesions that extend minimally on to the facial surface. Ferrier's design is therefore more commonly used on the distal surfaces of anterior teeth, which are less conspicuous compared to mesial.

The general outline form is roughly triangular in shape. With a No. 1 round bur, the carious lesion is approached from the facial surface. A No. 33½ inverted cone bur is used to extend the marginal outline form. End of the bur establishes the lingual wall using incisogingival strokes (The lingual wall may also be created using a wedelstedt chisel). End of the bur creates the gingival wall by it being moved labiolingually. The side of the same inverted cone bur can be used in incisogingival direction to form the facial wall.

From the facial view, gingival 4/5th of the facial margin is straight and parallel to the external contour, and in the incisal 1/5th it curves gently to meet the incisal margin. When viewed proximofacially, the facial outline follows the buccal contour of the tooth and meets the gingival margin in a slight obtuse angle. Gingival margin is straight facio-lingually and placed beneath the free gingiva if possible. It meets the facial margin in a slight obtuse angle and the lingual margin in a slight acute angle. Lingual margin is straight in its gingival 2/3rds and then curves abruptly in the incisal 1/3rd to meet the incisal angle.

The incisal margin is extended incisal to the contact area to provide access for instrumentation. It is not extended too far incisally such that it weakens the incisal edge. Incisal margin meets the facial and lingual margins in a smooth curve.

The axial wall extends 0.5 mm into dentin and is flat facio-lingually and inciso-gingivally. Resistance form is created by this flat axial wall, and slight divergence of the buccal and lingual walls to preclude any undermined enamel. Retention is provided by the inwards sloping dentinal portion of the gingival wall, i.e. an acute axiogingival line angle and an incisal undercut placed into dentin directed facio-incisally. Sharp line angles and point angles also improve upon the retention. A small bibevelled hatchet is used for establishing the incisal undercut. Small angle formers are used to sharpen the linguo-axio-gingival and facioaxio-gingival line angles and for creating the acute axio-gingival line angle.

Convenience for compaction is obtained by the abrupt linguoincisal curve and the sharp point angles. Final finishing involves planing all the preparation walls. A small hoe (6½-2½-9) is used for lingual and gingival walls, an angle former for the facial wall and an axial plane for the axial wall. Final planing of the cavosurface margins may be done with a wedelstedt chisel. A bevel is placed on all the enamel margins using a wedelstedt chisel.

Restoration

Restoration of the cavity is done with gold foil or a combination of mat gold and gold foil. The former method is described in detail. Small sized pellets (1/64 or 1/128) are selected, degassed and placed into the linguo-axio-gingival point angle with a carrying instrument. A holding instrument serves to stabilize the gold while compaction is done first by hand pressure and then by malleting. A small (0.4 mm) monoangle condenser is used for the purpose and directed from the facial surface of the adjacent tooth into the linguo-axio-gingival point angle. After the gold has been adequately compacted in this area, succeeding pellets are added onto the first pellet along the gingivo-axial line angle until 2/3rds of it is covered. A pellet of suitable size which will fit into the remaining portion of line angle is then selected and placed into position. The pellet is first cohered to the already condensed mass of gold using linguo-axiogingival forces and then wedged into the point angle using labio-axio-gingival forces. This area is best accessed and condensed with an offset plugger. In this way a completed gold tie on the gingival wall is formed.

The bulk of the restoration is built up with medium to large sized pellets (1/16-1/32) beginning in the linguo-gingival area. Bank the gingival wall and gingival half of the lingual wall using forces directed into the linguo-axio-gingival point angle. Gold is then added in a similar pattern, with the lingual wall being banked ahead of the labial. At this time, if a cavosurface margin is met with, it should be covered with gold because it would be very difficult to reach the margin at a later stage.

After the cavity has been two thirds filled, the incisal portion is restored. Building the incisal area is known as 'making the turn' and is accomplished as follows (1) Sufficient gold is built up on the remaining lingual wall such that it is very near to the incisal angle (2) Small sized pellets (1/128) are used to fill the incisal area with a right angled hand condenser (3) Gold foil pellets are compacted into the linguoincisal and incisal area with an offset condenser until the surface. In this way the incisal portion is restored from the lingual to the facial. A concavity is finally seen in the restoration facing labioproximally. This is filled with gold forces directed axially. Slight over contouring of the restoration allows for the final finishing and polishing.

A slight additional separation of the teeth may be done before beginning the finishing procedures. A spratley blade carver is moved from the restoration to the tooth surface for the purpose of burnishing. Excess gold at the contact area is removed with a gold knife thereby creating space for the introduction of interproximal finishing strips. Strips coated with cuttlefish or garnet is used in a descending grade of their abrasiveness for refining the contour and removing excess at the gingival margin. Excess at the facial and lingual proximal margins is removed either with a file moved in pull strokes or a gold knife moved in push strokes, in both cases from the restoration to the tooth. Cleoid discoid carver may also be employed. Burnishing is again performed and the final smoothening done with an extra fine cuttle strip that has been worn out. Polishing is avoided as a surface devoid of very high lustre will reflect less light and be more esthetic.

Loma Linda Design

The cavity preparation under this design is made with a lingual access. It is therefore best indicated in those areas where esthetics is the major concern and where the carious extent is such that the lingual marginal ridge is involved. Restoration of these cavities is primarily done with powdered gold and gold foil veneer.

Using a ½ round bur, the carious lesion is entered from the lingual surface and the tooth structure removed within the proposed outline at a minimum depth. Then the base of a 33½ inverted cone bur is used to establish the labial and gingival walls using incisogingival and labiolingual strokes respectively. Side of the same 33½ bur helps in creating the lingual wall. General outline of this cavity design is triangular with rounded corners. Facial outline is extended only minimally into the facial embrasure and parallels the facial contour of the tooth. Where the restoration demands high esthetics, the labial margin may be limited to within the contact area. To be precise, there is no lingual wall but just the lingual margin. It is placed far enough on to the lingual surface to include the marginal ridge and provide sufficient access to the preparation. Gingival margin is similar to the one in Ferrier's design. Incisal angle is rounded and placed on the lingual surface of the tooth.

Cavosurface bevels and flares are not needed for these preparations and the walls should terminate in butt cavosurface margins. Retention is provided by grooves in three opposing directions using a No ½ round bur to drill into the dentin. Incisal undercut is placed in an inciso-labio-axial direction. A No. 33½ inverted cone bur may also be used for placing incisal retention area in the incisal point angle. The other two grooves in the form of a cylinder (1.0-1.5 mm deep) are given on the gingival wall. Linguo-gingival retentive area is placed just inside the linguo-gingival dentino-enamel junction directed linguo-gingivoaxially. The other retentive point is placed at the facioaxio-gingival point angle and directed facially, axially and gingivally.

Planing of the walls is done with an angle former. Incisal hatchets are used in shaping and refining retentive areas. All the line angles in the cavity preparation are accentuated with the sharp end of an angle former.

Restoration

The following section describes restoration of the cavity with powdered gold and gold foil. A matrix is indicated only when the facial wall extends considerably facially. Matricing involves inserting a wedge from the labial embrasure apical to the gingival cavosurface margin. Heated and softened guttapercha is then inserted into the cavity from the lingual side until excess appears on the facial side. Self curing acrylic resin in the doughy stage is then adapted on to the facial surfaces of teeth. Facial portion of the acrylic should be approximately 4 mm thick, extending onto at least three teeth and slightly covering the incisal edges for retention. Guttapercha is then removed after the resin has hardened thereby leaving behind an acrylic matrix.

The first pellet of powdered gold is degassed and placed over the inciso-labio-axial point angle. The pellet is compacted with stepping and rocking hand pressure. Succeeding pellets are added along the labioaxial line angle until the opposing labio-gingivoaxial point angle is covered. This creates a gold tie between two opposing undercuts. Incisal half of the gold tie is condensed with forces directed inciso-labioaxially and the gingival half with forces directed labiogingivo- axially. Gold is firmly compacted against the labial wall. The bulk of the cavity is then filled in a labio-lingual direction, banking the incisal, labial and most of the gingival wall. A pellet of desirable size is then selected for the remaining portion of the gingivoaxial line angle and placed into position. It is adapted to the already condensed mass of gold using labioaxio- gingival forces and into the point angle using linguo-gingivo-axial forces. The pellet gets wedged into the retentive area and the remaining portion of the gingival wall is hence banked. Whenever a cavosurface margin is reached it is covered with gold at that time itself. A concavity is produced in the restoration which faces linguoproximally. It is best filled with gold foil using labio-inciso-axial pressure for the incisal half and linguo-axio-gingival pressure for the gingival half. The matrix is removed by cutting through the incisal portion of the acrylic. Restoration is finally finished and polished as mentioned before.

Ingraham Design

This cavity design is indicated primarily for the incipient proximal lesions in anterior teeth where esthetics is the major concern. Maintenance of oral hygiene and low caries and plaque indices are essential requirements when using this design.

The general form of the cavity is parallelogram in shape. Labial margin is placed within the contact area so that it is not visible externally. The gingival margin clears the contact area and extends minimally into the gingival embrasure. Incisal margin is also limited to within the contact area. The lingual margin extends on to the lingual surface past the lingual marginal ridge to provide access for instrumentation. Axial wall is flat, forms a right angle to the labial wall and opens directly on to the lingual surface of the tooth. Retention grooves are placed on the inciso-axial and gingivoaxial line angles such that their depth decreases towards the lingual surface. This would mean that the undercuts are deeper towards the labial position of the line angle compared to the lingual portions.

The carious lesion is entered with a No. 1 round bur from the lingual access. No. 168 bur is moved labially, inciso-gingivally and axially to remove tooth structure in the proposed outline (Figs 15.20A). The incisal and gingival walls are planed with a hatchet. Labial wall is flattened utilizing the same hatchet in lateral strokes. Incisal and gingival retention grooves are cut at the expense of incisal and gingival walls respectively with an inverted cone bur. The sharp end of a gingival marginal trimmer is used to accentuate the line angles and retentive grooves. Bevel may be placed on all the margins using the sides of a gingival marginal trimmer.

Restoration

The following restorative technique describes the use of mat gold and gold foil in the Ingraham cavity design. A piece of mat gold is cut to the shape and dimensions of the labial wall, degassed and placed onto it. Parallelogram condensers are used to lightly adapt the gold to the cavity wall. Heavy compaction with rocking motion followed by malleting wedges the gold firmly between two opposing walls. This is followed by placement of the gold foil in the incisolabial corner which is cohered to the already compacted gold in this area. Similarly, gold pellets are placed and cohered to the gold in the gingivolabial corner. In this way, all of the labial wall and most of the incisal and gingival walls are banked. Whenever a cavosurface margin is encountered during the process, it should be covered immediately, because it is difficult to be reached at a later stage. Finally a concavity in the gold is left facing linguoproximally. This is filled to a slightly higher level using incisoaxial and gingivoaxial pressure. The restoration is burnished, finished and polished (Fig. 15.20B).

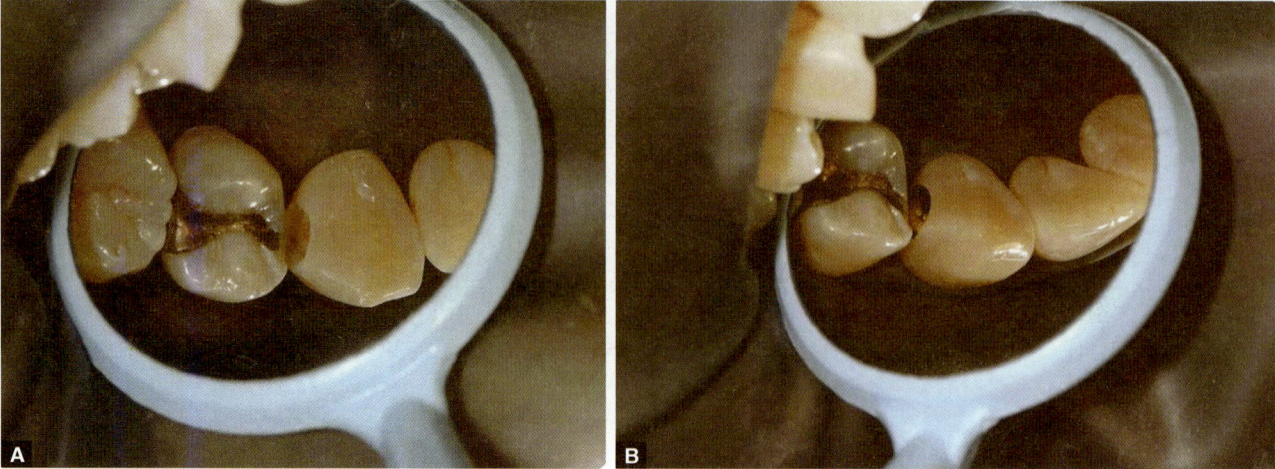

Figs 15.20A and B: **(A)** Preparation of class III cavity; **(B)** Restored class III cavity

Class II Cavity

Preparation

The outline form is similar in size and shape to the preparation for amalgam. Cavity extension is minimal but should be large enough to include all of the defect and allow proper instrumentation and manipulation. Marginal outline form is represented by straight lines and definite curves. It should cover all the faulty pits and fissures also. The occlusal portion of the class II preparation is similar to the class I cavity as described before. The tooth on the occlusal surface is entered with a No. 1 or 2 round bur and the cavity form extended with a No. 169 tapering fissure.

The proximal box is placed in dentin and is in the form of a cone. The width of the proximal box at the gingival portion is only slightly greater than at the occlusal portion. All the walls of the proximal box are extended minimally in their respective embrasures. With the same No. 169 bur, a drop is made at the dentinoenamel junction on the proximal part uptil the anticipated gingival depth. Moving the bur labiolingually and incisoaxially, the tooth structure is removed within the planned outline. The proximal walls are finally cut and planed with a No.10-7-8 binangled chisel for maxillary and 10-7-14 hatchet for mandibular preparations. A No. 33½ inverted cone bur establishes a flat gingival wall and a 10-4-8 hoe smoothens the pulpal and gingival floors.

Retention is provided by sharp line angles and point angles. Here it differs from an amalgam preparation which has slightly rounded angles. These angles are accentuated with Nos. 10-80-8-14 and 10-95-8-14 gingival marginal trimmers. Additional retention if desired is given at the facioaxial and linguoaxial line angles in the form a long triangular groove, i.e. base of the triangle is towards the gingival portion of the line angle and the apex is towards the occlusal portion of the line angle. Cavosurface bevels of 30–40° is placed on all the margins compared to an amalgam preparation which ends in butt joints (Fig. 15.21A).

Restoration

A matrix is necessary for restoring class II preparations which would serve as a proximal support. A small shim steel matrix band which extends 1.0 mm above the marginal ridge and 2.0-3.0 mm beyond the proximal contact is placed interproximally. T band is then wrapped around both the shim and the tooth. The matrix is secured with a wedge inserted from the lingual or palatal side. Acrylic resin in the doughy stage is adapted and wedged into the facial and lingual embrasures such that the matrix does not move. Finally, the shim band is removed with pliers so as to provide a small space at the margins where the gold can be condensed.

Restoration of the cavity is described using a combination of mat gold and gold foil. Piece of mat gold cut to the size and shape of the gingival wall is degassed and placed into position by a carrying instrument. It is thoroughly condensed first by hand pressure and later by malleting, into the line and point angles and against the margins. Another pellet is placed against the facial wall of the proximal box and condensed against the wall, cavosurface margin and retention groove. Similarly condensation is done on the lingual wall of the proximal box. This creates a concavity while building the restoration. Proximal portion of the cavity is continued to fill until just slightly above the pulpal floor. Next the occlusal portion is built together with the proximal portion.

Direct Filling Gold

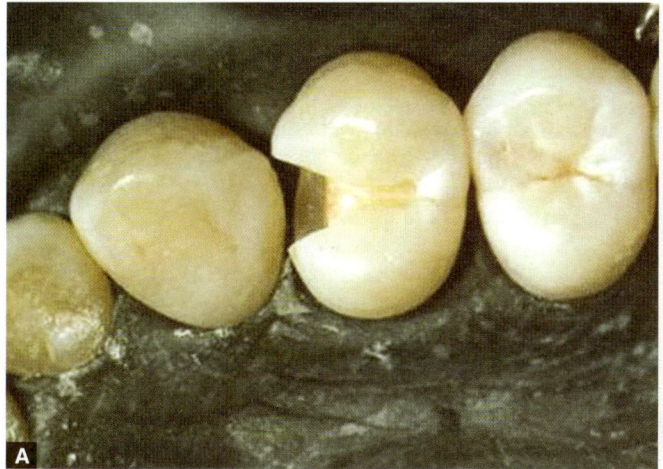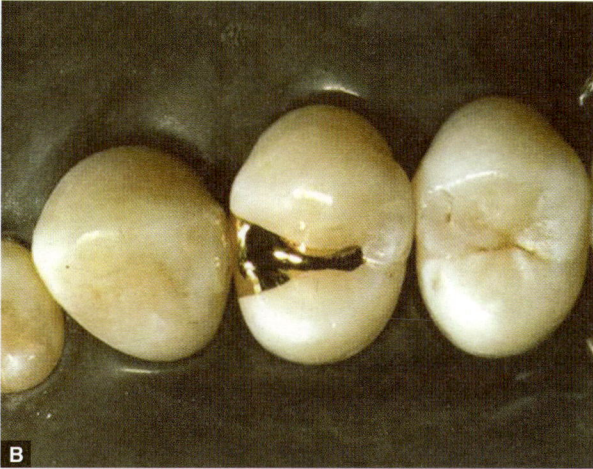

Figs 15.21A and B: **(A)** Preparation of class II cavity; **(B)** Restored class II cavity

Gold is placed and condensed over the entire pulpal floor. Small pieces are condensed against all walls of the occlusal step and the proximal matrix. Filling is continued in a concave form until the cavity is 2/3rd full. The remaining portion of the cavity is filled with gold foil to a slightly higher level using the same principles as mentioned before.

After the cavity has been completely filled, the acrylic is cut through and the two portions pushed apart. Wedge is removed followed by the band. The restoration is burnished, contoured and polished similar to as mentioned before for the class I and class III restorations (Fig. 15.21B).

Summarizing the Advantages and Disadvantages of a Direct Filling Gold Restoration

Advantages

1. A permanent method for repairing teeth, and the restoration can last as long as the tooth itself.
2. A noble metal hence does not tarnish and corrode in the oral cavity.
3. Insoluble and has a coefficient of thermal expansion close to that of tooth.
4. The cavity preparation when kept ideally small is atraumatic to the dental pulp and supporting structures.
5. Tooth discoloration does not occur around the margins because of good material adaptation and its noble and inert qualities.
6. No cementing medium is necessary for retention of the restoration.
7. The surface can be effectively polished and the smoothness can last indefinitely reducing the chances of plaque accumulation.
8. Pure gold is ductile and hence can be burnished to produce an accurate margin for the restoration.
9. The density and hardness of compacted gold enables the restoration to withstand compressive forces sufficiently.
10. The restoration procedure develops skills of the operator in other dental procedures also.
11. Most efficiently sealing permanent restorative material.

Disadvantages

1. Unesthetic
2. Expensive
3. Long chairside time required for restoration
4. Use limited to conservative cavities
5. High thermal conductivity could lead to postoperative sensitivity
6. Technique sensitive
7. High condensation forces may injure the tooth and supporting structures.

BIBLIOGRAPHY

1. Alperstein, K.S., Yearwood, L. and Boston, D.: E-Z Gold: The new Goldent. Oper. Dent. 21, 36, 1996.
2. Balzig, P. and Gagro, D.: The use of gold foil in restorative dentistry: Acta. Stomatol. Croat. 20, 239, 1986.
3. Baum, L.: Gold foil (filling gold) in dental practice. D.C.N.A., p. 109, 1965.
4. Baum, L.: Gold foil. Oper. Dent., 9, 42, 1984.
5. Billing, R.J. and Simmons, F.F. Jr.: A survey of gold foil use among Texas dentists. Tex. Dent. J., 99, 25, 1981.
6. Birkett, G.H.: Is there a future for Gold foil. Oper. Dent.: 20, 41, 1985.
7. Dowden, W.E. and Langeland, K.: An evaluation and comparison of the pulpal response to gold foil and indium alloy. J.P.D. 50, 497, 1983.
8. Ferrier, W.I.: The use of gold foil in general practice. J.A.D.A., 28, 691, 1941.

9. Germain, H.A.S.T., Jr. and Rusz, J.E. Jr.: Restoring Class 6 abrasion/erosion lesions with direct gold. Oper. Dent. 21, 49, 1996.
10. Harken, B.J.: Gold foil: A potential practice builder in the 80s. Oper. Dent. 10, 28, 1985.
11. Henry, D. : Gold foil restorations : An old friend whose time has come again. Todays FDA : 13, 24, 2001.
12. Hodson, J.T.: Structure and properties of gold foil and matgold. J.D.R. 42, 575, 1963.
13. Iwaku, M., Nagata, N., Hosoda, H. and Fusayama, T.: Edge strength of powdered gold fillings. J.D.R. 48, 1468, 1966.
14. Lambert, R.L.: A survey of the teaching of compacted gold. Oper. Dent. 5, 20, 1980.
15. Leach, C.D. and Grubb, R.: Diamond working faces on gold foil condenser points. Oper. Dent. 8, 42, 1983.
16. Lund, M.R. and Baum, L.: Powdered gold as a restorative material. J.P.D., 13, 1151, 1963.
17. Margetis, M. : Gold foil restorations. J.A.D.A. : 133, 686, 2002.
18. O'Connel, M.A.: Gold foil: Is it a health hazard or a superior material. Dent. Stud., 59, 41, 1980.
19. Richter, W.A. and Mahler, D.B.: Physical properties vs. Clinical performance of pure gold restorations. J.P.D. 29, 434, 1973.
20. Stibbs, G.D.: Manipulation of cohesive gold foil in dental restorations. Oper. Dent. 10, 49, 1985.
21. Stibbs, G.D.: Direct gold in dental restorative therapy. Oper. Dent. 5, 107, 1980.
22. Thomas, J.J., Stanley, H.R. and Gilman, H.W.: Effects of gold foil condensation on human dental pulp. J.A.D.A. 78, 788, 1969.
23. Thomas, J.J.: Gold foil as a teaching material. Oper. Dent., 7, 107, 1982.
24. Wolcott, R.B. and Vermetti, J.P.: Sintered gold alloy for direct restorations. J.P.D., 25, 662, 1971.

Bonding in Dentistry

One major problem in restorative dentistry is the lack of proper union between the restorative material and the tooth surface. The gap at the tooth-restoration interface may create problems such as sensitivity and recurrent caries, etc. subsequently failure of the restoration. The processes of inventions over a period of time have led to the development of various techniques and modalities, which help in adhesion/bonding. Bonding or adhesion may be physical, mechanical or chemical and such restorations are known as bonded restorations or adhesive restorations. However, the continuous search to minimize the restoration - tooth interface has not been able to achieve complete success because of many inherent weaknesses of restorative materials like setting/polymerization expansion/contraction, different coefficients of thermal expansion and modulus of elasticity, etc.

Bonding improves retention and stabilization of a restoration without excessive removal of sound tooth structure. The need for providing auxiliary retentive aids is eliminated. Adhesive restorations are better able to transmit and distribute functional stresses across the bonding interface thereby reinforcing weakened tooth tissue. Bonding also facilitates repair and replacement of deteriorated fillings with little or no additional removal of tooth structure.

Adhesive techniques have greatly expanded the horizon of aesthetic dentistry. Correction of shapes, positions, dimensions and shades of teeth is now possible with the adhesive restorative materials. Repair of fractured teeth can be carried out using the same fractured fragments thereby maintaining original aesthetics. Bonding successfully reduces the extent and amount of microleakage. Preventing the ingress of oral fluids and bacteria along the cavity-restoration interface reduces most clinical problems such as post-operative sensitivity, marginal staining and recurrent caries.

Adhesive agents are also useful in other clinical situations as in luting porcelain, composite or metal inlays, onlays, crowns, veneers, fixed partial dentures, resin bonded prosthesis, etc. These agents can also be employed for treating dentin hypersensitivity, as pit and fissure sealants, in direct pulp capping procedures and beneath amalgam restorations as insulators. Before studying the bonding agents, let us discuss the basic principles involved in bonding phenomenon.

DEFINITIONS

Adhesion is the force or the intermolecular attraction that exists between molecules of two unlike substances when placed in intimate contact with each other. The substance added to produce the adhesion is known as the '*adhesive*' and the material to which it applied is known as the '*adherend*' (Fig. 16.1). An interface is present wherever adhesion exists. Adhesion can be seen between any two phases, e.g. solid, liquid or gas with the exception of two gases where an interface is not present. Most commonly, a solid is the adherend and liquid is the adhesive.

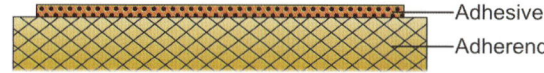

Fig. 16.1: Adhesive and the adherend

TYPES

Adhesion in dentistry is of three types and involves the following mechanisms:
a. *Chemical adhesion* is based on primary valence forces such as covalent, ionic or metallic bonds.
b. *Physical adhesion* relies on secondary valence forces. Such forces occur at molecular dipoles (van der Waals forces), the interaction of induced dipoles (dispersion forces) or electron clouds (hydrogen bonds).
c. *Mechanical adhesion* relies on penetration of one material into a different material at a microscopic level. The formation of hybridized dentin is regarded as a form of mechanical adhesion in the

sense that resin polymers become entangled with collagen fibrils.

Certain authors have the wrong conception that an adhesive bond is primarily a chemical bond. Most adhesives, however, rely on van der Waal's forces plus whatever mechanical adhesion they can achieve. If the surface is rough and porous, the mechanical adhesion will predominate. If the surfaces are smooth and polished, van der Waal's forces are effective. Although theoretically, an adhesive bond that sets up by primary chemical bonding should reveal higher adhesive strength than one that relies on van der Waal's bonds; but in practice, the primary bonds are susceptible to attack by water, and often prove weaker than the van der Waal's bonds.

FACTORS AFFECTING ADHESION

The phenomenon of adhesion is dependent upon certain factors. The three factors, surface energy, wetting and contact angle are important determinants of adhesion. Not only do they individually control adhesion but are also closely interrelated.

a. *Surface Energy*: The energy of a solid on the outer surface is comparatively higher than its interior. Inside the crystal, each atom is equally surrounded by atoms on all sides and the inter-atomic distances are equal, hence the energy is minimal; whereas, towards the periphery, the atoms are not equally distributed. The surface atoms get strongly attracted to each other resulting in surface tension. Because of this energy, substances are attracted to the substrate surface, for example, silver, gold and platinum attract oxygen molecules to their surface. With gold, oxygen adheres by secondary forces, whereas with silver chemical forces exist forming silver oxide. The adhesive can attach to the adherend either by physical or chemical force. Initially when the two substances are far apart, only physical forces exist between them but as the distance diminishes, chemical forces start becoming effective. In practice, when two attracting molecules are separated by a distance that exceeds their own approximate diameter, the distance usually being 3.0-4.0 nm, they no longer show any appreciable attraction. Hard solids have specific free surface energy values between 500-5000 ergs/cm². Harder the surface, higher is the surface energy and higher the adhesive properties.

b. *Wetting*: Wetting can be illustrated by a simple experiment in which two glass slides, however polished they may be, when placed in close contact with each other do not exhibit any attachment. This owes to the presence of micro irregularities on the slides and is responsible for the two surfaces contacting only at their 'high spots' or 'hills'. The total surface area in contact is decreased and hence no perceptible adhesion takes place. Whereas if a film of water is placed between them, it becomes increasingly difficult to separate the two. For producing such type of adhesion, the liquid must easily flow over the entire surface and adhere to the solid. This characteristic is referred to as *wetting*. The wetting ability of a liquid adhesive depends upon the surface energy and cleanliness of the adherend. Higher the surface energy, greater would be the wetting capability. Metals generally have a high surface energy. On the other hand, teflon (polytetra-fluoroethylene) synthetic resin has a comparatively very low surface energy. Contamination of the substrate surface also reduces wetting by the adhesive.

c. *Contact angle*: Contact angle is an important factor in controlling adhesion. *It is a measure of wettability and is the angle formed by the adhesive with the adherend at the interface* (Figs 16.2A to C). Smaller the contact angle greater is the wettability of the adhesive.

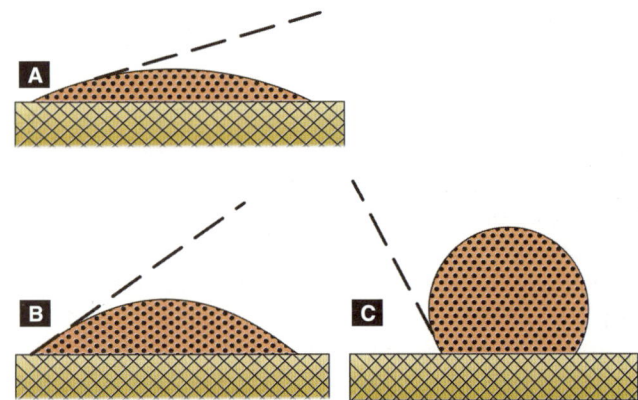

Figs 16.2A to C: Degree of contact angle influences the wetting of surface; **(A)** When contact angle is small, wettability of the adhesive is better; **(B)** and **(C)** When contact angle is large, liquid does not wet the surface completely

A low viscosity of the adhesive is imperative for better flow and bond formation. However, micro-irregularities and crevices still remain a limiting factor in close bond formation because air may be entrapped at the base of the pockets and serve as discontinuities in the adhesive joint (Fig. 16.3). Under continual thermal and mechanical loading, stress concentration occurs around these sites and a break could be initiated adjacent to the void, which could then propagate unhindered.

Many a times, there is only mechanical union between two surfaces. This type of union refers to the attachment of two substances by mechanical means rather than molecular bonding. At a gross

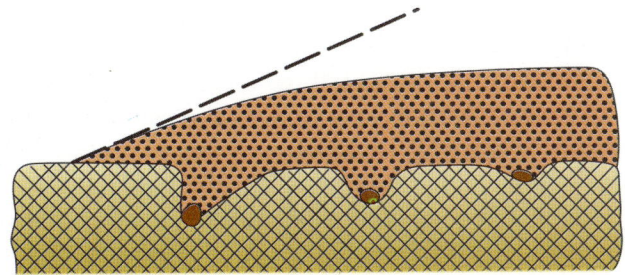

Fig. 16.3: Air incorporated in the irregularities at the interface despite low contact angle of the adhesive. Such areas are points of stress concentration and promote adhesive failure

level, examples include screws, bolts or undercuts. Retention of cast gold restoration using luting cement is also dependent on the amount of mechanical union between the two surfaces.

TOOTH AS A SUBSTRATE FOR BONDING

The tooth surface, when used as a substrate for bonding generally comprises of two components: enamel and dentin. Though bonding to enamel is effectively achieved in clinical practice, similar level of adhesion to dentin poses difficulties. Significant contrast in composition and structure of enamel and dentin greatly influence the prospects of bonding. Both organic and inorganic components vary in both the tissues.

Within the same tissue, nature of the substrate presented for bonding may vary with the location, e.g. enamel etched on its rod ends provide better area for bonding compared to enamel etched on the side of the prisms. Fluoridated enamel has a low surface energy and is more difficult to bond compared to the nonfluoridated enamel. Dentin in its superficial portion allows greater bond strengths than in the deeper portions. This might be because the superficial layer has more of solid dentin and less moisture contamination as compared to deeper portions. Sclerotic areas present difficulties in bonding compared to natural tubular dentin.

The presence of moisture in dentin is the major hurdle in achieving bonding. The inherent wetness owes to the outward flow of the dentinal fluid under positive pulpal pressure. Occasionally, moisture may be seen on the surface of dentin due to external factors like accidental contamination by saliva and/or air humidity. In order to obtain a stable and long lasting bond to wet dentin, it is essential that the adhesive displace or be miscible in the fluid in areas where the dentin is most permeable. Furthermore, such a bond must be maintained in a continuously aqueous environment. Dentin permeability is more towards the pulp horns and near the pulp because of an increase in tubule density and diameter respectively. Permeability reduces with the presence of intra tubular deposits, tubule irregularities, etc.

An important factor that influences the bonding to tooth surface is the presence of smear layer on cut dentin. The smear unit (smear layer + smear plugs) may serve as a contaminant and prevent adequate penetration of the adhesive into the underlying substrate. On the contrary, some believe that it acts as a protective barrier to the pulp by minimizing leakage of bacterial and other substances.

REQUISITE OF AN IDEAL BONDING AGENT

- Should be biocompatible
- Should bond effectively to both enamel and dentin
- Should have sufficient strength to resist failure as a result of masticatory forces
- Should have mechanical properties close to tooth structure
- Should be resistant to degradation in oral environment
- Should be easy to use

CONDITIONING ENAMEL AND ETCHING

Enamel surfaces generally have a low surface energy, are inert, reactive and under normal circumstances maintain homeostasis with the surroundings. Untouched enamel is covered by a predominantly organic layer, comprised of adsorbed proteins most of which originate from the saliva. This organic bio film is referred to as the *pellicle*. Enamel when ground, is also covered by a protein rich film called the *smear layer*. Both pellicle and smear layer are considered as surface contaminants which differ from their subsurface in composition and structural arrangement. In stagnant sites, these protein biofilms on enamel may attract micro-organisms forming plaque. It is, therefore, quite evident that untreated enamel presents a far less than ideal surface for establishing strong durable bonds. The objective is to remove the contaminants and subsequently raise the energy and reactivity of the enamel surfaces. *The procedure that leads to this removal of organic layer, making the enamel surface more reactive is known as 'conditioning'. The procedure that leads to demineralization of superficial calcium ion is known as 'etching'.*

A thorough dental prophylaxis for removing materia alba, plaque and other accretions is an important component of the conditioning etching regime. It has been observed that prophylaxis alone can double the bond strength. The prophylaxis pastes devoid of oils, flavouring agents and fluorides are recommended for this purpose. Rubber cups are preferred as they are less likely to damage gingival tissue or abrade enamel. After cleaning, the enamel is thoroughly washed with water, the treatment site dried and carefully isolated from oral fluids like saliva and gingival crevicular fluid. Ever since Buonocore (1955) used phosphoric acid for conditioning/etching enamel, researchers have tried various concentration of phosphoric acid in the form of liquid or gel, alternative acids and varying etching times. Less concentration of acid for smaller period of time is used for conditioning while the higher concentration of the same acid for longer period is used for etching. Following acid application for stipulated period, the area is thoroughly washed for 10–15 seconds to remove the acid, its reaction products and mineral hydroxyapatite. In case gels are used, the washing time is doubled so as to flush away its cellulose vehicle which otherwise might serve as a contaminant. An effectively etched surface on drying gives a matt white or frosted appearance. Since the etched surface at this stage has a very high surface energy, a contaminant can readily adhere to the surface. Even a minor exposure to saliva, blood or oil can ruin the potential for resin tag formation and bonding. All measures should therefore be taken to prevent any contamination. If accidental contamination occurs, the procedure should be repeated.

Acid conditioning/etching affects the enamel in the following ways:

- Removes residual pellicle to expose the inorganic crystallite component of enamel.
- Removes approximately 10 μm of surface enamel
- Creates a porous layer, the depth of the pores range from 5.0-50.0 μm. When a low viscosity resin is subsequently applied, it flows into the microporosities and polymerizes to form resin tags.
- Increases the wettability and surface area of the enamel substrate.
- Raises the surface energy of enamel with creation of reactive polar sites.

Three patterns of etching in enamel have been observed.

Type I: Most common etching pattern, involves the preferential removal of enamel prism cores with prism peripheries remaining relatively intact.

Type II: Etching pattern is the reverse of type I, i.e. the peripheries are removed leaving the cores intact.

Type III: Etching pattern is less distinct, and includes areas resembling type I and type II patterns as well as regions in which the etching pattern appears unrelated to prism morphology. This type of etching is generally associated with the presence of prismless enamel.

Recently type IV and type V patterns have been added. Type IV pattern displayed only a random distribution of depressions with no preferential destruction of either cores or peripheries. These pitted areas occasionally occurred in little patches over the enamel surface. This type of etching pattern is commonly seen in cervical areas and rarely on occlusal. Similarly to type IV pattern, type V etching shows no evidence of prism outline. The regions of enamel are flat and smooth and lack micro irregularities for penetration of resin. Such type is seen in high fluoride areas.

Resin tags which form in the enamel rod peripheries, i.e. between enamel prisms are known as *macrotags*. A much finer network of thousands of small tags form across the end of each rod where individual hyrodxyapatite crystals have been dissolved leaving crypts outlined by residual organic matter. These fine tags are called *microtags*. Both macro tags and microtags are the basis of micromechanical bonding to enamel (Figs 16.4 and 16.5). Microtags are essentially more important because of their larger number and also they offer greater surface area of contact. It is established that when enamel prisms are exposed perpendicularly, the bond strength is reduced to 50% compared with the parallel exposure of the prisms.

Phosphoric Acid as an Etchant

37% phosphoric acid is the most commonly used acid for etching. At concentrations greater than 50 percent, there occurs formation of a layer of monocalcium

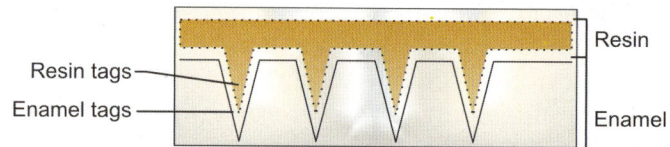

Fig. 16.4: Resin tags and enamel tags aid in microm-mechanical bonding

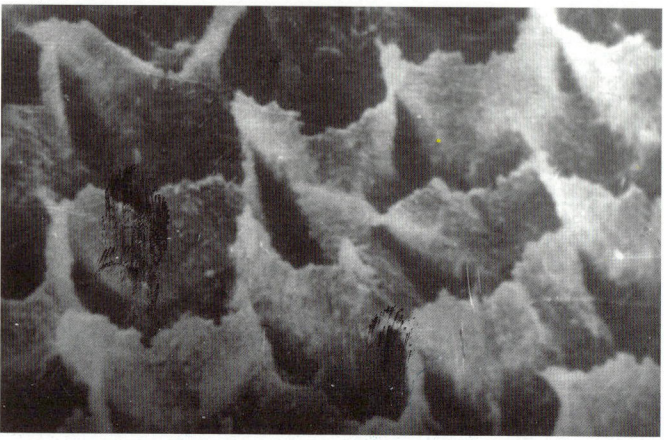

Fig. 16.5: Enamel tags in which resin tags will fit

phosphate monohydrate on etched surface which prevents any further dissolution, whereas below 30 percent there forms a precipitate of dicalcium phosphate dihydrate that cannot be easily removed. Higher concentration of acid produces deeper tags, which being brittle give way leaving 10–25 μm depth similar to as obtained with the lower concentration of the acid. It is accepted that 30–40% concentration of the acid is the most effective.

Acid etchants are available in liquid and gel form (Fig. 16.6). Gel etchants are preferred because of the ease and control of placement. However, etching pattern with gel and liquid remains the same. Gels are often made by adding colloidal silica or polymer beads to the acid. These additives change the pH of these acids. They are applied to the surface either with a brush or dispensed through a syringe onto the enamel.

The time for etching with 30% to 40% phosphoric acid has been recommended as 15 seconds. Studies with scanning electron microscopy have confirmed that 15 seconds etching provides the same surface roughness as 60 seconds. And also, similar shear bond strengths and marginal leakage values for 15 and 60 seconds have been observed. However, enamel which is acid resistant because of a high fluoride content can be etched for 60 seconds. Primary teeth also require longer etching time since the enamel is more aprismatic than that of permanent teeth.

Alternative acids have been tried as enamel etchants, mainly pyruvic acid and sulphuric acid. 2.0% sulphuric acid used for 30 seconds has shown to be as effective as phosphoric acid, where as higher sulphuric acid concentrations produce heavy crystal deposits which interfere with bonding and cannot be washed away easily. With the present concept of total

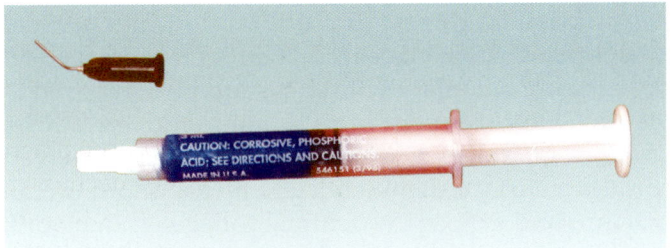

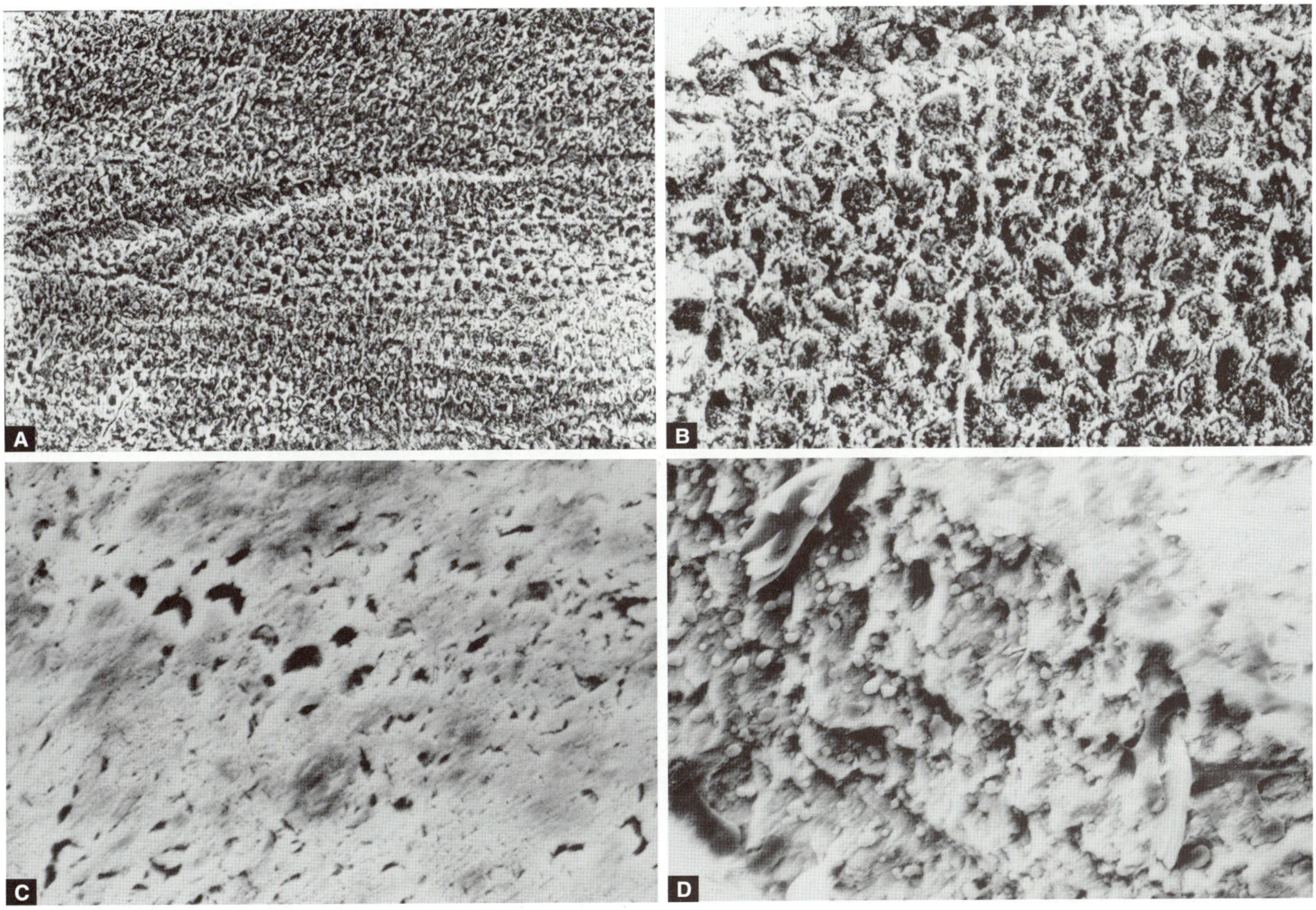

Fig. 16.6: Gel etchant

Figs 16.7A to D: SEM images of etched enamel surface: **(A)** SEM view of enamel surface etched for 15 seconds (surface view); **(B)** SEM view of enamel surface etched for 15 seconds (oblique section); **(C)** SEM view of enamel surface etched for 60 seconds (surface view); **(D)** SEM view of enamel surface etched for 60 seconds (oblique section)

etch techniques, acids such as 10% phosphoric acid, 10% maleic acid, 2.5% nitric acid, citric acid, oxalic acid, etc. are used to etch both enamel and dentin simultaneously. However, weaker acids provide significantly lower shear bond strengths.

The bonding agent and low viscosity monomers are then flown over the etched enamel. It is believed that when applied to clean, dried and conditioned enamel, the bonding agent because of its low viscosity rapidly wets and penetrates into the micro spaces forming resin tags. The resin also forms an extremely close physical relationship with the enamel crystallites and often encapsulates them to form a composite zone in the outer enamel. The bonding agent may be chemically cured or light cured. Subsequent application of composite restorative resin then becomes continuous with the resin bonding agent. Bond strengths to acid conditioned enamel using these early adhesive agents have been reported to be in the range of 16–21 MPa. Over the period, bond strengths have been greatly improved and may be attributed to better wetting solvent agents, improved resin chemistry that allow complete polymerization of the adhesive and better water stability at the interface. Enamel bonding agents have been replaced by the same systems that are used on dentin as they facilitate simultaneous bonding to both enamel and dentin.

Though acid conditioning remains the most popular method of bonding composite resin to enamel, other methods have also been tried. One such method which was tried was depositing calcium sulphate crystals on the surface of enamel by treatment with a solution of polyacrylic acid and potassium sulphate. It was suggested that these crystals trapped resin to retain it mechanically. However, subsequent work showed etched surface under the solution and these crystals to interfere with bonding. Recently, 'Lasers' have been used for enamel/dentin etching. Laser etching is a process of continuous vaporization and micro explosions due to vaporization of water trapped within the hydroxyapatite matrix. In general, more material is removed by the micro-explosion of entrapped water than by direct vaporization of the hydroxyapatite crystals. The amount of surface roughening is dependent upon the type and wavelength of the laser. CO_2 and Nd:YAG are most effective Lasers for etching. It is observed that changes in surface morphology and bond strength after Laser etching are similar to acid etching.

BONDING TO DENTIN

Dentin bonding is comparatively difficult because of the fact that dentin is a complex tissue and contains plenty of fluids. Because of the vast structural and functional variations between the dentin and enamel, bonding to each is not similar.

Dentin is a living tissue and is directly connected to the pulp through fluid filled channels that contain odontoblastic processes, the body of which lie in the pulp. Along with the chemical issue of adhesion, biologic concern of pulpal compatibility becomes exceedingly important when dentin is concerned. 37% phosphoric acid when used to etch both enamel and dentin did not lead to pulpal damage.

Treatment of Dentin for Optimal Bonding

The characteristics of successful bonding of a resin composite to dentin includes micromechanical attachment between resin and demineralized, primed layer of intertubular dentin. This complex, referred to as the *hybrid layer*, is best achieved by acidic conditioning agents which remove the smear layer, produce surface demineralization to a depth of 3.0-6.0 µms and expose the dentinal collagen framework. In some cases, the smear layer is not removed but rather dissolved or modified to include it within the bonding process. Application of hydrophilic resin primers facilitates subsequent penetration of low viscosity adhesive resins into the microporous collagen scaffold and dentinal tubules. Polymerization of this infilterated resin stabilizes the surface hybrid layer. Meticulous application of these steps lead to a gap free bond.

Other areas of concern during dentinal bonding are the complex histological structure and variable composition of dentin at different locations. It consists of 50 Vol% of inorganic content, 30 vol% of organic material, and 20 Vol% of fluid. The high protein content is responsible for the low surface energy of dentin (44.8 dynes/cm^2), which differentiates it from etched enamel. Wetting of such a low energy surface is difficult vis-à-vis the adhesion. Further, water is an essential component of natural dentin and surface drying is difficult to achieve. Rewetting of the surface, which may be subclinical, occurs instantaneously. The bonding is difficult in aqueous environment, since water competes effectively for all the adhesion sites.

Role of Smear Layer in Dentin Bonding

Smear layer is a product of dental instrumentation, which covers the normal structural components of dentin by 1-2 µms and penetrates several micrometers (1–5 µms) into the tubules to form smear plugs. It has two phases, a solid phase made up of cutting debris - primarily denatured collagen and mineral, and a liquid phase made up to tortuous fluid filled channels around the cutting debris. Smear layer, may also be a deterrent to the bonding process, since it may serve as a barrier to the penetration of resin to the underlying dentin substrate (Fig. 16.8). Bacteria entrapped in the smear layer can survive and multiply beneath the restoration. A few authors, however, believe it to be a protective barrier against bacterial and toxin penetration.

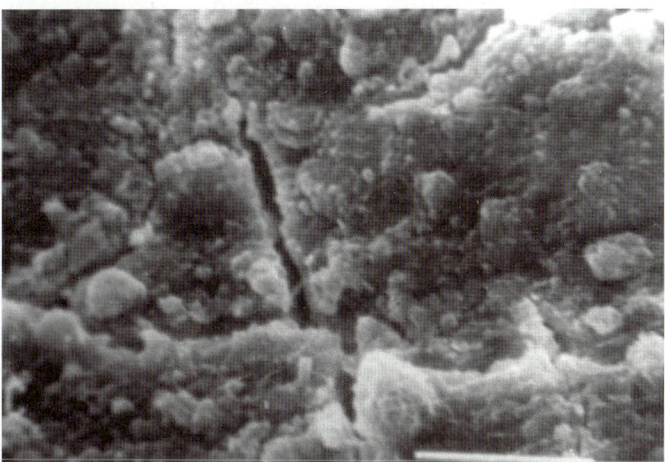

Fig. 16.8: Presence of smear layer on cut tooth surface

Reasons for retaining smear layer on the bonding substrate are:
- Retention of smear layer lowers dentin permeability
- Prevents decrease in bond strength seen with some bonding systems as deeper dentin is prepared
- Greatly lowers the effect of pulpal pressure on bond strength.

Recent generation of dentin adhesives involves modification of the smear layer as it is believed to greatly improve the bond strength to dentin. The removal of smear layer and demineralization of dentin matrix may facilitate bonding through a number of mechanisms like:
- The exposed collagen provides reactive groups that can chemically interact with primers.
- Amino groups may act as a catalyst to polymerization reactions.
- Exposed collagen promotes micro mechanical bonding to resin by providing a framework.

It is quite probable that all three mechanisms operate simultaneously to improve bonding.

Conditioning of Dentin

Conditioning of dentin is defined as an alteration of the dentin surface including the smear layer with the objective of producing a substrate capable of micromechanical and possibly chemical bonding to a dentin adhesive. The principal effects of conditioning on dentin can be physical or chemical. Physical effects are the alteration in the thickness and morphology of the smear layer and also the dentinal tubules whereas chemical effects are modifications of the fraction of organic matter and decalcification of the inorganic portion. Conditioning can be performed by chemical, thermal or mechanical means.

A. Chemical Conditioning

Both acids and calcium chelators, which rely on removing the smear layer are used as chemical conditioners.

i. *Acid conditioners*: Acid conditioners are employed with the objective of not only removing the smear layer but also simultaneously demineralizing superficial dentin (3-6 μms) to expose a microporous collagen scaffold into which the resin will penetrate. On intertubular dentin, the exposed collagen fibers are often additionally covered by an amorphous layer which is of variable thickness and has microporosities, having been ascribed to combined effect of denaturation and collapse of residual smear layer collagen. This '*collagen smear layer*' may reduce the permeability of underlying dentin to resin monomers, and is insoluble in acids. At the tubule orifices, peritubular dentin is often completely dissolved to form a funnel shape structure and expose collagen fibrils which are often additional retentive sites at the tubule wall (Figs 16.9 A to D). After conditioning, maintenance of a moist dentin surface is recommended, following the wet bonding technique to prevent collapse of unsupported collagen and promote wetting and infiltration of subsequently applied resin.

37% phosphoric acid is routinely used. 10% phosphoric acid appears to provide better bond strength than the higher concentrations. Dentin bonding agents (e.g. Tenure, Mirage bond) that use nitric acid conditioners are highly adhesive

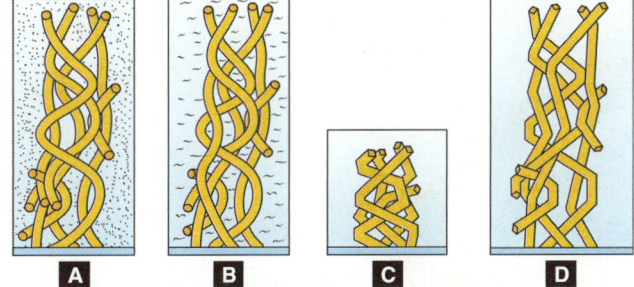

Figs 16.9A to D: Schematic representation of dentin matrix: **(A)** Mineralised dentin matrix; **(B)** Demineralised dentin matrix filled with water, i.e. in a plasticized state; **(C)** Collapsed, stiffened, air dried demineralized dentin matrix and; **(D)** Demineralized dentin matrix stiffened by organic solvent prior to air drying

and provide good tubule seals. 10% citric acid combined with 3% ferric chloride is used as a smear layer remover and etchant. Another combination etchant is 10% citric acid and 20% calcium chloride (e.g. Clearfil Liner Bond). Compared to the phosphoric acid etching (Figs 16.10A), this combination etchant decalcifies dentin to a lesser depth, and tubules do not open into a funnel shape (Fig. 16.10B). Maleic acid (e.g. Scotch bond) results in removal of the smear layer but not the smear plugs.

ii. *Chelators*: Contrary to the strong acid etchants, chelators remove the smear layer without decalcification or significant physical changes on the underlying dentin substrate. Also no funnel shaped changes are evident; instead, a chelate is formed. *A chelate refers to a compound with a central metal ion surrounded by covalently bonded atoms, ions or molecules called ligands which possess additional bonds for chemical reaction.* The best known chelator conditioner is Ethylene diaminotetra acetic acid (EDTA) adjusted to a pH of 7.4. It was developed for use in Gluma system. When used for 30 seconds, the smear plugs were not fully removed with this conditioner.

Certain bonding systems do not remove the smear layer but rather utilize it as a legitimate bonding substrate (Fig. 16.10B). These systems are utilized by so called self etching/self priming agents which are acidic monomer and can enlarge the channels and also remove mineral deposits from within the tubules; thereby promoting resin permeation. With this type of bonding there are less chances of incomplete resin penetration because both etching and priming occur simultaneously. Since the self etching/self priming solution is not rinsed from the surface, the demineralized smear layer is incorporated into the bonding interface.

B. Thermal Conditioning

Lasers are being used to condition dentin. The commonly used Lasers are CO_2 and Nd:YAG Laser. It is speculated that Lasers cause recrystallization of dentin resulting in a fungi form appearance that contributes to increased micro-retention or possible chemical adhesion of a restorative material to the tooth structure. The carbonized black spot that results after lasing is easily washed off with water.

C. Mechanical Conditioning

Micro-abrasion is used to mechanically condition the dentin.

PRIMING

Priming is the second step in bonding procedure. The primers are the agents that contain monomers with hydrophilic properties, which have an affinity for the exposed collagen fibrils, and hydrophobic properties for co-polymerization with adhesive resin. These monomers, usually HEMA and 4-META are dissolved in solutions of acetone or ethanol, which because of their volatile characteristics can displace water from the dentinal surface and the moist collagen network. The primer promotes resin diffusion into the moist, demineralized dentin with the aim of achieving complete resin penetration. Microscopic examination has however shown deficiencies in the spread of primer at three levels (i) incomplete surface coverage (ii) incomplete interfibrillar penetration and (iii) incomplete penetration to the full depth of demineralized dentin. In order to achieve the best bond strengths it is essential that the primer spreads uniformly over the surface.

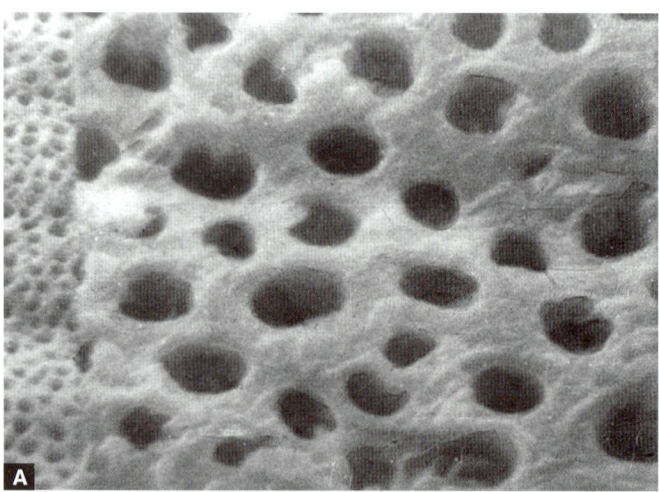
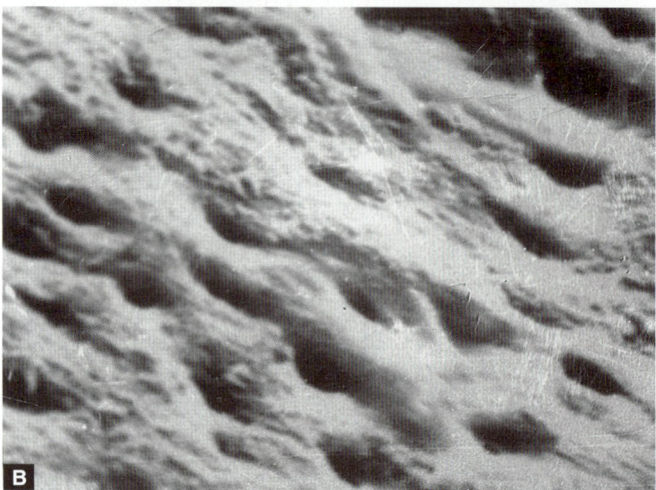

Figs 16.10A and B: SEM images of etched dentin surface: **(A)** Dentin surface after phosphoric acid etching (SEM); **(B)** Dentin surface after conditioning with a combination etchant of 10% citric acid and 20% calcium chloride (SEM)

To improve the surface coverage and diffusion of the primer it can be applied in multiple coats. When a second coat of Primer was applied, it was found that the shear bond strength improved significantly, but there was no further increase up to five additional applications. Second consideration for improving penetration is the condition of the dentinal surface. As described earlier, water is an essential component needed to keep the collagen fibrils suspended and hence creating space for subsequent penetration of primer and adhesive resin. Excessive drying of the conditioned dentin collapses the collagen network and the primer is prohibited from entry. On the other hand, an overwet surface results in separation of the primer components leading to emulsion polymerization of the adhesive resin. An ideal dentin surface for bonding is visibly moist, without any excessive water. This can be achieved clinically by blot drying with a damp cotton pledget. Third, short conditioning times of no longer than 15 seconds are considered adequate for allowing complete penetration of primer and resin. It is speculated that more stable bonds are formed if primer and resin permeate dentin less deeply and more uniformly rather than spotty and more deeply.

DENTIN BONDING AGENTS

Bonding resin is an unfilled or semifilled resin, which matches the resin of the composite but has a lower viscosity to permit easy flow and penetration. The major role of adhesive resin application is the formation and stabilization of hybrid layer, production of resin tags in the unplugged dentinal tubules and at the same time effectively sealing them to reduce the chances of increased permeability and thus pulpal irritation. When the adhesive resin is applied, a part of it penetrates into the microporous collagen scaffold of the intertubular dentin known as the intertubular penetration. Here it polymerizes and co-polymerizes with the primer to form an intermingled layer of collagen and resin and is termed as the *'resin reinforced layer'*, *'hybrid layer'* or *'resin interdiffusion zone'*. The rest of the adhesive resin enters into the dentinal tubules to a limited depth of 10-20 µms forming resin tags known as the *intratubular penetration*. Within the dentinal tubules, these tags are attached only at this point to the peritubular dentin and any further extension of resin tags into the dentinal tubules is passive. Tags do not appear to contribute to the attachment mechanism and it should be noted that prolonged conditioning is actually not needed. With the latest systems, resins have also shown to penetrate and hybridize the walls of lateral tubule branches forming sub micron resin tags and the phenomenon is called *lateral tubule hybridization*. Both intra tubular and intertubular permeabilities are critical to achieve optimal bond strengths and sealing of dentinal surfaces. At times the resin may not completely infilterate into the collagen meshwork and such microspaces are then open to microleakage referred to as *'Nanoleakage'*. In case of failure of the bond at the two common sites of top and bottom of hybrid layer, the intimate attachment of the resin tags to the tubule wall at their orifices keeps the dentinal tubules sealed and the pulp protected. The ability of resins to penetrate both dentinal tubules and intertubular dentin is dependent upon several variables. In superficial portions of dentin where tubules are fewer compared to deep dentin, intertubular penetration accounts for the major portion of the bond strength, whereas the reverse is true for deep dentin where intratubular penetration contributes to most of the retention and sealing. Difficulties encountered in the infiltration of resins into tubules are mainly because of the presence of dentinal fluid and mineral casts in sclerotic dentin. Resin infilteration into intertubular dentin is primarily dependent upon the porosity between collagen fibrils, which further depends upon the amount of moisture in this layer.

Adhesive resins can be either chemically cured or light cured. For light cured resins it is advisable to cure the bonding resin separately. In this way adequate light intensity is available to polymerize the hybrid layer, which will be able to counteract the polymerization shrinkage of the resin composite. During polymerization, an oxygen inhibited layer of 15 µm is formed on the top of the adhesive resin. The unpolymerized methacrylate double bonds present in this layer offer co-polymerization with the subsequently placed restorative resin. A thin uniform layer of adhesive resin is critical to bonding as it serves as an elastic intermediary for absorbing stresses of polymerization shrinkage. Use of air stream on adhesive resin should be avoided as it causes uneven thinning of the valuable intermediary layer.

MECHANISM OF DENTIN BONDING

Composite resins do not show an intimate microscopic contact with dentin when placed directly into the cavity. In order to overcome this, an intervening layer of fluid is used, which fills in the microscopic space, polymerizes and combines with the composite resin and components of dentin. The basic chemical composition of these dentin bonding adhesives can be conceived as illustrated in the Fig. 16.11.

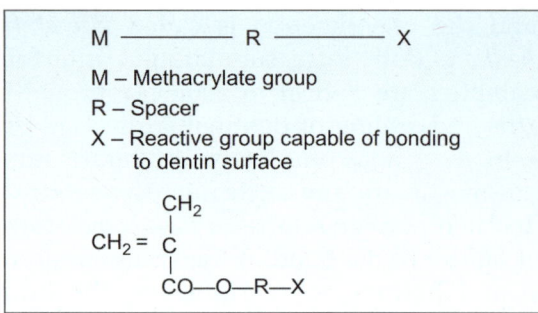

Fig. 16.11: Chemistry of dentin bonding agent

The adhesive molecule is bifunctional, one part of which (X) enters into chemical union with the tooth structure, and the other part (M) co-polymerizes to the resin through the double bond of methacrylate. Adhesion with dentin can occur either to the inorganic or organic components present on the surface of the tooth. The spacer group (R) is responsible for making the molecule large enough to keep the methacrylate groups spatially located for optimal chemical reaction with the composite. Ideally, dentin adhesives should be both hydrophilic and hydrophobic. It is required to be hydrophilic so as to be able to displace dentinal fluids and thereby wet the surface, permitting penetration into porosities with the dentin and eventually react with organic or inorganic components. Hydrophobic properties are needed to allow bonding to the composite resin, the matrix of which is hydrophobic in nature.

Bonding to Inorganic Portion of Dentin

Bonding to the inorganic part of dentin occurs through ionic interaction between positive Ca^{2+} ions on the surface of dentin and negative charges on the group X of the adhesive. Group X can be phosphates, aminoacids and amino-alcohols or dicarboxylates. The bonding mechanisms for all the three are presented in the Figs 16.12 a,b,c. To the left, Ca^{2+} ions are seen and to the right are adhesive molecules. Agents that use a phosphate group in their bonding to calcium ions are referred to as *phosphate bonding systems* and are the most common ones employed. The substituent 'Z' in the phosphate based adhesives may be chlorine, a hydroxy or a phenyl group.

The reported bond strengths of calcium bonding adhesives when used alone are moderate, seldom exceeding 6 MPa. However, when different Ca^{2+} bonding adhesives are combined or used in conjunction with dentin conditioning, bond strengths of 10-15 MPa have been seen. This is probably due to the phenomenon of interpenetration. Some adhesives that involve bonding to inorganic ions are: Bondlite,

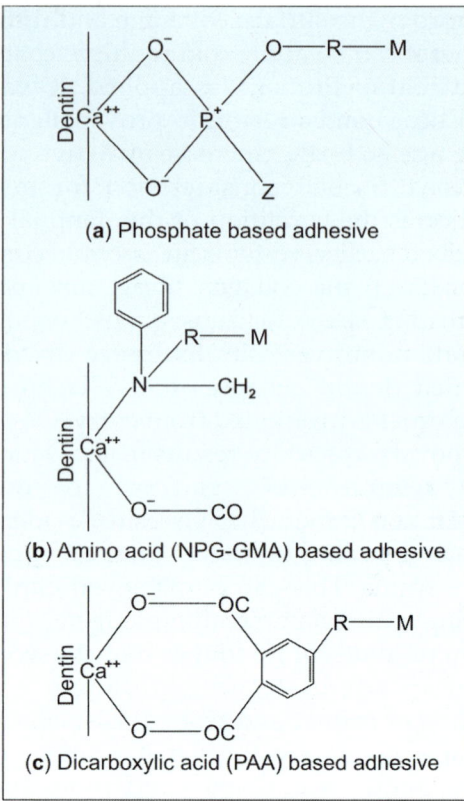

Fig. 16.12: Bonding to inorganic portion of dentin

Scotch bond, J&J Bonding agents, Clearfil, Prisma Universal Bond, etc.

Bonding to the Organic Portion of Dentin

Bonding to the organic part of dentin involves interaction with the amino (–NH), amido (-CONH), hydroxyl (–OH) or carboxylate (–COOH) groups present in the collagen of dentin. Removal of hydrogen from any of these groups allows combination with chemicals present in dentin bonding agents. Compounds that have a capacity to react with one or more groups of collagen are isocyanates, carboxylic acid chlorides, carboxylic acid anhydrides and aldehydes (Fig. 16.13).

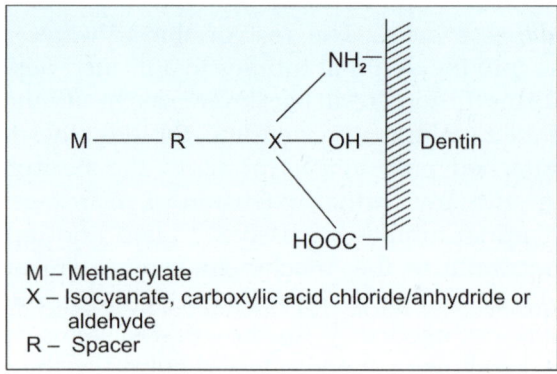

Fig. 16.13: Bonding to organic part of dentin

Examples of the adhesives that rely on bonding to organic part of dentin are Dentin Adhesit (isocyanate based), Gluma (aldehyde based), etc. Although the concept of chemical adhesion with early dentin bonding agents seemed reasonable, resultant bond strengths with these systems were not very attractive. Studies showed that dentin conditioning procedures like acid etching or demineralization with EDTA (ethylene diamine tetra acetic acid) greatly improved clinical results. Use of adhesives based on the concept of infiltration into moist collagen network to provide mechanical retention has started gaining more importance than their ability to form chemical bonds to the tooth surface. In brief, the key to adhesion presently is to use a hydrophilic monomer that could easily infiltrate the collagen meshwork produced by conditioning of dentin (Figs 16.14A, B).

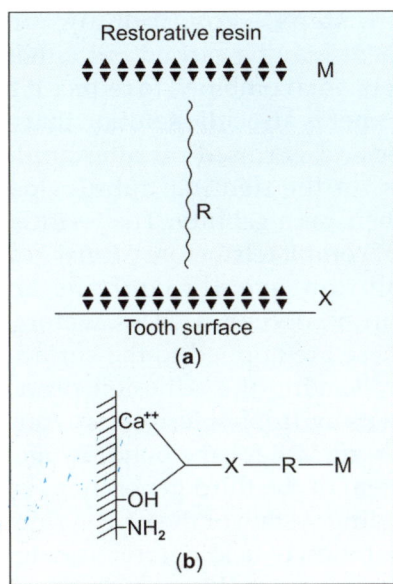

Fig. 16.14A and B: Mechanism of bonding: **(A)** Bonding mechanism with intervening adhesive and **(B)** Bonding to inorganic or organic portion of dentin.

EVOLUTION OF DENTIN BONDING AGENTS

For convenience, these agents have been divided into 'generations' depending upon the evolution of these agents.

1. First Generation Dentin Bonding Agents

The initial trial was using a surface active comonomer, N-phenyl-glycine-glycidyl methacrylate (NPG-GMA), which acted as a primer and adhesion promoter between enamel/dentin and resin materials by chelating with surface dentin (Fig. 16.15). Since calcium ions of the tooth substance are a mediator in the bond formation, agents of this type are expected to form stronger bonds to enamel than to dentin. Studies with this system have not shown good

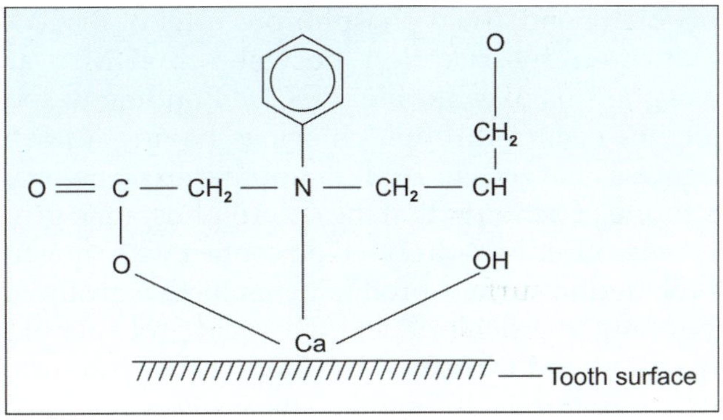

Fig. 16.15: Bonding of NPG portion to Ca^{2+} ions by chelation

retentive values. A commercially introduced system, Cervident (SS White) has shown bond strengths to dentin of only 2.8 MPa and no improvement in marginal leakage when compared to conventional unfilled bonding agent.

2. Second Generation Dentin Bonding Agents

Most of the second generation bonding agents were phenyl phosphorous, phosphorous/chloro phosphorous esters of unfilled resins such as BisGMA or HEMA. The bonding mechanism involved improved wetting of the surface and ionic interaction between the phosphate group and calcium of the tooth. Clearfil (Kuraray, Japan) was the first agent introduced in this series. It composed of an ethyl alcohol solution containing tertiary amine as the activator. The catalyst liquid was BisGMA monomer containing a phenyl phosphate ester, benzoyl peroxide and methyl methacrylate. The interfacial bond was established through attraction between the negative charges of the oxygen on the phosphorous group and the positively charged calcium ions in the dentin surface (Fig. 16.16).

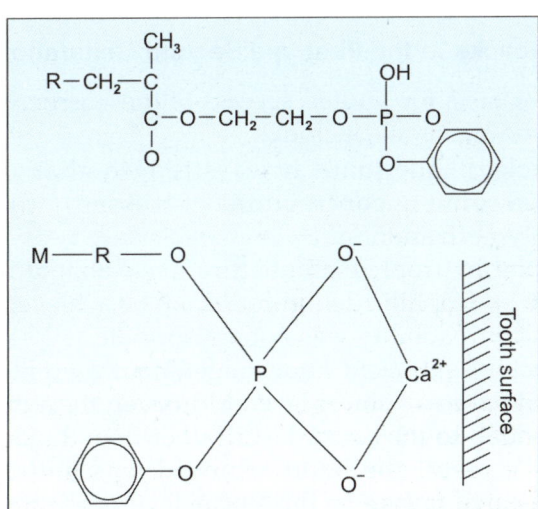

Fig. 16.16: Bonding mechanism in Clearfil

Scotch bond, (halo phosphorous ester of BisGMA) is formed by reaction between BisGMA and phosphorous oxychloride ($POCl_3$). Bonding to tooth calcium occurs through chlorines having a partial negative charge (Fig.16.17). Another explanation of its mode of action is that the chloro phosphate group becomes rapidly hydrolysed on contact with moisture at the dentin surface producing a reactive group and liberating hydrochloric acid. This acid probably plays a part in bond formation by altering the structure of surface dentin including the smear layer.

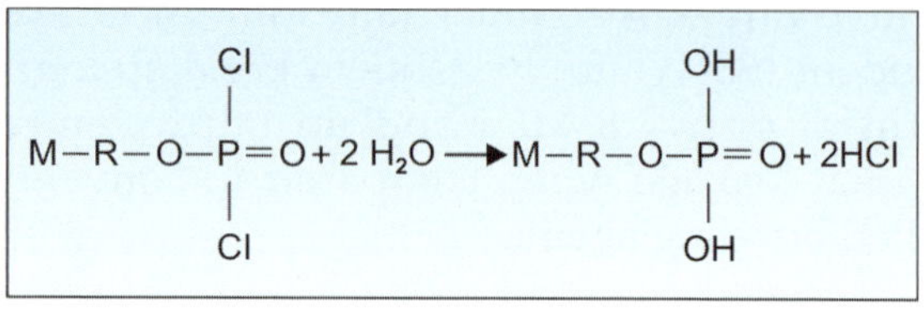

$$\begin{array}{c} Cl \\ | \\ M-R-O-P=O+2H_2O \\ | \\ Cl \end{array} \longrightarrow \begin{array}{c} OH \\ | \\ M-R-O-P=O+2HCl \\ | \\ OH \end{array}$$

Fig. 16.17: Bonding mechanism in Scotchbond

Dentin Adhesit (Vivadent) comprising of isocyanate monomer is also generally considered a second generation bonding agent. Chemical bonding with this agent is mediated through amino and hydroxyl groups on the dentinal surface. Other systems belonging to this generation are Prisma Universal Bonding Agent (Johnson and Johnson) and Dental Adhesive (Kulzer). Most of these systems are not available now. Mean shear bond strengths to dentin have been reported to be 2-7 MPa for the second generation bonding agents. Bond strengths in this range are considered to be quite weak to counteract the polymerization shrinkage of composite resins. Furthermore, evidences have shown hydrolysis of the bond between phosphonate esters and dentin, when immersed in water.

Drawbacks in the First and Second Generations

The reasons for limited success of these generations of bonding agents include:
- Lack of adequate bond strength that could overcome contraction stresses during polymerization.
- Being hydrophobic in nature, close adaptation to the hydrophilic dentin could not be achieved.
- Biocompatibility was not appropriate.
- Lack of sufficient knowledge about the presence and nature of smear layer. Moreover, the adhesive bonded to the smear layer rather than the dentin. As a result the bond achieved was limited by cohesive failure in the smear layer or a break at the smear layer-dentin interface.

3. Third Generation Dentin Bonding Agents

As further research ensued, it became evident that the smear layer had a negative influence on the performance of adhesive systems. To overcome this, third generation dentin bonding agents were introduced which differed from early materials in that an additional step was employed to either modify or remove the smear layer before the application of the actual adhesive. The extra step comprised of conditioning and priming of dentin but made the procedure more complicated and time consuming. The bond strengths to dentin with these agents were usually higher (9-15 MPa) and more durable thereby reducing microleakage. This might be because the agents relied primarily on mechanical means of bonding as opposed to the less reliable chemical adhesion used in earlier materials.

The three steps – conditioning, priming and bonding agent may be carried out either separately or the components combined to reduce it to two steps. The conditioner is an acidic solution that removes the smear layer and is rinsed off after application. The acid opens up the dentinal tubules partially and increases their permeability. The residual acid must be rinsed off completely before primer is applied. The primer solution usually contains an adhesion promoter in a solvent such as water, ethanol or acetone. These are applied to the surface and dried, presumably leaving the adhesion promoter on the dentin with its hydrophobic groups exposed to create a favourable surface for the bonding agent.

First system of the third generation, known as the oxalate bonding system or the FNP system (Fig. 16.18) utilized a solution of acidic ferric oxalate (2.5% nitric acid + ferric oxalate) on the enamel and dentin surface as a conditioner. The ferric ions are adsorbed onto the dentin to increase the number of positive ions on the surface. This is followed by the application of an acetone solution of NTG-GMA (reaction product of N p-toluidine glycine and glycidyl dimethacrylate) and then another acetone solution of PMDM (Pyromellitic dianyhdride + 2 HEMA). This technique gave bond strengths of about 15 MPa to both enamel and dentin. Tenure was the first commercial oxalate

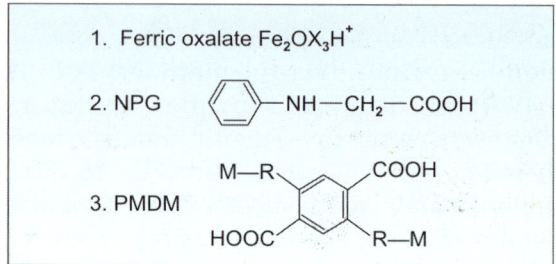

Fig. 16.18: Three-step oxalate system conceived by Bowen

bonding system, which utilized phosphoric acid in conjunction with aluminium oxalate and nitric acid as a dental conditioner. Later researchers replaced ferric oxalate with aluminium oxalate, to eliminate the possible risk of discoloration due to ferric ions. A third generation bonding agent called Gluma (Fig. 16.19) utilizes 0.5M EDTA at an approximately neutral pH to remove the smear layer and free collagen from embedding apatite.

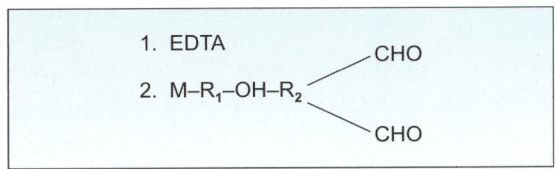

Fig. 16.19: Gluma bonding system

Drawbacks in the Third Generation Bonding Agents

Clinical studies showed decrease in retention with time. So the main problem was the longevity of the maintenance of the bond. These are technique sensitive and time consuming.

4. Fourth Generation Dentin Bonding Agents

Till now, the strategies for dentin adhesion were based upon the formation of resin tags penetrating into tubules of conditioned dentin, followed by chemical and mechanical bonding to inorganic or organic components of dentin. *Nakabayashi* (1982) proposed a concept in which the resin is impregnated into partially decalcified dentin followed by polymerization creating a resin reinforced layer or the 'hybrid layer'. Hybrid layer is defined as *'the structure formed in the dental hard tissues by demineralization of the surface and subsurface followed by infiltration of monomers and subsequent polymerization'*. The mineralized tissues of peritubular and intertubular dentin are dissolved by acidic action; the initial surface penetration exposes the collagen fibers. The advantages of this concept of bonding agents are:

- Reduced technique sensitivity.
- Similar bond strengths to enamel and dentin.
- No reduction in bond strength when applied to moist surface or under conditions of high humidity.
- Some systems can bond to mineralized tissue as well as metal, amalgam, porcelain and indirect composite restorations.

It has been suggested that excessive drying causes collapse of the collagen meshwork and prevents complete penetration of the subsequently applied primer and resin. A thin film of water present on the conditioned dentin helps suspend the collagen fibrils and create space between them for penetration. All Bond-2 and Scotch-bond multi-purpose are the earlier products.

All Bond-2 uses an etchant of 35% phosphoric acid on dentin and enamel followed by the application of hydrophilic primer containing 2% NTG GMA (N Tolyglycine – glycidyl methacrylate) and 16% BPDM (biphenyl dimethacrylate) in ethanol or acetone. Subsequently, an unfilled resin containing BisGMA and HEMA is applied. Mean bond strength for this system is seen to be 21.4+7.8 MPa.

Scotchbond Multipurpose uses 10% maleic acid to etch both enamel and dentin. Primer is an aqueous solution of HEMA and poly alkenoate copolymers. The adhesive resin is a BisGMA containing HEMA. The effectiveness of maleic acid as an enamel etchant is questionable. Therefore, some clinicians prefer phosphoric acid to etch enamel and maleic acid to condition dentin. Use of 35% phosphoric acid to etch both enamel and dentin has also been advocated. The bond strength achieved was 21.0MPa with wet dentin and 18.0MPa with dry dentin.

Other fourth generation bonding system include Imperva Bond (Shofu), Solid Bond (Kulzer), Opti Bond C & B, Metabond, etc. Mean shear bond strengths achieved with this generation of agents is 17-24 MPa. There are so many commercial preparations and the manipulation might vary from one type to another.

5. Fifth Generation Dentin Bonding Agents

This class of adhesives are also based on the concept of hybridization, and rely on the wet bonding technique. It differs from its predecessor in that it uses one component resin, i.e. after conditioning of enamel and dentin, the steps of priming and bonding are combined so that bonding is achieved with a one component formula (Fig. 16.20).

Prime and Bond (Dentsply, Caulk) and Prime and Bond 2.1 (with cetylamine fluorides) contain PENTA,

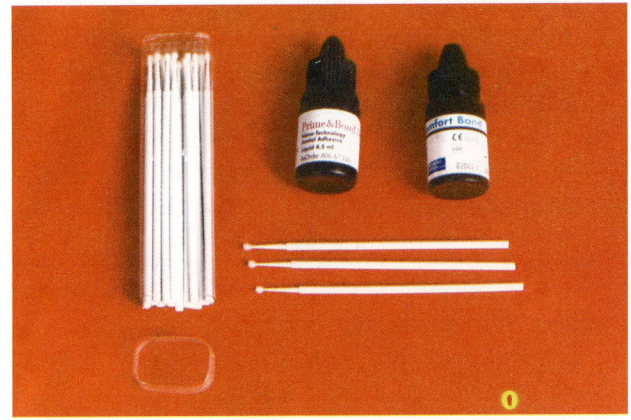

Fig. 16.20: Prime and Bond NT and comfort bond for which the priming and bonding steps are combined

TEGDMA and an elastomeric UDMA resin in acetone. The system is highly sensitive to even mild dessication of acid conditioned dentin. Bond strengths exceeding 20 MPa have been reported with it. Like other PENTA containing adhesives, Prime and Bond and Prime and Bond 2.1 do not necessitate dentin conditioning but require acid conditioning on enamel for optimal enamel bonding. PENTA is a multifunctional molecule and is believed to partially demineralize dentin, facilitating penetration of resins into it.

Opti Bond Solo (Kerr) is a recently developed one component version of Opti Bond and consists of HEMA, GPDM and BisGMA in an ethanol/water system. It also contains fillers like fumed silica and barium but at half the concentration of that found in Opti Bond.

Single Bond (3M) is also a recently developed one component version of Scotch Bond Multi-purpose. The material contains HEMA, BisGMA, dimethacrylate resin and a unique methacrylate functional copolymer of polyacrylic and polyitaconic acids in water and ethanol solvent base.

Bond strengths for fifth generation systems are almost equal to those of fourth generation agents, i.e. 17MPa-24 MPa. Although these systems have reduced the number of components, they are not necessarily faster or simpler procedures. None of these agents is truly a one component system because almost always they require a pretreatment with acid on enamel and sometimes on dentin. In addition, these materials are sensitive to even minor drying and may require multiple applications of the adhesive to ensure optimal penetration of resin.

Advantages of Fifth Generation Bonding System

- Bond strength is sufficient.
- Post-operative sensitivity is rare.
- Some agents have incorporated fluoride and elastomeric components to improve marginal integrity.
- Time saving and simple to use.
- Elimination of washing out of the acidic gel, therefore elimination of risk of collagen collapse.
- Combination of etching and priming steps decreases the working time.

Disadvantages

- Solution must be refreshed continuously and a residual smear layer remained between the adhesive material and dentin.

6. Sixth Generation Dentin Bonding Agents

To improve upon the bond strength and to make the manipulation easy, this generation of adhesives relied on the use of acidic primer (pH 2.5 – 4.5), eliminating the need for phosphoric acid as etchant (Figs 16.21 and 16.24). Though manipulation is quite easy with these materials and they show a sufficient bond to conditioned dentin, but bond with enamel has been shown to be less effective. This may be due to the fact that the sixth generation systems are composed of an acidic solution that cannot be kept in place for long and must be refreshed continuously. Moreover these systems have a pH that is not enough to properly etch enamel.

The diagrammatic representation of componenets of self-etching adhesive is depicted in Fig.16.22.

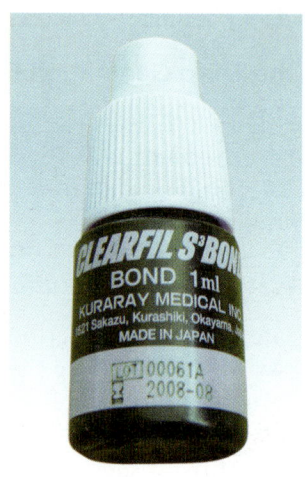

Fig. 16.21: Clearfil S³ bond

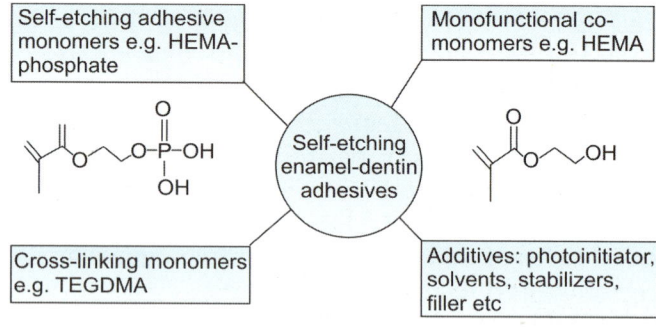

Fig. 16.22: Components of self-etching adhesives

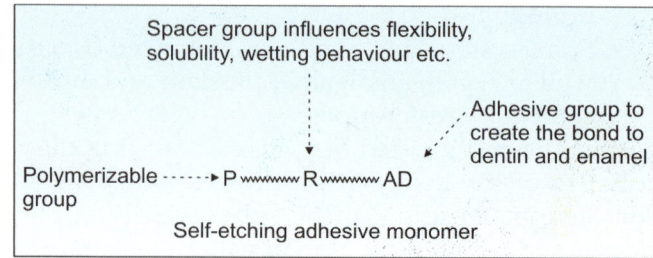

Fig. 16.23: General structure of self-etching adhesive monomer

Bonding in Dentistry

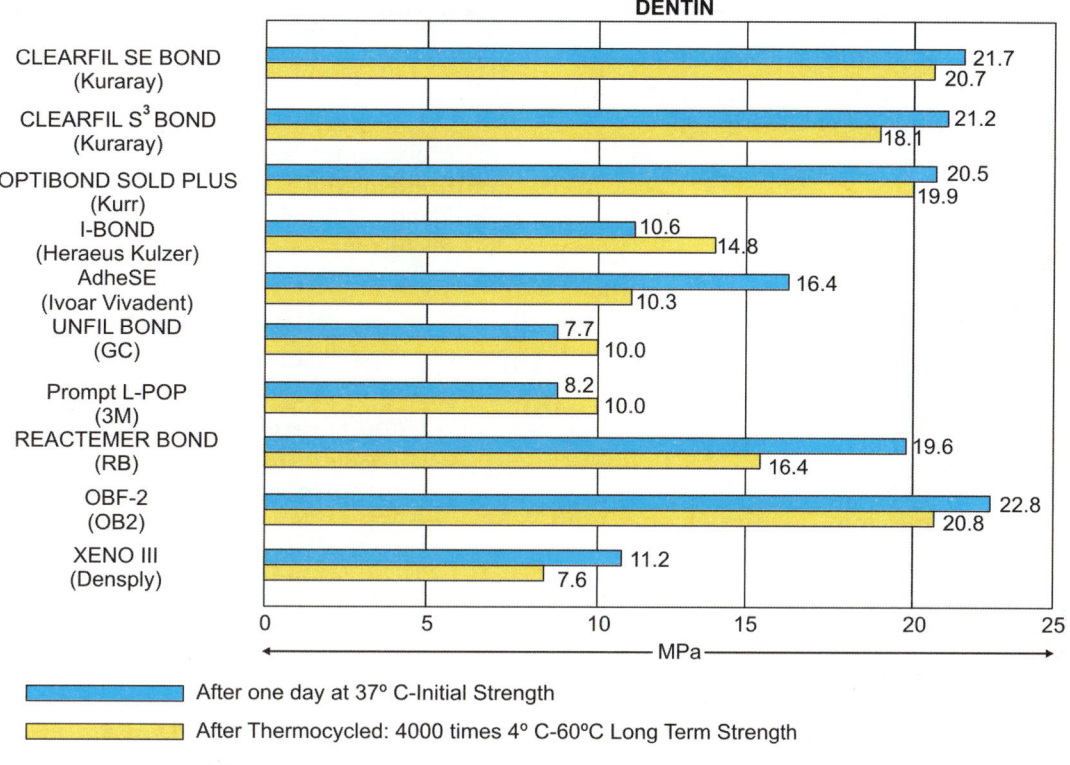

Fig. 16.24: Bonding strength of various self-etch systems.

Sixth generation dentin bonding agents are further of two types :

Type 1 (Self-etching primer and adhesive)

These are available in light cure or dual cure product. Self etching primer and resin adhesives are applied in separate layers.
- Two bottles, Liquid 1 (acidic primer), Liquid 2 (adhesive); acidic primer applied to tooth followed by adhesive
- Unprepared enamel may require etching with phosphoric acid
- Light cured/dual cured formulations
- Solvent is water, e.g. Nano Bond, Optibond, Prompt L-PoP (Fig. 16.25)

Type 2 (Self-etching adhesive)

Available only in light cure type. The self-etch primer and adhesive is mixed outside and applied (Fig. 16.23).
- Two bottles, containing acid primer and adhesive; a drop of each liquid is mixed and applied to tooth
- Unprepared enamel may require etching with phosphoric acid
- Light cured formulations
- Solvent is water, e.g. Xeno III (Fig. 16.26).

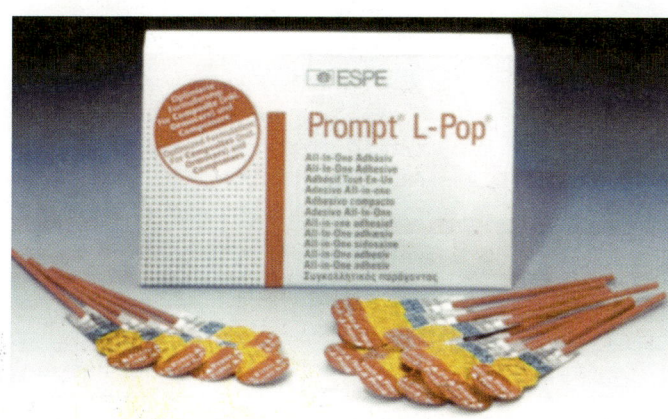

Fig. 16.25: Prompt L-PoP

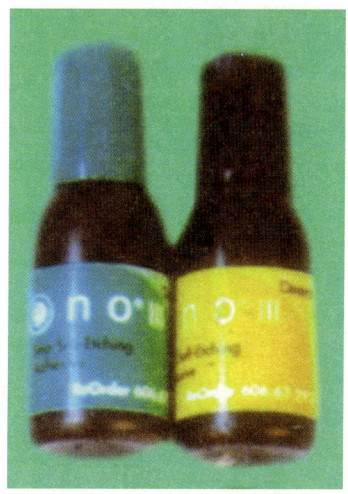

Fig. 16.26: Xeno III

Advantages
• They are designed to be used on dry dentin. • They do not etch very far into dentin beneath smear layers. This avoids removal of smear plugs.

7. Seventh Generation Dentin Bonding Agents

Available both as light cure and dual cure type. All three components are combined in a single bottle.

Seventh generation bonding agents (No mixing, Self-etch adhesive) are slight modification of type II sixth generation bonding agent.

The features are:
- More acidic (pH < 1)
- Single bottle containing acidic adhesive
- Unprepared enamel may require etching with phosphoric acid
- Solvent is water, e.g. G-Bond and i-Bond (Fig. 16.27)

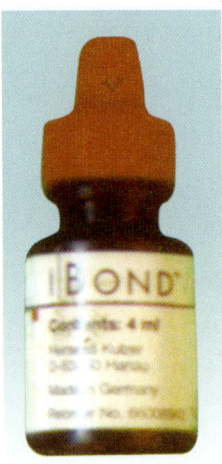

Fig. 16.27: i-Bond

Disadvantages
• Relatively short shelf life (acidity of maleic acid accelerated the breakdown of HEMA). • Their composition is very hydrophilic. They attract and absorb water leading to leaching of unpolymerized monomers or hydrolytic degradation products through water filled channels called water trees.

8. Eight Generation Bonding Agent

A modified version of seventh generation bonding agent is intorudced by Voco America as Futurabond DC. This is one-step dual-cured, non-filled, self-etch adhesive available in single use blister packs. The 'chemical cured' mode makes the product suitable to be used in root canals, avoiding blocking the root canals with cured boding agent.

Advantages
• Can be used with light-cure and dual-cure and self-cure composites • Provides high bonding strength • Moisture tolerant • Contains fluorides • Nano-fillers help in better cross linking of the bonding resin components.

Since the generations are becoming confusing, a simple classification is presented, which involves as the past and present adhesives.

I. Etch and rinse strategy
  A. Three steps (e.g. All-Bond 2, Syntac, Scotchbond multipurpose)
    • Acid
    • Primer
    • Bonding agent
  B. Two steps (e.g. Gluma, One step, Prime and Bond)
    • Acid
    • Primers + Bonding
II. Self-etch strategy
  A. Two steps (e.g. Clearfil Liner 2, Clearfil SE, Optibond plus, Optimbond Solo)
    • Acid + Primer
    • Bonding agent
  B. One step (e.g. Clearfils3, iBond, GBond, Xenov)
    • Acid + Primer + Bonding agent

The evolution of Dentin bonding systems is depicted in Table 16.1.

Table 16.1: Evolution of dentin bonding systems
1st generation → Cavity primers with low bond strength
2nd generation → Dentin-enamel bonding agents with improved bond strength to etched enamel
3rd generation → Etching of dentin and partially removal of smear layer
4th generation → Total-etch technique and formation of the hybrid layer and resin tags
5th generation → Simplification of clinical procedures: one-bottle systems and self-etching primers
6th generation → One-step bonding systems with proper bond to enamel and dentin; Type 1 are compatible with self-cured composites and Type 2 are not
7th generation → Single bottle no mix self-etching adhesive, not compatible with selfcured composites

Table 16.2: Use of individual component in self-etch adhesive systems

UDMA/HEMA	Conditioning of enamel and dentin Wetting agent, help in thin film formation Promotes infiltration
4-META	Binding to calcium of apatite Binding to collagen
Glutaraldehyde	Disinfectant Desensitizing agent
Acetone	Helps in removing humidity Solvent for monomer
Water	Helps in etching process Solvent for monomer

The use of individual component in self-etch adhesive system is given in Table 16.2.

Compositions of some of the bonding systems along with their advantages and disadvantages are given in Tables 16.3 and 16.4 respectively.

CATEGORIZATION OF ADHESIVES ACCORDING TO THE MODE OF APPLICATION

Modern dentin adhesive systems can also be classified on their clinical approach to smear layer. Based on this criteria, there are currently reported three mechanisms of adhesions.

i. One, in which the adhesives *modify the smear layer* and incorporate it into the bonding process. Their application can be completed in one or two steps using a single adhesive or primer and adhesive respectively. The smear layer in this adhesion process is retained based on the concept that it serves as a natural barrier to the pulp, prevents bacterial invasion and limits the outward flow of pulpal fluid that might impair bonding efficiency. Penetration of monomers into the smear layer and their subsequent polymerization reinforces the attachment of the smear layer to the underlying dentin and also forms a micromechanical and perhaps a chemical bond to the underlying dentinal surface. It is however observed that resin is able to penetrate only to a limited extent into the superficial dentin. Clinically, these systems require selective etching of enamel in a separate step.

ii. Two, in which the adhesives *completely remove the smear layer* and are subdivided into two and three step application. A two step process involves dentin conditioning followed by a combined primer and adhesive; whereas the three step process involves separate conditioning, priming and bonding agent application. Any of the processes results in complete removal of the smear layer by acidic conditioners that are simultaneously applied to enamel and dentin using the total etch technique. The action of these agents is principally based on the combined effect of hybridization and resin tag formation.

iii. Three, in which the adhesives *dissolve the smear layer rather than remove* it. The process is accomplished in two steps using a combined conditioner and primer (self etching primer) followed by application of the adhesive resin. The slightly acidic primers supplied with these systems partially demineralize the smear layer and the underlying dentin surface without removing the dissolved smear layer remanants and unplugging the tubule orifices. The rationale behind their use is to superficially demineralize dentin and simultaneously penetrate it with monomers, which can be polymerized in-situ. Examples of all the three systems of adhesives are given in Table 16.5.

ROLE OF WATER IN THE BONDING PROCESS

When prepared dentin is acid etched, the smear layer and plugs are removed and the underlying 2-7 μm layer of dentin is demineralized. Solutions used for etching are generally acidic and contain water to ionize the acids and dissolve the extracted minerals. Post-etching rinsing with water removes this dissolved mineral and leaves a demineralized dentin surface covered with water. About 70% of the demineralized dentin is occupied with water in areas from where the mineral has been removed. This water is responsible for maintaining the collagen in an expanded state and thereby preserving the spaces needed for infiltration of resin. In other words, water acts as a plasticizer for collagen and keeps it in a soft state. If the dentin is dried or exposed to air, water evaporates leaving collagen in a collapsed stiffened state (Fig.16.9C) because of surface tension forces. This reduces the ability of the subsequently applied agents to penetrate the collagen web. Also when the collagen fibrils are brought closer, secondary forces start becoming active between adjacent peptide chains in the collagen triple helix, which is not possible when water is present, thereby increasing the stiffness or modulus of elasticity for collagen. Total demineralization with air drying results in as much as 65 volume percent shrinkage. Upon addition of water, the collagen network reexpands to about 100 percent of its original volume. It is believed that a critical water concentration exists that prevents collapse of the network or allows re-expansion of the dried dentin over a period of 10-30 seconds.

Table 16.3: Dentin adhesive systems

Adhesive System	Etchant/Self-etching Primer	Adhesive
Single Bond	35% phosphoric acid gel	BisGMA, HEMA, polyalkenoic acid copolymer, ethanol, water, photoinitiator
Clearfil Liner Bond 2	Primer A Phenyl P, 5-NMSA, CQ, ethanol Primer B HEMA, water	MDP, HEMA, BisGMA, Microfiller
One Step	32% phosphoric acid gel	BPDM, BisGMA, HEMA, Acetone, photoinitiator
Imperva Fluoro Bond	Primer A Water, acetone, initiator Primer B 4-AET, HEMA, 4-AETA, initiator	4-AET, HEMA UDMA, glass-ionomer Filler, microfiller
Prime & Bond NT	34% Tooth conditioner gel	Di & Trimethacrylate resins, PENTA, acetone
OptiBond Solo	37.5% phosphoric acid	BisGMA, HEMA, ethyl alcohol
Scotch Bond Multi-purpose	HEMA, Polyacrylic acid, water	BisGMA, HEMA
Liner Bond 2V	Primer A MDP, HEMA, water, photoinitiator, accelerator Primer B HEMA, water accelerator	MDP, dimethacrylates, photoinitiator, accelerator, microfiller
Clearfil SE Bond	MDP, HEMA, Hydrophilic dimethacrylate di camphorquinone N-N-Diethanol-p-toluidine water	MDP, BisGMA, HEMA, Hydrophobic di-camphorquinone dimethacrylate N-N-Diethanol-p-toluidine silanated colloidal silica
Prompt L-Pop	Self etching	Water methacrylated phosphoric oxide fluoride complex with zinc photoinitiators
Tyrian, SPE	Self etching primer 2-acrylamido 2-methyl propane sulfonic acid BIS (methacryloyloxy ethyl) phosphate ethanol	Biphenyl dimethacrylate EMA, acetone glass filling photo-initiators
Reactmer Bond (RB)	Bond A Bond B	4-MET, 4-META HEMA, UDMA, water, photoinitiator, fluoride complex
XENO III	Universal catalyst	METP, UDMA, HEMA, Ethanol, water, silica, filler, photoinitiator, fluoride complex
OB2	Bond A Bond B	MAC-10, HEMA Phosphoric acid ester, photoinitiator, water, aluminosilicate glass filler
One up Bond F	Self-etching	HEMA, MMA, Methacrylolyoxy alkyl acid phosphate, fluorosilicate glass filler, water, photoinitiator
i Bond	Self-etching	Acetone/Water UDMA, 4-META, Glutaraldehyde

PENTA – dipenatacrylthritol penta acrylate monophosphate
BisGMA – Bisphenyl glycidyl methacrylate
HEMA – 2 Hydroxyethyl methacrylate
BPDM – Bisphenyl dimethacrylate
CQ – Camphorquinone

MDP -10 – Methacryloyloxy methacrylate
NMSA – N-methacryloxy-5-amino salicylic acid
Phenyl P – 2- methacryloyloxy ethyl –phenyl hydrogen phosphate
4 AET – 4-acryloxyethyl trimellitic acid
4-AETA – 4-acryloxyethyl trimellitate anhydride

Bonding in Dentistry

Table 16.4: Advantages and disadvantages of currently available bonding agents

Bonding agents	Advantages	Disadvantages
i. Self-etching primer (Clearfil SE Bond) Ep + B	• No rinsing, quick application • Less post-operative sensitivity total-etch adhesives • Results of clinical studies support their use on dentin • Bond very well to dentin etched with phosphoric acid	• May result in enamel microleakage due to deficient enamel etching • Slight degradation of the hybrid layer
ii. Self-etching all-in-one adhesive (Prompt L-Pop) Ep + B	• No rinsing, very quick applications • Results in enamel etch pattern similar to that of phosphoric acid • No bottles, no cross-contamination	• Has resulted in a wide range of bond strength values • Bonds better with compomers than with composites • May need multiple coats to bond effectively to dentin • Does not bond well to unprepared enamel • Not indicated for indirect restorations
iii. Total etch multi-bottle adhesives (All-Bond 2, Scotchbond Multi-Purpose, OptiBond FL) E + p + B	• In vivo and in vitro research back up their use on different substrates • The highest dentin bond strengths among all the adhesives • Generally contain a dual-cure option for indirect restorations and bonded amalgams	• Multiple bottles make their utilization cumbersome • Some bottles in the kit may never be used • Possibility of running out of Primer A before Primer B (or vice-versa) • Because primer and adhesive resin air dispensed into the same plastic container, their sequential application may be inverted
iv. Total etch one-bottle adhesives (Excite, One Step, OptiBond SOLO Plus, PQI, Prime & Bond NT) E + pB	• Laboratory research back up their use on enamel and dentin • Clinical studies show very positive results • The one-bottle concept makes them extremely user-friendly	• Generally, lower bond strengths than multi-bottle adhesives, Acetone-based adhesives may lose their efficacy with constant utilization • Acetone-based adhesives may need more coats than those recommended by the manufacturer (rule of thumb: to prevent the occurrence of dry spots not covered with adhesive, always apply one extra coat when using acetone-based adhesives) • Ethanol-based adhesives may pool easily around the preparation margin • Most one-bottle adhesives cannot be used as dual-cure materials • Have potential for excessive dentin decalcification and their reliance on very careful moisture control to achieve good bonding [E - Etching, P - priming, B - bonding agent]

When non-aqueous primers are applied onto dry dentin, the collagen is not rewetted by water and the network continues to exist in a collapsed stiffened state with little or no resin penetration because of the reduced porosity around collagen fibrils. Instead the resin is limited to the surface of collapsed layer. On the other hand when water based primers are applied to air dried, shrunken and demineralized dentin, two events may occur (i) If the water concentration of the primer is low, water soluble resin monomer and/or organic solvent will stiffen the collagen meshwork faster than the water can plasticize the collagen and it will not completely re-expand (ii) However, when the water content of the primer is large enough to plasticize the collagen faster than the resin/solvent stiffens it, the hydrophilic resin monomers infiltrate the network as it is gradually expanding. As a result more complete penetration can be expected with this *'self rewetting'* effect of water based primers used on dry dentin. Excessive water in the primer should be avoided as it dilutes the monomer concentration drastically. In dry bonding technique, if water free acetone based primers are used, they do not effectively infiltrate the exposed collagen network because of absence of water, forming the so called *'hybridoid regions'*. Well infiltrated areas under these

Table 16.5: Categorization of adhesives according to the mode of application

Systems	Smear layer modifying	Smear layer removing	Smear layer dissolving
One step	• Hytac OSB • Pertac Universal Bond • Prime & Bond 2.1 • Solist • Tokuso Light Bond		
Two step	• Optec Universal Bonding • Pro Bond • Tokuso Light Bond (two step) • Tripton	• Fuji Bond LC • Gluma 2000 • Optibond Solo • Prime & Bond 2.0 (total etch) • Scotch Bond 1 (Single bond) • Syntac Single component	• Clearfil Liner Bond 2 • Denthesive 11 • Opti Bond (No etch) • Imperva Bond (No etch) • Scotchbond 2 • Syntac • XR Bond
Three step		• All Bond 2 • Amalgam Bond Plus • Clearfil Liner Bond • Gluma • Imperva Bond (Total etch) • Mirage Bond • OptiBond (Total etch) • Scotchbond Multipurpose • Scotchbond Multipurpose Plus • Tenure	

Table 16.6: Current classification of adhesive systems

Classification	Acid	Primer	Bonding Resin
Etch-and-Rinse, 3 Steps	Phosphoric acid 32%-40%	Hydrophilic monomers, organic solvents	Hydrophobic monomers
Etch-and-Rinse, 2 Steps	Phosphoric acid 32%-40%	Hydrophilic monomers, organic solvents	Hydrophobic monomers
Self-Etch, 2 Steps	Acidic and hydrophilic monomers	Organic solvents	Hydrophobic monomers
Self-Etch, 1 Step	Acidic and hydrophilic monomers	Organic solvents	Hydrophobic monomers

primers are seen to be more electron dense and found only superficially along the walls of tubules and along the course of their lateral branches. When the dentin is kept moist, the collagen network is maintained in an expanded state and the inter fibrillar spaces are left open. Bonding to this moist surface could be efficient only if water within the dentin is completely eliminated and replaced by monomers during subsequent priming step. An effective wet bonding technique advocates use of primers that contain hydrophilic resin monomers dissolved in water miscible organic solvents like acetone and ethanol. On application of such primers on wet dentin, the water from it diffuses into the organic solvent, while the latter diffuses into the demineralized dentin matrix and tubules carrying with it the polymerizable monomers. The water is hence gradually lost as the solvents and resin monomers move further around the collagen fibrils. This probably explains the better bonding ability in the wet bonding technique (Gwinnett, 1992 and Kanca, 1992). If the water inside the collagen network is not completely displaced, polymerization of resin inside the hybrid layer may be affected or the remaining water will compete for space with resin inside the demineralized dentin. When the water from dentin is not completely removed by hydrophilic monomer, the phenomenon is referred to as *overwetting phenomenon*. In such overwet conditions, excess moisture decreases the concentration of organic solvents in the primer, thereby lowering the solubility of monomers. The monomers are present in the form of globules over

Table 16.7: Common dental adhesives	
Adhesive	Manufacturer
Three-step etch-and-rinse	
Adper Scotchbond Multi-Purpose	3M ESPE, ST Paul (MN), USA
All-Bond 2	Bisco Inc., Schaumburg (IL), USA
Optibond FL	Kerr, Orange (CA), USA
Syntac	Ivoclar Vivadent, Schaan, Liechtenstein
Two-step etch-and-rinse	
Excite	Ivoclar Vivadent, Schaan, Liechtenstein
Gluma Comfort Bond	Heraeus Kulzer, Hanau, Germany
Single Bond	3M ESPE, ST Paul (MN), USA
One Coat Bond	Coltene-Whaledent, Aistatten, Switzerland
One-step	Bisco Inc., Schaumburg, IL (USA)
One-Step Plus	Bisco Inc., Schaumburg, IL (USA)
Optibond Solo Plus	Kerr, Orange (CA), USA
Prime & Bond NT	Dentsply De Trey, Konstanz, Germany
Two-step self-etch	
Clearfil Liner Bond 2	Kuraray Medical Inc., Tokyo, Japan
Clearfil Protect Bond	Kuraray Medical Inc., Tokyo, Japan
Clearfil SE Bond	Kuraray Medical Inc., Tokyo, Japan
One Coat Self-Etching Bond	Coltene-Whaledent, Alsatten, Switzerland
Optibond Solo Plus Self-Etch	Kerr, Orange (CA), USA
Unifil Bond	GC, Tokyo, Japan
One-step self-etch	
Adper Prompt L-Pop	3M ESPE, ST Paul, MN, USA
AQ Bond	Sun Medical Co., Shiga, Japan
Clearfil S^3 Bond	Kuraray Medical Inc., Tokyo, Japan
G-Bond	GC, Tokyo, Japan
iBond	Heraeus Kulzer, Hanau, Germany
One-up Bond F	Tokuyama Dental Corporation, Tokyo, Japan
One-up Bond F Plus	Tokuyama Dental Corporation, Tokyo, Japan
Reactmer Bond	Shofu Inc., Kyoto, Japan
Xeno III	Dentsply De Trey, Konstanz, Germany
Xeno IV	Dentsply De Trey, Konstanz, Germany

the water layer. This is more common in the dentinal tubules where high content of water is present than in the intertubular dentin. They may present as *'blister like'* structures on the dentin surface with water being trapped beneath the resin layer. Many resin globules have been demonstrated inside the water droplets as well as tubules. An interesting feature occurred when the tubule orifice was blocked with water. No resin tags formed but several globules were present in the lumen. It is concluded that a critical amount of water is prudent for good bonding but an overwet condition decreases bond strength by lack of resin tags and formation of blister like structures at the interface.

The primer solvent should be either water or water miscible agent. The commonly used solvents are:
- Acetone (used in Prime & Bond NT, Bisco One step)
- Ethanol (used in Optibond solo, 3M Single bond)
- Water (used in Scotchbond Multipurpose Plus)

Acetone has a relatively high vapor pressure value (184 mmHg at 20°C) compared to ethanol (43.9 mmHg at 20°C) and water (17.5 mmHg at 20°C) a higher vapor pressure will allow the solvent to evaporate more easily. As the solvent evaporates, the viscosity of the dentin bonding agent increases, which decreases the ability of the bonding system to penetrate around the exposed collagen fibers and the opened dentinal tubules, consequently inhibiting the proper bond formation.

BONDING IN OTHER CLINICAL SITUATIONS

The spectrum of bonding is quite wide. Bonding at the microscopic level has been the subject of interest in recent years. Almost every material and technique has tried to achieve bonding between two variables. The possible bonding spectrum is illustrated in Fig. 16.28.

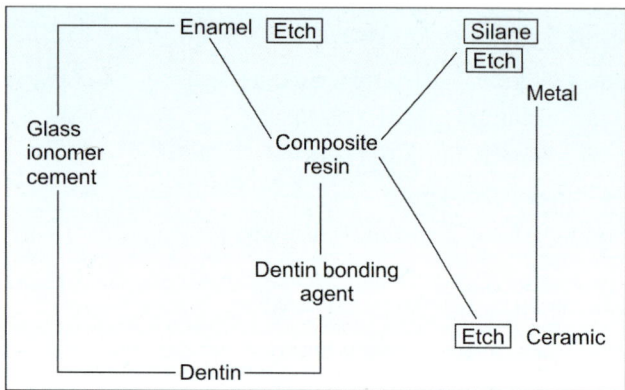

Fig. 16.28: Bonding spectrum in dentistry

Bonding of Glass-ionomers to Hard Tissue

Glass-ionomers possess an important property of adhering to enamel and dentin. They can also bond to other reactive polar substrates such as base metals. The primary mechanism in their bonding is chemical adhesion rather than micromechanical as seen in composites, hence acid etching or other surface roughening procedures are of no use with glass-ionomers. On placing the hydrophilic and highly ionic glass-ionomer cements on the tooth substrate, they compete successfully with water because of the multiplicity of carboxyl groups that form hydrogen bonds with the substrate. Water is either displaced or incorporated into the cement. Adhesion so obtained is permanent and resistant to water degradation. Also, an additional feature is that the ionic polar bonds that attach the glass-ionomer cement to the substrate can be re-established if broken, in contrast to covalent chemical bonds that cannot be reformed.

In the early stages of the chemical reaction, glass-ionomers are quite acidic because of the presence of unreacted caryboxylic acid groups in the material. These groups are hence free and offer an adhesive mechanism with the Ca ions of hydroxyapatite $(Ca_{10}(PO_4)_6(OH)_2)$ in enamel and dentin. As expected, bonding to enamel will be stronger than bonding to dentin because of the larger inorganic (hydroxyapatite) content in the former. Although it is quite certain that carboxyl groups of glass-ionomer can bond strongly to the multivalent Ca ions, yet no precise mechanism of adhesion can be elucidated.

Initially it was speculated that chelation of calcium in apatite by glass-ionomer was the primary mechanism involved in adhesion. Earlier, it was thought that interaction between apatite and polyacrylic acid resulted in polyacrylate ions which formed strong ionic bonds with the calcium ions in enamel and dentin surface. It has been suggested that when cement was initially applied to the tooth in a fluid consistency, wetting and adhesion occurred by hydrogen bonding mediated by carboxyl groups in the cement paste. As the cement set, hydrogen bonds were gradually replaced by ionic bonds. Later it was postulated that a series of complex ions exchanges occur during chemical reaction and adhesion. As the polyacrylate ions enter the molecular surface of hydroxyapatite, they displace and replace one phosphate and one calcium ion. As a consequence, an intermediate layer of calcium and aluminium phosphate and polyacrylate is formed at the interface between the cement and apatite. Chain length is also an important factor in adhesion of glass-ionomers. A simple assembly of cations and anions will not be expected to fill the gap at the interface whereas a polymer chain can bridge the gap and complete the bond.

Bonding of Composite to Glass-ionomer

Glass-ionomer invariably is used as a substitute for dentin under composite resins. This technique is commonly known as *bilayered technique (Sandwich technique)* in which the enamel and cement are etched prior to placement of the restorative resin.

Generally, 37% phosphoric acid is used to etch glass-ionomer and the enamel. Acid treatment of glass-ionomer improves its bond to composite by producing a rough surface in which glass particles stand out above the matrix. A thin liquid resin, which is then applied is able to penetrate into the micropores between the particles thereby providing mechanical interlocking.

Low viscosity resins are advisable as they have a lower contact angle and better wetting ability with the substrate. The cement should be allowed to fully set before it is etched otherwise the unreacted particles may dissolve and weaken the cement. A minimum delay of 20 minutes is therefore recommended prior to etching. The time for which etching needs to be done also deserves attention. Acid etching should be restricted to time periods that will remove just enough matrix material to provide a surface that is mechanically retentive and yet not harm the strength of the underlying cement. 15-20 seconds etching period is sufficient. Above 30 seconds of etching, the cement is excessively prone to degradation by the acid. Grinding of the set cement should be avoided as it might decrease the bond strength values.

The type of glass-ionomer cement has shown to influence the bond at the dentin surface and the glass-ionomer/composite interface. Higher the strength of the cement, better are the clinical results. The rate of set of the cement has also shown to affect bond strength values. A slow setting cement will be weakened considerably if etched prematurely. Faster setting cement can be etched after 2-5 minutes. Glass-ionomer cements should be used in adequate bulk under composite resin to avoid stresses from the shrinking composite. Use of light cure glass-ionomer lining materials have greatly reduced the chances of debonding. These achieve high early strength on photo-polymerization and also chemically bond to the resin composite without the need for etching. Should a layer of separating medium be applied at the glass-ionomer composite interface, remains controversial. A few authors advocate the use of varnish over glass-ionomer cement with the rationale that the polymerization shrinkage of composite will not disturb the underlying cement.

Bonding of Composite to Porcelain

Bonding of porcelain to composite is partly because of mechanical interlocking and partly because of chemical union. Such a situation occurs when porcelain inlays and onlays are cemented to the tooth using a resin based cement. Mechanical retention is obtained by etching the fitting surface of porcelain with dilute hydrofluoric acid or grit blasted with alumina to increase surface roughness. The optimal time for etching depends upon the etchant concentration as well as the type of porcelain used. To improve upon the mechanical attachment, gap between the bonding medium and the porcelain should be minimized by using an intermediate low viscosity resin which penetrates into the pores by capillary action.

Shear bond strengths have shown to increase by several times when porcelain is etched compared to when it is not etched.

Chemical union between porcelain and composite is made possible by treating the etched surface with a silane coupling agent. However, relatively low increase in bond strength has been observed with this additional treatment suggesting that mechanical interlocking is probably more important than chemical adhesion. Silane coupling agents have also shown to reduce the gap between porcelain and composite presumably by improving upon the wetting ability and hence promoting mechanical interlocking. Since concern still exists regarding the shelf life and durability of silane in moist conditions, it is preferable to use it as an aid to mechanical retention.

Bonding of Amalgam to Resin

Bonding of amalgam to resin is a relatively new treatment modality and has made bonding between amalgam and tooth structure, amalgam and amalgam or amalgam and metal quite a successful possibility. Bonding offers many advantages like:
- Increases retention without the use of additional retentive features like pins, grooves, dovetails, etc.
- Increases fracture resistance while conserving tooth structure
- Reduces microleakage and
- Decreases chances of recurrent caries

Agents that can be used for bonding amalgam to the substrate are All Bond, Liner Bond-2, Amalgam bond and Panavia. A specific feature desired in these materials is that they should have dual characteristics to achieve optimal wetting. Dental amalgam is strongly hydrophobic whereas enamel is hydrophilic, hence a wetting agent needs to be incorporated into the bonding resin that can wet both hydrophobic and hydrophilic surfaces. 4-META and MDP are commonly used for this purpose.

The nature of bond between resin and amalgam is mainly micromechanical, as amalgam interlocks with the fluid resin during condensation. Bond strengths with amalgam to dentin have shown to be relatively low (2-6 MPa). Failure generally occurs at the interface between bonding agent and amalgam, while the bond on the other side, i.e. between resin and tooth is sufficiently strong. Much clinical evidence is yet needed to establish the durability and superiority of bonded amalgam over conventional amalgam restorations.

ADDITIVES FOR DENTIN-ENAMEL ADHESION

The filler contents, though in minute quantity, play a vital role in dental adhesion. All types of fillers are being used in adhesion. The addition of fillers in total etch adhesives improves bond strength of these adhesives. The newer self-etching bonding systems, where adequate wetting and penetration of acidic monomer is essential, contain only small amount of fillers. In single step systems, silica fillers are often used as thickener to increase the viscosity, resulting in adequate film thickness. It also prevents over thinning and incomplete polymerization due to oxygen inhibition.

Recent adhesives contain fillers having properties of fluoride release and opacity. Polysiloxane encapsulated sodium fluoride particles are used as a source for fluoride ions. Fluoride is applied because of anticariogenic activity resulting in an increased resistance of enamel and dentin to acid attacks and inhibits the carbohydrate metabolism of dental plaque. The addition of fluoride definitely improves the bond strength.

Certain adhesives use dyes with the intention to clearly indicate the proper mixing of the components. One-up bond and Tyrian SPE are the examples of such adhesives. In one-up bond the color changes from yellow to pink. When the adhesive is light cured, the color fades. The addition of antibacterial agents in adhesives is showing promising results. Antibacterial components are added to adhesive systems to ensure biological sealing of the restoration. The total etch adhesive system use phosphoric acid to condition the prepared tooth surface by removing the smear layer. The phosphoric acid also exhibits antimicrobial activity, though for a shorter time. Glutaraldehyde has been used as disinfectant in earlier multi bottle systems such as Syntac or Gluma-bond as well in i-Bond (one step self etching system). Another product MDPB, (methacryl-oyloxydodecyl pyridinium bromide) is also used as antibacterial component in various adhesives.

SUCCESS/FAILURE OF ADHESIVES

Several variables can effect the clinical performance of adhesive systems vis-à-vis the success/failure of the system (Fig.16.29). These can be summarized as below:

1. *Material factors*: Thorough knowledge of chemistry of the material to be used is mandatory for successful bonding. Hydrophobic bonding agents do not provide sufficient bond. The manufacturer's instructions should be carefully followed regarding washing off the conditioner and mode of applying the primer and bonding.

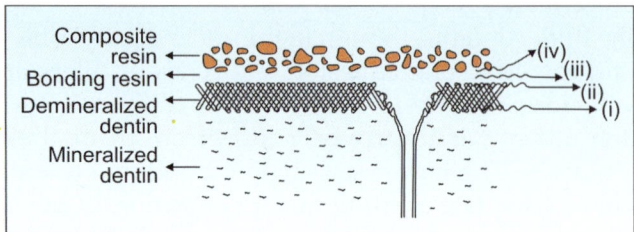

Fig. 16.29: Diagram illustrating different positions of failure at the resin-adhesive-tooth interface (i) Between the mineralized and demineralized dentin (ii) Between demineralized dentin and bonding resin (iii) Within the bonding resin; and (iv) Between the bonding resin and composite resin

2. *Substrate*: Variability of the substrate has shown to have a major effect on the clinical performance of adhesive systems. Its details have already been covered in the preceeding pages.

3. *Size and shape of lesion*: Size of the lesion or the area of dentinal substrate available for bonding is critical for adhesion. Less adhesion is seen in small sized cervical lesions. Deep wedge shaped lesions have also shown to better retain adhesive restorations than shallow saucer shaped lesions.

4. *Maxillary verus mandibular arch*: Better adhesion results are expected in the maxillary arch because of lesser chances of moisture contamination and lower tooth flexure effects in the upper jaws.

5. *Patient's age*: With age, the dentin becomes sclerosed and the sclerosis is associated with a decrease in clinical adhesiveness and hence a higher failure rate. Besides sclerosis, increased tooth flexure may also be a factor towards failure of restoration vis-à-vis adhesion. Recent trials however, have predicted no direct relation between retention failure and patient's age as sclerosis is pertinent not only to old age but is determined by the lesion age or the time period for which the dentin has been exposed to the oral environment.

6. *Tooth flexure*: More recently, tooth flexure is a probable factor in influencing the retention of adhesive restorations especially the cervical restorations. Heavy centric occlusal and eccentric forces are responsible for generating compressive and tensile forces in the cervical area, which may gradually dislodge and debond the resin restoration. The composites with adequate elastic capacity like microfilled composites are prefered in such lesions.

7. *Dentin wetness*: Basically the principle of good spreading of monomer on dentin is important for successful bonding. Along with the wetting, the permeability of the demineralized dentin to monomer also aids in dentin bonding. The bonding agents with effective wetting capability ensure successful bonding.

8. *Elastic bonding concept*: Composite resins shrink during polymerization. In order to protect the tooth composite interface from debonding during polymerization, the intervening adhesive resin should be sufficiently elastic to absorb the polymerization stresses. This can be achieved by using a relatively thick layer of separately polymerized, unfilled or semifilled bonding resins. Alternatively, the additional use of intermediate glass-ionomer liners under composites are known to reduce the total stiffness of the restoration.

'WATER TREEING' PHENOMENON

The adhesives normally contain hydrophilic and/or ionic monomers in order to improve their bonding to wet substrate of dentin. It is established that since the adhesives lack non-solvent resin coatings, they act as semipermeable membrane, permitting water movement across the polymerized adhesives. It implies that there are interconnected channels within the adhesives which are responsible for such movement. Usually these channels are not visible unless incorporated with silver nitrate, since the water is lost after dessication of the specimens. These water channels (revealed by silver staining) were seen at resin-dentin interface. These water channels within the adhesive layer is termed as 'water trees'. Water trees are generally located along the surface of the hybrid layer extending into the underlying adhesive layers (Fig. 16.30).

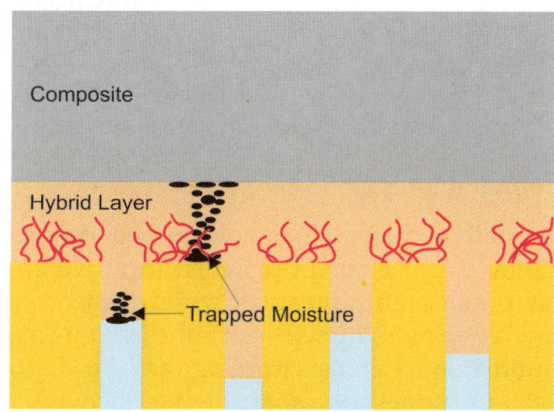

Fig. 16.30: Water tree formation

Tay and Pashley (2003) hypothesized that water trees in dental adhesives along with nanoleakage within the hybrid layer, represent water rich interfacial regions from which the leaching of hydrophilic resin components may occur readily, leading to degradation of resin-dentin bonds.

Two theories have been proposed as regards genesis of water treeing phenomenon.

a. *Remnant water theory:* Earlier authors belived that water trees were 'left out' water that was incompletely removed from water in dentin adhesives. Water trees were observed from resin-dentin interface bonded with ethanol-based adhesives and rarely in acetone-based adhesives. It was further observed that addition of HEMA to water lowered the rate of evaporation of water from the HEMA-water mixture.

   However, this theory does not account for following aspects of water free formation.
   i. Uneven distribution: Water trees are never uniformly described. Water trees were seldom seen in the central part of the adhesive layer; rather predominantly present at the surface of the hybrid layer.
   ii. Substrate dependence: Water trees have been frequently observed in sound dentin bonded with one-step self-etch adhesives; however, they were virtually absent when discs of composite resins were used as bonding substrate, if the adhesive was air dried before bonding. It implies that water tree contribute minimally by residual water derived from the dentin adhesive.
   iii. Reverse water trees: Different shapes and forms of water trees have been observed. Usually water trees originate from the surface of dentin, with their branching pointing upwards into the adhesive. In case of reverse water tree, they appear to originate from water trapped at the interface between the adhesive and the overlying resin composite; they spread downwards with the 'branches' pointing towards dentin.
   iv. Secondary water trees: Water droplets are entrapped and seen as clear holes within the adhesive layer. When observed under silver nitrate tracer, water trees were seen radiating circumferentially from the periphery of these water droplets creating a 'sunburst' effect around the droplets.

   As water trees seldom exist when water-containing adhesives are used to bond composite to composite. It is unlikely that water tree formation is caused by water, that is present within the adhesive formulations. Two features which could not be explained are:
   - From where the water is derived
   - What triggers the movement of this additional source of water

   These two features are explained in the water 'flux'.

b. *Water-flux theory:* The fluid movement in dentin can be of three types, viz. evaporative, osmotic or convective water fluxes. Evaporative is due to air drying. Touch of paper point induce capillary forces leading to outward movement of fluid. Non-vital dentin also contain water, evaporative water flux may occur irrespective of tooth vitality.

The high concentration of water soluble ionic monomer in the presence of water may also induce osmotic water flux from deep dentin. This may occur just prior to polymerization. As soon as the monomers are converted to polymers, the osmotically induced water flux is ceased.

Both osmotic and evaporative fluxes result in the permeation of water within the adhesive mixture. These explain the predilection of normally oriented water trees along the surface of the dentin. It has been shown that following the detection of outward evaporation water flux (reverse water tree) after air-drying of the adhesive coated dentin, additional inward fluid flux was induced by light activation of the adhesive. During light activation process some of the water that has reached the top of the adhesive layer cannot escape, as it is trapped by the initially polymerized surface of the adhesive. The heat generated by the curing lights reflect water back into the less polymerized subsurface adhesive matrix forming water tracks that are morphologically identified as reverse water tree. Water droplets trapped between the adhesive and the resin composite may account for their incompatibility. These droplets reduce the bonded surface area and increases interfacial stresses, subsequently leading to dislodging of the resin composite (Fig. 16.31).

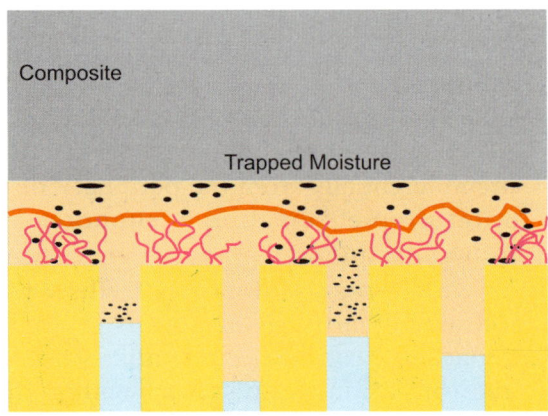

Fig. 16.31: Failure of Resin—dentin bond by hydrolytic degradation with passage of time

Absence of Water Treeing in Transparent Carious Dentin

Transparent carious dentin is heavily occluded with intratubular mineral deposits. These deposits account for relative impermeability of this layer. Both water treeing and nanoleakage were absent from hybrid layers of transparent dentin. The hybrid layer of transparent dentin is usually three times as thick as that of sound dentin. No nanoleakage can be because of both evaporative and convective water fluxes from dentin were blocked by heavily occluded dentinal tubules. This may result in excellent initial resin seal with the complete absence of water rich interfacial zones above a highly porous bonding substrate that is partially depleted of its mineral contents. Although these hybrid layer were thicker, it was not possible for any adhesive to completely diffuse through a zone of partially demineralized dentin that may be several hundred micrometer thick.

Nanoleakage and Water Treeing

The nanoleakage seen during bonding to sound dentin is demonstrated as the inward diffusion of acidic monomer demineralise the dentin and dissolve smear layer. The outward osmotically induced water fluxer may flush out the partially neutralized resin monomer from the demineralised dentin. The presence of such water in acidic adhesive may retard the polymerization of resin within the interfibrillar spaces. The water usually finds its way through the smear layer and is manifested as water trees within the adhesive matrix. Depending upon the chemical composition of the adhesive phase separation of the water may occur in the form of water droplets which is manifested as secondary water trees. The nanoleakage in self etch adhesives and the water trees formation occur along the surface of the hybrid layer. In the case of nanoleakage within the hybrid layer, the subsurface water moves preferentially to pre-existing channels.

Functional Implications of Water Treeing

Functionally reduction in nanoleakage and water tree formation may be achieved when multiple coats of one-step self-etch adhesives were used on sound dentin. When one step self-etch adhesives are applied to sound dentin water droplets may be deposited between the adhesive composite interface due to the rapid water movement across the adhesive. If sufficient layer of adhesive is present, the phenomenon of water blistering may be of minor implications. The adhesives can be rendered less permeable by treating the one step self-etch adhesive as a primer and covering it with a coat of less hydrophilic resin. The extra step converts one step into two step self-etch adhesive and render them less permeable to water movement.

BIBLIOGRAPHY

1. Arantha, A.C., Siqueira, Jr. S., Cavalcante, L.M., Pimenta, L.A. and Marchi, G.M.: Microtensile bond strength of composite to dentin treated with desensitizer products. J. Adhes. Dent.: 8, 85, 2006.
2. Belli, S., Ozcopur, B., Yesilyurt, C., Bulut, G., Ding, X. and Dorsman, G.: The effect of loading on MTBS of four all-in-one adhesives on bonding to dentin. Journal of Biomedical Materials Research Part-B Applied Biomaterials: 91, 948, 2009.
3. Bonillaguet, S. and Wataha, J.C.: Future direction in bonding resins to the dentin-pulp complex. J. Oral Rehab.: 31, 385, 2004.

4. Breschi, L., Mazzoni, A., Ruggeri, A., Cadenaro, M., Di Lenarda, R. and De Stefano Dorgio, E.: Dental adhesion review: aging and stability of the bonded interface. Dental Materials: 24, 90, 2008.
5. Carrilho, M.R.O., Tay, F.R., Pashley, D.H., Tjaderhane, L. and Carvalho, R.M.: Mechanical stability of resin-dentin bonds components. Dent. Mater.: 21, 32, 2005.
6. Chang, J.C., Hurst, T.L., Hart, D.A. and Estey, A.W.: 4-META use in dentistry: a literature review. J.P.D.: 87, 216, 2002.
7. Choi, K.K, Condon, J.R. and Ferracane, J.L.: The effect of adhesive thickness on polymerization contraction stress of composites. J. Dent. Res.: 79, 812, 2000.
8. DeMunck, J., Pneumuns, M., Poitevin, A., Lambrechts, P., Braem, M. and Van Meerbeek, B.: Durability of adhesion to tooth tissue: methods and results. J. Dent. Res.: 66, 1636, 2005.
9. De Munck, J., Van Landuyt, K., Peumans, M., Poitevin, A., Lambrechts, P. and Braem, M.: A critical review of the durability of adhesion to tooth tissue: methods and results. J. Dent. Res.: 84, 118, 2005.
10. Duke, E.S. and Lindemuth, J.: Variability of clinical dentin substrates. Am. J. Dent.: 4, 241, 1991.
11. Dunn, J.R.: i Bond – the seventh generation, one bottle, dental bonding agent. Compend. Contin. Educ. Dent.: 24, 14, 2003.
12. Erickson, R.L. and Glasspoole, E.A.: Bonding to tooth structure: A comparison of glass-ionomer and composite resin systems. J. Esthet. Dent.: 6, 221, 1994.
13. Fadaie P, Atai M, Imani M and Karkhareh A.: Cyanoacrylate –POSS nanocomposites: novel adhesives with improved properties for dental applications.: Dent Mater 29,6,2013.
14. Foxton, R.M., Melo, L., Stone, D.G., Pilecki, P., Sherriff, M. and Watson, T.F.: Long-term durability of one-step adhesive-composite systems to enamel and dentin. Oper. Dent.: 3, 651, 2008.
15. Haag, P.: Bonding between titanium and dental porcelain: A systematic review. Acta. Odont. Scand.: 68, 154, 2010.
16. Hanabusa M, Mine A, Kukobi T, Momoi Y, Ende AV, Meerbeek BV and Munck JD.: Bonding effectiveness of a new 'multi-mode' adhesive to enamel and dentin. J Dent: 40, 475,2012
17. Hashimoto, M., Nakamura, K., Kaga, M. and Yawaka, Y.: Crystals growth by fluoridated adhesive resins. Dent. Mater.: 24, 457, 2008.
18. Hitmi, L., Bouter, D. and Degrange, M.: Influence of drying and HEMA treatment on dentin wettability. Dental Materials: 18, 3, 2002.
19. Hotta, M. and Yamamoto, K.: Comparative radiopacity of bonding agents. J. Adhesive Dent.: 11, 207, 2009.
20. Inoue, N., Tsujimoto, A., Takimoto, M., Ootsuka, E., Endo, H., Takamizawa, T. and Miyazaki, M.: Surface free-energy measurements as indicators of the bonding characteristics of single step self-etching adhesives. Eur. J. Oral Sci.: 118, 525, 2010.
21. Ito, S., Hoshino, T., Iijima, M., Tsukamoto, N., Pashley, D.H. and Saito, T.: Water sorption/solubility of self-etching dentin bonding agents. Dent. Material: 26, 617, 2010.
22. Janda, R., Roalet, J.F., Wulf, M. and Tiller, H.J.: Resin-Resin bonding: A new adhesive technology. J. Adhesive Dent.: 4, 299, 2002.
23. Lee, Y.K., Pinzon, L.M., O'Keefe, K.L. and Powers, J.M.: Effect of filler addition on the bonding parameters of dentin bonding adhesive bonded to human dentin. Am. J. Dent.: 19, 23, 2006.
24. Leloup, G., D'Moore, W., Bouter, D., Degrange, M. and Vreven, J.: Meta analytical review of factors involved in dentin adherence. J.D.R.: 80, 1605, 2001.
25. Lima, G., da, S., Ogliari, F.A., da Silva, E.O., Ely, C. and Demarco, F.F.: Influence of water concentration in an experimental self-etching primer on the bond strength to dentin. J. Adhesive Dent.: 10, 167, 2008.
26. Lopes, G.C., Baratieri, C.M., Baratieri, L.N., Monteiro, Jr. S., Vieira, L.C.: Bonding to cervical sclerotic dentin: Effect of acid etching time. J. Adhesive Dent.: 6, 19, 2004.
27. Lopes, G.C., Vieira, L.C., Araujo, E., Bruggmann, T., Zucco, J. and Olieviera, G.: Effect of dentin age acid etching time on dentin bonding. J. Adhesive Dent.: 13, 139, 2011.
28. Lopes, G.C., Thys, D.G., Klauss, P., Mussi, G. and Widmer, N.: Enamel acid etching: a review. Compendium: 28, 662, 2007.
29. Lung C and Matinlinna J.: Aspects of silane coupling agents and surface conditioning in dentistry: An overview. Dent Mater: 28, 467,2012
30. Mine, A., De Munck, J., Van Laduyt, K.L., Poitevin, A., Kuboki, T. and Yoshida, Y.: Bonding effectiveness and interfacial characterization of a HEMA/TEGDMA-free three-step etch and rinse adhesive. Journal of Dentistry: 36, 767, 2008.
31. Moszner, N., Salz, U. and Zimmermann, J.: Chemical aspects of self-etching enamel dentin adhesives: A systemic review. Dent. Mater.: 21, 895, 2005.
32. Moura, S.K., Pelizzaro, A., Dal Bianco, K., de Goes, M.F., Loguercio, A.D., Reis, A. and Grande, R.H.: Does the acidity of self-etching primers affect bond strengths and surface morphology of enamel ? J. Adhesive. Dent.: 8, 75, 2006.
33. Munck J, Ende A, Suyania Y, Mine .: Bonding effectiveness of self-adhesive composite to dentin and enamel . Dent Mater 29,2 ,2013.
34. Nakabayashi, N., Nakamura, M. and Yasuda, N.: The hybrid layer as a dentin bonding mechanism. J. Esthet. Dent.: 3, 133, 1991.
35. Nakaoki, Y., Sasakawa, W., Horiuchi, S., Nagano, F., Ikeda, T., Tanaka, T. and Inoue, S.: Effect of double application of all-in-one adhesives on dentin bonding. J. Dent.: 33, 765, 2005.
36. Ohba, M., Manabe, A., Itoh, K., Hisamitsu, H. and Wakumoto, S.: 2-HEMA-free dentin bonding system to prevent contraction gap. Dental Materials J.: 17, 83, 2008.
37. Owens, B.M., Johnson, W.W. and Harris, E.F.: Marginal permeability of self-etch and total etch adhesive systems. Oper. Dent.: 31, 60, 2006.
38. Papadogiannis D. , Lakes R.S. , Papadogiannis Y. and Tolidis K.: Mechanical viscoelastic behavior of dental adhesives.: Dent Mater 29,6, 2013.
39. Pashley, D.H., Tay, F.R., Brechi, L., Tjaderhane, L., Carvalho, R.M., Carrilho, M. and Mutluay, A.T.: State of the art etch-and-rinse adhesives. Dent. Materials: 27, 1, 2011.

40. Perdigao, J., Frankenberger, R., Rosa, B., Breschi, L.: New trends in dentin/enamel adhesion. Am. J. Dent.: 13, 25, 2000.
41. Plasmans, P.J.J.M., Vollenbrockkuipers, I., Reukers, E.A.J., and Vollenbrock, I.I.R.: Air humidity: A detrimental factor in dentine adhesion. J. Dent.: 21, 228, 1993.
42. Penumas, M., Kanumilli, P, De Munck, J., Van Landuyt, K., Lambrechts, P. and Van Meerbeek, B.: Clinical effectiveness of contemporary adhesives: a systematic review of current clinical trials. Dental Materials: 21, 864, 2005.
43. Ricci, H.A., Sanabe, M.E., deSourza, C., Pashley, D.H. and Hebling, J.: Chlorhexidine increases the longevity of in vivo resin-dentin bonds. Eur. J. Oral Sci.: 118, 411, 2010.
44. Salz, U., Zimmermann, J., Zeuner, F. and Moszner, N.: Hydrolytic stability of self-etching adhesive systems. J. Adhes. Dent.: 7, 107, 2005.
45. Salz, U. and Bock, T.: Testing adhesion of direct restoratives to dental hard tissues – a review. J. Adhesive Dent.: 12, 343, 2010.
46. Schneider, D.J., Combe, E.C. and Martins, L.V.: The effect of washing water on bonding to etched enamel. J. Oral Rehab.: 31, 85, 2004.
47. Sharrock, P. and Gregoire, G.: HEMA reactivity with demineralized dentin. J. Dent.: 38, 31, 2010.
48. Shin, T.P., Yao, X., Huenergardt, R., Walker, M.P. and Wang, Y.: Morphological and chemical characterization of bonding hydrophobic adhesive to dentin using ethanol wet bonding technique. Dental Materials: 25, 1050, 2009.
49. Shirai, K., DeMunck, J., Yoshida, Y., Inoue, S., Lambrechts, P. and Shintani, H.: Efficacy of cavity configuration and ageing on the bonding effectiveness of six adhesives to dentin. Dent. Mater.: 21, 110, 2005.
50. Spencer, P., Wang, Y., Walker, M.P., Wielickza, I.M. and Swafford, J.R.: Interfacial chemistry of the dentin/adhesive bond. J. Dent. Res.: 79, 1458, 2000.
51. Taschner, M., Nato, F.;, Mazzani, A., Frankenberger, R., Kramer, N., Lenarda, R., Petscheldt, A. and Breschi, L.: Role of preliminary etching for one step self etch adhesives. Eur. J. Oral Sci.: 118, 517, 2010.
52. Tay, F.R. and Pashley, D.H.: Water treeing- a potential mechanism for degradation of dental adhesives. Am. J. Dent.: 16, 6, 2003.
53. Tay, F.R. and Pashley, D.H.: Resin bonding to cervical sclerotic dentin. A review. J. Dent.: 32, 173, 2004.
54. Tay, F.R., Pashley, D.H., Bi, Suh, Hiraishi, N. and Yiu, C.K.Y.: Water treeing in simplified dentin adhesives – Déjà vu ? Oper. Dent.: 30, 561, 2005.
55. Vaidyanathan, T.K. and Vaidyanathan, J.: Recent advances in the theory and mechanism of adhesive resin bonding to dentin: a critical review. J. Biomedical Materials Research B Applied Biomaterials: 88, 558, 2009.
56. Van Laduyt, K.L., Snauwaert, J., De Munck, J., Peumans, M., Yoshida, Y. and Poitevin et al.: Systematic review of the chemical composition of contemporary dental adhesives. Biomaterials: 28, 3757, 2007.
57. VanMeerbeck, B., Yoshihara, K., Yoshida, Y., Mine, A., De Munck, J. and Van Landuyt, K.L.: State of the art of self-etch adhesives. Dent. Material: 27, 17, 2011.
58. Wattanawongpitak, N., Yoshikawa, T., Burrow, M.F. and Tagami, J.: The effect of bonding system and composite type on adaptation of different c-factor restorations. Dent. Mater. J.: 25, 45, 2006.
59. Ye, Q., Park, J.G., Topp, E., Wang, Y., Misra, A. and Spencer, P.: In vitro performance of nanoheterogenous dentin adhesive. J. Dent. Res.: 87, 829, 2008.
60. Yoo, H.M., Oh, T.S. and Pereira, P.N.: Effect of saliva contamination on the micro shear bond strength of one step self-etching adhesive systems to dentin. Oper. Dent.: 31, 127, 2006.
61. Zanchi, C.H., Munchow, E.A. Ogliari, F.A.. Chersoni, S., Prati, C., Piva, E. and Demarcu, F.F.: Development of experimental HEMA-free three step adhesive system. J. Dent.: 38, 503, 2010.

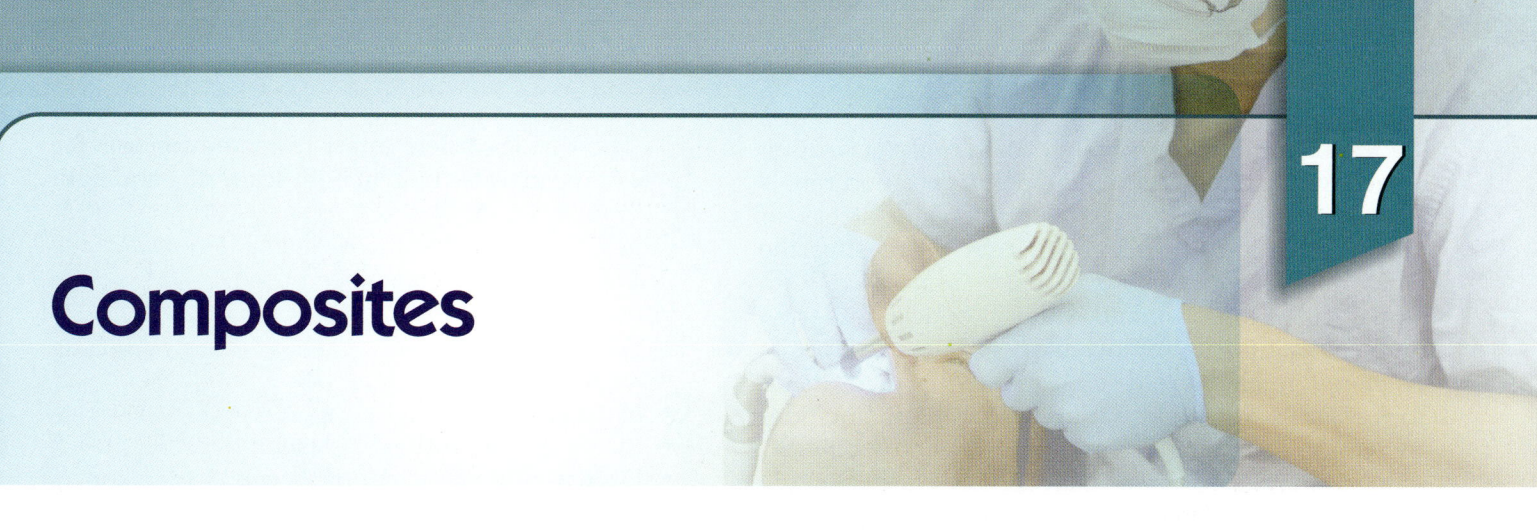

Composites

The concept of the esthetic restorations is not new. The translucent silicate cement used earlier had certain disadvantages such as their solubility, pulp irritation potential and dessication etc. These disadvantages lead to the advent of acrylics which could overcome some of the problems associated with silicates but did not last long because of inherent drawbacks of higher coefficient of thermal expansion and higher polymerization shrinkage. To improve upon these drawbacks, filler particles were added to the acrylic resin matrix. Various types of fillers ranging from plastic fillers to glass fillers were added, but the fillers could not bind with the matrix and remained isolated.

The course of inventions and developments lead to the introduction of composites by *R.L. Bowen* in 1962. *Composite* is basically a botanical term, where the clusters of flowers are clubbed giving shape to a different flower. Metallurgically, composite is a combination of two or more materials having chemically distinct interface between them.

However, the accepted definition is of Anusavice, which says '*Composite material is a compound of two or more distinctly different materials with properties that are superior to or intermediate to those of the individual constituent.*'

The resin matrix of Bowen's formulation was BiSGMA (Bisphenol Glycidyl methacrylate which is a reaction product of Bisphenol A and Glycidyl methacrylate). Bowen also gave the concept of coupling agents, which help the filler particles to bind with the resin matrix. The composites at this time were chemically cured, a reaction similar to monomer polymer reaction along with activators and inhibitors.

COMPOSITION

The components of composites are:
   a. Resin matrix
   b. Fillers
   c. Coupling agents
   d. Coloring agents

a. Resin Matrix

The initial resin matrix was Bisphenol Glycidyl methacrylate (BisGMA) and urethane dimethacrylate (UDMA).

The BiSGMA/UDMA was viscous and blending of filler particles was difficult, so other matrix were tried having lower viscosity, such as:

TEGDMA (Triethylene glycol dimethacrylate)

The mixture of two of these three resins provides appropriate viscosity needed for binding of filler particles. BisGMA and TEGDMA in the ratio of 3:1 is preferred as increase in TEGDMA substantially increases the polymerization shrinkage.

The methacrylate based systems were modified to create monomers with lower viscosity, such as hydroxyl free BisGMA, aliphatic urethane dimethacrylate, partially aromatic urethane dimethacrylate or highly branched methacrylates. Also, ring opening monomers such as spiro orthocarbonates and epoxy base resins like siloranes as well as a series of high molecular weight monomers like dimer acid based dimethacrylates, tricyclodecane urethane and organically modified ceramics (ormocers) were introduced to the market for the same purpose.

Expanding matrix composites are introduced with the idea to compensate for the polymerization shrinkage. Vinyl cyclopropanes as ring opening compounds are also used which help in reducing the polymerization shrinkage. Spiro-ortho-carbonates are the expanding matrix used. It is preferably used with epoxy resin, because when used with BiSGMA/TEGDMA, it could not produce the required expansion. A newer system containing a diepoxide monomer and polyol has substantially reduced the polymerization shrinkage.

Hydrophobic monomers containing fluorinated dimethacrylate is also used as matrix. The memory polymer, which expand and shrink according to that of tooth is also being tried.

Modification of the dynamics of the polymerization reaction by slowing down the polymerization rate is the further mechanism to compensate stress of polymerization shrinkage, thereby increasing the material flow capacity and being associated with lower stress build up and better interfacial integrity. A recently introduced flowable resin based composite material, intended to be used as liner in occlusal and approximal restorations (Surefil SDR Flow) includes a monomer having incorporated a photo activated group in a urethane based methacrylate resin, showing 60–70% reduction in shrinkage stress. The activated resin demonstrated a relatively slow radical polymerization rate, suggesting that the photoinitiator incorporated into resin is affecting the radical polymerization process. These resins are patented as being based on stress decreasing resin (SDR) technology.

b. Fillers

Different types of fillers have been tried (Fig. 17.1).

The size of the filler particles vary from composite to composite depending upon the requirements and needs. To ensure acceptable esthetics of composites, the translucency of the filler must be similar to tooth structure. Mostly glasses have refractive index 1.5 which is comparable to dentin 1.52 and enamel 1.62.

The routinely used fillers are:
i. *Quartz*: Quartz is extremely hard and to grind it in finer particles is difficult. These were used in early composites, which were difficult to polish and even abraded the opposing tooth structure.
ii. *Silica*: Silica has been used as filler in many forms as pure silica, fused silica and colloidal silica. Both pyrogenic and precipitated form of colloidal silica has been used. Glasses as aluminosilicates and borosilicates are also used.

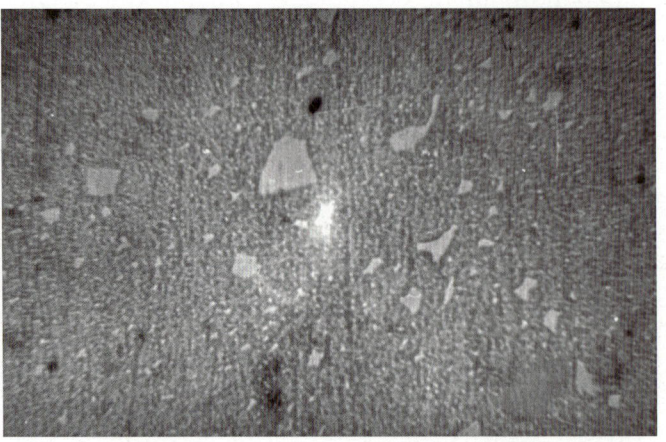

Fig. 17.1: Filler particles in Surefil

These silica fillers apart from reinforcing the composite, also help in light scattering and light transmission.

Other fillers such as *Tricalcium phosphate and Zirconium dioxide* have also been used.

Fillers provide:
- Strength
- Rigidity
- Hardness
- Increase in modulus of elasticity
- Decrease in coefficient of thermal expansion
- Decrease in contraction

The fillers containing fluoride such as *Yttrium trifluoride* and *Yitterbium trifluoride* have also been used.

Recent composites contain combination of Macro (Barium glass, particle size 0.7–2.0 µm) and micro (Pyrogenic silica, particle size 0.04–0.07 µm) fillers. These types of fillers provide:
- Better polishing
- Kindness to antagonist tooth
- Good esthetic and chameleon effect

The size of filler particles incorporated in the resin matrix of commercial dental composites has continuously decreased over the years from the traditional to nano-composite materials. When inorganic phases in an organic/inorganic composite become nanosized, they are called nano composites. Nanofillers can be prepared by various techniques such as flame pyrolysis, flame spray pyrolysis have dimensions below the wavelength of visible light, they are unable to scatter or absorb light. Thus, nanofillers are usually invisible and offer advantage of optical property improvement. Additionally, nanofillers are capable of increasing the overall filler level due to small particle sizes.

c. Coupling Agents

Coupling agents are used to bind filler particles to the resin matrix. Apart from binding, these allow the more flexible polymer matrix to transfer stresses to stiffer filler particles. These agents also provide hydrolytic stability by preventing the water from penetrating along the filler resin interface.

The silane molecule undergoes hydrolysis and forms a silanal group, which forms a bond with filler particles and carboxyl group, which help in polymerizing with the resin matrix.

It has been observed that coupling agents are best suited with silica particles. The combination provides appropriate translucency.

Organic silanes such as γ-methacryloxy propyl trimethoxy silane are commonly used as coupling agents.

Recently, 10–methacryloxy decyl-trimethoxysilane is being used, which is more hydrophobic and better suited as coupling agent.

In nanocomposites various coupling agents are used. Silanization with combination of methacryrloxy-propyltrimethaoxysilane (MPTS) and n-octyltrimethoxysilane (OTMS) was done. Dual silanization of silica particles offers several advantages compared to with MPTS alone.

Epoxy resin ERL4221 used γ glycidonypropyl-trimethoxysilane (GPS) as a coupling agent. With GPS as coupling agent, the tendency of agglomeration of silica particles reduces thus increasing the curing efficiency.

Organosilane acryltriethoxysilane (ATES) was used in TiO_2 nanoparticle reinforced nanocomposite, increases the dispersion and linkage of TiO_2 nanoparticles within the resin matrix.

d. Coloring Agents

Aluminium oxide and titanium dioxide in 0.001–0.007% by wt. are commonly used as coloring agents.

The earlier composites were chemically cured. Benzoyl peroxide as initiator was always been a part of resin matrix. An accelerator – a small amount of tertiary amines such as dimethyl-p-toluidine is added in the monomer. The polymerization starts by the release of free radicals from the reaction between benzoyl peroxide and the amine.

Because of degradation of amines, these composites show loss of color match after varying period of time. To improve upon this, more stable activator such as p-toluidine sulifinic acid is used.

Light cure composites were introduced which utilizes Benzoin methyl ether (UV light activated) and camphoroquinone (visible light activated) as initiator. Dimethyl amino ethyl methacrylate is used as activator.

Difference between chemically cured composites and light cured composites are given in Table 17.1.

The earlier UV light activated composites have been replaced by visible light activated composites. The difference between the two lights used for curing composite is given in Table 17.2.

EVOLUTION OF COMPOSITES

The evolution of composites vis-à-vis composition, filler particles, their size and percentage etc. is elaborated in Table 17.3.

PROPERTIES OF COMPOSITES

Physical properties vary between the three basic types of composites i.e. conventional or macrofilled, microfilled and hybrid (Table 17.4).

Table 17.1: Difference between chemically cured composites and light cured composites

Chemically cured	Light cured
Polymerization is central	Polymerization is peripheral
Curing is in one phase	Curing is in increments
Sets within 45 seconds	Sets only after light activation
No time for manipulation	Plenty of time for manipulation
More wastage	Less wastage
Not properly finished	Take better finish

Table 17.2: Difference between UV light and Visible light used for curing composites

UV light	Visible light
It works at 360–400 nm	Light range is 400–500 nm
Intensity falls with time	Intensity remains the same
Injurious to operator and patient eyes	Not injurious
Greater depth cannot be cured	Greater depth can be cured

ADVANCES IN COMPOSITES

i. Flowable Composites

The flowable composites are characterized by the presence of filler particles that have a particle size similar to that of the traditional hybrid composites but the filler content is reduced which results in a decrease in viscosity. These were launched to improve upon the handling characteristics of existing composites (Fig. 17.2). They serve as liner to absorb the shrinkage/contraction of the overlying composite restoration.

These materials have the following features:
- The filler content is 20–25% less than that of the traditional hybrid composites.

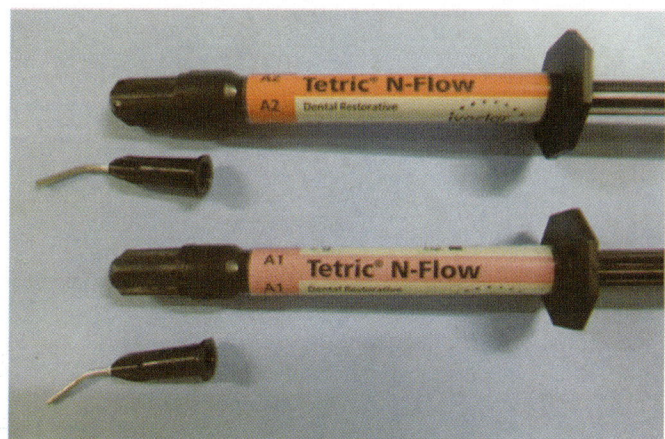

Fig. 17.2: Flowable composites

Table 17.3: Evolution of composites vis-à-vis composition, filler particles, size and percentage of filler

Year	Nomenclature	Resin matrix	Filler	Percentage and size of filler
1962	Conventional Type 1	Polymethyl methacrylate	Quartz	30–70% by wt., 25–30 mm
1968	Conventional Type II	BiSGMA (Bisphenol glycidyl methacrylate replaces PMMA)	Quartz (barium added in traces)	30–70% by wt., 7–10 μm
1975	Microfilled	BiSGMA	Silica replaces quartz	30–70% by wt., 0.05 μm
1978	Organic	BiSGMA	Quartz	10% by wt., 20–30 μm
1989	Hybrid	UGDMA/TEGDMA	Silica	50–70% by wt., 20–30 μm and 0.05 μm
1996	Flowable	TEGDMA	Silica	60% by wt., 0.05 μm
1996	Packable	Urethane Modified BiSGMA	Fumed silica and barium fluoroaluminoborosilicate	82% by wt., 0.8 μm
2000	Modified Hybrid	BisGMA and Propanal	Barium glass Pyrogenic silica	80% by wt. 0.07–0.7 μ

Table 17.4: Physical properties of conventional, microfilled and hybrid composites

Property	Conventional composite	Microfilled composite	Hybrid composite
Compressive strength (psi)	36000–43000	50,000	60,000
Tensile strength (psi)	7000	7500	10,000 to 13,000
Coefficient of thermal expansion	$25 \times 10^{-6}/°C$	$50 \times 10^{-6}/°C$	$30–40 \times 10^{-6}/°C$
Water sorption	0.5%	1.4%	0.5%
Polymerization shrinkage	1.2–1.3%	1.5–2.0%	1.0–1.5%
KNH	50–60	20–30	50–60

- Because of the lesser amount of fillers loading, the flow is increased.
- The depth of cure is approximately 6.0 mm.
- Stickiness to the instrument, which makes it difficult to smoothen the material.
- Mechanical properties like compressive strength, tensile strength, flexure strength and toughness values are generally much less than those of the conventional composites.

The flowable composites are useful as follows:
- As filling materials in low stress areas.
- As pit and fissure sealing and preventive resin restorations
- As liners in proximal boxes of class II preparations.
- For repairing porcelain.
- For rebuilding worn contact areas in composite restorations.
- Tunnel restorations.
- Core build-up.
- Cementing agents for porcelain restorations.

The inferior features are:
- Curing shrinkage
- Reduced compressive strength
- Low elastic modulus
- Increased wear resistance
- Water sorption

Flowable composites are generally contra-indicated for class I, II and IV restorations, because of the relatively high stresses in these areas.

Recently, self adhering flowable composite (Vertise Flow) was developed. It incorporates GPDM monomer, phosphate functional group of which forms chemical bond with the calcium ions of the tooth and micromechanical bond formation is there.

ii. Packable/Condensable composites

Packable/condensable composites are based on the newly introduced concept, called PRIMM (*Polymer Rigid Inorganic Matrix Material*). This system consists of a resin and a ceramic component. The filler/inorganic phase instead of being incorporated into composites as ground particles is present as a continuous network/scaffold of ceramic fibers. The fibers are composed of alumina and silicon dioxide. The diameter of the individual ceramic fiber is less than 2.0 μm.

The consistency of PRIMM based composites is similar to that of a freshly triturated mass of silver amalgam. The composite is inserted into the prepared cavity by carrying and ejecting from a carrier whose nozzle is preferably made from/coated with wear resistant teflon polymer (Fig. 17.3). The use of a

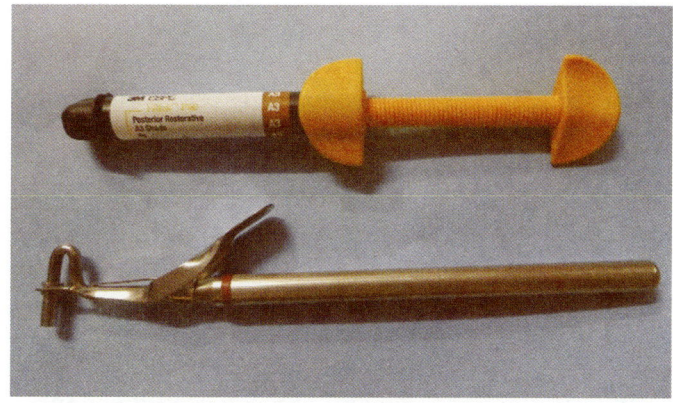

Fig. 17.3: Composite carrier and posterior composite

conventional amalgam carrier is not advised as the hard alumina fibers can scratch/damage the nozzle easily. Each ejected increment is then condensed. The preparation is filled to a point slight beyond the cavosurface margin, the excess removed with a cleoid/discoid or Hollenback carver and the restoration light cured for 30 seconds. It is then polished with appropriate instruments.

Packable composites present improved properties over conventional ones, like:
- *Increased flexural modulus*
- *Increased resistance to wear*
- *Non-stickiness* (Examples of condensable composites include Solitaire (Heraeus-Kulzer), Alert (Jeneric/Pentron), Surefil (Caulk, Dentsply), Filtek P60 (3M) and etc.)

iii. Antibacterial Composites

Several studies have shown that a greater amount of bacteria and plaque accumulate on the surface of the resin composites than on the surface of other restorative materials/enamel surface. The more the plaque accumulates, greater is the incidence of recurrent caries around these restorations. Antibacterial agents are being tried in the composite resins.

Initially, Chlorhexidine was tried in an attempt to reduce plaque accumulation around composite restorations. However, that was not successful since the release was not uniform and lead to certain disadvantages like:
- Toxic effects of the released material
- Population shifts of the micro-organisms
- Antibacterial activity is short-lived
- Deterioration of the physical and mechanical properties of the material.

Later, Silver was added in the composites to make it antibacterial.

The inhibitory effect of these silver containing composites is attributed to the direct contact with bacteria and not to the silver ion release. Because of the catalytic action of silver and the hydroxyl radicals under the effect of water and air, these products result in the structural damage of bacteria (phenomenon is referred to as the *oligodynamic action*).

The inclusion of silver into composite does not adversely affect the mechanical properties like strength, translucency, color stability and depth of cure. Silver do not disrupt the polymer network or impair polymerization of composite monomers. When silica gel is used as a carrier for silver ions, water is adsorbed and silver ions are released resulting in impaired mechanical properties. Another antimicrobial agent used is Halo, which is added up to 1% by weight to commercial composite.

A newly synthesized monomer, MDPB (methacryloxydecyl pyridinium bromide) with antibacterial properties has been incorporated into the resin composite The methacryloyl structure of the MDPB molecule co-polymerizes with other methacrylate monomers and hence is chemically bound to the matrix resin on curing. After the composite has been cured, there occurs no elution of the antibacterial components from the material. The antibacterial activity of this compound has been found to be comparable to that of triclosan. However, whether its antibacterial effect owes to the direct bacterial contact with the immobilized antibacterial component on the surface or to the anti-adhesion property of the surface is not clear. Inclusion of MDPB into composite had no adverse effects on the mechanical properties of BiSGMA based composites. MDPB was found to be effective against various streptococci. However, its activity against other important species in plaque formation like Actinomyces, Neisseria and Veilonella still needs to be investigated.

Zinc oxide powders have also been incorporated as opaque reinforcing fillers into the resin composites. ZnO powder also displays antimicrobial properties. Smaller particles of ZnO nanoparticles (ZnO-NPs) have been found to be more effective than larger particles both against gram negative and gram positive micro-organisms. One mechanism proposed to explain the antimicrobial properties of ZnO-NPs is that they generate active oxygen species such as H_2O_2 which inhibit growth of planktonic microbes. Another potential mechanism of ZnO-NP occurs via leaching of Zn^{2+} into the growth media. Toxicological mechanisms of zinc ions play an important role in biofilm inhibition by inhibiting the active transport and metabolism of sugars as well as disrupting enzyme systems of dental biofilms by displacing magnesium ions essential for enzymatic activity of plaque.

Caries prevention fillers – To increase the mineral content to control dental caries, Ca phosphate ion releasing fillers have been developed such as nanoparticles of dicalcium phosphate anhydrous (DCPA) and tetracalcium phosphate (TTCP) whiskers. Even fluoride releasing nanocomposites have been developed to increase remineralization and inhibit caries development. Addition of calcium fluoride nanoparticles (30%) and reinforcing whisker fillers (35%) to nanocomposites increased the fluoride release. Three types of fluoride releasing polymer Kaolinite nanocomposites was developed by Wang et al (2007) including C (K-diamine), C (K-acrylamide) and C (K-acetate).

The use of antibacterial composites is still under research.

iv. Expanding Matrix Resins for Composites

Composite resins that expand slightly during polymerization are highly desirable as these would facilitate bulk placement of the material, and reduce post operative sensitivity. Spiro-ortho-carbonates (SOCs) have been tried as a possible solution.

Earlier the SOCs were not found to be compatible with resins based on BiSGMA monomer. It was found that SOCs with lower melting points and other structural variations were compatible with BiSGMA-TEGDMA mixtures. These formulations exhibited less shrinkage than the conventional resins but still shrinkage could not be completely eliminated.

Epoxy resins show relatively low volumetric shrinkage compared to methacrylate based resins. Epoxy monomers can be initiated cationically and so are the SOCs capable to undergoing cationic ring polymerization with volume expansion. The epoxy resins contract approximately 3.4% and SOCs expand approximately 3.6%; therefore, combining these two will achieve a net polymerization expansion. It is observed that spiro-orthocarbonate in combination with epoxy resin decreases polymerization shrinkage, increases toughness and decreases water permeation.

v. Bioactive Composites

Calcium phosphate and its modified varieties are being used as filler in recent composites. These composites serve as bioactive liners and bases to enhance the remineralization. When the pH of saliva becomes less, the calcium and phosphate ions are released which act as remineralizing agent. Amorphous calcium phosphate hybridized with glass forming agents is also used as filler, known as 'Smart Composite'.

vi. Ormocer

Recently, a new material was developed improving upon the weaknesses of composites and compomers. *Ormocer*, the acronym of *organically modified ceramic*, can be used as a restorative material for both anterior and posterior teeth. Ormocer can virtually replace amalgam and composites.

Composites are based on a purely organic resin matrix, while Ormocers can be classified between inorganic and organic polymers and have an inorganic as well as an organic network. The monomeric molecular pre-stages are characterized by three structural segments. The inorganic condensing molecule segment is used to build up the inorganic network. An inorganic Si-O-Si network is produced through targeted hydrolysis and inorganic polycondensation in a sol-gel process. The organically polymerizing molecular segment has (meth) acrylate groups which form an additional highly cross-linked network matrix after induction of a radical-based polymerization. The inorganic poly-condensation and the organic polymerization result in the formation of an inorganic co-polymer.

These long ormocer molecule chains are very rigid, have extremely high molecular weight with a preformed structure, hence, exhibiting low shrinkage during polymerization. These are considered to be more biocompatible than the currently available composite resins owing to their cross-linked structure with least amounts of residual monomer. The bonding agent used with ormocers is an ormocer based agent with calcium complexing functional group for enhancing the bond strength to the tooth structure.

Chemically, it differs from composites in matrix constituent. Traditional composites are based upon BisGMA, TEGDMA and etc. The ormocer matrix consisting of ceramic polysiloxane (silicon-oxygen chains) presents a whole new approach. The polysiloxane is biocompatible and exhibits low shrinkage. It contains 20–25% of matrix and the rest is the fillers and coloring agents.

Physical Properties

The physical properties are tabulated in Table 17.5.

Table 17.5 Physical properties of ormocer	
Bending strength (3-point bending test)	100–160 MPa
Modulus of elasticity	10–17 GPa
Coefficient of thermal expansion	$17–25 \times 10^{-6} K^{-1}$
Water uptake	<1.2%

Composites

Advantages
i. Biocompatible
ii. Reduced polymerization shrinkage
iii. High abrasion resistance, can be used in stress bearing areas
iv. Esthetically pleasing, available in different shades
v. Anticaries properties due to fluoride release
vi. Safe handling and easy manipulation
vii. Cost effective

Ormocer is the most promising development of the decade. However, studies are still being carried out to assess the success of the material.

vii. Silorane

The name Silorane derives from the combination of its chemical building blocks siloxanes and oxiranes (Fig. 17.4). The siloxane backbone was introduced in order to provide a most hydrophobic nature, which is very important since too high water sorption limits the long term intraoral physical strength of the composite. The network of Siloranes is generated by the cationic ring opening polymerization of the cycloaliphatic oxiranes moieties, which stand for their low shrinkage and low polymerization stress. The cationic cure starts with the initiation process of an acidic cation which opens the oxirane ring and generates a new acidic center, a carbocation. After the addition to an oxirane monomer, the epoxy ring is opened to form a chain, or in the case of two-or multifunctional monomers a network is formed. The volumetric shrinkage of the Silorane composite was determined to be 0.94–0.99 vol%. Silorane is used with sixth generation bonding agent i.e. self-etching primer and adhesive.

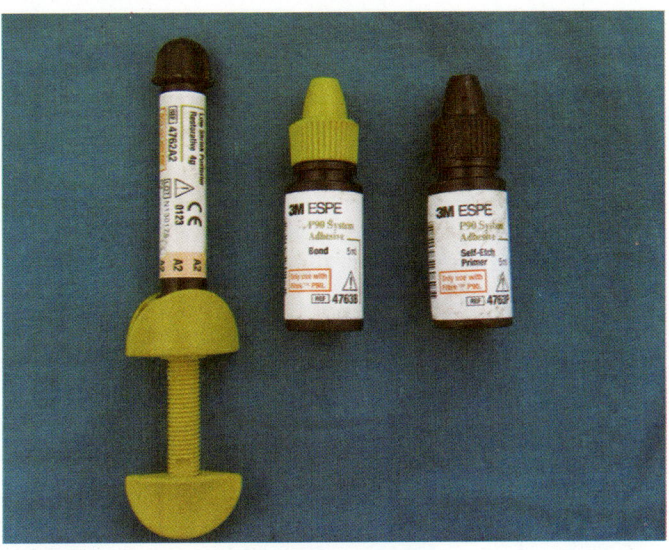

Fig. 17.4: Silorane

The Initiating System

The development of a photoactivated Silorane composite was realized with a three component initiating system comprising camphoroquinone, an iodonium salt and an electron donor (ethyl dimethylalminobenzoate). Camphoroquinone was chosen as a photo initiator to match the emission spectra of the currently used dental lamps. In this reaction path the electron donor acts in a redox process and decomposes the iodonium salt to an acidic cation which starts the ring opening polymerization process.

Filler

Silorane is filled with a combination of fine quartz particles and radiopaque yttrium fluoride. The silane layer is modified with epoxy functionality and is introduced by a silanization process. As it is known, the silane layer increases the hydrophobic character of the surface of the filler and acts as the interface between filler and resin facilitating the reinforcement of the resin with the hard filler particles. A very important function of the silane layer in the Silorane technology is to prevent an attack of the acidic Si-OH group of the quartz, potentially resulting in undesired initiation of the cationic polymerization process.

Filler content 76 wt%, Filler particle size is 0.04 – 1.7 μm.

Composition

Filler – 76%
Silorane – 23%
Initiator – 0.9%
Stabilizer – 0.13%
Pigments – 0.005%

viii. Fibre-reinforced Composite

Composites are reinforced by fibers. Fiber reinforced composites can be divided according to the reinforcement and polymer matrices used. Fiber reinforced composites are structural materials that have atleast two distinct constituents. The reinforcing component provides strength and stiffness, while surrounding matrix support the reinforcement and provides workability. Polymer matrix also protects the fibers from the effect of mechanical damage and moisture. Glass fibers are the most commonly used reinforcing fiber in dental applications. Carbon/graphite, aramid boron, metal fibers are also used. Fiber reinforced composites (FRCs) can also be divided into groups based on length and orientation. Long fibers containing FRCs are called continuous FRCs, but there are also short FRCs. The two main structural types of FRC products presently available are continuous unidirectional and bidirectional fibers (weaves). Unidirectinoal fibers give anisotropic mechanical properties to the composite. On the other hand, woven fibers have an equally reinforcing effect in two directions (orthotropic). FRCs have high favourable mechanical properties and their strength to weight ratios are superior to those of most alloys. They offer many advantages:

- Non-corrosiveness
- Translucency
- Good bonding properties
- Repair facility
- Facility for both office and laboratory preparation

Fiber reinforced composites have potential for use in many applications in dentistry:

- Periodontal splinting
- Orthodontic retention
- Fiber reinforced post crowns
- Reinforcement and repair of removable partial denture
- Repair of fixed partial dentine

Glass fibers have documented reinforcing efficiency and good aesthetic qualities compared with carbon or aramid fibers. The effectiveness of fiber reinforcement is dependent on many variable including the type of resin used, quantity of fibers in the resin matrix, fiber length, form, orientation, adhesion to the polymer matrix and impregnation with the resin. For improvement of bond between the matrix and the fiber, some manufacturers have produced machined-impregnated FRC materials. Polymethyl methacrylate based semi interpenetrating polymer network matrix is used to improve the bond between matrix and fiber. In this fiber structure can be reactivated in order to be bonded reliably.

For further reinforcement of dental composites, electrospun nyron 6 nanocomposites nanofibers containing highly aligned fibriller silicate single crystals were added in BisGMA/TEGDMA. Such composites contain 50 wt% nanofibers (SiO_2, 20 nm in size) and E-glass fibers (3 mm in length) with BISGMA-PMMA resin matrix and silane treated radiopacity fibers of $BaAlSiO_2$ (3±2 μm in size).

ix. Nanocomposite

When inorganic phases in an organic/inorganic composite become nanosized (range 0.1–100 nm), they are called nanocomposites. Nanofillers can be prepared by various techniques, such asflame pyrolysis, flame spray pyrolysis, and solgel processes. Nanofillers are extremely small filler particles, have dimensions belowthe wavelength of visible light (0.4–0.8 μm), they are unable to scatter or absorb visible light. Thus, nanofillers are usually invisible and offer the advantage of optical property improvement. Additionally, nanofillers are capable of increasing the overall filler level due to their small particlesizes. However, the increase in nanofillers also increases the surface area of thefiller particles, which limits the total amount of filler particles because of the wettability of the fillers. Increase in filler level results in significant reduction of polymerization shrinkage and dramatically improve the physical properties of nanocomposites. There are several products of nanocomposites on the market. Filtek Supreme contains nanometric particles (nanomers) and nanoclusters(NCs). Nanomers are monodispersed, non-agglomerated, and non-aggregated silica particles of 20 and 75 nm in diameter. Nanocluster fillers are loosely bound agglomerates of nanosized particles (less than 0.6 μm). Premise is a nanohybrid composed of 3 different types of filler components: nonagglomerated "discrete" silica nanoparticles, prepolymerized fillers (PPF), and barium glass fillers. The non-agglomerated discrete silica nanoparticles are spheroidal and 20 nm in size. The prepolymerized fillers (PPF) are about 30–50 μm in size, and the barium glass filler has an average particle size of 0.4 μm. Ceram-X is an ormocer-based, nanoceramic-composite. Ceram-X contains glass fillers (1.1–1.5 μm) and methacrylate modified silicon-dioxide-containing nanofiller (10 nm). Conventional resin matrix is replaced by a matrix full of highly dispersed methacrylate-modified polysiloxane particles (2–3 nm).

CURING OF COMPOSITES

After the discontinuation of chemically cured composites, various types of lights hae been used to cure composites. Light allowed 'cure on demand' feature, which was not attainable with self cure composites. A light curing unit with a minimal light output of 550 lux is considered appropriate for dental use. The amount of light radiation reaching a given point in the material depends on following factors:

a. *Lamp output intensity*. This is governed by lamp power rating and light guide diameter.
b. *Exposure time*. The energy output is the product of intensity multiplied by exposure time and can be consumed at high or low intensity. The exposure time is adjusted to maximize energy efficiency.
c. *Distance from light source to material*. It is established that part of the emitted light is

absorbed by the air through which it passes, thus decreasing the intensity reaching the target surface.

d. *Curing depth.* Light is gradually absorbed within the working material. For any given target depth, the amount of energy required will be equal to the intensity and the duration of exposure.

e. *Presence of elements between light source and target material.* The amount of light absorbed by intervening elements varies according to the thickness and optical behavior of those elements. Enamel is transparent and allows the passage of a great deal of light; however, dentin is considerably less transparent and allowing virtually no light to pass through. The passage of light through bands and preformed crown is similarly governed by transparency and thickness. When curing through dental structures, the best results are obtained by reducing the intensity.

Various modalities of light and light cure units are:

1. Ultraviolet Light Cure Units

Ultraviolet light cure unit utilizes the polymerization process accomplished by the energy derived from the ultraviolet light in the range of 365 nm. Benzoin ether type compounds were used as photoinitiator.

Disadvantages
• Prolonged exposure time (90 seconds)
• Harmful effects of ultraviolet radiation to human eyes (corneal burns and cataract formation)

2. Quartz Tungsten Halogen

Quartz tungsten halogen (QTH) devices are the most widely used light-curing units and contain a quartz bulb with a tungsten filament in a halogen environment. The units irradiate both UV and white light that must be filtered to remove heat and transmit light only in the violet-blue region of the spectrum that matches the photoabsorption range of Camphorquinone. Less than 0.5% of the total light produced in a QTH is suitable for curing, and most is converted to heat. To minimize heating, UV and infrared band-pass filters are inserted just before the fiber optic system. Orange filters are widely used because they are complementary to blue and absorb blue radiation. A small fan is employed to dissipate unwanted heat from the filters and reflector. Usually, filters degrade with time due to the heating and cooling cycles. QTH-curing lights work at wavelengths of 400 nm to 500 nm with output ranging from 400 mW/cm² to 800 mW/cm² (Fig. 17.5). The halogen bulb usually last for 50 hours and had to be replaced.

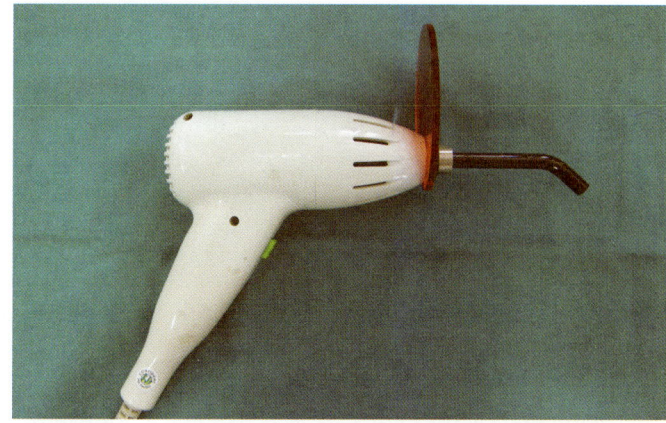

Fig. 17.5: Quartz tungsten halogen light cure unit

Advantages
• Easy to install
• Relatively inexpensive

Disadvantages
• They have a slower cure time (about 40 to 60 seconds).
• The units are relatively large and cumbersome.
• The lights (bulbs) decrease in output with time and thus need frequent replacement.
• They have low-energy performance and generate high temperatures.
• They require a filter and ventilating fan.
• Darker shades of composite have lesser degree of conversion as compared to light shades when cured at same intensity and for same duration.

Turbo tips provide greater curing intensity and faster curing than conventional QTH units; they become smaller at the site of the exit of curing light. Recently, enhanced halogen curing lights have been introduced. This unit has a special tungsten quartz halogen bulb whose performance does not degrade with time.

3. Light-Emitting Diode

Initially, low-power blue light emitting diodes using silicon carbide having a power output of 7µW per LED were utilized (Fig. 17.6A). The modified LEDs, were built on gallium nitride technology and had a power output of 3 mW (400 fold increase). These units are cordless, small, lightweight, and battery-powered (Fig. 17.6B). They do not require filters because they emit light at a specific wavelength within the range of 400 nm to 500 nm. All the emitted light is useful, resulting in high energy performance of the curing light. The spectral output falls between 410 nm and 490 nm.

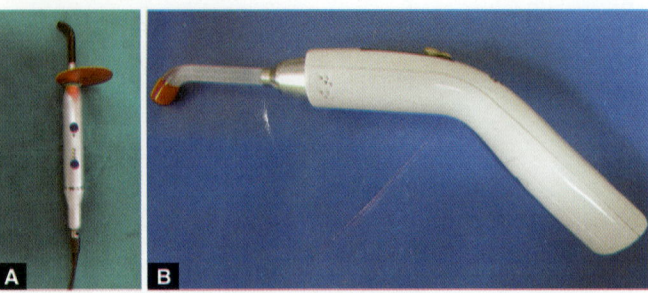

Figs 17.6A and B: Light emitting diode **(A)** with cord, **(B)** cordless

Advantages
• These units show a constant effectiveness without any drop in intensity with time because the diodes do not require frequent replacement. • Cooling fan is not needed because no heat generation occurs during curing. • Depth of curing with LED units is higher than QTH devices. • LED unit has no bulb or filter that require maintenance. • It has the potential lifetime of 10,000 hour. • Some units have integrated microprocessor to control the light intensity which remain constant at all times, irrespective of whether the battery is freshly charged or already running down.

Disadvantages
• The batteries must be recharged. • They cost more than conventional halogen lights. • The curing time is slower than that of plasma-arcuring lights and some enhanced halogen lights.

4. Plasma Arc

Plasma-arc curing lights are high-intensity light curing units (900mW/cm^2). They have more intense light sources (fluorescent bulb-containing plasma), allowing for shorter exposure times. Light is obtained from an electrically conductive gas (xenon) called plasma that forms between two tungsten electrodes under pressure. The light spectrum provided by plasma is limited. The wavelength of high-intensity light emitted is determined by the bulb-coating material and filtered out to minimize transmission of infrared and UV energy and to allow emission of blue light. This also helps remove the heat from the system. Because a high-intensity light is available at lower wavelengths, these units are able to cure composites with photoinitiators other than camphorquinone. An exposure of 10 seconds from a plasma arc light is equivalent to 40 seconds from a QTH light. These systems work at wavelengths between 370 nm and 450 nm.

Advantages
• These units have a high energy output and short curing time. • These units have been shown to have higher conversion rates and depths of cure for composites as compared with QTH units.

Disadvantages
• The heat production must be controlled. • They are expensive. • The lamp (bulb) replacement is costly. • Most devices are large, heavy, and bulky. • They have low-energy performance. • Filters and ventilating fan are required. • Composites cured with a PAC unit have shown more polymerization shrinkage than with QTH units.

5. Argon Laser

The emitted wavelength of Laser depends on the material used (Argon produces blue light having the highest intensity 800mW/cm^2). These lamps work within a limited range of wavelengths, do not require filters, and require shorter exposure times for curing composites. The devices generate little infrared output, so not much heat is produced. They work at specific bandwidths of light in the ranges of 454 nm to 466 nm, 472 nm to 497 nm, and 514 nm. Because a Laser is a narrow beam of coherent light, no loss of power over distance occurs as in seen in QTH units. Therefore, Argon laser curing lights are the units of choice for inaccessible areas. The intensity of laser required for curing is 250mW ± 50mW.

Advantages
• Curing time is very short (5–10 seconds) • Polymerization is uniform and is not affected by the distance between the material and the light source. • Uniform depth of cure • Degree of conversion of materials of all the shades is higher when cured by lasers as compared to the conventional halogen light

Disadvantages
• The curing tip is small, so more time is needed to cure the composites. • They have narrow spectral outputs. • They are expensive. • The size and weight of these units are very large.

Radiometer

The light intensity and output of a light-curing unit can be monitored using a portable or chairside built-in radiometer. A radiometer measures the number of photons, per unit area, and unit time through a standard 11-mm diameter window. Usually, a minimal output higher than 300mW/cm^2 is recommended. Also, the radiometer measures all light energies and cannot discriminate the light energy of the photoinitiator, limiting the measurement of the real value (Fig. 17.7).

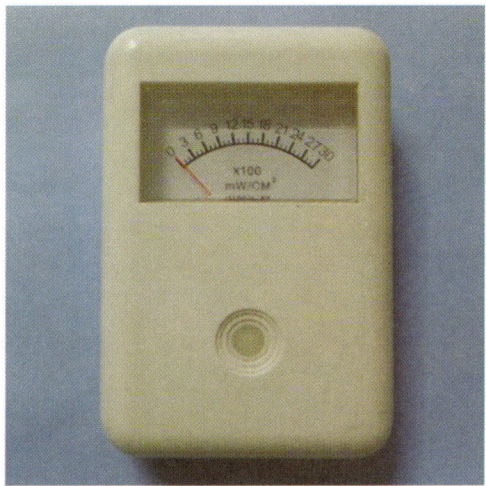

Fig. 17.7: Curing light meter

Light-curing Techniques

The techniques of curing composites are:

a. Soft Start

In Soft-start technique, low intensity curing is utilized initially followed by a high intensity curing. Various light curing units automatically provide one or more soft-start exposure sequences. Some produce a 100 mW/cm^2 output for 10 seconds, followed by an immediate increase to 600 mW/cm^2 output for 30 seconds. Soft-start polymerization is divided into three techniques: stepped, ramped, and pulse-delay.
- i. **Stepped:** The restoration is initially cured at low intensity to contour and shape the restoration. It is followed by second exposure to completely cure the finished restoration.
- ii. **Ramped:** In this method, intensity is gradually increased or "ramped up." The intensity is increased with time either by bringing the light toward the tooth from a distance or using a curing light designed to increase in intensity with time.
- iii. **Pulse Delay:** In the pulse-delay method, a series of exposure pulses is used, each separated by a rest period. An initial exposure of up to 1 J/cm^2 is considered to be most efficient in reducing shrinkage stresses. During the rest period, polymerization reaction occurs at a reduced rate.

b. High Intensity

High-intensity curing allows for shorter exposure times for a given depth of cure. A depth of 2.0 mm can be cured in 10 seconds with a Plasma arc light and 5 seconds with an Argon laser-curing light, as compared with 40 seconds by a Quartz tungsten halogen lamp. A high-intensity curing initiates a multitude of growth centers during an initial irradiation period along with a final polymer with higher cross-link density. Because the relationship between energy density and post-gel shrinkage strain is high-energy densities may translate into increased stress levels but do not result necessarily in high degrees of conversion or superior mechanical properties.

Disadvantages

- Short exposure times cause accelerated rates of curing and insufficient time for stress relaxation. This leads to greater shrinkage stresses and a poor interface.
- High-intensity light curing has a narrowed wavelength range for the output (the wavelength range of the light source must be coincident with the photoinitiator).
- Heat is a significant problem.
- It may not produce the same type of polymer network during curing.
- Using a higher intensity of light for shorter exposure time is reported to result in more cytotoxicity than a longer curing time with lower intensity.

c. Extra-Oral Curing

Usually, extra-oral curing is used for the fabrication of indirect composite restorations that are processed in the laboratory. These laboratory photocuring units work with various combinations of light, heat, pressure, and vacuum to increase the degree of polymerization and wear resistance of composites. It is reported that laboratory units, which provide light curing in conjunction with heat and nitrogen pressure, result in a significant increase in hardness and tensile strength of composites.

CONFIGURATION FACTOR

C-factor is the ratio of bonded surface area in a cavity to the unbonded surface area. It is an important clinical consideration regarding its effects on polymerization shrinkage. Throughout the entire polymerization process, plastic deformation or flow of the composite occurs along the unbonded surface that might partially relieve the induced shrinkage stress. Such compensation through flow is affected by the c-factor of the restoration. An increase in the number of bonded surfaces results in a higher c-factor and greater cxontraction stress on the adhesive bond.

CAVITY PREPARATION FOR COMPOSITES

Mostly composites are restored directly, though indirect inlays are also being fabricated.

Certain factors influence the choice of composite restoration such as:

- *Age of the patient*: In very young age, mostly during rampant caries stage, the composite restorations are avoided.
- *Caries index of the patient*: Composites are not preferred in higher caries index patients.
- *Abnormal occlusal contacts and stresses*: The ceramic filler composites can bear the stresses; however, composites are avoided in heavy occlusal stresses.
- *Areas, which cannot be isolated properly*, the composites are not preferred.
- Patient with poor oral hygiene; composite is not the right choice.

General Consideration for Composite Restorations

The cavity for composite restorations is usually conservative. It is advisable to shape the cavity following the principle of resistance and retention form. Preferably the outline form of the cavity should include the carious fissures/areas. The concept of extension for prevention is not implemented.

The steps followed for cavity preparation are:.

1. *Anaesthesia*: Anaesthesia is indicated in almost all the patients, more so, while restoring lesions near the gingival tissues. Anaesthesia acts in two ways, (i) it eliminates the apprehensions of the patient and (ii) it also help in isolation procedure. Anaesthesia also reduces salivation, thereby keeping the operator and the patient at ease. However, prior to anaesthesia, history of the patient and the possibility of toxic/allergic reactions must be looked into.

2. *Prophylaxis*: Thorough prophylaxis of the total oral cavity especially the area concerned is mandatory for composite restorations. Bleeding gums are one of the causes for failure of such restorations. Polishing with pumice powder and water is preferred since mixing of glycerine and other ingredient can hamper with the acid etch technique, subsequently the success of the restoration.

3. *Shade selection*: Color matching should be carried out in such a manner so that the restorations should not look isolated or an individual identity, but it should merge with the rest of the tooth.

For color matching following factors should be kept in mind:

- The selection of shade/color should preferably be carried out in day light. In case, the day light is not available, the light source should be kept at a distance of six feet.
- Patient and the attendant should not be involved in the process; only the operator, or if need be, the operator's helper can carry out the color matching.
- Ask the patient to rinse or sip water before shade selection (dry tooth appear lighter.
- Shade guide should also be wet during shade selection.
- Prior to shade selection, judge visually and think of the possibility of 2 or 3 shades. These 'possible' shades should be kept aside for final matching. There are plenty of shade guides available. Different manufacturers' have their own shade

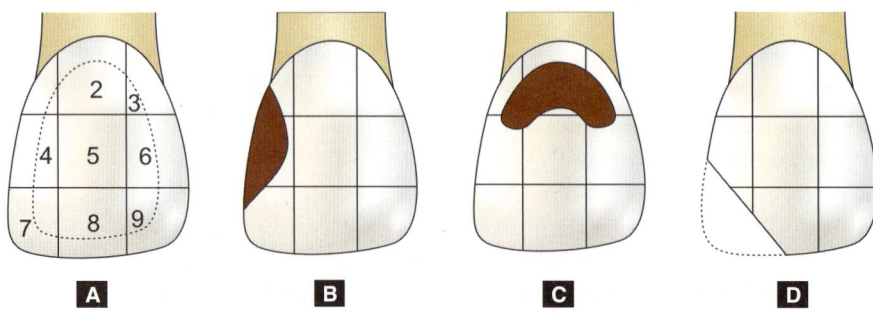

Figs 17.8A to D: Final shade is recorded on patient chart and the menu is prepared keeping in mind the cavity to be restored

guide, however VITA shade guide or VITA 3D is the most accepted one.

- Keep one selected shade on the lingual aspect of the teeth and move buccally. Examine the shade for 20 seconds only. If more time is needed, the eyes should be rested by looking at a blue or violet object for few seconds. The change in color at the cervical (darker) and incisal (translucent) can be made accordingly.
- For final checking the shade, place a small amount of selected composite on the adjacent tooth and cure. In case it matches, the cured composite is removed.
- The final shade is recorded on patient chart (Figs 17.8A to D).

Isolation

Composite resins are susceptible to moisture; therefore, complete control of moisture during composite restoration is mandatory. Isolation from moisture and also from soft tissues have been discussed in chapter 8. In brief, the isolation can be accomplished by rubber dam or cotton rolls. The choice of rubber dam or cotton rolls depends upon the anticipated time for the restoration. If longer time period is anticipated, rubber dam is indicated, otherwise cotton rolls are sufficient for the procedure.

a. *Rubber dam*: It is advisable to isolate one tooth mesial and one tooth distal to the one where cavity preparation is indicated in posterior teeth. In anterior teeth, preferably all the anterior teeth should be isolated so as to have clear access during lingual/facial approach. A wedge is usually needed where the proximal lesions are extended subgingivally, to expose the extent of the lesion at the gingival end. Similarly, in class V cavities, the retainer is pushed more gingivally to expose the gingival extension of the lesion. For placing the wedge or retainer, care should be taken not to injure the rubber dam or the gingiva.

b. *Cotton rolls*: Prefabricated cotton rolls or the available cotton drawn into rolls with the help of tweezers etc., can be used to isolate the area. The cotton roll is preferred if the anticipated treatment time is less. The moment, the cotton rolls are half soaked in saliva, these are changed and replaced with fresh cotton rolls. A few patients, especially children are non-cooperative with the placement of cotton rolls.

c. *Retraction cords*: Retraction cords are employed to facilitate better accessibility and to control gingival bleeding and the crevicular fluid seepage. These cords, mainly impregnated in astringents and other chemical agents help in receding the gingival tissue temporarily. Retraction cords are available in different shapes and sizes to suit the various clinical situations. The cord is gently placed in the sulcular area with the help of plastic instruments or any blunt instrument. Use of probes and sharp edged instruments should be avoided as these may injure the gingiva leading to more bleeding from the area.

The time for cord placement is usually dependent upon the chemical used and the retraction required. Mostly these are instructed on the commercial preparations. The cord should not be pressed unnecessarily and also should not be kept longer than required. This can lead to ischaemia of the gingiva.

The cord should be removed gently without injuring the gingival tissue and without leaving a loose strand. Loose strands will lead to defective restorations.

Cavity Preparation

The cavity preparation for composite is of following two types:

a. *Conventional cavity preparation*: The conventional form follows Black's principles of cavity preparation. The outline form includes extension of susceptible lesions, proper uniform depth and the external walls are in accordance with enamel rods. The retention locks etc. can also be given in such preparations. Whether bevel is to be given or not depends upon several factors such as:
   - Area required for etching
   - Area visible externally
   - Whether color matching is mandatory
   - Area prone to stresses
   - Accessibility and visibility of the area
   - Caries index of the patient

   Bevels are usually recommended on labial surfaces of anterior teeth so as to merge the color of the composite and the enamel. Lingual bevels can be avoided since that might lead to stresses and the color merging is not of paramount importance. Similarly in class V cavities, bevels are given only on occlusal walls and the gingival walls are spared. In posterior restorations, bevels are not indicated since the thin layers of composites might chipped off under stresses leading to marginal gaps.

b. *Modified cavity preparation*: Modified cavity preparation does not follow Black's principles. The retention part is totally dependent upon the etched enamel and bonding. The cavity preparation is usually kept in enamel, if otherwise dictated by the lesion. The individual pits are restored separately. There can be two, three or even more cavities in a single tooth. This type of cavity preparation conserves more tooth structure and the 'less deep' cavities maintain the strength of the tooth. No definite walls and line angles are visible and usually appear saucer shaped. Such type of cavity preparation is indicated only for smaller lesions or for correcting enamel defects. Whether beveling is indicated or not depends upon the factors already described.

Class I Cavity Preparation

The outline is planned keeping in mind the features as described earlier (Fig. 17.9). The surface is cleaned with water and air. A small round bur is used to enter into the caries from the deepest or more carious pit. The movement of the bur is kept parallel to the long axis of the tooth crown. The depth is kept inside the dentino-enamel junction. The uniformity in the depth can be achieved using flat fissure bur of appropriate size. The depth of the cavity can be kept only in enamel, but for better retention and function, extension into the dentin is advisable. The total depth can be kept as 1.5 mm. The buccolingual width of the cavity is kept as small as possible, only otherwise dictated by caries. The usual width is ¼th of the intercuspal distance.

The cavity walls may not be kept perpendicular and parallel. In deeper cavities, a base of light cure calcium hydroxide or glass-ionomer cement is indicated.

The cavosurface margins are kept at right angle to the cavity walls. No bevel is given. The butt joint preparation minimizes marginal breakdown and ditching of the composites. However, it may lead to marginal staining.

The pits and fissures on the occlusal two-third of the buccal and lingual surfaces of posterior teeth and lingual pits of anterior teeth can be restored with composites in a similar way. The pits are widened with flat fissure bur to remove undermining of enamel. The caries is removed and the walls of the restoration are not modified. Butt joint preparation is preferred. However, a short bevel can be given for merging the color of composites. The depth of such preparation is 1.0–1.5 mm and should be kept as shallow as possible. If otherwise dictated by caries the depth is increased and a base is indicated. In case of wide involvement of the surface, inspite of removing all the undermining enamel, bilayered restorations are preferred.

Class II Cavity Preparation

The occlusal part of the cavity is prepared as described for Class I cavity. The proximal box is prepared keeping in mind the extent of caries, convexity of the proximal surface, caries indices and the anticipating masticatory loads.

The matrix band is applied prior to cutting of the proximal box so as not to injure the adjacent tooth. Holding a flat fissure bur perpendicular to the pulpal floor, extend onto the marginal ridge, cutting the ridge and creating a width of 1.0–1.5 mm. The bur is then inserted deep towards the contact point. The buccal and lingual walls of the proximal box are kept slightly away from the contact area. These might not be in self cleansing areas, the idea is to involve the contact area. Preferably, the gingival wall is kept in enamel without injuring the underlying gingiva. The occlusal convergence, though not indicated, can be given to achieve better retention.

In case of class II preparation for composites, certain *modifications* have been suggested.
  i. Minimal occlusal part is involved along with the proximal box (conventional) (Figs 17.10A and B).
  ii. Box only preparation: In this case, only proximal box is prepared and the occlusal part is not involved. Grooves are not given (Figs 17.11A and B)
  iii. Proximal box preparation with retentive grooves (Figs 17.12A and B).

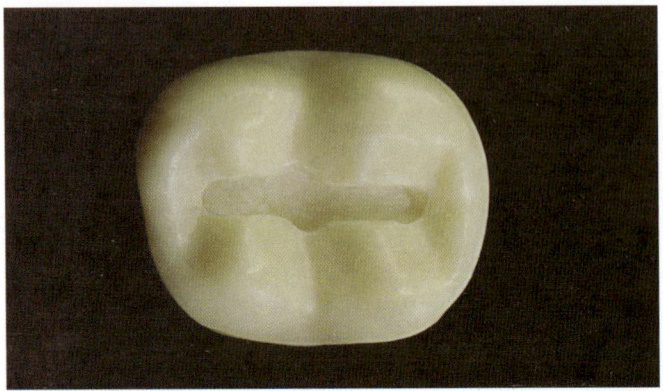

Fig. 17.9: Class I cavity preparation for composite in mandibular molar

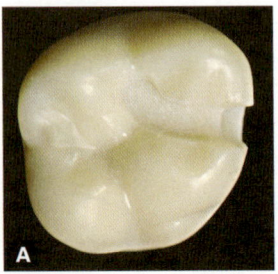 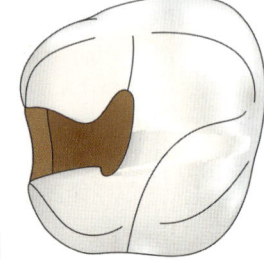

Figs 17.10A and B: Conventional conservative cavity preparation for composites **(A)** On model; **(B)** Diagrammatic

iv. Proximal box preparation with unsupported proximal enamel (Figs 17.13A, B).

The cavity walls are finished and a short bevel can be given on the cavosurface margins of the walls of the proximal box. No beveling is indicated on occlusal side. In case of deep lesions, a base of light cured calcium hydroxide or glass-ionomer cement can be given.

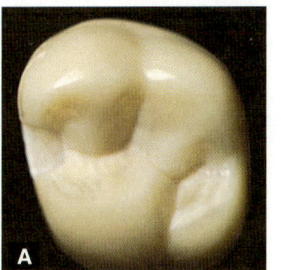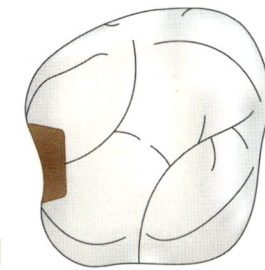

Figs 17.11A and B: Box only preparation without retention grooves. **(A)** On model; **(B)** Diagrammatic

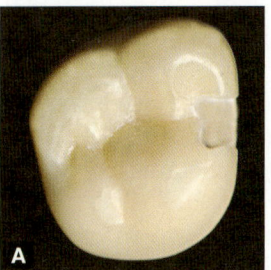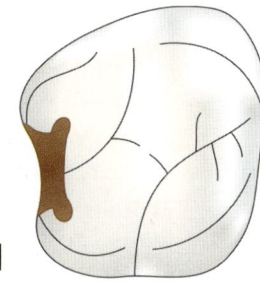

Figs 17.12A and B: Box only preparation with retention grooves. **(A)** On model; **(B)** Diagrammatic

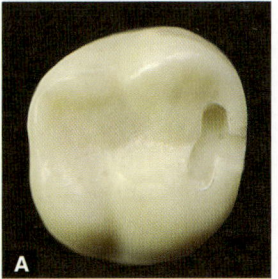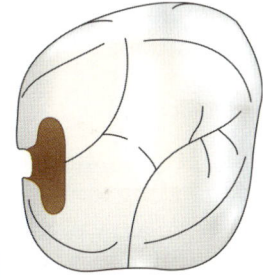

Figs 17.13A and B: Box only preparation with unsupported promixal enamel. **(A)** On model; **(B)** Diagrammatic

Class III Cavity Preparation

The outline of the cavity depends upon the extent of the lesion proximally and/or labially and lingually. The cavity preparation should always be started from lingual side, except in rare instances, labial approach can be initiated (Figs 17.14A and B).

The lingual approach preserves the labial enamel, vis-à-vis the esthetics. One can compromise in color matching and color merging in lingual approach.

Indications for labial approach are:

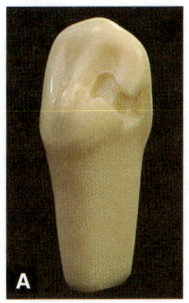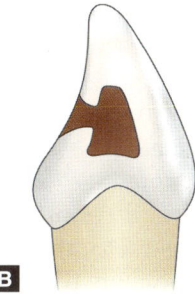

Figs 17.14A and B: Class III cavity preparation. **(A)** On model; **(B)** Diagrammatic

- Labial enamel is involved
- Malaligned teeth where lingual approach is difficult
- Rotated teeth where lingual side is hidden

In case labial approach is followed, beveling at the labial enamel wall is indicated to merge the color of the restoration with the enamel. In such cases judicious color matching is also very important to create pleasing esthetics.

The cavity preparation is started using no. ¼ or no. ½ round bur and piercing through the lingual marginal ridge of the concerned side. The direction of the bur is maintained perpendicular to the lingual surface of the tooth, moving the bur 0.5 mm inside the dentino-enamel junction.

With the small fissure bur extending incisally and gingivally, create incisal and gingival walls. The labial enamel is left intact as far as possible. The walls are kept at 90° with the cavosurface margins (bevels are not given). Such a preparation does not have lingual wall. If need be, small locks can be given at incisal and gingival walls using no. ¼ or no. ½ inverted cone bur. In certain teeth where the access from lingual marginal ridge is difficult, access can be gained through lingual side, creating lingual lock as usually given for silver amalgam restorations. Lingual locks in composite, is kept as small as possible, conserving the lingual aspect of the tooth. The isthmus between lingual and proximal axial walls should also be kept minimum, not exceeding 1.0 mm in routine.

If facial approach is utilized, then the outline form varies slightly. The small round bur is pierced into the caries lesion. Then with small fissure bur, gingival and incisal extensions are given. The cavity preparation is similar to the one described earlier with lingual approach, only difference is that a bevel is to be given on labial cavosurface margin. This bevel is continuous from incisal to gingival side.

The depth of the axial wall should be 0.5 to 1.0 mm. Usually the depth is more incisally and as we move gingivally the depth is decreased. The axial wall depth can be increased in case, where the gingival wall extends into the cementum i.e. on the root surface, sufficient axial depth is required for proper retention. Final finishing and shaping of the enamel is carried out using hand instruments (mostly marginal trimmer and chisels).

Any defective lesion or remaining caries is removed using small round burs. In cases of retreatment, the previous restoration should be thoroughly removed. The floor or the axial wall should be checked thoroughly for any signs of secondary caries.

A base of light cure calcium hydroxide or glass-ionomer can be given in deep lesions where the remaining dentin is very thin.

Class V Cavity Preparation

The choice of composite as a restorative material for class V cavities depends upon the features like caries index, oral hygiene and pattern of occlusal stresses.

Cervical lesion with one surface extending to cementum is a common feature. The prevalence of cervical lesions increases with advancing age. Tooth colored restorations are preferred in such lesions. In posterior teeth, where esthetics is not the prime consideration, silver amalgam restoration can be given.

The outline form is dictated by the extent of the lesion at these sites (Figs 17.15A and B). The caries or the abrasive/erosive lesion can extend to the cementum or can be totally in cementum. A fissure bur of appropriate size is used to enter the center of the lesion. The bur is kept perpendicular to the axis of the tooth and maintaining the pulpal depth of 0.5 mm below dentino-enamel junction, the bur is moved mesially and distally. The total depth from enamel is 1.0 mm and for cementum is 0.75 to 1.0 mm. The mesial/distal extension is kept within the line angles of the tooth. The gingival wall is contoured according to the cemento-enamel junction and the occlusal wall is more or less straight or slightly curved. The fissure bur shape the gingival and the occlusal walls keeping the axial wall perpendicular to the mesial, distal, occlusal and gingival walls. The axial wall contour

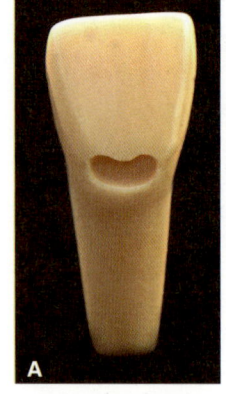
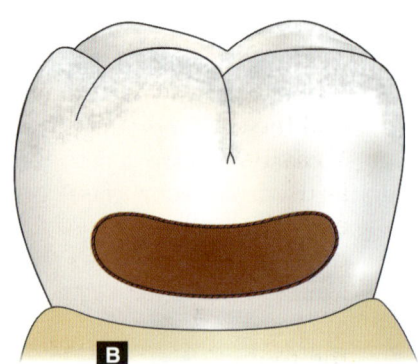

Figs 17.15A and B: Class V cavity preparation. **(A)** On model; **(B)** Diagrammatic

follows the pulp chamber or the outer surface of the tooth.

All the four walls of the cavity i.e. mesial, distal, occlusal and gingival are kept diverging outwards. The gingival wall, however, is kept straight if it falls in cementum. A short bevel is given on the occlusal wall so as to have better merging of the composite resin with the tooth.

The occluso-gingival width of the cavity is kept as minimum as possible, usually not exceeding 1.5 mm. In case the extension of the lesion dictates, the width can be increased accordingly.

The walls are finished with the help of chisel or marginal trimmers. The cavosurface margin of all other walls is kept at 90° except the occlusal wall where a bevel is placed.

Retention grooves are not required in composite restorations. In extra large cavities, bilayered (sandwich) restorations are preferred (Figs 17.16A to C).

Modification of the Cervical Cavities

The class V cavity preparation is modified in depending upon the location and extent of the lesion.
a. When the lesion is on the line angles of buccal/lingual walls of posterior teeth [preferably classified as class IV Div. II by the author]

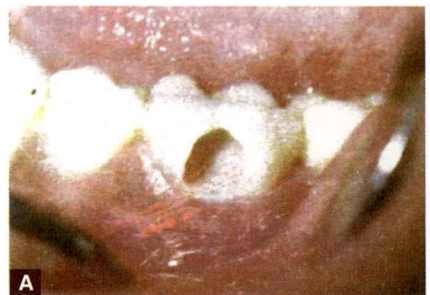
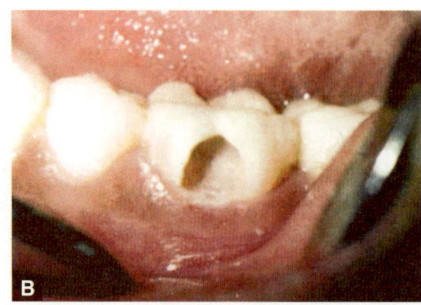
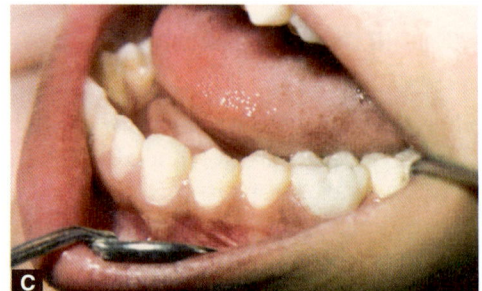

Figs 17.16A to C: Class V cavity preparation and restoration; **(A)** cavity preparation **(B)** application of glass-ionomer cement **(C)** completed restoration

(Fig. 17.17). Such lesions, as mentioned earlier, have not been included in Black's classification. The outline form depends upon the size of the lesion. The usual form given is rounded or oblong and the cavity is prepared as described for class V cavity. A small fissure bur of appropriate size is used to enter the center of the lesion and extending all around involving the caries. The depth is kept 0.5 mm into the dentino-enamel junction. The short bevel is given wherever the operator feels the necessity of color merging with the tooth. The cavosurface margins are finally finished with a small chisel or marginal trimmers.

b. In rare instances, cervical lesions extend occlusally along the sides. This extension can be unilateral or bilateral (Figs 17.18A, B & 17.19A, B). The cavity preparation remains the same with one side of the occlusal wall is raised accordingly. The bevel can be placed all along this wall. The depth and extension of walls is as described earlier. Final finishing can be carried out using hand cutting instruments, mostly straight chisel or marginal trimmers.

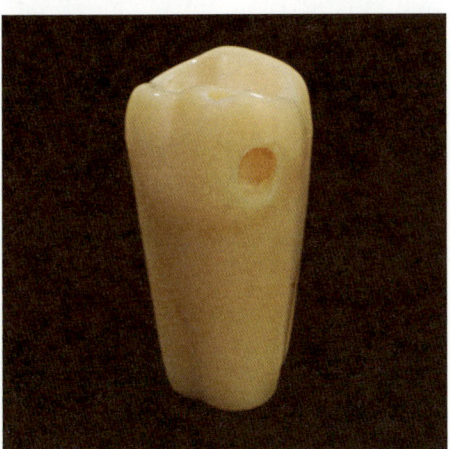

Fig. 17.17: Cavity on the line angle

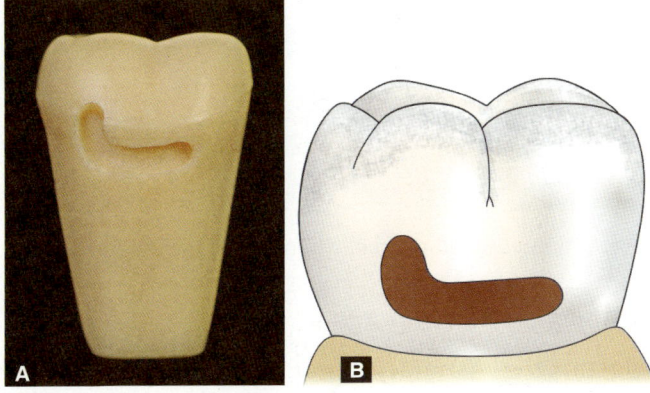

Figs 17.18A and B: Class V cavity with unilateral extension **(A)** On model; **(B)** Diagrammatic

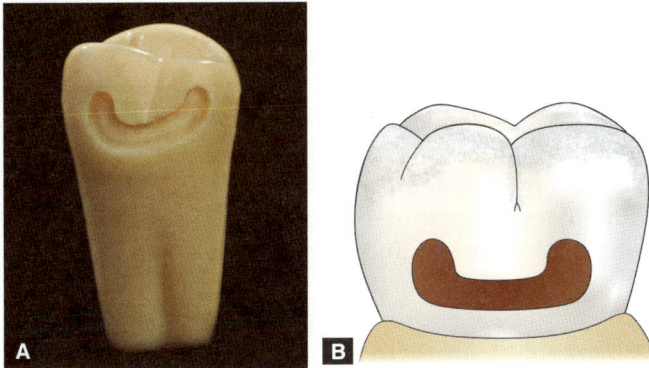

Figs 17.19A and B: Class V cavity with bilateral extension **(A)** On model, **(B)** Diagrammatic

Class VI Cavity Preparation

The outline form is dictated by the extent of caries. Usually these lesions are very small and not very deep. The occlusal aspect of the antagonist tooth should be looked into.

The center of the lesion is penetrated with a small fissure bur or inverted cone bur. The bur is extended all along to include the caries. The depth of the cavity is maintained inside the dentino-enamel junction. The surrounding walls should have definite dentin support (Figs 17.20A and B). The shape of the cavity is usually round in posterior teeth and squarish in anterior teeth. The cavosurface angle is usually 90° and bevels are not given. Finally the cavity is finished with straight chisel or marginal trimmer.

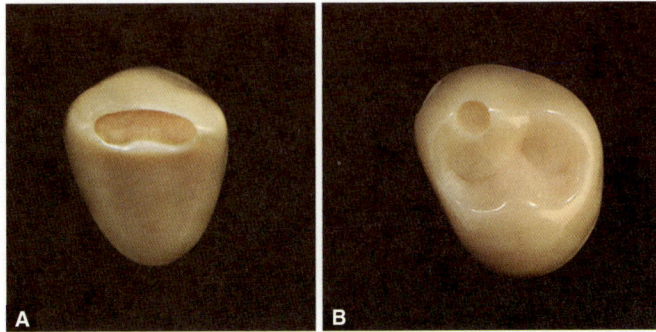

Figs 17.20A and B: Class VI cavity on **(A)** mandibular canine; **(B)** maxillary first molar

PLACEMENT OF COMPOSITES

The placement of composites is carried out following the sequence as given below:

a. Pulp Protection

After the cavity preparation is completed and the remaining caries is excavated, the depth of the cavity inside the dentino-enamel junction is thoroughly evaluated. In case where the depth is more, measures for pulp protection should be undertaken. Calcium hydroxide and glass-ionomers are preferred bases under the composite restorations. Zinc oxide eugenol is contraindicated since it hinders with polymerization of methacrylate group of composite resins. Light cure calcium hydroxide, and glass-ionomers are preferred since over these surfaces, etching is not required. Compomers are also being used as base under the composites. Glass cermets are preferred bases at the cervical wall of the proximal lesions. The release of fluoride ions at the cervical wall minimizes the chances of secondary caries.

b. Acid Etching

Isolate the tooth properly and make the area accessible for acid etching. Both liquid and gel etchants are available (Fig. 16.6). Gel etchants are preferred over liquid etchants since overflowing is common with liquid etchants. Liquid etchants can only be used where the area is large and the flow is not towards the gingival side, such as labial side of upper anterior teeth. The liquid etchants should not be used on the mandibular teeth since the liquid in all probability might trickle into the gingival sulcus area.

The liquid can be applied with cotton pellet or brush. The liquid is gently placed over the surface and should not be rubbed.

The gel etchants can be applied with the help of plastic instrument, brush or directly sprayed with the fine needle provided with the syringe. The syringe and needle system is efficient in applying the etchant at the selected surfaces. Care should be exercised not to etch the adjacent teeth and not let the etchant touch the gingival tissues. The etching time depends upon the area to be etched, caries susceptibility of the patient and the manufacturer's instructions. The etching time is doubled in deciduous enamel and decreased accordingly for caries susceptible patients.

After the stipulated time (usually 10–15 seconds), the etchant is washed thoroughly. Care should be taken not to leave any residual acid on the cavity walls. The area is dried preferably from chip syringe.

Compressed air should be avoided as it may injure the enamel tags.

The etched enamel will appear clean, white and frosted. Do not touch the etched surface with any instrument, cotton or hand (Figs 17.21, 17.22, 17.23 & 17.24). In case saliva or gingival fluid escapes isolation and touches the cavity preparation, repeat the procedure again.

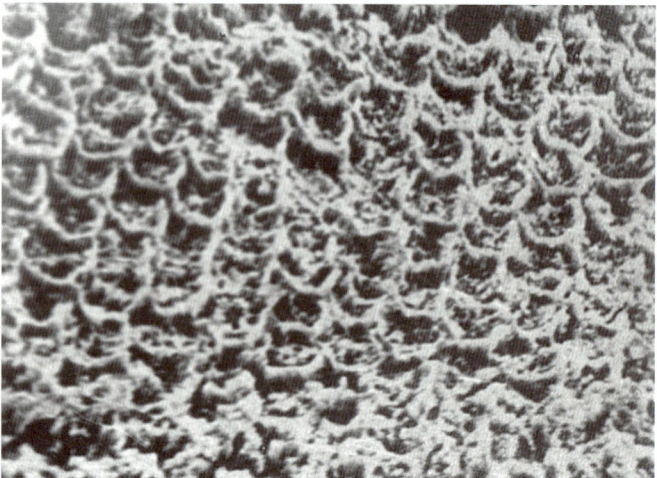

Fig. 17.21: Tooth surface after etching

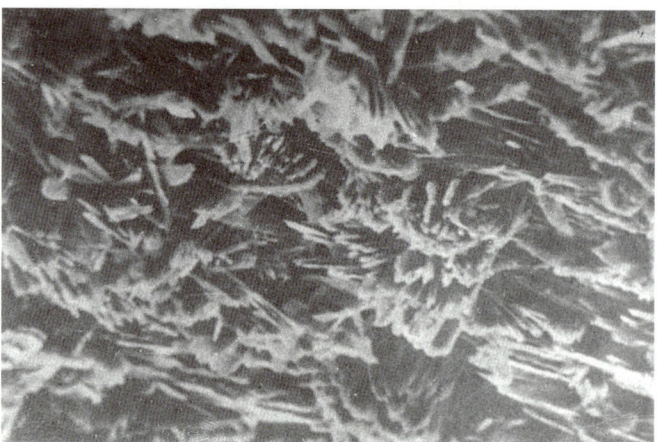

Fig. 17.22: Etched enamel without washing

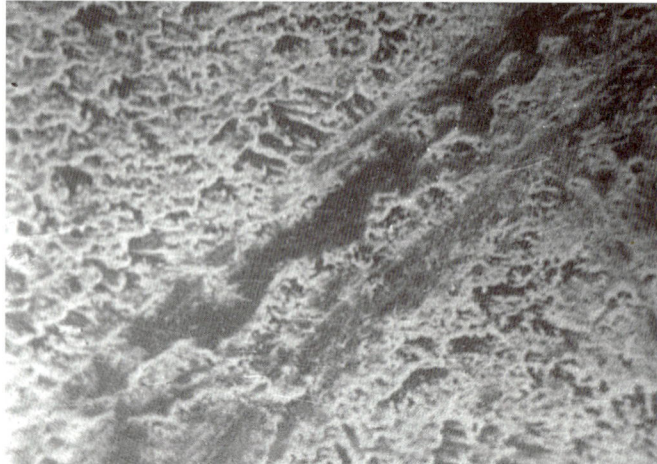

Fig. 17.23: Etched enamel when cotton has been touched

c. Applying Bonding Agent

Most of the manufacturers now supply primer and bonding agent in one step, one bottle container (Fig. 17.19). The bonding agent is applied over the etched

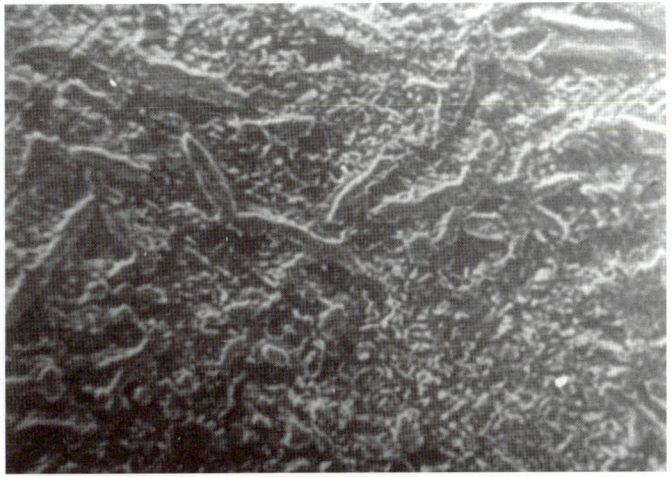

Fig. 17.24: Etched enamel when contaminated with saliva

surface carefully with the help of brush or the tip designed by manufacturers. Only one coat of bonding agent is to be applied. The bonding agent is made to flow uniformly all along the walls with the help of air from chip syringe. Air should be gently blown without any pressure otherwise there might be no bonding agent at certain areas of the cavity. Then it is light cured for 10 seconds.

Complete isolation should be maintained otherwise if saliva and/or gingival fluid trickle in, the whole process is to be repeated right from etching.

Double coat of bonding agent and overcuring should be avoided for optimal results. After bonding the area should not be touched with any instrument and the repeated checking whether bonding is completed or not is also to be avoided.

d. Placement of Matrix

Matrices are placed to achieve the proper contact and contour of the tooth. No matrix is required in teeth or restorations where contours can be controlled; such as, class V and VI cavities and cavities on the labial surfaces of anterior teeth etc.

Should matrix be placed before the etching/bonding step or after, remained controversial. The placement of matrix after the etching and bonding steps is preferred. In case the matrix is placed before these steps, the application and removal of etchant become difficult. However, authors who favour matrix placement before these steps are of the opinion that while doing so the matrix aids in isolation thereby increasing the accessibility especially at the gingival areas.

After placing the matrix, it is stabilized with the help of wedge or impression compound as the need be. Details regarding matrices and wedges are given in Chapter 8.

Two types of matrices are usually used for composite restorations
- Metal matrix
- Polyesyter strips

The strip or the metal matrix is shaped outside the oral cavity with the help of handle of the mirror or with contouring pliers. It can be suitably cut to suit the size and contour of the tooth. The matrix should be extended beyond the incisal end/marginal ridge area and the gingival area. Care should be taken not to impinge the gingival tissues. A properly shaped wedge is then inserted to make the matrix stable. Extra wedge can be cut so as not to injure the tongue and/or the cheeks.

Wedge helps in the following ways:
- Helps stabilize the matrix
- Provides slight separation of teeth
- Prevents overhangs at gingival areas
- Creates gingival embrasures effectively

Metal matrices, available in very thin metals (0.001–0.002 inch) can also be used for proximal lesion. The metal matrix is also stabilized with the help of wedges. In case the adjacent tooth is absent, impression compound can be used to stabilize the matrix and to produce required gingival embrasures.

For posterior teeth, relatively thick metal matrix is used since it can resist the condensation pressure with ease and will not give way while packing composite. Transparent matrices, which can reflect light are also used for proximal restorations. Though with the introduction of fine curing tips and the light reflecting wedges proper placement and curing of composite at gingival third area has become easier, even then the matrix hinders with the proper curing at that end. In case the transparent matrix is applied, it is exchanged with metal matrix after completing the gingival curing.

Since all composites (except a few with expanding matrix) contract after curing due to polymerization shrinkage, creating a proper contact at the proximal posterior restorations is always a challenge. How to produce better contact is described later in this chapter.

e. Restoration

In early days of chemically cure composites, manipulation time was minimum and the operator used to be in hurry to mix, carry, place and carve the restoration within 45 seconds. With light cure composites, these disadvantages are over and the operator has ample time to manipulate the composites.

Syringes with composites (usually flowable composites) are available with disposable needles to be applied directly at the surface. Guns with ampoules of composites are also available which manufacturers supply in various sizes and shapes (Fig. 17.25).

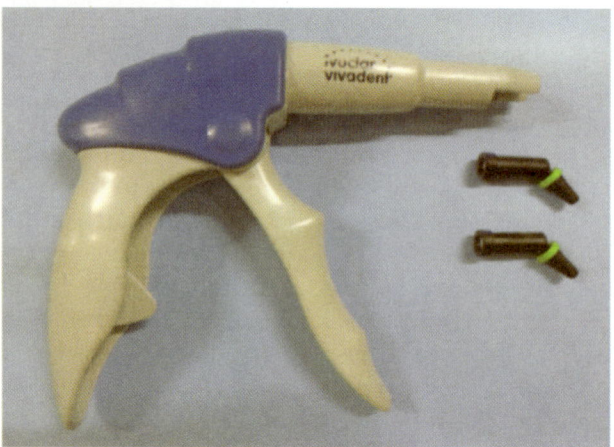

Fig. 17.25: Composite gun with ampoules of composite

Basically guns are used for viscous composites and the syringes for flowable composites.

Usually Teflon coated instruments are used to pick and insert the composite (Fig. 17.26). Stainless steel instrument should not be used since the composite will stick to the instrument. The instrument should be kept dry during manipulation and be wiped with cotton at every pick. In no case the instrument should be touched with hands or any moist object.

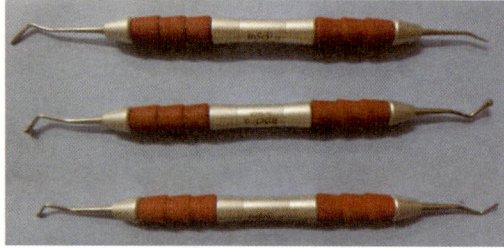

Fig. 17.26: Teflon-coated instruments for manipulating composite

i. Restoring Anterior Teeth (Class III & Class IV Cavities)

After etching, bonding and stabilizing the matrix, the composite in small increment is placed first at the gingival wall. Whether the approach of cavity preparation is labial or lingual, the gingival wall is first to be restored. Care should be taken so as to completely visualize the gingival cavosurface area. Use of retraction cords and pushing of rubber dam with plastic instruments can help visualize the area completely. The first increment should be kept small, approximately 1.0 mm thick and the subsequent increments of 1.0–1.5 mm thickness can be applied over the first. Each increment is cured for 20 seconds and final one cured for 40 seconds to one minute. If lingual approach is utilized, curing is preferred from labial aspect and vice versa in case labial approach is followed. Finally, the composite should be cured from all the surfaces. The complete stepwise procedure for the restoration of class IV cavity is shown in Figs 17.27A to P.

Blending of shades in these cavities class is important. The extent of the lesion and the labial involvement will dictate the amount of blending. As described in Fig. 17.7, from cervical to incisal area, color of the composite would be from dark to light and translucent. On labial enamel, since it is bevelled, blending will be followed in the same way i.e. darker shade at the cervical, less dark in the middle, lighter at the incisal and translucent at the incisal edge.

Similarly restoring teeth with fractured incisal edges or horizontal fracture of the tooth, care is taken to blend the color following the basic principles as shown in Fig. 17.7.

ii. Restoring Posterior Teeth (Class II Cavities)

Utmost care is necessary before restoring posterior proximal lesions whether on one side or both the sides of the tooth i.e. mesio-occluso-distal or only mesio/disto-occlusal lesions.

After the process of etching, bonding and the matrix placement, the restoration is initiated keeping in mind the volume of the cavity and the areas, which would come under stresses. The volume of the cavity will dictate the operator regarding number and locations of the increments and the future stress bearing areas will dictate the operator to use particular type of composites. The complete stepwise procedure for the restoration of class II cavity is shown in Figs 17.28A to K.

Initially the composites were given only in conservative class II preparation; however, with the recent technology), extensive lesions are also restored with composites.

The cavity for composite is always restored in increments. The increments can be given in a variety of designs, but the thickness of the increment should be kept as small as possible i.e. not exceeding 1.5 mm at a time. Each increment is cured for 20 seconds before placing the next over it. A few authors are of the view that partial curing of these increments would lead to better adaptation of each increment. This phenomenon is known as *'soft start polymerization'* in which the initial increments are cured for 10 seconds before placing the next The different designs of increment placement are:

- *Three increment design*: One flat increment at gingival and pulpal and two oblique increments both at proximal box and the occlusal box (Fig. 17.29A). This is the simple and accepted design. The first increment (usually less than 1.0 μm) is

Composites

Step-wise procedure for the restoration of class IV cavity

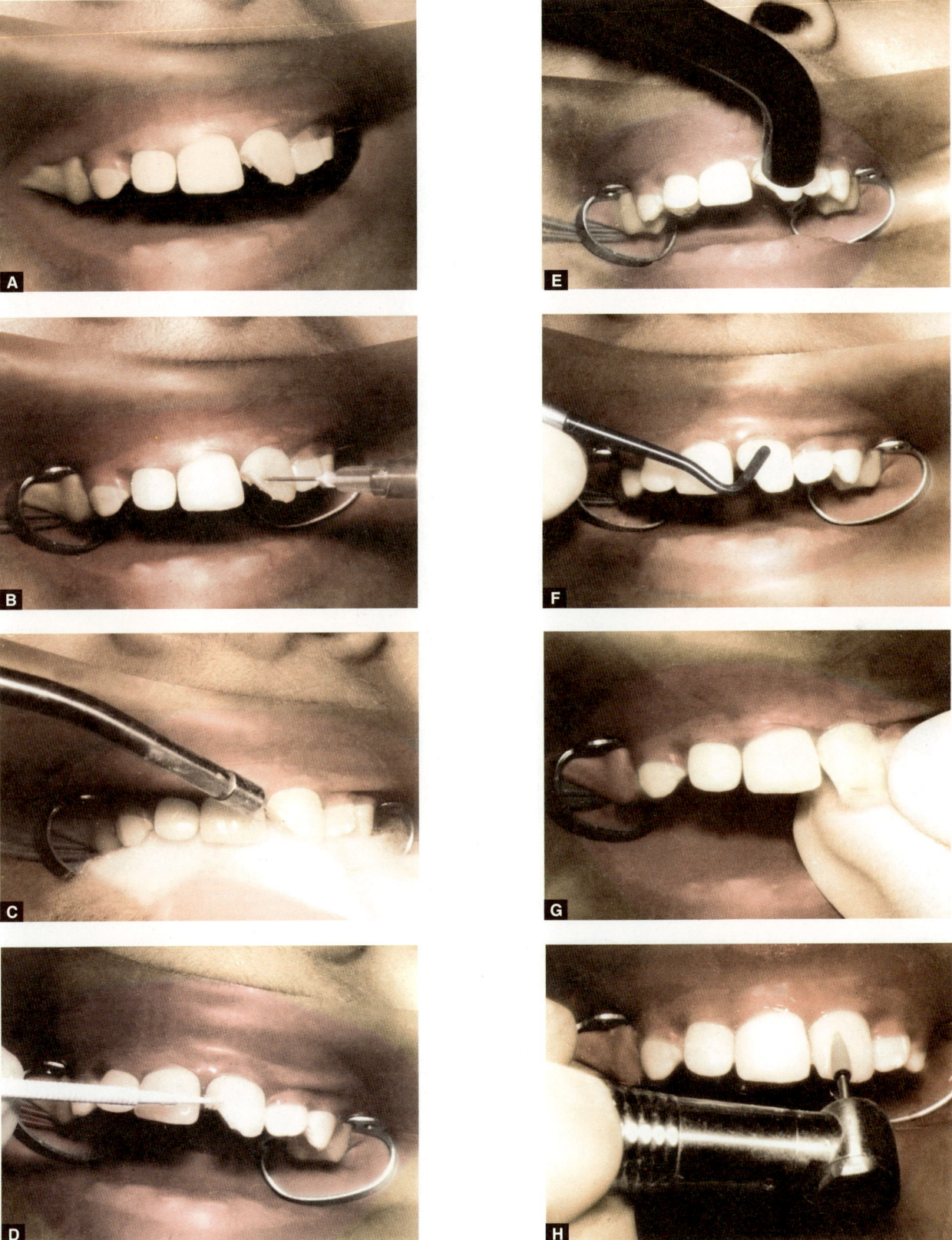

Figs 17.27A to H: **(A)** Prepared cavity; **(B)** Etchant applied in the cavity; **(C)** Washing with water spray; **(D)** Bonding agent application; **(E)** Curing with light; **(F)** Application of composite; **(G)** Using mylar strip when restoring interproximally; **(H)** Finishing with green tungsten carbide point

Step-wise procedure for the restoration of class IV cavity

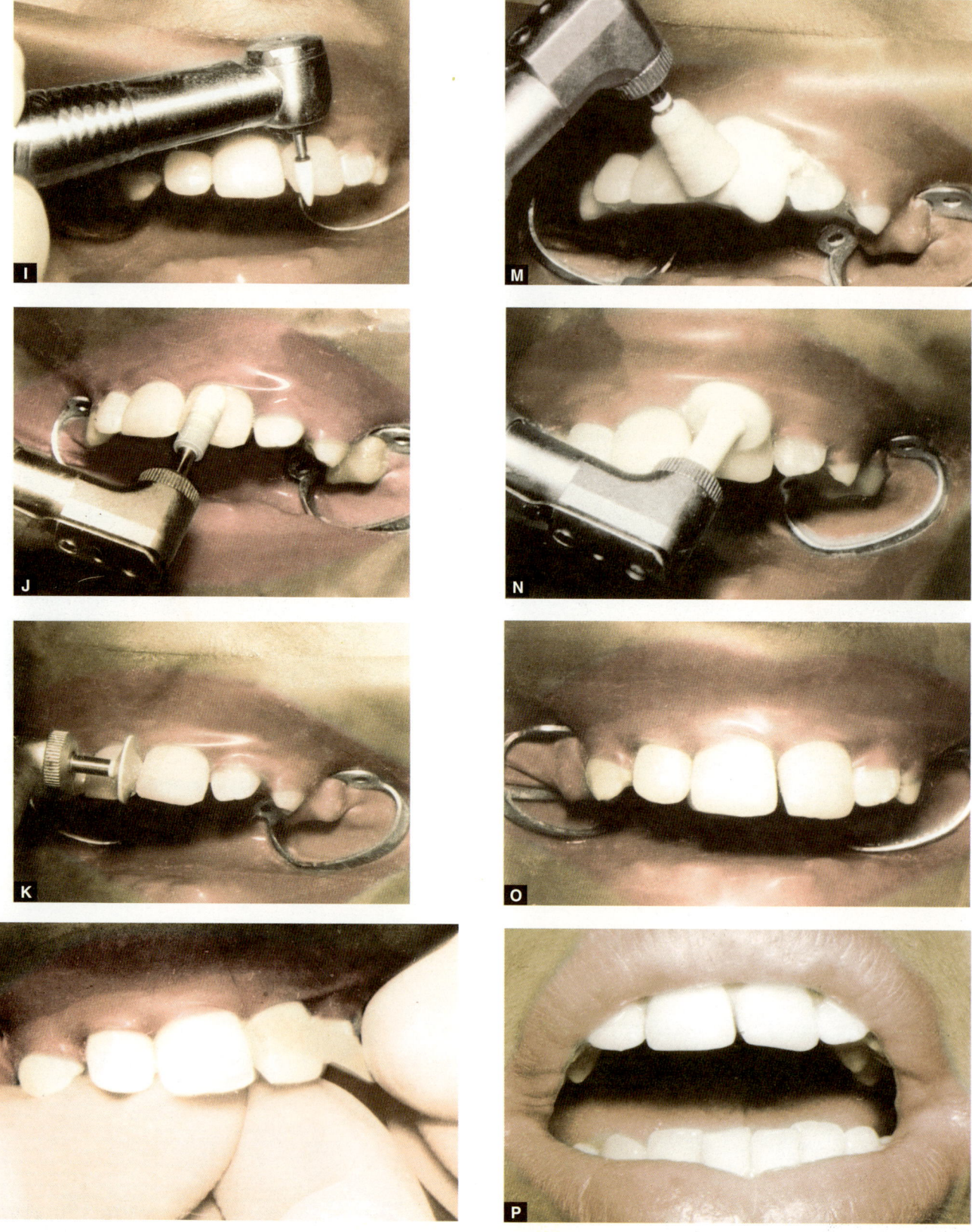

Figs 17.27I to P: **(I)** Finishing with white aluminium oxide stone; **(J)** Smoothening with rubber polishing point; **(K)** Interproximal smoothening with rubber disks; **(L)** Interproximal finishing with strips; **(M)** Polishing with rubber cup and aluminium oxide paste; **(N)** Polishing with a buff; **(O)** Completed restoration; **(P)** Final restoration without rubber dam

Composites

Step-wise procedure for the restoration of class II cavity

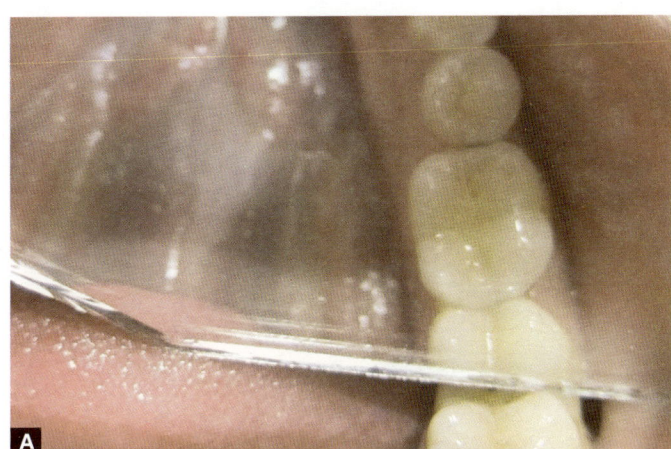

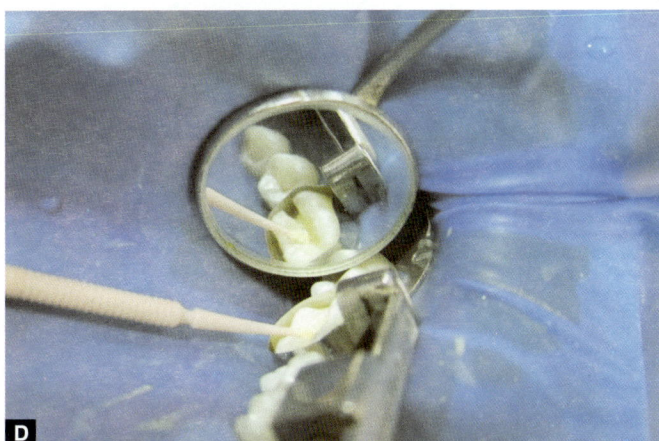

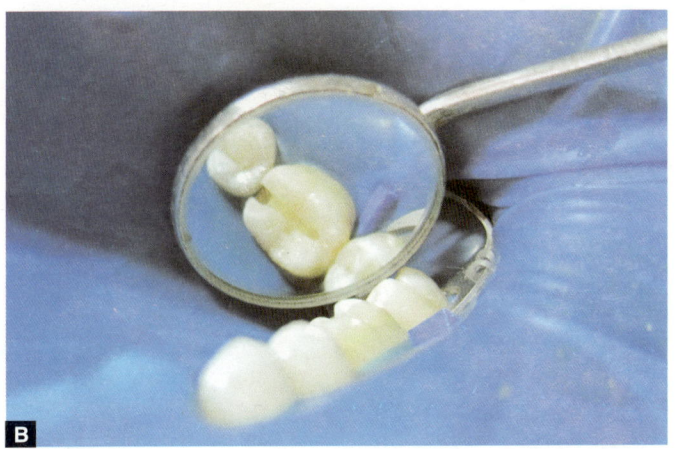

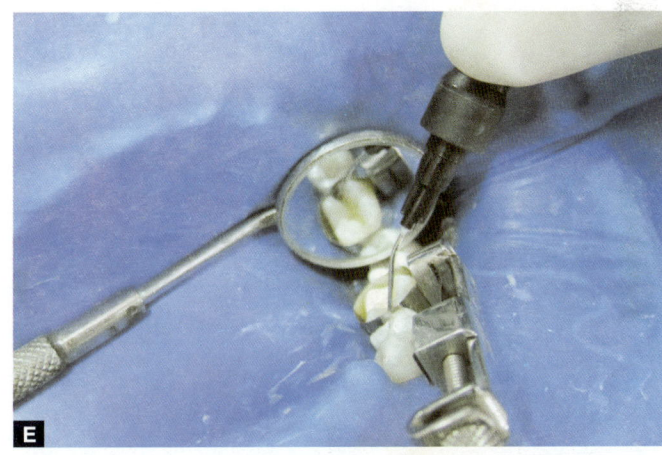

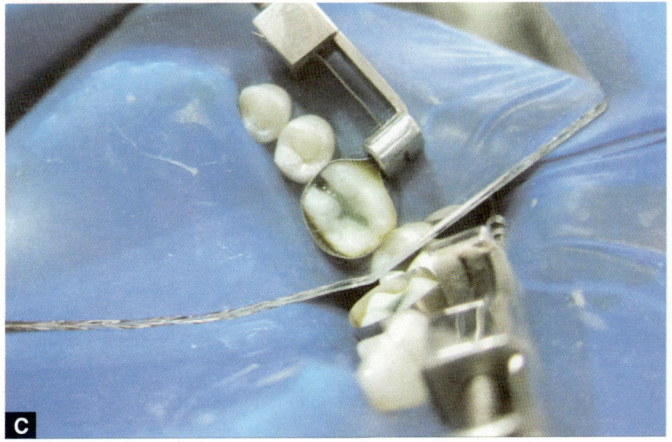

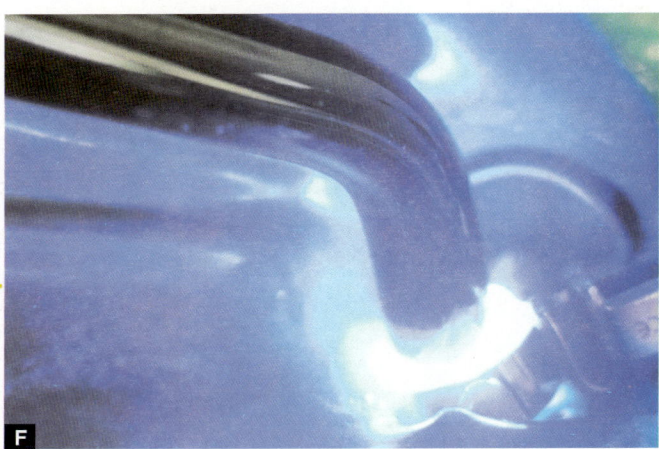

Figs 17.28A to F: **(A)** Pre-operative; **(B)** Cavity preparation; **(C)** Etchant application; **(D)** Bonding agent application; **(E)** Flowable composite application in the proximal box; **(F)** Curing with light

Step-wise procedure for the restoration of class II cavity

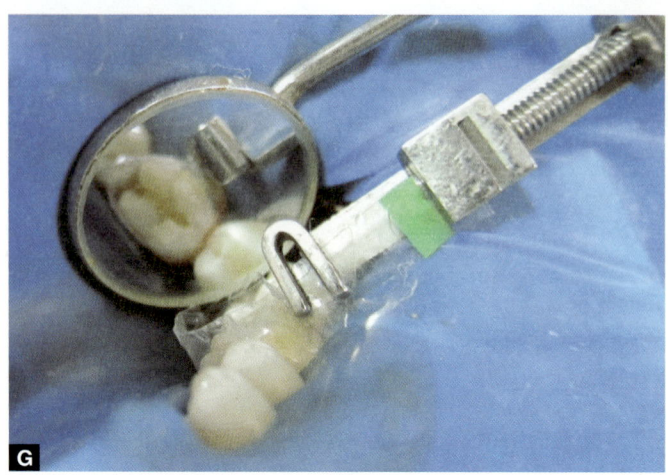

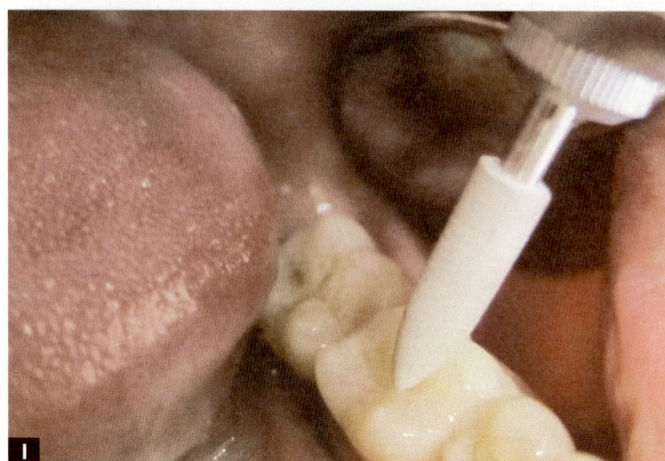

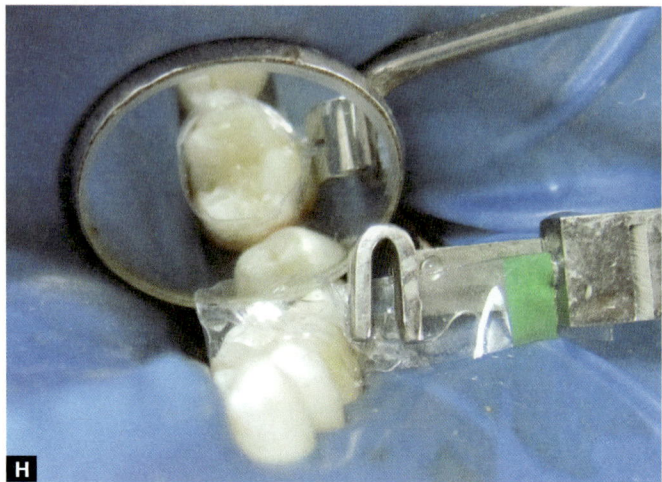

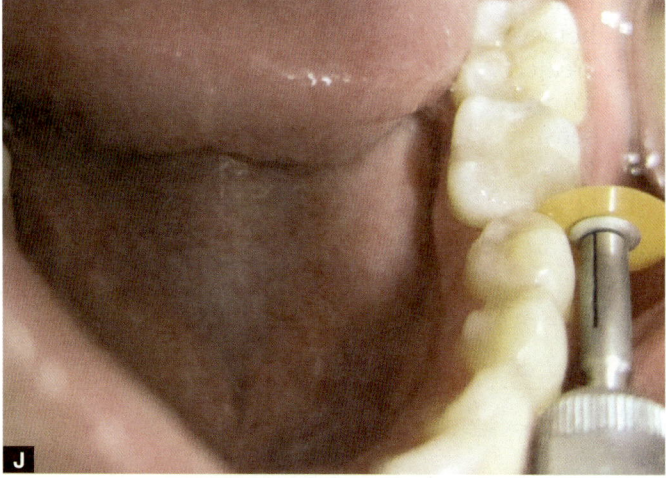

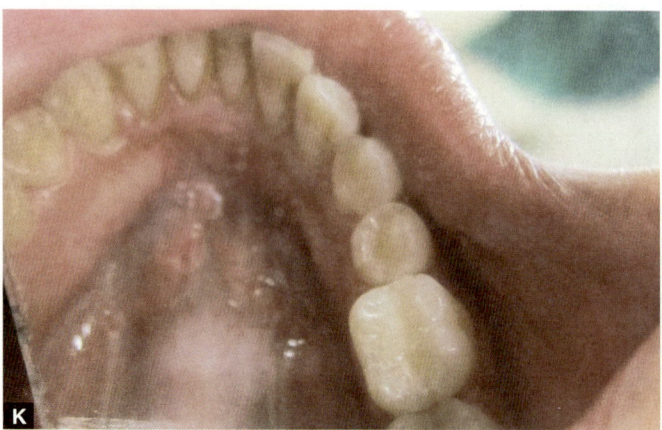

Figs 17.28G to K: **(G)** Change of matrix band after curing of gingival increment; **(H)** Curing completed; **(I)** Finishing of occlusal surface; **(J)** Finishing of proximal surface; **(K)** Completed composite restoration

always cured from the sides first rather from the occlusal end.
- *Horizontal layering design*: Small increments placed horizontally one above the other starting from gingival wall to occlusal end. The number of layers depends upon the depth of the proximal box (Fig. 17.29B).
- *Oblique layering design*: Each increment is placed obliquely starting from any side i.e. buccal or lingual (Fig. 17.29C).
- *U-shaped layering design*: At the base, both gingival and occlusal, U-shaped increment is placed first and over that horizontal and oblique increments are placed (Fig. 17.29D).
- *Vertical layering design*: The increments are placed in vertical fashion starting from one wall, i.e. buccal or lingual and carried on to other wall in small increments (Fig. 17.29E). The curing is started from behind the wall as the ease may be, i.e. if first increment is placed on the buccal wall, it is cured from outside the buccal wall. This type of technique helps in reducing the gap at the gingival wall created due to polymerization shrinkage, thereby minimizing the chances of post-operative sensitivity and the secondary caries.
- Layering technique in the proximal box and curing each increment by inserting the fiber-optic microtip into the composite (Figs 17.29F, G).

Whichever design may be used, care should be taken to compress the increments so as not to have any voids between the two increments. Teflon coated instruments can be utilized for this purpose. Use of bonding agent in between the increment, is not required since partially cured increments unite of their own. However, few authors advocate use of bonding agents after the last increment to have better marginal adaptability.

Establishing Proximal Contact

One of the problems with composite restoration is establishing proper contact at the proximal sides. Since composites shrink after setting, coupled with the gap created by matrix, this problem increases two folds. Though with the advent of newer composites and newer techniques along the ultra thin matrices, the problem is minimized, yet it is not completely solved.

Proximal contacts are restored in two ways:
i. After curing of the gingival increment up to the contact area, the wedge and the matrix is removed and rest of the restoration is carried out without the matrix though in increments. The final occlusal embrasures can be contoured with the instruments. A few authors are of the view that the minor separation created by the matrix placement and wedging is sufficient for the establishment of final contact. Therefore, the removal of matrix in between is not indicated according to their view.
ii. Duokoudakis (1996) devised a technique whereby proper contact can be established at the proximal areas. According to him, the width of the cavity preparation from the contact area to the opposing cavity wall is measured. The area of the contact, which is to be restored is also measured (Fig. 17.30).

A small tube, containing composite of the same width and slightly more in length is taken and cured. This composite rod will be slightly larger in size and

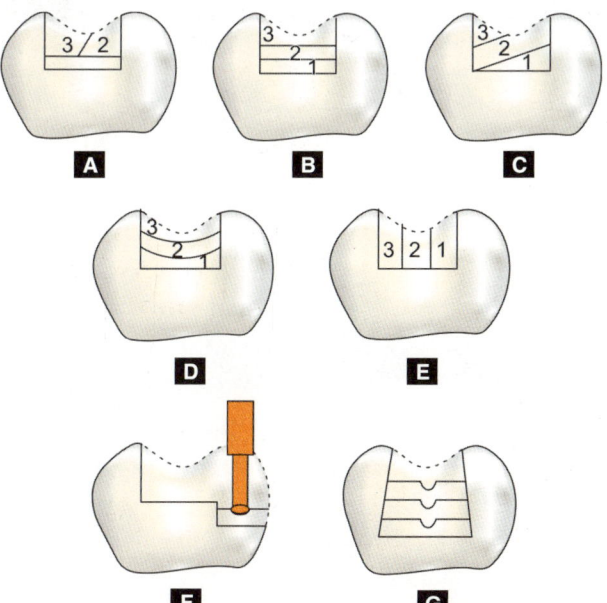

Figs 17.29A to G: Different designs of increment placement for composite **(A)** Three increment design **(B)** Horizontal layering design **(C)** Oblique layering design **(D)** U-shaped layering design **(E)** Vertical layering design **(F & G)** Curing each increment by inserting the fibre-optic microtip into the composite

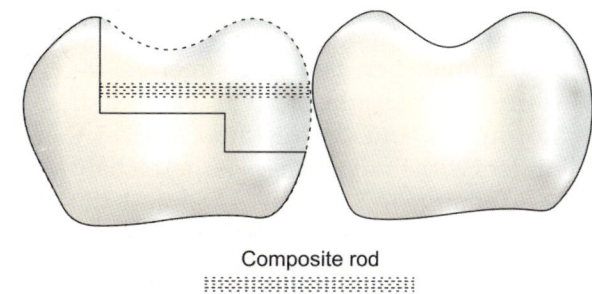

Composite rod

Fig. 17.30: Composite rod and its placement at the desired place adjacent to the contact area

finally adjusted by finishing at the margins (Fig. 17.30). The composite is restored as in routine keeping the matrix and the wedge in place and the rod is kept at the desired place adjacent to the contact area (Fig. 17.30). Finally the rest of the cavity is restored with the composite. This technique helps in maintaining the proper size and shape of the contact. Preferably the composite rods are fabricated in darker shades since after the final restoration, they provide better esthetic results.

FAILURES IN COMPOSITE RESTORATIONS

Composite restorations are very technique sensitive; therefore, utmost care is necessary before, during and after their placement. Care should be exercised during cavity preparation and each step of composite placement to avoid or minimize failures. The visible modes of failures seen in composite restoration are:

- Discoloration, especially at the margins (Fig. 17.31).
- Marginal fracture (Fig. 17.32).
- Recurrent caries (Fig. 17.33).
- Post-operative sensitivity
- Gross fracture of restoration (Fig. 17.34).
- Lack of maintaining contact (Fig. 17.34).
- Accumulation of plaque around the restorations

The following features usually lead to failure in composites:

a. *Incomplete excavation of caries*: The caries if not thoroughly removed (Fig. 17.35), the left over caries may hinder with the bonding mechanism. Similarly, if zinc oxide eugenol is not removed thoroughly from the base of the cavity and the walls, this will also lead to failure.

b. *Incomplete etching or failure to remove residual acid from the enamel tags:* Proper concentration of acid along with proper etching time is mandatory to achieve the requisite tags. Fluorosed enamel require more etching time; however, the total etching time should not be more than 60 seconds. Repeated touch after etching, blowing with compressed air under pressure and/or sweeping the etched surface with cotton can lead to fracture of tips of the tags leading to lack of proper union between the enamel tags and resin. Many a times, the acid is not washed out thoroughly and the residual acid in the tags hinders with the bonding. The gel etchant should be washed for 20–30 seconds and the liquid etchant washed for 10–15 seconds. For drying, air from chip syringe should be used. Three-way syringe should be avoided as the air could be contaminated by machine oils or water which condenses in the pipelines.

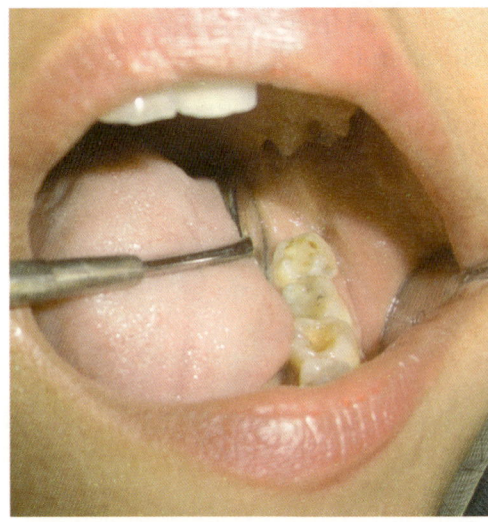

Fig. 17.31: Marginal staining and ditching aroung composite restoration

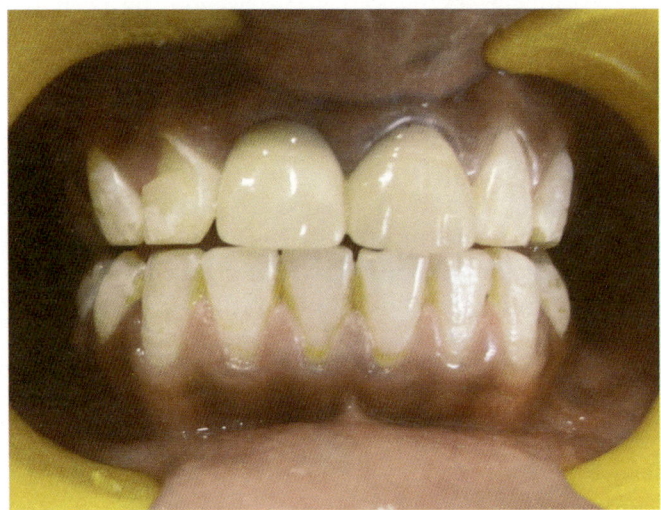

Fig. 17.32: Fractured composite restoration

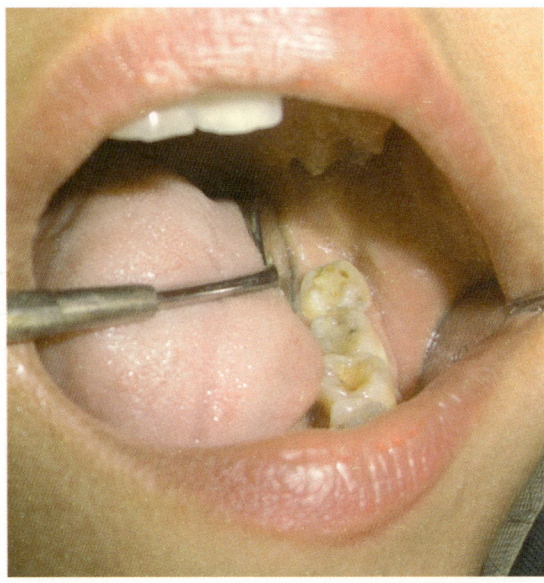

Fig. 17.33: Recurrent caries adjacent to composite restoration

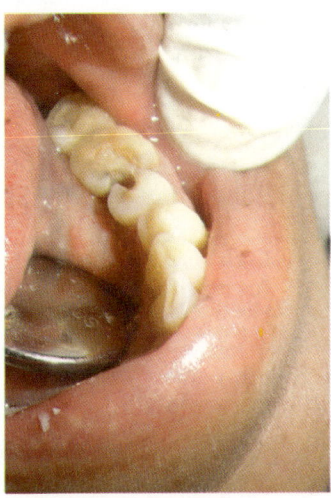

Fig. 17.34: Gross fracture of composite restoration leading to loss of contact

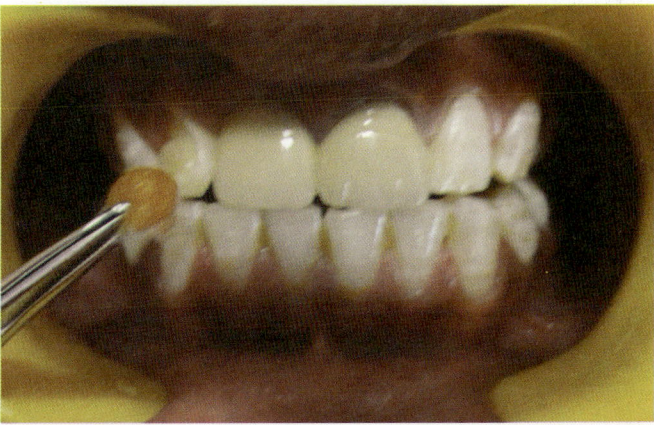

Fig. 17.36: Excess bonding agent applied in the cavity preparation

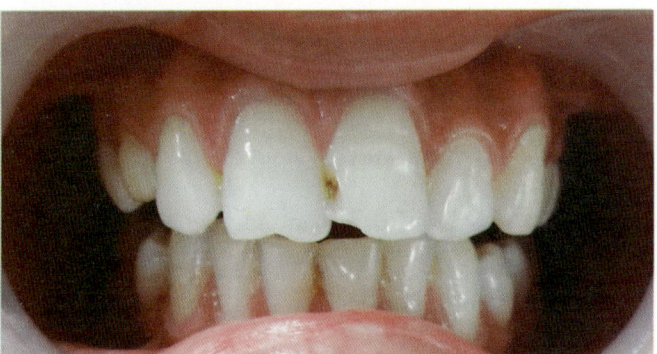

Fig. 17.35: Caries not thoroughly removed during cavity preparation

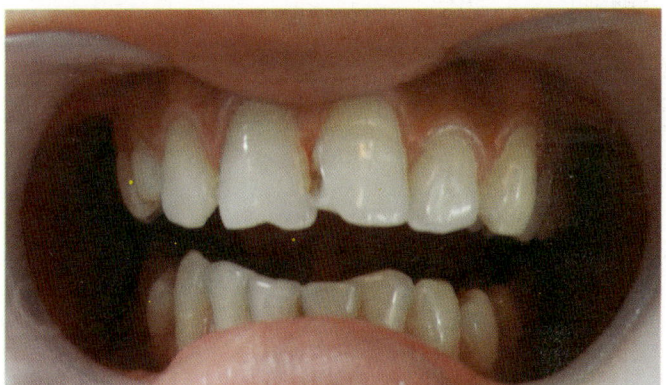

Fig. 17.37: Lack of isolation during restoration

c. *Excess or non-uniform application of bonding agent* (Fig. 17.36): Bonding agent is to be applied uniformly all around the cavity walls. Excess of bonding leads to marginal leakage and also, non-uniform bonding at certain areas hinders the union of material with the bonding agent.

d. *Lack of isolation:* A rubber dam isolation is mandatory; however, cotton rolls can be used if the time consumption is less. Gingival retraction cords can be utilized in class III and class V cavities and also in composite laminates (Fig. 17.37). The touch of saliva and the gingival fluid is to be avoided even after etching and bonding phenomenon. In patients with uncontrolled salivation, antisialogouge drugs can be used.

e. *Touch of composite with fingers:* The composite in any case should not be touched with fingers (Fig. 17.38). Many a times, the operator uses his finger to pack or keep the material in place. This practice is to be avoided. Always pick and hold the composite with Teflon-coated instruments. Sometimes the composite falls over the tongue and the operator picks it up and pack the same into the cavity. This will lead to failure (Fig. 17.39).

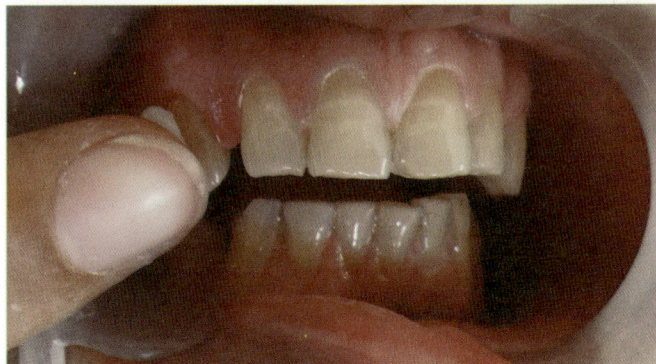

Fig. 17.38: Composite being touched with fingers

f. *Avoid bulk placement of composites* (Fig. 17.40): The composite is to be placed in increments and each increment should be as small as possible, since the contraction after polymerization leads to gaps at the tooth restoration interface. These gaps consequently lead to post-operative sensitivity, marginal leakage and secondary caries.

g. *Improper curing:* The curing of the composite should be from all the sides and for stipulated period. The filter and the bulb vis-à-vis the

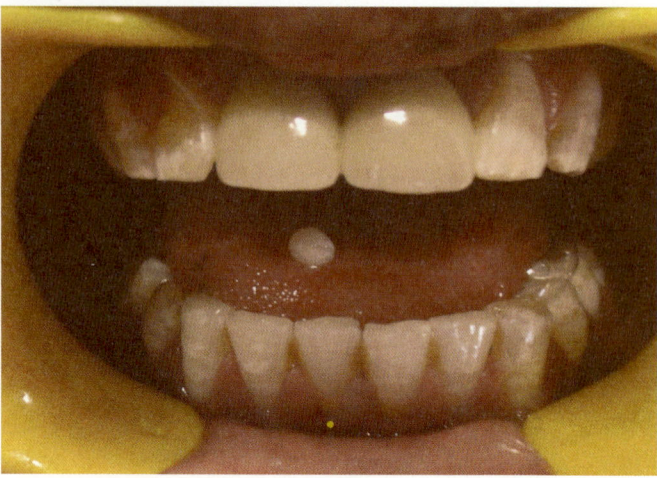

Fig. 17.39: Composite fallen on the tongue

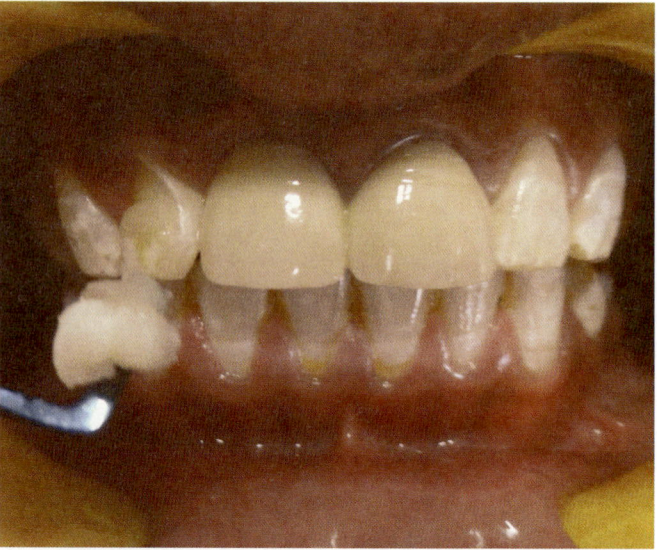

Fig. 17.40: Composite being placed in bulk

- Use small increments, holding each increment with Teflon coated instruments.
- Fill proximal box separately and create proper contact areas.
- Composite, especially at the bevelled areas, should be finished and polished properly.

COMPOSITE LAMINATES AND VENEERS

The laminates and veneers are interchangeable terms; the only difference is in laminates, the overall shape is not changed while in veneers the shape of the tooth is changed. Laminates are given only where the teeth are discolored but their shape, size and position in the arch is normal whereas veneers are given where the teeth need change in their shape, size and the position in the arch.

The laminates are preferred in maxillary anterior teeth since these teeth play a predominant role in smile and esthetics of a person. Mandibular anterior teeth are rarely laminated because of lack of space and more so, the teeth are hidden under the lower lips.

Composite laminates/veneers can be partial or complete depending upon the area involved. These can be direct and indirect depending upon whether the laminate is fabricated inside or outside the oral cavity.

Indirect laminates are advantageous since they provide better esthetics, less fatigue to the patient and easily manipulated. However, the procedure is completed in two steps. Direct laminates, though save patient's visits, are tiring and more technique sensitive.

Tooth Preparation for laminates/veneers

i. *Preparation for partial veneers:* In case of partial veneers, the concerned patch is removed using appropriate burs. There can be only one patch or more than one. Each patch is restored individually. The stained area is involved keeping the depth 0.5–0.75 mm preferably only in enamel. In case the stains are very dark and deep, the preparation can be extended into the dentin. Such lesions require opaquer while restoring. A slight involvement of the normal enamel is necessary to achieve better esthetics. A short bevel is placed all along the cavosurface margins to provide better color mixing.

ii. *Preparation for full veneers:* Preparation for full veneers varies depending upon whether it envelopes the marginal ridges and the incisal edge or not. In deeply darkened stains, which extend towards the incisal enamel, the preparation involves the incisal edge. Otherwise the preparation ends slightly away from incisal edge. Similarly whether to extend the

intensity of the light should be checked in routine to ensure the proper curing. For proximal restoration, fine curing tips can also be used.

h. *Improper finishing and polishing:* Composites should be finished and polished thoroughly. The occlusion should be checked before final polishing. Antagonist tooth, if impinging can be grinded off.

Certain *guidelines* should be followed which can minimize the chances of failure:
- The cavity preparation should be kept as small as possible since composite in bulk leads to failure.
- Avoid sharp internal line angles in cavity preparation, which increases stresses.
- Deeper cavities should be given base of calcium hydroxide or glass-ionomer cement.
- Strict isolation regime is to be followed.
- Avoid inadequate curing, since it leads to hydrolytic breakdown of composites.

composite veneer is also etched with weak acid. In case the veneer or the prepared tooth is contaminated, this is thoroughly washed, dried and the etching and bonding procedure is repeated. After completely placing the veneer, the margins are checked thoroughly. The veneer is cured for 40 seconds both from the labial and the lingual sides.

Though the veneers are directly polished, minor finishing and polishing may be required at the margins. The occlusion, particularly the protrusive movement is checked to restore occlusal harmony. Patients are instructed not to try reverse bite with these veneers.

COMPOSITE INLAYS (INDIRECT TOOTH COLORED RESTORATIONS)

An inlay is intracoronal restoration. A composite inlay is defined as a restoration which is cemented into a cavity prepared specifically for the composite material. A solid mass simulating the cavity shape is fabricated from composite resin, outside the oral cavity.

Need for a Composite Inlay?

Direct posterior composite restorations have certain limitations viz.

- Despite the incremental build-up and techniques polymerization shrinkage of the resin during curing is a major problem which contributes to marginal defects, cuspal distortion, crack formation and propagation within the tooth tissues resulting in post-operative sensitivity.
- An adequate bond, especially in areas where the cavosurface margin is situated in dentin may not be achieved.
- Inadequate polymerization in deep interproximal areas may lead to partly cured restoration.
- Increased wear in load bearing situations.
- Water sorption with resultant hydrolytic instability.
- Contour, contacts are not proper.

To overcome these clinical problems, the indirect composite inlay system was introduced. Most clinical studies have demonstrated a dramatic improvement in their clinical performance. It has been established that heat treatment enhances the resin hardness and wear resistance and also reduces the microleakage.

Indications

- Regular dental patients requiring tooth colored restoration of better quality.
- Moderate to large sized lesions, where sufficient tooth tissue remains following preparation.
- Where there is no evidence of excessive tooth wear.
- Restoration not overloaded occlusally.
- When better control over contacts and contours is desired.

Contraindications

- Patients who do not maintain oral hygiene.
- Uncooperative patients.
- Teeth broken down to the extent that inadequate tooth tissues remain to create adequate resistance and retention forms for the purposes of bonding.
- Teeth in which outline form includes marked under-cuts.
- Teeth which show excessive wear.
- Situations where moisture control cannot be secured and maintained.
- Teeth that experience heavy occlusal forces like in bruxism, clenching etc.

Advantages

Enhanced physical properties such as:
- Better compressive strength, tensile strength and hardness
- Better visco-elastic stability
- Increased creep resistance to occlusal stresses
- Better control of Contacts and contours
- Improved control over marginal adaptation
- Soft and gentle to nearby tooth
- Less technique sensitive
- Saves patient's as well as doctor's chair time.
- Can easily be adjusted in the oral cavity

Disadvantages

- The fabrication of an inlay usually requires two appointments and a temporary restoration. The overall cost is increased.
- Preparation of the cavity may necessitate removal of sound tooth structure to create parallelism and other features.
- Chances of luting agent washing out of (The success of the restoration depends largely upon the bond between the inlay and tooth using a luting material).
- Temporary restoration, if not proper, may lead to bacterial contamination etc.
- Stain more readily than porcelain
- Durability is not established

Classification of Composite Inlays

Inlay may be classified according to the method of construction, method of curing and type of composite.

Method of Construction

Composite inlays can be constructed by
a. Direct technique
b. Indirect technique

Method of Curing

Composite inlays can be classified on the basis of curing as:
- Superficial inlays
- Conventional cured inlays
- Secondary cured inlays
  a. *Superficial inlays*: The inlays are cured at elevated temperature and under pressure in one stage. The composite employed is heat cured rather than light cured, e.g. SR Isosit system where inlays are cured at 120°C and under pressure.
  b. *Conventional cured inlays*: One mode of curing only e.g. light curing (EOS system), where the inlay is cured by light only.
  c. *Secondary cured inlays*: Initial curing at room temperature by light followed by additional curing by heat and light e.g. Coltene Brilliant Aesthetic Line system in which secondary curing is done under high intensity light at 120°C for 7 minutes. Kulzer inlay system in which secondary curing is done in an enclosed light activating unit.

Evolution of Composite Inlays

First generation composite inlays—introduced in the early 1986.

SR Isosit Inlay System

SR Isosit (Microfilled composite) is a homogeneously filled composite containing 55% by weight colloidal silica plus 20% lanthanum fluoride. Available in 7 non-vita shades.

Coltene Brilliant

The Coltene-Brilliant system (fine hybrid composite) incorporates a fine particle size (0.5 µm) hybrid composite containing 78.5% (by mass) glass fiber. Available in four Vita shades, the inlay is cured on a fabricated die and further polymerized in the Coltene DI500 light/heat curing oven for 7 minutes at a temperature of 120°C. The system can be employed for both direct and indirect techniques.

Kulzer Inlay

Kulzer system (Coarse hybrid composite) employs a glass ceramic filled composite containing 80% filler by mass. The inlays are light cured and then tempered for either 180 seconds in the Dentacolor XS light unit, or 6 minutes in the light box.

Visio Gem

Visio Gem was initially introduced as a material suitable for anterior composite veneers, but its use was expanded to include indirect inlays. The inlays are initially light cured followed by a 15 minute light cure under vacuum.

Second Generation Composite Inlay

Incorporated ceramic fillers with particle size less than 1.0 µm diameter. It reduces the polymerisation shrinkage while increases the modulus of elasticity. For example: 1. Sculpture: Advanced light, heat and vaccum cured polymer glass restorative material 2. Herculite: Bis-GMA micro-hybrid light activated composite with an average particle size of 0.6 µm 3. Art glass 4. Bella glass

Art Glass

The filler content of Art glass is essentially a radiopaque barium glass with a mean particle size of 0.7 µm. A moderate amount of colloidal silica is also incorporated for the purpose of enhancing handling characteristics.

Art glass is photocured in a special unit using a xeno stroboscopic light. The system emits a total of 4.5 watts as usable luminus power, while the emission range is between 320 and 500 nm. This range is significant because excitation of the initiator, camphoroquinone is optimized at about 470 nm.

The manufacturer proposed that the short excitation time followed by a longer period of nonexposure allows the already cured resin molecules to partially relax. Consequently, more non reacted double bond carbon groups are made available for reaction.

Belleglass HP

The resin matrix in Belleglass HP is chemically similar to that of the BiSGMA restorative systems. Belleglass HP is polymerized under pressure at an elevated temperature (138°C) and in the presence of nitrogen.

The use of a nitrogen during the polymerization process plays the most important role since it relates to an increase in wear resistance. It produces an oxygen free environment which results in higher level of polymerization.

Cavity Preparation

It is generally agreed that a directly placed composite is suitable for a small or medium sized posterior cavity while a composite inlay is suitable for a medium or large sized posterior cavity. Preparation for inlays, as usual, requires creating a withdrawal form. The cavity design may vary from a '*saucerized*' preparation

to a *'modified traditional gold inlay cavity preparation'*. The cavity preparation includes the following features:
- Remove existing restoration and/or caries.
- Assess occlusion and identify occlusal contacts.
- Adjust the extension of preparation to optimize the form and location of margins.
- Manage undercuts by blocking them with a suitable material like glass-ionomer cement.
- A taper, 6–8° can be given on the opposing walls.
- A minimum cavity depth of 1.5 mm.
- A typically cavity usually has an interproximal box width of ½ the buccolingual and an occlusal isthmus width of 1/3rd the bucco-lingual width.
- Rounded internal line angles to reduce stress concentration.
- Cavosurface bevels are not indicated.

Direct Posterior Resin Inlay Technique

A direct inlay is fabricated and inserted during the same appointment without the need for any laboratory procedures.

Technique

After securing local anaesthesia and isolating the field with a rubber dam, a conventional cavity is prepared. Internal line angles are rounded slightly to ensure maximum adaptation of the restorative resin. A base can be given if the cavity is deep.

The prepared cavity is then lined with tinfoil using a cotton pledget and pressing the foil against the preparation walls and line angles. The tin foil will serve as a separating medium allowing for removal of the inlay to accomplish refinement procedures. The use of petroleum jelly or liquid separating medium, is discouraged because of uncertainty about their effects on polymerization of the resin. Additionally, the capability of these materials to be completely removed from the enamel in order to procure maximum benefits from enamel etching procedures is also questionable.

A light cure resin restorative material designed for posterior inlay is placed in the cavity preparation over the tinfoil and polymerized according to the manufacturer's specifications.

The inlay is then removed from the prepared cavity and separated from the tinfoil liner. Proximal contact and contours are established. The inlay is finished and polished.

The tooth is cleaned, dried and enamel etching procedures are carried out. A photoactivated unfilled resin is placed over the etched enamel and dispersed with a gentle air stream. The thin resin layer can now be cured.

The inlay is tried into the cavity preparation. If the adaptation of the restoration is acceptable, it is cemented with dual cure resin cements. Following placement of the unfilled resin into the cavity, the restoration is seated and the unfilled/filled resin complex is polymerized.

After polymerization, the occlusal anatomy is refined with carbide finishing burs and sof-lex discs. The occlusal surface is polished to a high luster using appropriate polishing points. The rubber dam is then removed and occlusion checked and adjusted if necessary.

Indirect Posterior Resin Inlay Technique

The Isosit-crown and bridge material is commonly used for indirect inlays. After the cavity preparation, rubber base impression is taken and two dies are made. The complete stepwise procedure for indirect composite inlay is shown in Figs 17.43A to 17.43O.

- Proper shade is selected
- The second die which might be less accurate, is used for the first polymerization. Body material is packed at the base of the die and the rest is covered with a layer of clear and incisal Isosit. The material is then polymerized at 100°C at 6 atmospheric pressure for 3 minutes. Isosit shrinks less than 1%.
- The inlay is now relieved on the first poured die and the material added where necessary. The second polymerization is then completed at 120°C and 6 atmospheric pressure for 6 minutes in an oven (Fig. 17.44). The small shrinkage has been controlled and finally checked on the first die. Final shaping and detailing is completed and repolymerized if need be. The prepared inlay is then polished with fine pumice and tin oxide.

Cementation

Indirect inlay can be cemented by either:
- Conventional cements
- Self cure composite
- Light cure composite
- Dual cure composite

Light cure composite is the material of choice. It offers superior esthetics and unlimited working time. Dual cure composite allows polymerization to continue in areas difficult to reach by light. When using light cure composite, a light that cures to a depth of 6.0 mm is required and many light cures are reliable only up to 3.0 mm. Recently, manufacturers claim light curing to a depth of 12.0 mm. Such units can be utilized for the purpose.

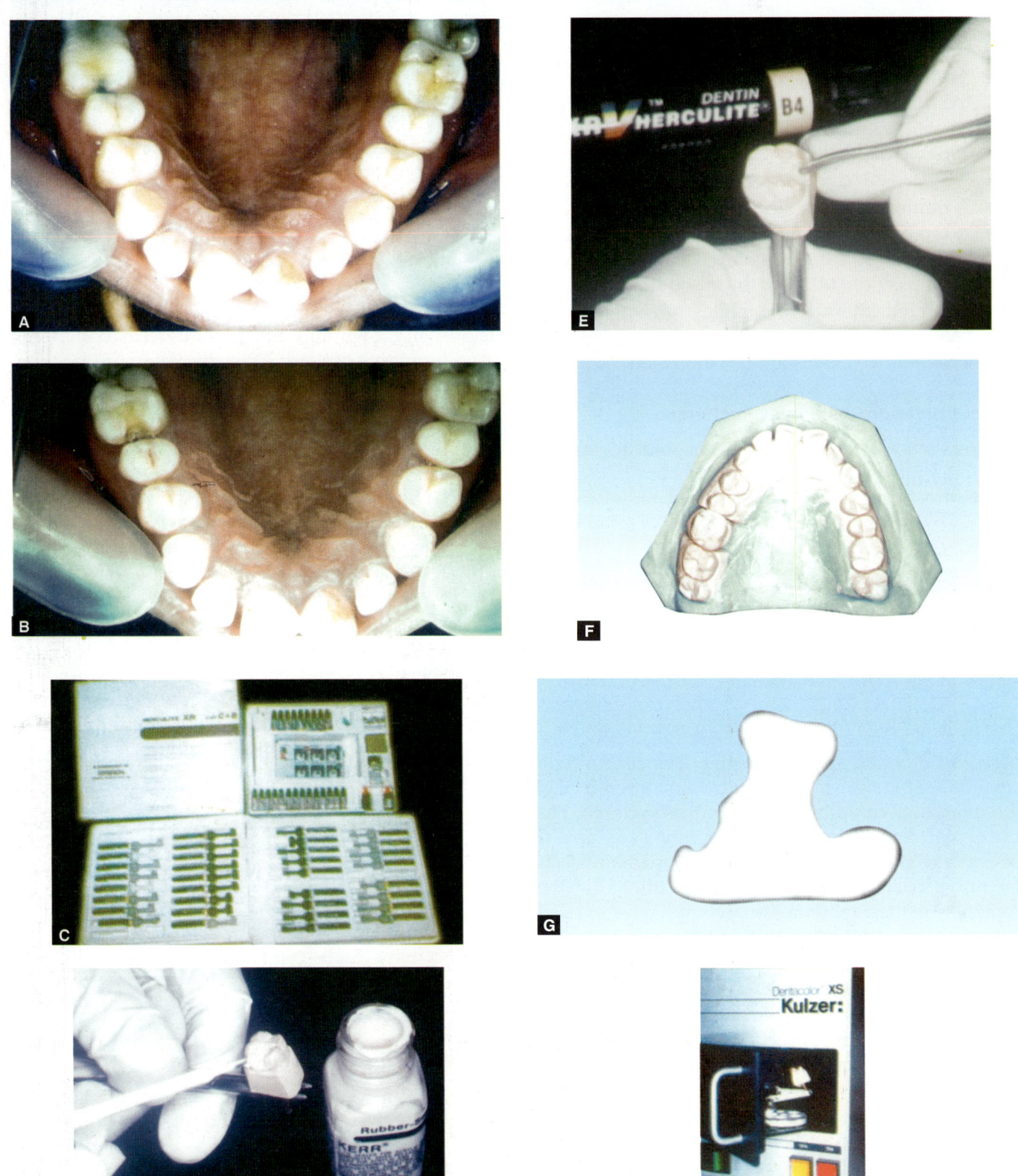

Figs 17.43A to H: **(A)** Pre-operative; **(B)** Cavity prepared; **(C)** Composite kit for indirect composite inlays; **(D)** Die spacer being applied on cavity preparation; **(E)** Composite being applied on cavity preparation; **(F)** Cavity on die filled with composite; **(G)** Cured composite restoration retrieved from the die; **(H)** Additional curing being done in an oven

Composites

Step-wise procedure for indirect composite inlay restoration of class II cavity on maxillary right first molar

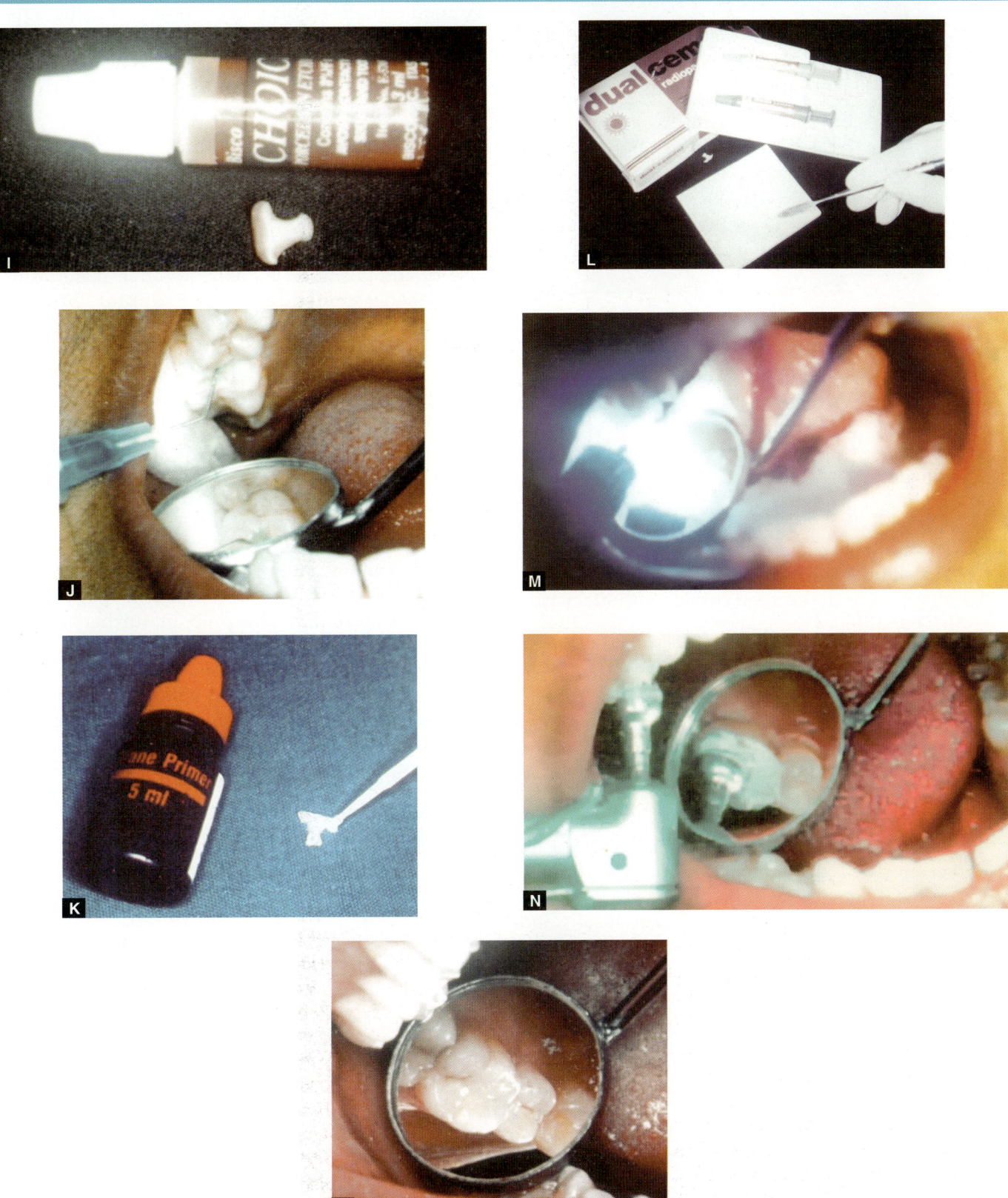

Figs 17.43I to O: (I) Composite inlay is etched; **(J)** Etchant applied in cavity preparation; **(K)** Primer being applied on composite inlay; **(L)** Dual cure resin being mixed for cementation; **(M)** Resin lute being cured after the inlay has been seated in the cavity; **(N)** Polishing of composite inlay being done; **(O)** Completed composite inlay restoration

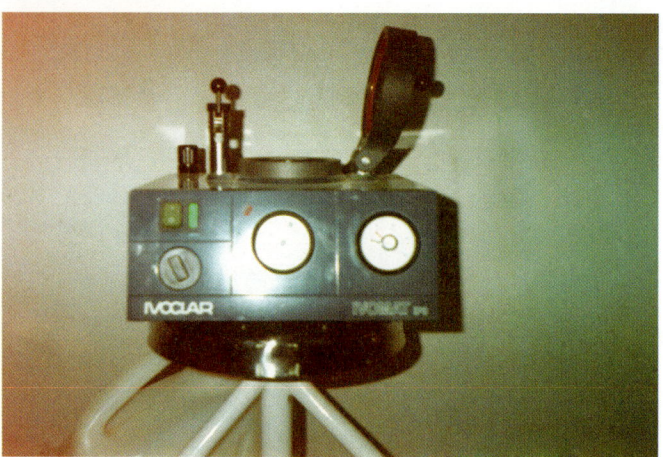

Fig. 17.44: Ivoclar oven for curing indirect inlay

Following *steps* are followed for *cementation:*
- The inlay is examined for flash at the gingival margin, if any, is carefully finished.
- The inlay is seated and proximal contacts are adjusted.
- Occlusion is adjusted.
- A rubber dam is applied for moisture control.
- The tooth is etched and dried.
- The dentist affixes one half of a bent plastic toothpick to the occlusal surface with sticky wax for handling of the inlay during cementation.
- After verifying that all instruments and materials are ready, a thin layer of unfilled resin is applied to the internal surface of the preparation and cured. A thin layer of unfilled resin is also applied to the cavity surface of the inlay and cured.
- The inlay is placed firmly on the tooth and the excess cement removed with a blunt instrument.
- The cement is cured for a minimum of 40 seconds with the light cure unit placed directly on the inlay surface. If box forms are involved, light should be applied buccally, occlusally and lingually.
- After composite has polymerized, margins are finished using 12 fluted carbide burs, Soflex finishing discs and finishing burs. Occlusion is rechecked and the restoration polished.

Advantages of Indirect Inlay Technique
- Esthetically more pleasing
- Improves resistance to breakage by bonding to the etched walls
- More durable, accurate, porosity free than conventional composites
- When cemented with a composite cement to acid etched enamel, good marginal seal is achieved
- Restoration can be repaired in the mouth

Composite or Porcelain?

A good esthetic result may be obtained using either system i.e. composite or porcelain. However, each inlay system has its own advantages and disadvantages. The comparative properties of composite and ceramic inlays are given in Table 17.6.

REPAIRING COMPOSITE RESTORATIONS AND PORCELAINS FUSED TO METAL RESTORATIONS WITH COMPOSITE RESINS

With increased concern and demand for esthetics, the use of composite resins as restorative material has increased tremendously in dental practice. Innumerable attempts have been made to improve the bonding systems, and mechanical-physical properties of the resin systems, but they tend to undergo degradations under various mechanical and chemical insults in oral environment. Wear, abrasion, fatigue, hydrolytic and acidic actions or temperature related changes lead to discoloration, microleakage, ditching at margins, delaminations or fractures of composite restorations quite often, demanding replacements or repair.

As directed by conservative philosophy, repair as an alternative to complete removal would preserve the tooth and spare the pulp of further damage. Repair is defined as the partial replacement of the composite restoration allowing preservation of that portion of the composite restoration which presents no clinical or radiographic evidence of failures.

Rationale for Restoration Repair
- Preservation of tooth structure
- Increased longevity of the restoration
- Reduction of potentially harmful effects on the dental pulp
- Reduction in treatment time
- Reduced cost to the patient
- Good patient acceptance
- No need of local anesthesia, provided the repair is not extensive
- Less risk of iatrogenic damage to the adjacent tooth

Bonding of New Composite Resin to Old Composite Restoration and Need of Surface Treatments

Repair of old composite restorations with a new composite resin requires a sufficient bonding between the two. Bonding to the resin matrix relies on the unconverted carbon-carbon double bonds remaining of the surface of the aged composite. It has been studied that in an old composite restoration the degree of unreacted carbon double bonds is lower, impairing

Table 17.6: Comparative evaluation of composite and ceramic inlays

	Composite	Ceramic inlays
Advantages directly placed composite	• Controlled polymerization shrinkage • Improved mechanical properties • Reduced microleakage	• Same as for composite inlay except marginal seal is better
Cavity design	• Medium to large • 8 to 10 degree taper • Minimum depth 1.5 mm • Isthmus width 2.0 mm minimum • Cusp reduction 1.5–2.0 mm minimum for onlays • No cavosurface bevel • No undercuts	• Same as for composite inlays except depth is more
Laboratory procedures	• Relatively simple • Initial outlay needed	• Costly, complex and time-consuming • Initial outlay need
Finishing	• Convenient	• Slightly
Aesthetics	• Good	• Excellent
Toxicity	• Unknown	• Biocompatible
Wear resistance	• Possibly material wear	• High level of wear resistance
Intraoral repair	• Possible	• Not possible
Cost compared to amalgam	• Six times	• Eight times
Clinical studies	• Promising	• Promising
Brittleness	• Not much	• Greater liability to fracture during try in
Strength	• Good, as required	• High compressive strength than composite but may be less in tensile strength

the chemical bond between the old and new resin matrices. Meanwhile with increasing polymerization, there is decrease in solubility and permeability of polymer that delimits the bonding with resin monomer of newly introduced composite resin. Moreover, in case of indirect composite restorations, the number of unreacted carbon double bonds is further reduced due to dual system of polymerization viz. light cure and heat cure. Thus the bond of repair is not a reliable bond and is often found to be lower (25–80%) than the cohesive strength of the composite.

Various methods have been suggested to establish adequate bond strength between the existing composite and the new composite. These treatments include surface roughening and the use of intermediate bonding agents to enhance repair bond strength. The roughening of the surface through acid etching, burs or abrasives, promotes mechanical interlocking through microretentive features and application of bonding agent improves surface wetting and chemical bonding with the new composite. In addition to surface roughening, silane treatment of the exposed filler particles can be carried out as silane acts as a binfunctional molecule that chemically binds to silica particles (through formation of siloxane bonds) of older composite and methacrylate groups of organosilane forms covalent bonds with resin monomer of newer composite.

Various methods of mechanical surface treatments:

1. Abrasion
   a. Air abrasion with 50 μm aluminium oxide particles
   b. Sandblasting with Co-Jet and system – 30 μm silanated silica coated aluminium oxide particles
   c. Abrasion with diamond bur
2. Acid etching
   a. 37% phosphoric acid etching for composites
   b. 6–10% or 1.23% APF acid etching for all ceramic or porcelain fused to metal crowns repair with composites

Clinical procedures for repair of direct composite restoration

1. Many marginal defects can be simply managed using refurbishing procedures that include recontouring and refinishing or resurfacing of the composite restorations. Minor superficial stains and defects can be removed using a fine-

grit diamond finishing bur followed by polishing and application of unfilled resin to seal over any marginal cracking and provide surface glaze.

2. Extensive repair procedures can be accomplished with following steps, using any of the surface treatment methods:
   - Administer local analgesia, as indicated clinically.
   - Clean the tooth or teeth to be repaired, together with the adjacent teeth using pumice.
   - Remove the defective part of the composite restoration and any adjacent lesions of secondary caries.
   - Ensure adequate moisture control (rubber dam isolation)
   - Pulp protection given, if indicated.
   - Bevel the margins of the preparation, as indicated clinically, and place a long (1.0 mm wide) deep bevel on the margin of the composite resin to be repaired. Appropriately prepared bevels increase the surface areas for bonding and facilitate a more esthetic clinical outcome.
   - Acid etching the composite resin substrate together with the adjacent tooth tissue preparation margins with 37% phosphoric acid for 15–30 seconds and wash thoroughly and dry the area using three-in-one syringe. Acid etching, in addition to producing a roughened area for bonding, provides a cleansing effect.
   - Sandblast the composite resin substrate and, exposed adjacent tooth tissue using the Co-Jet micro-blaster, according to manufacturer's instructions. After a brief (approximately 5 seconds) blasting of the silica particles, excess powder is dispersed.
   - The silica-coated composite substrate surface is silanized by the application of the silane (allowed to dry for one minute).
   - An adhesive bonding system should be applied to the acid-etched composite substrate and adjacent tooth tissues and preparation margins, according to manufacturer's instructions.
   - Composite resin restorative material, compatible with the adhesive bonding system, is applied using an incremental technique to repair the defect with adequate photopolymerization. The same type and brand of composite materials should be used as the composite substrate. Alternatively commercially available composite repair systems can be used.
   - Carefully contour and finish the repair composite with proper occlusal assessment of the restoration.

Repair of All Ceramic or Porcelain Fused to Metal Crowns with Composite Resin

Preparation of the Fracture Site

1. The fractured site needs to be enlarged by atleast 3–4 times the original size to increase the surface area. This increased surface area is critical for a more predictable and longer lasting repair.
2. Surface treatment of metal and porcelain substrate surfaces:
   a. Surface roughening of metal and porcelain
      i. Air abrasion unit using 50 µm aluminium oxide particles provide adequate roughening of both metal and porcelain surfaces. It is followed by cleaning with phosphoric acid etchant for ten seconds, rinsed off and dried from the surface. The phosphoric acid does not etch the porcelain surface, but leave residual hydrogen ions that enhance silane porcelain primer bonding.
      ii. Surface roughening using Co-Jet Sandblasting surface treatment.
   b. Porcelain surface can be acid etched.
      i. Using Hydroflouric acid
         - 6–10% concentration
         - Gel form for controlled placement
         - 30 seconds to ten minutes etching time depending upon type of porcelain
         - Very caustic
         - Injurious to oral tissue, soft tissue must be protected and isolated with either dental dam or light cured resin based paste.
      ii. Using Acidulated phosphate fluoride
         - 1.23% concentration
         - 5–15 minutes etching time
         - Safe to oral tissues
   c. Using Diamond burs – copious water spray is to be used always with diamond abrasives to cool the diamond.
   d. Chemical metal bonding: The air abraded or surface roughened metal is then covered with an opaque metal adhesive bonding agent that facilitates metal bonding to composites, e.g. Gold Link or 4-meta containing metal adhesive agents, followed by application of a resin opaque.
   e. Chemical porcelain bonding: A silane primer is applied to all exposed treated porcelain surface

for 30 seconds to one minute and dried from the surface.

3. Apply the adhesive system to the treated metal-porcelain surface followed by incremental placement of composite resin with subsequent photopolymerization.
4. Contour and finish the restored fractured segment.

Repair of Composite Laminates with Composite Resin

The repair procedures remain essentially the same as direct composite restoration repair. Additionally mechanical locks may be placed in remaining composite material with small round bur.

BIBLIOGRAPHY

1. Alessandro, D.L., Reis, A. and Ballester, R.Y.: Polymerization shrinkage: effects of constraint and filling technique in composite restorations. Dent. Mater.: 20, 236, 2004.
2. Althoff, O. and Hartung, M.: Advances in light curing. Am. J. Dent. 13, 77, 2000.
3. Anjum, A., Matin, K., Uchida, R. and Tagami, J.: Influence of aging on direct resin composite repair bond. Int. Chin. J. Dent.: 8, 35, 2008.
4. Avcangelo, C., Vanini, L.: Effect of three surface treatments on the adhesive properties of indirect composite restoration. J. Adhes. Dent.: 9, 319, 2007.
5. Baratieri, L.N., Monteiro, S. Jr., Correa, M. and Ritter, A.V.: Posterior resin composite restorations: A new technique. Quint. Int.: 27, 733, 1996.
6. Baratieri, L.N. and Ritter, A.V.: To bevel or not in anterior composites. J. Esthet. and Restorat. Dent.: 17, 264, 2005.
7. Blank, T.J., Latta, M.: Composite resin layering and placement techniques: Lase Presentation and Scientific Evaluation. Pract. Proced. Aesthet. Dent.: 17, 2005.
8. Boulden, J.E., Cramer, N.B., Schreck, K.M., Couch, C.LO., Troconis, C., Stansbury, J.W. and Bowman, C.N.: Triolane – methacrylate composites as dental restorative materials. Dent. Material: 27, 267, 2011.
9. Browning, W.D. and Dennison, J.B.: A survey of failure modes in composite resin restorations. Oper. Dent.: 21, 160, 1996.
10. Bruke, F.J.T. and Qualtrough, A.J.E.: Aesthetic inlays: Composite or ceramic ? B.D.J.: 176, 53, 1994.
11. Bryant, R.W.: Direct posterior composite resin restorations: A review. Part I and II. Factors influencing case selection. Aust. Dent. J.: 37, 81 and 161, 1992.
12. Burgess, J.O., Walker, R. and Davidson, J.M.: Posterior resin based composites. Review of the literature. Pediatric Dent.: 2, 465, 2002.
13. Burke, F.J.T. and Shortall, A.: Posterior Composites: A practical guide revisited. Dent Update: 4, 211, 2012.
14. Can Say, E., Kayahan, B., Ozel, E., Gokce, K., Soyman, M. and Bayirti, G.: Chemical evaluation of posterior composite restorations in endodontically treated teeth. J. Contemp. Dent. Pract.: 7, 17, 2006.
15. Cardoso, P.C., deOliviera, A.R., Lopes, L.V., Cabral, S.C. and Beatriz, M.: In vivo evaluation of different techniques for establishment of proximal contacts in posterior resin composite restorations. Braz. J. Oral Sci.: 10, 12, 2011.
16. Carvalho, R.M., Garcia, F.C.P., Silve, S.M.A. and Castro F.L.A.: Adhesive- composite incompatibility, part 1. J Esthet Restor Dent.: 17, 12, 2005.
17. Carvalho, R.M., Garcia, F.C.P., Silve, S.M.A. and Castro F.L.A.: Adhesive- composite incompatibility, part 2. J Esthet Restor Dent.: 17, 3, 2005.
18. Carvalho, R.M., Garcia, F.C.P., eSilva, S.M.A. and Castro, F.L.A.: Adhesive-composite incompatibility: Part I, II. J. Esthet. Restorat. Dent.: 17, 129 and 191, 2005.
19. Carvalho, R.M., Pereira, J.C., Yoshiyama, M. and Pashley, D.H.: A review of polymerization contraction: the influence of stress development versus stress relief. Oper. Dent.: 21, 17, 1996.
20. Charlton, D.G.: Effect of humidity on the volumetric polymerization shrinkage of resin restorative materials. Gen. Dent.: 54, 113, 2006.
21. Chen, M.H.: Update on dental nano-composites. J. Dent. Res.: 89, 549, 2010.
22. Correa, M.B., Peres K.G., Horta, B.L., Barros A.D. and Demarco F.F.: Amalgam or composite resin? Factors influencing the choice of restorative material. J Dent.: 40, 703, 2012.
23. Cramer, N.B., Stansbury, J.W. and Bowman, C.N.: Recent advances and developments in composite dental restorative materials. J. Dent. Res.: 90, 402, 2011.
24. Devoto, W., Saracinelli, M. and Manants, J.: Composite in everyday practice: How to choose the right materials and simply application techniques in anterior teeth. European J. Esthetic Dent.: 5, 102, 2010.
25. Doukoudakis, S.: Establishing approximal contacts in Class-II composite resin restorations. Oper. Dent.: 21, 182, 1996.
26. Efes, B.G., Dorter, C., Gomec, Y. and Koray, F.: Two year clinical evaluation of Ormocer and nanofill composite with and without a flowable liner. J. Adhes. Dent.: 8, 119, 2006.
27. Fan, C., Chu, L., Rawls, H.R., Worling, B.K., Cardeon, H.L. and Whang, K.:: Development of an antimicrobial resin – a pilot study. Dent. Material: 27, 322, 2011.
28. Felippe, L.A., Monteiro, S. Jr., De Andrada, C.A. and Rittu, A.V.: Clinical strategies for success in proximo-incisal composite restorations. Part II: composite application technique. J. Esthet. Rest. Dent.: 17, 11, 2005.
29. Ferracan J.L.: Resin-based composite performance: Are there some things we can't predict? Dent Mater: 29, 51, 2013.
30. Ferracane, J.L.: Resin composite – state of the art. Dent. Material: 27, 29, 2011.
31. Fusayama, T.: Posterior adhesive composite resins: a historic review. J.P.D.: 64, 534, 1990.
32. Garoushi, S.K., Lasilla, L.V.J. and Vallittu, P.K.: Fiber reinforced composite in clinical dentistry. Chinese Jr. Dent. Res.: 12, 7, 2009.
33. Goldberg, M.: In vitro and in vivo studies on the toxicity of dental resin components: a review. Clin. Oral Invest.: 12, 1, 2008.

34. Harrero, A.A. and Dannison, J.B.: Polymerization shrinkage and depth of cure of packable composites. Quint. Int.: 36, 25, 2005.
35. Hickel, R., Brüshaver, K. and Illie N.: Repair of restorations – Criteria for decision making and clinical recommendations. Dent Mater: 29 ,28, 2013.
36. Ho, E. and Marcolongo, M.: The role of interfacial mechanics in the prediction of global mechanical behaviour of a bioactive composite: an in-vitro study. J. Oral Implantol.: 32, 63, 2006.
37. Ilia, N. and Hickel, R.: Investigations on mechanical behaviour of dental composites. Clin. Oral Invest.: 13, 427, 2009.
38. Imazato, S.: Antibacterial properties of resin composites as filled adhesives. Dent. Mater: 18, 227, 2002.
39. Imazato.S., Tarumi, H., Kato, S and Ebisu, S: Water sorption and color stability of composites containing antibacterial monomer MDBP. J.Dent., 27 279, 1999.
40. Jagger, D.C. and Wilson, N.H.F.: Defective dental restorations: to repair or not to repair ? Part I: Direct Composite Restorations. Dent. Update: 38, 78, 2011.
41. James, A., Mackenzie, L. and Sanch, P.: The current status of materials for posterior composite restoration: the advent of low shrink. Dent. Update: 36, 401, 2009.
42. Kawai, K., Tantbirojn, D., Kamalawat, A.S., Hasegawa, T. and Retief, D.H.: In vitro enamel and cementum fluoride uptake from three fluoride - containing composites. Caries. Res.: 32, 463, 1998.
43. Kirtley, G.E.: Metal-composite copings in the aesthetic restoration of the severely compromised patient. Pract. Proced. Aesthet. Dent.: 18, 105, 2006.
44. Kuijs, R.H., Fennis, W.M.M., Kreulen, C.M., Barink, M. and Verdonschot, N.: Does layering minimize shrinkage stresses in composite restorations? J.D.R.: 82, 967, 2003.
45. Kuijs, R.H., Fennis, W.M.M., Kruelen, C.M., Roeters, F.J.M. and Burgersdijk, N.H.J.: Fracture strength of cusp replacing resin composite restorations. Am. J. Dent.: 16, 13, 2003.
46. Kuijs, R.H., Fennis, W.W.M., Kreulen, C.M., Roeters, F.J.M., Verdonschot, N. and Creugers, N.H.J.: A comparison of fatigue resistance of three materials for cusp-replacing adhesive restorations. J. Dent.: 34, 19, 2006.
47. Landuyt, K.L.V., Yoshiara, K., Geebelen, B., Peumans, M., Godderis, L., Hoet, P. and Meerbeek, B.V. Should we be concerned about composite nano-dust? Dent Mater.: 28, 1162, 2012.
48. Lee, Y.K., Lu, H. and Powers, J.M.: Measurement of opalescence of resin composites. Dent. Mater.: 21, 1068, 2005.
49. Lien, W. and Vandewalle, K.S.: Physical properties of a new silorane-based restorative system. Dent. Material: 36, 337, 2010.
50. Liebenberg, W.H.: The axial bevel technique: A new technique for extensive posterior resin composite restorations. Quint. Int.: 31, 231, 2000.
51. Loguercio, A.D., Alessandra, R. and Battester, R.Y.: Polymerization shrinkage: Effect of constraint and filling technique in composite restoration. Dent. Mater: 20, 236, 2004.
52. Loguercio, A.D., Reis, A. and Ballester, R.Y.: Polymerization shrinkage: effect of constraint and filling technique in composite restorations. Dent. Mater.: 20, 236, 2004.
53. Loomans, B.A.C., Opdam, N.J.M., Roeters, F.J.M., Bronkhorst, E.M. and Burgersdijk, R.C.W.: A randomized clinical trial of proximal contacts of posterior composites. J. Dent.: 34, 292, 2006.
54. Loomans, B.A., Opdam, N.J., Roeters, F.J., Bronkhorst, E.M. and Plasschaert, A.J.: The long-term effect of a composite resin restoration on proximal contact tightness. J. Dent.: 35, 104, 2007.
55. Lopes, G.C., Vieira, L.C.C. and Araujo, E.: Direct posterior composite resin restorations: a review of some clinical procedures to achieve predictable results in posterior teeth. J. Esthet Restorat Dent.: 16, 19, 2004.
56. Lung, C.Y.K. and Matinlinna, J.K.: Aspects of silane coupling agents and surface conditioning in dentistry: an overview. Dent Mater.: 28, 467, 2012.
57. Mehl, A., Hickel, R. and Kunzelmann, K.H.; Physical properties and gap formation of light cured composites with and without 'Soft start polymerization'. J. Dent.: 25, 321, 1997.
58. Morces, R.R., Garcia, J.W., Barros, M.D., Lewis, S.H., Pfeiler, C.S., Liu, J. and Stansbury, J.W.: Control of polymerization shrinkage and stress in nanogel-modified monomer and composite material. Dent. Material: 27, 509, 2011.
59. Motisuki, C., Santos-Pinto, L. and Giro, E.M.A.: Restoration of severely decayed primary incisors using indirect composite resin restoration technique. Int. J. Pediat. Dent.: 15, 282, 2005.
60. Musanje, L. and Darvell, B.W.: Polymerization of resin composite restorative materials exposure reciprocity. Dent. Mater.: 19, 531, 2003.
61. Nomoto, R., Mcabe, J.F., Niva, K. and Hirano, S.: Relative efficiency of radiation sources for photopolymerization. Odontology: 97, 109, 2009.
62. Oca, S.D., Papacchini, F., Radovic, I., Polimeni, A. and Ferrari, M.: Repair potential of a laboratory-processed nano-hybrid resin composite. J. Oral Sci.: 50, 403, 2008.
63. O'Hara, J.W., Reeves, G.W. and Quiroz, L.: Posterior composites: A review of current clinical concepts. Gen. Dent.: 36, 207, 1988.
64. Palin, M. W.: Advances in light- curing units: four generations of LED lights and clinical implications for optimizing their use: part 2. From present to future. Dent Update.: 1, 13, 2012.
65. Pallesen, U. and Qvist, V.: Composite resin fillings and inlays. An 11-year evaluation. Clinical Oral Investigations: 7, 71, 2003.
66. Peumans, M., Kanumilli, P., Munck, J.D., Landuyt, K.V. and Lambrechts, P.: Clinical effectiveness of contemporary adhesives: A systemic review of the current clinical trials. Dent. Mater.: 21, 864, 2005.
67. Peutzfeldt, A. and Asmussen, E.: Resin composite properties and energy density of light cure. J.D.R.: 84, 659, 2005.
68. Pires, J.A.F., Cvitko, E., Denehy, G.E. and Swift, E.J.: Effects of curing tip distance on light intensity and composite resin microhardness. Quint. Int.: 24, 517, 1993.
69. Pontes, A.P., Oshima, H.M.S., Pacheco, J.F.P., Martins, J.L. and Shinkari, R.S.: Sheer bond strength of direct

composite repairs in indirect composite systems. Dent. Mat.: 343, 2005.
70. Puy, M.C.L., Navarro, L.F., Lacer, V.J.F. and Ferrandez, A.: Composite resin inlays: A study of marginal adaptation. Quint. Int.: 24, 429, 1993.
71. Ram, D. and Fuks, A.B.: Clinical performance of resin bonded composite strip crowns in primary incisors: a retrospective study. Int. J. Pediat. Dent.: 16, 49, 2006.
72. Rees, J.S., Jagger, D.C., Williams, D.R. and Brown, G.: A reappraisal of the incremental packing technique for light cured composite resins. J. Oral Rehab.: 31, 81, 2004.
73. Roberts, H.W., Hermesch, C.B. and Charlton, D.G.: The use of resin composite pins to improve retention of class IV resin composite restorations. Oper. Dent.: 25, 270, 2000.
74. Rueggeberg, F.A.: State of the art: Dental photocuring – a review. Dent. Material: 27, 39, 2011.
75. Safty, S., Akhtar, R., Silikas, N. and Watts, D.C.: Nanomechanical properties of dental resin-composites. Dent Mater.: 28, 1292, 2012.
76. Sahafi, A. and Pentzfeldt, A.: Effect of pulse delay curing on invitro wall-to-wall contraction of composites in dentin cavity preparations. Am. J. Dent.: 14, 295, 2001.
77. Saleh, R., Gallab, O., Zaaaou, M. and Niazi, H.: The influence of different surface pretreatments on the shear bond strength of repaired composite. J. Am. Sci.: 7, 705, 2011.
78. Saunders, S.A.: Current practibility of nanotechnology in dentistry Part I: Focus on nanocomposite restoratives and biomimetics. Clinical, Cosmetic and Investigational Dentistry: 1, 47, 2009.
79. Shortall, A.C., Uctasli, S. and Marquis, P.M.: Fracture resistance of anterior, posterior and universal light activated composite restoratives. Oper. Dent.: 26, 87, 2001.
80. Tabatabaei, M.H., Alizade, Y. and Taalim, S.: Effect of various surface treatment on repair strength of composite resin. J. Dent. TUMS: 1, 5, 2004.
81. Thomsen, K.B. and Pentzfeldt, A.: Resin composites: strength of the bond to dentin versus mechanical properties. Clin. Oral Invest.: 11, 45, 2007.
82. Unterbrink, G.L., Liebenberg, W.H.: Flowable composites as 'filled adhesive' literature review and clinical recommendations. Quint. Int.: 30, 249, 1999.
83. Van Dijken, J.W.V.: Direct resin composite inlays/onlays: An 11-year follow up. J. Dent.: 28, 299, 2000.
84. Versluis, A., Tentbirojn, D. and Douglas, W.H.: Do dental composites always shrink towards the light? J.D.R.: 77, 435, 1998.
85. Versluis, A, Tenbirojn, D., Lee, M.S., Tu, L.S. and Delong, R.: Can hygroscopic expansion compensate polymerization shrinkage ? Part I. Deformation of restored teeth. Dent. Material: 27, 126, 2011.
86. Wassell, R.W., Walls, A.W.G. and McCabe, F.: Cavity convergence angles for direct composite inlays. J. Dent.: 20, 294, 1992.
87. Wassell, R.W., Walls, A.W.G. and McCabe, J.F.: Direct composite inlays vs. conventional composite restorations: 5 year follow up. J. Dent.: 28, 375, 2000.
88. Wataha, J.C., Lockwood, P.E., Lewis, J.B., Rueggerberg, F.A. and Messer, L.W.: Biological effects of the light from dental curing units. Dent. Mater: 20, 150, 2004.
89. Wilson, E.G., Mandradjieff, M. and Brindock, T.: Controversies in posterior composite resin restorations. D.C.N.A.: 34, 27, 1990.
90. Wilson, N.H.F.., Cowan, A.J., Unterbrink, G., Wilson, M.A. and Crisp, R.J.: A clinical evaluation of class II composites placed using a decoupling technique.: J.Adhesive Dent. 2, 319, 2000.
91. Xu, H.H.K., Eichmiller, F.C., Antonucci, J.M., Schumacher, L.K. and Ives, L.K.: Dental resin composites containing ceramic whiskers and procured glass-ionomer particles. Dent.Mater. 16, 356, 2000.
92. Yap, A.U.J., Chew, C.L., Teoh, S.H. and Ong, L.FKL: Influence of contact stress on OCA wear of composite restorartives. Oper. Dent.: 26, 134, 2001.
93. Yousef, K.M., Khoja, N.: Repair and replacement perception of dental restorations. JKAV Med. Sc.: 16, 75, 2009.

18

Glass-Ionomer Cement

Glass-ionomer cement was developed by *Wilson* and *Kent* in England in the year 1972. This material has been in general clinical use in dentistry in Europe since 1975 and was introduced in the U.S. as ASPA (Alumino Silicate Poly Acrylate) in 1977.

The glass-ionomer cement has been evolved as a hybrid from the Silicate cement and the polycarboxylate cement. The term glass-ionomer cement was coined by Wilson and Kent though the ISO terminology for the cement was Polyalkenoate Cement (Fig. 18.1). The glass-ionomer was introduced as a potential replacement for the silicate cement. Because of the extensive use of this cement as a dentin replacement material it has also been referred to as *'Man Made Dentin'* and *'Dentin Substitute'*. The greatest advantage of this new cement was its adhesion to enamel and dentin and the fluoride release for anticariogenic effect. And the most useful clinical applications of glass-ionomer cements have been in restoring erosion lesions, without cavity preparation and the restoring or sealing of pit and fissure defects. Though, glass-ionomer was originally aimed to be a restorative material, soon it was modified as luting cement also. The composition of the powder particle, particularly the type of glass, could be altered to achieve different characteristics. The early cement was slow setting and highly technique sensitive. But since its introduction it has undergone many changes. The inclusion of tartaric acid was the first change just after a year of the presentation of the material for dental use. Thereafter maleic acid, itaconic acid etc. were added to decrease the viscosity of the liquid polyacrylic acid. Today there are a variety of glass-ionomer cements each designed and developed for different applications in dentistry, such as restoration, luting, base-liner, core build-up, geriatric and pedodontic restoration, ART (Atraumatic Restorative Treatment), cementation of orthodontic bands and brackets etc.

COMPOSITION

The glass-ionomer powder basically contains silica, alumina and fluorides of Calcium, Sodium and Aluminium. Fluorides are fundamentally used as flux. From the set cement, fluorides are leached out that provide anti-cariogenicity to the tooth. Hence it is added to get the best benefit from it. The mixture is fused at high temperature of about 1,100 to 1,500 degrees centigrade and the molten mass is then shock cooled. This mass is then finely powdered to required sizes. Particle size depends upon its use. Restorative cements have a particle size of about 50 μm and for luting it is about 20 μm.

Traditional Glass-Ionomer

Powder

Constituents	% by weight
Silica [SiO_2]	35–50
Alumina [Al_2O_3]	20–30
Aluminium Fluoride [AlF_3]	1.5–2.5
Calcium Fluoride [CaF_2]	15–20

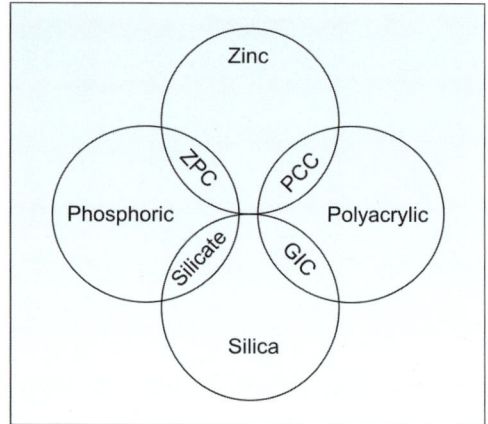

Fig. 18.1: Evolution of glass-ionomer cement. (ZPC - Zinc Phosphate Cement, PCC - Polycarboxylate Cement, GIC - Glass-Ionomer Cement.)

Sodium Fluoride [NaF]	3.0–6.0
Aluminium Phosphate [$AlPO_4$]	4.0–12
Lanthanum, Strontium, Barium (for Radio opacity.) [Fluorides act as Ceramic Flux]	in traces

The powder of traditional glass-ionomer cement is a calcium-fluoro-alumino-silicate glass (SiO_2-Al_2O_3-CaF_2-Na_3AlF_6-$AlPO_4$). This powder is referred to as an *ion leachable glass*.

Modifications in Powder

Traditional glass-ionomer powder has been undergoing modifications ever since its introduction and the various benefits of the cement came to be understood. The modifications were to improve upon the existing property in the manipulation and the area of clinical use.

Some of the modifications of the powder are:
- Dried Poly Acrylic Acid (anhydrous GIC).
- Silver-Tin alloy (Miracle Mix).
- Silver-Palladium/Titanium (Cermet cement).
- BiSGMA, TEGDMA and HEMA (Light/Dual cure GIC).

Liquid

• Polyacrylic acid	45%
• Itaconic acid	
• Maleic acid	5% (Decreases viscosity)
• Tricarballylic acid	
• Tartaric acid	Traces (Increases working time & decreases setting time)
• Water	50% (Hydrates reaction product)

Polyacrylic acid co-polymer provided by the different manufacturers vary within a wide range of composition of the components. The liquid is usually a 45% solution of co-polymer of polyacrylic acid and rest are modifiers and water. The modifiers constitute one or more of the following acids: Itaconic acid, Tartaric acid, Maleic acid, Tri carballylic acid. The ratio of polyacrylic acid to modifiers is about 2:1. The average molecular weight of the copolymer is 10,000.

The itaconic acid co-polymer reduces the viscosity of the liquid. It also inhibits the gelation caused by the intermolecular hydrogen bonding. As a result it increases the shelf life of the liquid. The 5% optically active dextro isomer of tartaric acid is incorporated for ideal manipulative property. It is also a hardener that controls the pH of the cement during setting process, which in turn controls the rate of dissolution of the glass. It facilitates extraction of ions from the glass. It typically increases the working time and also aids in a snap set (Fig. 18.2).

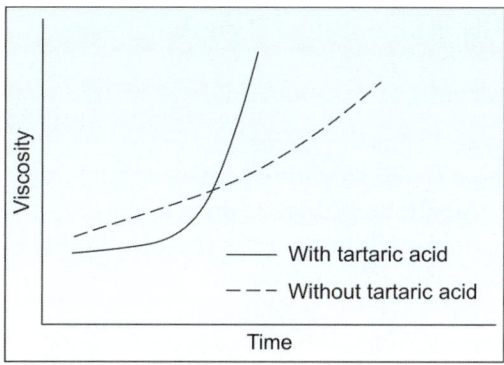

Fig. 18.2: Effect of tartaric acid on the viscosity of the glass-ionomer cement.

Modifications in Liquid

- Only water and Tartaric acid [anhydrous cement].
- HEMA [Light cure components].

DISPENSING

Glass-ionomer cements were supplied by manufacturers as a bulk of powder and liquid for hand mix version. They were also supplied in multiple bottles of three or more shades. The cement is supplied in convenient pre-proportioned capsules form for mixing in mechanical mixers. These come with nozzles for dispensing directly into the cavity from a gun. Anhydrous glass-ionomer cements are supplied as powder that may be mixed with water. The powder is modified by the addition of freeze-dried liquid in it. There appears to be no advantage in this over the traditional cement dispensed as powder and acid independently. In fact the shelf life of the anhydrous cement appears to be shorter during clinical use. Moreover the dispensing of correct quantity of water is difficult and the different quality of water used has a negative effect on the properties of the cement. Compomers that are polyacid modified resins are supplied as single pastes in bulk as tubes or compules (cavifils) for single use. The cavifils also are shaped to dispense directly into the cavity using a dispensing gun. They are also dispensed in clicker dispensers for quantum dispensing.

CLASSIFICATION

A. According to Wilson and McLean

1. Type I - Luting Cements.
2. Type II - Restorative cements.
   - Restorative aesthetic.
   - Restorative reinforced.

B. According to McLean

1. Glass-Ionomer Cements [Traditional]
2. Resin modified glass-ionomer cements.
3. Poly acid modified Composite resins.

C. According to Application

1. Type I - Luting Cements.
2. Type II - Restorative cements.
    - Aesthetic filling materials.
    - Reinforced materials (Fuji IX, Fuji II LC).
3. Type III - Lining Cement.
4. Type IV - Fissure sealant.
5. Type V - Orthodontic cement.
6. Type VI - Core build up cement.

D. According to Chararcteristics Specified by the Manufacturer

1. Type I - Luting Cement. e.g. Fuji I, Ketac Cement.
2. Type II - Restorative material. e.g. Ketac Fil, Fuji II, Fuji IX etc.
3. Type III
    a. Bases & Liners - Weak with low acidity. e.g. GC Lining Cement, Shofu Liner.
    b. Bases & Liners - Stronger but more acidic. e.g. Ketac Bond, Shofu base, GC Dentin cement.
    c. Bases & Liners - Strong even in thin layer - Light cure e.g. Vitrebond.
4. Type IV - admixtures. e.g. ketac silver, miracle mix.

E. Newer Classification

1. Traditional glass-ionomer
    - Type I - Luting Cement.
    - Type II - Restorative Cements.
    - Type III - Liners & Bases.
2. Metal Modified glass-ionomer
    - Miracle Mix
    - Cermet Cement.
3. Light Cure glass-ionomer
   HEMA added to liquid.
4. Hybrid glass-ionomer/Resin modified glass-ionomer
    - Composite resin in which fillers are substituted with glass-ionomer particles.
    - Pre-cured glasses blended into composites.

SETTING REACTION

1. Acid – Base Reaction
2. Light activated Polymerization.

1. Acid-base Reaction

The glass-ionomer cement is formed by the reaction of three materials. A fluoro alumino silicate glass powder, an ionic polymer of poly acrylic acid and water. An acid base reaction occurs between the glass powder and the ionic polymer. Water is essential because that is the medium through which ion transfer take place. While mixing the powder and liquid the acid slowly degrades the outer layer of glass particles, calcium ions and aluminium ions. During the early stages of setting, divalent calcium ions are released more rapidly and are primarily responsible for reacting with the poly acid, cross-linking with the adjacent carboxyl ions on polymer chain to form a reaction product, that is, calcium polysalts. The initial set is due to this reaction. At this stage it has a critical relationship with water. Hence the cement needs to be protected from coming in contact with extraneous moisture as well as drying. If the cement comes in contact with moisture, then the aluminium ions that are slowly leached out may get washed out of the cement before it combines with the cement network. This will result in a weak cement as well as a more soluble cement which will get more rapidly eroded by the oral fluids. If the cement is dried, then the water, which is essential for ion transfer to take place, will prevent further progression of the reaction to completion. In this case also the material is weak and crumbles easily. It also appears dull and white and exhibits poor esthetics. Trivalent Aluminium ions are released more slowly and become involved in setting at a later stage often referred to as *secondary reaction stage*. The aluminium ions also replace divalent calcium ions and form tighter network of crosslink between polymer chains. The set material consists of unreacted glass cores embedded in a matrix of cross linked polyacid (Fig. 18.3). The second stage of setting reaction hence involves the incorporation of significant quantities of aluminium in the matrix structure resulting in a marked maturation of the physical properties of the material. This stage requires about 24 hours and occurs when a polysalt matrix completely surrounds all of the initial reaction products. Although it may appear to be hard and set after the first 5 minutes it truly takes at least one full day (24 hours) before the material is set to a stable form. It is the

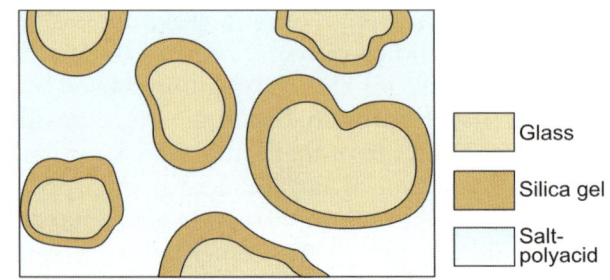

Fig. 18.3: Diagrammatic representation of final set cement

aluminium ions that provide the strength to the set cement. For a complete reaction to take place, it may take as long as seven days (Fig. 18.4). Once the replacement reaction is complete the solubility of the cement in water also decreases. Silica ions react with the available water and form covalent silica network around the glass particles. The fluoride in the cement exists in a dynamic relationship with the oral environment. There is a continuous leach of fluoride throughout the lifetime of the cement. The initial release is high followed by a gradual decrease to reach a constant level. But whenever there is an increase in the fluoride level in the environment the cement imbibes the lost fluoride and stores it like a reservoir to release gradually over a period of time.

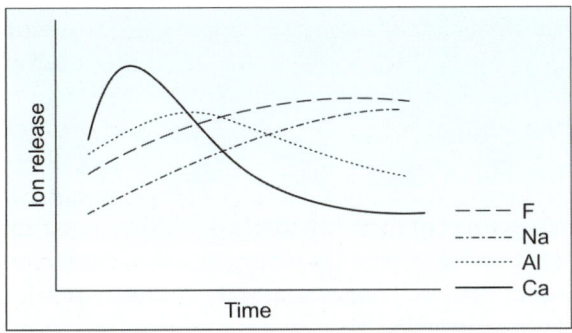

Fig. 18.4: The effect of time during setting on the release of different ions

The above reaction is also described in three overlapping stages such as dissolution, gelation and hardening.

2. Setting Reaction by Light Polymerization

The setting reaction in light cure glass-ionomers is basically a two stage process. Since the powder component of light cure glass-ionomer cements consist of initiators for light curing and the liquid component is modified with hydroxy ethyl methacrylate (HEMA), these ingredients are responsible for polymerization by light. The initial reaction lead to the polymerization of methacrylate groups and subsequently followed by the acid-base reactions of the glass component of powder and polyacrylic acid of the liquid. This is also known as dual cure cement.

Tri Cure Cement

In addition to the light curing mechanism and the acid/base reaction, some of the resin modified glass-ionomer cements harden by a chemical "dark cure" catalyzed by a reduction/oxidation reaction. The dark cure is perhaps important in deeper restorations in which light beam penetration may not be sufficient for completion of the light-hardening phase and chemical reaction is also insufficient. These materials are termed "tricure" as these resin modified glass-ionomer cements set by three phenomena.

1. Acid base reaction between the components of conventional glass-ionomer cement.
2. Light cure reaction stimulated by light application.
3. Autocure reaction, which is a reduction oxidation (Red-Ox) reaction that takes place between the initiator-catalyst system of resin that gets activated when the powder and liquid components are mixed together. The exact mechanism of action is not well described but this reaction ensures that over time there will be a complete cure throughout the entire restoration with no free resin remaining.

PHYSICAL AND MECHANICAL PROPERTIES

Powder is finely ground to a particle size of 15 µm or less. The working time of traditional cements is 2–3 minutes. The water settable systems tend to have somewhat longer working time. It is less stiff and more vulnerable to elastic deformation. Solubility in water during the first 24 hours is high. Glass-ionomer has a co-efficient of thermal expansion close to that of dentin. It also inhibits bacterial growth. This may be due to fluoride release by the cement, which is a metabolic poison for the micro-organisms. The glass-ionomer cement is only a mild irritant to pulp tissue especially when placed over dentin. The biocompatibility of the cement is due to the large molecular size of the cement, which does not travel through the narrower dentinal tubules. The initial pH of the mixed cement is close to 2 but soon reaches a value between 6 and 7. However glass-ionomer should not be placed over a direct exposure of the pulp. In cases where the remaining dentin is less than 0.5 mm, it is prudent to protect the dentin and pulp with calcium hydroxide.

Physical and mechanical properties are given in Table 18.1.

OTHER PROPERTIES

1. Sensitivity to Moisture

Glass-Ionomer cements are very sensitive to moisture, especially during initial setting phase. Both sorption of water and over drying are deleterious to the mechanical properties of the set cement. Absorption of water lead to weak cement and the over drying will lead to cracks in the cement. Therefore, protection of the cement during and after placement is mandatory.

Table 18.1: Physical and mechanical properties of glass-ionomer cement

	Traditional GIC	Glass cermet	Light cure GIC	Compomer
Compressive strength	16000–22000 psi	27500 psi	23200 psi	29000 psi
Tensile strength	900–960 psi	950–1000 psi	2000–3000 psi	2000–3000 psi
Modulus of elasticity	2900000 psi	–	906175 psi	1217900 psi
Coefficient of Thermal expansion/°C	10–11×10^{-6}	15×10^{-6}	18×10^{-6}	18×10^{-6}
Solubility	0.3–0.5%	0.1%	0.08%	0.08%
Opacity	90%	95%	85%	80%
Hardness (KHN)	48	39	40	38
Film Thickness (µm)	22–25	–	30–40	30–40

2. Post-operative Sensitivity

Post-operative sensitivity is usually associated with poor manipulation and/or poor powder/liquid ratio. This is also related with moisture contamination during setting of the cement leading to hydraulic effect on dentinal fluid. However, the menace of post-operative sensitivity is less affected with light cure glass-ionomers and compomers.

3. Adhesion

Ion-exchange adhesion with tooth structure: One of the most important characteristics of glass-ionomer cement is their ability to adhere chemically to mineralized tooth tissues. This requires the tooth surface to be cleaned of debris and smear layer and proper conditioning prior to placement of a glass-ionomer material. On placement of the mixed cement there will be an immediate ion exchange between the cement and the mineralized tissues. The probable mechanism of adhesion is said to be based upon both diffusion and adsorption phenomena. The polyalkenoic acid of the glass-ionomer will penetrate the tooth structure, releasing phosphate ions, each of which will take with it a calcium ion from the tooth surface to maintain electric neutrality. These ions will combine with the surface layer of cement and from an intermediate layer of new material which is firmly attached to the tooth surface. This has been described as a 'diffusion based adhesion'. There is also a degree of adhesion available to the collagen of dentin through either hydrogen bonding or metallic ion bridging between the carboxyl groups on the polyacid and the collagen molecules. This means the dentin does not have to be fully mineralized to achieve a chemical union with a glass-ionomer.

Advantages
- Adhesive aesthetic restorative
- Liberates fluoride: anti-cariogenic
- Biocompatible
- Low oral solubility

Disadvantages
- White and crazed surface
- Clinically poor aesthetics
- Opaque
- Debonds readily
- Highly technique sensitive
- Poor strength

4. Fluoride in Glass-Ionomer Cement

Incorporation of fluoride in glass-ionomer is useful in all stages. It acts as a flux during the sintering of the powder particle. The cement may contain up to 28% of fluoride. Fluoride also helps prolong the working time of the cement. Fluoride release in glass-ionomer can continue for years after the cement hardens. There is an initial rise in fluoride release from the cement for about a week and then gradually decreases within few months and levels off to a low release for years. The most advantageous phenomenon of the cement is that it can also take up fluoride from the environment and replenish itself functioning like a reservoir of fluoride in the mouth. It has been observed that two restored surfaces may release about 0.4 ppm fluoride in saliva over a period of 10 weeks.

Fluoride releasing esthetic materials that also provide microbial inhibition have attracted considerable attention. Some restorative techniques using GIC employ an incomplete removal of the carious tissues and consequently enhance the risk of secondary caries. Various additives with the ability to enhance the antimicrobial effect of these materials without counteracting their physical and fluoride releasing properties have been tried. The addition of zinc sulphate to glass-ionomer has shown significant inhibition of Streptococcus mutans growth and also increased fluoride release.

Anti-cariogenicity

Fluorides reduce the metabolic activity of the cariogenic micro flora resident in the oral cavity and grown in the dental plaque. This reduces the number of micro-organisms in the adherent plaque. It converts the typical calcium hydroxyapatite crystals of the dental tissues to acid resistant calcium fluorapatite crystals that resist acid attack from caries producing micro organisms.

There have been reports about the validity of anticariogenic property of glass-ionomer. There are increasing suspicions that the fluoride release has little or no real effect in reducing dental caries. A survey of general practitioners participating in continuing education at the University of Florida reported on types of restoration failures observed and the types of materials involved. Secondary caries was the leading reason for failure. Glass-ionomer restorations were replaced slightly more frequently than amalgams and almost twice as frequently as composites. Almost half of the glass-ionomer restorations were replaced for reasons of secondary caries. This calls into question the value of the fluoride being released.

5. Aesthetics

Various shades of glass-ionomer cements are manufactured by the addition of pigments, which are generally metal oxides, such as ferric oxide and carbon black. What lacks in the traditional glass-ionomer is the translucency to simulate natural enamel. It is inferior to composites and ceramics in this aspect of aesthetics. It is opaque and may become dull and lifeless in course of time. Esthetically, compomers are better than light cure glass-ionomer and traditional glass-ionomers. The relative percentage of opacity in traditional glass-ionomer cement is 90% whereas light cure glass-ionomer cement is 85% and compomer is 80%.

USES OF GLASS-IONOMER CEMENT

1. *Restoration of permanent teeth*
   - Class V & Class III cavities.
   - Abrasion/Erosion lesion.
   - Root Caries.
2. *Restoration of deciduous teeth*
   - Class I - Class VI cavities.
   - Rampant caries, nursing bottle caries.
3. *Luting or cementing*
   - Metal restorations viz. inlays, onlays, crowns.
   - Non-metal restorations viz. composite inlays and onlays
   - Veneers.
   - Pins and Posts.
   - Orthodontic bands and brackets.
4. *Preventive restorations*
   - Tunnel preparation.
   - Pit and fissure sealants
5. *Protective liner,* under composite and amalgam
6. *Bonding agent.*
7. *Dentin substitute.*
8. *Core build up.*
9. *Splinting* of periodontally weak teeth.
10. *Glazing* (Fuji Coat LC)
    - Glazing of traditional GIC filling.
    - Improving aesthetics of old GIC filling.
    - Protection of new GIC filling.
11. *Other restorative technique*
    - Sandwich technique/Layered restorations/Laminated restorations/Bilayered Restorations.
    - Atraumatic Restorative Treatment [Fuji VIII and Fuji IX].
    - Co-cure technique.
    - Bonded Restorations.
12. *Endodontics*
    - Repair of external root resorption.
    - Repair of perforation.
    - Retrograde filling.

MODIFIED GLASS IONOMER CEMENTS

Metal Modified Glass-Ionomers

i. Miracle Mix or Silver Cermet

Silver cermet was introduced by *Simmons* in the year 1983. Initially it was prepared by the incorporation of Silver-Tin alloy into the glass-ionomer cement powder. Glass is generally brittle and addition of silver was expected to improve the toughness of the cement by silver acting as a stress absorber. It was also expected to improve the abrasive resistance of the cement. But most properties of the cement including the compressive strength, flexural strength, solubility and abrasive resistance remained without improvement. In fact it gave a grey or blackish color to the cement that was aesthetically unacceptable (Fig. 18.5). It did not exhibit promising results, due to metal-carboxylate interface failure.

ii. Glass Cermet

Glass cermet was introduced by *McLean* and *Gasser* in the year 1985. Glass and metal powders were sintered at high temperature. This could be made to react with polyacrylic acids to form improved glass-ionomer cement. This was attempted to improve the wear resistance and flexural strength, at the same time maintaining the aesthetics. Sometimes other metals like Titanium oxide are added in smaller proportion (approximately 5%) as whitening agent. The suggested application of these cements was in small class-I cavities, in restoration of deciduous teeth and for core

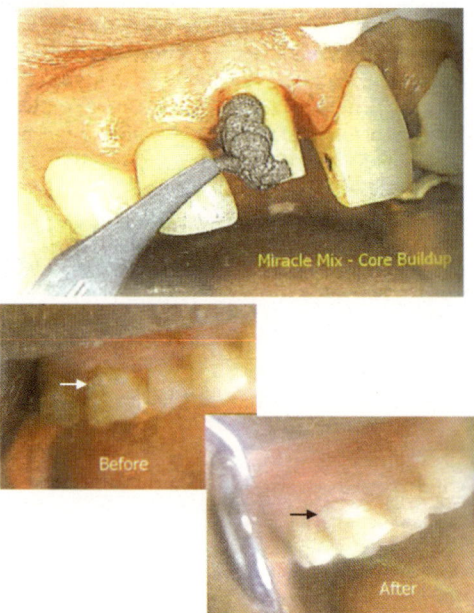

Fig. 18.5: Miracle mix (clinical use)

build-ups. This cement produced good radiopacity and was a cement of choice for application as cement base under composites.

Resin Modified Glass-Ionomer Cements

A dimethyl methacrylate monomer, hydroxyethyl methacrylate (HEMA) is grafted in the polyacrylic acid. The presence of unsaturated carbon-carbon bonds enables the covalent cross-linking of the matrix. With the exposure of light, polymerization is initiated along the methacrylate groups. After that the polyacrylic acid reacts with glass particles though acid base reaction. As these are water based, the main reaction is the acid base reaction. They maintain the ability to bond to hard tooth tissues via the carboxylic group of polyalkenoate component. The fluoride release is also optimum. Fuji II LC is one commercial preparation of resin modified glass-ionomer (Fig. 18.6).

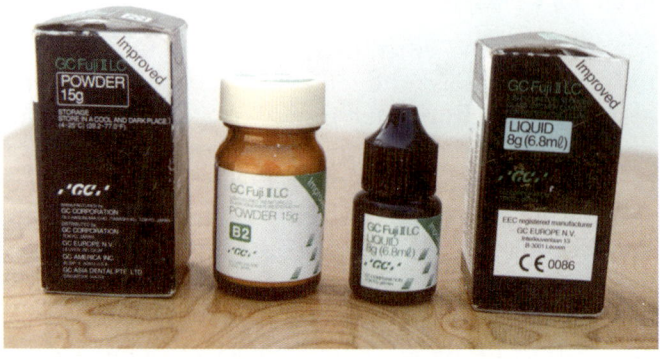

Fig. 18.6: Light cure glass-ionomer cement

These are widely used in class V, erosion/abrasion cavities and also in rampant caries. They are well tolerated by the pulp and can continually be finished and polished. Various studies have confirmed their suitability as restorative material, as luting cement and also as base under different restorative materials.

Advantages
• Stronger
• Nearly insoluble
• Fluoride release
• Good radio opacity
• Easy manipulation
• Satisfactory wear resistance
• Better aesthetics
• Early resistance to water attack
• Bonding to tooth-chemical and micromechanical
• Bond strength - excellent
• Minimal or no post-operative sensitivity
• Condensable viscosity
• Light/dual cure setting
• Long working time and a snap command set by photoactivation
• Can be finished and polished immediately after set
• Repair of fractured restoration possible as the bond between old and new material is very strong
• Exhibits increased adhesion to composite when used as a base

Compomers (Polyacid Modified Composite Resins)

Compomers are the combination of composites ('comp') and glass-ionomers ('omer'). With the idea of improving upon the mechanical properties of glass-ionomer cements, various modifications were tried viz, addition of silver-tin-copper alloy particles and addition of silver particles in the filler component. Resin modified glass-ionomer cements were developed with the addition of dimeth-acrylate monomer in the matrix. The unsaturated carbon-carbon bond enables the crosslinking of the matrix via free radical polymerization reaction. Compomers contain dimethacrylate monomer and two carboxylic groups along with ion leachable glass. There is no water in the composition of these materials and the glass particles are partially silanated to ensure some bonding with the matrix. These materials set via free radical polymerization reaction and do not bond to hard tooth tissues. There is insignificant acid-base reaction between the glass particles not silanated and sparse carboxylic groups.

The physical and mechanical properties of compomers are inferior to hybrid composites (Table 18.1).

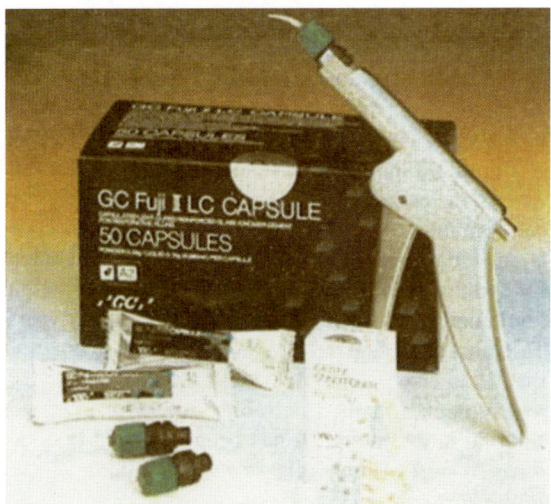

Fig. 18.7: GC Fuji II™ LC. Resin reinforced glass-ionomer cement

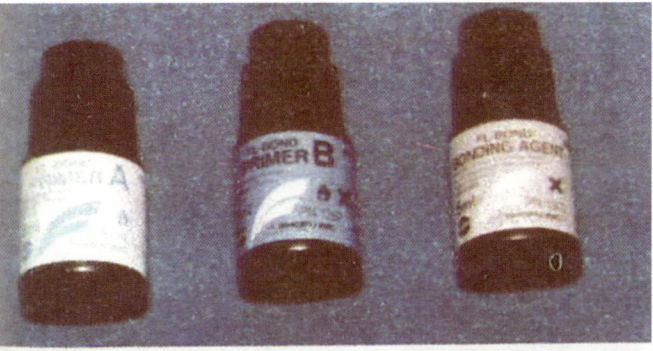
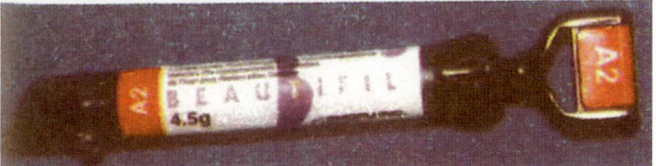

Fig. 18.8: Giomers

The bond strengths are however comparable to glass-ionomer cements and resin modified Glass-Ionomer cements. The roughness values are also comparable to glass-ionomers and composites.

These materials are well tried in class V restorations and are as successful as composites and glass-ionomers. These are also being used in class II restorations. The authors were of the view that the use of conditioner along with compomer improves the marginal adaptability as compared to composites. Alternatively, these can also be tried in bilayered technique giving base of compomer and finally restoring with composites.

Long term studies are required before compomers are recommended for routine clinical use.

Giomers

Conventional glass-ionomer cements, though accepted as a luting and restorative material, has some limitations, such as moisture sensitivity, low initial mechanical properties and inferior translucency. To overcome these limitations, resin modified GICs and polyacid modified composites (compomers) were developed. These two are better in certain clinical situations; however, even the modified versions could not overcome the total short-comings of GICs. Recently, a new category of hybrid aesthetic restorative material, which differs from both resin modified GICs and compomers has been introduced known as GIOMERS.

Giomers are available in the market as one paste form. They are light polymerizing and require bonding agents for adhesion to tooth structure. Currently available Giomers are: Reactmer (Shofu, Japan) and Beautifil (Shofu, Japan) (Fig. 18.8).

Chemical Nature

Giomers are hybrid restorative materials which employ the use of pre-reacted glass-ionomer (PRG) technology to form a stable phase of GIC, also known as PRG composites. The fluoroalumino silicate glass in these materials is reacted with polyalkanoic acid in water prior to inclusion into silica filled urethane resin. This technology differs from compomers, in which a variable amount of dehydrated polyalkenoic acid is incorporated into the resin matrix and the acid does not react with glass until water uptake occurs into the restoration. Giomers do contain glass-ionomer components, but cannot be classified as compomers as the acid base reaction has already occurred. Therefore the term PRG composite is suggested to describe giomers. Like compomers, giomers are light polymerized and require bonding system. Recently single application bonding system that combine the function of self-etching primer and bonding agent have been developed. Reactmer (Shofu-Japan) bond is a single application bonding agent. It is glass-ionomer based, all-in-one filled adhesive based on PRG technology consisting of 4 AET, 4 AETA, UDMA, HEMA, PRG filler, fluoro-alumino silicate glass, acetone, water and initiator. The adhesive in the one application bonding system is a hydrophilic solution that is extremely effective in wetting the tooth surface.

The etching effect of these systems relate to acidic monomers or organic acids that may interact with the mineral component of tooth substrate and enhance monomer penetration. The adhesive etches and penetrates the etched enamel and hardens on evaporation of the solvent and exposure to light. Giomer based adhesives create a thick hybrid layer as compared to other single step adhesives between the restorative and tooth substrate, though their bond strengths are lower than two step bonding system.

Indications

- Restoration of root caries
- Non-carious cervical lesions
- Class V cavities
- Caries in deciduous teeth

Advantages

- *Fluoride release:* The giomers release substantial amount of fluoride and are effective in prevention of secondary caries. It has been recently established that giomer adhesive is more permeable and this permeability of adhesive layer in bonded dentin affects the potential of caries inhibition by these materials.
- *Fluoride recharging:* The fluoride recharging effect on giomer significantly reduces the incidence of recurrent caries and also increases thickness of caries inhibition zone.
- *Biocompatibility:* It is established by various authors that giomers are biologically compatible with vital pulps.
- *Smooth surface finish and esthetics:* The giomers have better surface finish than conventional GIC and resin modified GICs. The surface finish is comparable to composites. That is why the giomers have better esthetics.
- *Excellent bonding:* The single step bonding agents provide excellent bonding and minimize tissue and manipulative intricacies. It is suggested that duration of single application of bonding was not crucial even though morphological changes such as demineralization of dentin with longer application duration is observed. The bond strength of single application bonding system were comparable to those of compomer but lower than those of the two step resin-composites bonding system.
- *Clinical Stability:* The giomers are clinically stable materials. It has been observed recently that giomers perform better than composites. The hardness of PRG composites was found to be significantly greater than polyacid modified composites and resin modified Glass-Ionomer cements.

Limitations

- Not of much benefit to patients who are at a risk for recurrent caries.
- Giomers exhibit rapid and extensive expansion and should be avoided in tooth preparation involving thin unsupported enamel.

Antibacterial GIC

Among all the dental restoratives, glass-ionomer cements are found to be the most cariostatic and somehow antibacterial due to release of fluoride. However, it has been found that the main reason for glass-ionomer cement failure is secondary caries indicating that fluoride release from GICs is not potent enough to inhibit bacterial growth. Numerous efforts have been made on improving antibacterial activities of dental restoratives, most of them have been focused on release or slow release of various incorporated low molecular weight antibacterial agents such as antibiotics, zinc ions, Ag ions, iodine and chlorhexidine. Recently a new antibacterial GIC has been formulated using 'Poly Quarternary Ammonium Salts (PQAS)' containing polyacid. QAS disrupts the surface membrane of bacteria by changing membrane permeability.

Theoretically, high positive charge density, substitute chain length and the surface exposure of QAS are directly proportional to the antibacterial activity of QAS e.g. the QAS with 16-carbon substitute shows higher antibacterial activity than the one with 2-carbon chain. But the drawback of such long chain lengths is a resultant decrease in compressive strength of GIC. To keep compressive strength values above 200 MPa and streptococcus mutans viability below 30%, GIC with 5% PAQs loading with 6-carbon substitute chain is considered to be the best formulation.

This experimental cement is a clinically attractive dental restorative due to its high mechanical strength and antibacterial function, although future research is required on the material.

Fluoride Recharge Material

This is a new development of a fluoride release material to overcome the shortcomings faced by fluoride releasing material.

- Greater the fluoride release in a material more open is the structure resulting in low strength.
- In order to improve the strength of these fluoride containing materials, if they are made more dense and strong then the efficacy of F release is decreased. Soon after placement there is sudden burst of fluoride release followed by a rapid decline in ion release rate.
- To overcome this, fluoride recharge material was developed.

This modified GIC is in 2 parts
1. Restorative part.
2. Charge part

The restorative part is used the usual way when the 1st burst of Fluoride is expelled the therapeutic potential of the restoration spent.

The material is given a second fluoride charge by using a gel material – charge part that replenishes the fluoride site in the restoration by ion exchange and recovers the fluoride release and therapeutic potential of the restoration. This is achieved without replacing the material.

Low PH Smart Materials

This material is based on that fact that fluoride release should be at a low pH, i.e. when caries attack may be more threatening. These are developed to release F at a low oral pH. Hence, they are known as "SMART MATERIALS". Fluoride is not released all the time, the episodic release prolongs usefulness of the material.

CLINICAL PLACEMENT OF GLASS-IONOMER

The clinical placement of glass-ionomer cement requires the following steps.
  I. Isolation.
  II. Tooth Preparation.
  III. Cement placement.
  IV. Finishing and Polishing.
  V. Surface Protection.

I. Isolation

Saliva control is an essential step in the restoration of glass-ionomer cement. The cement is very sensitive for water loss as well as contamination. Saliva, sulcular fluid and gingival haemorrhage, have to be controlled during the restoration procedure. Rubber Dam, retraction cords and cotton rolls with saliva ejectors are generally used and are rather mandatory in the restoration of lesions close to the gingival margins of the tooth. Details are given in Chapter 8.

II. Tooth Preparation

Tooth preparation for glass-ionomer restoration may be divided into
  A. Mechanical preparation.
  B. Chemical preparation (conditioning).

A. Mechanical Preparation

Glass-Ionomer cements are used extensively for restoration of Class V cavities and also for hidden Class III cavities. The class V cavities mostly presents in two types. A 'V' shaped notch with definite sharp boundaries or a 'Saucer' shaped lesion with merging boundaries. The latter one is usually restored with laminated Ionomer-Composite resin restoration. With the improvement of the mechanical and physical properties of the cement its use is extended to restoration of small Class I and Class II cavities in adults and in geriatric and paediatric practice. A high strength glass-ionomer cement, Atraumatic Restorative Treatment (ART) material is also manufactured for universal use in the under-developed parts of the world where regular dental treatment with mechanised tooth preparation is not possible.

The steps in cavity preparation and fundamentals laid for amalgam restorations hold good to an extent in the mechanical tooth preparation with glass-ionomer cements too, particularly in the restoration of carious defects. But the tooth preparation is not dictated by all the rules specified by G V Black for amalgam restorations. This is so because of the adhesive nature of the cement, the poor abrasive resistance, the beneficial anti-cariogenic and limited mechanical properties of the cement.

In class III the access is gained through the lingual marginal ridge using small sized inverted cone bur, the bur is extended towards incisal and gingival area depending upon the extent of caries. The labial enamel is preserved as far as possible (Figs 18.9A, B).

In class V cavities the lesion can be only in enamel or both in enamel and cementum. The cavity preparation follows the access opening through the lesion and extending towards the occlusal, gingival, mesial and distal walls. In case the extent of lesion is too wide, a groove on the occlusal/gingival wall can be given. Similar grooves on all the four sides can be given, if lesion so dictates (Figs 18.10A to D).

a. Outline Form

Mechanical preparation is concentrated basically in the removal of carious and defective tooth structure.

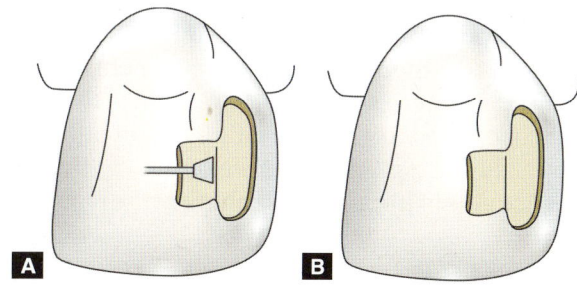

Figs 18.9A and B: Class III cavity. **(A)** Access through lingual marginal ridge **(B)** Preparation and cavity

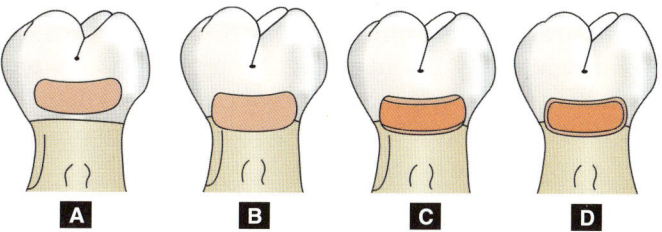

Figs 18.10A to D: (A) Cervical cavity only in enamel **(B)** Cervical cavity both in enamel and cementum **(C)** Grooves on the occlusal and gingival wall **(D)** Grooves on all the four walls

Hence the outline form is dictated primarily by caries, discoloration and aesthetics only.

In proximal lesions no attempt should be made to break the contact to bring the restoration to a self cleansing area. Whatever unaffected tooth material is available, should be left behind to keep as much contact as possible even if it is not well supported by the dentin. This may leave portions of tooth restorative interfaces within the contact areas and is acceptable, as the remaining tooth structure affords better wear resistance and strength than the glass-ionomer cement. Only point to be considered while leaving such thinned enamel is that it should not come under direct loading by an opposing tooth during mastication.

Ragged peripheries may leave an unsightly geographic outline if the interface of the tooth and restoration get stained. Hence it is prudent to prepare the tooth and leave the wall exposed facially along the axis of the tooth and in contour with the axial angle. This would mask the unsightly appearance that attracts attention and help blending with the geometric and textural pattern of the natural tooth.

The gingival extent of the tooth preparation is generally dictated by the extent of the lesion. It is often close to or extending into the sulcus. Care should be taken to manage the sulcular fluid during the placement of the restoration.

b. Retention and Resistance Form

The retention of glass-ionomer cement is essentially chemical in nature or by true adhesion to tooth structure. Any step to create undercuts and dovetails are unnecessary and considered unwarranted destruction of sound tooth material. It is definitely desirable to have a bulk of the material for the cement to be self supported and resistant to fracture. Hence the outline may be deepened to give at least 1.0 mm of bulk for the cement. This also gives a definite outline to the cavity and hence aids in improved finishing of the restoration.

c. Convenience Form

In class III cavities the lingual wall is broken for access in the maxillary teeth. Teeth may be mechanically separated for convenience of operation too. Smallest drills are used that will aid in the removal of decayed tooth material without over cutting of sound enamel and dentin. In the preparation of Class V cavities the lip and cheek retractors and tongue guards are useful for convenience of operation.

d. Prophylaxis and Debriding

Glass-Ionomer bonds to dentin and enamel. The bonding is enhanced if the surface is clean and conditioned. Prophylaxis is usually performed by pumice slurry carried in rubber cups, bristle brush or Burlew's brush. This will remove plaque and pellicle. Care is taken to see that the juxtaposing soft tissue is not injured which may present a difficult situation to control the bleeding and staining of the restoration. Haemorrhage from gingival tissue may be cauterized with a very light application of trichloro-acetic acid.

B. Chemical Preparation

After a thorough prophylaxis the surface is conditioned using chemical agents. Several conditioning agents have been tried and some of them are still in use. Citric acid 50%, phenolic acid, hydrogen peroxide 3%, Tannic acid 25%, Dodicin 0.9%, mineralizing solutions, EDTA 10% and polyacrylic acid 20% are some of the conditioning agents suggested for better bonding of the cement to the enamel and dentin. Of these, polyacrylic acid 10% to 20% is still the most commonly used and that which has been supplied and advised by the manufacturers for best adhesion. The acid is applied for about 10 to 20 seconds and then washed away.

Light activated glass-ionomers have an additional step of priming the tooth surface. The proprietary priming agent is applied in two or more coats as suggested by the manufacturers. It is then spread to a thin layer with gentle blast of air and light activated for 20 seconds.

III. Cement Placement

a. Mixing of the Cement

The best method of mixing and placing glass-ionomer cement is to use the capsulated cement that can be used with a syringe technique.

Hand mixing has to be done with great care. Correct ratio of powder to liquid is ensured and the mixing technique should be followed assiduously according to the manufacturer.

Mixing can be done on either a paper pad or a glass slab. The advantage of a glass slab is that it can be cooled a little to prolong the working time. Though for restorative cements the type of spatula used is not considered very important provided it is recognized that the cement should not be over spatulated, it is prudent to use an agate or plastic spatula. The primary objective of mixing the cement is to merely wet the surface of the powder particles with the liquid and not to aid in dissolving them entirely in the liquid. It should be noted that there is not enough liquid to dissolve all the powder particles in the powder/liquid ratio suggested for restorative cement. The core of every particle remains unreacted like filler particles in composite resin.

When dispensing the powder shake the bottle lightly first to fluff up the powder. See that the spoon is quite full of powder and level off the surface using the lip on the bottle, which is provided for the purpose.

The powder is dispensed first on to the slab and divided into two halves with the spatula. The liquid bottle is then tilted horizontal to allow the liquid to displace the air through the nozzle and occupy the nozzle. Now the bottle is oriented vertically and gently squeezed to dispense the required ratio of liquid at only one drop at a time, without the inclusion of an air bubble (Figs 18.11 A, B and C).

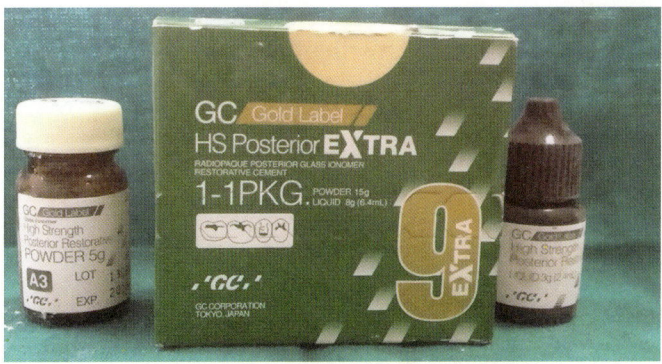

Fig. 18.11C: Correct power/liquid ratio

If the liquid has become more viscous over time it can be thinned down by immersing the bottle in water at 70 degrees centigrade for 15 minutes. Allow it to cool again before using the liquid.

With both the powder and the liquid dispensed on the pad, one half of the powder is mixed at a time by rolling the powder into the liquid to wet the surface of the powder particles. **Do not vigorously spatulate**. The first half of the powder should be all wet within 10 to 15 seconds. Roll the remaining powder into the mass. Do not spread the mix around the pad. The mixing is then completed in about 30 seconds.

b. Loss of Gloss or Slump Test

This test helps to recognize if cement is properly mixed. The mixed cement is placed in a glass slab. Lift the top of the pile of the cement with a spatula. The cement breaks and slumps back. There will be a point when the cement breaks but does not slump. Working time is normally 60–90 seconds for traditional glass-ionomer and about 3 minutes for resin modified glass-ionomer. Moisture sensitivity during the first hour is very critical, therefore the cement is coated with either varnish, cocoa butter, copal ether or unfilled resin.

c. Restoration

The technique for placement of an auto-cure or resin-modified glass-ionomer restoration is essentially the same. After mixing, both the chemical cure cement and the light cure cement are carried in one bulk for placement into the cavity. The gross excess is quickly removed and the filling contoured. The use of a matrix is always desirable because it will assist in positive placement of the cement on to the tooth surface and will also lead to a reduction of voids and porosities within the restoration.

A syringe dispenser like the Centrix syringe is an excellent and superior alternative. Syringing out the cement into the prepared cavity help to fill the cavity without entrapment of air bubbles in the cement and

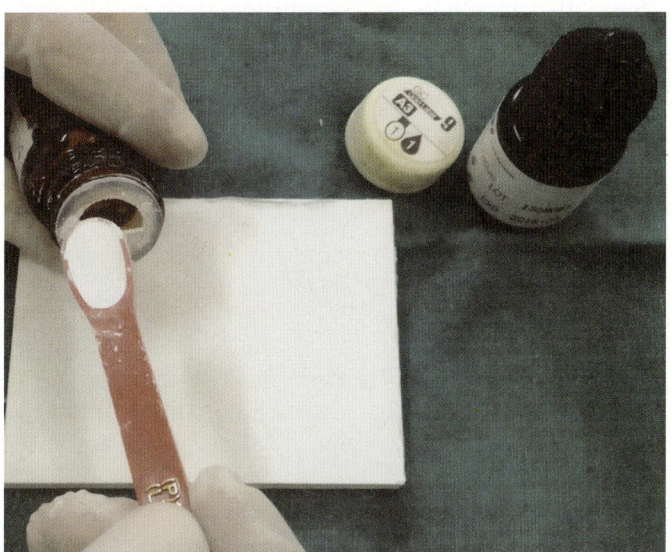

Fig. 18.11A: Dispensing of powder

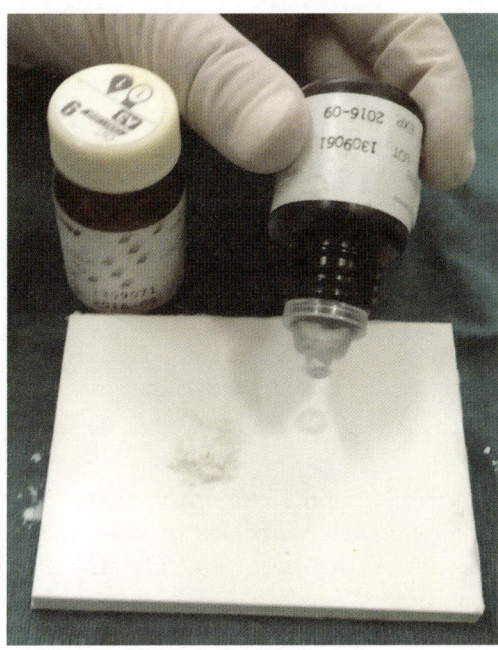

Fig. 18.11B: Dispensing of liquid

give absolute control of the quantity of the cement placed in the tooth. The tip of the syringe is placed to the floor of the cavity and the cement ejected into the cavity as the nozzle is withdrawn out. The chemical cure cement is held with matrix till it attains initial hardness and the light cure cement is photo-activated for rapid set. It is not possible to over cure by excessive light activation. So a restoration should be subjected to longer exposure than suggested to avoid deficient light activation due to the distance of the light from the restoration. Large restorations are exposed again for a total of 60 seconds. A fully light activated resin-modified glass-ionomer is resistant to water uptake after completion of light activation, but it is still possible to dehydrate the cement.

A material which is supplied in a compule or as single paste and does not require mixing, it cannot have an acid/base reaction and is therefore not a glass-ionomer. There will be no chemical adhesion to tooth structure with such a material and the fluoride release will be limited.

IV. Finishing and Polishing

The best finish is necessarily the matrix finish. Initial contouring may be done using sharp instruments like Bard parker blades, gold foil knives or diamond points in high speed. Final polishing is done after 24 hours. Many clinicians prefer to do even the initial contouring after 24 hours to avoid water from affecting the cement. The final finishing is done using 'Sof-lex' discs or discs with different gradation of abrasives from coarse to fine, in a series. Super fine diamond points, silicon abrasives embedded in rubber in various shapes and abrasive strips are available to finish the various areas of the restorations (Fig. 18.12). The finishing using abrasive has to be carried out in moist condition. Dry cutting will dehydrate the surface and give it a porous and mottled appearance and result in early disintegration of the cement. At the end of the initial contouring as well as final finishing of the surface the cement surface has to be protected with varnish, proprietary coats or resinous glaze material. Details are given in Chapter 22. The scanning electron microscopic picture of finished surface of conventional glass-ionomer is shown in Figs 18.13A and B, and C and light cure glass-ionomer is shown in Figs 18.14A, B and C.

V. Surface Protection

Resins such as enamel bonding agents afford the best surface protection to the cement. It fills the irregularities on the surface and gives a smooth finish for a longer period compared to varnish and petroleum jelly. Resins are also more impermeable compared to even varnish. Cocoa Butter and petrolatum are easily washed away in a short period while optimum period of protection is 24 hours.

The newly placed cement should be sealed immediately after removal of the matrix to prevent water exchange. If the seal remains for the first 24 hours

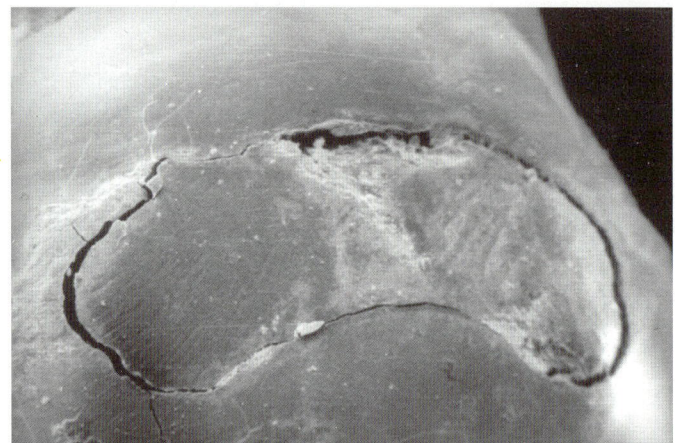

Fig. 18.13A: SEM photograph of finished conventional GIC (Magnification 25x)

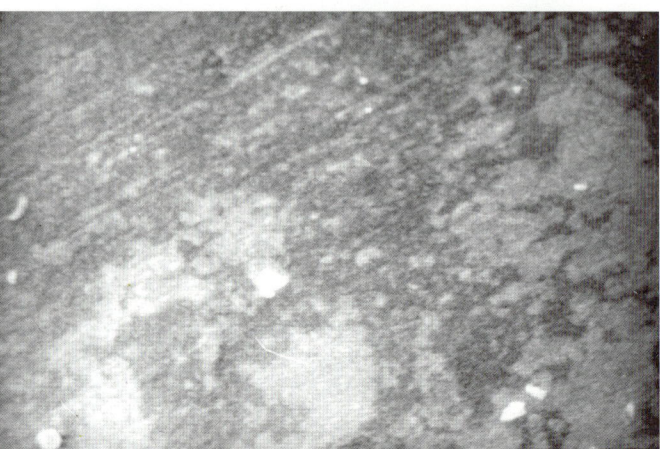

Fig. 18.13B: SEM photograph of finished conventional GIC (Magnification 200x)

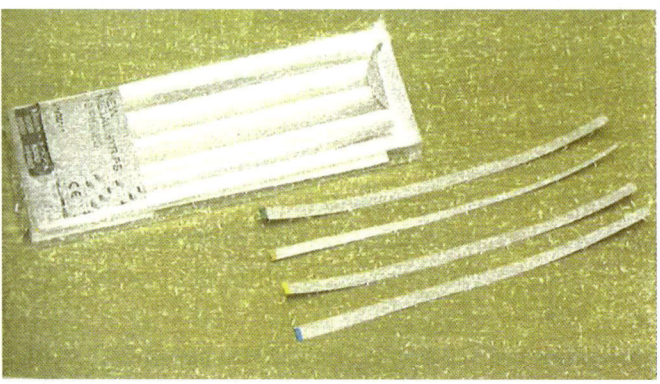

Fig. 18.12: Metal finishing strips for glass-ionomer restorations

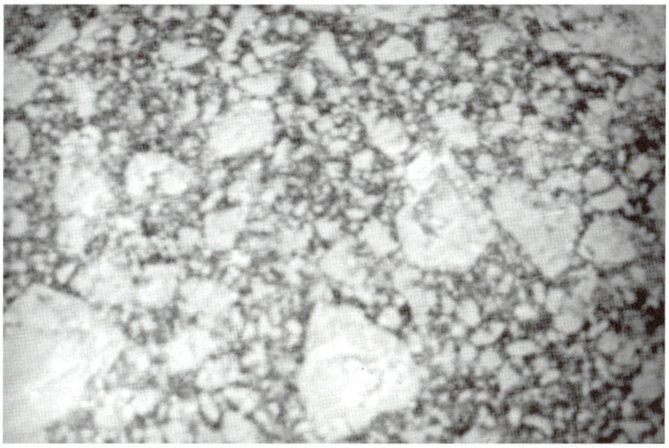

Glass-Ionomer Cement

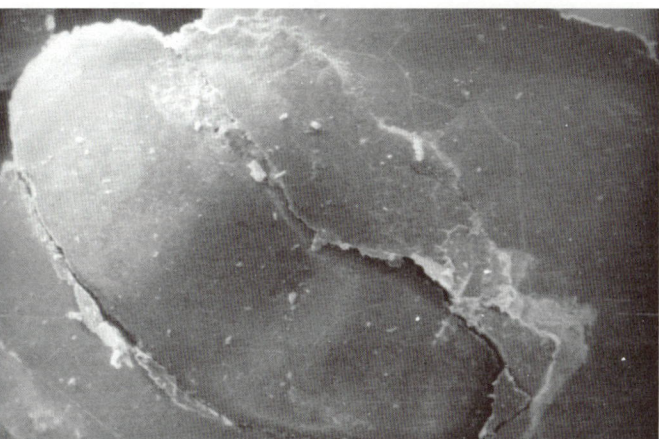

Fig. 18.13C: SEM photograph of finished conventional GIC (Magnification 1000x)

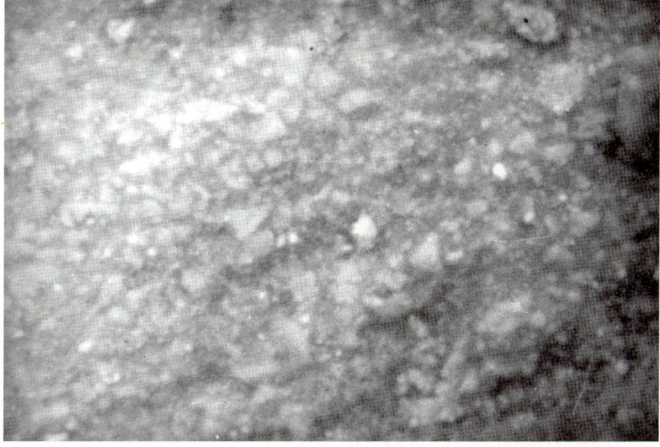

Fig. 18.14C: SEM photograph of finished light cure GIC (Magnification 1000x)

the cement will have matured sufficiently to develop full translucency. In case the surface is not protected during maturation, it will lead to the crack formation at the surface (Fig. 18.15). The problem of developing full translucency and aesthetics was solved with the use of a very low viscosity, light activated, resin enamel bond as a sealant rather than the recommended varnish, which is likely to allow some transmission of water.

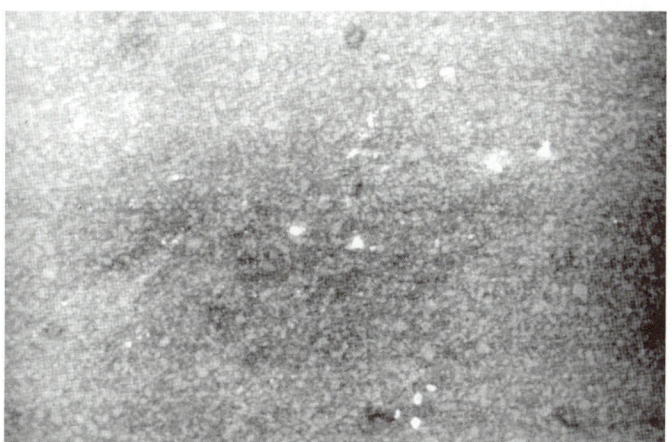

Fig. 18.14A: SEM photograph of finished light cure GIC (Magnification 25x)

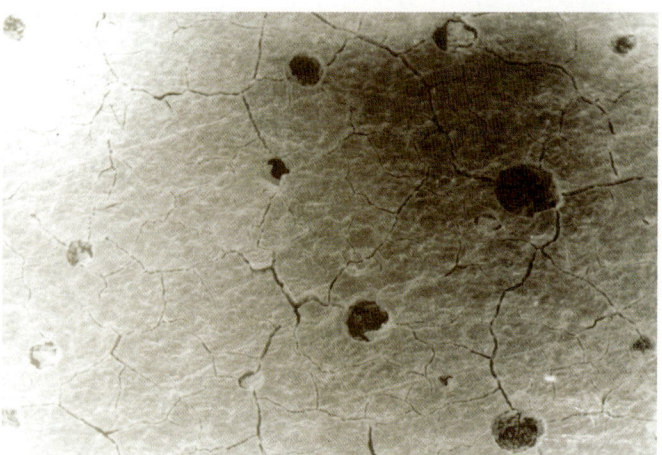

Fig. 18.15: Cracks at the surface of glass-ionomer restoration.

CLINICAL APPLICATIONS

a. Restorative Cements

i. Lesions at the Cervical Margin of Teeth

In Fig. 18.16A, note the diffuse outline at the cervical portion and the well defined margin at the occlusal extent with involvement more towards the distal of the root surface. Though the defect looks large and deep and the teeth are mildly stained, the oral hygiene of this patient was not poor. The cause of this defect would have been placed as abrasion defect but for the fact that it also shows fair amount of glossy appearance and appears to be invading into the sulcus, it would be appropriate to diagnose the defect as a combination of *abrasion* due to the notch like deep defect at the occlusal

Fig. 18.14B: SEM photograph of finished light cure GIC (Magnification 200x)

margin, *erosion* as the surface is also smooth and glossy, and *abfraction* as the lesion extends into the sulcus where the cemento-enamel junction was present. The photographs also demonstrate and concur with the fact that the most flexural teeth are the premolars in the posterior segment. Examining the occlusion for contacts during the lateral and protrusive excursion and modifying the same is mandatory in such cases. The restoration of choice would be a glass-ionomer because there is less likelihood of loss of restoration than if composite resins were placed. The ion exchange adhesion of glass-ionomer is superior and the cement appears to be sufficiently flexible to withstand the stresses of flexion in these teeth.

Figs 18.16B shown in the text was taken immediately after it had been filled with a Type-II glass-ionomer cement. The cement is not yet mature and lacks its ultimate translucency and hence the cavity outline form can just be perceived.

a 'V' shaped and notched defect that is typical of an abrasion lesion. However, it must have arisen through '*abfraction*' also. Fig. 18.17B shows the restoration of these teeth with glass-ionomer cement.

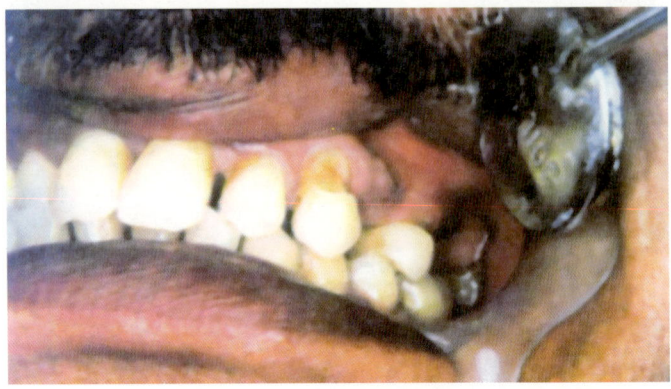

Fig. 18.17A: Abrasion/erosion lesions with caries

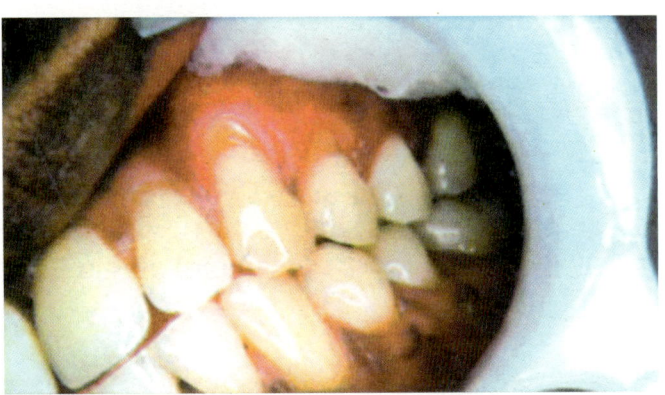

Fig. 18.16A: Cervical lesions on maxillary canine and first premolar

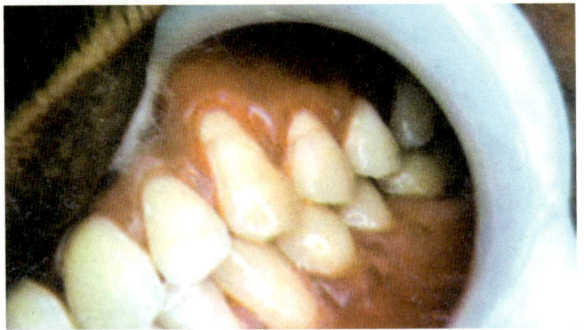

Fig. 18.16B: Restored lesions

ii. Abrasion-Erosion Lesion with Caries

The photograph in Fig. 18.17A shows erosion-abrasion lesions in maxillary canine and first premolar with caries superadded. Glass-ionomer is the restoration of choice in such defects as the anti-cariogenic effect and the ability to bear the flexural change in the tooth will be better borne by this cement. The premolar has

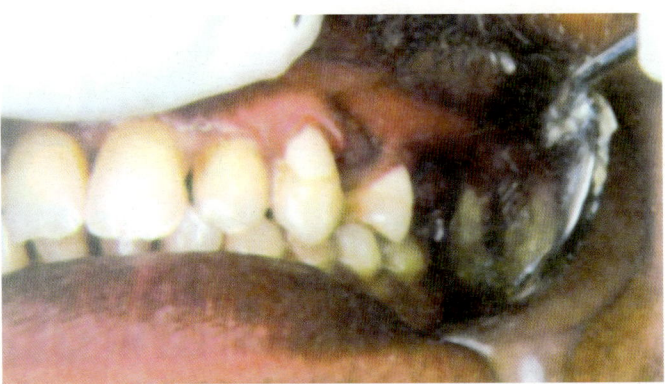

Fig. 18.17B: Restored lesions

If a root surface lesion on the exposed root of a tooth is found, the remainder of the dentition should be carefully explored for other root surface lesions because they generally do not occur in isolation.

An atypical cervical carious defect is seen in the photograph displayed in Figs 18.18A to D. The occurrence does not readily fit into what can be termed as "Rampant" caries. These caries appear to have developed without any predetermination that will aptly define a rampant caries.

A typical erosion lesion will leave a diffuse outline that leads to difficulty in determining the cavity margin at the time of restoration.

iii. Abfraction Lesions

Abnormal physical forces many a times lead to microcracks at the cementoenamel junction. These cracks subsequently help in development of caries or in case the forces remain active for a longer period of time the lesions become wider and deeper. Figs 18.19A, B show the restoration of multiple abfraction lesions in the maxillary teeth.

Glass-Ionomer Cement

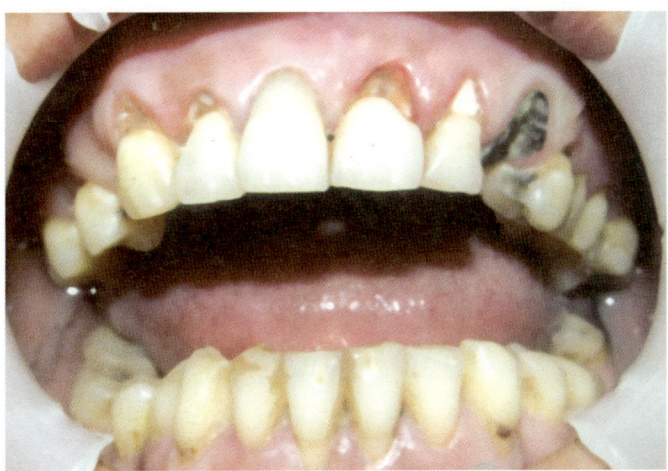

Fig. 18.18A: Cervical caries (pre-operative)

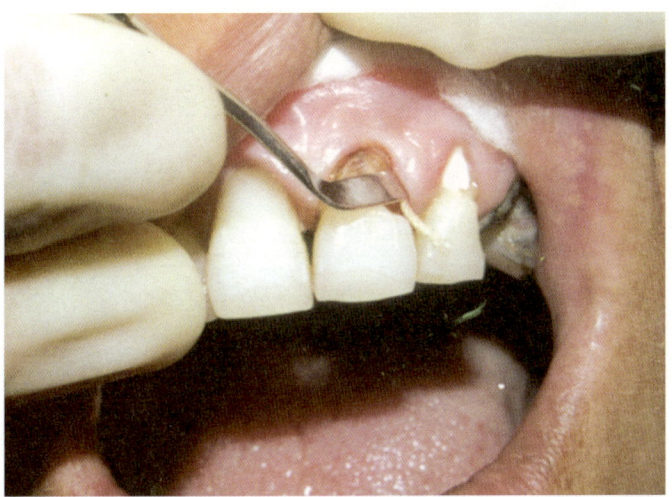

Fig. 18.18B: Placement of cord

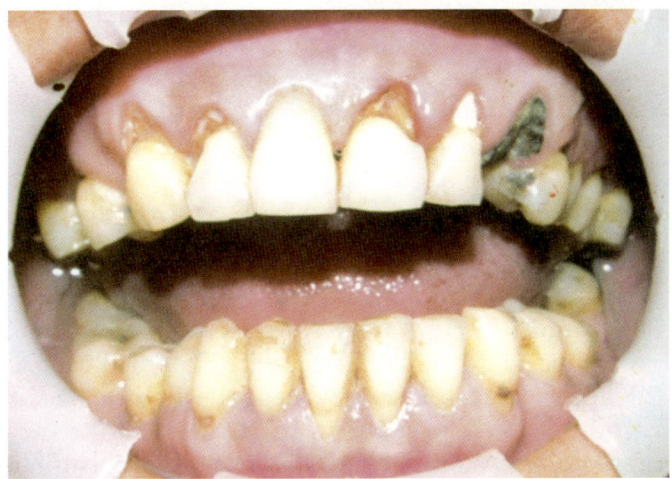

Fig. 18.18C: Tooth with gingival cord in place

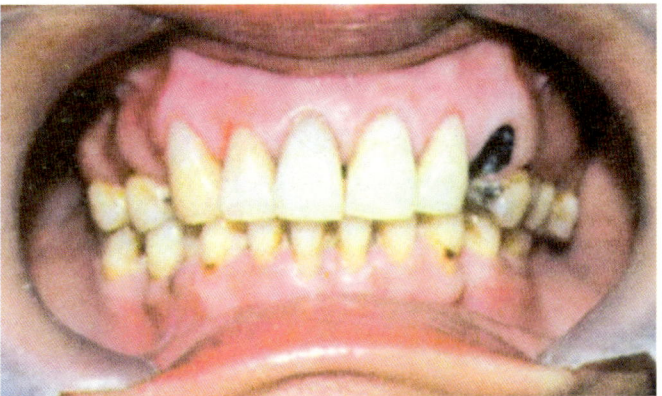

Fig. 18.18D: Restored lesion.

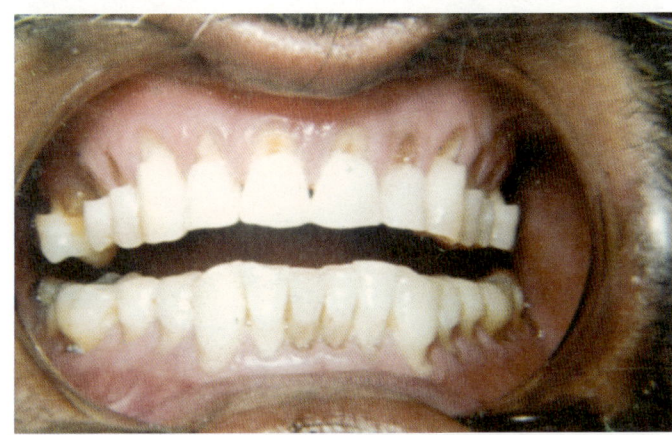

Fig. 18.19A: Multiple abfraction lesions.

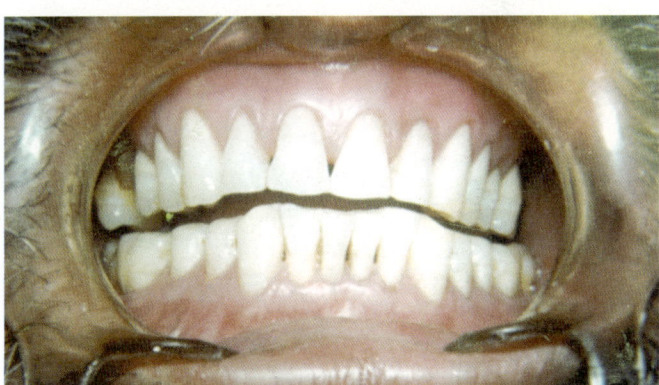

Fig. 18.19B: Restored lesions

iv. Class-III Cavities

Class-III cavities are best restored with light cure glass-ionomer for better aesthetics than with conventional chemical cure cement. Only hidden lesions may be restored with the ion exchange cement. The auto cure cements positively have superior fluoride release than the light cure cement. For adjacent lesions, a "T" shaped matrix is fabricated as shown in Figs 18.20A to D.

The restoration is light activated through the matrix for 20 seconds, then the matrix is removed and cured further.

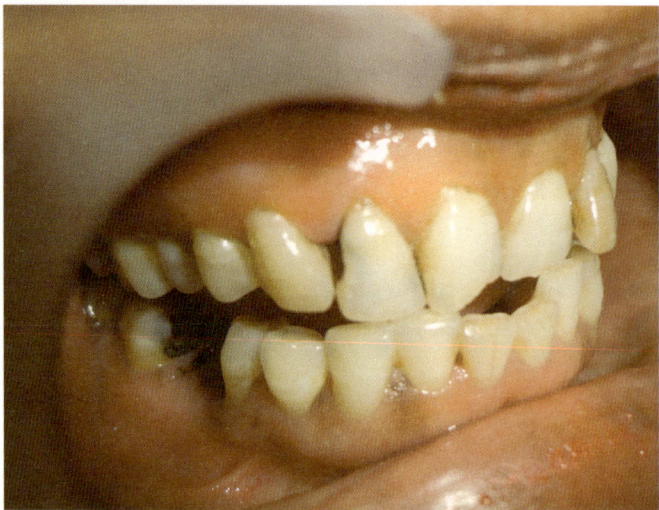

Fig. 18.20A: Class III lesion in maxillary lateral incisor

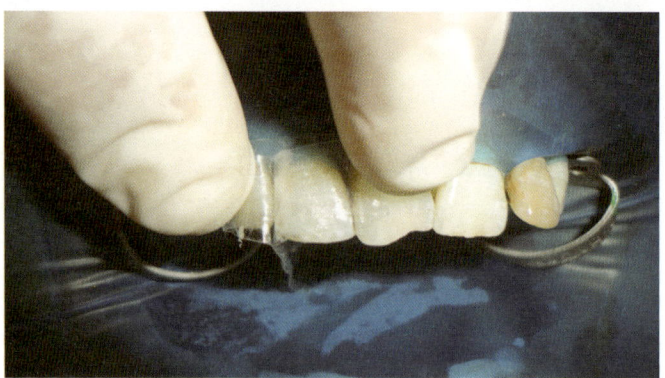

Fig. 18.20B: Mylar strip in place ('T' shaped)

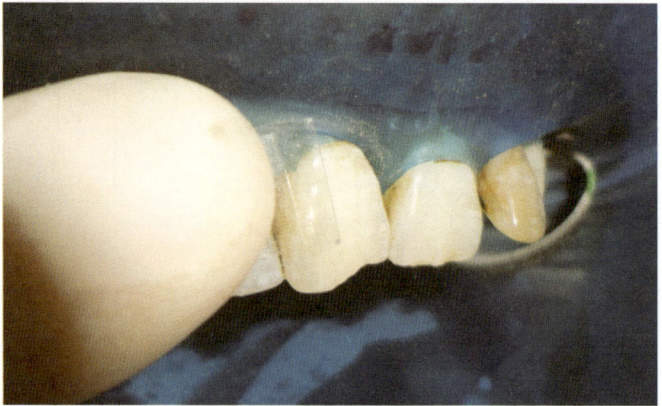

Fig. 18.20C: Holding the strip tight after insertion of the restorative material

The resin seal will wear off quite rapidly but will presumably leave the porosities and scratches filled and smooth.

v. Class I Cavities

In conservative class I preparations glass-ionomer cement can be given, especially in individuals with high caries indices (Figs 18.21A and B).

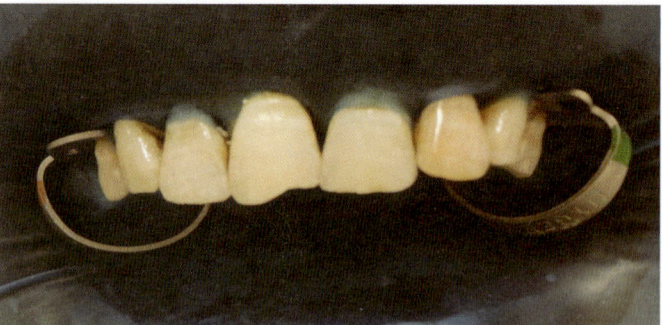

Fig. 18.20D: Finished restoration. adhesive property and tooth color

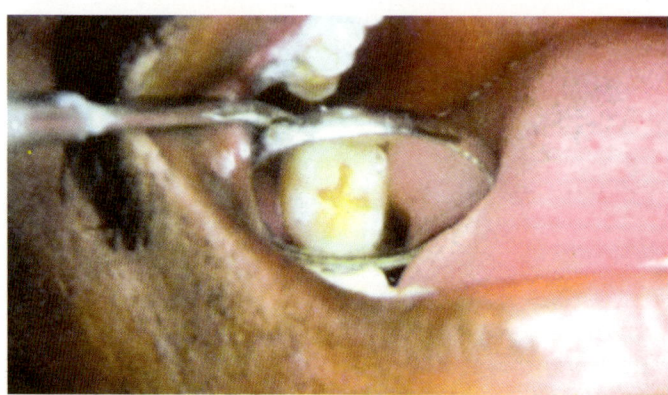

Fig. 18.21A: Prepared class I cavity

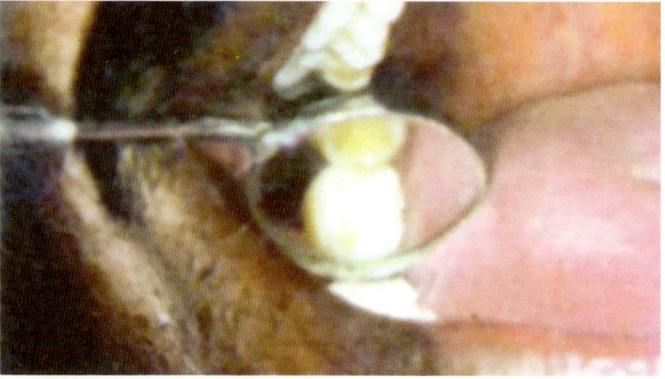

Fig. 18.21B: Restored class I cavity

b. Lining

Glass-ionomer is also used as lining cement. A lining is designed to be a thin layer placed under a metallic restoration, which is intended to afford thermal protection to the pulp-dentin organ. It is also used to fill up undercuts in cavity design where a line of withdrawal is required as in an inlay cavity or crown preparation. A luting cement will set rapidly and has a positive fluoride release. The Type-III lining cement has rather limited physical properties and hence should not be relied upon as a base for a composite resin in the lamination technique. If a glass-ionomer is to be used as a base under a composite a Type-II restorative or a light-cure cement must be used.

c. Bilayered/sandwich Restorations

Traditonal Type-II and Light-cure glass-ionomer cements are used as cement base and more rightly called as bilayereded restorations. Due to the comparatively better adhesion of the cement it is used to bond to the dentin in erosive lesions that leave out only a small area of enamel that can be used for bonding composites. It is also used for bonding dental amalgam to posterior teeth where there is compromised retention form due to loss of walls to support the amalgam. It is also used as laminated restoration along with composite or dental amalgam in the proximal cavities in posterior teeth where the gingival seat is not well defined to provide retention or when the cervical extension of the defect is subgingival. A glass-ionomer is easier to place in these locations than the more exacting and very technique sensitive composite (Figs 18.22A to D).

d. Luting

Glass-ionomer is a very useful material for luting all crowns and bridges as well as orthodontic appliances. The advantages of using this cement for luting are its anticariogenic property, low solubility in oral environment, pulp compatibility, good thixotropic flow, low film thickness, and to lesser extent the adhesive property and tooth color.

The tensile strength of the cement is not sufficient to enhance retention. So adhesion from the cement alone should not be relied upon to retain the restoration in place. Moreover to ensure adequate flow properties, the cement is mixed at a low powder to liquid ratio. It therefore, does not have proper physical properties also.

The luting cements are fast setting and can therefore be exposed to water contamination within five minutes of the start of mix.

Some patients experience severe sensitivity on seating of the restoration with this cement. The reason attributed is the hydraulic displacement of dentinal fluid. Hence it is desirable to seal the dentin tubules by painting the prepared surface with a low viscosity resin enamel bond or apply a remineralizing solution.

The correct mix of the cement for luting is demonstrated by the string test. When mixed it should be able to string out from the pad to about 3.0 cm or before it breaks and slumps back into the body of the mix. Following mixing to the correct consistency, some prefer to paint a small quantity of the cement on to the prepared tooth surface, using a small stiff bristle brush, to minimise the chances of air inclusions under the crown. Then coat or fill the restoration with the cement and seat it in place with continuous heavy pressure. If a coat of cement is applied over the tooth then there should be no delay in the placement of the restoration as the cement painted on to the tooth surface will set faster due to the increase in the oral temperature than the ambient temperature.

Glass-ionomer does not have an elastic memory and the restoration will not retreat from the tooth as it is likely to do with a zinc phosphate cement.

The luting cement is fast setting cement and hence is not affected by moisture in about 5 minutes after the mixing. Hence excess cement may be removed immediately upon initial set with a sharp instrument. These luting cements are radio opaque and any proximal residue can generally be detected with a radiograph.

Recently, glass-ionomer cements for luting purposes have been introduced in a paste form, which can be either a premixed paste in capsules or a two paste form which is mixed on the paper pad, each of which is available with a special dispenser.

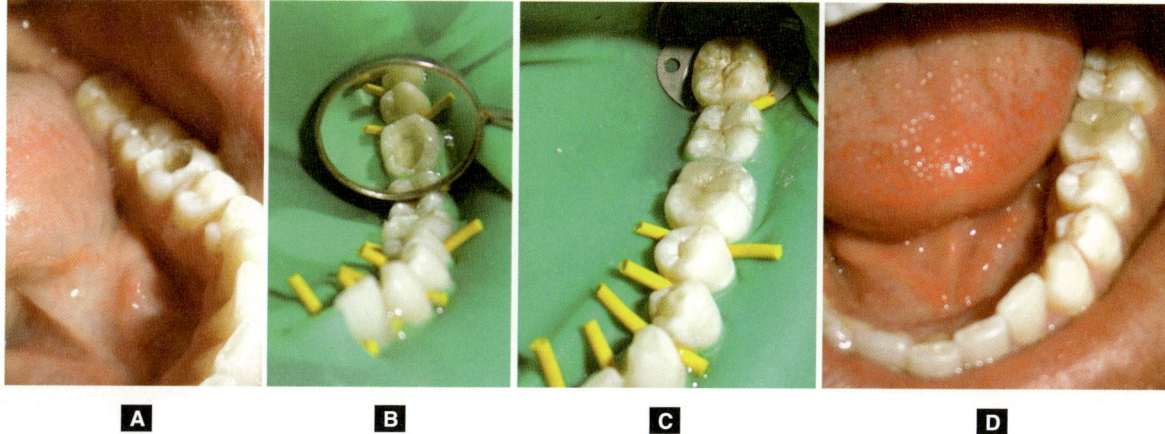

Figs 18.22A to D: (A) Prepared cavity for bilayered technique; (B) Base of glass-ionomer cement given; (C) Cavity restored with composite; (D) Finished restoration

LOSS OF RESTORATION

Loss of restoration may take place by the following means.
- Dissolution of the immature cement.
- Long term erosion.
- Loss of cement by abrasion.
- Fracture of restoration.

Dissolution of some amount of cement occurs from the surface during the first 24 hours because the surface is not sufficiently matured. Temporary protection with a layer of nitrocellulose, methyl methacrylate or amide resins in the form of varnish applied over the restoration will help prevent this loss to a great extent. Cocoa butter and vaseline help to a lesser extent. Long term erosion and loss of cement by abrasion is to be expected without much surprise especially if it is a restoration of an area of the natural, hard and highly resistant tooth structure, which had undergone a similar change. This can be reduced to a large extent by the correction of faulty cleansing habit, diet counselling, etc. Fracture of restoration, which is not due to improper manipulation is said to occur as a result of flexural change in the tooth. The cervical areas of the teeth, which undergo maximum flexural change, and beveling are likely to dislodge the restoration. It is also observed that the fracture often occurs within the body of the restoration – cohesive failure. The cement often leaves an acid resistant hybrid surface layer when it fractures from the defective area.

REACTION OF PULP TO GLASS-IONOMER CEMENT

Reaction of pulp-dentin organ to glass-ionomer cement is milder than composites. When the effective dentin depth is about 1.5 mm, a healthy reparative reaction is seen. When the effective dentin depth is about 0.5 mm to 1.0 mm, unhealthy or doubtful reparative changes may be observed. And when the effective dentin depth is less than 0.5 mm there is often a destructive reaction of the pulp dentin organ. The occasional mention about GIC being beneficially used over pulp may be considered anecdotal and cannot be recommended for regular clinical practice. Calcium hydroxide is the most recommended pulp protection agent under glass-ionomer cements (details in Chapter 24).

BIBLIOGRAPHY

1. Abdalla, A.I. and Garcia-Godoy, F.: Bond strengths of resin modified glass-ionomer ionomers and polyacid modified resin composites to dentin. Am. J. Dent.: 10, 291, 1997.
2. Beneli, E.M., Serra, M.C., Rodrigues, A.L. and Cury, J.A.: In situ anticariogenic potential of glass-ionomer cement. Car. Res.: 27, 280, 1993.
3. Billington, R.W., Williams, J.A., Dorban, A. and Pearson, G.J.: Glass-ionomer cement: evident pointing to fluoride release in the form of monofluoro phosphate in addition to fluoride ion. Biomaterials: 25, 3399, 2004.
4. Bourke, A.M., Walls, A.W. and Mccabe, J.F.: Light activated glass polyalkeonate cements: the setting reaction. J. Dent.: 20, 115, 1992.
5. Browning, W.D.: The benefits of glass-ionomer self-adhesive materials in restorative dentistry. Compend. Cont. Educ. Dent.: 27, 308, 2006.
6. Coutinoho, E., Van Landuyt, K., Munck, J.D., Poetevin, A., Yoshida, Y., Inoue, S. and Pneumans, M.: Development of a self-etch adhesive for resin modified glass-ionomers. J.D.R.: 85, 349, 2006.
7. Croll, T.P. and Nicholson, J.W.: Glass-ionomer cements in pediatric dentistry: review of the literature. Pediat. Dent.: 24, 423, 2002.
8. Culbertson, B.M.: New polymeric materials for use in glass-ionomer cements. J. Dent.: 34, 556, 2006.
9. El-Kalia, I.H. and Garcia Godoy, F.: Mechanical properties of compomer restorative material. Oper. Dent.: 24, 2, 1999.
10. Iehim, I., Schmidlin, P.R., Keiser, J.A. and Swain, M.V.: Mechanical evaluation of cervical glass-ionomer restorations: 3D finite element study. J. Dent.: June, 2006.
11. Knight, G.M. and Mc Intyre, J.M.: Bond strength between composite resin and anti-cure glass-ionomer cement using the co-cure technique. Aust. Dent. J.: 51, 175, 2006.
12. Millet, D.T., Doubleday, B., Alatsaris, M. and Love J.: Chlorhexidine-modified glass-ionomer for band cementation ? An in vitro study. British Orthodontic Society: 32, 36, 2005.
13. Mount, G.J.: Glass-ionomers: A review of their current status. Oper. Dent.: 24, 115, 1999.
14. Nicholson, J.W.: Chemistry of glass-ionomer cements – a review. Biomaterials: 19, 485, 1998.
15. Prentice, L.H., Tyas, M.J. and Burrow, M.F.: The effect of boric acid and phosphoric acid on the compressive strength of glass-ionomer cements. Dent. Mater.: 22, 94, 2006.
16. Walls, A.W.G.: Glass polyalkeonate (glass-ionomer) cements: a review. J. Dent.: 14, 231, 1986.
17. Weng, Y. et al: A novel antibacterial dental glass-ionomer cement. Eur. J. Oral Sci.: 118, 531, 2010.
18. Xie, Dong, Weng, Y. and X. Guo et al: Preparation and evaluation of a novel glass-ionomer cement with antibacterial functions. Dental Materials: 27, 487, 2011.
19. Yap, A.U.J., Mudambi, S., Chew, C.L. and Neo, J.C.L.: Mechanical properties of an improved visible light cured resin modified glass-ionomer cement. Oper. Dent.: 26, 245, 2001.
20. Yli, U.H., Lassila, L.V., Narhi, T. and Vallittu, P.K.: Compressive strength and surface characterization of glass-ionomer cements modified by particles of bioactive glass. Dent. Mater.: 21, 201, 2005.
21. Yosida, Y., Van Meerbeek, B., Nakayama, Y., Snauwaert, J., Hellemans, L. and Lambrechts, P.: Evidence of chemical bonding at biomaterial hard tissue interfaces. J.D.R.: 79, 709, 2000.

Minimal Invasive Dentistry

In the recent past, scientific developments in cariology, dental materials and diagnostic armamentarium have revolutionized operator's approach in managing caries. The previous surgical approach requiring removal of diseased portion of tooth along with extension of cavities to the areas prone to caries is no longer used. The *'extension for prevention'*, which was commonly taught has been changed to *'prevention for extension'*. The tooth weakened by extensive surgical approach leads to frequent retreatment and replacement, subsequently resulting in more complex treatment modalities and even extraction. The emerging technologies have paved the way for preventive aspects vis-à-vis remineralization of the existing lesions. Though this concept might not be fully practical, however the early trials are promising. Alternatively the treatment of the existing lesion is to be carried out, which includes minimum involvement of the healthy tooth structure.

Often, the terms 'Minimal Intervention Dentistry' and 'Minimal Invasive Dentistry' are used interchangeably, although they describe different concepts. Minimal Intervention dentistry implies patient care that deals with the cause of dental disease and not just the symptom. Minimal intervention is based entirely on prevention and control of oral disease; whereas, Minimal invasive dentistry embraces operative restorative procedures. The excavation of caries is performed with the objective of preserving not only sound tooth tissues but also that tissue which has potential to remineralize. The use of adhesive biomaterial is preferred. Minimal invasive dentistry is merely a component of minimal intervention treatment (care) plan. Ultraconservative and microdentistry are terms further incorporated within minimal invasive dentistry that implies use of optical magnification aids and other sophisticated devices other than traditional rotary instruments such as chemo-mechanical, air abrasive, sono-abrasion and laser systems.

The *'minimal intervention (minimally invasive)'* approach in managing dental caries incorporates detecting, diagnosing, intercepting and treating dental caries on the microscopic level. This approach of treating dental caries includes mostly non-surgical modalities or minimum possible surgical intervention. However, the basic concept of dental caries being infectious disease is followed.

Over the years, modern dentistry has adopted this approach, avoiding surgical approach as long as possible. The focus is on maximum conservation of demineralized, non-cavitated enamel and dentin. The development of adhesive dentistry and scientific knowledge in understanding the progress of caries coupled with recently introduced diagnostic aids has enabled the operator to do more than just mechanical removal and preparation.

The minimally invasive approach includes the following concepts:
 I. Early diagnosis of caries
 II. Assessment of individual caries risk
 III. Radiographic assessment of depth of caries and its progress
 IV. Decreasing the risk of further demineralization and arresting existing lesions
 V. Remineralization of the existing lesions
 VI. Restoring cavitated lesions using minimal tooth preparation
 VII. Repair rather than replacement of defective restorations

I. EARLY DIAGNOSIS OF CARIES

The early diagnosis of caries involves early detection of carious lesions and also determination of caries activity. Caries activity must be determined by monitoring the lesion over time. Various caries activity tests are available.

Different kinds of diagnostic tools are being utilized to detect caries. Some are preferred for detecting occlusal caries while others detect proximal or smooth surface lesions in a better way. The emerging technologies in diagnostic armamentarium include electrical conductance methods, quantitative laser fluorescence, tuned-aperture computed tomography and optical coherence tomography.

There is still a need for research to increase the accuracy of diagnostic methods. Though indices for progress of caries activity are also used but certainly improved versions are required to analyze the progress of the caries. The on-the-spot assessment of caries activity is required in the profession.

II. ASSESSMENT OF INDIVIDUAL CARIES RISK

Risk assessment helps professionals supervise individual's oral health. The frequency and type of oral health supervision needed by any individual depends on the likelihood that specific diseases may develop. It is a process that attempts to identify those individuals who are at greater risk of caries attack. These features are helpful in early treatment of the caries and also the possibility of reversal phenomenon.

The procedure involves examining risk factors that may negatively impact a child's oral health, and protective factors that promote oral health. Using risk assessment, the dentist is better able to make specific preventive and treatment recommendations to reduce a child's risk and improve overall oral health. This also contributes to efficient management of case by eliminating unnecessary interventions.

The risk factors are:

Physical
- Variations in tooth enamel, deep pits and fissures, anatomically susceptible areas
- Gastric reflux
- High Mutans streptococci count
- Previous caries experience
- History of baby bottle tooth decay

Behavioural
- Feeding bottle used at night for sleep or 'at will' while awake
- Taking frequent snacks
- Inadequate oral hygiene
- Eating disorders, including self-induced vomiting (Bulimia)

Socio-environmental
- Inadequate fluoride
- Poor family oral health
- High parental levels of Mutans streptococci

Disease or treatment related
- Special carbohydrate diet
- Disturbed saliva flow due to medication or irradiation
- Orthodontic appliances

III. RADIOGRAPHIC ASSESSMENT OF DEPTH OF CARIES AND ITS PROGRESS

The radiographs, especially the bitewing radiographs are helpful in detecting and analyzing the depth of caries. Follow up radiographs can also describe the progress of the caries. Though further advancement is required in dental radiology to analyze the radiolucencies and the opacities in a better way, yet the method is reasonably dependable and accurate. The digital radiographic procedures are helpful in analyzing the depth as well as the progress. However, radiographic techniques are not of much help in detecting early caries.

IV. DECREASING THE RISK OF FURTHER DEMINERALIZATION AND ARRESTING EXISTING LESIONS

It involves use of chemical and other agents, which can decrease the rate of progress of the carious lesion. Such agents, mostly fluorides, can be utilized in arresting the existing lesions. These agents are utilized for remineralization of the affected part of the dentin (Fig. 19.1) and arrest the progress of the lesion.

One such agent for arresting caries that has shown promise is silver diamine fluoride ($Ag(NH_3)_2F$). It is a combination of silver nitrate and sodium fluoride that when applied to carious tissues inhibits carious lesion progression. 38% silver diamine fluoride has been used in cavitated carious lesions. Twice yearly application of this concentration might be able to arrest the carious process. This non-invasive treatment

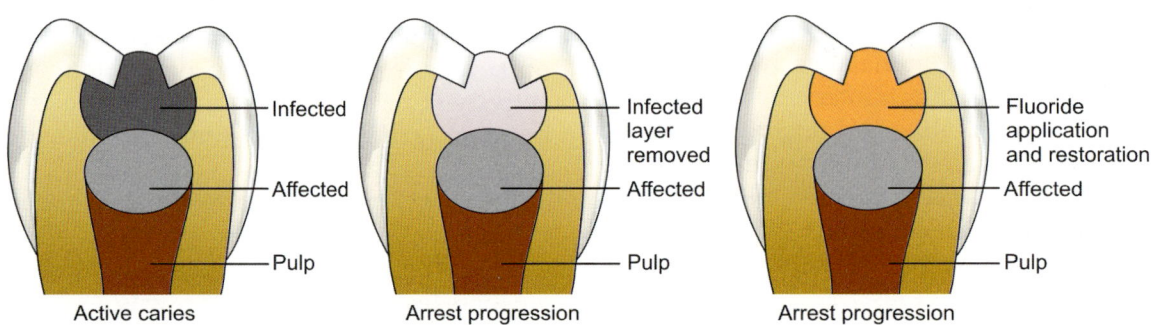

Fig. 19.1: Arresting caries progression

has the advantage that trained dental auxiliary personnel can also apply the solution.

Also, Ozone gas was proposed as an antimicrobial agent that could reduce the number of microorganisms on tooth surfaces. It is naturally produced in the presence of light or by different industrial processes. In dentistry, Ozone is claimed to have a sterilizing effect, killing cariogenic bacteria and subsequently leading to arrest of carious lesion. A Ozone generating system 'KaVo Healozone' that delivers ozone gas at a concentration of approximately 2100 ppm has been developed. The application procedure normally takes between 20–120 seconds per tooth surface.

V. REMINERALIZATION OF THE EXISTING LESIONS

It has been established that it is possible to arrest and even reverse the mineral loss associated with caries at an early stage, before cavitation takes place. Depending upon the oral environment, the tooth alternatively loses and gains calcium and phosphate ions. This cyclic loss and gain forms the basis of demineralization and remineralization. The pH of the oral environment matters in this regard.

Taking advantage of the tooth's ability to remineralize, the balance can be tipped in favour of remineralization by altering the oral environment. The phenomenon of alteration includes:

- Decreasing the frequency of intake of refined carbohydrates
- Following optimum plaque control measures
- Maintaining salivary flow
- Motivating and educating the patient

The chlorhexidine and topical fluorides encourage remineralization. Chlorhexidine acts by reducing the number of cariogenic bacteria and topical fluorides by formation of fluorapatite, which increases the resistance of the tooth to demineralization and also increasing local fluoride concentration, which favours remineralization.

The newer technologies for enamel remineralization include casein derivatives, tricalcium phosphate, NovaMin, enamelon, dicalcium phosphate dehydrate and ion exchange resins.

Casein Derivatives

Casein is the predominant phosphoprotein in bovine milk and accounts for almost 80% of its total protein. Under alkaline conditions the calcium phosphate is present as an alkaline amorphous phase along with calcium phosphate, referred to as casein phosphopeptide-amorphous calcium phosphate (CPP-ACP). They have the ability to stabilize high concentrations of calcium and phosphate in metastable solutions. CPP-ACP is a useful cariostatic agent for the control of dental caries as it contains calcium and phosphate in a bio-available form. CPP-ACP can be used as an:

- Adjunct preventive therapy to reduce caries in high risk patients
- Reduce dental erosion in patients with gastric reflux
- To repair enamel involving white spot lesions
- Orthodontic decalcification
- Desensitizing agent

Tricalcium Phosphate (TCP)

It has been established that a substantial increase of calcium and phosphate concentration occurred in plaque and saliva in subjects who used a chewing gum that incorporated tricalcium phosphate. This increases the pH which further increases tooth mineral saturation during an acidic challenge and thus decreases demineralization.

NovaMin

It is a bioactive glass ceramic (calcium sodium phosphosilicate) material that when exposed to aqueous medium provides calcium and phosphate ions that form hydroxyl-carbonate apatite (HCA) with time. NovaMin is able to fill in small surface defects in tooth enamel and thereby help stop erosion from acidic foods and beverages. By filling the surface defects it allows remineralization of these defects.

Enamelon

Enamelon consists of unstabilized calcium and phosphate salts with sodium fluoride. Enamelon toothpastes have shown to be beneficial in reduction of white spot lesions and remineralization of tooth enamel by acidic beverages.

Dicalcium Phosphate Dihydrate

Dicalcium Phosphate Dihydrate (DCPD) slurries were shown to be effective in preventing plaque pH drop and allowing higher degree of saturation for an extended period of time.

Ion-Exchange Resins

Ion-exchange resins (IER) have been used in pharmaceuticals as drug delivery systems. Toothpastes containing mixture of IER which supply calcium, fluoride, phosphate and zinc ions promoting remineralization are under research.

VI. RESTORING CAVITATED LESIONS USING MINIMAL TOOTH PREPARATION

It is established that caries progression through the enamel, even in active lesions, is slow. Therefore, early treatment of lesions confined to inner half of enamel and even slightly into the dentin is not indicated. By focusing on infection control measures coupled with application of remineralizing agents it is estimated that the restoration placement can be reduced to approximately 50%.

Cavitation makes plaque control difficult especially at the affected site; therefore, surgical approach is more reliable. The technological improvement in techniques of tooth preparation allow much more conservative preparation designs than those used earlier.

The classification conceived by Mount and Hume (Chapter 2) based on site and size of the lesion is considered the basis for minimal cavity preparation, though the advanced and extensive lesions do not fall under such regimes. Secondly the classification is also subjective, the size of the lesion is not well defined.

The tooth can be restored by one of the following:
a. Preparation with hand instruments
b. Preparation with high speed instruments
c. Air abrasion
d. Chemo-mechanical cavity preparation
e. LASER cavity preparation
f. Sonic oscillating system

a. Preparation with Hand Instruments

Atraumatic Restorative Treatment (ART)

This technique involves the removal of affected tooth tissues with hand instruments, followed by restoration of the cavities with a specially designed glass-ionomer restorative material (GC Fuji VIII) (Fig. 19.2).

The ART approach to managing caries lesions was first tried in the mid 1980's and is being used widely. Long term studies supporting its efficiency are not available.

Early authors described the success of ART restorations in one to three years evaluation. Single surface restorations were found to have a better success rate than multisurface restorations.

Later, a few authors indicated that there was no difference between restoration survival data for children and adults. Marked operator effects were found on the survival rate of restorations.

Clinical Technique

With the patient sitting on desk or bed of bamboo, the lesions are removed following the steps as (Figs 19.3A to E):
- Undermined enamel is broken off with hand instruments.
- The soft dentin is excavated.
- Glass-ionomer material is applied to the cavity and to any confluent pits and fissures.
- Vaseline coated finger is pressed over the restoration.
- Hand instrument is used to finish the restoration.

Advantages of ART
• No sophisticated dental equipment is needed (can be used in rural areas).
• Treatment is not dependent on electricity.
• Minimal discomfort to the patient.

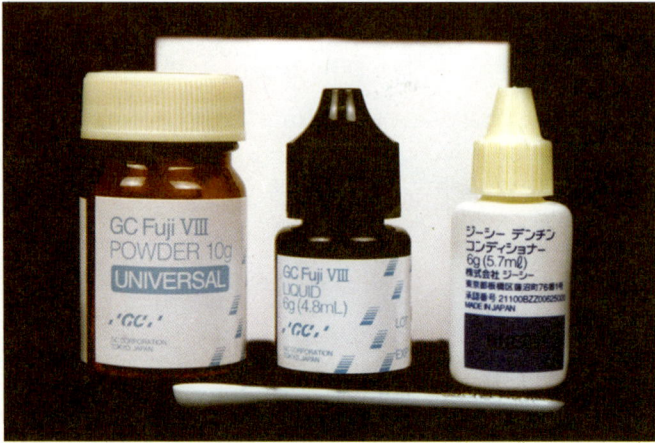

Fig. 19.2: GC Fuji VIII powder and liquid

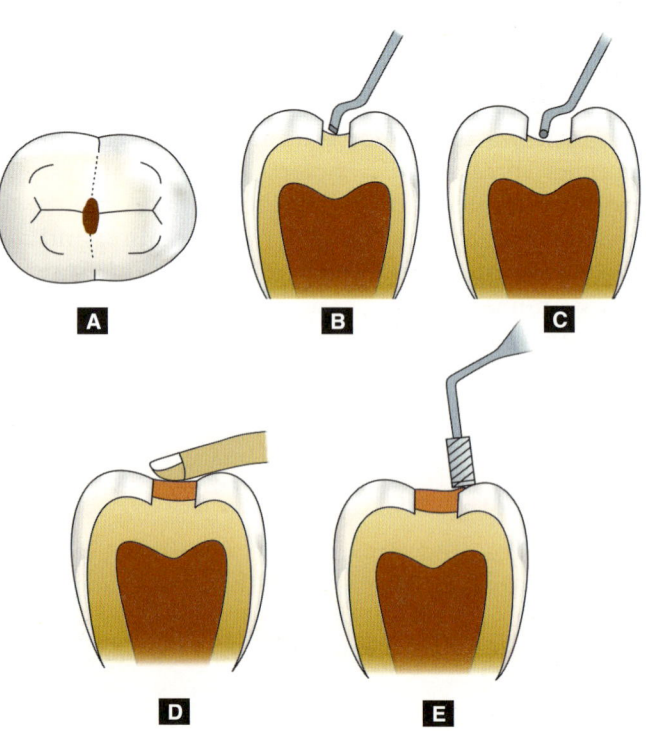

Figs 19.3A to E: ART approach

- The operator requires minimal training.
- Fluoride release from glass-ionomer cement will have a cariostatic effect.
- Cost is very low.
- If this treatment fails, a more radical approach may be used.
- Less time consuming.

Hall Technique

Hall technique is a newer method for managing carious lesions. Pre-formed metallic crowns are used to seal decay by cementation over carious primary molars with a glass-ionomer luting cement. Tooth preparation and caries excavation is not required for this technique.

b. Preparation with High Speed Instruments

Some modified designs include tunnel and internal preparations for proximal surface lesions. A high speed handpiece and small burs are used to prepare the cavity.

i. Tunnel Preparation

The tunnel preparation is performed by accessing the proximal carious lesion from the occlusal surface, while preserving the marginal ridge.

When caries is present only on proximal side, usually the access is gained through occlusal side. Conventionally, after making occlusal dovetail and breaking the marginal ridge, proximal box is prepared. Such restorations lead to more of tooth loss and jeopardize the integrity of marginal ridges. In tunnel preparations, the access is gained through occlusal side without involving the marginal ridge.

Tunnel restorations were designed with the idea of preserving the marginal ridge during posterior proximal restorations. For convenience, the tunnel restorations are divided into three types, viz. internal, partial and total (Fig. 19.4). The internal tunnel is the cavity preparation touching the lesion and the objective is to help remineralization. This is also known as 'Terminated tunnel' preparation. In partial tunnel preparation the enamel is smoothened around the periphery and the remaining lesion in touch with restoration can remineralize. In total tunnel preparation, all demineralized enamel is removed.

The adjacent tooth is protected with matrix bands before cavity preparation. The access is gained through the mesial/distal pit depending upon the side involved. A small round bur is pierced through the pit, directing the bur at 45° towards the proximal contact area (Figs 19.5A and B). Once the lesion is approached, the access can be slightly widened using tapering fissure burs. The carious lesion is thoroughly excavated by moving the bur in occlusal and gingival directions. Till the completion of the cavity preparation and the restoration, the band is maintained stable so as not to injure the adjacent tooth and the underlying gingiva. Various studies conducted on tunnel restorations could not show promising results. The strength of the marginal ridge is not maintained. The chances of leakage and secondary caries is more with these preparations. However, these are indicated in small lesions, especially in deciduous teeth.

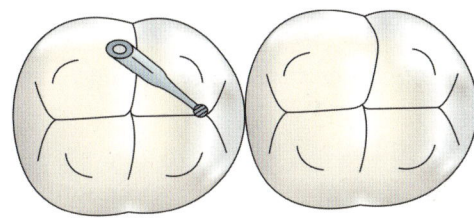

Fig. 19.5A: Direction of the bur (occlusal view)

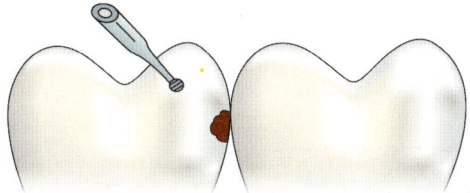

Fig. 19.5B: Direction of the bur (cross-sectional view)

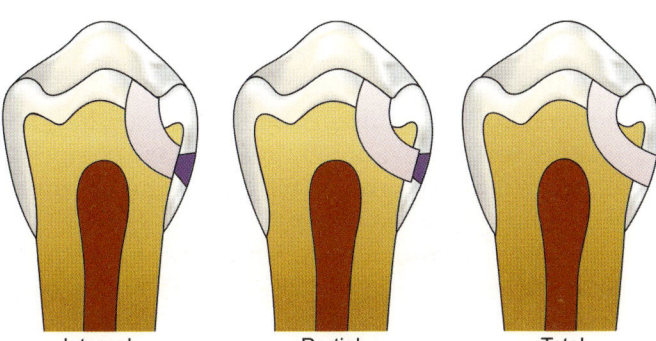

Fig. 19.4: Tunnel preparation

Advantages
- Preservation of tooth structure
- Maintenance of marginal ridge and proximal contacts
- Avoidance of iatrogenic damage to the adjacent tooth during cavity preparation
- Fluoride supply to adjacent tooth
- Negligible effect on gingival tissue
- Cost effective
- Aesthetic appearance
- Risk of overhang is minimal

Disadvantages
• Limited accessibility • Risk of incomplete removal of caries • Marginal ridge being undermined, may break • Risk of pulpal involvement • Marginal adaptability of the restoration is poor • Difficulty in insertion and finishing of the restorative material

ii. Minibox or Slot Preparations

These involve the removal of the marginal ridge, but do not include the occlusal pits and fissures if caries removal in these areas is not necessary. These cavities may have either a box or saucer shape and may be restored with resin-based composite or amalgam. (Fig. 19.6).

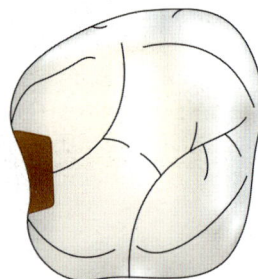

Fig. 19.6: Minibox slot preparation

c. Air Abrasion

The concept of air abrasion was given with an idea to replace belt driven hand pieces. The air abrasive technique might not work as an alternative to rotary instruments; however, this can be utilized as a supplement in the treatment of caries.

With the evolution of bonding mechanism and the related materials, the air abrasive concept finds a potential in today's restorative dentistry.

Air abrasion is non-rotary method of cutting hard tissues. The technique uses pseudo-mechanical kinetic energy from a stream of abrasive particles thrown at the tooth surface at a certain velocity.

The commonly used abrasive particles are aluminium oxide with an average particle size of 25–30 µm. Recently bio-active glass is being used in place of aluminium oxide. The particle size varies with the requirement of the cavity design and the morphology of the tooth. The normal exit pressure utilized is between 60–120 pound per square inch. The velocity of the particle exit will depend upon the diameter of the nozzle tip. The particles escape from the tip in a conical manner; the height and width of the cone depends upon the size of the nozzle. The dimension also increases as the distance between the nozzle tip and the tooth increases. The more near the tip is placed the more precise the cavity preparation is. The internal line angles are usually rounded by air abrasive technique; however if the tip is placed within 1.0 mm from the tooth surface, the line angles can be sharp. In case when beveled preparations are required, the nozzle tip is kept at a distance of 5.0 mm. For the preparations requiring a butt joint, the tip is placed 1.0 mm from the tooth surface. Since air abrasion follows end cutting pattern, the depth of the cavity can be more than required. The size and type of the particles, speed and the distance and length of the time play an important role in the cutting efficiency.

Uses

- *Minimal cavity preparation:* It requires minimum cavity preparation and also the prepared cavity is at the requisite location.
- *As an adjunct to acid etching:* Authors are of the view that abraded enamel surfaces are irregular, the pattern dissimilar to the acid etched enamel. Air abraded dentin shows only smear layer with no open dentinal tubules. The air abrasion alone cannot be used as a substitute of acid etching. It is established that the use of air abrasion along with acid etching gives good results.
- *As a repair modality:* The repair of fractured restorations pose difficulty for the operator. The composite to porcelain union is enhanced using hydrofluoric acid. It is established that use of air abrasion followed by application of hydrofluoric acid provides much better union. In case of composite repair, the contamination of surface layer by polishing agents and then environmental debris make it difficult to achieve bonding at the repair site. The silicate ceramic particles with and without alumina particles have shown better results in providing the necessary roughened surfaces. Certain authors, however, are of the view that such roughening does not provide better bonding during composite to composite repair.
- *As preventive measure:* Air abrasion technique has also been tried in preventive measures such as application of pit and fissure sealants, and small tunnel preparations. The technique has also the potential of use during composite veneering. The enamel surfaces are air abraded and the composite is applied keeping in view the esthetic requirements of the patient.
- *Detecting early carious lesions:* The air abrasive technique has been used in detecting the early carious lesions, mostly pit and fissure caries. For detecting caries, air polishing using sodium bicarbonate powder is utilized to remove the

surface stains, plaque etc. The sodium bicarbonate powder does not disturb the enamel surfaces. The tooth can be washed and dried and examined for any opacity on the surface of the enamel. Air abrasion with routine alumina powder is avoided in detecting caries, as alumina abrasive can damage the surface and lead to microscopic cracks on to the enamel surface.

Advantages
- Relatively pain free as compared to dental drill
- No problem of heat generation, vibration etc.

Disadvantages
- Lack of tactile sense
- May over prepare cavities
- Inhalation of particles may lead to systemic problems

d. Chemo-mechanical Cavity Preparation

The carious lesion is softened/dissolved using chemical means and then the softened material is excavated using sterilized excavators. The routinely used chemical agent is 'Carisolv'. The material is available in two tubes. One tube contains the amino acids leucine, lysine, glutamic acid and carboxylmethyl cellulose and sodium hydroxide. The other tube contains sodium hypochlorite.

The active gel is formed by mixing equal parts of these two components. Once the gel is mixed, the amino acids bind chlorine and form chloramines at high pH. The chloramines bind to different areas of protein in the carious dentin. The porous nature of the demineralized dentin allows the gel to penetrate. Degraded collagen of carious dentin has an open structure and is more susceptible to breakdown by chloramines.

The unaffected collagen is more resistant to degradation but the framework of degraded collagen is the porous mineral, which is broken down and can be easily penetrated. With the result the healthy tissues remain unaffected. The carious dentin is much easy to dislodge than the sound dentin.

The cavity preparation using carisolv includes:
- Local anaesthesia is not required, however, it can be administered if patient is apprehensive.
- The enamel lesion can be removed with small round bur. The agent is applied to the carious dentin.
- After waiting for 30 seconds, the caries is excavated using excavators. The lesion is kept soaked with the gel and during subsequent application no waiting period is required.
- The excavation is continued till the gel no longer turns cloudy.
- The remaining part of the cavity is checked for any left out debris. After removal of caries, the surface of the cavity has frosted appearance.

Advantages
- Painless, comfortable for the patients
- Conservative cavity preparation
- Patient's acceptance

Disadvantages
- Time consuming
- Rotary instruments may be required

e. LASER Cavity Preparation

LASERS have been widely used in dentistry since long. The Er: YAG and Nd: YAG lasers have been used to cut dental tissues, whereas CO_2 lasers facilitate sealing of fissures. Laser treatment reduces the number of carious bacteria and also volatilizes the water in the caries. With the use of Lasers, the effect of vibrations, pressure and unfavourable temperature changes associated with the use of rotary cutting instruments is eliminated. The cavity cutting by Lasers are clean with minimum debris and smear layer. The morphology of enamel prisms and dentinal tubule is preserved. Lasers can allow the dentin to remove caries selectively by maintaining healthy enamel and dentin. Preparations are similar to those made with air abrasion; adhesive materials are preferred for restoration.

Advantages
- Safe and efficient treatment modality for caries removal
- No need for anaesthesia, thus avoiding any numbness
- No vibration, little noise
- No smell

Disadvantages
- Cost factor
- Need to learn the technique

f. Sonic Oscillating System

The sonic oscillating system was devised for cutting and preparing proximal cavities. The device utilizes air driven oscillating handpiece and partially diamond coated working tips. Rotary instruments usually damage the adjacent tooth. The placement of bevels using rotary instruments is also difficult. The one sided torpedo shaped diamond tips in a sonic device allows the beveling of the proximal walls. As compared to hand instruments, the sonic tips allow for significantly better finishing of proximal bevels. The small tips are best suited for minimal cavity preparation. The caries removal can be carried out using small round burs rotating at low speeds. In no case the beveling be tried using rotary instruments as the chances of damaging the adjacent tooth increases many folds.

The minimal invasive techniques managing the carious substrate are summarized in Table 19.1.

Table 19.1: Minimal invasive management of carious substrate

Mechanism	Technique
Mechanical (rotary)	Burs/diamond points
Mechanical (non-rotary)	Hand instruments, Air-abrasion Ultrasonics, Sono-abrasion
Chemomechanical	Caridex, carisolv gel, Pepsin-based solutions/gels
Photo-ablation	Lasers
Disinfection	Photo-active disinfection, Ozone

Restorative Materials

Adhesive dental materials make it possible to conserve tooth structure using minimally invasive cavity preparations because they do not require the inclusion of mechanical retention features. Examples of such materials are glass-ionomer cements, composite/dentin bonding agents, resin based glass-ionomer cement and the bonded amalgam.

i. Glass-ionomer Cements

The conventional cavity preparation for glass-ionomer cement (GIC) has been modified in the form of Atraumatic restorative treatment (ART) and also the tunnel/internal preparation for the proximal lesions without disturbing the marginal ridge area as described above.

The advantages of GICs include adhesion to tooth structure and release of fluoride and other ions. They perform well in low stress areas. Set GIC is 'rechargeable', meaning it can take up fluoride from the environment, which is provided by exposure to fluoride varnishes and fluoride containing tooth pastes.

The disadvantages include technique sensitivity and their opaque nature. The handling properties and bitterness of the material can be overcome by adding resin to the material resulting in resin-modified GICs, which are easier to place, are light cured, and have improved esthetics.

ii. Composite Resins

The cavity preparation for composite widely depends upon the surface area of the tooth, which can be utilized for bonding. Cavity preparations designed to conserve maximum enamel can eliminate the need for macromechanical retention. Bonding, both to dentin and enamel is required for composite restorations. Various types of composites are available for use in anterior and posterior teeth. Flowable composites with lower filler loading have also been developed which are preferred in inaccessible areas. These materials have low modulus of elasticity and higher polymerization shrinkage, therefore not used in routine.

Box/slot form of the cavities or the saucer shaped cavities are preferred for composites. The detail is given in Chapter 19.

iii. Bonded Silver Amalgam

The bonded silver amalgam was introduced with an idea to improve the bonding of amalgam to the cavity walls. A chemically active, resin based luting material is placed along the cavity wall and at its base before condensing the silver. Though the adhesion is definitely improved, the other physical properties might be compromised since proper depth required for silver is not provided. The thickness of the oxygen inhibited layer in dentin bonding agents create difficulty in bonded amalgam.

Advantage
- Amalgam can be used in short clinical crowns
- Marginal leakage is checked
- Conservative approach is maintained
- Sealed and bonded restorations prevent further progress of caries

Disadvantage
- Increased cost
- Proper strength may not be achieved, especially in minimal cavity preparation

VII. REPAIR RATHER THAN REPLACEMENT OF DEFECTIVE RESTORATIONS

The replacement of existing restoration because of varied reasons is a common feature. Such replacements become necessary with almost all the materials. It is established that with every replacement, the loss of tooth structure increases. This loss is much more in case of composites and other tooth colored materials. The repeated restoration replacement leads to the need of more complex treatments, may be indirect restorations. The repair process, earlier considered as patchwork, is being accepted in the profession with the evolution of composites and bonding agents.

Cavity preparations should ensure independent retention and resistance form for the repair. The decision to repair rather than replace a restoration always must be based on the patient's risk of developing caries, the professional's judgment of benefits vs. risks and conservative principles of cavity preparation.

The composite has shown promise in re-attachment of the fractured anterior teeth. The fracture of anterior crowns is very common in young age and the technique of re-attachment with composite produce requisite strength and adequate aesthetics. The repair of fracture of ceramic crowns, both metal ceramic and all ceramic has also been attempted using an abrasive silica impregnated technique. Repair with glass-ionomer cement may be preferable in cervical areas, because of the potential for fluoride release and GIC's excellent adhesion.

BIBLIOGRAPHY

1. Alonso, R.C., Correr, G.M., Borges, A.F., Kantovitz, K.R. and Rontani, R.M.: Minimally invasive dentistry: bond strength of different sealants and filling materials to enamel. Oral Health Prev. Dent.: 3, 87, 2005.
2. Ardu, S., Perround, R. and Krejci, I.: Extended sealing of interproximal caries lesions. Quint. Int.: 37, 423, 2006.
3. Banerjee A.: Minimal invasive dentistry: part 7. Minimal invasive operative caries management: rationale and techniques. B.D.J.: 214,107,2013.
4. Banerjee, A., Kidd, E.A.M. and Watson, T.F.: In vitro evaluation of five alternative methods of carious dentin excavation. Caries Res.: 34, 144, 2000.
5. Banerjee, A., Watson, T.F. and Kidd, E.A.M.: Dentin caries excavation: a review of current clinical techniques. Br. Dent. J.: 188, 476, 2000.
6. Banerjee, A. and Watson, T.F.: Air abrasion: its uses and abuses. Dent. Update: 29, 340, 2002.
7. Banerjee, A., Thompson, I.D. and Watson, T.F.: Minimally invasive caries removal using bio-active glass air-abrasion. J. Dent.: 39, 2, 2011.
8. Beelay, J.A., Yip, H.K. and Stevenson, A.G.: Chemomechanical caries removal: a review of the techniques and latest developments. B.D.J.: 188, 427, 2000.
9. Bernardon, J.K., Gondo, R. and Baratieri, L..N.: Minimal invasive restorative treatments of hyopplastic enamel in anterior teeth. Am. J. Esthet. Dent.: 1, 10, 2011.
10. Burke FJ.: Ozone and caries: a review of the literature. Dental update: 39,271,2012.
11. Burke, F.J.T.: From extension for prevention to prevention of extension: (Minimal Intervention Dentistry). Dent. Update: 30, 492, 2003.
12. Christensen, G.J.: The advantages of minimally invasive dentistry. J.A.D.A.: 136, 1563, 2005.
13. Czarmecka, B.: The use of ART technique in modern dental practice: a personal view. J. Dent.: 34, 620, 2006.
14. Czarrnecka, B., Limanowksa, S.H. and Nicholson, J.W.: Microscopic-evaluation of the interface between glass-ionomer cement and tooth structure prepared using conventional instruments and the atraumatic restorative treatment (ART) technique. Quint. Int.: 37, 557, 2006.
15. daFranca, C., Colares, V. and Amerongen, E.: The operator as a factor of success in ART restorations. Braz. J. Oral Sci.: 10, 60, 2011.
16. Ericson, D., Kidd, E., McComb, D., Mjor, I. And Noack, M.J.: Minimally invasive dentistry: Concepts and techniques in cariology. Oral Health Prev. Dent.: 1, 59, 2003.
17. Ericson, D.: What is minimally invasive dentistry ? Oral Health Prev. Dent.: 2, 287, 2004.
18. Featherstone J.B.D and Domejean S.: Minimal invasive dentistry: part 1. From 'compulsive' restorative dentistry to rational therapeutic strategies. B.D.J.: 213,441,2012.
19. Frencken Jo E ,Peters MC , Manton DJ, Leal SC, Gordan V and Eden E.: Minimal intervention dentistry for managing dental caries – A review. Int Dent J: 62,223,2012.
20. Garcia G. F., Marshall, T.O. and Mount, G.J.: Microleakage of glass-ionomer tunnel restorations. Am. J. Dent.: 1, 53, 1998.
21. Hamilton, J.C., Gregory, W.A. and Valentine, J.B.: Diagnodent measurement and correlation with the depth and volume of minimally invasive cavity preparation. Oper. Dent.: 31, 291, 2006.
22. Innes N.P.T , Evans D.J.P and Stirrups D.R.: Sealing caries in primary molars: Randomized Control Trial , 5 year results. J Dent Res 12, 90, 2011.
23. McComb, D.: Systematic review of conservative operative caries management strategies. J. Dent. Educ.: 65, 1154, 2001.
24. McDonald, S.P. and Sheiham, A.: A clinical comparison of non-traumatic methods of treating dental caries. Int. Dent. J.: 44, 465, 1994.
25. Mickenautsch, S. and Grossman, E.: Atraumatic restorative treatment (ART): factors affecting success. J. Appl. Oral Sci.: 14, 34, 2006.
26. Mickenautsch, S., Yengopal, V. and Banerjee, A.: Atrauamtic restorative treatment versus amalgam restoration longevity: a systematic review. Clin. Oral Invest.: 14, 233, 2010.
27. Milnar, F.J.: Sequencing three conservative minimally invasive treatments. Contemporary Esthetics: P1, 24, 2007.
28. Mjor, J.A. and Gordan, V.V.: A review of atraumatic restorative treatment (ART). Int. Dent. J.: 49, 127, 1999.
29. Momesso, M.G.C., deSilva, R.C., Imparato, J.C.P., Molina, C., Navarro, S. and Ribeiro, L.: In vitro surface roughness of different glass-ionomer cements indicated for ART restoration. Braz. J. Oral Sci.: 9, 77, 2010.
30. Moune, G.J. and Ngo, H.: Minimal intervention: A new concept for operative dentistry. Quint. Int.: 31, 527, 2000.
31. Muniz, M, Quioca, J, Dolei, GS, Reis, A and Loguercio, AD.: Bonded amalgam restorations: Microleakage and tensile bond strength evaluation. Oper. Dent.: 30, 228, 2005.

32. Paolinelis, G., Banerjee, A. and Watson, T.F.: An in-vitro investigation of the effects of variable operating parameters on alumina air abrasion cutting characteristics. Oper. Dent.: 34, 87, 2009.
33. Papa, J., Wilson, P.R. and Tyas, M.J.: Tunnel restorations: A review. J. Esthet. Dent.: 4, 4, 1992.
34. Peng J.J.Y, Botelho MG and Matinlinna J.P.: Silver compounds used in dentistry for caries management: A review. J Dent:40,531,2012.
35. Renne WG and Mennito AS .: A simplified technique for restoring interproximal root surface lesions. Oper Dent: 37, 211, 2012.
36. Reston EG, Corba VD, Broliato G, Saldini BP and Busato ALS.: Minimally invasive intervention in a case of non carious lesion and severe loss of tooth structure. Oper Dent: 37,3 2012.
37. Smales, R.J. and Yip, H.K.: The atraumatic restorative treatment (ART) approach for the management of dental caries. Quint. Int.: 2, 97, 2002.
38. Staninec, M. and Sectcos, J.C.: Bonded amalgam restorations: current research and clinical procedure. Dent. Update: 30, 430, 2003.
39. Tyas, M.J., Anusavic, K.J., Frencken, J.E. and Mount, G.J.: Minimal intervention dentistry: A review. FDI Commision Project. I.D.J.: 50, 1, 2000.
40. Vant Hot, M.A., Frenken, J.E., Helderman, W.H. and Holmgross, C.J.: The ART approach for managing dental caries: A meta-analysis. Int. Dent. J.: 56, 345, 2006.
41. Wearheim, K.I. and Groen, H.J.: The residual caries dilemma. Comm. Dent. Oral Epid.: 27, 436, 1999.
42. White, J.M. and Eakle, W.S.: Rationale and treatment approach in minimally invasive dentistry. J. Am. Dent. Assoc.: 131, 13S, 2000.
43. Whitehouse, J.: Minimally invasive dentistry: Clinical application. Dent. Today: 23, 56, 2004.
44. Yip, H.K., Smales, R.J., Yu, C., Gao, X.J. and Deng, D.M.: Comparison of ART and conventional cavity preparation for glass-ionomer restorations in primary molars: 12 months results. Quint. Int.: 33, 17, 2002.

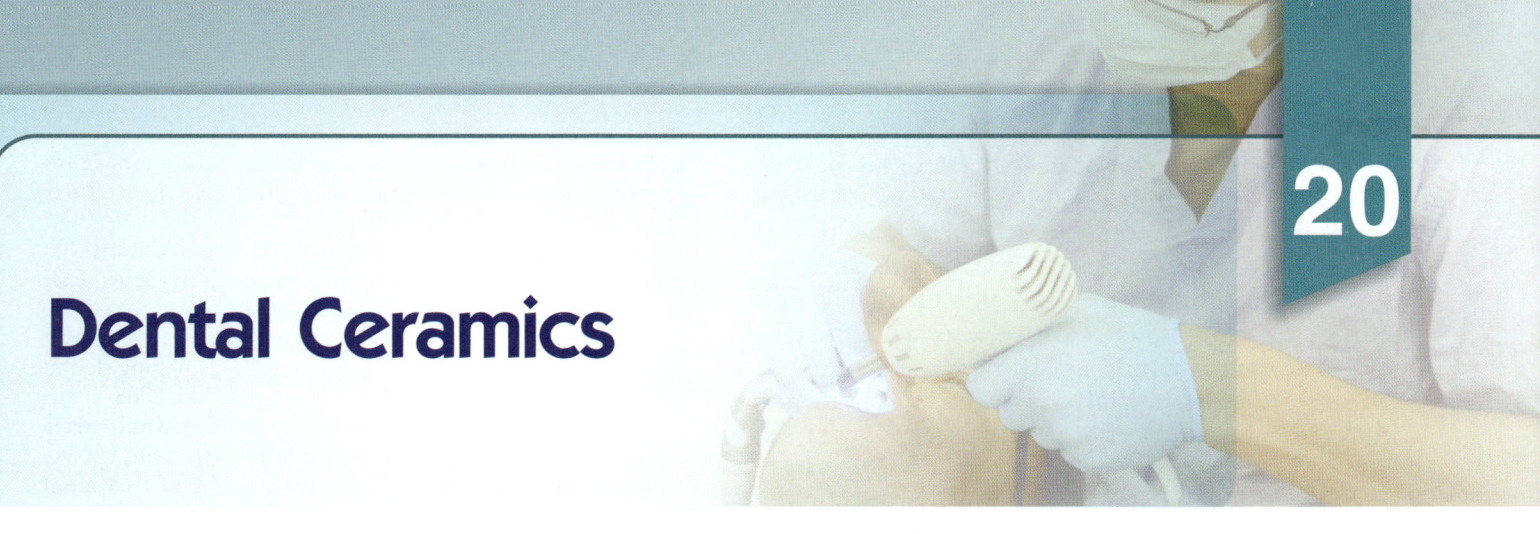

20

Dental Ceramics

Ceramic was probably the first material to be artificially made by humans, and has held the attention of dental profession for more than two hundred years. Early fabrication of ceramic articles dates back to 23,000 BC. The use of porcelain in dentistry was first mentioned by **Pierre Fauchard**. The word *'ceramic'* is derived from the Greek word *'Keramikos'* which means *'earthern'* and some believe it to have been derived from *'Keramos'*, which means pottery or burnt stuff.

Ceramic is a product manufactured by the action of heat on earthern materials in which silicon and silicates predominate. Porcelain, glass, refractories, some cements, silicon carbide, clay products such as brick, tile and terracota are some of the principal ceramic objects.

Ceramics on the other hand is the art of forming, i.e. modelling and processing objects made of clay or similar material.

The wide popularity of ceramic dental restorative materials owes to their life like optical properties, biocompatibility, low thermal conductivity, coefficient of thermal expansion close to that of tooth structure, durability and etchability. However, two major problems associated with its use are the potential for brittle fracture and the ability to cause abrasive wear of opposing tooth surfaces. With recent advances, these limitations have also been overcome to a large extent. In the following chapter, dental ceramic is first briefly described as a material and then its restorations are discussed.

TERMINOLOGY

Alumina core - a ceramic containing sufficient crystalline alumina (Al_2O_3) to achieve adequate strength and opacity when used for the production of a core for ceramic jacket crowns.

Aluminous porcelain - a ceramic composed of a glass matrix phase and 35 vol % or more of Al_2O_3.

CAD-CAM ceramic - a machinable ceramic material formulated for the production of inlays and crowns through the use of a computer-aided design, computer-aided machining process.

Castable dental ceramic - a dental ceramic specially formulated to be cast using a lost-wax process.

Ceramic - a compound of metallic and non-metallic elements.

Ceramic, dental - a compound of metals (such as aluminium, calcium, lithium, magnesium, potassium, sodium, tin, titanium, and zirconium) and nonmetals (such as silicon, boron, fluorine, and oxygen) that may be used as a single structural component, such as when used in a CAD-CAM inlay, or as one of several layers that are used in the fabrication of a ceramic-based prosthesis. Dental ceramics are formulated to provide one or more of the following properties: castability, moldability, injectability, color, opacity, transluency, machinability, abrasion resistance, strength, and toughness. *Note:* all porcelains and glass ceramics are ceramics, but not all ceramics are porcelains or glass-ceramics.

Copy-milling - a process of machining a structure using a device that traces the surface of a master metal, ceramic, or polymer pattern and transfers the traced spatial positions to a cutting station where a blank is cut or ground in a manner similar to a key-cutting procedure.

Core ceramic - a dental ceramic material that provides a mechanically strong base onto which a body ceramic (also called *dentin* or *gingival ceramic*) can be veneered.

Cracking - the formation of large or minute fissures (microcracks).

Crazing - the formation of one of the more minute cracks as an immediate or delayed result of thermally induced stresses.

Feldspathic porcelain - a ceramic composed of a glass matrix phase and one or more crystal phases. An important crystal phase is leucite ($K_2O \cdot Al_2O_3 \cdot 4SiO_2$), which is used to create a high-expansion porcelain that is thermally compatible with gold-based, palladium-based, and nickel-based alloys. A more technically correct name for this class of dental ceramics is leucite porcelains, because feldspar is not present in the final processed porcelain nor is it necessary as a raw material to produce leucite crystals.

Glass-ceramic - a soild consisting of a glassy matrix and one or more crystal phases produced by the controlled nucleation and growth of crystals in the glass.

Glass-infiltrated dental ceramic - a minimally sintered Al_2O_3 or $MgAl_2O_4$ core with a void network that has been sealed by the capillary flow of molten glass. Examples include In-cream (Al_2O_3) and In-cream Spinell ($MgAl_2O_4$) core.

Injection-molded ceramic - a glass or other ceramic material that is used to form the ceramic core of an inlay, veneer, or crown by heating and compressing a heated ceramic into a mold under pressure. An example is IPS Empress.

Shade guide, ceramic - a series of ceramic tooth-shaped tabs mounted on metal or plastic strips that is designed for comparison of hue, value, and chroma characteristics with those of natural teeth or existing ceramic restorations. The letter and number code on the metal strip allows the dentist to communicate the perceived appearance properties to a dental technologist who may not be able to observe the teeth to be restored.

Shoulder porcelain - a porcelain that is formulated to be sintered at a lower temperature than that of opaque porcelain and higher than that of body porcelain to produce an esthetic porcelain margin as an alternative to a metal margin on a metal-ceramic crown.

Sintering - the process of heating closely packed particles to achieve interparticle bonding and sufficient diffusion to decrease the surface area or increase the density of the structure. For products such as In-Ceram and In-Ceram Spinell surface contact sintering and minimal density change are required.

Spinel or spinelle – a hard crystalline mineral ($MgAl_2O_4$) consisting of magnesium and aluminum. Also, any of the group of mineral oxides of ferrous iron, magnesium, manganese, or zinc.

Stain - a mixture of one or more pigmented metal oxides and usually a low-fusing glass that when dispersed in an aqueous slurry or monomer medium, applied to the surface of porcelain or other specialized ceramic, dried or light cured, and fired will modify the shade of the ceramic-based restoration. One product is supplied in a light-curable binder. These stain products are also called 'surface colorants' or 'characterization porcelains'.

CLASSIFICATION

There are several categories of dental ceramics: conventional leucite-containing porcelain, leucite-enriched porcelain that may contain leucite, glass-ceramic, specialized core ceramic (alumina, glass-infiltrated alumina, magnesia, and spinel), and CAD-CAM ceramics. Dental ceramics can be classified:–

- *By type*: feldspathic porcelain, leucite-reinforced porcelain, aluminous porcelain, alumina, glass-infiltrated alumina, glass-infiltrated spinel, and glass-ceramic.
- *By use*: denture teeth, metal-ceramics, veneers, inlays, crowns and anterior bridges. \
- *By processing methods*: sintering, casting, or machining.
- *By substructure material*: cast metal, swaged metal, glass-ceramic, CAD-CAM porcelain, or sintered ceramic core.

Dental porcelains can also be classified on the basis of their maturing temperature, i.e. the temperature at which a product with satisfactory physical properties and esthetic qualities is obtained. These are as follows:

High fusing	>1300°C
Medium fusing	1101°C–1300°C
Low fusing	850°C–1100°C
Ultra low fusing	<850°C

High and medium fusing porcelains are used for making porcelain teeth for dentures whereas low and ultra low fusing ones are used for crown and bridge construction. Since porcelain teeth are no more used, the classification is now being reduced to high fusing (850°C–1100°C) and low fusing (850°C). Because this classification is not very popular, it is beneficial to always mention the firing temperature range when discussing porcelain.

COMPOSITION

The various ingredients used in different formulations of ceramics are:

- Silica (Quartz or Flint) – Filler
- Kaolin (China clay) – Binder
- Feldspar – Basic glass former
- Water – Important glass modifier
- Fluxes – Glass modifiers
- Color pigments
- Opacifying agents
- Stains and color modifiers
- Fluorescent agents
- Glazes and Add-on porcelain
- Alumina
- Alternative Additives to Porcelain

Silica

It can exist in 4 different forms:
- Crystalline quartz,
- Crystalline cristobalite
- Crystalline tridymite
- Non-crystalline fused silica

Pure quartz crystals (SiO_2) are used for manufacturing dental porcelain. Quartz (crystalline silica) is used in porcelain as a filler and strengthening agent. Because it has a high melting point, it also provides a high strength framework for other ingredients during firing and helps to maintain the form (shape) of a freestanding object during firing.

Kaolin (White China Clay)

Its functions are:-
- It increases the mouldability of the plastic porcelain
- Acts as a binder and helps in maintaining the shape of the unfired porcelain during firing.
- At high temparature, it fuses and reacts with other ingredients to form the glassy matrix.

Kaolin has properties of opaqueness even when present in very small quantities. It is the main drawback of Kaolin.

Feldspars

They have a crystalline structure and are opaque in nature with an indefinite color between gray and pink.

Natural feldspar mixed with quartz in the proportion of 75–85%, feldspar 12%, quartz 22% and upto 4% of Kaolin was commonly used in dental porcelain until the advent of 'fluxed glasses'. The larger the proportion of feldspar, greater the translucency and glass like appearance of the resultant ceramic material. Feldspar is of two types 1) Soda feldspar 2) Potash feldspar. Soda feldspar decreases the fusion temperature and potash feldspar increases the viscosity of glass. The type of feldspar used can effect the coefficient of thermal expansion (mainly soda spar); thus, low or medium fusing dental poercelain can be formulated by the appropriate addition of balancing oxides.

Role of Feldspar

- *Glass phase formation:* During firing, the feldspar fuses and forms a glassy phase that softens and flows slightly allowing the porcelain powder particles to coalesce together. The glassy phase forms a translucent glassy matrix between the other components in the dense solid.
- *Leucite formation:* Another important property of feldspar is its tendency to form the crystalline mineral leucite when melted, which is exploited to advantage in the manufacture of porcelain suitable for metal bonding.

Leucite

Is a potassium-aluminum-silicate mineral with a large coefficient of thermal expansion ($20–25 \times 10^{-6}/°C$) compared to feldspathic glasses ($10 \times 10^{-6}/°C$). It is an artificial crystal feldspathoid ($K_2O.Al_2O_3.4SiO_2$) formed by the incongruent melting (Incongruent melting is the process by which one material melts to form liquid plus a different crystalline material) of feldspar ($K_2O.Al_2O_3.Al_2O_3–4SiO_2$). In most dental porcelains, the leucite crystals are created by transforming feldspar crystals into glass and leucite crystals (precipitate) by a special heat treatment. When feldspar is heated at a temperature between 1150°C and 6530°C, it undergoes incongruent melting to form crystals of leucite in liquid glass. The leucite forms a refractory skeleton and the glass fills the spaces in between adding special qualities required for dental porcelain.

Feldspar Crystals $\xrightarrow{\text{Special heat treatment}}$ Glass & Leucite Crystal

Functions of Leucite

- To raise the coefficient of thermal expansion (CTE) of porcelain and bring it closer to that of the metal substrate; consequently increasing the hardness and fusion temperature. Leucite is a high expansion (or high contraction) crystal phase whose volume fraction in the glass matrix can greatly affect the CTE of porcelain. Adding leucite (35–40%) to porcelain creates a high expansion porcelain to match thermal expansion of the alloys used in dentistry (crown and bridges) preventing a thermal mismatch, which could lower the strength.
- Strengthening of porcelain in high strength ceramics, e.g. Optec HSP, Cerinate, & IPS Empress. High Leucite percentage results in an increase in CTE, hardness, fusion temperature, abrasive effect, and strength possibly due to stress being developed at the glass crystal interface during cooling.

Glass Formers

Glass is basically composed of silica (SiO_2) with oxides of Sodium, Potassium, Calcium, Barium etc. The principal anion in all glasses is O_2 ion, which forms very stable bonds with small multivalent cations such as Silicon, Boron, Germanium or Phosphorus resulting in formation of random networks of SiO_4 tetrahedrals in glass. These ions are thus termed as Glass Formers. The essential component that allows the formation of glass is silica, thus it is also called the network former. Oxides of Titanium, Zinc, Lead and Aluminum can all take part in the formation of the glass network and produce stiff network structures. However, for dental purposes only two glass forming oxides – Silicon and Boron oxides are used to form the principle network (B_2O_3 can form Boron Glasses). Although not on its own, under certain circumstances Alumina (Al_2O_3), may also be regarded as a glass network forming oxide (when used in conjunction with other oxides); for this reason it is termed a Glassy intermediate.

Devitrification

'Vitrification' in ceramic terms is the development of a liquid phase by reaction of melting, which on cooling provides the glassy phase, resulting in a vitreous structure. However, a small amount of crystallization always occurs during glass formation, although the rate of crystal growth is very low. When a glass begins to crystallize, the process is called **Devitrification**. It may occur when the glass is held at an elevated temperature in the molten form for a long time, allowing some reorganisation of the molecules. The glass tends to take on a translucent appearance due to the scattering of light from the surfaces of the newly formed small crystals. This is the basis of the formation of 'glass-ceramics'

Alkalis such as soda (Na_2O) and lime (CaO) lower the viscosity, and thus the glass transition temperature, considerably, by causing extensive disruption of SiO_4 tetrahedral network. This slows the production of glass and when too many of the glass forming SiO_4 tetrahedrals are disrupted, the glass may crystallize or devitrify. Devitrification is often associated with high expansion glasses, (used in metal-ceramics) since the usual way of increasing the thermal expansion of a glass is by introducing more alkalis, particularly soda. Devitrification may be seen when cloudiness develops in dental porcelain and this can be accentuated by repeated firing. Once the porcelain has devitrified, it becomes increasingly difficult to form a glaze surface. In contrast to high expansion glasses, the regular or aluminous porcelains are less susceptible to devitrification due to their higher silica to alkali ratio, lower soda content (Low thermal expansion) and their high combined alumina content which tends to neutralize the effect of excessive quantities of Na^+ ion.

Glass Modifiers

They can be defined as elements that interfere with the integrity of the SiO_2 (glass) network and alter their three-dimensional state. Their functions are:

- To decrease the softening point
- Decrease the viscosity (flux action increasing the flow)

The main purpose of a flux is principally to lower the softening temperature of a glass by reducing the amount of cross-linking between the oxygen and glass forming elements, e.g. Alkali metal ions such as Na, K or Ca (usually as carbonates) [Fig. 20.1]. However, higher concentration of glass modifiers could result in reduced chemical durability (resistance to attack by water, acids and alkalis) and devitrification due to disruption of too many tetrahedral networks (crystallization occurs when the modifiers act as nucleating agents for the process of crystal growth). Manufacturers employ glass modifiers to produce dental porcelains with different firing temperature such as high medium and low fusing ceramics.

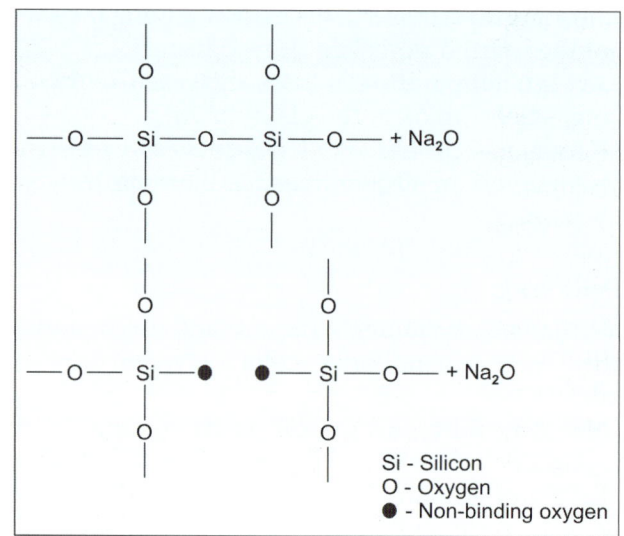

Fig. 20.1: Diagram showing interruption of silica tetrahedra by sodium oxide

Intermediate oxides: Addition of glass modifiers to reduce the softening point also decreases the viscosity, resulting in slump or pyroplastic flow; hence it is necessary to produce glasses with high viscosity as well as low firing temperature. This can be done by the incorporation of an intermediate oxide such as alumina (Al_2O_3), to increase hardness and viscosity of glass.

Boric oxide fluxes: Boric Oxide (B_2O_3) although a powerful flux (glass modifier), it can also act as a glass former and form its own glass network, producing Boron Glasses. When added to a glass, it forms a separate lattice interspersed with the silica lattice, resulting a structure, that is a three-dimensional continuous network of strong SiO_4 tetrahedral and BO_3 triangles. An additional oxygen atom results in formation of strong BO_4 tetrahedral, which is low expansion, more stable glass with good chemical resistance. Hence, Boric oxide is used in quantities of about 12%, above which the less stable form BO_3 takes over. (This phenomenon is termed as *boron anomaly*).

Water: Although not an intentional addition, water is an important glass modifier. The hydronium ion, H_3O^+ can replace Na^+ or other metal ions in a ceramic that contains glass modifiers. This replacement is responsible for the phenomenon of "slow crack growth" of ceramics that are exposed to tensile stresses and stored in moist environment. It may also account for the occasional long-term failure of porcelain restorations after several years of service.

COLORING AND OPACIFYING DENTAL PORCELAIN

The greatest color problem encountered, with porcelain if not colored is the slightly greenish hue exhibited by all glasses. In addition, some porcelains assume a greenish hue after firing, and this inherent greenness can be further accentuated by overfiring (over-vitrification). In order to dampen down this effect and produce life-like dentin and enamel colors; the basic dental porcelain frit must be colored. Dental porcelains colored by the addition of concentrated color frits which are prepared by fritting high-temperature resistant coloring pigments (generally metallic oxides) into the basic glass. The glass thus obtained will be highly color saturated and when ground to a fine powder, can be used in small amounts to modify the uncolored porcelain powder. The color pigments used are:

Color pigments	Metal oxides
Pink	Chromium or chrome-alumina
Yellow	Indium or praseodymium
Blue	Cobalt salts in the form of oxides
Green	Chromium oxide, Copper oxide
Grey	Platinum grey
Lavender	Manganese oxide
Black	Iron oxide
Brown	Iron/nickel oxide

Opacifying Agents

The translucency of porcelain is not suitable to produce dentin colors in particular, which requires greater opacity than that of enamel colors. An opacifying agent may be incorporated, which generally consists of a metal oxide.

The common metallic oxides used are –
- Cerium oxide,
- Titanium oxide,
- Tin oxide, and
- Zirconium oxide (ZrO_2)- most popularly used opacifying agent (usually added with the concentrated color frit to the porcelain during final preparation).

Stains & Color Modifiers

The stains and color modifiers supplied with dental porcelain are prepared in much the same way as color frits.

Stain is a mixture of one or more pigmented metal oxides, and usually composed of a low fusing glass that when dispersed in an aqueous slurry or monomer medium applied to surface of porcelain or other specialized ceramic, dried or light cured, and fired will modify the shade of the ceramic-based restoration. These stain products are also called as *surface colorants or characterization porcelain* (Fig. 20.2).

Internal staining: One method for ensuring that the applied characterizing stains will be permanent is to use them internally. Internal staining and characterization can produce a very life-like result, when built into porcelain rather than when it is merely applied to the surface. However, if unsuitable the porcelain has to be stripped completely.

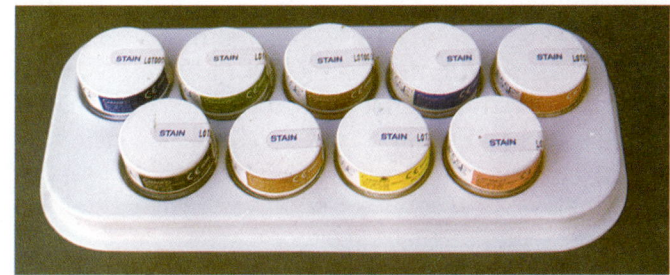

Fig. 20.2: Stains used to imitate markings like enamel craze lines, calcification spots, fluoresced areas etc.

Color modifiers – are used to obtain gingival effects or to highlight body colors at the same temperature as the dental porcelain (Fig. 20.3).

Special Effects in Dental Porcelain

Human teeth vary considerably in texture, color and form. In order to duplicate a natural tooth, the structural defects, degrees of calcification and varying thickness in enamel should be reproduced in the porcelain build up. 'Special effects' in dental porcelain are created with the use of supplementary colors of the basic dentin porcelain, translucent or colorless porcelain and color frits.

Translucency

It is the property of a material that allows the passage and scattering of transmitted light. In dental porcelain it refers to the ability to accurately simulate the surface structure and lifelike appearance of natural teeth.

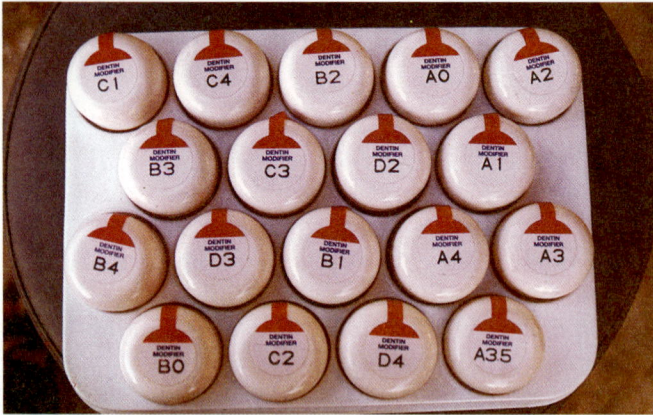

Fig. 20.3: Color modifiers used to obtain gingival effects or highlight body colors.

Fluorescence

It is the absorption of radiation of a particular wavelength and its re-emission as a radiation of longer wavelength. Fluorescence adds definite contribution to the brightness and the vital appearance of a human tooth.

The production of fluorescence in dental porcelains has assumed greater prominence in recent years due to the use of lamps, which emit the blue end of the spectrum, in addition to some U-V radiation. When a non-fluorescent material is used it tends to exhibit a grayish appearance and will appear as a black hole when seen under ultraviolet or 'black-light' illumination such as that commonly used in nightclubs.

Fluorescing agents
- Cerium oxide produced a bluish-white fluorescence,
- Spinels (Magnesia alumina compounds)
- Lanthanide Earths

Opalescence

Opalescence in dental porcelains is a light – scattering effect achieved with the addition of minute concentrations of oxides with high refractive index, in a size range near the wavelength of visible light. Teeth display some opalescence, and incorporation of this effect in dental ceramic restorations can provide an additional subtle vitality in concert with natural translucency, hue, value, chroma and surface texture. But excessive use of opalescent materials can lead to a bluish-grey appearance of the restoration.

Glazes & Add-On Porcelain

Glazes are low fusing uncolored glass powders that are applied on the surface of a porcelain restoration and fired at a maturing temperature lower than that of the restoration to produce a transparent glossy layer on the surface. They are also referred to as *Overglazes or Applied glazes*. The purpose of glazing is:

- To seal the open pores on the surface of a fired porcelain.
- To impart an impervious smooth surface and develop greater translucency in the porcelain restoration.

Self glaze: After all the constituents of the porcelain frit have completely melted to form a single phase glass, the porcelain is further heated to reach glazing point at which the surface becomes plastic and flows to form a shiny continuous surface. This property is known, as Self-glazing and dental porcelain can be easily self glazed, by careful control of temperature cycle during firing. Self-glazing is exhibited by all porcelains except those containing high quantity of strengthening agents such as alumina or opaquing materials.

Add-on porcelain: These are generally made from materials similar to that of glaze porcelain except for the addition of less finely ground powder of opacifying and coloring pigments. These are used sparingly for repairs, addition and simple corrections to tooth contour or contact points.

ADDITIVES IN DENTAL PORCELAIN

Alumina

Refers to aluminium oxide (Al_2O_3) one of hardest and probably the strongest oxides of aluminium known, prepared from alumina trihydrate by calcination.

$$\text{Alumina Trihydrate} \xrightarrow{600°C} \lambda-\text{alumina} \xrightarrow{1250°C} \alpha-\text{alumina}$$

(The α-form of alumina is used in ceramic applications as a fine powder in some dental porcelains such as aluminous porcelain).

Types of alumina used: Calcined alumina (α type), Fused alumina and Alumina whiskers.

Alternative Additives in Dental Porcelain

During fritting, small quantitites of alternative modifying agents can be added to dental porcelains.
- Lithium oxide (LiO_2) – as an additional fluxing agent
- Magnesium oxide (MgO) – used in minute quantities to replace CaO.
- Phosphate pentoxide (P_2O_5) – sometimes added to induced opalescence and is also a glass forming oxide.

PROPERTIES OF PORCELAIN

The different properties of porcelain have been cited in Table 20.1.

The compressive strength of porcelain is quite high compared to the porcelain's tensile or shear strength.

Dental Ceramics

Table 20.1: Different properties of porcelain

Properties	Values
Compressive strength	50000 psi
Tensile strength	5000 psi
Shear strength	16000 psi
Elastic modulus	10×10^6 psi
Knoop Hardness Number	460
Linear coefficient of thermal expansion	$12 \times 10^{-6}/°C$
Thermal conductivity	$0.0050°C/cm$
Diffusivity	$0.64\ mm^2/sec$
Specific gravity	2.2–2.3
Linear shrinkage - High fusing	11.5%
Linear shrinkage - Low fusing	14.0%
Refractive Index	1.52–1.54

The tensile strength is low because of the unavoidable surface defects and the shear strength is low because of the lack of ductility in the material. Voids and blebs greatly reduce the strength of porcelain. Both underfiring and overfiring are also deleterious to its strength. When porcelain is underfired, i.e. firing done at temperatures lower than normal or for inadequate periods, the desired amount of vitrification does not occur; whereas when overfired, i.e. firing done at temperatures above normal or for longer periods, excessive vitrification is seen.

Blebs or internal voids tend to reduce the specific gravity of porcelain. The true value of specific gravity is approximately 2.4 but the apparent value is reduced to 2.2 to 2.3.

Porcelains are extremely hard materials and because of this property offer considerable resistance to abrasion. This could be a disadvantage in that it causes excessive wear of the opposing natural tooth structure or the restorative material.

One major drawback with porcelain is its brittleness. Dental ceramic is inherently fragile in tension, and the susceptibility to fracture is most common because of stress concentration areas like cracks, voids, defects etc. Unlike ductile materials which can dissipate stresses by slip and plastic deformation, brittle materials like ceramic have only a very limited capacity for distributing localized stresses. The critical strain of dental ceramic is low and the material can withstand a deformation of only 0.1% before fracture. Failure (fracture) intraorally occurs by a combination of bending and torsional forces.

Life like translucency is another critical property of dental porcelain. Opaque, body and incisal porcelains differ considerably in their translucencies. Opaque porcelain has a very low translucency needed to mask the color of the underlying metal. Body porcelain has a translucency from 20–35%, whereas incisal porcelain has the highest translucency ranging from 45–50%. In order to match the fluorescence of porcelain to that of enamel, oxides such as uranium oxide or cerium oxide are added.

Porcelain is relatively inert, chemically stable and corrosion resistant which renders it highly biocompatible. Its ability to attain highly smooth and polished surfaces does not allow plaque accumulation and hence is conducive to gingival health. The response of the pulp to these restorations is largely determined by the intervening cementing medium. The solubility of dental porcelain is extremely low and is probably the most resistant material to attack by oral fluids.

STRENGTHENING DENTAL PORCELAIN

Dental ceramic is a brittle material and its strength is largely dictated by the presence of flaws inside it. Both the number and severity of flaws are important determinants. These flaws act as *'stress concentration areas'* such that localized stress at a particular point causes inter atomic bonds to be broken and a crack to be initiated. Once the crack starts propagating, the concentration of stresses continues to exist at the tip until it travels completely through the material or meets another flaw or a crystalline particle. Regarding stress concentration around flaws, tensile stresses are more damaging than the compressive stresses. The latter tend to close the crack.

Flaws of greatest importance are ones which are located in surface areas and are in the range of 100 μm in diameter. Surface flaws have higher stress concentrated around them than do the internal flaws of similar dimensions. Microcracks, one of the commonly seen flaws on the porcelain surface, may be a result of condensation, melting and sintering process, cooling of ceramic after maturing, high contact angle of ceramic on metal, differences in the coefficient of thermal expansion between alloy/core and veneers, grinding and abrasion, tensile stresses generated during manufacture, function and trauma etc. Other areas of high stress concentration are:

a. Porosity, roughness and machining damage.
b. Sharp line and point angles.
c. The interface region of a bonded structure where the elastic modulus of the two components is quite different. Ideally, the more brittle material should have a lower elastic modulus so that stresses are transferred to the one which has a higher modulus of elasticity.
d. The interface region of a bonded structure where a large difference in the thermal coefficient exists between the two materials. Ideally, the two coefficients should match. If this is not possible, the weaker and more brittle material should have a lower thermal coefficient so that a

protective compressive stress is generated in the structure next to the interface.

e. Areas of sharp point contacts on the brittle material. Roundening of the opposing cusp tips is hence advocated so that the occlusal contacts are large areas.

Effect of moisture contamination: Another factor that weakens the ceramic is the water produces a time dependent reduction in strength. This can be explained by a process in which the alkali ions are replaced by hydrogen ions, which attract water molecules into the spaces originally occupied by the alkali. Water hence serves as a network modifier in weakening the glass.

Measures to Strengthen Dental Porcelain

Methods employed to overcome the brittleness of porcelain fall into two main categories (1) *strengthening the material* (2) *designing components such that stress concentration and tensile stresses are minimized*. As noted by now, flaws are a major contributor in reducing the strength of the ceramic. Hence the best efforts should be directed in reducing the size and number of flaws. Surface flaws can be reduced in depth by fine polishing and glazing however little can be done for the internal flaws.

Strengthening the Material

Methods used for strengthening dental porcelain are based on the following mechanisms:

- Development of residual compressive stresses
  - ❏ Ion exchange (Chemical tempering)
  - ❏ Thermal tempering
  - ❏ Thermal compatibility (Thermal expansion coefficient mismatch)
- Interruption of crack propagation
  - ❏ Dispersion of crystalline phase
  - ❏ Transformation toughening

Dispersion strengthening with second phase crystals was used in Dicor, Cerapearl, Cerestore introduced in the 1980's, but have been restricted in their use in fabrication of Porcelain Jacket Crown due to the following drawbacks – Expensive equipment and materials, High laboratory fees, not strong enough for Fixed Partial Denture, Drawbacks of dispersion, Technique sensitivity, and High fracture/failure rates.

Designing the Dental Prosthesis

Any prosthesis requiring ceramic should be designed such that direct exposure to high tensile stresses, stress concentration at sharp line angles and point angles or marked changes in thickness are avoided. Full coverage of posterior teeth with conventional porcelain jacket crowns is contraindicated because heavy occlusal forces can concentrate large tensile stresses on the internal surface of the crown. Tensile stresses may also develop under a porcelain jacket crown in the anterior teeth where there is deep bite with minimal overjet.

All areas of stress concentration should be minimized in the restoration. Sudden or large changes in the shape or thickness of ceramic can create areas of stress concentration and so can the sharp line angles and point angles. A platinum foil when used as a substrate for the fabrication of porcelain jacket crown, if inadvertently gets folded and the fold is embedded in the porcelain, it could leave a notch in the final restoration, which could serve as a stress raiser. A stray particle on the internal surface of a porcelain restoration could greatly increase the tensile stress concentration, when the restoration is being seated. In any porcelain restoration, occlusion should include contact areas and not contact points.

CONDENSATION OF DENTAL PORCELAIN

Porcelain powder is mixed with a liquid binder so that the particles are held together, and the thick creamy paste can be worked and built to the desired shape. *The process of bringing the particles closer and of removing the liquid binder is known as condensation.* Distilled water is the liquid binder used most commonly. However, glycerine, propylene glycol or alcohol have also been tried. The liquid because of its surface tension property serves as the binder. During subsequent firing it is eliminated, and the porcelain particles fill the space formerly occupied by the binder, thereby resulting in shrinkage.

The aim of condensation is to pack the particles as close as possible, in order to reduce the amount of porosity and shrinkage during firing. Two important factors, which determine the effectiveness of condensation are the size and shape of the powder particles. If only one sized particles are used, even the greatest condensation is expected to leave a void space of 45 percent between the particles. With two sized particles, the void space is reduced to 25 percent, and with three or more sized particles, the void space comes down to 22 percent. System that uses three sizes of powder is known as the *gap grading system*. In addition, the shape of the powder particles also governs the packing density. Round particles produce better packing compared with angular particles. The most important factor in condensation is the effect of surface tension. As the liquid is withdrawn, surface tension causes the powder particles to pack closely together. However, sufficient amount of liquid should be present so as to wet all of the powder particles.

Several methods of condensation are employed (1) In the *vibration method*, the paste is applied on to the platinum matrix and vibrated slowly. This brings the excess water on to the surface, which is then drawn away with a linen or clean tissue. Excessive vibration should be avoided as it can cause slumping of the mass. (2) In the *spatulation method*, a small spatula is used to apply and smooth the wet porcelain. The smoothening action disturbs the particles bringing them closer and also the water rises to the surface, which is removed as described earlier. (3) *Dry brush technique* involves placement of dry powder onto the wet surface. The excess water moves from mixture to the dry powder by capillary action and the wet particles are pulled together. (4) In the *whipping method*, a large soft brush is moved in a light dusting action over the wet porcelain. This brings excess water to the surface, and the same brush can be used to remove any coarse surface particles along with the excess water. A combination of the vibration and the whipping methods can also be used. The mix is first vibrated and then whipped with a brush.

FIRING PROCEDURE

Most of the thermochemical reactions in porcelain are completed during the manufacturing process. The role of firing is simply to sinter the particles of porcelain powder together to form a dense restoration. Some chemical reaction may however occur during prolonged firing or multiple firings, like the formation of leucite crystals in porcelain. During firing, the following changes are seen in the porcelain. The first change involves the loss of water, which was added to the powder to form a workable mass. The excess water is partially removed by slightly warming the mix before it is placed in the preheated furnace. This prevents the sudden production of steam that could result in voids or fractures. After the mass is placed in a furnace, both the free and combined water are lost until a temperature of 480°C is reached. The second change occurs with a further rise in temperature, when the particles fuse together by sintering. As a continuous mass is formed, there occurs a decrease in volume referred to as firing shrinkage (32–37% for low fusing and 28–34% for high fusing). The third change seen is glazing which occurs at temperatures of 955–1065°C. Glazing results in the formation of a glossy surface. After the mass has been fired, it is cooled very slowly because rapid cooling might result in surface cracking and crazing.

Porcelain restorations may be fired either by the *temperature method* or the *temperature-time method*. In the former, the furnace temperature is raised at a constant rate until a specific temperature is reached. In the latter, the temperature is raised at a given rate until certain levels are reached, after which the temperature is maintained for a measured period of time until the desired reactions are completed. Different media can be employed for firing like:
   a. Air
   b. Vacuum
   c. Diffusible gas

Air Firing Procedure

All porcelain powder mixes have a certain amount of porosity present in them. When these porcelains are placed in the air furnace, the furnace atmosphere occupies these void spaces. Once the softening of glass begins, the grains of porcelain start lensing at their contact points. Surface tension causes some of the porosity to be swept out via the grain boundaries, but some of it gets entrapped by the flowing ceramic around the air voids. With the increase in temperature, the void spaces containing air assume a spherical appearance under the influence of surface tension. Still further rise in temperature increases the pressure of the entrapped air and the bubbles enlarge. Cooling decreases the pressure and hence the size of the bubble. The surface of air fired porcelain is generally devoid of bubbles because interstitial air near the surface can escape easily. Whenever air firing methods are employed, a very slow maturation period is preferred to allow for the maximum amount of entrapped air to escape. The porcelain should not be exposed to its full maturing temperature and it is advisable to stay 30°C to 50°C below the maximum firing temperature.

Porosity

Bubbles or voids in the fired porcelain are caused by inclusion of air during firing or in some cases as a byproduct of vitrification of feldspar. Porosity reduces both translucency and strength of dental porcelain. Translucency depends on the number and size of the entrapped air bubbles. Large sized particles have fewer but larger air voids between them compared to small sized particles. Fewer bubbles, even of large size, give improved translucency. On the other hand, fine sized particles have multiple small air bubbles present in between them, which makes them highly opaque. Therefore porcelain powders fired in air should preferably be of necessarily coarse nature.

Vacuum Firing

This technique is used to reduce porosity in dental porcelains. It works on the basis of removing air or atmosphere from the interstitial spaces before surface sealing occurs. Although the vacuum (760 torr) removes most of the air from interstitial spaces, some of it is left behind. With the increase in temperature and because of surface tension, the remaining air spaces assume a spherical appearance. When air at normal atmospheric pressure is allowed to enter the furnace, it exerts a compressive effect on the surface skin, which further compresses the internal voids to one tenth of their original size. This results in a very dense porcelain with very few remaining bubbles and that too of extremely small size.

Factors to be kept in mind while firing porcelain in vacuum are:

1. Porcelain powders must be dried slowly to eliminate the water vapours, and vacuum should be applied before the placement of porcelain in the hot zone of furnace. The interstitial spaces are hence reduced before the surface skin seals off the interior too rapidly.
2. Vacuum should not be applied after the surface skin has sealed and the porcelain has matured. Prolonged application can force the residual air bubbles to rise to the surface and cause surface blistering. Additionally, high temperatures can cause swelling of these blisters.
3. The vacuum should be broken while the work is still in the hot zone of the furnace. This permits the dense skin to hydraulically compress the low pressure internal voids.
4. Vacuum firing cannot reduce the large sized bubbles to any significant degree. Hence, it is necessary to avoid porcelains with large interstitial spaces, i.e. porcelain powders with small sized particles are preferred.

Diffusible Gas Firing

In this technique, a diffusible gas like helium, hydrogen or steam is substituted for the ordinary furnace atmosphere. Air is driven out of the porcelain powder bed and replaced by the diffusible gas. With these gases, the interstitial spaces do not enlarge under the influence of increasing temperature, but decrease in size or disappear. This occurs because these gases diffuse outward through the porcelain or actually dissolve in porcelain.

Various Stages of Maturity

Several stages of dental porcelain have been identified when it is 'sintered' or 'fired'. The common terminology used for describing the surface appearance of an unglazed porcelain is 'bisque'.

Low bisque: The surface of porcelain is quite porous. The grains of porcelain begin to soften and 'lense' at their contact points. Shrinkage is minimal and the fired body is extremely weak or friable.

Medium bisque: Pores still exist on the surface of porcelain, but the flow of glass grains is increased. As a result, any entrapped furnace atmosphere that could not escape via the grain boundaries becomes trapped and sphere shaped. A definite shrinkage is evident.

High bisque: The flow of glass grains is further increased, thereby completely sealing the surface and presenting a smoothness to the porcelain. In the case of non-feldspathic porcelains, a slight shine appears at this stage. The fired body is strong and any corrections by grinding can be made prior to final glazing at this stage.

ALL CERAMIC SYSTEMS

Porcelain is the most natural appearing synthetic replacement material for missing tooth substance, available in an extensive range of shades and translucencies for achieving life-like results. However, its esthetic appearance was compromised when it was fused to a metal substrate in an effort to strengthen porcelain (due to the relatively low tensile strength and brittleness of porcelain). In addition some patients have allergic reactions or sensitivity to various metals. These drawbacks together with the material and labor costs associated with metal substrate fabrication have prompted the development of new all ceramic system that do not require metal, yet have the high strength and precision fit of ceramo-metal systems.

The term *"All-Ceramic"* refers to – *Any restorative material composed exclusively of ceramic, such as feldspathic porcelain, glass-ceramic, alumina core systems and certain combination of these materials.*

Compared to Metal-ceramics, the advantages of All-ceramic restorations include:
- Increased translucency
- Improved fluorescence
- Greater contribution of color from the underlying tooth structure
- Inertness
- Bio-compatibility
- Resistance to corrosion
- Low temperature / electrical conductivity

Newer types of all-ceramic restorations developed may prove to have a lower incidence of clinical fracture for 3 important reasons:
- All-ceramic restorations today consist of stronger materials and involve better fabricating techniques
- Most all-ceramic restorations can be etched and bonded to the underyling tooth structure with the new dentin adhesives

- With greater tooth reduction than what was previously used for PJC's, clinicians now provide laboratory technicians with enough room to create thicker and stronger restorations.

Various all ceramic restorations based on their fabrication process are classified as follows:

1. Conventional powder slurry ceramic
   - Hi-Ceram – Alumina reinforced porcelain
   - Optec HSP – Leucite reinforced porcelain
   - Duceram LFC – Hydrothermal low fusing ceramic
2. Pressable ceramic
   - IPS Empress
   - Optec pressable ceramic
3. Infiltrated ceramic
   - In-ceram
4. Castable ceramic
   - Dicor
5. Machinable ceramic
   - Cerec Vitablocs Mark I and Mark II
   - Celay blocks
   - Dicor MGC

A brief comparison of these materials is given in Table 20.2.

Aluminous Porcelain (Hi Ceram)

High strength alumina reinforced feldspathic porcelains were introduced by *Mclean and Hughes* in 1965[42]. These are based on the principle of dispersion strengthening, i.e. dispersing *alumina* (Al_2O_3) crystals of high strength and elasticity in a glass matrix. A cored structure is formed that has an increased flexural strength, elasticity and fracture toughness compared to conventional porcelains. High strength crystalline alumina particles serve as a reinforcing phase which is able to bear majority of the load applied onto the ceramic body. For dental purposes, single crystals of alumina are preferred over fine powdered alumina. This is to avoid excessive opacity which occurs because of the difference in the refractive indices of the glassy porcelain and the alumina crystals. Two important requirements when using these filler reinforced porcelains are: (1) a bond between filler particles and the matrix and (2) an identical coefficient of thermal expansion (CTE) of the two phases. If there occurs a mismatch between the coefficient of thermal expansion of the two phases, e.g. the glass matrix having a coefficient of thermal expansion higher than the alumina crystals, there would occur a radial compression and tangential tension in the glass matrix on cooling, resulting in markedly reduced elasticity and strength (Fig. 20.4). Alumina has a coefficient of thermal expansion in the range of 6.4 to 7.8 × 10^{-6}/°C.

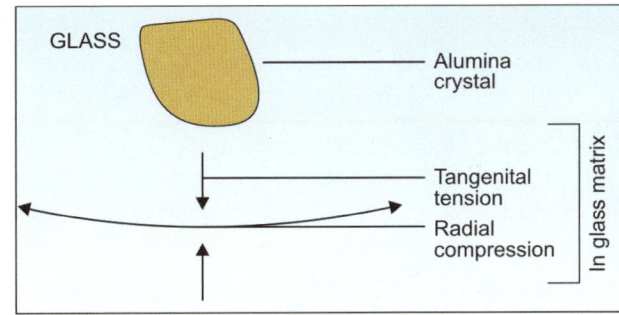

Fig. 20.4: Diagram showing development of radial compression and tangential tension in glass when coefficient of thermal expansion of glass matrix is higher than that of alumina crystals.

The glass used for incorporating alumina crystals is generally borosilicate glass containing silica (62.0–65.0 wt%), alumina (17.0–20.0 wt%), potash (6.5–7.7 wt%), soda (4.2–4.7 wt%), lime (1.6–1.8 wt%) and boric oxide (6.7–7.3 wt%).

The strength and opacity of aluminous porcelain is dependent upon the size, shape and concentration of the alumina crystals. Finer the grain size, greater is the strength; but at the same time there occurs an increased opacity due to the high difference in the refractive index of the two components, which causes increased scattering of light. Very opaque porcelains are not desirable as they would increase the amount of light reflected, defeating the esthetic appearance of the translucent porcelains, which are used as veneers. Coarse grains of alumina on the other hand reduce strength because of the 'notched effect' created on the grain boundaries. These however show increased transmission of light and are less opaque. Hence, it can be understood that there exists a compromise between the strength and opacity of the material. For this reason, grain size on an average should be 25 μms (maximum being 37 μms), that would allow light transmission of atleast 10–15% on 1 mm thick discs and be fine enough to give sufficient strengths. The size range of glass powder is also important (<40 μms), as this sized powder softens and flows more easily around the alumina grains producing high sintered densities. Filler shapes also influence the strength. Rounded grains are preferable over angular ones as the latter interfere with the flow of the glass phase producing flaws around the grains and reducing strength. The concentration of alumina crystals should range from 40–50% by weight. Concentrations higher than this would prevent complete flow and wetting by the glass matrix. This would result in a weak interface between the filler and the matrix. Any crack would then be deviated along the crystal boundary rather than through the crystals, which have been incorporated for bearing stress.

Table 20.2: Comparison of ceramic restorative systems

Product Name	Flexural strength	Abrasiveness vs. natural tooth Hardness	Special equipment needed	Other characteristics
Traditional powder-slurry ceramic				
Optec HSP (Jeneric/Pentron)	146 MPa	Higher than that of conventional feldspathic porcelain due to high leucite content	Special die material	No core material; uniform translucency and shade throughout; etchable for bonding to tooth
Duceram LFC (Degussa)	110 MPa	Close to hardness of natural tooth owing to absence of leucite	Special die material	Low fusing temperature; can be characterized by surface stains
Castable ceramic				
Dicor (Dentsply, L.D. Caulk Division)	152 MPa	Same as that of tooth and softer than conventional feldspathic porcelain; Dicor Plus is however as hard as conventional feldspathic	Special investment and casting equipment	Dicor has reported less plaque accumulation compared to other ceramic restorations; because of the lost wax casting procedure anatomy can be very precise; porcelain etchable core for bonding, surfacestains (esthetics) can be lost to abrasion or acidulated fluoride (Dicor Plus is more stable)
Machinable ceramic				
Cerec Vitablocs Mark I (Vident)	93 MPa	Similar to that of conventional feldspathic porcelain	Siemens; milling of a ceramic ingot from a digitized optical scan	Can be characterized with surface stains; however they may be lost to abrasion.
Cerec Vitablocs Mark II (Vident)	152 MPa	Similar to that of enamel	Same as above	The gap between the restoration and tooth is wider than that in all other ceramic systems
Dicor MGC (Dentsply L.D. Caulk Div.)	216 MPa	Between those of Cerec Vitablocs Mark I and Mark II	Same as above	Wear of the resin cement may have a clinical significance
Celay (Vident)	152 MPa	Similar to that of enamel	Celay copy milling system; milling of a ceramic ingot from a direct pattern	Etchable for bonding to tooth structure
Pressable ceramic				
IPS Empress (Ivoclar North America)	126 MPa initially; 160–182 MPa after heat treatment	Possibly higher than that of conventional feldspathic porcelain owing to increased leucite content after	Special oven, die material and moulding procedure	Core material is shaded and translucent; etchable for bonding to tooth
Optec Pressable Ceramic (Jeneric/Pentron)	165 MPa	Same as above	Same as above	Same as above
Infilterated ceramic				
In-ceram (Vident)	450 MPa	Same as that of conventional feldspathic porcelain	Special die material, high temperature oven	Core material is more opaque than other types; not etchable for bonding to tooth

In case of aluminous porcelains, when the alumina crystals are more than 50% by weight, densities can be improved by pre-fritting the alumina crystals and glass powder at 1200°C and then regrinding the crystal-glass composite to be incorporated into the glass matrix. This process allows thorough wetting by the glass and strong chemical bond formation despite the high percentage of alumina bodies. Unfortunately, these are very opaque and their use is limited to construction of lingual reinforcements or all ceramic bridge substructures. Commercially, a product based on this is Hi-Ceram (Vita).

Alumina crystals increase the strength by two mechanisms (1) crystals reduce surface area of the matrix where microcracks might form (2) crystals increase fracture resistance in body porcelain.

Properties	
Compressive strength	3,16,000 psi
Transverse strength	20,000 psi
Shear Strength	21,000 psi
Modulus of rupture	15,000 psi

Uses
Because of reduced translucency, aluminous porcelain is limited to forming a refractory framework capable of supporting weaker, more translucent dentin and enamel porcelains.

Leucite Reinforced Porcelain (Optec HSP)

Leucite porcelain, is commercially available as Optec HSP. These porcelains contain dispersed *leucite* [potassium alumino silicate ($KAlSi_2O_6$) crystals] in a glassy matrix. Earlier, leucite was added to the feldspathic porcelain compositions to match the thermal contraction of the ceramic to the metal when cooled. However, later they began serving as reinforcing fillers because of their very high tensile strength. This rendered leucite reinforced porcelains to be stronger compared to conventional feldspathic porcelains. The leucite and glassy components are fused together during the baking process at 1020°C. The buildup, condensation and contouring is done using the powder slurry technique on a special semipermeable die material. Leucite concentration in Optec HSP has been reported to be 50.6 wt% which is appreciably greater that that of the IPS Empress Ceramic (23.6 wt% or 41.3 wt%). The leucite porcelains can be used for both the body and incisal portions as the esthetics provided by the leucite crystals does not necessitate the employment of a translucent porcelain. Surface stains or pigments can be applied to give the desired shade and translucency. To reduce mismatch between coefficients of thermal expansion, potassium ions in the leucite have been exchanged for rubidium or cesium ions.

Advantages
• Lack of metal or opaque substructure, good translucency.
• Moderate flexural strength, higher than conventional feldspathic porcelains.
• Ability to be used without special laboratory equipment.

Disadvantages
• Margin inaccuracy caused by porcelain sintering shrinkage
• Potential to fracture in posterior teeth
• Increased leucite content may cause relatively high in-vitro wear of opposing teeth.

Uses
Employed for inlays, onlays, crowns for low stress areas and veneers.

Duceram LFC

This is a relatively new category of restorative material, referred to as '*hydrothermal low fusing ceramic.*' It is composed of an amorphous glass containing hydroxyl ions. Properties claimed by the manufacturer for this noncrystalline material are greater density, higher flexural strength, greater fracture resistance and lower hardness than feldspathic porcelain. Because of the absence of leucite crystals, the hardness of the material and its ability to abrade the opposing natural tooth structure is reduced. However, there are no clinical studies to substantiate the manufacturer's claim that the material is less abrasive than feldspathic porcelain.

The restoration from Duceram LFC is made in two layers. The base layer is Duceram Metal Ceramic (a leucite containing porcelain), which is placed on a refractory die using the powder-slurry technique and then baked at 930°C. The second layer, which is Duceram LFC is applied over the base layer using powder-slurry technique and baked at 660°C. This material is available in a variety of shades and can be characterized with surface stains and modifiers. No special laboratory equipment or techniques are required for the fabrication process.

Uses
Can be employed for the fabrication of ceramic inlays, veneers and full contour crowns.

Injection Moulded Glass Ceramic/Leucite Reinforced Hot Pressed Glass Ceramic (Optec OPC)

This system was first described by Wohlwend, et al. in 1989[76] and became available commercially as IPS Empress and Optec OPC. The former is more popular of the two. The ceramic is primarily a precerammed glass reinforced with leucite, that prevents crack propagation without significantly diminishing its translucency. It is available in the form of ingots (Fig. 20.5). These ingots are heated and injected under pressure and temperature into a mold created by the lost wax technique to produce a restoration.

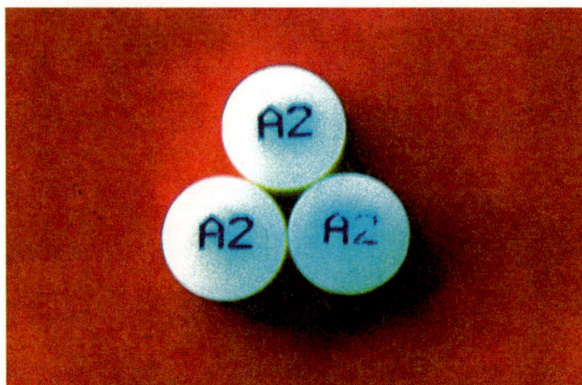

Fig. 20.5: IPS empress ingots

Fatigue parameter testing indicates this material to be less susceptible to fatigue failure than conventional feldspathic porcelain. However, it shows a lower compressive strength than metal ceramics or In-ceram restorations. Flexural strength is higher than Dicor and conventional porcelain, and improves under subsequent heat treatment as a result of growth of additional leucite crystals.

Advantages
• Lack of metal or opaque ceramic core
• Moderate flexural strength
• Excellent fit
• Excellent esthetics

Disadvantages
• Potential to fracture in posterior areas
• Need for special equipment (pressing oven and die material)

Uses
Indicated for single anterior crowns, inlays, onlays and veneers.

Infiltrable Ceramic/High Alumina Ceramic (In Ceram)

The strength of alumina reinforced porcelain is dependent upon the volume fraction of alumina present inside the glassy matrix. However, its incorporation is limited by the introduction of porosity. To overcome this disadvantage and simultaneously improve upon the strength, a system was introduced known as infilterable ceramic that utilized alumina as the core material.

Infiltrable ceramic is supplied as two components: a powder (aluminium oxide) which is fabricated into a porous substrate, and a low viscosity glass which is infilterated at high temperature into this three dimensional porous network. The fine grained alumina powder particles are mixed with water to form a suspension or slurry referred to as a 'slip'. This slip is painted onto an absorbent refractory die. The die draws water from the slurry thereby, depositing a layer of solid alumina on the surface, which is subsequently sintered at 1120°C for 10 hours to produce an opaque porous core. At this stage, careful handling is a must as the material is very fragile. Also during baking, the slip (aluminous core) undergoes a shrinkage, which should be compensated for by the expansion in die stone. In the second phase, glass infiltration material of appropriate shade is applied onto the core and fired at 1100°C for 3–5 hours. The molten glass infilterates into the residual pores by capillary action, and results in a dense composite structure, which has 20 times the strength of the core material. The final infilterated core has about 85% of the crystalline component which confers a three times increase in its flexural strength (450 MPa) compared to any other dental ceramic. The core is then veneered with dentin and enamel conventional feldspathic porcelains (Fig. 20.6) using the conventional powder-slurry technique. A compositional analysis has revealed alumina to be 99.56 wt% and the infilterated glass to be lanthanum aluminosilicate with small amounts of sodium and calcium. Lanthanum decreases the viscosity of the glass to assist infiltration and increases its index of refraction to improve the translucency of ceramic. One notable disadvantage with these high alumina ceramics is their high opacity, which limits their use to the construction of high strength substructures.

A further development in this system is the In-ceram Spinel, which uses a spinel instead of alumina. Spinel is a composition containing aluminum and magnesium oxide, $MgAl_2O_4$. Because of the lower refractive index of spinel compared to alumina, the translucency of ceramic is improved but has a comparatively lower flexural strength. The fabrication process is similar to In-ceram.

Dental Ceramics

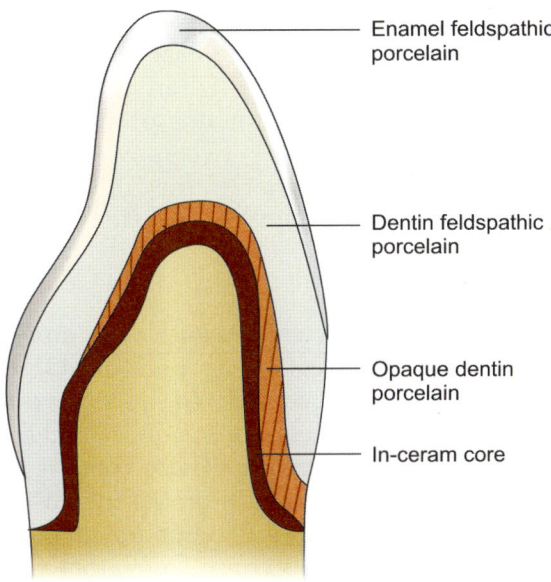

Fig. 20.6: In-ceram crown restoration

Properties

The densely packed alumina particles limit crack propagation, and glass infiltration eliminates residual porosity. Spinel strengthens the ceramic by deflecting the crack. Infilterable ceramic has an extremely high flexural strength of about 450 MPa. Tensile strength is 3–4 times greater than that for the other dental ceramics. The density of these ceramics is high hence the traditional etching of internal surface to improve its bond to tooth structure is not possible. Alternatives for improving its bond are sand blasting, silica coating or application of low fusing glazed powder on the internal surface. Marginal fit is similar to that of metal ceramic units.

Fabrication

In brief, the steps for fabricating an In-ceram prosthesis are as follows:
1. A heavy circumferential chamfer of >1.0 mm is prepared on the concerned tooth.
2. Make an impression and pour two dies or duplicate one die in refractory die material.
3. Apply Al_2O_3 on duplicate dye using the slip cast method as described before. Heat the die material at 120°C for 2 hours to dry the Al_2O_3.
4. Sinter coping for 10 hours at 1120°C.
5. Apply slurry of glass infiltration material.
6. Fire at 1100°C for 3–5 hours to allow the glass to melt and infilterate.
7. Trim any excess from coping with diamond burs.
8. Add dentin and enamel porcelain on the core.
9. Fire in the oven, grind in anatomy and occlusion, finish and glaze.

Advantages
a. Has the highest flexural strength amongst all ceramic systems
b. Excellent fit, comparable with metal ceramics

Disadvantages
a. Opacity of the material; hence can be used only as a core
b. Unsuitable for conventional acid etching

Uses
Indicated for both single unit anterior and posterior crowns and three unit bridges.

Castable Glass Ceramic (DICOR)

A glass ceramic is a material that is formed into the desired shape as a glass and subsequently heat treated under controlled conditions to induce partial devitrification or crystallization. This conversion process, which involves crystal nucleation and growth is referred to as 'ceramming' and is accompanied by a small and controlled volume change. The crystalline particles, needles or plates formed during the ceramming process constitute an interlocking network, which increases the strength of the material by interrupting crack propagation. The first description of DICOR castable ceramic was given by *Adair and Grossman* in 1984.

The glass ceramic material is composed of SiO_2, K_2O, MgO, MgF_2, minor amounts of Al_2O_3 and Z_rO_2 incorporated for durability, and a fluorescing agent for esthetics. The fluoride acts as a nucleating agent, and improves the fluidity of the molten glass. After ceramming, the material is approximately 55% crystalline and contains tetrasilicic fluoride crystals ($K_2Mg_5Si_8O_{20}Fl$), which closely resemble mica. The refractive index of these crystals is close to that of the surrounding glass matrix, helping to maintain translucency in the devitrified body. Mica crystals are achromatic and the desired shade in final restoration is developed by adding external colorants. The disadvantage behind the use of these colorant stains is that they may be lost during occlusal adjustment, during routine prophylaxis or through the use of acidulated fluoride gels.

The fabrication method for DICOR restorations uses the lost wax and centrifugal casting techniques similar to those used for fabricating alloy castings. A wax pattern similar to the final restoration is made and invested in a phosphate bonded refractory material. Molten glass is then cast into the heated mould after dewaxing. The cast restoration is freed from the investment, covered by a protective 'embedment' material and subjected to ceramming. Addition of 2.5% lithium fluoride to the embedment material may promote crystallization of mica and increase the fracture toughness of glass ceramic. The completed restoration is acid etched on its fit surface to enhance bonding to the underlying tooth. Surface stains and colored luting cements are employed to improve upon the esthetics.

Properties

The physical properties of DICOR are given in the Table 20.3.

Table 20.3: Physical properties of DICOR			
Property	Dicor	Enamel	Feldspathic Porcelain
Density, g/cm^3	2.7	3.0	2.4
Translucency	0.56	0.48	0.27
Modulus of rupture, psi	22000	1500	11000
Compressive strength, psi	120000	58000	50000
Modulus of Elasticity, psi × 10^6	10.2	12.2	12.0
Microhardness	362	343	450

Esthetic Qualities

DICOR restorations are highly esthetic because of their translucency, which closely matches that of natural tooth enamel. The numerous small mica crystals that constitute castable ceramic closely match in their index of refraction to the surrounding glass phase. In addition, the castable ceramic permits a one piece restoration made entirely of the same material, and no opaque substructure exists to impede light scattering. A *'chameleon effect'* is seen with DICOR restorations in which the restoration acquires a part of the color from adjacent teeth, fillings as well as the underlying cement lute. Application of an external coloring system allows independent control over hue, chroma and value. However, as mentioned before, there are chances of losing this external layer thereby defeating the best of esthetics.

Precision of Fit

DICOR crowns and veneers have been demonstrated to fit accurately in the clinical and laboratory studies and their precision of fit has been found to be better than with metal ceramic restorations.

Durability

DICOR can withstand 20 years of simulated tooth brush abrasion without any changes. The resistance of DICOR to chemicals and staining agents also compares favourably with conventional feldspathic porcelains. Little wear of the cast ceramic or the opposing dentition occurs when using DICOR restorations. Two reasons for this property are: (a) closely matching hardness between the cast ceramic material and natural enamel (b) the DICOR shading porcelains contain minimal abrasive opacifying agents.

Tissue Acceptance

DICOR is chemically inert and has shown to pass all thebiocompatibility tests. The periodontal tissue reaction to DICOR is considered quite favourable because (i) there is no need for opaquer porcelains to mask the metal substructure. These coarse grained opaque porcelains generally promote the adherence of plaque. (ii) the absence of an opaque layer allows the technician to obtain natural translucence in the gingival area, avoiding overcontouring often found in metal ceramic restorations. Little discomfort occurs on contact with hot or cold foods because of its extremely low thermal conductivity and a coefficient of thermal expansion, which closely matches that of natural enamel.

Radiographic Qualities

The radiographic density of DICOR is similar to that of enamel allowing proper evaluation of the underlying structures and the margins.

Advantages
1. Excellent marginal fit
2. Relatively high strength
3. Surface hardness and occlusal wear is similar to enamel
4. Can reproduce wax patterns precisely by using the lost wax technique
5. Simple uncomplicated fabrication from waxup to casting, ceramming and coloring
6. Ease of adjustment
7. Excellent esthetics resulting from natural translucency
8. Inherent resistance to plaque accumulation (seven times less than on the natural tooth surfaces)

Disadvantages
Chances of losing low fusing feldspathic shading porcelains, which have been applied for good color matching.

Uses
Inlays, onlays, complete crowns and possibly partial tooth coverage restorations. It is not indicated for fixed partial denture or removable partial denture abutments with deep rests or internal attachments.

Castable Apatite Ceramic (Cera Pearl)

Castable apatite ceramic was first developed by *Hobo and Bioceram Group* as $CaO-P_2O_5-MgO-SiO_2$ glass ceramic. This material can be cast similar to the dental metal alloys. Its casting once obtained has an amorphous structure but when subjected to ceramming, at a temperature of 870°C for one hour *crystalline oxylapatite*, $Ca_{10}(PO_4)_6O$ results. This apatite is chemically unstable but becomes stable when exposed to moisture by forming *crystalline hydroxyapatite*. Compared to normal enamel, the crystals of Cera Pearl show a somewhat irregular arrangement and this different arrangement probably accounts for its superior mechanical properties.

Cera Pearl is composed of CaO, P2O5, MgO, SiO2 and traces of other elements. CaO (45%) and P_2O_5 (15%) are the main ingredients in glass formation. They are essential for formation of hydroxyapatite crystals as well. MgO (5%) helps in the formation of hydroxyapatite and alongwith CaO decreases the viscosity of the compound when melted. SiO_2 (34%) in combination with P_2O_5 forms the matrix. Further, SiO_2 regulates the thermal properties.

Because the crystalline constituent is similar to natural enamel, Cera Pearl is also expected to be quite biocompatible. The Young's modulus, tensile strength and compressive strength of Cera Pearl are appreciably higher than conventional porcelains and most restorative materials where as hardness compares favourably with the natural enamel. The values for these mechanical properties are given in the Table 20.4. Cera Pearl is indicated for both crowns and inlays. Another castable lithium containing glass ceramic Olympus Castable Ceramic(OCC) was introduced shortly after Cera Pearl. After crystallization it produces mica crystals to increase its physical strength.

Machinable Ceramic

These products are supplied in the form of ceramic ingots in various shades and with the help of a machine, are fabricated into inlays, onlays, crowns and even veneers. The fabrication process involves exposing the ceramic ingot to a machining apparatus, which produces the desired contours. This is followed by occlusal adjustment, polishing, etching and bonding the final restoration to the prepared tooth. The machined restoration may be stained and glazed after the adjustment has been done to obtain the desired characteristics. The various types of ingots used for the purpose are as follows:

a. *Cerec Vitablocs Mark I*: This is feldspathic porcelain and was the first composition used with Cerec system (Siemens). Its composition, strength and wear characteristics are similar to the feldspathic porcelain used in porcelain fused to metal restorations.

b. *Cerec Vitablocs Mark II*: This is a high strength feldspathic porcelain and has a grain size which is finer than the Mark I composition. Laboratory evaluation has shown less abrasive wear of the opposing tooth structure with this material, but there is no clinical evidence to document the finding.

c. *Dicor MGC*: This is a glass ceramic with fluorosilicate mica crystals in a glass matrix. Its flexural strength is higher than the castable Dicor and earlier described Cerec compositions. Additionally, they have been shown in-vitro to be softer and less abrasive than Cerec Mark I but probably, causing more wear than Cerec Mark II.

d. *Celay*: It is a fine feldspathic porcelain with a composition, which the manufacturers claim is

Table 20.4: Comparative data of properties of Cera Pearl and other common materials

Material	Young's modulus (GPA)	Tensile strength (MPa)	Compressive strength (MPa)	Knoop hardness number (KHN)	Coefficient of thermal expansion (10–6/°C)	Thermal conductivity (Cal cm/cm²sec°C)
Cera Pearl	103	150	590	350	11.0	0.0023
Gold Alloy	95	140		220–240	14.4	
Enamel	80	14	390	390	11.4	0.0022
Dentin	20	70	280	70	7.0	0.0014
Porcelain	70	80	170	590	12.0	0.0024
Amalgam	58	70	360	120	25.0	0.0540
Composite resin	18	18	185		39.0	0.0026

similar to Cerec Mark II. On this basis, the physical and clinical properties of the two can be expected to be similar. It is believed that these cause less wear of the opposing tooth structure but there is no clinical evidence to prove the claim.

POLYCRYSTALLINE CERAMICS

Ceramics (based on composition) fall into three main categories: predominantly glass – esthetic ceramics (aluminosilicate glass); particle-filled glass–structural ceramics (special silicate glasses like IPS and In-Ceram) and polycrystalline ceramics (Table 20.5). For polycrystalline ceramics, which contain no glass, the matrix is aluminum oxide or zirconium oxide, and the fillers are not particles but modifying atoms called 'dopants'. All of the atoms in Polycrystalline ceramics are packed into regular crystalline arrays through which it is difficult to drive a crack. Hence, polycrystalline ceramics are much tougher and

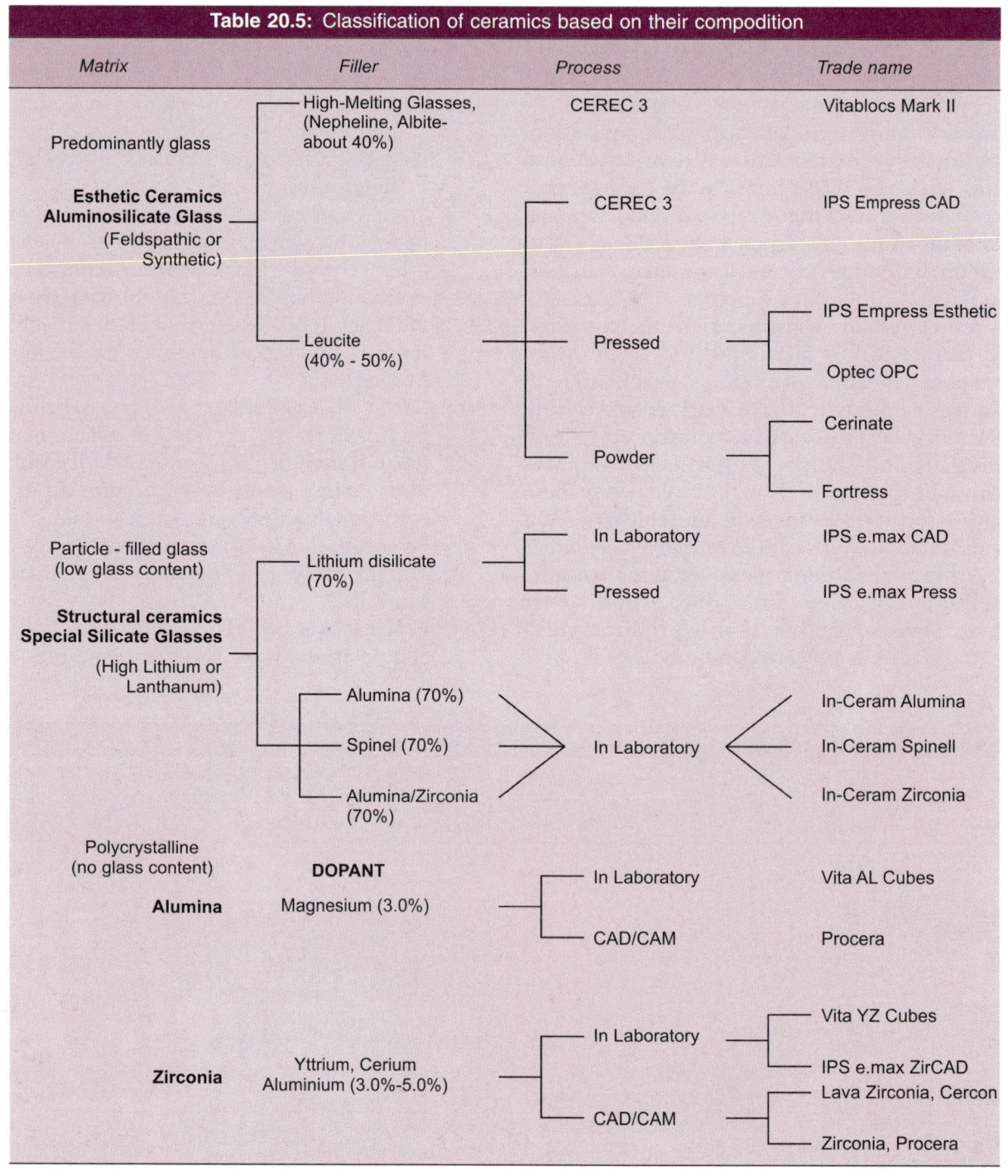

Table 20.5: Classification of ceramics based on their compodition

Matrix	Filler	Process	Trade name
Predominantly glass **Esthetic Ceramics Aluminosilicate Glass** (Feldspathic or Synthetic)	High-Melting Glasses, (Nepheline, Albite- about 40%)	CEREC 3	Vitablocs Mark II
		CEREC 3	IPS Empress CAD
	Leucite (40% - 50%)	Pressed	IPS Empress Esthetic / Optec OPC
		Powder	Cerinate / Fortress
Particle - filled glass (low glass content) **Structural ceramics Special Silicate Glasses** (High Lithium or Lanthanum)	Lithium disilicate (70%)	In Laboratory	IPS e.max CAD
		Pressed	IPS e.max Press
	Alumina (70%)	In Laboratory	In-Ceram Alumina
	Spinel (70%)	In Laboratory	In-Ceram Spinell
	Alumina/Zirconia (70%)	In Laboratory	In-Ceram Zirconia
Polycrystalline (no glass content) **Alumina**	**DOPANT** Magnesium (3.0%)	In Laboratory	Vita AL Cubes
		CAD/CAM	Procera
Zirconia	Yttrium, Cerium Aluminium (3.0%-5.0%)	In Laboratory	Vita YZ Cubes / IPS e.max ZirCAD
		CAD/CAM	Lava Zirconia, Cercon / Zirconia, Procera

stronger than glass-based ceramics. Well-fitting prostheses made from polycrystalline ceramics were not practical before the availability of computer-aided manufacturing.

PORCELAIN INLAYS

The use of porcelain in constructing individual inlays and crowns started in the late 1800's. The first successful fused porcelain inlays were made by Land of Detroit in 1886. He also earned a patent in 1887 for burnishing of platinum foil in order to form a matrix for fusing porcelain. Jenkins in 1898 introduced the first low fusing porcelains for making inlays and Wain in 1923 used the method of casting dental porcelain by the lost wax technique. For the past few years, employment of computers have resulted in restorations with precise details. The modern inlay provides the best esthetics, has a good marginal fit, retention, sealing, shade matching and fracture resistance. No doubt, ceramic restorations are now a viable alternative to conventional restorations.

Indications

The general indications for a porcelain restoration are:

1. Patients who maintain good oral hygiene.
2. Patients requesting for tooth colored restorations in posterior teeth.
3. In the cervical and proximal regions of an anterior tooth where esthetics is the prime concern.
4. Restoration will not be overloaded occlusally.
5. Teeth in which strengthening/protection of remaining structure is required.
6. No evidence of excessive attrition in relation to patient's age.
7. Cavity free from marked undercuts.
8. Ideally where all cavity margins are in enamel.
9. Sufficient tooth structure is available for bonding.
10. Lesions on the occlusal or proximal surfaces of posterior teeth.

Contraindications

1. It is not a restoration of choice if an anterior tooth is grossly involved either proximally or cervically. There must be adequate tooth structure to support the restoration.
2. When access to the lesion is poor and overcutting of tooth structure would be required, e.g. in rotated teeth. In such situations other restorations should be considered.
3. Patients with poor oral hygiene/inadequate motivation.
4. When short teeth preclude developing adequate resistance and retention forms, e.g. heavily worn down teeth.
5. Teeth with insufficient tooth substance for bonding.
6. Preparations with excessive undercuts.
7. In bruxers, where heavy occlusal forces have worn down natural teeth.
8. Where adequate isolation is not possible.
9. Teeth with large pulp chambers, which limit the reduction of tooth structure.
10. Where posterior group function and reduced vertical dimension apply strong lateral forces on the restoration.

Advantages of porcelain inlays

a. Good esthetics – color harmonious with that of tooth structure.
b. Low thermal conductivity.
c. High tolerance of the soft tissues to its presence.
d. Chemically inert and relatively insoluble in oral fluids.
e. A coefficient of thermal expansion close to that of natural tooth.

Disadvantages

a. Increased cost and time for fabrication when compared with a direct restoration.
b. Technique sensitive. Restorations usually require a high level of operator skill.
c. Some newer type of ceramic restorations require a special and expensive laboratory equipment.
d. Restorations made from porcelain are brittle and can fracture, if inadequate thickness is present to resist occlusal forces. Fractures can occur during try-in or post cementation, especially in patients who generate unusually high forces.
e. Because of their very high hardness, they can cause abrasion of the opposing teeth or restorations.
f. Lack of perfect adaptation to cavity walls exposes the cement line.

CAVITY PREPARATION

Earlier, porcelain was widely used in class III, class IV and class V cavities, but with the advent of other tooth colored restorative materials, their use in this regard has virtually disappeared. They are gaining more popularity for class II inlays and onlays. Before any cavity preparation is begun, shade of the tooth is obtained and recorded followed by the application of rubber dam.

Class III Cavity Preparation with Access from the Labial Surface

Access is gained from the labial when the tooth is involved by caries proximo-labially and the lingual marginal ridge is intact and not undermined by caries. A separator is applied to obtain a separation of 0.75 mm between two adjacent proximal surfaces. The cavity is prepared such that a labioproximal path of withdrawl is established. Initial entry is made with a #56 (or #57) straight fissure bur. The inclination of the bur should be in the direction of the projected path of withdrawl. Maintaining this bur inclination, the labial wall is established. The same bur is used to establish the gingival wall in a direction approximately perpendicular to the long axis of the tooth. For establishing the lingual wall, the bur is kept parallel to the proximal surface. The cavosurface line angle is carried into the lingual embrasure, and the incisal extent of the wall situated incisal to the contact area. The gingivoincisal direction of the lingual and labial walls is approximately parallel to the lingual and labial surfaces respectively. The axial wall is smooth and flat.

After the gingival, lingual and incisal walls have been established, the labial wall is refined to obtain the correct path of withdrawl, labioproximally. The junction of these outline walls should be smooth and rounded. The bur, which is used should have a rounded end to avoid any sharp angles in the preparation. All cavosurface line angles should be well defined and as near to right angles as possible, while being consistent with the direction of the enamel rods.

The labial and lingual walls in the cavity exhibit considerable divergence hence, no resistance to displacement is offered from lingual and labial walls. The gingival and incisal walls exhibit only minimal divergence therefore provide the major part of the resistance to displacement.

The completed cavity preparation as seen from the proximal view is shown in Fig. 20.7.

Class III Cavity Preparation with Access from the Lingual Surface

This cavity form is indicated on the proximal surfaces of all anterior teeth when the lingual marginal ridge is weak or missing and the labial aspect demands an esthetic restoration.

The shade of the tooth is selected, rubber dam applied and separation obtained. Entry to the proximal lesion is made through the lingual marginal ridge with a No. #170 carbide bur. The basic cavity form is completed with this bur. The incisal and gingival

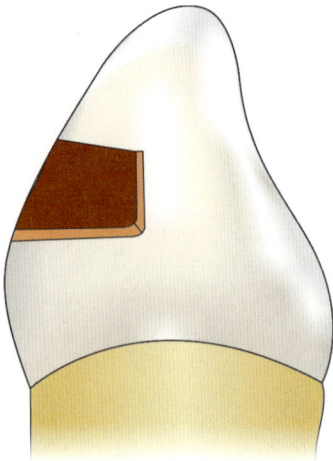

Fig. 20.7: Completed class III cavity preparation as seen from the proximal view

walls have a slight divergence labio-lingually. The line angles between the incisal and labial wall as well as between the gingival and labial wall are rounded. The axial wall is flat labio-lingually. This creates a definite box form.

The cavosurface line angles are refined so as to place them at right angles. Also, the axial line angles should be rounded to avoid stress concentration. With a No.169 L carbide bur, a retention groove is placed in the incisoaxial and gingivo-axial line angles at the expense of the incisal and gingival walls respectively. These grooves should be consistent with the labio-lingual path of withdrawl that has already been established.

Resistance to displacement in a lingual direction is offered by the near parallelism of the incisal and gingival walls labio-lingually.

A completed class III cavity with lingual access is shown in Fig. 20.8.

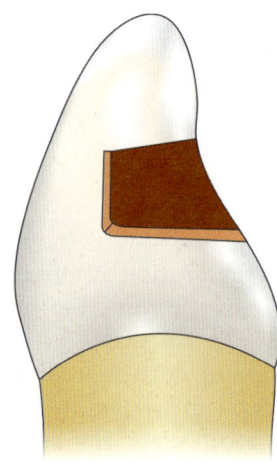

Fig. 20.8: Completed class III cavity with lingual access

Class V Cavity Preparation

The shade of the tooth is obtained and recorded. Rubber dam and Ferrier cervical clamp are applied to aid in isolation, access and gingival retraction. If necessary, low heat modeling compound is used to support the clamp. Since esthetics is a major concern when restoring a class V cavity, all cavosurface margins except the incisal/occlusal should be extended to beneath the free gingiva.

The lesion is entered in its center with a no. 56 or no. 57 carbide bur. Generally, the outline form includes the area affected by caries, erosion, abrasion or existing restoration; and if need be is further extended for convenience and placement of gingival, mesial and distal margins beneath the gingiva. Incisal/occlusal outline is longer than the gingival outline and both are parallel to each other mesiodistally. The mesial and distal margins follow the proximal contours of the crown of the tooth. The outline form is hence trapezoidal with the junction of the four walls rounded to the extent of the curvature of the #56 or #57 bur.

In establishing the mesial and distal walls, the mesiodistal inclination of the bur is such that it is perpendicular to the respective surface being cut. This avoids any undermining and the walls follow the approximate direction of the enamel rods. The axial wall is prepared with a slight mesiodistal convex curvature, so that the entire wall is of the same depth into dentin. The depth of the axial wall should be approximately one and a half times deeper axially than the corresponding depth in a class V gold foil preparation. This ensures better esthetics because of thicker section of porcelain and also the retentive quality of the preparation is increased.

The gingival wall is established by positioning the bur perpendicular to the long axis of the tooth. The gingival cavosurface margin is kept 0.5–0.75 mm occlusal to the buccal jaw of the clamp and mesiodistally its extent is restricted to less than that of the clamp jaw. The gingival wall in the mesiodistal direction is approximately parallel to the occlusal surface of the tooth. The occlusal wall shows a slight divergence from the pulpal floor to the surface. This divergence guides the path of withdrawl in the cavity preparation. The occlusal wall is also prepared parallel to the occlusal surface mesiodistally, and is extended to just include the occlusal extent of the lesion. Its mesiodistal length is such that mesial and distal ends are slightly subgingival, when the retracting effect of rubber dam is removed. The mesial ends of the occlusal and gingival walls are joined by the mesial wall and the distal ends by the distal wall. All walls are finally planed.

The critical relationship of the gingival and occlusal walls linguolabially provides the main resistance to displacement of the restoration. All line angles and point angles should be rounded to avoid stress concentration prior to cementation. Retention can be improved by grooving incisoaxial and gingivoaxial line angles. If the axial wall is quite deep, a base for protection is recommended.

A completed cavity preparation is shown in Figs 20.9A and B.

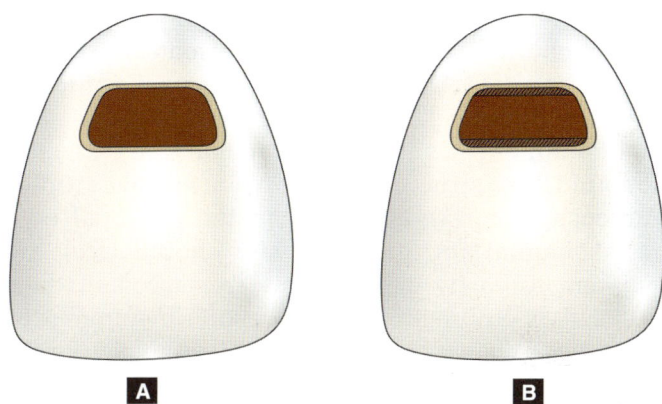

Figs 20.9: Completed class V cavity preparation; **(A)** Without grooves, **(B)** With grooves.

Class II Cavity Preparation

In brief, the cavity preparation for a porcelain inlay is similar to that for cast metal, minus beveling and secondary flaring (Fig. 20.10).

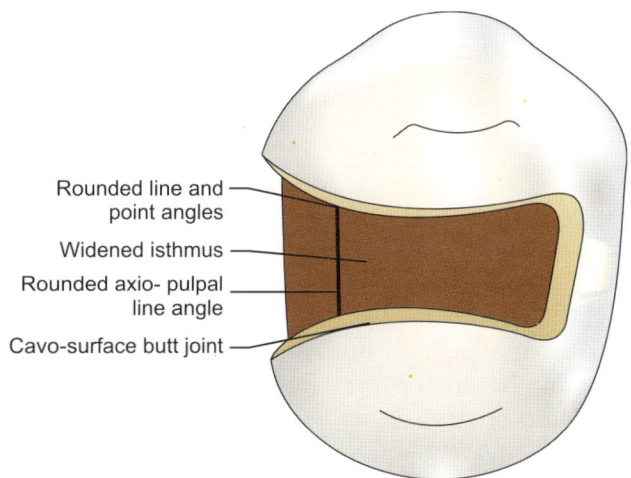

Fig. 20.10: Class II cavity preparation for a porcelain inlay

A tapering carbide bur is used for the cavity preparation, which allows for divergence of the walls towards the occlusal and hence eases insertion and removal of the restoration. The occlusal divergence per wall of the cavity preparation for porcelain restorations is kept at 6–8° compared to the conventional 2–5° for cast metal restorations. The reasons for this are (a) porcelain inlays will adhesively bond to the tooth structure and (b) minimal pressure is to be applied during its try in and cementation. Throughout the cavity preparation, the instruments must be oriented to a single path of 'draw'.

Ceramic requires a minimum of 1.0 mm thickness for its strength. It is recommended that the depth of the occlusal step be in the range of 1.5–2.0 mm for all types of ceramic systems (Fig. 20.11). Width of the isthmus should be a minimum of 1.5 mm and the axial reduction in the proximal box also on an average be 1.5 mm. For DICOR restorations, the axial reduction can be reduced to 1.2 mm and for Optec systems even to 1.0 mm. The facial and lingual walls are extended to sound tooth structure and are made to move around the cusps in graceful curves. In the proximal box, facial, lingual and gingival walls should clear the adjacent tooth by 0.5 mm and are placed in their respective embrasures for ease of finishing after bonding. Whenever possible, the gingival margin should be placed at levels where adequate enamel is present for bonding. Also deep gingival margins are difficult to isolate during cementation.

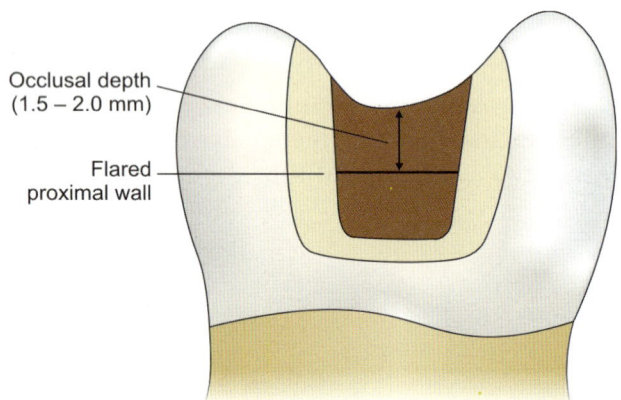

Fig. 20.11: Cavity preparation for porcelain inlay showing occlusal depth of 1.5–2.0 mm and flared proximal walls

The tapering bur used for cavity preparation should have a rounded end to avoid sharp line angles and point angles in the preparation. No undercuts are permitted in the cavity and if present, should be blocked out using GIC. Pulpal floor should be smooth and flat. In case the floor is rough or deep, a glass-ionomer composite base is recommended. In very deep preparations, a subbase of calcium hydroxide is given. All cavosurface margins should terminate in a butt joint, i.e. 90° angle. Final finishing is done with diamond points. All stains are removed from the walls as they may appear as black or grey lines at the margin after cementation.

Cusp capping is needed when a cusp has fractured or is hopelessly undermined. It should also be considered when the margin of the preparation approaches to within 1.5 mm of the cusp tip. For the functional cusps, reduction is 1.5 mm on premolars and 2.0 mm on molars. Nonfunctional cusps require less protection and 1.0–1.5 mm seems to be adequate. When capping functional cusps, a 'collar' is prepared to move the margins of the preparation away from any possible contact with opposing teeth. The width of the collar should be 1.0–1.5 mm.

If a large portion of facial or lingual surface is affected by caries or any other pathology, then the preparation is extended around the transitional line angle of the tooth to include the defect. A gingival shoulder with a minimum width of 1 mm should be created whenever extension is made onto the facial/lingual surface.

FABRICATION OF A PORCELAIN INLAY

Ceramic inlays can be classified into four groups according to their material composition and fabrication.

- Inlays fired on a platinum foil
- Inlays produced on a refractory die material
- Inlays made by the lost wax technique
- Machined ceramic inlays

Inlays Fired on a Platinum Foil

A satisfactory porcelain restoration can be produced only, if careful attention is given to the principles and details of the process from the very beginning. The stages in the construction of a porcelain inlay include (a) preparation of the cavity (b) making a platinum matrix, which closely fits the cavity (c) fusing porcelain into the matrix to restore the tooth form (d) glazing (e) removing the matrix from the inlay and (f) cementing the inlay into the cavity.

A cavity is prepared as discussed earlier. In order that the porcelain inlay conforms to this cavity, a matrix or mold is required into which the porcelain powder can be built and fused. Several materials can be used for the formation of this matrix, e.g. metal, silicon compounds etc. The metal matrix is usually made of platinum although other metals like palladium, pure gold or platinum-gold alloy may also be used. The matrix must have a softening point well above the temperature at which the porcelain fuses to ensure its stability during the making of an inlay. Platinum and Palladium can be used in the fusing of any of the dental porcelains available, while gold and palladium-gold alloys, because of their lower fusing points permit the use of low fusing porcelains only.

Hence platinum is the material most commonly used. Palladium is not very popular because it cannot be easily worked and also takes on a surface discoloration, which is objectionable. Platinum foil may be obtained in gauzes of 0.0013", 0.00153" and 0.0023". Most preferred thickness is 0.001". When using thinner gauzes, care must be exercised to prevent any distortion. The platinum is supplied in an already annealed state by the manufacturer, and during the initial stages of matrix construction, annealing need not be done by the dentist. After it has been worked for sometime, it becomes stiff and requires annealing. This is done by holding the matrix in a flame until it becomes cherry red in color and then quickly quenching it in water or alcohol.

The matrix can be obtained in several ways:

1. Direct, i.e. making it directly in the tooth cavity.
2. Indirect, i.e. by taking an accurate impression of the cavity, and then proceeding on the impression or a model made out of it.
3. Indirect-direct, i.e. by making the matrix on the model and then reburnishing it directly in the tooth cavity to complete it.

1. Direct Method

A well annealed, 0.001 inch foil is cut into proper size and shape such that sufficient excess extends 3–4 mm beyond the margins of the cavity. The foil is placed over the cavity and carefully forced inside it and adapted, beginning in the center of the axial or pulpal walls using wet cotton/chamois, with smooth burnishers or blunt orangewood stick. Further adaptation is done by moving a ball burnisher over a cotton pledget, from the center to the lateral walls. The burnisher should not contact the foil directly until it is well adapted, hence the need for an intervening cotton or chamois. After the foil has been well adapted in the deeper parts of the cavity, it is burnished over the margins and the adjoining surfaces. Care should be taken to avoid folding or tearing during the adaptation process. Now, with the matrix full of cotton and partially adapted, stretch a cellophane tape over it. Holding it firmly in position, burnish over the tape with a ball burnisher to improve adaptation of the platinum foil to the cavity walls, margins and adjacent tooth surfaces. Now remove the tape and the cotton pledget, and stretch a piece of rubber dam over the matrix. Burnishing is again done to adapt it more completely to the underlying tooth structure.

The matrix is removed at this stage and examined. There should be no tears at the margins. Tears in the interior parts of the matrix and away from a margin are of little concern, unless they are large enough to destroy anchorage. The foil is annealed, replaced back into the cavity and burnished with a ball burnisher and cotton. The matrix is swaged with an orangewood stick so that it accurately reproduces every surface detail. If swaging has been correctly executed, there should be no movement of the matrix in the cavity. The matrix is touched at various places with an explorer point and observed for any movement. If any movement is seen then reswaging is done.

The matrix is carefully removed by filling it with sticky wax. The wax is burnt off and the matrix stored in a small covered receptacle filled with water, till it is needed.

2. Indirect Method

This method is much more safe and convenient compared to the direct method, as it precludes any contamination with moisture and difficulty in obtaining access. Moreover, tooth separation is not required. No doubt, the indirect method is preferred over the direct one. For this method, first an impression is made. Various materials can be used for taking impression – Impression compound, a suitable hard wax or elastic impression materials. At present, the impression materials of choice are elastic impression materials.

For Class III Cavities with Labial Access

Separation of the teeth is done. Lingual embrasure is blocked out using utility wax. The lingual cavosurface margin should be clear of wax by approximately 0.5 mm. A strip of 26 gauge perforated brass screening is trimmed to approximately 1½ inches in length and 1/4 to 1/3 inches in width. A slight 90° bend in the strip facilitates access to the area. The brass screening is bent at the edges so that it serves as a tray for the heavy bodied rubber base impression material. Alternatively, impression compound may be adapted at the borders of the screening to form a tray. The tray should cover approximately half the labial surfaces of the prepared tooth and the tooth approximating it. A small amount of light bodied impression material is mixed and a small bead of this is carried with the tip of an explorer into the cavity. The explorer is used to vibrate the material into all the line angles. The cavity is then filled with excess of the light bodied material. A small amount of heavy bodied rubber base material is now placed on one end of the perforated brass tray. The tray loaded with material is attached to the previously placed light bodied material. When the material has set, the impression is removed and examined for discrepancies.

For Class III Cavities with Lingual Access

The instruments, materials and technique are the same as described above, except that the labial embrasure instead of the lingual needs to be blocked out to permit impression taking from the lingual aspect.

For Class V Cavities

A strip of 25 gauge perforated brass screening is trimmed to approximately 1½ inch in length and same width as the prepared tooth. It is bent to an angle of 45° at approximately half its length. This produces a handle that does not interfere with the lips. The end where the impression material is to be placed is contoured and shaped to the outline of the prepared cavity but slightly larger than it. To prevent the tray from touching the margins of the cavity, an impression in low fusing impression compound is taken of the incisal/occlusal half of the labial surface. This prevents the tray material from touching any cavity margin and thereby, ruining the impression. A small amount of light bodied material is mixed and carried to the cavity on an explorer tip. The impression material is vibrated into the preparation. The cavity is filled to excess with the light bodied material. Heavy bodied impression material is then carried on the tray and attached to the light bodied material. After the material has set, the impression is removed and examined.

For Class II Cavities

Impression can be taken using impression compound in seamless copper bands or elastomeric impression materials. The method is similar to that used for a gold inlay. The same holds true for proximoincisal cavities with an incisal step.

Making a Model/die

After having obtained an acceptable impression, there are numerous materials with which the die can be formed:
- Copper plated dies
- Silver plated dies
- Stone dies
- Phospho-silicate dyes (e.g. Model Kryptex)
- Amalgam
- Inlay metal

Use of phospho-silicate (Model Kryptex) for constructing a die has proved to be quite popular.

Advantages of this material are as follows:
- Convenient to use. The die can be poured immediately at the chairside.
- Accuracy.
- Reproduction of very fine surface detail.
- Sufficient abrasion resistance for use as a working die.
- A crushing strength capable of resisting various technical procedures.
- Does not require special procedures.

12 drops of Model Kryptex liquid are placed on a glass slab alongwith adequate powder. The cement is mixed to a thick creamy consistency. On the tip of an explorer, a bead of the mixture is carried to the region of the impression close to the cavosurface line angle. With the tip, the material is vibrated into the cavosurface line angle. The material should flow ahead of the tip so that no voids are created in the die. When the cavosurface line angle is completely filled, more material is added until the thickness of the material covering the cavity surface is approximately ¼ inch. After the initial set of the material, the die is covered with petroleum jelly to prevent surface dehydration. The die should not be separated from the impression for a minimum of 4 hours and preferably be kept overnight. It is advised to separate the die just prior to its use. Support should be given to the die by backing it with low fusing compound.

Platinum Matrix Adaptation

For this, the end of a 2 inch length of balsa wood is trimmed with a no.15 B.P blade, such that the cross-sectional shape is slightly larger than the outline of the cavity. With sufficient hand pressure, the trimmed end is forced into the cavity preparation. Thus it takes the form of the cavity. It is around this stick that the platinum foil is initially adapted. The stick carrying the platinum foil is forced into the preparation. The excess foil at the margins is adapted using a small burnisher. The stick should be held in the cavity during burnishing because there is a tendency for the foil pulling away from the pulpal (axial) line angles.

Swaging is done so as to obtain a closer adaptation of the foil to the die. For swaging, pressure is exerted using a moldine swager. A second swaging is done to obtain a very close adaptation. A sticky wax transfer aids in removing the matrix from the die without distortion. The matrix is separated from the sticky wax by softening the wax over the flame. Heating the matrix over a flame to red-hot burns off any residual wax. **Another indirect method is to utilize the impression itself for platinum matrix formation.** Two ways can be employed for accomplishing this: One, by taking the impression in blue inlay wax and then converting it into gold by the casting process. Two, the impression may be taken in silicate or zinc phosphate cement and the same used as a model for the formation of a matrix. To take impression by the latter method, the cavity is lubricated to prevent adhesion of the cement. When initially a small amount of material is worked into the cavity, the mix should not be too heavy. The remaining amount is then mixed heavily, kneaded between the fingers to a suitable shape and inserted into the cavity under pressure. After the cement has fully set, it is loosened and removed.

Platinum Matrix Adaptation on the Impression

The technique of forming a matrix on the impression varies slightly from the earlier described. Tears can develop in the marginal areas of the matrix when using such a model. Adapting the foil loosely, and then burnishing it onto the outer areas of the model from the sides at about 45° angle overcomes tearing. This creates folds in the foil, but since only the inside of the matrix is of concern, the thickness of the foil and the folds make little difference as long as the matrix interior is smooth and continuous. If tears do develop on some margin, folding over some of the excess foil at that point can cover them. The matrix is again burnished and swaged into place. Before removing the matrix from the die, it is lubricated and an impression taken with impression compound which would serve as a support for the matrix. It is then carefully separated from the impression, annealed, placed back on the model and re-swaged. The matrix is removed with utmost care and if difficulty is experienced, a sticky wax transfer is best employed. It is quite evident that this method is more accurate than the earlier described, because in this the inside of the matrix is the same size as the preparation whereas in the former technique, the outside of the matrix corresponds to the cavity.

3. Indirect-Direct Method

The impression of the tooth is taken. A model is poured and a matrix is adapted in much the same way as in the indirect procedure. The matrix is subsequently removed and annealed and adapted inside the oral cavity by the direct method. This technique has the advantage of overcoming difficulties encountered in making the matrix by the direct method and yet, enables one to verify the fit and obtain the best of accuracy.

Porcelain Build up and Firing

Complete cleanliness is required at this stage. Unclean environments can easily contaminate the porcelain with dust, plaster or any other material and injure the work. The basic armamentarium which is needed includes: a clean glass slab, one Camel hair brush (size 8), one or more round sable brushes (size 4 and less), mixing spatula, porcelain carver, tissue, a receptacle for distilled water and locking tweezers. Additional instruments may be added as per the individual's requirements.

Two drops of distilled water are placed on a glass slab and along side it are placed porcelain powder/s of selected shades. The matrix is prepared by holding it in locking tweezers and heating in a flame to render it clean. Previously dispensed powder and water are now mixed to a creamy consistency. An adequate consistency is attained when the mix tends to run on tipping the glass slab. The pointed end of a porcelain carver serves to transfer this mix to the cavity area of the matrix. Rubbing the carver across the locking pliers holding the matrix, causes the mix to flow across the pulpal/axial wall of the cavity into the line angles. The material is condensed by any of the methods described earlier in the section. An even thickness of porcelain is maintained and the cavity filled to one half. Any excess is carefully wiped off with a sable hair brush. Porcelain that may have run through the tears, if any exist in the matrix, must also be definitely removed each time before firing the work. Overcontouring is not permissible except in areas of contact points or incisal angles, and that too only by amounts equal to the contraction that will take place during firing. It is to be remembered that porcelain even when well condensed shrinks by approximately one sixth on firing and shrinkage occurs towards the bulk. In order to compensate for this shrinkage, a number of methods can be employed, details of which are covered later in the chapter.

The matrix along with the condensed porcelain is now subjected to firing. For this, it is placed on a low heat absorption tray. This tray is constructed from a double thickness of 0.001 inch platinum foil with its three edges upturned. The approximate dimensions of the tray are 1 inch front to rear, ¾ inch side to side and 1/8 inch in height. A thin layer of crystalline alumina (90 mesh) mixed with a luting cement in 50:50 concentration is fired in the tray to render it rigid and resistant to heat during subsequent firings. The mixture also has the property to withstand sudden and major heat changes. In order to dry the wet porcelain, the tray along with the matrix is placed in front of a preheated furnace muffle. The furnace is preheated and held at the fusing temperature of the particular porcelain being used. After drying, the tray and the matrix are introduced into the rear of the muffle. When the door of the furnace is opened, the temperature drops by about 100° F. The temperature is brought back to its firing temperature, and the porcelain held at this temperature for 25 to 30 seconds, depending on the individual recommendations of the furnace and then quickly removed. The porcelain should exhibit an underglaze, i.e. a medium biscuit (bisque) bake. Cooling takes about one minute.

Some amount of shrinkage and distortion of the matrix occurs. The matrix and first bake of porcelain are placed back on the die, swaged and a sticky wax transfer performed. This permits re-adaptation of the matrix to the die cavity. However, fractures are produced in the fused porcelain during the procedure.

Small amount of porcelain present on the glass slab is remixed and deposited into the fractures by adequately vibrating the mix, so that no air is entrapped. The second build up is performed in the same manner as the first build up. The cavity is filled upto about seven eights at this stage. A cut is made deep down to the previously fused porcelain to bisect the build up. Firing is done in the same way as before. The matrix with the fused porcelain is again swaged and a sticky wax transfer performed.

The third porcelain build up is carried out, care being taken to obtain the correct contour and marginal apposition. Slight over-contouring is beneficial at this stage since the porcelain will shrink on fusion. The porcelain is subjected to firing, and if slight discrepancies develop in contour and/or marginal adaptation, they are corrected by adding small amounts of low fusing porcelain and 'refiring'. The inlay is tried in the mouth and ground to proper contour and occlusion with a fine stone, if required. Glazing is done by heating the inlay for an additional 2–3 seconds at the firing temperature.

Removal of the Matrix

The matrix is removed by immersing the inlay along with the matrix in alcohol or water for approximately one minute, then carefully peeling away the matrix with the aid of locking tweezers, by moving from the margins to the center. Some matrix may remain adherent in the region of tears, which can be ground off with a sharp stone or a sharp bur (used in critical areas). Small attached pieces of foil are also easily removed after acid etching by hydrofluoric acid or by dissolving it in aquaregia.

Methods for Reducing the Firing Shrinkage in Porcelain

There are generally four methods, which may be used either singly or in combination.

Ditching: A ditch is cut into the porcelain around the inner margins of the matrix, leaving some porcelain on the margins (Fig. 20.12). Because porcelain shrinks towards the center, the ditch is enlarged but the

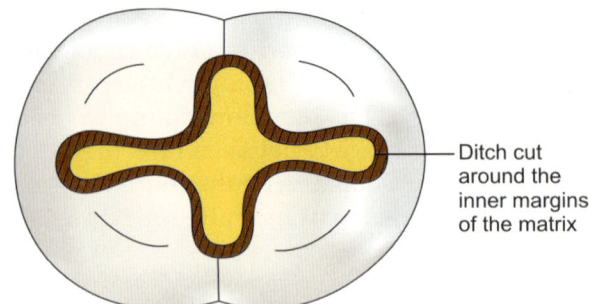

Fig. 20.12: Ditching method for reducing shrinkage in porcelain

margins will remain partially covered. The ditch is then filled with fresh porcelain and refired.

Crosscutting: A cut in the form of a cross is made with some sharp instrument through the porcelain to the platinum matrix (Fig. 20.13). This creates four sections in porcelain, which shrink individually during firing. Hence, distortion of the platinum matrix resulting from porcelain shrinkage is minimized. The contraction voids are then filled with fresh porcelain and fired again.

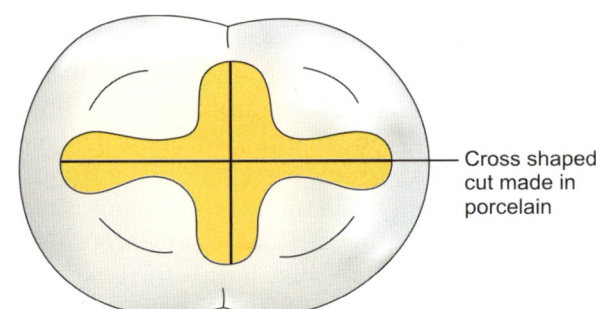

Fig. 20.13: Crosscutting method for reducing shrinkage in porcelain

Etching and Cementation

The cavity surface of the restoration is etched prior to cementation to aid in mechanical retention. Soft wax is applied on the areas that need protection from etchants. The restoration is then dropped in hydrofluoric acid (10%) and left there for about 30 seconds. Any acid remaining on the inlay is neutralized by placing it in a sodium carbonate solution. After etching, the etched surface can be treated with a silanating agent, which further improves the bond to the luting composite. An alternative procedure is sand blasting with 20 µm aluminium oxide particles under 40 psi pressure.

After this surface treatment, the inlay is now ready for cementation. Mylar strip is positioned in the affected proximal surface and wedged. The preparation surfaces are conditioned and a bonding agent applied in a thin film. A dual cure composite resin luting agent is selected, so that curing is not hampered in areas difficult to be reached by light. It is mixed and inserted into the cavity with a suitable instrument or a syringe. The cavity side of the restoration is also coated with the mix. The inlay is inserted into the cavity using minimal pressure and slightly vibrated into the cavity using a ball burnisher. The excess composite is removed with a bladed instrument or with the tip of an explorer, taking care not to remove any cement from between the interface. The restoration is then light cured from all three directions, i.e. occlusal, facial and lingual for a minimum of 40 to 60 seconds in each direction. Excessive care is mandatory while handling ceramic restorations because they are extremely fragile and can easily fracture. Resin modified glass-ionomers are also a good alternative to composite resin for cementation. Both these luting agents have replaced the traditional zinc phosphate or silicate cements used for cementation.

After the curing has completed, matrix strips and wedges are removed. All the margins are inspected both visually and with an explorer for hardness of cement, any deficiency or excess. The restoration is finally finished and polished. The procedure for try in, cementation, finishing and polishing is the same for all types of ceramic inlays whether fired, cast or machined.

Porcelain Inlays Fired on Refractory Dies

Currently, most of the ceramic inlays and onlays manufactured in the dental laboratory are by firing dental porcelain on refractory dies. This method eliminates the use of a platinum foil, which in part causes inaccuracy and deformation. After the cavity has been prepared, an impression is taken and a master working cast is poured in die stone or epoxy resin. Die pins aid in forming a die (Figs 20.14 and 20.15). The master cast is separated and trimmed (Fig. 20.16). A die spacer is applied in the cavity preparation usually on the pulpal and axial walls (Figs 20.17 and 20.18). Prepared master model is then duplicated with a silicone impression and poured in refractory investment capable of withstanding porcelain firing temperatures. After hardening, the cast is fired at 1000°C to eliminate accumulated gas, which may be generated during the first porcelain firing. It is then soaked in a conditioning solution until completely saturated. This solution enables porcelain contraction to be directed towards the cavity itself.

Dental porcelain is added into the cavity preparation on the refractory die and fired in an oven. A two to

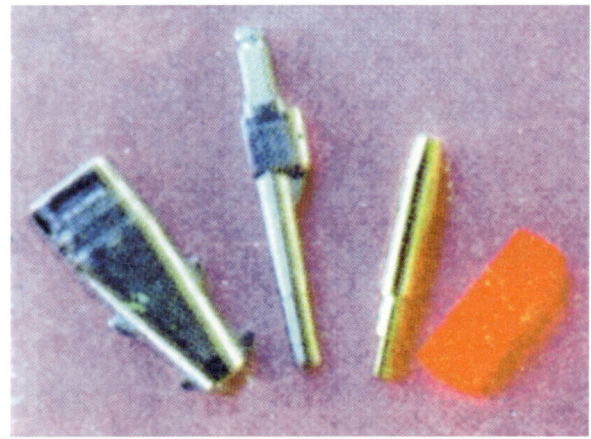

Fig. 20.14: Die pins used in forming a die

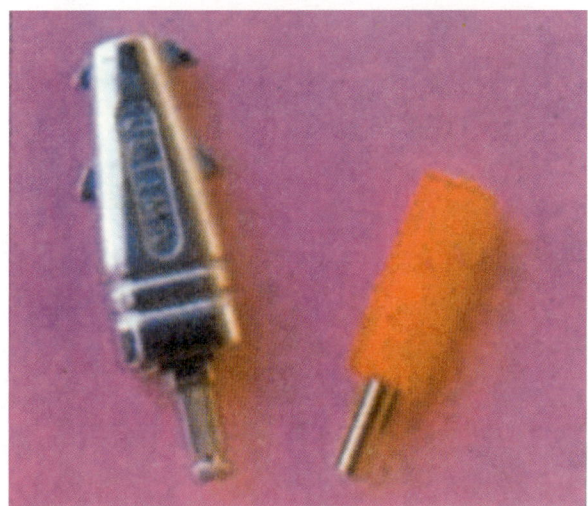

Fig. 20.15: Die pins used in forming a die

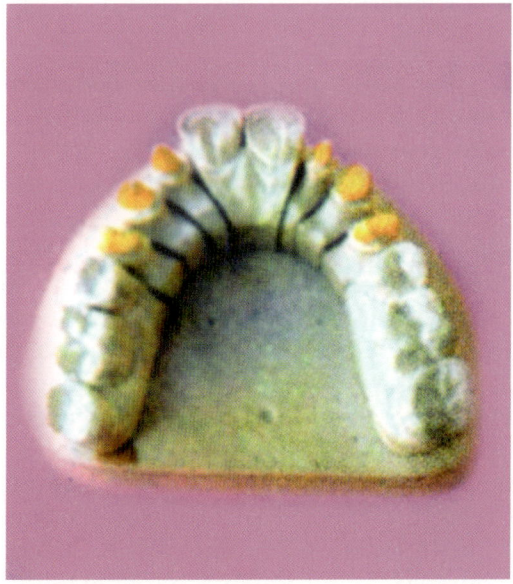

Fig. 20.16: Master cast separated and trimmed to form separate dies

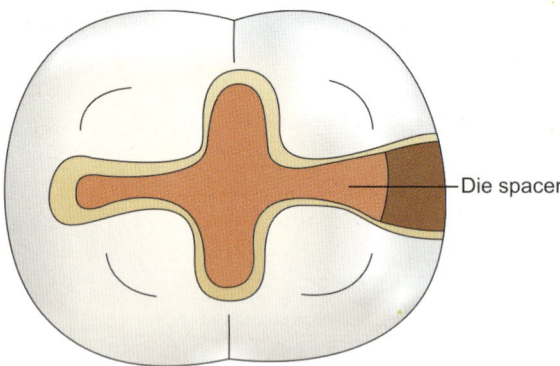

Fig. 20.17: Die spacer applied on the pulpal and axial walls of the cavity preparation

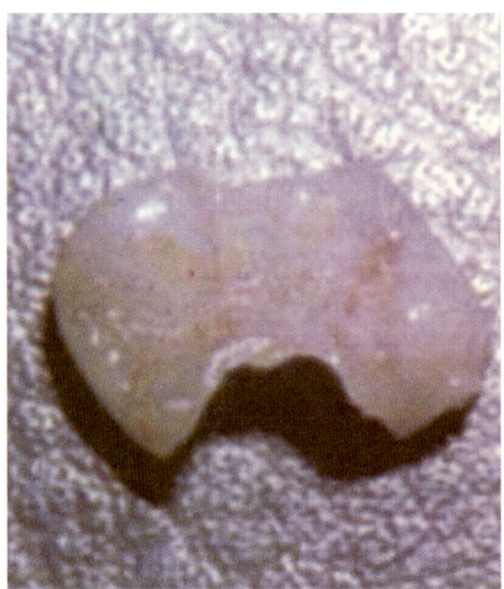

Fig. 20.19: Porcelain inlay

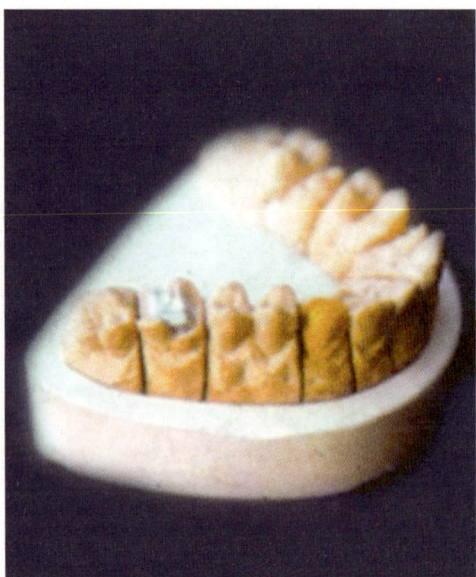

Fig. 20.18: Die spacer applied on the die of maxillary first motar for forming porcelain inlay

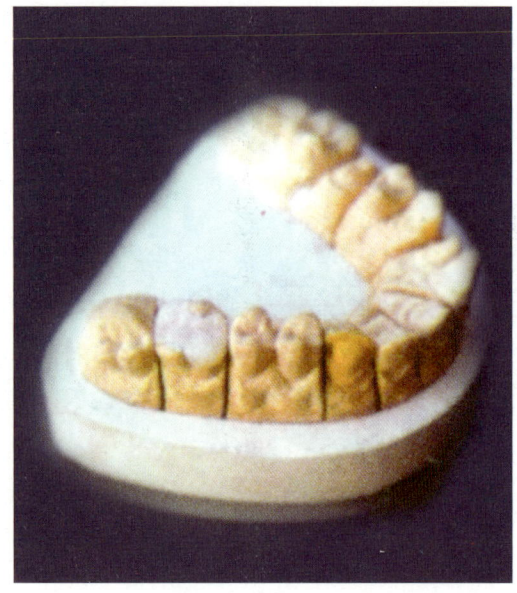

Fig. 20.20: Porcelain inlay

three step build up technique is necessary to compensate for the sintering/firing shrinkage. The ceramic restoration is retrieved from the die (Fig. 20.19), cleaned and seated on the master die for adjustment and finishing (Fig. 20.20). Occlusal contacts are adjusted and proximal overhangs, if any, are removed. After an accurate finishing of the margins, the product can be finally glazed. The restorations fabricated with this technique must be carefully handled during the try-in to avoid any fracture. Etching is done on the restoration's cavity surface followed by application of a luting agent for cementation.

The chief advantage with this technique is the relatively less expensive set up and compatibility with most existing ceramic ovens used in the laboratory. Major disadvantages of the technique are its technique sensitivity and a higher incidence of fracture compared to other ceramic systems. Problems may be encountered in the fit and marginal integrity of these restorations.

Inlays Made by the Lost Wax Technique

Castable Glass Ceramic (DICOR)

Cast glass ceramic restorations require a minimum reduction of 1.0 mm. The recommended axial reduction is 1.2–1.5 mm and the incisal/occlusal reduction is 1.5–2.0 mm. The degree of taper recommended for axial surfaces is 6–8°, consistent with the path of withdrawl for the wax pattern. Ideal margin form for a crown is either a 90–120° shoulder with a rounded gingivo-axial line angle or a deep 120° chamfer.

After tooth preparation, standard impression procedures are applied and a master working cast in improved die stone is poured. Epoxy resin die materials are acceptable as they provide increased hardness and wear resistance. A tooth shaded die spacer is then chosen from the shading chart and applied in two thin coats, avoiding the margins. Die lubricant is applied directly over the die spacer, and a wax pattern is made using conventional techniques. Occlusal detail can be carved into the pattern and retained throughout the subsequent process. The completed wax pattern is sprued, usually an eight gauze sprue is used. Length of the sprue should be such that the pattern is positioned 1/4 to 1/8 inch from top of the ring. The spruing technique uses a long casting ring (13/16 inches) and a generous reservoir to ensure complete emptying of the molten glass into the mould during casting.

One layer of Kaoliner investment ring liner is lined on the inside of the ring. The lined ring should be placed in water for 10 seconds before seating the ring around the pattern. A special type of phosphate bonded investment that produces 1.6% thermal expansion is employed for investing. 60 gms investment powder is mixed with 8 cc of distilled water for 30 seconds with an electric vacuum mixer at low speed. The mix is then vibrated for an additional 20–30 seconds. A small amount of investment is painted on the pattern without trapping air. After the ring has been filled with investment, it is allowed to set for one hour before placing it in the oven for burn out.

A two stage burnout is recommended. The ring is placed in a cold furnace and temperature slowly raised to 480°F. At this temperature it is heat soaked for 30 minutes. The temperature is then again raised further to 1750° F (950°C) and heat soaking given for 2 hours. For more than three rings placed together, an additional 10 minutes is added for every extra ring. The casting machine features a platinum electrical resistance type muffle mounted on an electrically driven straight centrifugal casting arm. It is maintained at an ideal temperature of 2010°F (1100°C) for 10 minutes to preheat the muffle. The rear muffle door is opened and the crucible loaded with 4gm ingot placed inside the muffle. The door is closed and the temperature raised to the casting temperature of 2476°F (1358°C). At this temperature, the ingot melts and this temperature is maintained for six seconds. The front door of the muffle is then opened and the muffle assembly is slid forward towards the casting ring until it is seated. The casting machine cover is closed and the 'cast' switch is turned on. The casting arm spins and the casting is completed. The casting ring is allowed to bench cool for 45 minutes.

The casting is then divested and any attached investment is removed with an air abrasive tool and 25 µm aluminium oxide. A finger should always be used to support the margin areas to prevent chipping. The sprue is separated using a double sided diamond disk, and the excess removed and finished with a white point running at slow speeds. Presence of any inclusion bodies, porosities or voids renders the restoration unacceptable. Adjustments if needed should be made at this stage.

The non-crystalline casting is now placed in the embedment material for the ceramming process (50 gms of the embedment material is mixed with 18 cc of distilled water). It is allowed to set for 15–30 minutes, after which it is placed in the ceramming furnace. The furnace takes approximately 114 minutes to reach the ceramming temperature of 1960°F (1075°C) and maintains the temperature for 6 hours. After this time elapses, the furnace is cooled for one hour and when the temperature has lowered to 392°F, the embedment material containing the casting is removed.

The embedment material is allowed to cool to room temperature and then broken apart using finger pressure. The retrieved crystalline glass ceramic restoration is subjected to grit blasting as described before. Any irregularities on the internal surface of the restoration that may interfere with seating are checked. These can be removed with extra fine diamond points. Overextensions are removed with a fine white point or a rubber wheel at slow speed. Correction of occlusal interferences is done with a fine diamond bur. Anatomy can be defined with a No. 0 or No. 1 round carbide bur followed by a light reblast with 25 µm aluminium oxide at 40 psi. The casting is cleaned ultrasonically in distilled water. Any void in the casting can be corrected by grinding and air abrading in that specific area. After cleaning it ultrasonically, DICOR add-on porcelain mixed in distilled water is applied on the desired location and condensed. The casting is dried in front of an oven at 1290°F (700°C). It is then placed in the muffle and fired in vacuum from 1290°F to 1775°F (700–900°C). The vacuum is released and the temperature maintained at 1775°F for one minute. The added fused porcelain is shaped and adjusted.

After all fit and contour adjustments have been made, feldspathic shading porcelains (Dicor Plus) are applied on the surface. The addition of shading porcelain determines the hue. More than one shading porcelain may be necessary to obtain the desired hue. The number of applications control the chroma. Generally four applications are considered satisfactory. The applied shading porcelain is dried by holding the restoration in a preheated furnace muffle of 1290°F (700°C). The additional color applications are fired at 1725°F (940°C) without hold time. For the final color cycle, firing is done in air at 1725°F by holding the temperature for 30 seconds to one minute. The thickness of the coloring porcelain after four applications is approximately 125 μm. Acidulated fluoride has the potential to damage these surface colorants, and hence if a fluoride mouthwash is prescribed it should be a neutral fluoride. The restoration is finally tried on the preparation and any necessary adjustments made. Polishing is completed with abrasive rubber wheels.

The cast glass ceramic restoration can be acid etched (with ammonium bifluoride) on its internal surface to aid in retention. The restoration is then cemented with a translucent glass-ionomer cement. If a metallic restoration like silver amalgam forms a part of the preparation, colored opaque cements should be considered.

Standard dental radiographs can verify the accuracy and fit of the restoration to the tooth. DICOR inlays are stronger than porcelain inlays fired on refractory dies. After cementation, the incidence of fracture for these inlays is lower than those of ceramic inlays fabricated on refractory dies, but higher than for inlays made with the CEREC system.

Castable Apatite Ceramic (Cera Pearl)

The required tooth reduction for Cera Pearl crowns is 2.0 mm on the occlusal or incisal surfaces, 1.5 mm on the axial surfaces, and 1.2 mm on the margins. The finish line may be a heavy chamfer or shoulder. All sharp angles should be rounded to minimize stress concentration. For class I and class II inlays, the desired reduction is 2.0 mm on the occlusal surface and 1.5mm from the proximal surface. Class III and Class V inlays since are subjected to a minimum force, do not need more than 1.5 mm thickness. All internal angles of the cavity preparation should be rounded, and no bevels placed on the cavosurface margin.

A full arch impression is taken and a sectional working cast poured in Type IV dental stone. Prior to wax up, a die spacer, 25 μms in thickness, is applied on every surface of the die except within 1.0 mm of the margins. A wax pattern is fabricated on the die. One end of the sprue is attached to the thickest portion of the die and the other end to the ceramic crucible. Phosphate bonded high heat investment material, which shows an expansion of 0.6% at 400°C and 0.9% at 800°C is used in this system. Its strength after heating is 90 kg/cm². A firing shrinkage of 0.53% is seen in Cera Pearl. The sprued wax pattern is located inside the preformed silicone mold. The investment is mixed for one minute under vacuum and poured into the silicone mold. After sixty minutes, the silicone mold can be easily separated from the set investment. The ringless investment is then dried in an electric oven at temperatures of less than 100°C for at least 30 minutes. Over the next 30 minutes the temperature is raised to 500°C. Finally, the oven temperature is held at 800°C for 30 minutes. The investment mold is then transferred to a high heat processor. 8–10 gms of raw Cera Pearl is placed in the ceramic crucible, melted at 1460°C under vacuum and cast into the mold. After the casting process has completed, the ring is removed from the processor and transferred to the crystallization oven.

Crystallization makes the casting highly dense and turns it into a more stronger, harder and chemically stable structure. The crystallization process is started at 750°C and the temperature maintained for 15 minutes. Oven temperature is then raised at 50°C per minute until the temperature of 870°C is reached. After one hour at this temperature, sufficient amount of crystal formation occurs. Above 870°C, crystals grow excessively and result in too white an appearance.

The investment ring is removed from the oven and cooled to room temperature. The casting is divested and cleaned of adhered investment by sand blasting with 20 μm aluminium oxide powder. The sprue is cut with a carborundum disk and the surface smoothened with a carborundum stone. At this stage, the internal and marginal fit of the restoration is checked on the die. Any minor adjustment if needed is done with a small round diamond point/carborundum stone using light pressure and less speed. Occlusal and proximal contacts are similarly adjusted using diamond points after placing the restoration on the working cast. Undue stresses can induce microcracks, therefore Cera Pearl should always be seated with light finger pressure. The restoration is then seated onto the prepared tooth and the final adjustments done with diamond points.

The crystallized CeraPearl casting is very white, hence requires the application of an external stain. Cera stain especially formulated for the purpose consists of B_2O_3-SiO_2-Al_2O_3-K_2O and traces of metal oxides. It is available in 14 cervical shades and 3 incisal shades. Selected shades of Cera Stain are mixed and applied evenly on the restoration surface. The stained restoration is dried and preheated in front of a glazing oven for 2–3 minutes, and then placed in the oven at 500°C. The temperature is raised 35–50°C per minute in air, until 790°C is reached.

Glass ionomer cement is considered the best choice for a luting agent, because it would adhere both to the tooth structure and CeraPearl restoration. However, CeraPearl must be made conducive for adherence to glass-ionomer cement. Activation is the process by which a casting is treated mechanically and chemically to improve its bond to the tooth structure. The cavity surface of the restoration is sandblasted with 20 µm alumina powder and cleaned in an ultrasonic bath. Acetone is used to remove any oil residue. Chemical activation is done by applying a liquid UHK 001 for 5 minutes. It is then rinsed away with distilled water, and the restoration subjected to heat at 140°C in an oven for 10 minutes. After cooling to room temperature, the restoration is ready for cementation. The activation process aids in adhesion by liberating calcium ions from the apatite and these form hydrate bonds.

Pressed Glass Ceramic (IPS Empress)

This system also utilizes the lost wax technique but differs from the earlier described castable ceramics in that the material is pressed into the mold under pressure and not centrifugally driven. Here also, a wax pattern of the proposed restoration (inlay, veneer or crown) is first fabricated and then invested in a phosphate bonded investment material. Following the burnout procedure, the ring along with the investment is placed in a specialized mold that has an alumina plunger (Fig. 20.21). The ceramic ingot is placed under the plunger, the entire assembly is heated to 1150°C and the plunger presses the molten ceramic into the mold. The final shade of the restoration is adjusted by surface staining or veneering. In the veneering technique, the original wax up is cut back by 0.3 mm. After moulding and baking have been carried out as described, feldspathic porcelains are then added on the surface to obtain full contour and the correct shade. In some cases, the pressed core itself is ground to produce a core, which represents the dentin onto which the incisal porcelain and glaze are added (Fig. 20.22). When using the lost wax technique, total shrinkage is reduced as the only shrinkage, which occurs, is during cooling, that can be controlled with an investment having an appropriate expansion.

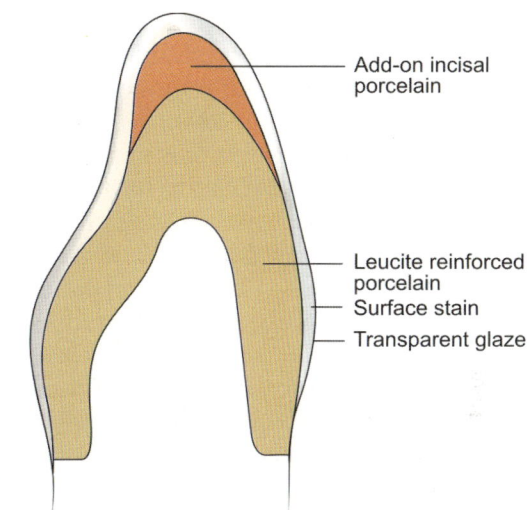

Fig. 20.22: Ceramic furnace for IPS Empress restorations

Machined Ceramic Inlays

Until 1988, ceramic restorations were fabricated mainly by sintering and/or casting techniques. Machined restorations have thereafter gained in popularity. There are two principle machining approaches for dental restorations.

Analogous Systems

- Copy milling/grinding technique: automatic (Ceromatic II) and manual (Celay)
- Erosive technique

Digital Systems

- CAD-CAM technology

Since the digital systems are more popular, these will be discussed in greater detail.

Copy Milling Technique

In this technique, it is possible to mill a restoration from ceramic materials using special systems like Celay, Ceromatic II, DCP etc. The best known copy grinding system is Celay (Mikrona, Switzerland), which was introduced commercially in 1991. Originally, the system was developed to produce

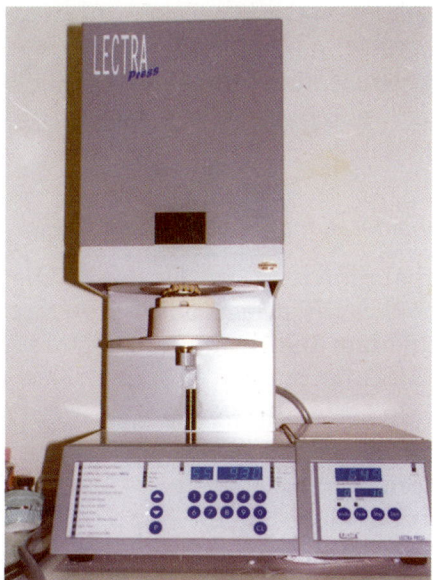

Fig. 20.21: Ceramic furnace for IPS Empress restorations

inlays and onlays, however recent modifications in this system allow for production of crown copings, bridge substructures and veneers. The materials, which can be subjected to milling, are Celay blocks and copings of InCeram and InCeram Spinel.

The copy milling technique is based on the idea of first fabricating a prototype inlay (proinlay), which is then copied using a scanning tool or micropalpation (finger) method. The final restoration is then milled from a preformed ceramic block. It is highly necessary to stress here that any cavity or tooth preparation receiving a porcelain restoration should be free of any undercuts. One approach is to remove the undercut but this would involve large destruction of sound tooth tissue. A more conservative approach is the blocking of undercuts in the cavity by using a resin modified glass-ionomer on the die if an indirect method of manufacturing is used. The proinlay is fabricated with a blue resin based composite (Celay Tech) made either directly on a prepared tooth or indirectly on a die made from the impression. The prototype is fixed into the Celay unit. As the surface of the proinlay is scanned with a tracing tool (smooth discs), a coarse diamond coated disc (124 μm grain size) simultaneously roughs out the shape of the ceramic restoration (A finger guide may also be used to trace the surface of the pattern). A fine white powder is applied to the proinlay and the scanning is again done using a smooth disc and fissured and tapered burs. Matching fine diamond discs and burs (60–70 mm grain size) refine the shape of the gross ceramic restoration. Once the white powder has been completely traced off, the milling of ceramic inlay is considered complete. Stains and glazes may be added before the inlay is etched and silanized. The time taken to mill the restoration depends upon the experience of the operator, complexity of the restoration and sharpness of the cutting disks. The average time taken for the milling procedure is 20–30 min. One problem, which may be frequently encountered during the use of the copy milling technique is the difficulty in obtaining accurate proinlays.

Erosion Method

Ultrasonic/sono erosion (DFE, Erosonic) used for grinding ceramic requires a metal based negative form of the interior and exterior contours of the restoration, which are produced by wax moulding and casting or by intensive copper plating of the impression. These are called 'sonotrodes'. Both sonotrodes fitting exactly together are guided onto a ceramic blank after connecting to an ultrasonic generator under slight pressure. The ceramic blank is surrounded by an abrasive suspension of hard particles such as boron carbide, which on acceleration by ultrasonics erodes the restoration out of the ceramic block.

CAD-CAM Generated Porcelain Inlays

Mormann and Brandestini for the first time used a CADCAM device to digitize and store cavity parameters, and a computer milling device to then shape a restoration out of the ceramic block. This method was made commercially available as an integrated CAD-CAM unit for dental use in 1988 by Siemens, known as *Cerec*. The original system came to be known as Cerec-1, when in September 1994 an improved version Cerec-2 was introduced. The unit consists of a three dimensional video camera (scan head), an electronic image processor memory unit and a processor (computer) which is connected to a miniature milling machine.

Cerec-1 cannot prepare the occlusal anatomy of the restoration whereas Cerec-2 can. In addition to the grinding wheel, the Cerec-2 unit is also equipped with a cylindrical diamond stone which is able to finish off undercuts at buccal extensions, curved shoulders at cusp preparations and the proximal areas. Also when comparing the camera systems and image processing of Cerec-1 and Cerec-2 units, Cerec-2 is a definite improvement over the former.

Briefly, a CAD-CAM system uses digital information about cavity preparation or a pattern of the restoration to provide a computer aided design (CAD) on the video monitor for inspection and modification. Once the three dimensional image of the restoration is accepted, the computer translates that image into a set of instructions to guide a milling tool (Computer Assisted Manufacturing CAM) in cutting the restoration out of the ceramic block. In a way, the computerized unit serves as an automated mini dental lab.

Cavity Considerations for CAD-CAM Inlays

Tooth preparation for a ceramic inlay/onlay requires conventional cavity design with slight modifications to accommodate the computerized milling device. These modifications are:

- No convexities should be present on the pulpal and gingival walls. They may be flat or concave buccolingually.
- The occlusal step should be prepared 1.5–2.0 mm in depth and any isthmus or groove extension should be at least 1.5 mm wide to decrease the possibility of fracture of the restoration.

- The buccal and lingual walls of the occlusal portion of the preparation may converge towards the occlusal. This feature is unique to the Cerec system as it can automatically block out any undercuts during the optical impression. A more conservative cavity preparation is therefore permissible along the occlusal aspect, especially when replacing old amalgam restorations where undercuts were purposely given for retention. The facial and lingual walls in the proximal box are prepared in the usual fashion with slight divergence towards the occlusal. Convergence is not given here so as to avoid excessively thick composite cement lines.
- Axial walls should be straight and not follow the convex contour of the proximal surface of the tooth.
- No cavosurface or marginal bevels should be given.

Technique for CAD-CAM Fabricated Inlays

Five steps are basically involved in any type of CADCAM system. These include:

- Computerized surface digitization
- Computer aided designing
- Computer aided manufacturing
- Computer aided esthetics
- Computer aided finishing

The last two steps are very difficult and hence as yet are not a feature in commercial systems.

Surface digitization: After the dentist has prepared the tooth, a scanning device is used to collect information on the shape of the preparation. This step is referred to as the *'optical impression'*. An image of the preparation is displayed on the monitor and the camera orientation corrected accordingly. Repeated optical impressions are taken until the most ideal is found and stored in the computer.

The scanning devices can be either mechanical or optical (infrared video camera). The optical sensors are not able to measure highly transparent or reflective surfaces and so enamel has to be covered with a powder or a water soluble color. The mechanical scanning conducted by a profilometer or pinpoint sensors are very precise, however they have several shortcomings. The scanning tip produces errors in measurement on steep flanks (cusp slopes) and distorts easily. Undercut areas and narrow gaps like fissures also cannot be explored and have to be blocked out.

The 3-D scanning methods can be applied either directly onto the tooth or indirectly onto a model fabricated from an impression of the cavity or a provision. The advantages of the direct technique are: (1) From cavity preparation to bonding, the entire procedure is completed in one session and eliminates the need for impressions, stone casts and dies and hence the associated inaccuracies (2) Adjustments are done in the mouth obviating the need for an opposing cast and articulator mounting. Laboratory facilities are also not required (3) Because the procedure is completed in one visit, an interim restoration is not necessary and the chances of lost temporaries, sensitivities between appointments and microleakage are greatly diminished. The disadvantages in the direct technique include a waste of expensive chair time in case of a difficulty during milling or designing. Also since, the adjustments and polishing need to be done at the chair side, the time required for the procedure is significantly increased. In offices where multiple practitioners are sharing the same CAD-CAM unit, simultaneous appointments cannot be given.

The indirect method of scanning overcomes the limitations of direct method. An impression of the prepared tooth as well as adjacent teeth is taken in elastomeric or hydrocolloid impression materials. A quadrant tray is acceptable. The impression is poured in die stone and a split cast model made. Temporization needs to be done in between the appointments, with Dura Seal best serving the purpose. It is an autopolymerizing polymethyl methacrylate resin with plasticizers; available as a powder liquid system, mixed and applied directly onto the tooth without a cementing medium. It does not contaminate bonding surfaces and also does not require shaping or adjustment. Because the material contains plasticizers, it remains elastic throughout the temporization period and is easy to remove at a later stage.

Computer Aided Designing (CAD)

This step involves three dimensional image processing. The operator enters data and confirms the features of the preparation like boundaries of the restoration, position of the gingival margins, proximal contacts and contours, buccal and lingual extensions etc. The collected data is further processed by curve smoothening and if necessary by data reduction. Undercuts can be blocked at this stage.

Computer Aided Manufacturing (CAM)

The cavity surface of inlays, onlays or crowns are milled to the dimensions of the scanned image with diamond disks or other instruments that are electrically driven and lubricated with water. The occlusal surface cannot be ground with CEREC-1 whereas CEREC-2 can form the occlusal surface also. The occlusal anatomy when using CEREC-1 is completed later by the operator using diamond burs. Controlled cutting of the ceramic is done by: rotation of the block; horizontal movement of the block into the wheel and vertical movement of the cutting wheel. The fit of the restoration is confirmed in the patient's mouth and any necessary adjustments made. Proximal contours and contacts can also be provisionally adjusted.

At the cementation visit, rubber dam is applied and fit of the inlay verified on the tooth. Proximal adjustments are done with diamond abrasive disks run from coarse to fine. Proximal surfaces should be polished at this stage itself, as these would be difficult to be reached later. The inlay is then prepared for bonding which includes preparation of both the restoration and the tooth. Etching is done on the cavity surface of the inlay either with a microetcher and/or ammonium bifluoride or hydrofluoric acid. After etching, a silane bonding enhancer is painted onto the surface. Surface preparation of the tooth follows the usual procedure. The cavity surface is etched for 15–30 seconds with 30% phosphoric acid. Depending on the bonding system used, the appropriate primer and bonding agent are applied to the tooth surface. The cementation procedure and subsequent finishing and polishing are similar to as in other ceramic inlays. Glazing may not be required in these restorations as they can be easily polished.

Disadvantages of the CAD-CAM system include (1) initial high cost for the purchase of Cerec unit (2) time and cost must be invested to master the technique and (3) contouring of the occlusal surface may still have to be carried out by the clinician.

Recently, a newer version of Cerec – Cerec 3 has been introduced. This system simplifies and accelerates the fabrication of ceramic restorations compared to former systems. It accommodates advances in computer technology thus allowing numerous simplifications and increased automation. Cerec 3 software simplifies occlusal and functional registration. Proper occlusion is established accurately and quickly, manual adjustment is reduced to a minimum. The separate branding device, which provides greater detail and is fitted with two finger cutters is connected via radio control wave to control unit. The grinding unit receives data from the control unit independent of its location in the practice. The second restoration can be designed while the first is being milled. The grinding unit is also equipped with a laser scanner and can be used for indirect applications through a personal computer. Since it is equipped with an intraoral video camera or a digital radiography unit, it can also be used for patient education and for user training.

Cicero Dental Systems B.V. (Hoorn, The Netherlands) has recently introduced a Cicero System for fabrication of ceramic restorations. The Cicero (computer integrated ceramic reconstruction) method for producing ceramic restorations uses optical scanning, ceramic sintering and computer assisted milling techniques to fabricate restorations with maximal static and dynamic occlusal contact relations. The technique consists of optically digitizing a gypsum die, designing the crown layer build up, and subsequent pressing, sintering and milling consecutive layers of a shaded high strength alumina core material, a layer of dentin porcelain, and a final layer of incisal porcelain. Final finishing is performed in the dental laboratory. The Cicero method allows efficient production of all ceramic restorations without compromising on esthetics or function.

PORCELAIN LAMINATES/VENEERS

Glazed porcelain has a long-standing history of use as one of the most esthetic and biocompatible materials available in dentistry, surpassed only by enamel. Porcelain's abrasion and stain resistance is excellent and it is well tolerated by gingival tissues.

The advent of porcelain labial veneers as a permanent esthetic restoration marked the progress in acid-etch, bonding and esthetic restorative techniques. The concept of acid etching porcelain was cited in the dental literature in 1975 when Pouchette described the innovative restoration of a fractured incisor with an "etched silanated porcelain block".

In the early 1980s, key pioneers in American laminate dentistry were instrumental in the development of porcelain veneers and the associated techniques of their fabrication and placement.

Features of Porcelain Laminate/veneers

The advent of bonding has provided the concerned dentist with a means to attach composite resins to the unsightly tooth in order to create an esthetic illusion. A recent breakthrough that facilitated retention of porcelain to the tooth surface has added a new dimension to esthetic dentistry (Figs 20.23A, B and 20.24A, B).

Advantages

- *Color*: Porcelain offers better color control, color stability and natural appearance.
- *Bond strength*: The bond of etched porcelain veneer to enamel is considerably stronger than any other veneering system.
- *Periodontal health*: Highly glazed porcelain surface provides less plaque accumulation.

- *Resistance to abrasion*: The wear and abrasion resistance is exceptionally good.
- *Inherent porcelain strength*: The bond strength and the actual strength of porcelain is greater than other materials.
- *Resistance to fluid adsorption*: Porcelain adsorbs less fluid than any other veneering material.
- *Esthetics*: Esthetics is considerably better than any other veneering material because of the ability to control color and surface texture with ceramic.

Disadvantages

- *Time:* The placing of veneers is technique sensitive and time consuming.
- *Repair:* The veneers cannot be easily repaired once they are luted to the enamel.
- *Technique sensitive:* The process of making veneers is an indirect one requiring impression making and laboratory phase.
- *Color:* It is difficult to modify the color once the veneers have been luted in position on tooth surface.
- *Tooth preparation:* Tooth preparation is required to prevent potential problems associated with overcontouring.
- *Fragility:* The veneers are extremely fragile and difficult to manipulate.
- *Cost*: Expensive for the patient.

Indications

Porcelain veneers are indicated in the following circumstances.

Discoloration: Due to fluorosis, tetracycline staining etc.

Enamel defects: Various types of enamel hypoplasias and enamel hypocalcification.

Diastemata: Diastema closure can be done.

Malpositioned teeth: The esthetic illusion of straight teeth can be developed when teeth are malpositioned.

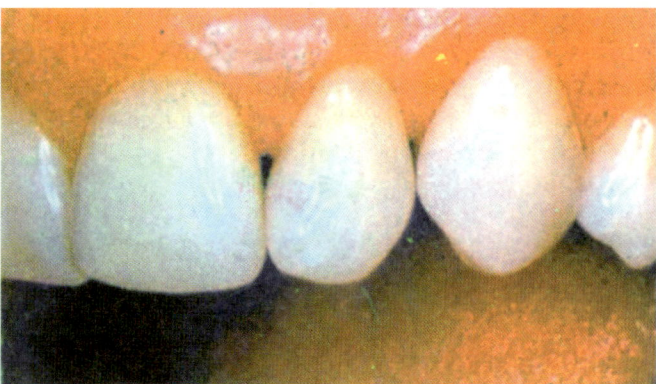

Fig. 20.23B: Maxillary left canine restored with porcelain laminate

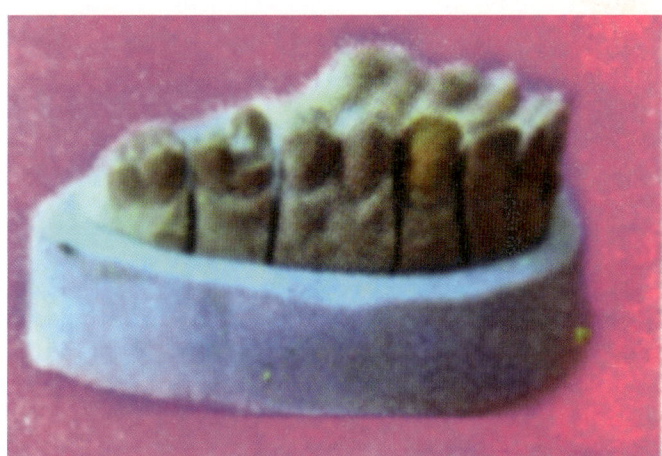

Fig. 20.24A: Maxillary left canine prepared for laminate

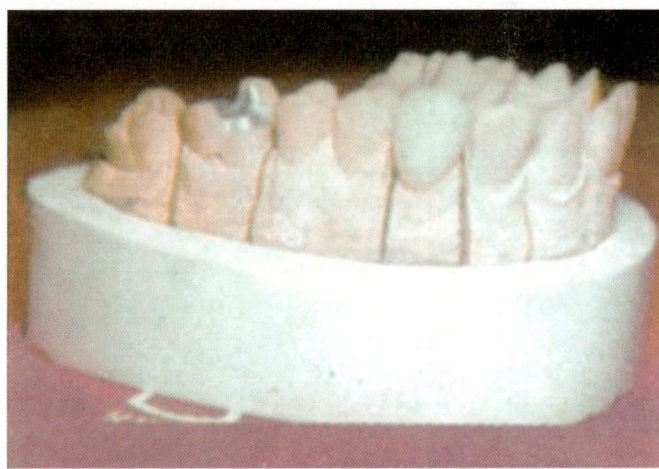

Fig. 20.24B: Laminate placed on maxillary left canine

Malocclusion: The configuration of lingual surfaces of anterior teeth can be changed to develop incisal guidance or centric holding in malocclusions or periodontally compromised teeth.

Poor restorations: Teeth with numerous, shallow, unesthetic restorations on labial surfaces can be dramatically restored.

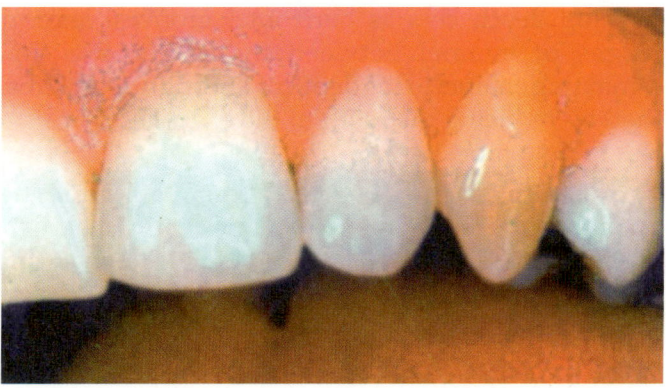

Fig. 20.23A: Discolored maxillary left canine (preoperative)

Aging: Color changes brought about by the ongoing process of aging can be masked.

Wear patterns: Porcelain laminates are also useful in those cases that exhibit slowly progressive wear patterns.

Contraindications

The contraindications are as follows:

Available enamel: There should be sufficient enamel around the whole periphery of the laminates not only for adhesion but more importantly to seal the veneer to the tooth surface. Bonding to dentin is generally much less retentive than to enamel. If the tooth surface is composed predominantly of dentin and cementum, crowns will be the treatment of choice.

Ability to etch enamel: Deciduous teeth and teeth that have been extensively fluoridated may not etch effectively.

Oral habits: Patients with certain habit patterns such as bruxism or biting on foreign objects may not be ideal candidates for veneers.

Enamel Reduction

There is no single way to prepare teeth for porcelain laminates. The decision of whether to reduce enamel should depend on the following biological and technical factors.

- Esthetics
- Relative tooth position
- Masking of tetracycline stains
- Margin placements
- Age and psyche of the patient
- Periodontal health

Rationale for Enamel Preparation

Enamel preparation may be performed for several reasons:

- To provide adequate space for the porcelain material.
- To remove convexities and provide for a path of insertion in above situations where either the incisal or the interproximal are to be included in the veneer; the best path of insertion is that which will require the least amount of enamel reduction, as modified by esthetic demands of the patient.
- To provide space for an opaquer where necessary and for the composite resin luting cement.
- To provide a definite seat to help position the laminate during placement.
- To obtain an enamel surface conducive for etching and bonding the laminate.
- To facilitate margin placement in the sulcus in severely discolored teeth.

Procedure for Enamel Reduction

It is extremely difficult for the ceramist to fabricate a laminate that fits accurately to a feather edge finish line, or to work with a thickness less than 0.3 mm. In broad sense, the amount of enamel reduction considered necessary to suit the technician's needs is in the range of 0.3 to 0.6 mm or about half the thickness of the available enamel.

Enamel reduction should be considered from five distinct aspects:

a. Labial reduction
b. Interproximal reduction
c. Sulcular extension and margin placement
d. Incisal or occlusal modification
e. Lingual reduction

a. Labial Reduction

The labial preparation should encompass the amount of reduction necessary to facilitate the placement of an esthetic restoration. Ideally, one would like to replace the same amount of enamel that is removed by the preparation. The preparation should remain within the enamel wherever possible and more certainly at all the peripheral marginal areas to ensure an adequate seal to enamel.

There may be situations when in small areas, to facilitate cosmetic alignment; some amount of dentin will be exposed by the preparation of the tooth. This is not very critical when limited only to small areas and if the margins remain on enamel.

Depth Guide: The depth cutting diamonds come in two sizes, LVS no. 1 and LVS no.2 (Fig. 20.25). These dimensions are 0.5 mm for the most situations and 0.3 mm for small teeth. The appropriate cutter is selected. Gently draw the diamond across the labial surface of the tooth in a mesial to distal direction. This will develop depth cuts as horizontal grooves, leaving ridges of enamel between them. Remove this remaining enamel to the depth of the original grooves, thereby reducing the tooth to the exact amount – no less and no more.

Alternative method is to use a round bur no.1. The bur should be held at the same angle every time when indentations are made into the enamel to the full depth of the bur head. These indentations are created randomly across the surface of the enamel, thereby ensuring that subsequent reduction to the depth of these indentations will create uniformly equal preparation on the labial aspect of the tooth.

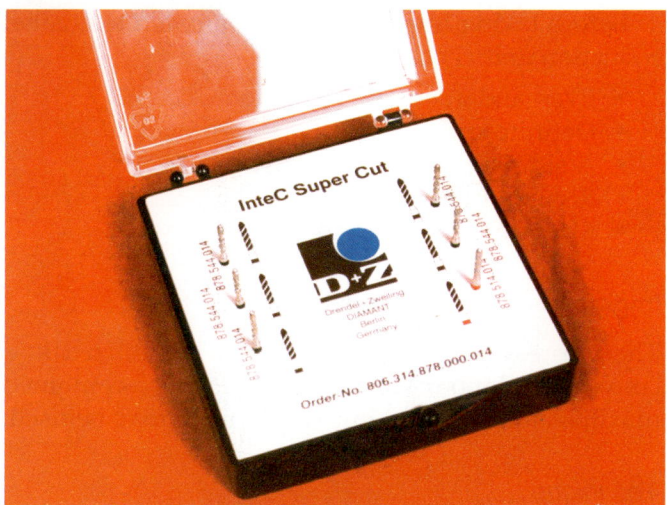

Fig. 20.25: Depth cutting instruments for laminate preparation

The problem with this type of approach is that these depth cuts can vary, depending on the angle that the bur is held at, and hence the amount of time necessary for this process might be greater.

Reduction of Remaining Enamel: The remaining enamel must be removed to the depth of these initial cuts. The labial reduction should encompass two aspects.

- The unique LVS two-grit diamond is specifically designed to do this simultaneously with only one bur. The instrument has 1.3 mm of fine grit diamond at the tip and a hybrid mixture of rapidly cutting diamond above.
- Move the diamond across the labial surface from mesial to distal direction, following the curvature of the gingiva from the top of the mesial interproximal papillae down to the most apical extent of the free gingival margin and back up to the tip of the distal interproximal papillae. The finish line should preferably be right at the gingival margin.

b. Interproximal Extension

The margin of the porcelain laminate proximally should generally be hidden within the embrasure area. Depending on the individual form of the tooth, it is usually desirable to extend this margin about half way into the interproximal contact area.

Extension of the laminate beyond the mesiobuccal and distobuccal line angles also ensure the wrap around effect, with etched resin bonds at right angles to the labial surface for increased bond strength. This is achieved with the LVS two grit diamond – moving the margin into the embrasure area and just lingual to the buccal surface of the interproximal papillae so that it will not be visible from the lateral oblique view or directly from the front. For the technician it is also useful to have extra reduction in the embrasure area so as to facilitate porcelain bulk which aids in the strengthening of the laminate around the whole periphery and promote proximal translucency.

c. Sulcular Extension and Margin Placement

At this stage the preparation ends right at the gingival margin. It is, however, desirable to place it just within the sulcus. There is no need to extend it deep and hide it sub gingivally as in crown and bridge procedures. The porcelain with the underlying composite resin will blend in harmoniously with the rest of the tooth without showing a cement line or metal margin. There is really no need to go any more than 0.05 to 0.1mm into the sulcus or even to remain supragingival if a dramatic color change is not a priority.

Sulcular extensions are carried out by LVS two grit diamonds described earlier. Place a gingival displacement cord in the sulcus for about 8–10 seconds. This procedure of first developing a preparation line confluent with the gingival margin and then placing a retraction cord prior to refining and extending the finish line into the sulcus ensures:

i. access for the diamond
ii. less gingival damage
iii. direct vision of the margin

This sulcular preparation remains at a considerable distance from the biologic width so there is little potential for violating it and developing untoward gingival reactions. The margin must remain at a point where after tissue displacement, it will once again be visible for finishing of the porcelain laminate and the resin-luting agent.

The fine diamond at the tip of the LVS two grit diamond cuts very slowly, thus reducing the risk of over preparation when finishing the sulcular extension of the preparation. The diamond merely refines and defines the finish line, and in doing so it moves the finish line from being right at the gingival margin to being 0.2 mm or less into the sulcus.

Finish Line Configuration

A feather or knife edge finish line is the most conservative preparation but is not advocated because of:

i. The difficulty in fabricating porcelain to the required degree of thinness accurately.
ii. The inevitable increased thickness subgingivally results in potential gingival problems.
iii. Laboratory problems in delineating the exact end of preparation line.

So a chamfer or a bevelled shoulder is the most acceptable finish line.

d. Incisal or Occlusal Reduction

The fabrication of a porcelain veneer overlapping an incisal edge makes placement of the restoration much easier by virtue of having a definite stop during seating. This incisal overlap can be fabricated purely as a positioning device and then later removed once the veneer is bonded in place. This latter type of incisal extension requires no incisal preparation because the overlap will be ground away following luting and placement of the laminates.

The reduction should be at least 1 mm if it is desired to restore the original length. Simple reshaping at the edge without vertical reduction will suffice if the teeth are to be lengthened. If the incisal edge is to be included it is useful to increase the amount of horizontal tooth reduction at the periphery of the preparation, the interproximal areas, and the incisal edges. This will give the technician extra space to stack porcelain and so develop a thicker periphery for strength.

In general, never end the incisal edge reduction in positions where excursive movements of the mandible will cause shearing stress across the junction of porcelain laminate and the tooth. This potentiates fracture of the porcelain causes debonding, and ongoing exposure of the composite resin in the crucial area.

e. Lingual Reduction

Any reduction of the incisal edge may necessitate some lingual enamel modification so that there is no butt joint at the incisal/lingual junction but rather a rounded chamfer. This modification will help to prevent the porcelain from shearing away from the incisal edge during function. It also ensures:

 i. increased thickness of porcelain in this critical lingual area that is being used for incisal guidance.
 ii. Enamel bonds at right angles to those on the incisal edges, and increased strength

Excessive buccal convexity in a tooth makes it difficult to overlap the incisal edge and still maintain an incisal path of insertion. An excessive amount of labial tooth structure may have to be removed to facilitate a path of insertion, but this increases the chances of exposing large amounts of dentine. In these situations, the veneer should be designed to rotate about a more rounded incisal preparation in seating it.

Before taking impressions, reevaluate the enamel reduction and check:
- Even and adequate reduction
- Definite smooth finish line
- A simple path of insertion
- Rounded line angles
- Modification of the contact areas

Impression and Temporization

The impression material either can be utilized in a conventional type of tray or, to save time, a combined maxillary-mandibular bite tray system may be used.

Technique

Prior to impression taking, the gingival tissue should be displaced adequately so that the final finish line can be placed in the sulcus. Tissue displacement is readily achieved with fine cotton impregnated with an astringent such as aluminium sulphate. Gently tuck the retraction cord into the sulcus. Excess force should not be employed to prevent disrupting the integrity of the junctional epithdium. The cord should extend from the interproximal mesial surface around the labial surface and into the distal interproximal surface.

It is kept in place for 5–8 minutes before being removed. Remove wet to avoid tearing the friable junctional epithelium and precipitate bleeding.

Rubber base impressions are the materials of choice. They should be of two consistencies: light and heavy. The tray material should be of the heavy type. The light bodied material should be syringed into the sulcus and over the preparation. The heavy body facilitates moving the light body into the sulcus and embrasures, to pick up the periphery of the preparation. The impression material should have high tensile strength as well as accuracy. Insert the tray from an oblique buccal direction to make sure that all labial and lingual relationships are properly recorded.

Temporizations

Temporizations for laminates are usually unnecessary because, in most situations, only half of the enamel surface is removed and the dentinal tubules are not exposed. Chances of sensitivity are reduced and there is minimal esthetic compromise.

Indirect acrylics are generally utilized for fabrication of temporary laminates (details given in Chapter 11).

The restoration is fabricated as described earlier. The technique may vary depending upon the material choosen.

Feldspathic and leucite reinforced porcelains have been commonly used for the fabrication of laminates. An inherent disadvantage when fabricating laminates of 0.3 mm thickness is that they are fragile and demand excessive care when manipulating them in the laboratory or clinics. Their thinness may also predispose to the development of flaws. To overcome this problem, Procera has developed an industrial procedure to fabricate individual ceramic shells of densely sintered, high purity alumina with a thickness of 0.25 mm. The shell is used as a core for a ceramic laminate and manufactured in the same way as a Procera Allceram core. Porcelain is baked on the shell and fired without a refractory model. These are simple to use and provide excellent esthetics.

CAD-CAM/CAD-CIM

Computer-aided design (CAD) is the use of computer terminology for the process of design and design-documentation. Computer-aided manufacturing (CAM) is the use of computer software to control machine tools and related machinery in the manufacturing of workpieces. Computer-integrated manufacturing (CIM) is the manufacturing approach of using computers to control the entire production process. This integration allows individual processes to exchange information with each other and initiate actions. Through the integration of computers, manufacturing can be faster and less error-prone, although the main advantage is the ability to create automated manufacturing processes. The CAD-CAM can be carried out at chairside or in the laboratory.

All CAD/CAM systems consist of three different steps:
 a. Scanner: A digitalization tool/scanner that transforms a present geometry into digital data that can be processed by the computer.
 b. Design software: Software that processes data and, depending on the application, produces a data set for the product to be fabricated.
 c. Processing device: A production technology that transforms the data set into the desired product.

CAD/CAM Components

a. Scanner

The term scanner in dentistry means data collection tools that measure three-dimensional jaw and tooth structures and transform them into digital data sets. There are two different types of scanners:
 i. Optical scanners
 ii. Mechanical scanners
 i. Optical scanner: The basis of this type of scanner is the collection of three-dimensional structures in a so-called 'triangualtion procedure'. Here, the source of light and the receptor unit are in a definite angle in relationship to one another. Via this angle the computer can calculate a three-dimensional data set from the image on the receptor unit. The recently introduced Nobel Procera scanner uses conoscopic holography technology. The manufacturer describes this technology as superior to triangulation as projected and reflected beams travel the same pathway. This allows scanning of steep slopes of up to 85^0.
 ii. Mechanical scanner: In this scanner, the master cast is read mechanically line-by line by means of a ruby ball measuring the three-dimensional structure. The disadvantage is the complicated mechanics, which make the apparatus very expensive and long processing times compared to optical systems.

b. Design Software

Special software is provided by manufacturers for designing various kinds of dental restorations. With such software, crown and fixed dental prostheses can be constructed. Some softwares also offer the possibility of designing full crowns, partial crowns, inlays, onlays, adhesive prosthesis and implant abutments.

c. Processing Devices

The construction data produced with the CAD software are converted into milling strips and loaded into the milling device. Processing devices are distinguished by means of the number of milling axes:
- 3-Axis devices
- 4-Axis devices
- 5-Axis devices

Milling device has degrees of movement in the three spatial directions. Thus, the mill path points are uniquely defined by the X -, Y -, and Z – values. In addition to three spatial dimensions, 4th axis is the rotable tension bridge and rotating the milling spindle is 5th axis. This enables milling of complex geometries with subsections.

The CEREC System

CAD-CAM device to digitize and store cavity parameters, and a computer milling device to shape a restoration was made commercially available for dental use by Siemens, known as Cerec. The original system was Cerec-1 (indications: single and dual-surface inlays). Later an improved version Cerec-2 was introduced (indications: inlays, onlays, veneers). The unit consists of a three-dimensional video camera (scan head), an electronic image processor memory unit and a processor (computer) which is connected to a miniature milling machine.

Cerec-1 cannot prepare the occlusal anatomy of the restoration whereas Cerec-2 can. In addition to the grinding wheel, the Cerec-2 unit is also equipped with a cylindrical diamond stone which is able to finish off undercuts at buccal extensions, curved shoulders at cusp preparations and the proximal areas. With enlargement of the grinding unit from three to six axes and upgrading of the software for the occlusion and the complex machining of the floor parts, the previous limitations have been eliminated.

Recently, a newer version, Cerec 3 has been introduced. This system simplifies and accelerates the fabrication of ceramic restorations compared to former systems. It accommodates advances in computer technology thus allowing numerous simplifications and increased automation. Cerec 3 software simplifies occlusal and functional registration. Proper occlusion is established accurately and quickly, manual adjustment is reduced to a minimum. The separate branding device, which provides greater detail and is fitted with two finger cutters is connected via radio control wave to control unit. The grinding unit receives data from the control unit independent of its location in the practice. The second restoration can be designed while the first is being milled. The grinding unit is also equipped with a Laser scanner and can be used for indirect applications through a personal computer. Since it is equipped with an intraoral video camera or a digital photography unit, it can also be used for patient education and for user training.

The newest model, known as CEREC AC (powered by BlueCam) also has the ability to take half-arch or full-arch impressions and create crowns, veneers, and bridges. The current acquisition system employs intense blue light from blue light-emitting diodes. To use the system, the entire tooth preparation to be scanned is coated with a layer of titanium dioxide powder, which makes translucent areas of the teeth opaque and permits the camera to register all of the tissues. Several optical impressions are then taken from an occlusal orientation, being sure to obtain images of the tooth to be restored as well as the adjacent and opposing teeth. After the impression is complete, a 3-D rendering of the tooth to be restored appears on the monitor. The dentist is able to mark where the die should begin and end based on this image. The software program then generates a proposed restoration based on comparisons to the surrounding teeth, which can then be altered or fine-tuned as needed. After the design is approved, the milling process can begin.

The Cadent iTero

Cadent introduced iTero as the first digital impression system for conventionally manufactured crowns and bridges. iTero acquire images using parallel confocal imaging. Specifically, the device projects 100,000 parallel beams of red laser light at the teeth and transforms the reflected light into digital data through the use of analog-to-digital converters. This technology allows scans to be taken without coating the teeth in powder. The absence of powder means that the scanner can be rested directly on the teeth during scanning. One disadvantage is that the scanner head is large.

The Lava Chairside Oral Scanner

The Lava Chairside Oral Scanner includes a mobile cart, a touch screen display, and a scanner with a camera at the end. The camera, which contains 192 LEDs and 22 lens systems, employs active wavefront sampling to capture images at video rate. After preparing the tooth and retracting the gingival tissue, the dentist dries the arch and gives it a light dusting of titanium dioxide powder. The scan is obtained by moving the wand first over the occlusal surfaces, then over the buccal surfaces, and finally over the lingual surfaces. An additional scan is taken of the occlusal surfaces. The monitor image, which appears instantly, can be rotated and magnified to ensure that all areas have been scanned properly and no holes appear. The dentist also has the ability to switch between 3-D and 2-D images. Finally, the system is compatible with 3-D glasses for a true 3-D experience. After signifying off on the scans, the data is send wirelessly to the laboratory, where the die is cut and the margin marked digitally.

Cavity Considerations for CAD-CAM Inlays

Tooth preparation for a ceramic inlay/onlay requires conventional cavity design with slight modifications to accommodate the computerized milling device. These modifications are:

- No convexities should be present on the pulpal and gingival walls. They may be flat or concave buccolingually.
- The occlusal step should be prepared 1.5–2.0 mm in depth and any isthmus or groove extension should be at least 1.5 mm wide to decrease the possibility of fracture of the restoration.
- The buccal and lingual walls of the occlusal portion of the preparation may converge towards the occlusal. This feature is unique to the Cerec system as it can automatically block

out any undercuts during the optical impression. A more conservative cavity preparation is therefore permissible along the occlusal aspect, especially when replacing old amalgam restorations where undercuts were purposely given for retention. The facial and lingua walls in the proximal box are prepared in the usual fashion with slight divergence towards the occlusal. Convergence is not given here so as to avoid excessively thick composite cement lines.

- Axial walls should be straight and not follow the convex contour of the proximal surface of the tooth.
- No cavosurface or marginal bevels should be given.

At the cementation visit, rubber dam is applied and fit of the inlay verified on the tooth. Proximal adjustments are done with diamond abrasive disks run from coarse to fine. Proximal surfaces should be polished at this stage itself, as these would be difficult to be reached later. The inlay is then prepared for bonding which includes preparation of both the restoration and the tooth. Etching is done on the cavity surface of the inlay either with a microetcher and/or ammonium bifluoride or hydrofluoric acid. After etching, a silane bonding enhancer is painted onto the surface. Surface preparation of the tooth follows the usual procedure. The cavity surface is etched for 15–30 seconds with 30% phosphoric acid. Depending on the bonding system used, the appropriate primer and bonding agent are applied to the tooth surface. The cementation procedure and subsequent finishing and polishing are similar to as in other ceramic inlays. Glazing may not be required in these restorations as they can be easily polished.

Advantages of CAD/CAM technology include speed, ease of use, and quality (ceramic blocks free from internal defects). Patients can receive their permanent restoration the same day they come in, without making a second appointment. Patients no longer need to have provisional restorations, which take time to fabricate and fit. Scans can be stored on the computer.

Disadvantages of CAD/CAM system include initial high cost for the purchase of unit, time and cost must be invested to master the technique and contouring of the occlusal surface may still have to be carried out by the clinician.

BIBLIOGRAPHY

1. Adair, P.J. and Grossman, D.G.: The castable ceramic crown. Int. J. Periodont. Rest. Dent.: 2, 33, 1984.
2. Andair, P.J. and Hoekstra, K.E.: Fit evaluation of a castable ceramic. I.A.D.R.: 61 (Abstr. 1500), 345, 1982.
3. Anderson, M. and Oden, A.: A new all ceramic crown. A densely sintered, high purity alumina coping with porcelain. Acta. Odont. Scand.: 51, 59, 1993.
4. Anderson, M., Razzoog, M.E., Oden, A., Hegenbarth, E.A. and Lang, B.R.: Procera: A new way to achieve an all ceramic crown. Quint. Int.: 29, 285, 1998.
5. Anusavice, K.J.: Degradability of dental ceramics. Adv. Dent. Res.: 6, 82, 1992.
6. Anusavice, K.J.: Recent developments in restorative dental ceramics. J.A.D.A.: 124, 72, 1993.
7. Anusavice, K.J. and Zhang, N.Z.: Chemical durability of Dicor and lithia based glass ceramics. Dent. Mater.: 13, 13, 1997.
8. Banks, R.G.: Conservative posterior ceramic restorations: A literature review. J.P.D.: 63, 619, 1990.
9. Barnes, D.M., Blank, L.W., Gingell, J.C. and Latta, M.A.: Clinical evaluation of castable ceramic veneers. J. Esthet. Dent.: 4, 21, 1992.
10. Blatz, M.B., Sadan, A. and Kern, M.: Resin-ceramic bonding: A review of the literature. J.P.D.: 89, 268, 2003.
11. Burke, F.J.T. and Qualtrough, A.J.E.: Aesthetic inlays: Composite or ceramic? B.D.J.: 176, 53, 1994.
12. Burke, F.J.T., Qualtrough, A.J.E. and Hale, R.W.: The dentine bonded ceramic crown: An ideal restoration? B.D.J.: 179, 58, 1995.
13. Calamia, J.R. and Simonsen, R.J.: Effects of coupling agents on bond strength of etched porcelain. J.D.R. (Spl. Issue): 63, 179, 1984.
14. Christensen, G.J.: Ceramic v/s porcelain fused-to-metal crowns: give your patients a choice. J.A.D.A.: 125, 311, 1994.
15. Christensen, G.J.: Veneering of teeth: State of the art. D.C.N.A.: 29, 373, 1985.
16. Christensen, G.J.: Why all-ceramic crowns? J.A.D.A.: 128, 1453, 1997.
17. Counil on Dental Materials, Instruments and Equipment: Porcelain repair materials. J.A.D.A.: 122, 124, 1991.
18. Daily, B., Gateau, P., Covo, L.: The double inlay technique: A new concept and improvement in design. J. Prosth. Dent. 85, 624, 2001.
19. David, S.B. and LoPresti, J.T.: Tooth-colored posterior restorations using cerec method (CAD/CAM) generated ceramic inlays. Compend. Contin. Educ. Dent.: 15, 802, 1994.
20. Denry I.L.: Recent advances in ceramics for dentistry. Crit Rev Oral Biol Med.: 7, 134, 1996.
21. Eidenbenz, S., Lehner, Ch.R. and Scharer, P.: Copy milling ceramic inlays from resin analogs: A practicable approach with the CELAY system. Int. J. Prosth.: 7, 134, 1994.
22. Fairhurst, C.W., Lockwood, P.E., Ringle, R.D. and Thompson, W.O.: The effect of glaze on porcelain strength. Dent. Mater.: 8, 203, 1992.
23. Ferrari, M., Mason, P.N., Fabianelli, A., Cagidiaco, M.C. and Davidson, C.L.: Influence of tissue characteristics at margins on leakage of class II indirect porcelain restorations. Am. J. Dent.: 12, 134, 1999.
24. Fuzzi, M. and Rapelli, G.: Ceramic inlays: clinical assessment and survival rates. J. Adhes. Dent.: 1, 71, 1999.
25. Geller, W. and Kwiatowski, S.J.: The Willi's glass crown: A new solution in the dark and shadowed zones of esthetic porcelain restorations. Quint. Int. Technol.: 11, 233, 1987.

26. Haywood, V.B., Heymann, H.O., Kusy, R.P., Whitley, J.Q. and Andreaus, S.B.: Polishing porcelain veneers: An SEM and specular reflectence analysis. Dent. Mater.: 4, 116, 1988.
27. Hager, B., Oden, A., Andersson, B., Andersson, L.: Procera allceram laminates: A clinical report. J. Prosth. Dent. 85, 231, 2001.
28. He L.H and Swain M.: A novel polymer infiltrated ceramic dental material. Dent Mater:27,527, 2011.
29. Heymann, H.O., Bayne, S.C., Sturdevant, J.R., Wilder, A.D. and Roberson, T.M.: The clinical performance of CAD/ CAM- generated ceramic inlays: A four year study. J.A.D.A.: 127, 1171, 1996.
30. Ibsen, R.L. and Yu, X.Y.: Establishing cuspid, guided occlusion with bonded porcelain. Esthet. Dent.: 1, 80, 1989.
31. Ironside, J.G.: Alternatives to amalgam - The role of bonded porcelain. NZ. Dent. J.: 87, 46, 1991.
32. Isenberg, B.P., Essig, M.E. and Leinfelder, K.F.: Three year clinical evaluation of CAD/CAM restorations. J. Esthet. Dent.: 4, 173, 1992.
33. Jensen, M.E., Redford, D.A., Williams, B.T. and Gardner, F.: Posterior etched porcelain restorations: An in vitro study. Compend. Contin. Educ. Dent.: 8, 615, 1987.
34. Juntavee, N., Giordano, R. and Nathanson, D.: Porcelain shear bond strength to a new ceramo-metal system. J.D.R.: 74, 159, 1995.
35. Kelly, J.R., Nishimura, I. And Campbell, S.D.: Ceramics in Dentistry: Histological roots and current perspective. J.P.D.: 75, 18, 1996.
36. Kelly J.R. and Nishimura I.: Ceramics in dentistry: historical roots and current perspectives. J. Prosthet. Dent: 75, 1, 1996.
37. Kelly J.R.: Dental ceramics: Current thinking and trends. Dent. Clin North Am:48, 513, 2004.
38. Kelly J.R.: Dental ceramics... what is this stuff anyway?. JADA: 139, 4s, 2008.
39. Krejci, I., Krejci, D. and Lutz, F.: Clinical evaluation of a new pressed glass ceramic inlay material over 1.5 years. Quint. Int.: 23, 181, 1992.
40. Krejci, I., Lutz, F. and Reimer, M.: Marginal adaptation and fit of adhesive ceramic inlays. J. Dent.: 21, 39, 1993.
41. Leinfelder, K.F., Isenberg, B.P. and Essig, M.E.: A new method for generating ceramic restorations: A CAD/CAM system. J.A.D.A.: 118, 703, 1989.
42. Loper, L.M.P., Leitao, J.C.M. and Douglas, W.H.: Effect of a new resin inlay/onlay restorative material on cuspal reinforcement. Quint. Int.: 22, 641, 1991.
43. Maruyama, T., Koh, N. and Hino, T.: Clinical use of a new castable glass - ceramic material. Int. J. Prosth.: 4, 138, 1991.
44. May, K.B., Razzoog, M.E., Lang, B.R. and Wang, R.F.: Marginal fit: The Procera All Ceramic Crown. J.D.R.: 76 (Abst. 2379), 311, 1997.
45. Mclean, J. W.: Evolution of dental ceramics in the 20th century. J.P.D., 85,61,2001.
46. McLean, J.W.: The science and art of dental ceramics. Oper. Dent.: 16, 149, 1991.
47. McLean, J.W. and Hughes, T.H.: The reinforcement of dental porcelain with ceramic oxides. B.D.J.: 119, 251, 1965.
48. McLean, J.W. and Seed, I.R.: The bonded alumina crown I. The bonding of platinum to aluminous dental porcelain using tin oxide coatings. Aust. Dent. J.: 21, 119, 1976.
49. Mormann, W.H., Brandestini, M., Lutz, F. and Barbakow, F.: Chairside computer aided ceramic inlays. Quint. Int.: 20, 329, 1989.
50. Mormann, W. H., Bindl, A.: The cerec 3-A quantum leap for computer-aided restorations: Initial clinical results. Quint. Int. Ind. Ed. 5,74,2001.
51. Mormann W.H. and Bindl A.: All-ceramic , chair –side computer-aided design/computer-aided machining restorations. Dent Clin North Am: 46, 405, 2002
52. Moscovich, H. and Creugers, N.H.J.: The novel use of extracted teeth as a dental restorative material - the 'Natural Inlay'. J. Dent.: 26, 21, 1998.
53. Narcisi, E. M., Culp, L.: Diagnosis and treatment planning for ceramic restorations. D.C.N.A. 45, 127, Jan., 2001.
54. Nasedkin, J.N.: Porcelain posterior resin bonded restorations: Current perspectives on esthetic restorative dentistry - Part III. J. Can. Dent. Assoc.: 54, 499, 1988.
55. Nathanson, D., Rus, O.N., Cataldo, G.L. and Ashayeri, N.: CAD-CAM inlays and onlays using an indirect technique. J.A.D.A.: 125, 421, 1994.
56. Nawabi, S. and Freidbank, W.: Porcelain inlays in restoration of vertical dimension. Gen. Dent.: 39, 25, 1991.
57. O'Brian, W.J.: A new small color difference equation for dental shades. J.D.R.: 69, 1762, 1990.
58. Otto, T. and De Nisco, S.: Computer aided direct ceramic restorations: A 10 year prospective clinical study of cerec CAD/CAM inlays and onlays. Int. J. Prosthodont.: 15, 122, 2002.
59. Piddock, V. and Qualtrough, A.: Dental ceramics – an update. J. Dent.: 18, 227, 1990.
60. Probster, L.: Survival rate of In-ceram restorations. Int. J. Prosth.: 6, 259, 1993.
61. Qualtrough, A.J.E. and Piddock, V.: Ceramics update. J. Dent.: 25, 91, 1997.
62. Qualtrough, A.J.E., Wilson, N.H.F. and Smith, G.A.: The porcelain inlay: A historical review. Oper. Dent.: 15, 61, 1990.
63. Quinn, F. and Byrne, D.: Porcelain laminates: A review. B.D.J.: 161, 61, 1986.
64. Rekow, D.: Dental CAD-CAM systems: What is state of the art? J.A.D.A.: 122, 43, 1991.
65. Richter, J. and Mehl, A.: Evaluation for the fully automatic inlay reconstruction by means of the biogeneric tooth model. Int. J. Comput. Dent.: 9, 101, 2006.
66. Rosenblum, M.A. and Schulman, A.: A review of all ceramic restorations. J.A.D.A.: 128, 297, 1997.
67. Roulet, J.F. and Harder, S.: Bonded ceramic inlays. Chicago Quint.: pp18, 1991.
68. Sadan, A., Blatz, M.B. and Lang, B.: Clinical considerations for densely sintered alumina and zirconia restorations. Part I, II. Int. J. Period. And Restorat. Dent.: 25, 213 and 343, 2005.
69. Scheibenbogen, A., Manhart, J., Kunzelmann, K.H. and Hickel, R.: One year clinical evaluation of composite and ceramic inlays in posterior teeth. J.P.D.: 80, 410, 1998.
70. Seghi, R.R., Rosenstiel, S.F. and Bauer, P.: Abrasion of human enamel by different dental ceramics in vitro. J.D.R.: 70, 221, 1991.

71. Seghi, R.R., Sorenson, J.A. and Engelman, M.J.: Flexural strength of new ceramic materials. J.D.R.: 69, 299, 1990.
72. Shearer, A.C., Thordrup, M., Bindslev, P.H. and Wilson, N.H.F.: A milled ceramic inlay/onlay system: A report from a series of cases. B.D.J.: 185, 283, 1998.
73. Southan, D.E.: Strengthening modern dental porcelain by ion exchange. Aust. Dent. J.: 15, 507, 1970.
74. Stangel, I., Nathenson, D. and Hsu, C.S.: Shear bond strength of composite bond to etched porcelain. J.D.R.: 63, 179, 1984.
75. Stenberg, R. and Matsson, L.: Clinical evaluation of glass ceramic inlays (Dicor). Acta. Odont. Scand.: 51, 91, 1993.
76. Thordrup, M., Isidor, F. and Bindslev, P.H.: A prospective clinical study of indirect and direct composite and ceramic inlays: ten year results. Quint. Int.: 37, 139, 2006.
77. Thordrup, M., Isidor, F. and Horsted, B.: One year clinical study of indirect and direct composite and ceramic inlays. Scand. J. Dent. Res.: 102, 186, 1994.
78. Trushkowsky, R.D.: Ceramic optimized polymer: the next generation of esthetic restorations - Part I. Compend. Contin. Educ. Dent.: 18, 1101, 1997.
79. Van der zel, J.M., Vlaar, S., De ruiter, W.J., Davidson, C.: The Cicero system for CAD/CAM fabrication of full ceramic crowns. J.P.D.: 85, 261, 2001.
80. Van Dijken, J.W.V., Hoglund, A.C. and Olofsson, A.L.: Fired ceramic inlays: A 6 year follow up. J. Dent.: 26, 219, 1998.
81. White, J.M., Goodis, H.E., Marshall, S.J. and Marshall, G.W.: Sterilisation of teeth by gamma radiation. J.D.R.: 73, 1500, 1994.
82. Wohlwend, A., Strub, J.R. and Scharer, P.: Metal ceramic and all-porcelain restorations: current considerations. Int. J. Prosth.: 2, 13, 1989.
83. Zalkind, M. and Hochman, N.: Esthetic considerations in restoring endodontically treated teeth with posts and cores. J.P.D.: 79, 702, 1998.
84. Ziskind, D., Avivi-Arber, L., Haramati, O. and Hirschfeld, Z.: Amalgam alternatives - microleakage evaluation of clinical procedures. Part I: Direct composite/composite inlay/ceramic inlay. J. Oral Rehab.: 25, 443, 1998.

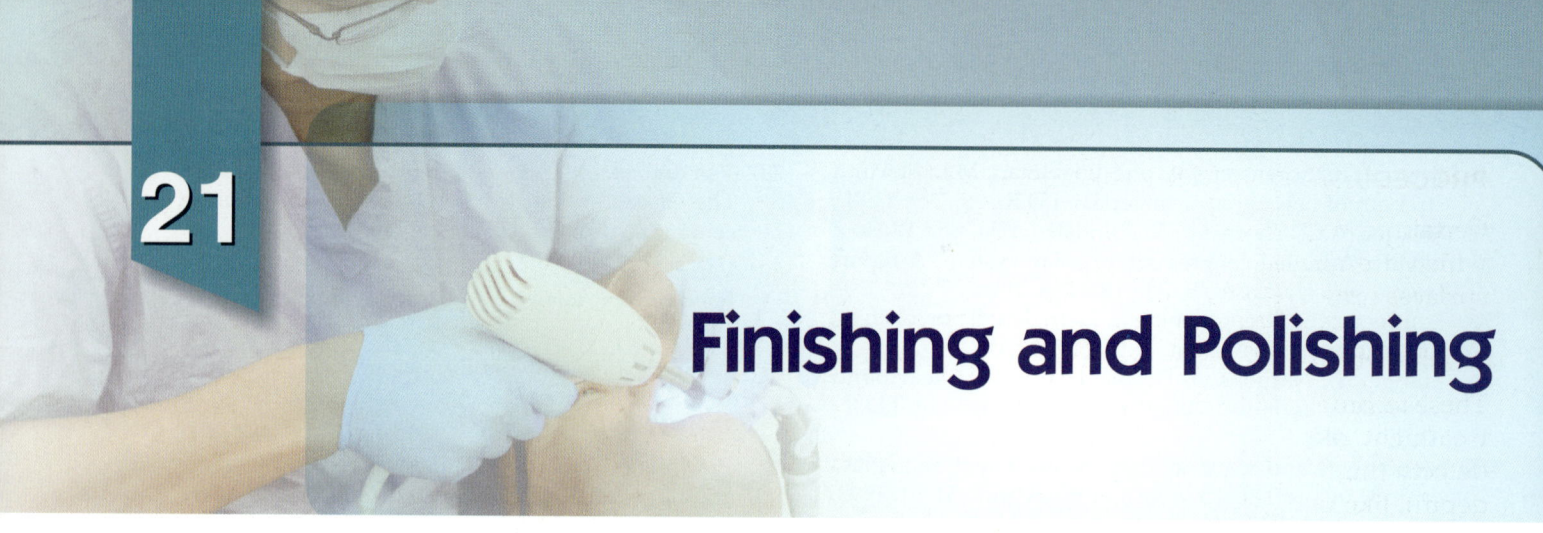

21. Finishing and Polishing

The main objective of an operative dentist is to restore the individual tooth to its form and functions along with imparting pleasing esthetics and maintaining periodontal tissues in good esteem. Many a times, the form and function is restored but the surface may not be smooth. It has been established that rough or uneven surfaces invite microbial flora and also the light reflected by these surfaces may not be uniform. A restored tooth should be evenly smooth and reflect light uniformly. The process of making the surface smooth so as to enable them to reflect light evenly is known as finishing and polishing. Several definitions have been given to define finishing and polishing.

Finishing is the removal of surface irregularities, whereas polishing is the creation of surface layer which can reflect light as good as enamel surface.

'Finishing' is defined as *'the transformation of an object from a rough to a refined form. The procedure involves removal of surface irregularities and shaping the restoration according to functional occlusion'*. **'Polishing'** is defined as *'the production of a shiny, mirror like surface, which reflects light similar to enamel without creating supplemental films by the addition of wax or lacquer'*.

Finishing can also be described as a process whereby substrate particles are removed by the action of cutting and/or grinding. The surface of the substrate is made to come into frictional contact with a comparatively harder material. This contact generates enough tensile and shear stresses to overcome the forces of atomic bonds and thereby release particles from the substrate. In a *'cutting operation'*, the substrate particles are removed by the use of any instrument which acts in a blade like fashion. A *'grinding operation'* on the other hand removes small particles of the substrate through the action of bonded or coated abrasive instruments. These instruments contain randomly arranged abrasive particles. Each particle has a sharp point that runs along the substrate surface and removes particles of the substrate. Both cutting and grinding procedures produce unidirectional scratches.

Finishing involves:

- Gross reduction of excess restorative material
- Contouring, which includes reproduction of size, shape, groove and other details of the tooth form.
- Establishes a well-adapted junction between the tooth surface and the restoration
- Removes scratches to produce smooth and shiny surface.

'Polishing' is the most refined process and acts on an extremely thin region of the substrate surface. It produces very fine scratches that can be visible only under very high magnification. An ideally polished surface does not have any surface imperfections, but this condition is very difficult to achieve because most of the restorative materials are brittle and get damaged even during fine grinding.

Basically 'polishing' is the process in which the polishing material does not cut or grind, but fills fine scratches and produces a perfectly smooth surface. During the polishing of metals, a highly stressed microcrystalline layer is formed on the surface called the 'Beilby layer'. This layer is composed of non-oriented crystals and is 20–40 Å thick. It is believed that because of rapid movement of the polishing agent, top layer of the material gets heated up causing it to flow and fill the scratches.

The optimum speed for polishing varies with the hardness of material. The harder the material, higher should be the speed (chrome cobalt alloys require higher speed than gold alloys). *'Buffing'* refers to the polishing process in which the abrasives are applied via bristle brushes, treated leather and cloth materials.

The final surface character achieved on a restorative material is the combination of finishing and polishing. The polished surface can also be obtained by a coating. Electroplated deposits, pit and fissure sealants, unfilled resin glazes and overglazes on porcelain are some examples of polish produced by coatings.

Finishing and Polishing

PROCEDURE TO ATTAIN SMOOTH SURFACE

Certain procedures in addition to cutting and grinding, which are also used to achieve smooth and shiny surfaces are:

A. Microabrasion and Macroabrasion

These techniques are conservative alternatives for the treatment of superficial discolorations or enamel defects (limited to a few tenths of a millimetre in depth), like in fluorosis, amelogenesis imperfect, etc. The technique can also be used for carious lesions that are incipient and have a rough surface. In case, the defect or stain still exists after the treatment, a restoration can be planned.

a. Microabrasion

McClosky (1984) recommended a technique for removing brown stains of fluorosis which were limited to enamel by applying 18% hydrochloric acid to stained surfaces. Later, the technique was modified (known as microabrasion) by using a paste made of 18% hydrochloric acid, pumice and water. The paste is then applied to the desired surface with a hand device like tongue blade or a slow driven rubber cup. The rubber cup should be rotated at very slow speed to avoid removing any excess tooth structure and to prevent spatter. If the defect is only confined to the superficial 0.2–0.3 mm of enamel, the acid pumice paste strips away the affected surface, resulting in improved appearance with clinically unrecognizable enamel loss. Acid causes dissolution of enamel and the abrasive causes removal of superficial stains and defects. After application of a topical fluoride solution and final finishing and polishing, normal enamel surface characteristics are established.

The technique was further modified by reducing the concentration of the acid to approximately 11% and increasing the abrasiveness by using silicon carbide particles instead of pumice, in a water-soluble gel paste. This product is marketed as 'Prima' and is comparatively safer because of its low acid concentration.

Recently, EMS introduced **Air-flow handy** system, which uses sodium bicarbonate as an abrasive agent. The powder is passed through a narrow nozzle of specially designed handpiece with the help of compressed air. This technique is utilized to remove extrinsic stains on the tooth surface (Fig. 21.1).

b. Macroabrasion

Macroabrasion utilizes a 12-fluted carbide bur or a micron diamond point revolving at high speed to remove the surface stains. Adequate air/water spray

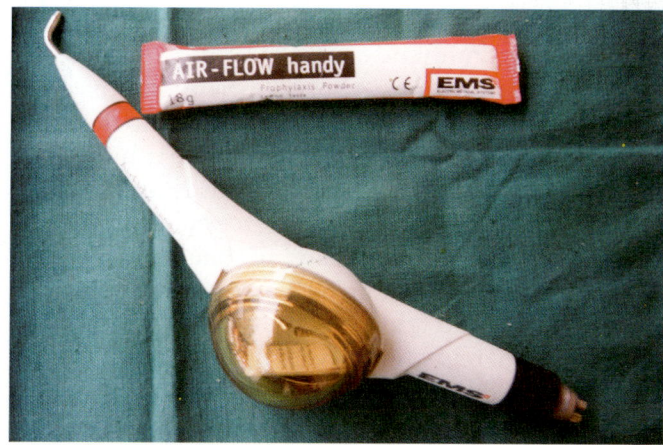

Fig. 21.1: Air flow polishing system

should be used not only as a coolant, but also to facilitate proper visibility of the defect. Certain defects are normally not visible when the teeth are hydrated, but become visible on dehydration. Light intermittent pressure is also recommended to avoid irreversible damage to the tooth structure. Following the removal of defect, or if it is decided that the defect can no more be removed, then the remaining part is finished with a 30 fluted carbide bur. Final polishing is carried out with an abrasive rubber point.

B. Burnishing

'Burnishing' is defined as the process of rubbing a metal over the restorative material to make it shiny or lustrous. Further, it aids in adaptation and compaction of the material at the margins.

'Burnishing' has also been described as a procedure in which the surface of a metallic restoration is smoothened by rubbing it with another small, highly polished, hard metal surface. It is most commonly employed for amalgam and gold foil restorations and is always carried out from the restoration surface to the tooth surface.

The metal of the burnishing instrument should not combine easily with the metal or alloy being burnished; otherwise some metal may be transported either on to the restoration or on to the instrument. Stainless steel or chromium-plated instruments are commonly employed either by hand, or in the form of smooth rotating engine burnisher. Instrument nibs for burnishing are smooth faced and are available in various shapes such as bell shaped, egg shaped, apple shaped, etc. Special burnisher, like 'Spratley burnisher' is used for proximal gingival marginal burnishing of metallic restorations.

a. Burnishing of Amalgam Restorations

In amalgam, 'burnishing' can be carried out by rubbing a smooth metallic instrument over setting, or indeed set material to produce a smooth shiny surface.

Comparatively little force is required to burnish a setting amalgam than set amalgam.

A round burnisher of appropriate size is often moved in light strokes from the amalgam to the tooth surface. Proximal portions can be similarly burnished using a beaver tail burnisher and/or Spratley burnisher. Caution should be exercised against using excessive pressure leading to heat generation. Temperature greater than 60°C can damage the pulp beyond repair and release mercury to the surface. The presence of mercury rich layer at the margins promotes corrosion and may lead to fracture.

It is demonstrated that burnishing increased the relative content of residual alloy grains and decreased the residual mercury. Burnishing also remarkably decreases the number of micropores. It has been established that burnishing improves the marginal seal.

The appropriate time for burnishing amalgam restorations may be divided as the '*precarve burnishing*' and the '*post carve burnishing*'. *Pre carve burnishing, as the name suggests, is carried out before the carving is initiated and is in fact a continuation of the condensation process*. Large egg shaped or ball burnisher is used with a pressure equal to that used for condensing amalgam (Fig. 14.32). The burnisher is moved mesiodistally and faciolingually taking care that its head contacts only the cuspal slopes and not the margins. Thereafter the burnishing is stopped. Pre carve burnishing is more effective in reducing the mercury content of amalgam compared to conventional polishing and also improves its carving characteristics. It is demonstrated that systematic overfilling and burnishing of margins and by subsequent removal of the excess by carving can obtain an optimum structure of the restoration margins. Many authors have also stated that precarve burnishing increases the resistance to marginal failure by producing denser amalgams at the margins, however consensus is that burnishing during condensation improves marginal adaptation both for the conventional and high copper amalgams.

'*Post carve burnishing*' *is carried out after the carving is completed*. Instruments used for amalgam carving are shown in Fig. 21.2. Small sized burnisher is used with light strokes. A satin or velvet finish should be the aim at this stage and not a highly reflective surface. The properties achieved by post carve burnishing are: increased surface hardness, decrease in the size and number of voids on the surface and marginal areas, a slower rate of corrosion, denser amalgam at the margins and improvement in the marginal seal. With the high copper amalgams, post carve burnishing can be avoided, as it has shown no clinically significant effect on their performance.

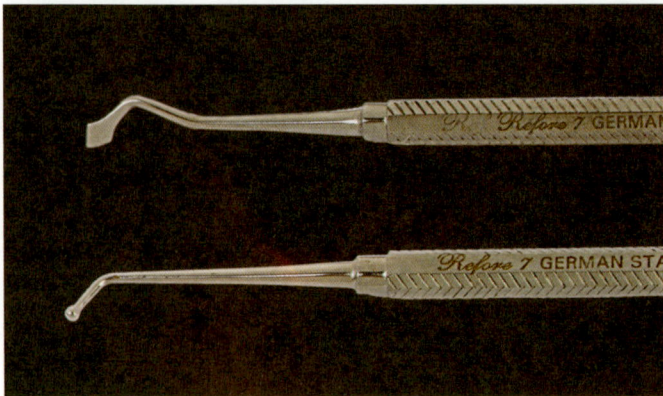

Fig. 21.2: Instruments used for carving and finishing amalgam

b. Burnishing of Direct Gold Restorations

The ability of pure gold to be malleted forms the basis for burnishing a direct filling gold restoration. It is the first step in finishing a direct gold restoration. Spratley burnisher is pushed with considerable pressure across the metal surface to the tooth. The metal is pushed to close the voids and to ride over the enamel margins. The pressure and rubbing gives the gold its shine, even though the surface is not ideally smooth. For proximal surfaces, Spratley blade carver can be used in the embrasure area. Burnishing also increases the hardness of the surface by cold working.

c. Burnishing of Cast Gold Restorations

Burnishing of cast restoration is performed at all peripheries of the casting until no interruption is felt on running an explorer over the tooth-casting interface. Hand burnisher is commonly used and occasionally rotary burnisher may be employed for alloys with high yield strength.

The time of burnishing a cast gold restoration varies with the type of cementing medium used. When zinc phosphate cement is used for cementing the cast inlay, burnishing should be done after 24 hours. The burnishing is delayed so as to let the cement dissolve at the margins. Once the cement is dissolved, burnishing is carried out to have the gold-tooth interface rather than gold-cement-tooth interface. On the other hand, if the cementing medium is glass-ionomer cement or resin cement, the burnishing can be carried out immediately after setting, since these cements are less soluble in oral fluids.

OBJECTIVES OF FINISHING AND POLISHING

The objectives of finishing and polishing are:
- Preservation of signs of decay in visible areas and at tooth margins.
- Obtaining adequate adaptation and continuity of the restoration margins with the tooth

- Optimum restoration contour, proper occlusal contacts
- Surface free of any scratches or irregularities to make it biologically acceptable
- Adjustment of any morphological or marginal defects

A restoration that is well finished and polished promotes oral health, especially at the gingival margins, by preventing the accumulation of food debris and pathogenic bacteria, thereby minimizing gingival inflammation, secondary caries, periodontal destruction and many related problems. A rough surface on the restoration contains microscopic pits in which small food particles tend to lodge and encourage galvanic action, which may lead to tarnish and corrosion. Smooth surfaces are also easy to clean during the daily oral hygiene regime.

Oral function is enhanced because food glides over the finished restoration more freely. Smooth and flowing surfaces are also polite to the cheeks, lips, tongue and gingiva. Moreover, smooth restoration contacts minimize wear on adjacent teeth.

Finally, a well-finished and polished restoration, which is in harmony with the natural tooth, is esthetically pleasing. It is desirable to achieve a surface smoothness that will result in reflecting light similar to that of tooth enamel. (A surface becomes reflective only when the surface imperfections are well below 1.0 μm, as this is below the resolution of the wavelength of light).

HEALTH HAZARDS DURING FINISHING AND POLISHING

a. *Production of aerosol:* An aerosol is a dispersion of fine solid or liquid particles (e.g. tooth structure, restorative material or micro-organisms) in air. Dental aerosols, which are usually produced during finishing and polishing procedures, pose a major health hazard both to the dental personnel and the patients. These are the potential sources for chronic and infectious diseases of the lungs, eyes and skin. Aerosols may remain suspended in the air for even more than 24 hours, thereby promoting cross contamination. A major pulmonary disease that may occur with the chronic exposure to aerosols containing silica is the 'Silicosis' or 'Grinder's disease'. Silica is a very common component of restorative and polishing materials. Aerosol hazards can be minimized by following procedures like:
   - adequate ventilation or a simple exhaust system in the operatory that filters harmful particles from the extracted air
   - self-protection by safety glasses with side shields, disposable face masks and gowns
   - use of rubber dam protects the patient against oral inhalation of aerosols
   - use of infection control procedures and high vacuum suction.

b. *Production of vapours:* During cutting of amalgam, high temperature that is generated may form mercury vapour. Thermal decomposition of polymeric materials like acrylic resins and composites produces monomer vapours. These vapour particles may be inhaled leading to alveolar irritation and tissue reactions. The production of vapours can be minimized by using low speeds and intermittent cutting. If using high speeds, copious air-water spray should be used as a coolant. Inhalation of these vapours can be prevented following the same procedures as given for aerosols.

c. *Pulpal reactions:* Temperature rise by as much as 20°C may occur during the use of rotary finishing and polishing instruments. If the remaining dentin and enamel thickness is less, this heat is rapidly conducted to the underlying pulp resulting in various pulpal ailments. Proper use of coolants such as water, air and air/water spray protects against excessive rise in temperature. Cup brushes should be preferred for polishing compared to rubber appliances as the former generate less heat. Also, use of intermittent polishing at low speeds is advocated to prevent excessive heat production.

d. *Soft tissue injuries:* Soft tissues like lips, cheeks, tongue and gingiva may be injured if adequate care is not taken to protect them.

FINISHING AND POLISHING INSTRUMENTS

a. *Finishing burs:* 12–30 fluted carbide burs are usually recommended for finishing depending upon the restorative material. Plain burs are also used before final polishing. Burs are available in various sizes and shapes such as straight fissure, tapering, flame shaped, rounded, wheel, etc. (Fig. 21.3).

b. *Diamond instruments and pastes:* Diamond is a transparent material composed of carbon. It is considered as a super abrasive because it is the hardest material known and is capable of abrading almost any other material. It is available commercially in the form of bonded abrasive rotary instruments, metal backed abrasive strips and polishing pastes. Finishing diamonds of medium-fine grit contain diamond particles of 8.0–50.0 µm in diameter (Fig. 21.4). They should always be used with a light speed (less than 50,000 rpm) and copious water spray to preserve the very fine diamond coatings. Diamond polishing pastes are also available with particle sizes ranging from 2.0–5.0 µm. Diamond abrasives are preferably used on ceramic and composite materials.

c. *Brushes:* Brushes can be used either alone or in combination with the abrasive particles. Most of the brushes have synthetic bristles; others may have wire bristles for polishing cast restorations. Various types of brushes are available which may be screwed into an extension, inserted into a handpiece or attached to a mandrel (Fig. 21.5).

d. *Cloth:* Cloth carried on a metal wheel may be used for final polishing, with or without a polishing medium.

e. *Felt:* Felt is used to attain lustre for the metallic restorations usually with a polishing agent. It is available in different shapes of wheels, cones and cylinders.

f. *Rubber instruments:* Rubber ended tools are commonly used for polishing procedures. They can be obtained in various shapes of cups, wheels, cones, etc. and are commonly used with other abrasives or polishing pastes (Fig. 21.5). These should not be used with heavy pressure, since excessive heat is produced. Most of these products contain latex (potentially causing allergic reaction and often leaves a residue on the surface of the restoration.

g. *Coated discs:* The abrasives particles such as sand, cuttle, garnet, boron carbide, silicon carbide, etc. are held on to a flexible heavy weight paper or mylar strips with a suitable adhesive material. The disks may be attached to a mandrel for rotary finishing (Fig. 21.6).

h. *Strips:* Abrasive strips are used by hand in a back and forth motion especially for finishing proximal areas (Fig. 21.7). They are available with metal or

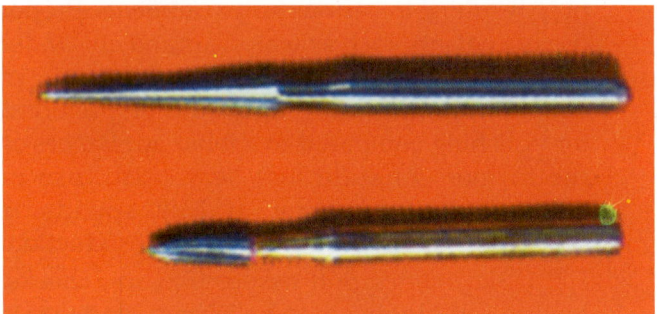

Fig. 21.3: Finishing burs

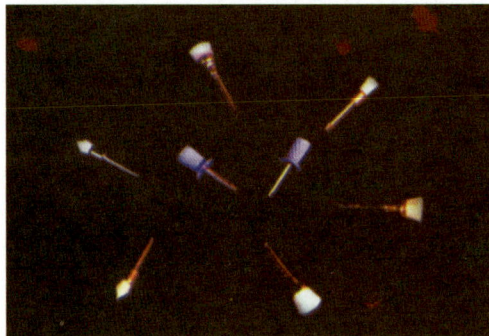

Fig. 21.5: Brushes and cups

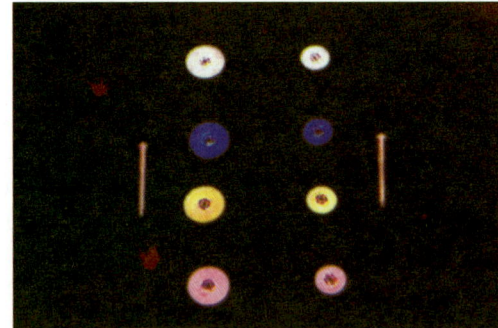

Fig. 21.6: Polishing disks

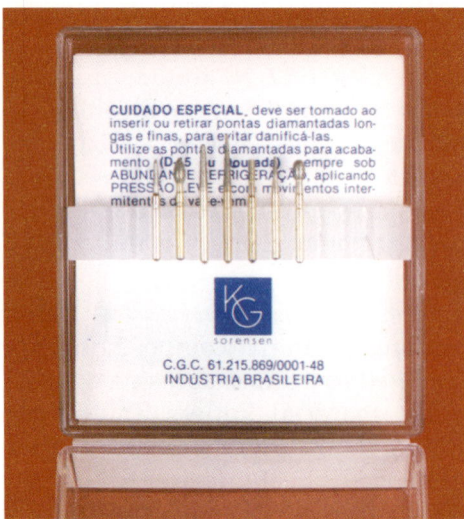

Fig. 21.4: Finishing diamonds

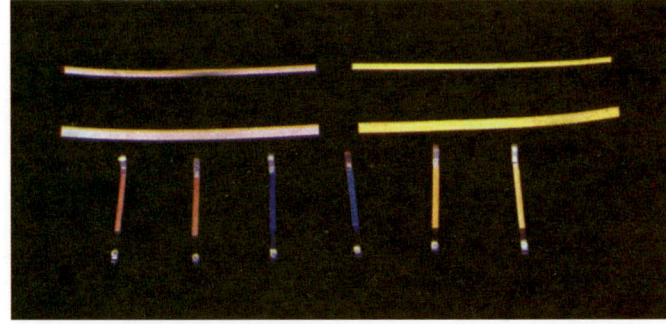

Fig. 21.7: Inter-proximal strips for finishing

plastic backing with different abrasiveness. Metal strips can be autoclaved, whereas plastic strips are for single use.
i. *Stones:* Stones are used for contouring and finishing where maximum abrasion is needed, such as adjusting the occlusion.

ABRASIVE MATERIALS

a. *Chalk:* It is a white colored abrasive composed of calcium carbonate. It serves as a mild abrasive for polishing tooth enamel, gold foil, amalgam and plastic materials.
b. *Pumice:* It is the most common fine abrasive used in dentistry. Its abrasive action is only for softer materials. Flour of pumice can be used for polishing tooth enamel, gold foil, amalgam and acrylic resins. Pumice powder is mixed with water or glycerine and carried to the surface by a revolving brush. Slow speed is recommended during its use; otherwise the centrifugal force throws out most of the pumice from the brush. Pumice slurry is a mix of pumice and water where as a pumice paste is a mix of pumice and glycerine.
c. *Corundum:* This is a form of aluminium oxide and is usually white. Corundum is used primarily for grinding metal alloys and is supplied in the form of bonded abrasives. White stone is the most common form of corundum.
d. *Emery*: This abrasive is greyish-black corundum and is a mixture of aluminium oxide and iron. Emery is commonly used as an abrasive coating on a cloth or paper disk. It may be used for finishing metal alloys and plastic materials.
e. *Garnet:* Garnet includes a number of different materials such as silica or aluminium, cobalt, iron, magnesium and manganese. Its color is dark red and is extremely hard making it a highly effective abrasive. It is used in grinding metal alloys and plastic materials.
f. *Sand:* Sand is predominantly silica. Irregularly shaped particles are bonded to the paper with glue or resin. It is supplied in the much familiar form of sand paper. Sand particles under air pressure are also used to remove the investment material from base metal alloy castings.
g. *Tripoli:* The grey and red colored tripoli are most commonly used in dentistry for polishing metal alloys and some plastic materials.
h. *Kieselguhr*: In addition to its use as a fine abrasive on paper disks, it is also used as filler in various impression materials. The coarser form is called 'diatomaceous earth'. Chronic exposure to this material can cause respiratory silicosis.
i. *Cuttle fish bone:* It is available as coated disks and strips for polishing metal margins and amalgam restorations.
j. *Quartz*: It is very hard, colorless and transparent. Sharp angular particles of quartz are used for coating abrasive disks. Quartz abrasives are mostly used to finish metal alloys.
k. *Zirconium silicate:* It is an off-white mineral used to make coated disks and strips. It forms an important component of the dental prophylaxis pastes.
l. *Silicon carbide (Carborundum)*: Mounted points, coated disks and grinding wheels are the most common form of this material. It has a green and blue-black color. Carborundum wears away rapidly at high heat; therefore it should always be kept wet when in use. Boron carbide is used similarly as an abrasive.

FINISHING AND POLISHING OF AMALGAM RESTORATIONS

Finishing and polishing of amalgam restorations is an important step in the ultimate clinical success of the restorations.

It has been shown that the Vickers hardness of the surface of amalgam improved from 75 to 90 after polishing. Finishing and polishing definitely increase the life of an amalgam restoration.

Procedure

The cavity is slightly overfilled during amalgam condensation. The mercury rich layer of the last increment is removed during carving. Usually within 3–5 minutes, the amalgam is sufficiently hardened and carving can be initiated. Setting time varies with the different brands of silver alloys. Clinically, when a ringing sound appears during carving that is the ideal period for carving. Whether burnishing should be done prior to carving or after carving or not done at all remains a debatable question. It is opined that burnishing should be carried out both prior to and after carving to smoothen the surface as it prepares the restoration for finishing and polishing. Burnishing alone has shown to produce a ten-fold decrease in surface roughness.

The restoration is then left undisturbed for a minimum period of 24 hours before it is finally finished and polished. 24 hours is the usual time period required for setting, hardening and dimensional changes of amalgam.

After 24 hours, the surface of the restoration is usually rough due to the heterogenous structure of amalgam on setting. The scanning electron microscopic picture of unpolished and polished amalgam is shown in Figs 21.8 and 21.9. Finishing is now begun with the use of steel finishing burs or stones (Figs 21.3, 21.10 and 21.11). This includes trimming any overextended and excess margins, creating adequate contour and correcting any occlusal disharmonies that may have been overlooked during the carving process. A high point in an amalgam restoration appears as a shiny area, which is reduced with carborundum stones or finishing burs. A common error in the trimming of amalgam is that of leaving fins or flashes at the margins. Since amalgam has a low tensile strength, thin sections of amalgam can easily get fractured resulting in marginal ditching.

For the proximo-occlusal restorations, careful evaluation of the cervical margins is mandatory. Despite the fact that matrix bands and wedges are used during restorations, gingival overhangs of varying degree may be created. These overhangs are

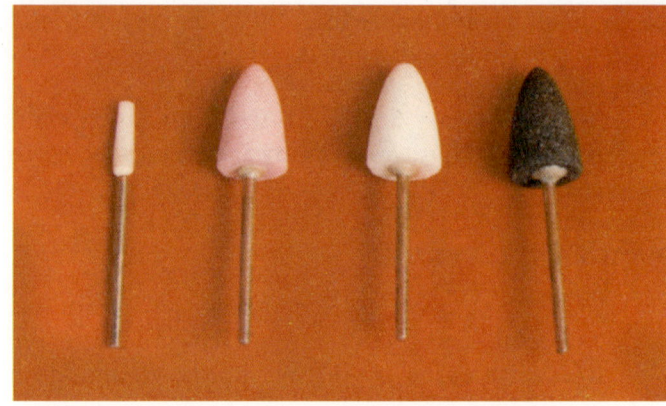

Fig. 21.10: Rotary finishing stones

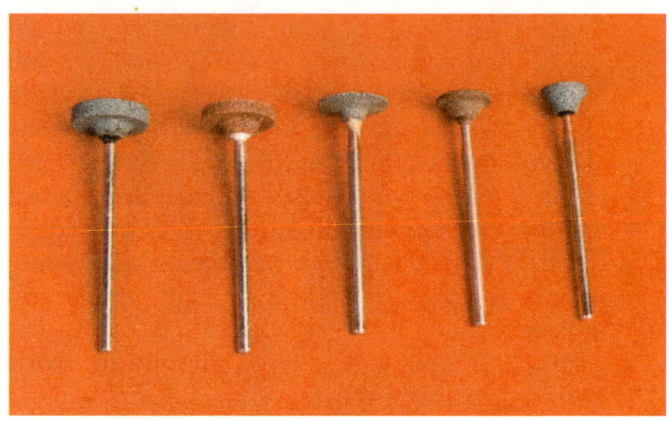

Fig. 21.11: Rotary finishing wheels

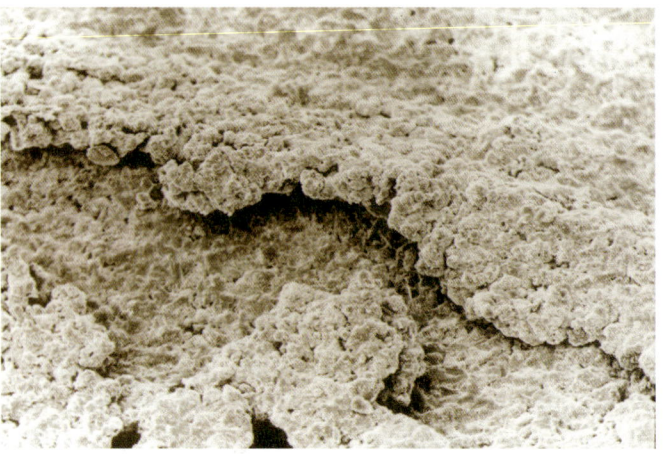

Fig. 21.8: Scanning electron microscopic view of the surface of unpolished amalgam

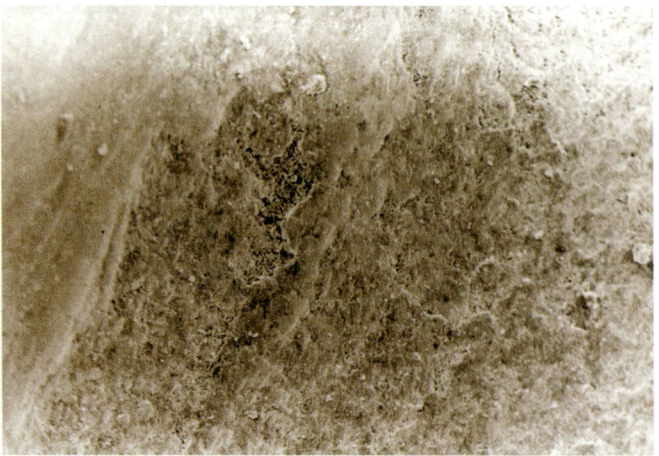

Fig. 21.9: Scanning electron microscopic view of the surface of polished amalgam

removed by using periodontal files or gold foil knives. Finishing of cervical areas is carried out by inserting fine water resistant strips cervical to the contact area through the interdental space and moving them to and fro. The facial and lingual proximal margins can be marginated with light cuttle fish sandpaper disks.

Removal of superficial scratches and irregularities is accomplished simultaneously. It should be remembered that abrasives always should be applied through a descending grade, i.e. coarse, medium, fine and ultra fine to achieve the final finish. The final polish or the metallic lustre is obtained by the application of a suitable polishing agent like tin oxide, zinc oxide, chalk, pumice, etc. carried with a soft rotating brush or rubber cup. For polishing in the contact areas and gingival embrasures, the abrasive is introduced through polishing strips and dental tape. It should be kept in mind that a high luster will show only if the restoration has been perfectly smoothened prior to the application of a polishing agent.

During polishing, the restoration should be kept moist and only low rotational speeds with light intermittent pressure should be used, to avoid any overheating. Excessive heat can damage the pulp and also tends to bring mercury to the surface causing early staining of the filling. The mercury vapours so formed are injurious both to the individual and the environment.

With the advent of high copper amalgams, it is now possible to finish the restorations much earlier. It is an established fact that the high copper alloys can be polished 15–30 minutes after condensation. High copper amalgams have a rapid setting tendency and achieve high early compressive strength, allowing them to withstand the forces of finishing quite earlier.

A few authors are of the view that polishing of high copper amalgam is less important than conventional amalgam, because the former is less susceptible to tarnish and marginal breakdown.

Hazards During Finishing and Polishing of Amalgam Restorations

- Production of aerosols
- High temperatures may damage pulp
- May bring mercury to the surface and produce mercury vapours

FINISHING AND POLISHING OF COMPOSITE RESTORATIONS

Finishing and polishing is mandatory for the surface quality and natural appearance of the composite restoration. Finishing also removes the smear layer from the composite. This is surface layer prevented from polymerizing properly by the oxygen. The surface smoothness varies with the type of composite resin, owing to the nature of the filler particles:

- Conventional composites pose difficulty in achieving a smooth surface because of the difference in hardness of organic and inorganic phases. The resin matrix is soft and filler particles are hard. If fine grit polishing methods are used, the softer resin matrix abrades away easily leaving behind the harder filler particles, which gives it a rough surface. If coarse abrasives are used on the other hand, the organic and inorganic phases are removed equally but the abrasive leaves behind rough marks. The unequal surfaces of conventional composites lead to unequal wear, which may further disturb the occlusal harmony thereby creating problems in the temporomandibular joint.
- Hybrid composites can be polished to a semigloss but the surface is somewhat hydrophobic which makes it quite unpleasant for the patient
- Microfilled composite materials can be polished to the highest gloss and are considered to be esthetically best amongst all composites. The surface of these restorations is highly smooth and the chances of extrinsic staining are minimal. Finish obtained on microfilled composites is a glossy one whereas that obtained on conventional composites is a satin finish.

A surface finish attained with the use of a plastic matrix band is the most desirable finish for resin restorations, but this is rarely obtainable because of the need for contouring and removal of excess material. Hence, it is advisable to contour the unpolymerized composite with hand instruments, so that the need for removal of large amounts of set resin leading to surface damage are minimized. The scanning electron microscopic picture of unpolished and polished composite resin is shown in Figs 21.12 and 21.13.

The composite resins may be filled directly into the cavity (direct restoration) or may be fabricated outside the oral cavity and cemented into the cavity (indirect restoration). The polishing of composite restoration involves three phases:

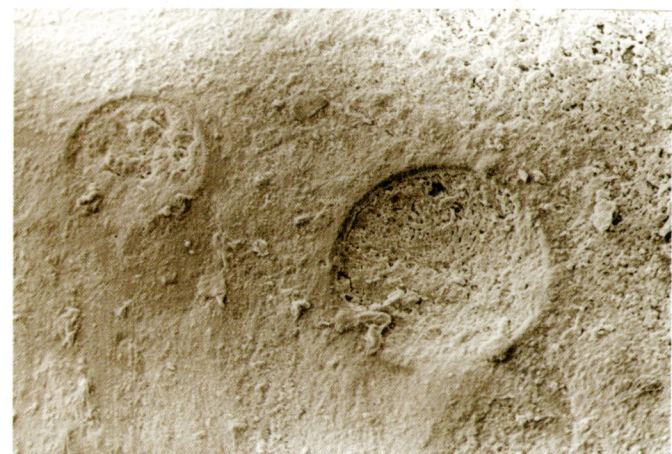

Fig. 21.12: Scanning electron microscopic view of the surface of unpolished composite

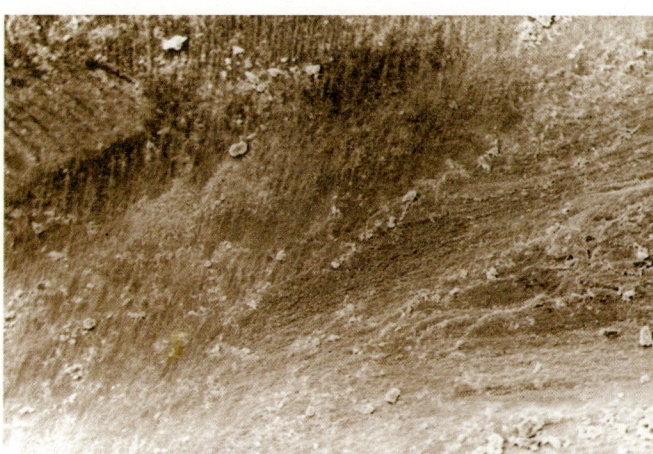

Fig. 21.13: Scanning electron microscopic view of the surface of polished composite

- Contouring the restoration
- Fine finishing of the restoration
- Actual polishing to provide the restoration a high lustre

The procedures for finishing and polishing of the two types of restorations are described separately.

a. Direct Composite Restorations

Excess composite at the cavosurface margins is scraped away using a scalpel or a sharp gold knife. The use of stainless steel instruments should be avoided, as these tend to leave grey marks on the restoration. For gross contouring and finishing of the comparatively non-accessible areas on the occlusal surface, the alpine stone, 12–30 fluted carbide burs and diamond points (15–45 μm size) are recommended (Figs 21.3, 21.14). Rotary instruments should always be used with a stream of water and little pressure. High pressure tends to loosen and dislodge the filler particles. The margins of the restoration should be spared of the rotary instruments. In the accessible areas of the occlusal surface, agents such as aluminium oxide, cuttle fish or silicon dioxide coated disks and strips are used in a descending grade of their abrasiveness. These instruments are used at very low speeds. Coarse disks are utilized for the gross reduction of excess composite and establishment of contour. Finer disks are used for producing a smooth surface texture and refined marginal adaptation (Fig. 21.15). Vaseline or petroleum jelly should be used as lubricant with these disks and strips. The strips are used in to and fro motion (Fig. 21.16).

For the proximal surfaces, the matrix is removed and the restoration inspected for any voids or faulty contour. Any excess from the margins is removed using sharp gold universal knife. The knife is moved from the restoration to the tooth with short, light cutting strokes in order not to disturb the adaptation of resin. The surface and margins of the restoration

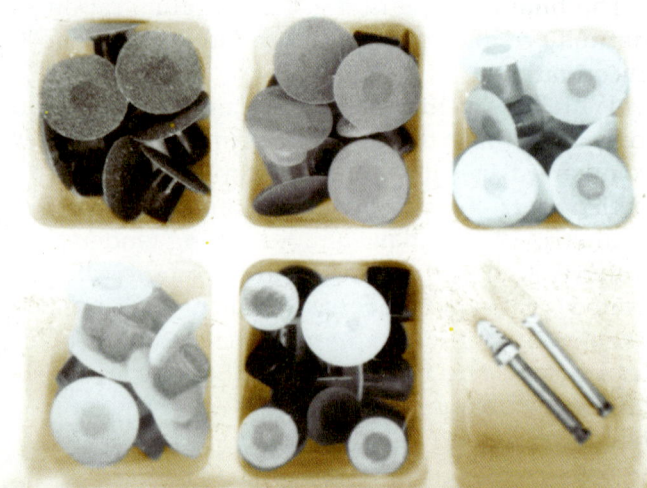

Fig. 21.15: Various types of discs used for finishing and polishing composite

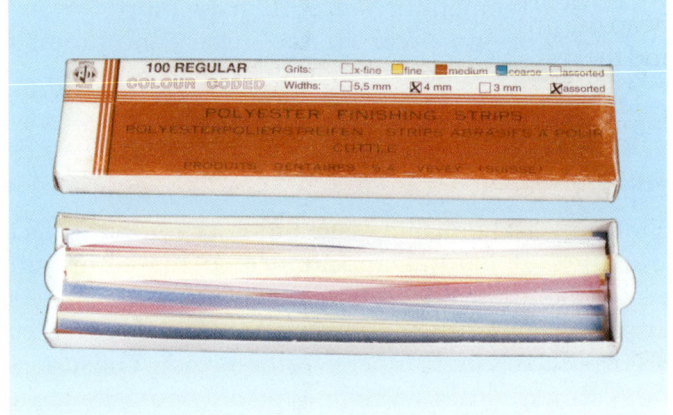

Fig. 21.16: Inter-proximal finishing strips

are then smoothened with a cuttlefish finishing strip. Strips are used with short strokes rather than rapid lengthy strokes in the embrasures.

For a class V composite restoration, almost all the finishing is accomplished with rotary instruments. The use of sandpaper disks may damage the gingiva and nick the cementum of the tooth. A finishing bur of adequate shape is moved quickly to remove any excess material. As the margins and approximate contours are approached, the bur is slowed down and used with light pressure, so as not to disturb the final shape.

The instruments used for finishing are:
- Manual instruments for removing small amount of marginal excesses (Scaler, curette)
- Coarse (30–40 μm) and Fine (15 μm) grit diamond burs for occlusal adjustment
- Tungsten carbide burs for finishing
- Finishing strips for proximal surfaces
- Waxed dental floss for checking

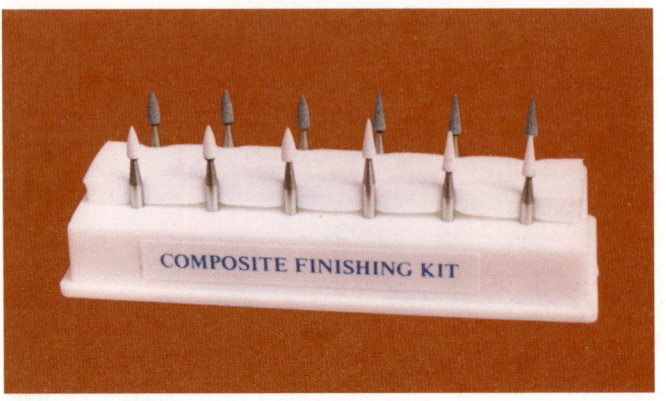

Fig. 21.14: Composite finishing kit

The final lustre is obtained with polishing pastes that may contain pumice, silica, alumina, tin oxide, silicon carbide, zirconium silicate etc (Figs 21.17, 21.18 and 21.19). The commonly used abrasives on composites are pumice and silica. The paste is made by mixing the abrasive with water or glycerine and carried to the restoration with brushes, rubber cups, linen strips or dental tapes. White rubber cups are preferred to avoid discoloring the resin and should be rotated slowly with light pressure. Care should be taken when polishing gingival margin because here the cementum is soft and easily abraded resulting in sensitivity. Some polishing pastes are now available that have the same ingredient as the reinforcing particles present in the composite resin. After the polishing is completed, air is used to blow away any remaining abrasive particles. An explorer may be used on the occlusal surface to remove any deeply seated debris in the grooves. Dental floss is used to clean the proximal embrasures of any remaining paste and the restoration finally inspected for any deficiency.

After the final polishing of the composite is completed, a thin layer of glaze may be applied to

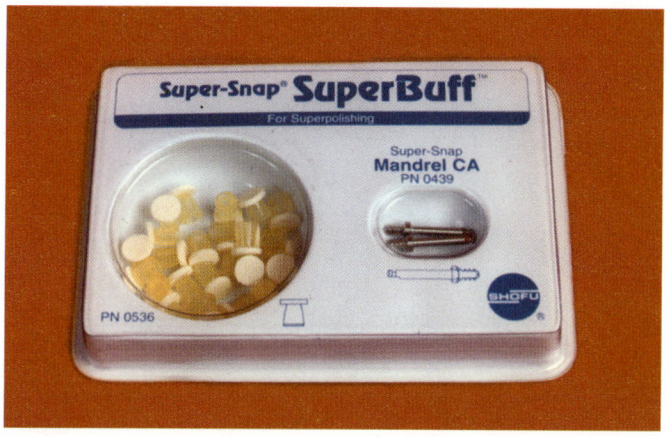

Fig. 21.19: Composite polishing disks

improve surface smoothness. Glaze is a film of unfilled polymers with a composition similar to the resin matrix. The restoration and adjoining enamel are acid etched to condition the enamel and provide a clean surface prior to its application. However, because of its poor adhesion to the composite and the ability to abrade away easily, the life of a glaze is very short ranging from one day to four months.

The following instruments used for polishing composites in descending order:

- Tungsten carbide bur (12 fluted) or diamond point (30–40 μm) for gross removal of excess material.
- Silicone polishers at slow speed
- Medium or fine grit finishing discs for proximal areas
- Silicone brushes with impregnated bristles for polishing pits and fissures
- Polishing pastes using 3.0 μm brushes followed by 1.0 μm brushes
- Felt wheel and aluminium oxide polishing pastes

Recently, a new material (Fortify, Bisco) has shown promising results. Functionally, this material acts as a surface penetrating sealant. The finishing process creates microstructural defects or cracks that extend below the surface. This type of surface decreases the wear resistance appreciably. Because of its extremely low viscosity and wetting ability, the material readily flows across the surface and then penetrates into the microstructural defects. After polymerizing for 20 seconds, it causes resolidification or refortification of the defective surface, thereby increasing the wear resistance of the composite resin appreciably and eliminating marginal defects. Stepwise procedure for finishing of composite restoration of maxillary central incisor is shown in Figs 21.20A to D; and for mandibular first molar is shown in Figs 21.21A to G.

The concept of megafilled composite resin restorations was first put into practice with the

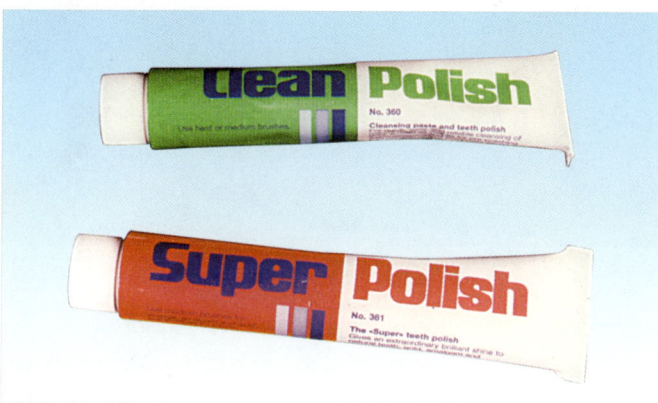

Fig. 21.17: Polishing paste

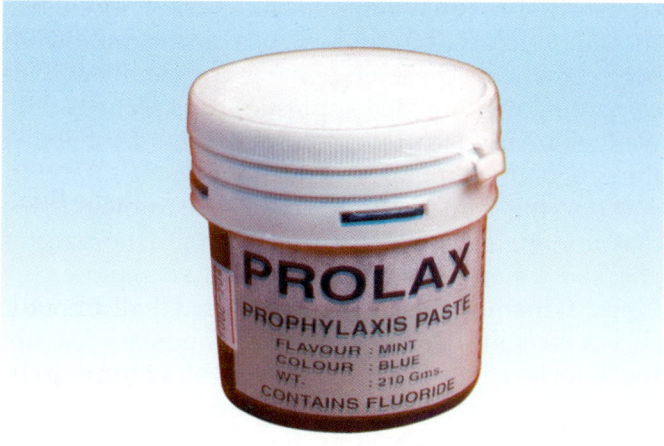

Fig. 21.18: Polishing paste

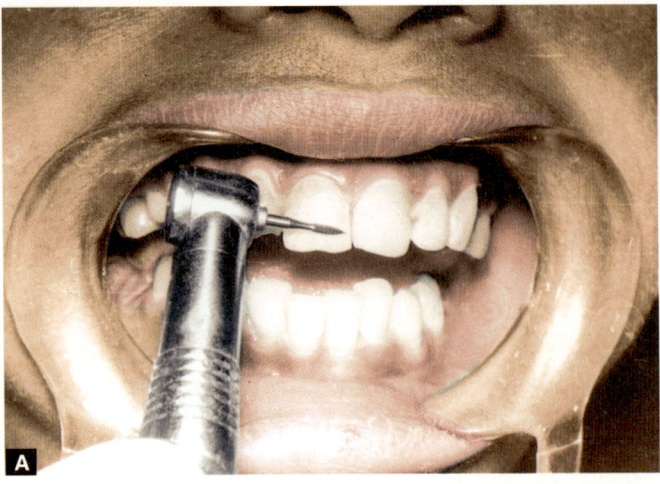
Gross finishing with tungsten carbide bur

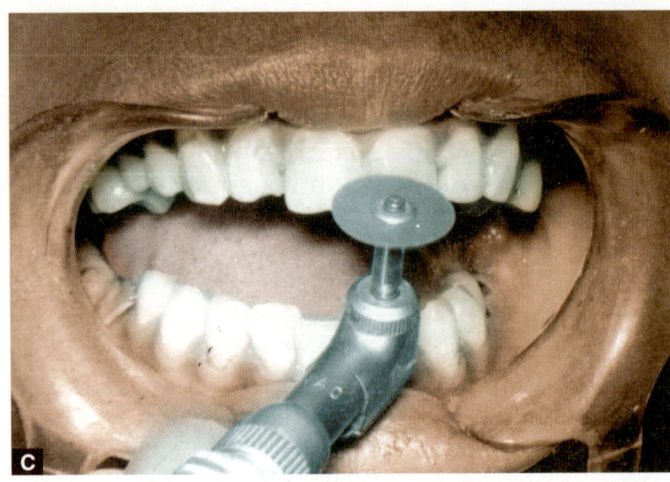
Finer finishing with finishing disk

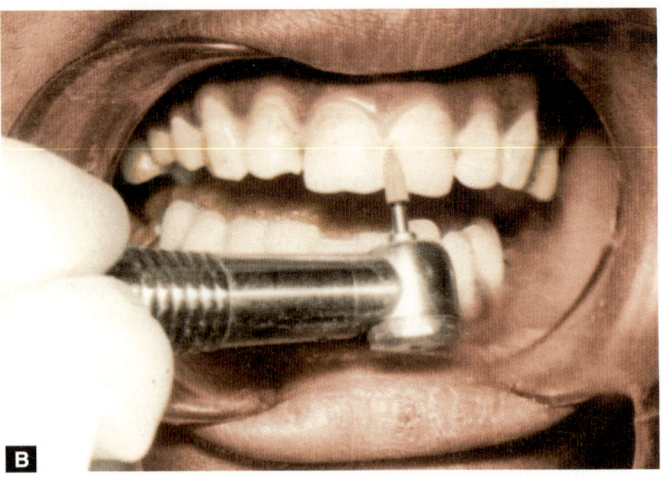
Further finishing with silicon carbide stone (green)

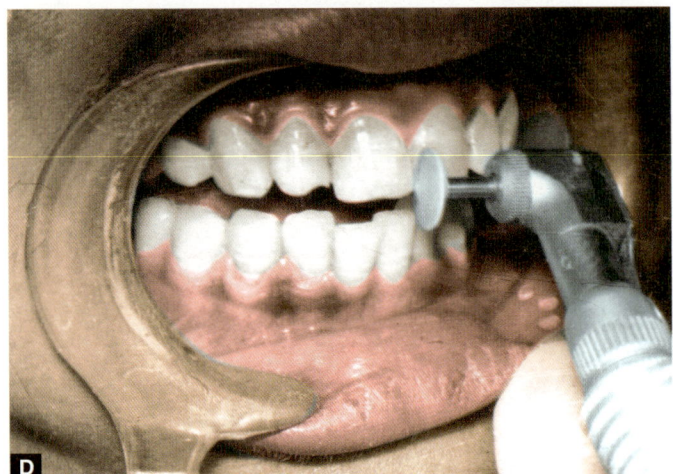
Final finishing with rubber disk

Figs 21.20A to D: Stepwise procedure for finishing of composite restoration of maxillary central incisor

introduction of glass ceramic inserts. These inserts are introduced into the uncured composite resin which become a part of the restoration surface. Because of the difference in composition and hardness between the glass ceramic and composite materials, an unequal polishing of the two surfaces is expected.

b. Indirect Composite Restorations

The cured composite inlay/onlay is primarily trimmed and finished on the die, using the same armamentarium as in a direct composite restoration.

Chairside Finishing Procedure

At the try-in stage of the restoration, excessive pressure should not be applied while seating, because of the high fragility of composite material. In case where the restoration fails to seat completely, the most probable cause is an excessive proximal contact. With the aid of dental floss, the contact is judged as to where it is tight and needs to be modified. Abrasive disks in a descending order of their abrasiveness are used to adjust the proximal contour and contact. Occlusion should preferably be checked once the restoration has been cemented. The resin cements are usually used as cementing medium. Clear plastic strips secured with wedges are used to prevent flow of excess cement into the gingival embrasures.

After the cementation has been completed, the matrix strips and wedges are removed and the margins checked for any excess cement with an explorer tip. Fine grit diamond instruments are used to remove the excess cement. Flame shaped diamonds are used in the interproximal region, while oval or cylindrical shapes are used occlusally. Finishing with diamond instruments is followed by finishing with 30 fluted carbide burs to obtain a smooth finish. Abrasive strips can also be applied in the interproximal region to

Finishing and Polishing

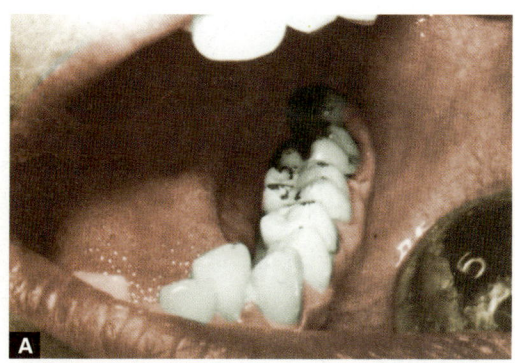

Checking the occlusion of restored posterior tooth with articulating paper

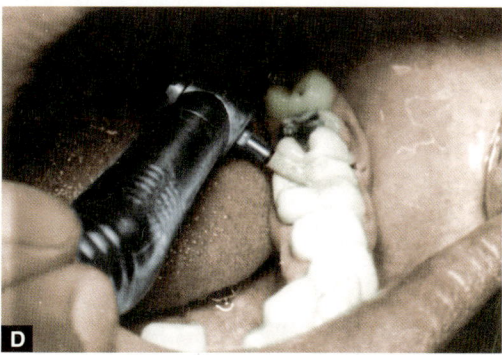

Finishing with fine stone

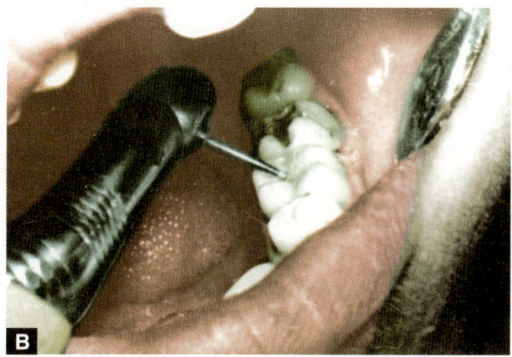

Initial finishing with carbide burs

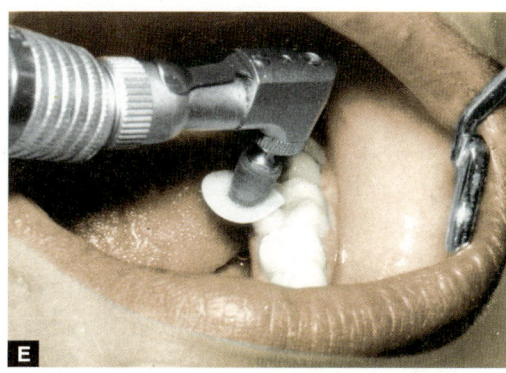

Finishing with disc

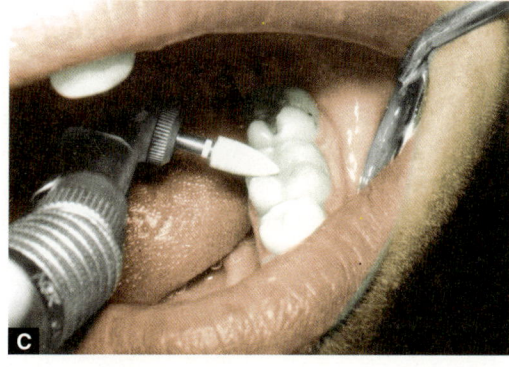

Finishing with alpine

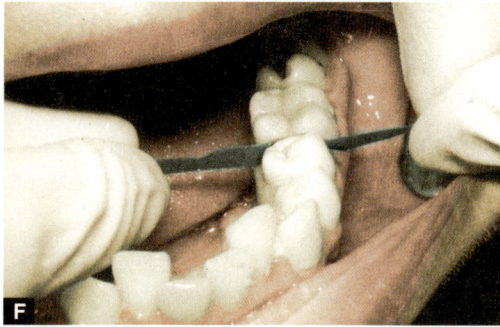

Inter-proximal strip used for finishing inter-proximal area

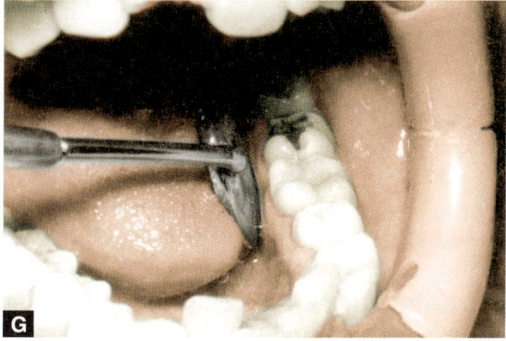

Finished restoration

Figs 21.21A to G: Stepwise procedure for finishing of composite restoration of mandibular first molar

remove any excess. Care must be taken to prevent any damage to the gingiva or root surfaces during their use.

Occlusal adjustments, if needed, are made using fine grit diamond instruments followed by 30 fluted carbide burs. The final polishing is carried out in the areas of adjustments, with the same instruments and materials as used for direct composite restorations.

Hazards During Finishing and Polishing of Composite Restorations

- Production of aerosols
- Excessive rise in temperature: May cause destruction of the underlying resin matrix and loss of filler particles. High temperatures may also damage pulp and produce monomer vapours.
- High-speed impact of the instrument may damage the filler particles.
- Microstructural defects or cracks can extend below the surface.
- Voids incorporated during the filling process may be exposed, lodging unsightly strains.
- The edges of the inflexible disks tend to scratch the surfaces and the central metallic mounting hub of certain disks also have a tendency to cut the surface.
- Composites can be lodged in the oral soft tissues during finishing and shaping procedures, which can lead to persistent chronic inflammation of those tissues.

FINISHING AND POLISHING OF GLASS-IONOMER RESTORATIONS

The ideal surface finish for glass-ionomer cements is produced by the matrix strip and any interference with hand or rotary instruments inevitably disrupts the surface. However, clinically it is almost impossible to place a restoration that adequately fills the cavity, without requiring any excess to be trimmed. It is, therefore, essential to have satisfactory procedure for finishing. Standardization of any one procedure for finishing of glass-ionomer cements is difficult since the handling characteristics as well as finishing procedures varies with each brand of glass-ionomer cement.

The surface of glass-ionomer cement is sensitive to both dehydration and water contamination during the initial setting phase. The scanning electron microscopic picture of dessicated glass-ionomer cement is shown in Fig. 21.22. If the restoration is exposed to air during this period, it loses water and develops crazing and cracks. Water contamination on

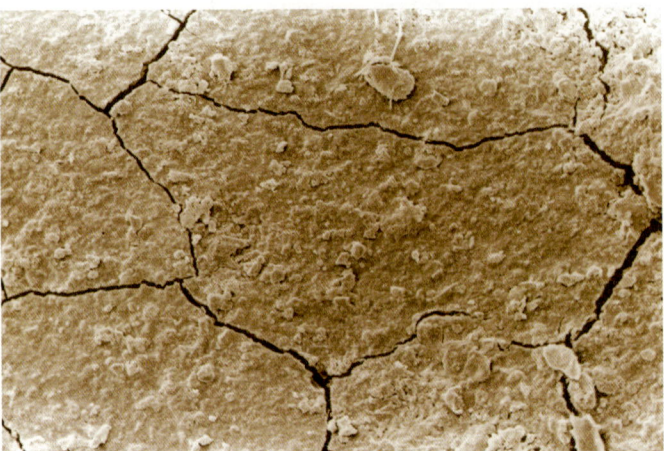

Fig. 21.22: Scanning electron microscopic picture of the surface of desiccated GIC

the other hand dissolves the matrix forming ions, resulting in weak and more soluble cement. A damaged restoration stains and dissolves very readily. The finishing and polishing of the restoration is delayed for at least 24 hours after insertion so that the setting reaction is not disturbed. After 24 hours, the surface of the material reaches ionic equilibrium with the oral environment. With some faster setting cements and light cure glass-ionomer cement, finishing can be started earlier, approximately within 10 minutes. Delaying finishing process for at least 6 minutes after placement of cement is recommended to prevent excessive desiccation of the surface.

Procedure

The gross finishing is carried out immediately after the strip or matrix is removed. The surface should be coated with a protective layer while the excess is being trimmed. A sharp gold finishing knife is used to shape the surface where the excess cement exists. The trimmed restoration is then again coated with cavity varnish or petroleum jelly to protect the cement from moisture during the initial setting phase (30 minutes). Rotary instruments can also be used at slower speeds to remove excesses at the margins. It is believed that manual cutting instruments tear the material at the margins causing marginal breakdown that may lead to staining and recurrent caries.

Restoration is given the final finish at a subsequent appointment. The final contours and embrasures are produced with fine diamonds or with 12 fluted carbide finishing burs. Margins are finished by using 1/2–3/8 inch fine cuttle fish disks. Aluminium oxide coated disks have also shown to achieve a very smooth surface. It is observed that Soflex disks with Vaseline produced the smoothest surface; whereas, the use of a tungsten carbide bur disrupted the surface of even mature glass-ionomer cements. A lubricant such as cocoa butter or petroleum jelly should be used along with finishing and polishing instruments to avoid excessive heat generation and dessication. Water spray appears to give a rough surface because of dissolution of the matrix and so, is not desirable as a coolant. Air coolants may be used. Polyacrylic gel has also been used for polishing glass-ionomer restorations. The scanning electron microscopic picture of polished glass-ionomer cement is shown in Fig. 21.23.

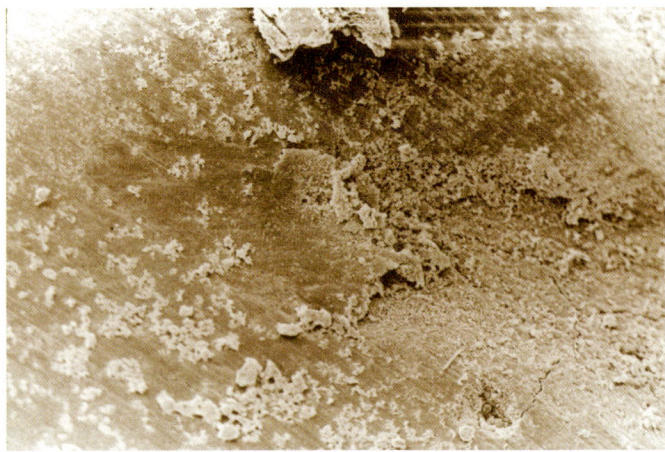

Fig. 21.23: Scanning electron microscopic picture of the surface of polished GIC

Hazards During Finishing and Polishing of Glass Ionomer Restorations

- Production of aerosols
- Excess temperature, dehydration and moisture contamination may damage the restoration surface.
- Use of sharp hand instruments before the material has fully set can produce marginal defects.

FINISHING AND POLISHING OF DIRECT GOLD RESTORATIONS

Finishing improves the qualities of pure gold. A smooth and polished gold surface is kind to the oral environment and will not tarnish or corrode in the oral fluids.

Procedure

Burnishing is the first step in finishing a gold restoration. For the occlusal surfaces, a Spratley burnisher or ball burnisher is moved with considerable pressure from the metal to the tooth surface (Fig. 17.13). A Spratley blade carver is used in the embrasures for proximal restorations.

The next step is giving an optimum contour to the restoration. Instruments used for this purpose include Morse Scaler, Jones Knife or Cleoid discoid carver. The instrument is moved on the occlusal surface from the centre to the margins. In the proximal portions, there is a need to remove any excess. The excess is removed and the remaining contoured by the use of abrasive strips and disks. The disks should be small to prevent any damage to the gingival tissue. Abrasives (mostly cuttlefish) used on the disks need to be in a descending grade. Only light pressure should be used and care should be taken to confine the instruments to the restoration. The disks are rotated from the filling to the tooth surface to achieve smooth exacting margins and surfaces. Lubricants and air coolants are used to prevent rise in temperature. The interproximal finishing strips coated with garnet or cuttlefish are also used in a sequence of descending abrasiveness.

Excess gold in the gingival area of the restoration is removed using the contrabevel end of a Wedelstedt chisel. A No. 12 Bard-Parker blade or Wilson's knife may also be used. Disks should not be used in the cervical areas for the fear of damaging cementum.

After the surface has been smoothened, burnishing is repeated once again on all the margins. Polishing with tin oxide or extra fine silex applied with a rubber cup gives the restoration a high metallic lustre and satin finish. Polishing instruments should be confined to the restoration surface and used with air coolants.

FINISHING AND POLISHING OF CAST GOLD RESTORATIONS

Initial finishing of a gold inlay is carried out on the die and most of the finishing is completed within the laboratory. The casting is separated from the investment (a fine bristle toothbrush helps in cleaning the casting of any remaining investment). It can also be cleaned using steam at pressure (Fig. 21.24). It is critical to examine the casting carefully, preferably with a magnifying glass, for any defects such as nodules or voids and even for any adherent investment before it is tried onto the die. If the casting is defective, it should be rejected and a new casting fabricated. Nodules or blebs if present are removed carefully with chisels, disks or small burs. The casting is then pickled in 50% hydrochloric acid and neutralized in sodium bicarbonate. It is only after all these procedures have been carried out, trial seating of the casting on the die is allowed. Initially, the sprue serves as a handle and helps in manipulating its insertion and removal. Once satisfied with the accuracy of the casting, the sprue is separated as close to the surface as possible using a separating disk or cutting pliers. The stub of the sprue is then smoothened back to the existing curvature on the casting.

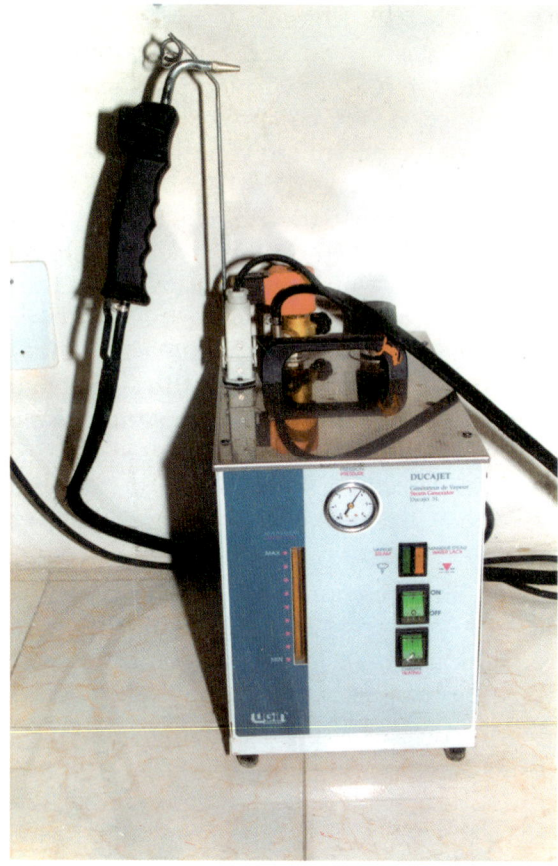

Fig. 21.24: Steam cleaner

Procedure

Any extension of the casting beyond the margins is removed upto the finish line with a small cylindrical diamond point rotating away from the operator. The remaining thick margin is carefully thinned with fine disks. Occlusal surface is then finished using abrasive stones and discs in an order of descending abrasiveness (Fig. 21.25).

The proximal surface is contoured lightly with a 1/2"–5/8" carborundum disk followed by smoothening with medium and fine cuttle paper disks. The disks should always be moved slowly and confined to the gold to prevent any abrasion of the stone die.

The occlusion is checked with an articulating paper, and premature contacts, if any, are refined by selective grinding. The roughness so created is finally finished with a rubber-polishing wheel in the accessible areas whereas pits, grooves and most inaccessible regions are finished by a fine rubber polishing points (Fig. 21.26B).

The entire occlusal surface is burnished lightly. Polishing is carried out with a No. 11 Robinson bristle brush and Tripoli. The brush should always be moved from the casting to the tooth surface. For achieving a very high lustre, a chamois wheel with rouge may be used (Fig. 21.26A). Over polishing should be avoided as it may ruin the anatomical contours or break the thin margins leading to an open casting.

Now the inlay/onlay can be tried in the cavity. Isolation the tooth properly and a throat screen (3" × 3" gauze sponge) (Fig. 8.12) placed to prevent any

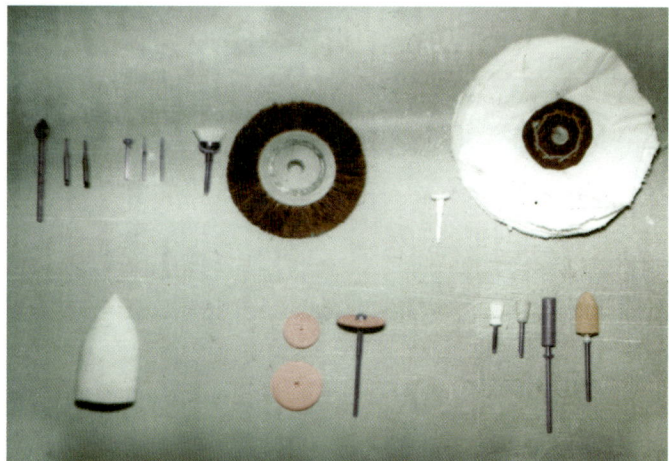

Fig. 21.26A: Polishing cast gold restoration with brushes and buffs

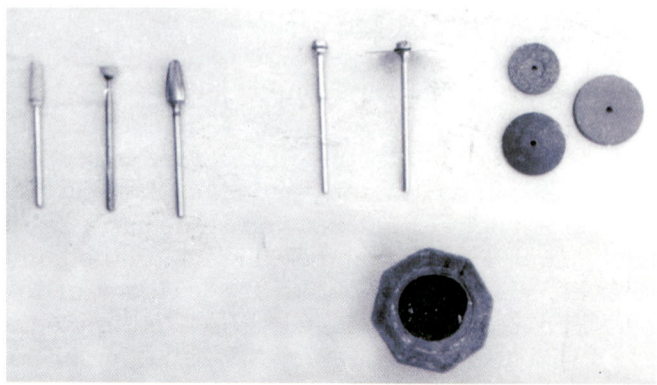

Fig. 21.25: Finishing instruments for cast gold restoration

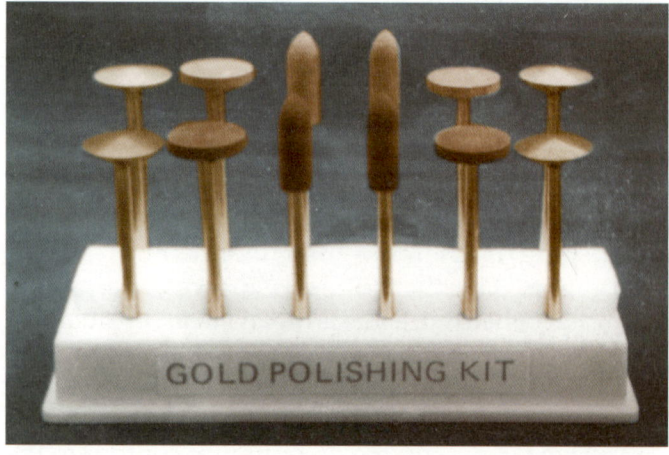

Fig. 21.26B: Polishing kit for cast gold restoration

accidental ingestion of the casting. With only little finger pressure, the inlay is seated into the prepared cavity. Heavier forces or malleting should not be applied to seat the inlay. If the casting does not seat completely, it is most likely because of heavy proximal contacts. Other causes may be, uneven internal surface of the casting or an actual distortion. A dental floss passed through the contact area gives an idea of where the contact is tight and should be accordingly reduced incrementally to prevent any over reduction. Bonded rubber abrasives or rubber wheels are the preferable instruments for adjusting the proximal contact. Seating of the casting is considered adequate, when it can be first inserted with hand pressure to within 0.2 mm of the final position; and then can be completely seated with a wooden peg or a burlew wheel placed on the occlusal surface with the patient biting onto it.

After the casting has been completely seated into the cavity, the occlusion is checked with an articulating paper. The occlusal contacts are first verified in the intercuspal position followed by lateral working and non-working positions and finally the protrusive and retrusive positions. Make sure that:

 i. Any heavy contact is reduced
 ii. The desirable position of the contacts are obtained and
 iii. There is an even distribution of contacts on the casting and adjacent tooth surfaces.

The next step is to check the marginal relationships under a magnifying glass by running a probe across the metal tooth interface. In cases where the margins of the inlay are bulky or override the unprepared tooth surfaces, the excess is reduced with a carborundum disk, stone or medium and fine cuttle disks. These instruments should be used at slow speed with light pressure and rotated either parallel to the margin or from the metal to the tooth surface. The surfaces are smoothened with preshaped fine grit stones and finished with fine waterproof disks. All those areas that have been adjusted intraorally are polished similarly as mentioned before.

The inlay is now cemented in the cavity and burnished.

FINISHING OF NON-PRECIOUS ALLOY RESTORATIONS

The most commonly used non-precious alloys are chrome cobalt and nickel chromium alloys.

These alloys have gained much popularity because of their high resistance to corrosion, which owes to the presence of large percentage of chromium. Chromium quickly forms an 'inert' or 'passive' oxide layer on the surface and thereby protects the underlying metal from environment. However, because of the increased hardness of these alloys compared to the gold alloys (about 1/3rd greater), it needs the use of special equipment to trim and polish these restorations. Difficulties during their finishing process are mainly because of two reasons:

First, chrome cobalt alloys have a very high hardness and are extremely resistant to abrasion. This necessitates the use of a higher speed for polishing. The dental stones of size 3.0–12.0 mm in diameter are rotated at the speed of 7000–20,000 rpm. The rotational speed may be reduced if larger abrasive wheels are used. However, the abrasion resistance of chrome cobalt alloys has a clinical advantage once the polishing is completed, as the polished surface can be maintained for longer periods of time in the oral cavity. The instrument kit required for finishing nonprecious alloy is shown in Fig. 21.27.

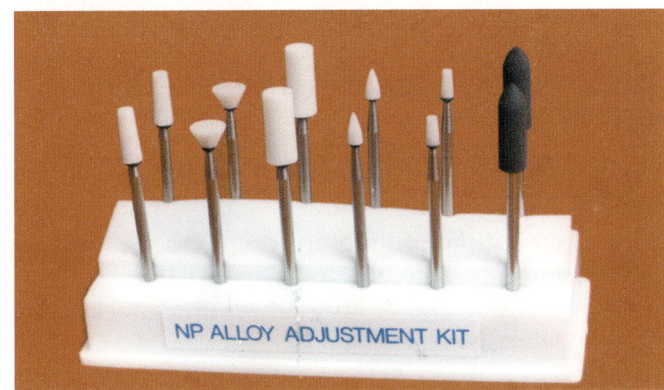

Fig. 21.27: Instrument kit for finishing non-precious alloys

Secondly, the difficulty in finishing is because of the coarse nature of the investment powder, which produces a rough surface on the casting. At times, in order to avoid such a rough surface, a thin layer of fine powdered refractory material may be sprayed on to the wax pattern to improve the cast metal surface.

Procedure

The casting is separated from the investment and cleaned under steam to remove adherent investment material and the oxide film. It is advisable to achieve the maximum shape and contours on the wax pattern itself so as to minimize any trimming of the casting. Trimming of the edges and abrading the surfaces with a fine flexible wheel is necessary before the final polishing.

Electrolytic polishing is commonly used as a part of the finishing process for chrome cobalt alloys as it reduces the time and effort for mechanical finishing. Electrolytic polishing works on the principle of reverse electroplating in which the restoration acts as the anode. The electrolyte is usually a mixture of sulphuric acid, phosphoric acid, glycerine and water. A current density of 0.5–1.0 amps/mm^2 at voltage of 4–10 V is passed for a few minutes at room temperature. The anode, i.e. the restoration ionizes and is depleted of a very small amount of alloy (a few angstroms) more readily on the rough surfaces than the smooth surfaces. These first products of electrolysis are collected in the hollows of the rough metal surface. The prominences are gradually dissolved and a smooth surface results.

Hazards During Finishing and Polishing of Non-Precious Alloys

- Production of aerosol.
- Beryllium fumes could be formed when finishing chrome cobalt alloys containing beryllium. Beryllium is also a known carcinogenic.
- Nickel, which is also a component of chrome cobalt alloys, has an ability to produce allergy.

FINISHING AND POLISHING OF PORCELAIN RESTORATIONS

There are three methods of fabrication available for ceramic inlays and onlays:

i. Conventional filling on a refractory die using firing porcelain,
ii. Milling from a preformed ceramic block using machinable ceramic and
iii. Casting by the lost wax technique using castable and pressable ceramic. The second and third methods do not use the application of a glaze layer to attain the final surface finish.

The technique for finishing and polishing of the restoration by each method is as follows:

i. Restoration Formed by Firing Porcelain

The desired finish on the fired ceramic restoration is obtained preferably by glazing and to a smaller extent by polishing. Any adjustment of the fabricated restoration needs to be done at the expense of the glaze layer; thus it is hoped that the restoration should be accurately processed and placed without adjustment. A glazed surface of porcelain is comparatively much stronger than the unglazed porcelain. Once the glaze layer is removed, transverse strength of the restoration almost reduces to one half. This situation has a clinical significance since the restoration often requires occlusal adjustment after placement. Any adjustment makes the surface rough and may lead to loss of glaze layer, thereby reducing the strength of the restoration. However, the results of recent studies have shown comparable strengths between highly glazed surfaces and those that are not glazed but only polished. Hence, with the use of polishing systems like Soflex disks, Shofu Porcelain laminate polishing kit, etc. it is now possible to minimize the damage caused by intraoral adjustment. Glazing the surface is also known to reduce flaws and eliminate crack propogation.

Glazing is of two types: *Autoglazing* and *Overglazing*. *'Autoglazing' is a process in which a smooth surface is obtained without the use of an additional glaze.* By careful control of the furnace temperature (955°C–1065°C), a glaze is created. At this temperature, the surface porcelain melts slightly, flows and glazes with a little roundening of the corners. The disadvantages with this technique are that any excessive glazing would completely destroy the shape of porcelain, increase porosity, reduce the strength and alter the color. This technique requires great precision but provides a more esthetic appearance.

'Overglazing' is the application of an external glaze layer over the surface of the porcelain. Such a glaze contains silica and low fusing fluxes and increases translucency.

The fabricated ceramic restoration is separated from the die and cleaned of any adherent investment with a coarse toothbrush or sandpaper. Metallic instruments should be avoided, as they tend to leave grey marks on the restoration. The restoration is then seated on the master die for any final adjustments and finishing. Extensive care should be taken during their handling as ceramic is very much brittle and susceptible to fracture.

Chairside Finishing and Polishing

Before the ceramic inlay/onlay is cemented into the cavity, the cavity side of the restoration is etched. After etching, the etched ceramic surface is treated with a silanating agent to improve its bond with the cementing medium. A dual cure composite is preferred for luting so as to ensure complete polymerization in any area where light may not reach. The finishing methods and equipment used are similar to those described earlier for an indirect composite restoration. During the process, care should be taken to preserve the glazed surface as much as possible. After all adjustments have been made, the areas where the glaze has been damaged is repolished. The following sequence is recommended to attain a smooth finish comparable to a glazed surface:

- Use of fine grit diamonds.
- 30-fluted carbide finishing burs.
- Rubber abrasive points and cups at slow speed with air water spray.

- Diamond polishing pastes applied with a bristle brush.

ii. Restorations Formed by Milling Ceramic Blocks

Computers are widely used in the fabrication of high precision ceramic inlays and onlays. The commercially available system which utilizes the CAD-CAM technology (Computer Assisted Designing – Computer Assisted Manufacturing) is the CEREC system. The other system which utilizes highly precise milling machine is the CELAY system.

The CEREC unit utilizes a CAD-CAM device to digitize and electronically store the cavity parameters and then a computerized milling device to shape the restoration from a ceramic block. The optical impression of the cavity is obtained either directly from the oral cavity or indirectly from a prepared die. The indirect technique reduces chair time, since most of the adjustments are performed extraorally. Checking for any seating interferences and correcting the occlusion are also carried out on the die thereby reducing the chairside finishing and polishing time.

The CELAY system uses a 'proinlay' made of composite as a template. The proinlay may be fabricated either directly in the oral cavity or indirectly in the dental laboratory. The proinlay is then manually traced with a stylus. This stylus is fixed to a turbine, which mills the inlay out of a ceramic block.

The milled restoration is adjusted on the occlusal surface using coarse to medium to fine diamond instruments with air - water spray as coolant. Since these systems mill the ceramics with diamond burs, a rough surface is produced on the casting initially. The dentist needs to polish these surfaces to a high gloss with soflex disks impregnated with diamond particles.

Chairside Finishing and Polishing

Mylar strips and wedges, which were inserted prior to cementation, are removed. These were used to avoid flow of composite lute in a gingival direction. Any excess composite in the proximal embrasure is removed with finishing diamonds and polishing strips. The final occlusal adjustments if needed are carried out with rotary diamonds followed by 30 fluted carbide finishing burs. Areas of adjustment are repolished using the same procedure as mentioned before, i.e. flexible polishing disks and diamond polishing pastes.

iii. Restorations Formed by Castable Ceramic

The fabricated restoration is finished and polished on the master die similarly as described earlier for other ceramic restorations. Care should be taken during handling of any ceramic restoration because of its extreme fragility. After all the adjustments have been made, the colorant shades are applied on the exterior surfaces and baked. The disadvantage with castable ceramic is the loss of external stains and esthetics, when restoration is adjusted for occlusion and marginal fit during the try-in. The restoration is cemented into the cavity and chairside finishing and polishing is carried out as described before.

Hazards during Finishing and Polishing of Ceramic Restorations

- Production of aerosols.
- An excess of glazing may lead to complete loss of anatomy.
- Loss of external stains may occur during finishing of castable ceramic restorations.
- Excessive heat generation may damage the pulp or tooth tissue.

Different systems used for finishing and polishing are given in Table 21.1.

Table 21.1: Different systems used for finishing and polishing

Abrasive used	Trade name	Manufacturer
Aluminium oxide	Soflex XT discs • Coarse grit • Medium grit • Fine grit • Superfine grit	3M Health Care
Aluminium oxide	Shofu super snap disks • Medium grit • Fine grit • Ultrafine grit	Shofu Dental Co.
Silicon carbide	Moore's X and XX (Waterproof) disks	E.C. Moore Co.
Rubber wheels and points	Composite and quasite	Shofu Dental Co.
Alumina pastes	Enhance finishing and an polishing strips	LD Caulk Dentsply
Alumina porcelain paste	Hawe Neos Neos system	Hawe Neos Dental Schweiz
Rubber abrasive points and cups	Porcelain laminate polishing kit	Shofu Dental Co.
Diamond polishing paste	Porcelain polishing system	Brassler

The well-finished and polished restorations are not only esthetically pleasing but are also conducive to the oral environment. Finishing and polishing of both the occlusal and proximal areas is important, since the proper marginal adaptability of the restoration, by and large, saves an individual from periodontal problems thereby achieving better clinical success of the treatment.

BIBLIOGRAPHY

1. Ashe, M.J., Tripp, G.A., Eichmiller, F.C., George, L.A. and Meiers, J.C.: Surface roughness of glass ceramic insert composite restorations assessing several polishing techniques. J.A.D.A.: 127, 1495, 1996.
2. Banerjee, A., Hajatdoost-Sani, M., Farrell, S. and Thompson, I.: A clinical evaluation and comparison of bio-active glass and sodium bicarbonate air polishing powders. J. Dent.: 38, 475, 2010.
3. Bergmann, P., Noack, M.J. and Roulet, J.F.: Marginal adaptation of class I composite restorations using different finishing techniques. J.D.R.: 69, 127(Abstr. 127), 1990.
4. Bower, C.F., Reinhardt, R.A. and DuBois, L.M.: Evaluation of interproximal finishing techniques for silver amalgam restorations. J.P.D.: 56, 274, 1986.
5. Bryant, R.W.: Marginal fracture of amalgam restorations – a review. Part I. Aust. Dent. J.: 26, 162, 1979. Part II: Aust.Dent. J.: 26, 222, 1979.
6. Carr, M.P., Mitchell, J.C., Seghi, R.R. and Vermiljen, S.G.: The effect of air polishing on contemporary esthetic restorative materials. Gen. Dent.: 50, 238, 2002.
7. Chan, D.C.N., Howell, M.L., Carraway, K.B. and Garcia, G.F.: Polarized and transmitted light microscopic study of enamel after micro-abrasion. Quint. Int.: 26, 57, 1995.
8. Chan, D.C.N., Lemke, K.C., Mowell, M.L. and Barghi, N.: The effect of micro-abrasion on restorative materials and tooth surface. Oper. Dent.: 21, 63, 1996.
9. Dutta,S., Maria, R.: The Effect Of Various Polishing Systems On Surface Roughness Of Nano and Microhybrid Composite Restoratives : An In Vitro Surface Profilometric Study. Indian J Basic Applied Med Res.: 1, 214, 2012.
10. Eide, R. and Tveit, A.B.: Finishing and Polishing of composites. Acta. Odont. Scand.: 46, 307, 1988.
11. Egilmez, F., Ergun, G., Nagas, I., Vallittu, P. and Lassila, L.V.J.:Short and long term effects of additional post curing and polishing systems on the color change of dental nano-composites. Dental Materials : 32, 107,2013.
12. Ergucu, Z., Turkun, L.S. and Aladag, A.: Color stability of nanocomposites polished with one-step systems. Oper. Dent.: 33, 413, 2008.
13. Goldfogel, M.H. and Bomberg, J.T.: Gingival margin finishing on castings: current teachings. J.P.D.: 55, 510, 1986.
14. Hondrum, S.O. and Fernandez, R. Jr.: Contouring, finishing and polishing class V restorative materials. Oper. Dent.: 22, 30, 1997.
15. Jefferies, S.R.: Abrasive finishing and polishing in restorative dentistry: a state-of-the-art review. Dent. Clin. North Am.: 51, 379, 2007.
16. Jeffrey, I.W.M. and Pitts, N.B.: Finishing of amalgam restorations: to what degree is it necessary ? J. Dent.: 17, 55,1989.
17. Jones, C.S., Billington, R.W. and Pearson, G.J.: The in vivo perception of roughness of restorations. Brit. Dent. J.: 196, 42, 2004.
18. Jung, M.: Finishing and polishing of a hybrid composite and a heat pressed glass ceramic. Oper. Dent.: 27, 175, 2002.
19. Jung, M., Eichelberger, K. and Klimek, J.: Surface geometry of four nanofiller and one hybrid composite after One-step and multiple-step polishing. Oper. Dent.: 32, 347, 2007.
20. Jung, M., Hornung, K. and Klimek, J.: Polishing occlusal surface of direct class II composite restorations in vivo. Oper. Dent.: 30, 139, 2005.
21. Jung, M., Wehlen, O., Klimek, J.: Finishing and polishing of indirect composite and ceramic inlays in vivo. Occlusal surfaces. Oper. Dent. 29, 131, 2004.
22. Korkmaz, Y., Ozel, E., Attar, N. and Aksoy, G.: The influence of one-step polishing systems on the surface roughness and microhardness of nanocomposites. Oper. Dent.: 33, 44, 2008.
23. Lovadino, J.R., Ruhnke, L.A. and Consani, S.: Influence of burnishing on amalgam adaptation to cavity walls. J.P.D.:58, 284, 1987.
24. Marghalani, H.Y.: Effect of finishing/polishing systems on the surface roughness of novel posterior composites. J. Esthet. Restor. Dent.: 22, 127, 2010.
25. Schmidlin, P.R. and Gohring, T.N.: Finishing tooth colored restorations in vitro: An index of surface alternation and finish line destruction. Oper. Dent.: 29, 80, 2004.
26. Schmitt, V.L., Puppin-Rantani, R.M., Naufel, F.S., Ludwig, D., Veda, J.K. and Sobrinho, L.C.: Effect of finishing polishing techniques on the surface roughness of a nanoparticle composite resin. Braz. J. Oral Sc.: 10, 105, 2011.
27. Schmitt, V.L., Puppin-Rontani ,R.M., Naufel F.S., Ludwig M, Ueda,J.K. and Sobrinho LC.: Effect of finishing and polishing techniques on the surface roughness of a nanoparticle composite resin. Braz J Oral Sci.: 10, 5, 2011
28. Turkum, L.S. and Turkum, M.: The effect of one step polishing system on the surface roughness of three esthetic composite materials. Oper. Dent.: 29, 203, 2004.
29. Tursi, C.P., Ferracane, J.L. and Serra, M.C.: Abrasive wear of resin composites as related to finishing and polishing procedures. Dent. Mater.: 21, 641, 2005.
30. Venturini, D., Cenci, M.S., Demarco, F.F., Camacho, G.B. and Powers, J.M.: Effect of polishing techniques and times on surface roughness, hardness and micro-leakage of resin composite restorations. Oper. Dent.: 31, 11, 2006.
31. Yap, A.U.J., Yap, S.H., Teo, C.K. and Nag, J.J.: Comparison of surface finish of a new aesthetic restorative materials. Oper. Ent.: 29, 100, 2004.

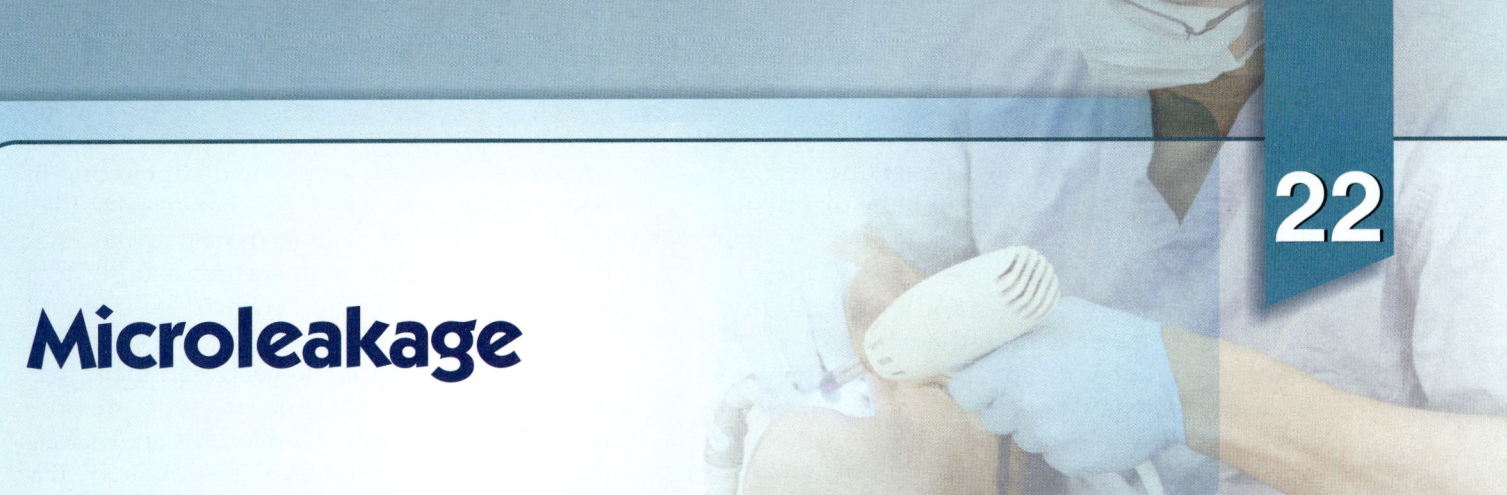

Microleakage

The goal of Operative Dentistry, undoubtedly, is to restore the tooth to its form and functions. One of the requisites of a restorative material is to adapt itself to cavity walls. Among the various restorative materials currently used, and despite of the tremendous improvements in means and technologies, none of the material could actually bond chemically with the tooth surface. The gap left between the cavity walls and the restorative material plays an important role in the prognosis of the restorative treatments. In the past, pulpal reactions to dental procedures were thought to be induced by mechanical irritation like heat, vibration, galvanism, etc. and/or chemical irritation by the restorative material and its components. Research by various authors demonstrated that probably bacterial leakage was a greater threat to the pulp than the toxicity of restorative materials. Since then the concept of microleakage has drawn widespread attention, especially so, in the clinical dentistry. Different authors have termed it as marginal percolation, liquid diffusion, fluid exchange, capillary penetration and, etc.

Microleakage can be defined as *'the clinically undetectable passage of bacteria and bacterial products, fluids, molecules or ions from the oral environment along the various gaps present in the cavity restoration interface'*. This interface is composed of the tooth, smear layer, filling and the cementing medium, if any. There are three possible routes of microleakage (1) within or via the smear layer (2) between the smear layer and the cavity varnish/cement and (3) between the cavity varnish/cement and the restoration (Fig. 22.1). It has also been emphasized that the cavity restoration interface was not a fixed, inert or an impenetrable border, but a dynamic microcrevice which allows free movement of ions and molecules. It has been established that a minimum of 10.0 μm space is definitely left at the tooth-restoration interface even after employing the adhesive liners and materials. Microleakage is hence a serious clinical problem that requires thorough analysis and discussion because all restorative materials exhibit varying degrees of leakage at the margins.

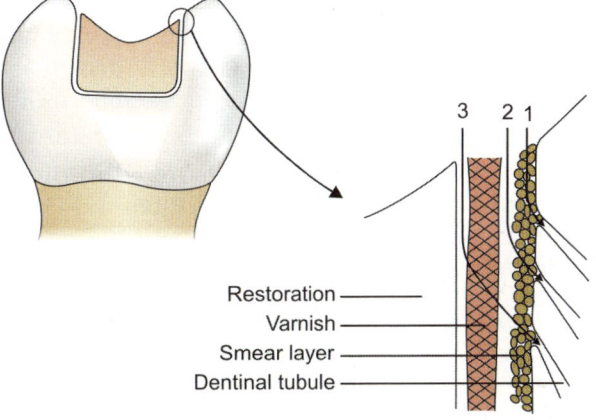

Fig. 22.1: Diagram showing cavity restoration interface and the possible routes of microleakage (1) within or via the smear layer (2) through the gap between the varnish and smear layer (3) between the varnish and restoration

CLINICAL IMPLICATIONS OF MICROLEAKAGE

1. *Post-operative sensitivity*: Microleakage often results in dentin sensitivity by creating a direct communication between oral fluids and the pulp. Change in local ionic concentrations caused by leakage of acids, basic materials and other substances along the dentinal walls produce movement of fluids in the tubules leading to pain in pulp. Dentin sensitivity is more pronounced in proximal and cervical cavities at the gingival wall and more common with resin restorations because of polymerization shrinkage.
2. *Secondary caries/recurrent caries*: Carious lesions that exist along the walls of a restored cavity can be attributed to the microleakage occuring at the tooth restoration interface. Bacteria with an average diameter less than 1.0 μm, can easily penetrate such gaps. At gap widths of 50 μm,

the space is large enough to house nutrients for the thriving of bacteria, hence inviting recurrent caries.

3. *Pulpal pathology*: Marginal gaps around restorations may become sufficiently wide to allow in-growth of bacteria. These bacteria may produce a number of inflammation inducing components, which penetrate the unprotected dentinal tubules affecting the underlying dental pulp, thereby creating pulpal diseases.
4. *Marginal discoloration*: This effect of microleakage is most commonly evidenced in aesthetic restorative materials. It leads to the accumulation of subsurface interfacial staining which cannot be eliminated by any means. A marked boundary is created around the restoration defining its shape which necessitates its replacement.
5. Hastening of the breakdown and dissolution of certain materials like cement lutes.

RESTORATIVE MATERIALS AND MICROLEAKAGE

Microleakage is a useful indicator of the microscopic and anatomic aspects of bond between the restorative material and the tooth. *Black* has stressed that the filling materials should be closely adapted to the cavity walls and should withstand thermal changes once placed in the oral environment. However, no restorative material can chemically bond to the tooth structure providing perfect seal which is capable of withstanding the wet oral environment and its temperature fluctuations. Good marginal adaptation requires adequate physical and mechanical properties of the filling material and its careful manipulation. Three properties of restorative materials that contribute largely to microleakage are:

　i. Coefficient of thermal expansion
　ii. Polymerization shrinkage
　iii. Property of adhesion

Other properties like creep, elasticity, resistance to fatigue failures, solubility, etc. also contribute to a minor extent.

　i. *Coefficient of Thermal Expansion (CTE)* is the change in length per unit length of a material per degree change in temperature. Both linear and volumetric coefficient of thermal expansion are important in restorative materials. On cooling or with a reduction in temperature, there occurs contraction of the material and conversely when the temperature is raised there occurs an expansion. Ideally, a restorative material should have a C.T.E. which closely matches that of tooth structure so that there occurs an equal expansion and contraction of both. In case of varying C.T.E. between the two, one may expand or contract more than the other during a change in temperature leading to a leaky restoration margin, i.e. micro-leakage, and in severe cases permanent debonding can occur. The greater the difference between the C.T.E. of two materials, greater will be the microleakage. From the Table 22.1, one can see that an acrylic restoration will show a greater microleakage compared to the glass-ionomer or pure gold restorations. It has also been proposed that marginal percolation may occur because of the changes in volume of fluid occupying the space between the tooth and restoration, subsequent to thermal changes.

Table 22.1: Linear coefficient of thermal expansion of dental materials relative to tooth enamel

Material	C.T.E. ($\times 10^{-6}/°C$)
Tooth (crown)	11.4
Dentin	8.3
Aluminous porcelain	6.6
Pure titanium	8.5
Type II glass-ionomer	11.0
Pure gold	14.0
Silver amalgam	25.0
Composites	20.0–25.0
Denture resin	81.0
Inlay wax	400.0

　ii. *Polymerization shrinkage* or volumetric shrinkage occurs with polymeric materials. When the monomer chains are polymerized to form polymer chain, there occurs a decrease in volume and an increase in density. (For the same mass, if density increases, volume has to reduce since Density = Mass/Volume). This shrinkage tends to pull the material away from the cavity walls. If an intermediate adhesive resin is used to bond the restorative resin to the tooth and the contraction stresses generated are very high, there may occur a break in the adhesive bond resulting in promotion of microleakage. The polymerization shrinkage of different polymeric materials is given in Table 22.2.

　iii. *Adhesion* is the attraction of the molecules of two different substances to each other, when they are brought in close contact. Lack of adhesion between the restorative material and the tooth may allow penetration of the external materials

Table 22.2: Polymerization shrinkage of different resins	
Resin	Polymerization shrinkage
Acrylic heat cure	7%
Acrylic cold cure	3.5%
Conventional composite	1.5–2.0%
Organic composite	2.5–3.5%
Microfilled composite	1.3–1.5%
Hybrid composite	2.2–2.5%

at a microscopic level. Adhesion is influenced by the wetting capabilities, surface energy, presence of water and smear layer, difference in composition of enamel and dentin, surface roughness, etc. Adhering of two solid surfaces is very difficult. This can be overcome to a small extent by using an intermediate layer of fluid or a low viscosity material to fill the irregularities and the space existing between the two (Figs 22.2A and B).

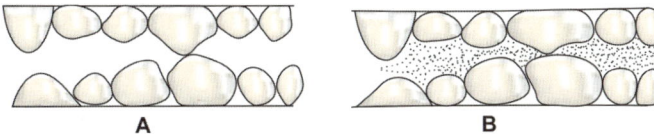

Figs 22.2A and B: (A) Inadequate contact because of suface irregularities could lead to microleakage (B) A low viscosity material fills the gap and reduces microleakage

The leakage pattern at the tooth restoration interface is to a large extent also influenced by the operator's care in placing the material. Poor packing, condensation and insertion of restorative materials and/or poor cavity design may lead to increased dimensional changes, early dissolution of the materials and poor marginal fit. Microleakage occurs unrestricted around such restorations. Hence, all restorative materials require the operator's discipline in adapting the material to the cavity walls, retention areas and the cavosurface margins. Various situations in which microleakage is promoted because of the negligence of the operator can be cited in our day to day practice, e.g. leaving the margins of a cast inlay unburnished, exposing a thin cement line to the oral cavity. Another common example is the failure to properly isolate the cavity during insertion of a composite resin. Surface contamination results in an inadequate bond between resin and the tooth resulting in microleakage.

Role of Smear Layer

Subsequent to instrumentation of the tooth, the natural deposits composed of microcrystalline cutting debris embedded within the denatured collagen are formed on the cut surfaces known as '*Smear layer*'. It is generally 1.0–2.0 µm thick and may consist of blood, saliva, bacteria, enamel and dentin particles. Some of the initial cutting debris may also be pushed into the dentinal tubules by almost 1.0–5.0 µm forming the '*smear plugs*'. Together the smear layer and the plugs serve as a functional unit (Figs 22.3 and 22.4) to reduce dentin permeability and thereby protect the pulp. However, the role of smear layer in preventing or promoting microleakage is still unclear. There is divergence of opinion as regard the role of smear layer in microleakage.

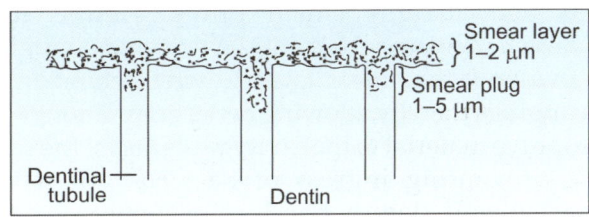

Fig. 22.3: Smear layer and plugs

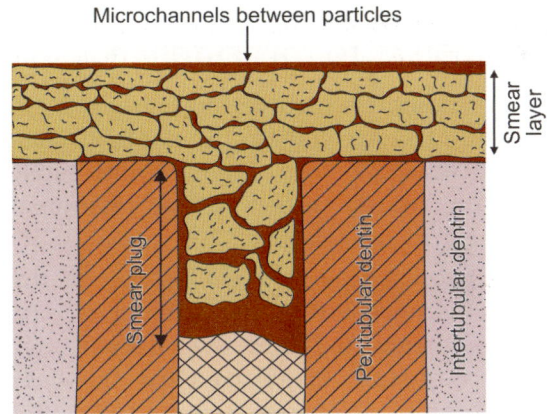

Fig. 22.4: Enlarged view of smear layer and plug around peritubular and intertubular dentin

One opinion is to leave the smear layer intact on the tooth surface because it is thought to act as a physical barrier in preventing the ingress of bacteria and their products into the underlying dentin. Pashley (1991) have reported a decrease of 86% in the permeability of dentin, when the smear layer is present. Clinicians supplementing this view should keep in mind that the smear layer is acid labile at a pH of 6.0–6.8 and less. It is inadvertantly destroyed when the pH drops, e.g. around plaque accumulated areas, or by proteolytic enzymes excreted by certain microorganisms or by acid etching. Smear layer on an exposed root surface dissolves more readily compared to one present on the occlusal surface.

The other school of thought is to remove the smear layer because of the belief that the smear layer itself may contain many bacteria. It has been demonstrated that the smear layer may be capable of preventing diffusion of bacteria as such, but not the bacterial products. Studies by some authors have also shown a decrease in microleakage when the smear layer is absent probably because removal of smear layer permits a good adaptation of the restorative material to the cavity walls.

The best way is to remove the natural smear layer and replace it with a *'sterile, inert and non-toxic'* synthetic smear layer. Research in this area has shown promising results. The smear layer is partially removed with weak acid leaving smear plugs. Tannic acid, polyacrylic acid and 0.04% EDTA are mild enough to remove only the smear layer leaving behind intact smear plugs thereby allowing better adaptation of the restorative material to the cavity walls and at the same time preventing ingress of bacteria. All newer generation of dentin bonding systems advocate treatments that remove only the smear layer while retaining intratubular plugs.

FACTORS CONTROLLING THE BACTERIAL PENETRATION AT TOOTH RESTORATION GAPS

Bacterial entry into the tooth restoration gaps is affected by the nature and size of the gap, defence mechanisms of the tooth and the nature of the restorative material. A schematic representation of this relationship is shown in Fig. 22.5.

1. *Size and nature of the gap*: The size of the gap varies around different restorative materials ranging from 10–50 µm. Even a small gap of 10 µm is quite a large area for the entry of lactobacilli. At times the gaps may be sufficiently wide to house bacteria, provide continuous nutrition and facilitate their growth. After establishing themselves in this area, the organisms may produce a number of components, which on penetration through the dentinal tubules could adversely affect the underlying dental pulp.

   Nature of the gaps cannot be described in physiochemical terms. However, the self sealing capabilities of the restorative material to a certain extent can reduce bacterial penetration. Self sealing may occur because of deposition of mineral salts of low solubility in the space, accumulation of corrosion products, calcification of the plaque like debris around the margins, etc.

2. *Host defense factors*: Natural defense mechanism of the tooth like sclerosis of dentinal tubules and reparative dentin formation decrease bacterial penetration. The hydrostatic pressure of the pulp is higher compared to the outside pressure of the oral cavity. This pressure difference moves the dentinal fluid outwards which opposes the bacteria and their products moving inwards, though only to a negligible extent. Some plasma proteins in the dentinal fluid may act as antibacterial substances and large molecular weight proteins like fibrinogen make dentin less permeable to bacteria.

   Presence of smear plugs also decreases the diffusion of bacteria to the pulp. Hence, the process of acid etching which removes these plugs and opens dentinal tubules increases their chances of penetration. Alteration of the chemical structure of dentin by leaching of tin or mercury ions from amalgam or fluoride ions from Glass Ionomer and silicate cement also checks bacterial diffusion.

3. *Restoration*: Certain restorations like Glass ionomers, silicates, compomers, etc. may release fluorides into the gaps. Fluorides are known to have an antimicrobial effect and thereby reduce entry of bacteria into the gaps. Other elements released from fillings may be silver, tin, mercury, etc.

A. MICROLEAKAGE AROUND AMALGAM RESTORATIONS

Amalgam when freshly condensed does not adapt closely to the walls of the prepared cavity. Generally, a gap of 10–15 µm width exists around the restoration. However, amalgam has the unique property that is the adaptation of the restoration to the cavity wall improves with time, hence referred to as a *'self sealing restoration'*. This is by virtue of the formation and accumulation of corrosion products in the interface with the passage of time. The corrosion products are the oxides and chlorides of tin mostly occurring in

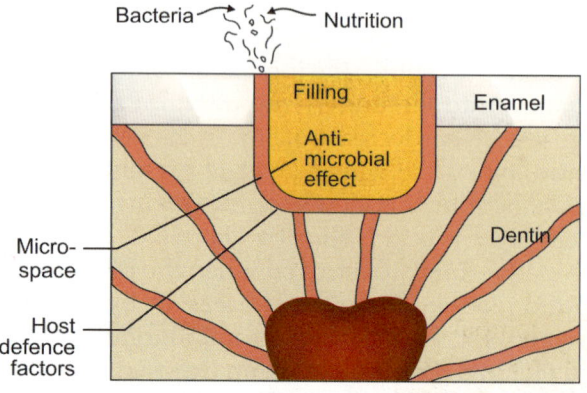

Fig. 22.5: Factors affecting bacterial penetration into marginal gaps

the low copper alloys. However, high copper alloys confer a greater resistance to corrosion. Because of this increased resistance and a slower rate of forming corrosion products, microleakage in the high copper restorations continue for a longer period of time.

Microleakage occurring as a result of dimensional changes in amalgam is quite minimal. During setting of the conventional mercury/alloy mix, a small contraction is seen initially when the mercury is consumed. This is followed by a small expansion as the crystalline matrix is formed. Modern alloys including high copper alloys undergo very little net dimensional change of approximately ± 0.2% by volume. Studies have shown that amalgam contracting by 2–40 µm/cm fails to reveal any marginal gaps. According to the ADA specification No.1, a dimensional change of 20 µm/cm is allowable for a set amalgam. The coefficient of thermal expansion of amalgam (25×10^{-6}/°C) is also not very much different from that of the tooth structure (11.4×10^{-6}/°C). Hence the change in dimensions of the gap because of thermal changes is moderate for amalgam.

Prevention of Microleakage

1. *Different types of silver alloys* exhibit different levels of microleakage. Spherical alloys display more microleakage and postoperative sensitivity compared to lathecut or admixed alloys. This might be because of the difficulty in obtaining a close adaptation with spherical alloys and/or more shrinkage of spherical amalgam as it sets. Lateral condensation helps to overcome this problem to a great extent for spherical amalgams.
2. *Condensation of amalgam* should be carried out immediately after trituration. A longer time lapse results in the loss of plasticity and increases the chances of internal voids and layering. Insertion of amalgam should be done in increments, so as to allow proper condensation and adaptation of each increment, especially so in large cavity preparations. Thorough condensation with adequate pressure removes voids and promotes adaptation of the material to the cavity walls. A pressure of 10 pounds is considered optimal when using a 2.0 mm condenser point, however the amount of force required varies with the shape of the alloy particle. Condensation should be first begun in the centre and the condenser point gradually worked towards the periphery using the stepping process. This removes any air space and pushes the material against the cavity walls, thereby decreasing the incidence of microleakage. Mechanical (pneumatic) means of condensation has shown to be superior to hand condensation in controlling marginal leakage.
3. *Burnishing of amalgam* after condensation can reduce microleakage by aiding adaptation of the material at the margin and enhancing homogenity. The effect of burnishing on the degree of marginal leakage varies with the particle shape of amalgam. With spherical alloys, no reduction of leakage results from the burnishing procedure compared to lathe cut and admixed alloys, probably because the spherical shape of the alloy allows the particles to be 'pushed aside' during the process.
4. *Alloys with lesser creep values* show a smaller degree of marginal leakage. A creep rate of less than 3% is considered acceptable under the ADA specification No. 1. Low copper alloys show a creep value ranging from 0.8–8.0% compared to high copper alloys which have much lower values of 0.1–1%.
5. *Sealing the cavity walls with a varnish* under an amalgam restoration prevents microleakage at least until the corrosion products of amalgam begin to fill the microspace. However the benefits offered by a varnish do not exist as long as the life of the restoration. Because of the solubility in the oral environment, its effectiveness is limited to approximately six months and by the end of one year almost all the benefits are lost. This time lapse is sufficient for the corrosion products to replace the varnish and permanently seal the interface. Application of a varnish layer under high copper amalgams did not prove to be effective in reducing any microleakage.

   It has been shown that the use of glass-ionomer liners can significantly reduce microleakage under an amalgam restoration but their placement involves an additional procedure.
6. *Sealed amalgam restorations*: In these types of restorations, a coating of unfilled resin is placed over the restoration margins and the adjacent enamel after having etched the enamel surface. Although the resin may finally wear away, it delays microleakage until the corrosion products are accumulated in the interface. It is established that sealed amalgam restorations offered fewest marginal deficiencies and best survival rates compared to traditional amalgam and composite restorations.
7. *Introduction of clinical techniques that bond amalgam to enamel and dentin* have shown to overcome the

problems of microleakage. Use of amalgam bonding agents have proved to be quite effective in this regard.

8. *Use of gallium alloys*: Gallium alloys as an alternative to amalgam alloys were introduced long ago but did not gain much popularity. These are alloys of Gallium-Tin-Indium (liquid) and a silver based alloy similar in composition to the high copper amalgam alloy (powder). Many of its physical and mechanical properties and handling characteristics are similar to silver amalgam. One major advantage with the use of these alloys is that because of their very high wetting ability, the final restoration is highly resistant to microleakage. They have such a high wetting characteristic that when the gallium rich mixture is inserted into the cavity, some of it tends to move up along the sides of the instrument.

B. MICROLEAKAGE AROUND GLASS-IONOMER RESTORATIONS

Glass-ionomer cement adheres to the tooth structure by forming chemical bond between carboxyl groups of the cement and calcium ions of the tooth. Since glass-ionomer is hydrophilic in nature, it can bond even in the presence of a slightly wet surface. In addition to this important property of chemical adhesion which contributes to decreasing microleakage, others properties are (a) a coefficient of thermal expansion which closely matches that of tooth structure (b) fluoride releases into the surrounding environment and (c) the ability to renew broken ionic bonds. All these features help to have long term cavity sealing properties.

Glass-ionomer cement is highly technique sensitive and the most critical aspect is isolation from moisture for the first 30 minutes after placement. On exposure to water the matrix forming ions are easily leached out during the initial set which could interfere at tooth restoration interface. Solubility in oral fluids continues to be a problem for 24 hours following insertion of the material. Excessive dehydration/dessication can result in a chalky, crazed or a cracked surface which if extends to the margins could result in considerable marginal leakage. Coating the restoration with surface protective agents like cavity varnishes or unfilled resins is highly recommended for protecting against dehydration. Once the cement has attained full maturity, it becomes highly resistant to solubility and disintegration in the oral fluids. Another factor that harms the marginal integrity of the restoration is the use of sharp hand instruments for finishing before the material has completely set.

Measures to Reduce Microleakage

- Proper manipulation and placement of glass-ionomer cement on dentinal surfaces only after they have been adequately cleaned. Formulations of lower powder: liquid ratio than recommended increase the solubility of the cement.
- Use of rotary instruments over manual instruments is advocated for finishing restoration margins. The latter have shown to tear away the material at the margins resulting in marginal ditching.
- During finishing, restoration surfaces should always be coated with vaseline or petroleum jelly to protect from moisture contamination and dessication
- Final protection of the cement while it is setting, is done by two coats of varnish or a layer of unfilled resin. Varnish is semi-permeable in nature compared to unfilled resin which is more resistant to water contamination. Despite of this fact, a varnish application is preferred as it closely adheres to the surrounding surface enamel also, preventing any moisture from reaching the glass-ionomer tooth interface.
- Prior conditioning of the tooth surface before insertion of GIC increases the bonding and possibly reduces microleakage scores. Various agents advocated for the purpose are tannic acid, polyacrylic acid, citric acid, etc.

Resin modified glass-ionomer cements, because of rapid initial setting, reduces the effect of moisture contamination. Unfortunately, resin modified glass-ionomers have occasionally shown increased levels of microleakage compared to the chemically cured ones. This is probably because of the resin component in the former that causes it to shrink during polymerization and setting. In contrast to the slow setting chemically cure glass-ionomer cements which permit stress relief, the resin modified systems exhibit more rapid setting contraction through light polymerization. Moreover, less water and less carboxylic acid content also decrease the wetting ability of light cure Glass ionomer cements to the tooth substance promoting marginal leakage. To a certain extent, expansion due to water uptake which is a function of the resin component of the cement compensates for the initial resin shrinkage and reduces microleakage.

C. MICROLEAKAGE AROUND COMPOSITE RESTORATIONS

Composite resins on their own do not possess the capability of bonding to either enamel or dentin. The inability to bond coupled with marked polymerization shrinkage and thermal expansion/contraction predispose to marginal leakage. Prior treatment of the tooth surface like acid etching, priming/conditioning and the use of enamel and dentin bonding agents therefore becomes a necessity for composite restorations. In enamel such treatment leads to an unparalleled success in preventing microleakage. Hence microleakage at the enamel restoration interface can be eliminated almost completely if sufficient enamel thickness is present. Conversely, the bond to dentin though substantially reduces microleakage but does not protect the dentin restoration interface completely. The tight adhesion to dentin is limited by a number of factors like vitality of the dentin, difference in physical and chemical composition of dentin compared to enamel, presence of dentinal fluid, smear layer and, etc. Development of internal stresses from polymerization shrinkage and thermal effects also have a detrimental effect on the bond. Microleakage therefore continues to be a problem in almost all composite restorations.

The most notable factors that contribute to marginal leakage of composites are:

1. Composite resin restorations are very much technique sensitive. Any step that goes beyond the actual procedure will lead to failure including an increase in marginal leakage.
2. Marginal gaps formed at the tooth restoration interface primarily result from dimensional changes like polymerization shrinkage of the setting resin. After the resin has set, the size and shape of the gaps are further affected by masticatory forces, thermal changes and water sorption.
   a. All the composite restorative resins shrink during polymerization. The volumetric polymerization shrinkage usually is in the range of 1.67–5.68%, the lesser being for the light activated ones.
      In case of a bonding agents being used to bind the restorative resin to the tooth structure, shrinkage results in the development of tensile and/or shear stresses at the tooth restoration interface. Within certain limits, the adhesive bond is able to withstand these stresses. Once the stresses exceed the bond strength and the plastic or elastic deformation of the combined system, a separation at the tooth restoration interface may occur leading to microleakage. It is usually the bond with dentin which is compromised during shrinkage where as the bond with enamel is sufficiently strong to withstand the same amount of forces.
   b. Functional stress incurred on restorations by cyclic mastication is another factor in inducing microleakage of resin restorations Occlusal stresses enhance leakage because of repeated plastic or elastic deformation of the restoration.
   c. The marked difference in the coefficient of thermal expansion of restorative resins and tooth structure also has a detrimental effect on adhesion. The composites have a coefficient of thermal expansion ranging from $22–55 \times 10^{-6}/°C$ comparatively higher than the tooth. Combined thermal and occlusal stresses have shown to induce more microleakage as compared to leakage induced by individual stresses.
   d. Composite resin restorations have a tendency to absorb water from the environment, causing the restoration to expand. Thus the property of water sorption is able to counteract polymerization shrinkage to a little extent. In contrast to the polymerization contraction stresses, which are generated at a rapid rate, relief of stresses by hygroscopic expansion proceeds more slowly. The resins with the largest quantity of filler have the least water sorption (water uptake is the property of the resin component of the matrix). It should be stressed here that though water sorption may improve marginal adaptation of composite resin, it impairs its mechanical properties.
   e. Incidence of marginal gaps are higher on the cervical margins of a class II restoration, the reasons being:
      i. Placing the restorative material at these areas is difficult.
      ii. Entrapment of air during placement.
      iii. Difficulty during condensation because of the pull back of sticky material.
      iv. Inadequate bonding to the gingival wall due to polymerization shrinkage.

Measures to Reduce Marginal Leakage

A number of techniques have been advocated to enhance marginal adaptation and reduce microleakage of composite restorations. These include:

1. Choice of Composite Material

Microfilled composite resins provide a better marginal adaptation over the macrofilled composite resins. This can be attributed to two reasons (a) Greater flexibility of the microfills during polymerization shrinkage decreases the contraction forces that tend to threaten the forming dentinal bond and (b) These show a larger absorption of water resulting in an expansion which counteracts some of the polymerization shrinkage. These facts indicate the use of microfilled resins in all situations where strength is not a major requirement.

2. Cavity Design

Cavity designs for composites should be as conservative as possible to overcome the disadvantages of polymerization shrinkage and wear under occlusal stresses. Moreover, composites are adhesive to the underlying tooth structure thereby limiting the need for retentive and extensive preparations. Modified cavity designs, placement of bevels, reduced depths and rounded internal angles are very effective in providing good marginal adaptation and reducing leakage (Fig. 22.6).

Not only the size but the shape of the cavity is also an important factor in determining the width of the marginal gap. This is illustrated in Fig. 22.7, which shows three dentin cavities of identical diameter but of different shapes. The cavity to the right is V shaped and the cavity to the left is box shaped. When the cavities are filled with composite resin without any intermediate bonding agent, the marginal gap is seen to reduce from 13 µ to 4.0 µ from left to right. Whereas when an intervening dentin bonding system is applied, the gap width is in the order of 3.0 µ to almost nil. This can be explained on the decreasing ratio of volume/bonded area from 1.0 for the box shaped cavity to 0.4 for the V-shaped cavity.

The role of bevels on cavosurface margins in reducing leakage remained controversial. The principle behind giving bevels is to increase the surface area for enamel bonding and reduce microleakage. Owing to the well known fact that etching rod ends rather than the sides of the prisms is beneficial makes it conducive to place bevels only in selected areas. Occlusal beveling is usually not required because of the enamel rod direction and the possiblity of extending the material to load bearing areas. Beveling of cervical margins in extensive class II preparations may result in removing the remaining enamel. Placement of bevels is recommended mainly on the accessible facial and lingual margins of the proximal box. In a study by Opdam, et al. (1998), bevels were placed on all the margins of a minimal class II composite preparation. Microleakage was limited to enamel of facial and palatal margins in 75% of the bevelled restorations compared to 30% of not beveled surfaces. Beveling gingival margin of class V preparations is not advocated as it usually increases microleakage.

3. Acid Etch Technique and Bonding

Acid etching removes surface contaminants, raises the surface energy and reactivity of enamel and increases the surface area for bonding. Subsequently, the bonding agent is drawn by capillary attraction into the micro-porosites created by acid etching. These polymer tags provide micro-mechanical interlocking with enamel thereby reducing microleakage to almost nil.

A shortcoming with this technique is its dependence on the presence of thick enamel at the cavity walls. The effectiveness of marginal seal is compromised by the position and surface structure of enamel as it anatomically varies in different areas of the same tooth. The results are obvious when the restoration margins are located in the cervical enamel. Cervical enamel is thin, irregular in prism structure and devoid of characteristic prism markings. Therefore the bond to cervical enamel is not very intimate compared to the more occlusally placed enamel. This is reflected in the microleakage scores, which are almost negligible on the occlusal cavosurface margins but are significant on the gingival margins.

Acid etching on dentin was traditionally discouraged because etchants were thought to open and widen the dentinal tubules resulting in increased

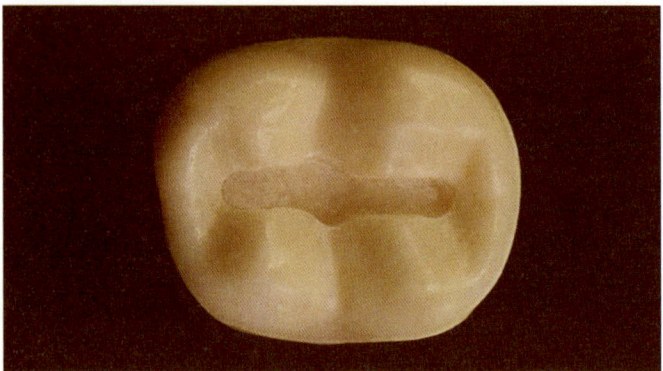

Fig. 22.6: Class I cavity preparation for composite in mandibular molar

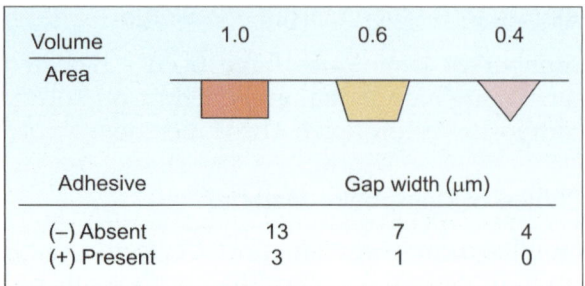

Fig. 22.7: Width of the marginal gap in relation to the shape of the dentin cavity

permeability and bacterial ingress to the underlying pulp. However, with the introduction of the newer and better hydrophilic resins over the earlier hydrophobic ones, the concept has now changed. Many authors now propose deliberate etching of dentin to create open tubules and a porous intertubular layer. It is believed that a close adhesion can then be attained between the resin adhesive and treated dentin preventing the penetration of toxic materials leading to pulpal irritation.

It has been reported that the leakage was not uniform along the interface. While some areas may show no microleakage, others may leak entirely from the cavosurface margins to the pulp. The non uniformity of bonding may be attributed to various factors like differences in the thickness of smear layer, different degrees of etching, wetness, force of polymerization contraction, etc. which may vary on the same surface.

New bonding agents based on glass-ionomer technology have been developed (e.g. Scotch bond Multipurpose). These have carboxylic acid groups incorporated inside them that become available for attachment to dentin. They are also useful in attaching composite resins to glass-ionomer cement surfaces. These agents can be separately grouped as 'glass-ionomer bonding agents.'

Another newly advocated material is the diluted version of the resin modified glass-ionomer cements such as Fuji Bond II LC which can be used to completely replace the conventional bonding agents under a composite resin. These would be advantageous in reducing leakage because of high chemical adhesion and a coefficient of thermal expansion close to that of tooth structure. Significantly better sealing ability with resin modified ionomers as a bonding agent on both enamel and dentin has been observed when compared to the commonly used agents like Scotch bond MP, Prime and Bond and Bisco.

4. Cavity Filling Technique

Volumetric contraction of thick layers or bulk material in a cavity can induce significant shrinkage of the entire mass and subsequently the high stress generated may debond some adhesive systems leading to microleakage. Placing composite resin in small multiple increments to fill the cavity is therefore recommended to control polymerization shrinkage and the contraction gap at the margins. Thickness of one increment should preferably be limited to 1.0–1.5 mm of the material. Different incremental placement designs have been described in the Chapter 17. Applying the material in layers assumes importance especially in class II and class V cavities where the resin does not adequately bond to the gingival margins.

The amount of polymerization shrinkage can be markedly controlled if the resin to filler ratio is decreased. This phenomenon led to the introduction of the concept of *beta quartz glass inserts* used as '*mega fillers*' in composite restorations. Inserts are made of lithium aluminosilicate glass, containing modifiers to give it a natural tooth appearance, and are available in various sizes and shapes. The choice of an insert is controlled by the cavity dimensions. Shrinkage in a composite restoration is a function of the resin matrix. Inserts tend to increase the filler content relative to the amount of resin, decreasing this contraction. They also have a low coefficient of thermal expansion of $4 \times 10^{-6}/°C$ and exhibit no polyermization shrinkage and water sorption.

Prepolymerised composite ball, have also been substituted for the glass insert. Prepolymerised composite ball containing restorations however showed significantly greater microleakage. This was probably because of the high cumulative internal stresses generated during thermal changes. Beta quartz insert has a coefficient of thermal expansion close to that of dentin, which is therefore expected to reduce additional stresses on the interface.

Recently, the method of '*Soft start polymerization*' has been advocated to reduce marginal gap and improve marginal integrity. The procedure involves a short prepolymerization at low intensity followed by the final cure at high intensity. This allows composite resin to flow during the initial setting period, thereby minimizing the stresses induced at the interface. Prolonging the curing time of a composite resin improves upon the microleakage by allowing a greater inversion rate of the monomer component.

5. Direction of the Light Source

It is presumed that the polymerization shrinkage vectors of setting composite resin are directed towards the light source. This has a practical importance especially when curing proximal restorations. Because of the inadequate access of the light guide in proximal areas and also since the curing tip is usually directed from the occlusal aspect, the gingival increment shrinks occlusally. Use of curing aids like light directing wedges, flexible light guides and focusing tips can facilitate better curing in areas of poor access and invert the shrinkage vectors of composite resin towards the gingival floor in proximal areas. A three sited light curing technique for better adaptation of conventional class II composite restorations has been advocated (Fig. 22.8).

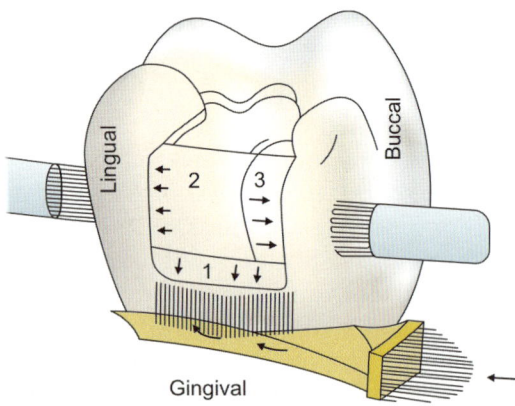

Fig. 22.8: Three sited light curing technique

6. Sealing the Marginal Gaps

An unfilled low viscosity resin is applied to the margins by slowly brushing the resin laterally from one side to another after the composite restoration has been finished and polished. It has been seen that the sealed composite restorations placed over frank cavitated lesions were successful in arresting the clinical progress of the carious lesions. Materials used for the purpose of sealing gaps are the commercially available pit and fissure sealants.

7. Delaying the Finishing Process

Finishing techniques and their timings have shown to affect the ability of restorative materials to resist leakage. Most of the authors advocate finishing of composites to be delayed for 24 hours, until the polymerization is complete. If done before the initial setting, it seems to break the bond between the resin and the tooth. It is established that finishing the restoration after three minutes of insertion resulted in a considerable microleakage at the enamel and dentinal/cemental margins, more so in the latter. Finishing after five minutes and one day after insertion was considered acceptable as it resulted in almost no microleakage. However, according to different authors, the delayed finishing after one week does not improve but instead can be detrimental to the already formed marginal seal of the restorations. Stresses which may disrupt the adhesive bonds are almost always generated during the finishing of restorations.

Variations in the finishing techniques have also shown to affect leakage. Increased leakage occurs with the use of dry finishing techniques, suggesting a detrimental effect of high heat on the marginal adaptation. It is therefore recommended that rotary instruments while finishing and polishing be run at slow speeds using light intermittent strokes and with generous air coolants. Use of Soflex disks for contouring and finishing have shown to provide the best marginal quality for composite restorations.

8. Use of Cavity Liners and Bases

Calcium hydroxide and glass-ionomer cements are the most commonly used base materials in a composite restoration. The two reasons advocated for their use in deep cavity preparations are (a) they serve as protective agents for the pulp and (b) their presence reduces the bulk of composite resin in the cavity and subsequently the polymerization shrinkage.

Glass-ionomer cements under composite resins have shown to be quite successful in reducing microleakage and its consequences. Bond of Glass ionomer cement to enamel is weaker as compared to composites; however, the bond to dentin is stronger. The bond between etched GIC and composite is also stronger than the tensile strength of the resin or the cement itself. It shows a chemical union with dentin even in the presence of dentinal fluid because of its hydrophilic nature, possesses a coefficient of thermal expansion close to that of tooth structure, acts as a fluoride reservoir and is kind to the pulp. All these properties make it logical to expect that Glass-ionomer cements would serve an excellent lining material under the composite restoration. This is also the basis for *Bilayered Restorations*, previously known as '*Sandwich Restorations.*' Criticism is however levelled for these restorations because it is believed that the polymerization shrinkage of composite resin breaks the seal of glass-ionomer cement to dentin. The contraction tends to pull the base away from the cavity floor resulting in a gap not less than 5 µm at the cavity restoration interface. Any gap created has a potential for leakage and fluid percolation. In shallow cavities the loss of seal is often related to the strength and thickness of the base used, and thin linings of less than 1.0 mm are considered unsatisfactory. Light cure glass-ionomers when used as bases show a slightly better performance compared to their chemically cure counterparts. Though gaps are also created with the former, yet their sizes are smaller. This is probably because of their ability to adhere immediately to the dentin and achieve high early tensile and compressive strengths. The hardened cement resists stresses that tend to disrupt the dentinal seal in a better way.

9. Use of Composite Inlay Restorations

Composite inlay restorations bond to the tooth structure using composite as a cementing medium. The resins employed may be either chemical cure or dual cure. Light cure composite luting agents are usually not advocated as it is difficult to cure them through a preprocessed resin restoration which exceeds 2.0 mm in thickness. Composite inlay seems to be a very efficient way of managing polymerization shrinkage since the bulk of the contraction occurs prior to cementation. Less leakage with inlay systems compared to direct resin restorations have been shown, but no significant difference in leakage between the direct and indirect methods of inlay fabrication.

However, shortcomings still exist in their use and the most vulnerable part of the resin inlay continues to be the cement lute. Since the luting cements are less heavily filled than the actual resin restorative materials, they tend to lose earlier by the wear mechanisms. The hybrid luting resins are more susceptible to wear than microfilled ones. Hence microfilled resins should be preferred for the cementation purposes.

Another drawback in their use is that the cement often fails to bond chemically with the inlay. This is attributed to the curing procedure which induces a very high conversion rate of the inlay and greatly reduces the availability of remaining unconverted monomers for co-polymerization with the resin lute. A passage for microleakage is hence created resulting in marginal staining. Studies have demonstrated failure of composite to cement bond by almost 60% after 6 months. For improving the bond between processed composite restorations and the resin cements, different methods have been advocated like (a) use of a solvent such as ethyl acetate to soften the cavity side of the restoration prior to cementation (b) sand blasting the cavity surface of the restoration with aluminium oxide abrasive particles so as to increase the surface area for bonding and (c) etching the cavity side of the composite restoration with 10% hydrofluoric acid.

10. Expanding Matrix Resins for Dental Composites

Composite resins that expand slightly during polymerization may be the future of restorative resins. These would facilitate bulk placement of the material, reduce post-operative sensitivity, secondary caries and microleakage. The concept of expanding matrix resins is still in a pioneering stage and may require lots of research.

D. MICROLEAKAGE AROUND DIRECT GOLD RESTORATIONS

Direct gold restorative materials adapt to the cavity walls most efficiently. When properly placed, they serve better than other materials and prevent recurrence of decay. The decreased marginal leakage can be attributed to the good adaptability of gold to the preparation walls because of inherent qualities as:

- High malleability and ductility of gold provides burnishing which contributes to reducing leakage by riding the gold over the marginal voids.
- A short bevel on the cavosurface margins facilitate the burnishing, contouring and polishing thereby promoting close adaptation at the cavity restoration interface.
- Complete insolubility in the oral fluids.
- The method of condensation induces elastic compression of the underlying and surrounding dentin, which adapts the material strongly after completion of the condensation.

If gold is improperly compacted into the cavity, air spaces/voids may be left behind at the gold tooth interface enhancing microleakage. Voids at the margins are particularly common when a convex surface in the centre is formed during the building of a gold restoration. Other reasons for the existence of voids in the restoration can be attributed to the type of gold selected, non-uniform method of stepping, improper lines of force and inadequate condensation pressure.

Measures to Reduce Leakage

1. In general, mat and powdered golds are porous and hence less effective than regular cohesive gold foils in obtaining a good cavity seal. It is therefore recommended that the former should be used for forming the internal bulk of the restoration of the gold foil and the latter be used as a veneer on the surface to prevent leakage.
2. Uniform stepping of the condenser point in individual steps as well as lines of steps by half or one fourth is indicated to drive away all air spaces and closely adapt the material to the underlying surface. Stepping should always proceed from the centre to the periphery.
3. Lines of force should be directed at 90° to the pulpal floor in the centre of the cavity preparation and then changed to 45° to the cavity walls at the periphery.
4. Average force of 10 pounds applied with a 1 mm condenser point is considered optimal for proper adaptation of the material to the cavity walls and cohesion of two gold surfaces.
5. Building of the restoration should be done in a convex form, i.e. material should always be banked on the cavity walls ahead of the centre. This allows application of forces in a right direction and thorough adaptation.
6. Surface procedures like burnishing, finishing and polishing bring the metal closer to the tooth structure improving the marginal seal.

E. MICROLEAKAGE AROUND CAST RESTORATIONS

Generally, the cast restorations do not offer close adaptation to the cavity walls. A gap ranging from 10 to 160 µms has been reported in various cast restorations. An intermediate layer of dental luting cement is therefore necessary to seal the interface and aid in retention. The low viscosity luting cements are able to penetrate the irregularities on both the tooth and the restoration surface creating micro-mechanical retention. With the rising popularity of adhesive cements being employed as luting agents, added chemical retention is also now possible.

The intermediate cement layer used for sealing intervening gaps, might sometimes promote leakage. Though the recent cements are less soluble in oral fluids, (the Zinc phosphate cement earlier used with cast gold restorations was highly soluble), yet none of the materials totally resist the solubility in oral fluids. In case of gold, the placing of bevels and burnishing the margins to reduce exposure of this cement line and hence leakage is illustrated in Fig. 15.11. The interfacial space is closed primarily by elongating and/or compressing the cast gold because of the ductility and malleability. The external forces applied to these margins are mediated by a number of factors like burnishing, abrasion, torquing, etc. Permanent deformation of the gold alloy occurs which results in a physically closing the discrepancy at the margins. Type II and type III gold alloys allow a percentage elongation of 20–35%. For the highly soluble cements (i.e. cements that have a solubility greater than the ADA recommendation of 0.04–0.10%) like zinc phosphate, silicate or silicophosphates, burnishing should be delayed for 24 hours. This gap of time period allows for the superficial few microns of the cement to dissolve leaving behind metal margins that can be burnished. For the non-soluble resin cements like resin lutes, burnishing can be performed immediately. Marginal gaps which exceed 0.1 mm should not be burnished, rather the castings remade.

Despite the efficient use of these methods to reduce leakage, it continues to be a problem in areas where the cement line is inadvertently exposed to the oral environment. This condition exists when the margins are not adequately bevelled and/or burnished, e.g. in regions difficult to be reached by the burnisher like the gingival margins of a class II inlay, or when harder golds used for crowns are not easily burnished. So this would mean that a thin layer of cement would continue to be exposed at the gingival margins of a cast inlay and subgingival margins of a crown restoration. Restorations that have a close fit (within 20 µms) to the adequately designed preparation surfaces resist degradation of the cement lute and increase life of the restorations for longer periods. Many a times, it is seen that the novice operator feels satisfied on sealing large marginal discrepancies with the cement lute.

But it should be stressed here that in no way is the cement a compromise for sealing these large marginal gaps as this could only increase the chances of microleakage and secondary caries.

Another cause of promoting leakage in cast restorations is the excessive taper of the underlying preparation. Under the continuous application of loads, the restoration gives away by rotating on the preparation surfaces. This results in a break in the cement lute and fracturing of the thin metal margins, leading to leakage and even dislogement.

F. MICROLEAKAGE AROUND PORCELAIN RESTORATIONS

Dental porcelain is a brittle material with low tensile strength and fractures easily if the strain exceeds 0.1%; therefore it requires adequate bonding to the underlying tooth surface for gaining structural and functional integrity. Earlier, ceramic inlays/onlays/crowns were bonded to the tooth structure using conventional luting cements like zinc phosphate, polycarboxylate, silicate, silicophosphate, etc. only to be met with high rates of failure. With the growing advancements in adhesive technology resin systems have now almost completely replaced the earlier luting cements for bonding and supporting the restoration to the cavity surface. The resin cements employed should preferably be dual cure to allow polymerization to be completed in areas inaccessible to light.

An adequate bond of the ceramic inlay and the resin luting agent is attained by treating the surface of the former both mechanically and chemically. First, acid etching of the inlay surface is done using hydrofluoric acid for fired porcelain and ammonium bifluoride for milled and cast ceramics. This provides a surface for micro-mechanical retention of the luting resin. The etched surface is then silanated to promote wetting with the resin thereby, improving chemical retention. However the chemical bond between silane and luting composite improves only the initial bond strength. Later on, this bond is weakened severely, probably by hydrolysis, which leads to marked decrease in bond strength after one year. Resin luting cements should not be applied without prior tooth bonding procedures because significant microleakage could occur due to inherent polymerization shrinkage.

Microleakage has been considerably reduced with the use of resin luting agents over conventional cements but not eliminated. The most vulnerable site continues to be the wear of cement lute itself and its interface zones with the inlay and the tooth (Fig. 22.9).

Interfacial gap widths have shown to vary amongst the different systems used for fabrication of inlay probably because of the technique sensitivity. In general, it is difficult to prepare ceramic inlays that

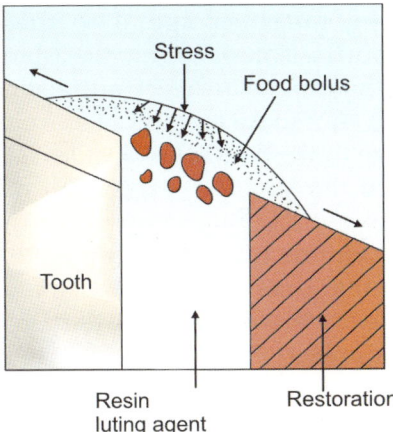

Fig. 22.9: Diagram showing wear related to resin lute

will precisely fit the cavity preparation. For the fired ceramic restorations the fit is highly dependent upon the patience and skills of the dental technician. Glass ceramic restorations (DICOR) have shown excellent marginal behaviour in-vitro with virtually no marginal openings. Naturally, closer the fit of the restoration to the preparation surface better will be the resistance to marginal leakage.

Conflicting results continue to exist regarding the microleakage performance of ceramic and resin inlay systems. It is difficult to affirm any conclusive results at this stage, since not many studies have been carried out till date. The interfacial marginal gaps, so formed after the loss of cementing medium have shown to be both wider and deeper for the ceramic inlays compared to the composite inlays, so microleakage is definitely higher for the ceramic inlays than composite inlays.

Another possible route for microleakage is between the ceramic and composite material, which could lead to marginal staining. This insufficiency in bond could be either because of the carelessness on part of the operator or gradual degradation on contact with water/oral fluids.

METHODS TO DETECT MICROLEAKAGE

Many different methods of demonstrating microleakage have been developed and applied to restorative materials. Most of these methods are employed in vitro. Though in-vitro tests tries to simulate oral conditions by thermo-cycling, etc., yet the dynamic nature of pulpo-dentinal complex and its defense mechanisms cannot be easily simulated in vitro. More so, the accumulation of plaque and other agents might vary the microleakage results in vivo. The methods are classified as below; however, none of these methods are considered perfect as of now.

1. Penetration Studies
   a. Dye penetration
   b. Chemical tracers
   c. Radioactive isotopes
   d. Neutron activation analysis
   e. Bacterial studies
2. Air pressure method
3. Fluid filtration method
4. Electrochemical method
5. Microscopic examination
   a. Scanning Electron microscope
   b. Fluorescent microscopy
6. Miscellaneous
   a. Artificial caries
   b. Pain perception
   c. Reverse diffusion method
   d. Three dimensional method
   e. Laser microspectral analysis
   f. Resin infiltration method

1. Penetration Studies

a. Dye Penetration

The use of colored agents like organic dyes is one of the oldest and most commonly used methods for detection of microleakage. The dye has a contrasting color vis-à-vis the tooth and the restoration (Figs 22.10 A, B). Agents most frequently used for this purpose are: Methylene blue, India ink, Crystal violet, Fluoroscein, Rhodamine B, Eosin, Basic fuschin, Erythrosin and, etc. These dyes are available either as solutions or particle suspensions of different particle

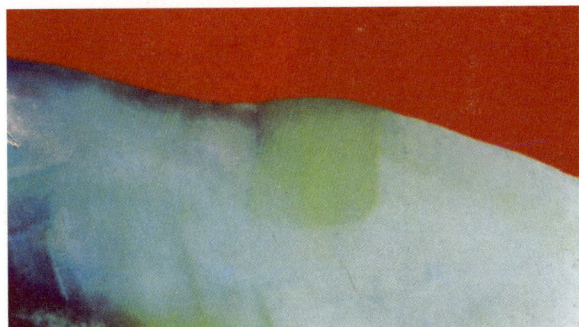

Fig. 22.10A: Detection of marginal leakage (cervical wall)

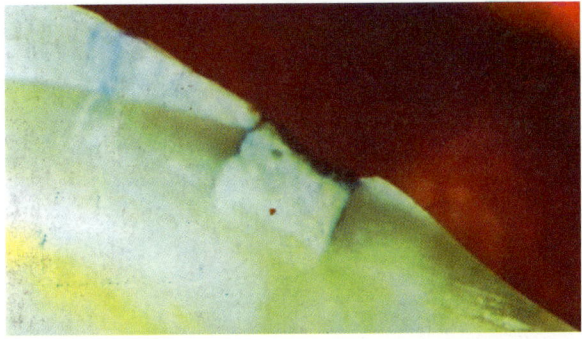

Fig. 22.10B: Detection of marginal leakage (occlusal and cervical walls)

sizes. They should not bond either with the tooth substance or the restoration and should be color stable under all conditions of investigation.

The technique involves immersion of extracted and restored tooth in a dye solution for a pre-determined period. After some time, the tooth is removed, washed, sectioned and examined under a microscope to establish the extent of penetration of dye. The results are then quantified by assigning numbers to the defined depths of penetration.

The validity of using dyes is however often questioned because of the various reasons as:

a. With a variety of dyes having different particle sizes, it cannot be expected that consistent results will be obtained even if standardized techniques are used. It has been shown that different concentrations of two dyes can vary in penetration times from 5 minutes to 1 hour.
b. A potential source of error exists when the dye binds to the tooth substance or restorative material, e.g. Basic fuschin dyes have shown to preferentially bind with the carious dentin Therefore, when attempting to demonstrate a space between the tooth and restoration, an area of stained carious dentin can potentially be mistaken for a larger gap than actually exists.
c. Dyes that are not color stable may lead to misinterpretation of results. For example, aniline blue becomes colorless in alkaline conditions such as in presence of a Calcium hydroxide. The assessment of results is only subjective, which is a major disadvantage with this method.

b. Chemical Tracers

Chemical tracers differ from dyes in that these rely upon the reaction between one or more chemicals used. The technique usually involves reaction of two colorless compounds to produce an opaque precipitate, usually a Silver salt. In all cases, it is essential that both the chemicals penetrate the margin, otherwise precipitation will not occur if only one of the two molecules penetrates.

The most common method used is - immersing the specimen, i.e. extracted tooth with restoration in a 50% Silver nitrate solution, which is subsequently reacted with a photographic developer such as benzene 1, 4-diol (hydroquinone). 1% Silver chloride has also been used. The *limitations* of chemical tracers are normally similar to dye penetration studies.

c. Radioactive Isotopes

Radioactive isotopes such as ^{45}Ca, ^{131}I, ^{32}P, ^{14}C, ^{35}S, ^{86}Rb, etc. are used in a manner similar to that of dyes for assessing microleakage. The specimens are removed from the isotope solution, washed, sectioned and autoradiographed to detect the tracer. The isotope can detect even minute amount of marginal leakage, since the size of the isotope molecules is only 40 nm compared to the smallest size of the dye particles (120 nm).

Limitations in the use of this technique are:

i. Subjective assessment of results; however, with the use of stereomicroscope the subjectivity can be minimized.
ii. A high energy isotope produces more scatter on the film leading to an increase in apparent leakage. Hence isotopes with low energies should be preferred for resolution.
iii. Isotopes such as ^{45}Ca, which have an affinity for the tooth or restorative material, may lead to misleading results.
iv. The isotopes are comparatively expensive and technique sensitive. All precautionary measures are to be taken to satisfy safety requirements.

d. Neutron Activation Analysis

This test has been used to test the microleakage both in-vivo and in-vitro. The restored tooth is soaked in an aqueous solution of a non-radioactive manganese salt. The tooth is then placed in the core of a nuclear reactor, where bombardment with neutrons activates the ^{55}Mn to ^{56}Mn. The radiation subsequently emitted by the tooth is measured to quantify the volume of the tracer present.

Limitations of this technique include:

i. Inability to identify the points where the restoration has leaked.
ii. Heavy experimental costs.
iii. A combined effort required from both nuclear engineers and dentists.
iv. Manganese may be absorbed by the tooth or restorative material.

e. Bacterial Studies

The use of bacteria in microleakage studies was performed testing the possibility of bacteria penetrating through or around the filling materials. Studies were performed, which involved the immersion of restored teeth in cultured broths and subsequently, the filling was removed and the dentin shavings from the base of the cavity cultured. The *disadvantage* with this method is that the results are qualitative and not quantitative. Moreover, marginal gaps that allow passage of bacteria are usually 0.5–1.0 mm or larger. These techniques are not valid for the gaps smaller than this size which could allow penetration of harmful toxins.

2. Air Pressure

Compressed air was used to test the marginal seal of restorations in early 20th century. One system which uses air pressure to test marginal leakage is shown in (Fig. 22.11).

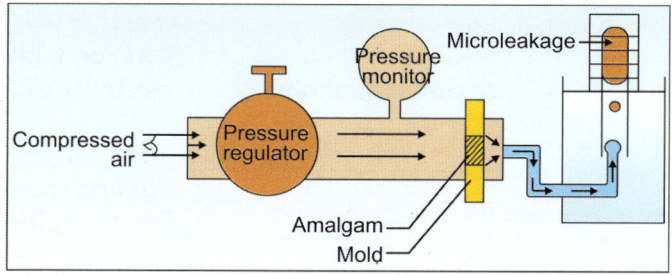

Fig. 22.11: Device used to measure microleakage at the amalgam mold interface. Air leakage is measured in μm/minute

Compressed air is introduced through the root canal and pulp chamber of the tooth and the loss of pressure measured within a static system. Microscopic examination of the release of air bubbles at the margins may in addition provide a subjective view of marginal integrity. The *disadvantages* with this technique are: inability to use in-vivo, does not represent the clinical situation and also does not take into account the drying effect of compressed air. It is possible that some air may leak before it enters the tooth. One *advantage* is that the tooth need not be destroyed and the result can be quantified.

3. Fluid Filtration Method

The fluid filtration method was developed on the principle of an air pressurization technique where instead of using pressurized air, a pressurized-liquid was applied to the pulp chamber of a restored tooth with a constant pressure generated by a gas system. The teeth are sectioned after the placement of a restoration. The sectioned teeth are connected to plastic tube. The plastic tube is filled with de-ionized water. A standard glass capillary tube is connected to the plastic tube at the outlet of the specimen. Using a syringe the water is sucked back approximately 3.0 mm in to the open end of the glass capillary, creating an air bubble in the capillary. The whole set up is then placed in water bath at a constant temperature. Using syringe, the air bubble is adjusted to a suitable position within the capillary, a required head speed pressure is applied from the inlet side to force the water through the void along the filling, thereby displacing the air bubble in the capillary tube. The volume of fluid transported is measured by observing the movement of the air bubble.

4. Electrochemical Studies

The use of electrochemistry in detecting microleakage involves the insertion of an electrode into the extracted tooth in such a way that it contacts the base of the restoration. Once restored, the tooth is suitably sealed to prevent any electrical leakage through natural tooth structure and then immersed in an electrolytic bath. A potential is applied between the tooth and the bath, and the leakage assessed by measuring the current flowing across a serial resistor. The major *drawbacks* with this technique are unsuitability for metallic restorations and inability to use in in-vivo situations.

5. Microscopic Examination

a. Scanning Electron Microscopy

The scanning electron microscope (SEM) provides a means of direct visual observation of the adaptation of restorative materials to the cavity margins because of its high magnification and depth. The method can be used both in vivo and in vitro. The early technique was to use the replicas of the teeth. Recently, the low vacuum SEM, evaluates the rubber base impression directly thereby, decreasing the number of steps and in effect chances of inaccuracy. The major *limitation* with the use of SEM is the potential to induce artefacts during specimen preparations.

b. Fluorescent Microscopy

Fluorescent microscopy uses UV radiation on selected dye, which are capable of absorbing these radiations at one wavelength and emitting at different wavelength.

Fluorescent dyes are detectable in dilute concentrations sensitive to UV light, easy to photograph, permitted more reproducible results and not expensive. The contrast of the natural fluorescence of the tooth against that of dye provided a contrast that made it easy to detect the path of dye penetration under UV light.

6. Miscellaneous

a. Artificial Caries

Artificial secondary caries like lesions have been produced in-vitro using either bacterial cultures or a chemical system, the acidified gelatin gel technique. Both the techniques are interlinked. The histological appearance of lesions under polarized light shows two parts: an *'outer lesion'* and a *'cavity wall'* lesion. The outer lesion exhibits the features of primary attack, while the cavity wall lesion was formed by microleakage of ions from the caries inducing medium into the tooth restoration interface.

The *advantage* with this method is that microleakage can be directly related to the development of artificial lesion. Quantification of results is possible using depth of the lesion as the measurable parameter. If degree of demineralization is used as a measure, it provides only subjective assessment.

b. Pain Perception

In this method the suspected margins of the restorations are painted with calcium chloride and kept there for few minutes. If there is an open communication to exposed dentin from tooth restoration interface, the patient will complain of pain within 30–60 seconds. The response is delayed because it takes time for the fluid to move osmotically through that space. The *disadvantage* of this method is the subjectivity regarding the pain perception of the patient.

c. Reverse Diffusion Method

This method involves placing a certain amount of tracers on the cavity floor prior to insertion of the restorative material. After a stipulated period of time the tooth is immersed in a definite volume of the medium. The amount of the tracers which leaks into the medium is measured (Fig. 23.12). This method is also modified by using calcium hydroxide in place of tracers at the base of the cavity. The pH of calcium hydroxide is seen on litmus papers which are placed at the possible gaps at tooth restoration interface. Reverse diffusion method is considered a better method as it reveals time dependent leakage at any given time; however the limitations of this method are:

i. Minimum amount of tracer necessary at a given time; and
ii. How to quantify marginal leakage with the numbers of tracers.

It is suggested that the '*microleakage coefficient*' should be considered which take into account all factors including marginal gaps during diffusion process.

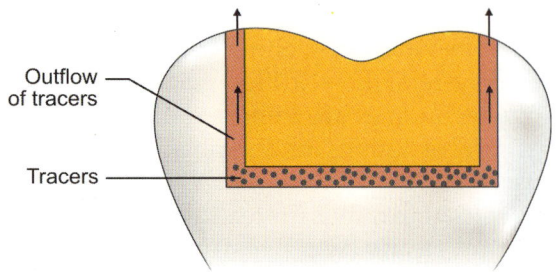

Fig. 22.12: Reverse diffusion method

It is concluded that no restorative material till date is capable of perfectly bonding to the tooth structure. The microleakage is an inherent shortcoming of all the restorative materials, the degree however varies. The aim of the operator should be to minimize this dilemma, by careful selection of the material, by employing prudent, disciplined techniques and that too under the umbrella of sound theoretical principles.

d. Three-dimensional Methods

The three-dimensional analysis is the technique of producing serial sections using a water cooled wire saw. Each section was approximately 200 μm thick and separated by 280 μm. Three dimensional models were then created by hand tracing projected transparencies and reconstructed by computer aided tools. Computer image analyzer was then applied to count the surface areas of dye leakage but the volume of leakage was calculated manually. It was reported that microleakage in this three dimensional analysis was significantly greater than that of the two dimensional analysis.

e. Laser Microspectral Analysis

Laser microspectral analysis device consists of an infrared pulsed laser, usually with ruby or neodimium doped glass as active medium. The laser pulse can be generated by population inversion with flash lamp, connected to high voltage pulse generator, Laser pulse is directed by prism and focalized with a mirror objective on the probe sited on the microscopic table. The energy of the laser used is around 0.5–2 J/pulse. This energy is sufficient to produce a crater of 20–300 μm diameter on the surface of the probe at the point of incidence of the laser pulse by vaporization of the probe. Vapors ejected from the crater having high temperature (20000°K), initiate an electric discharge between the electrodes which are situated above the crater and connected to a high voltage source. This discharge will excite the atoms from the plasma, after which, by transition from the excited states, it will emit photons. The radiation produced by the discharge is focused to the input slit of spectrophotometer. The spectrophotometer will give the emission spectrum of the atoms contained in the plasma. From this spectrum it can be established the content of atoms and their concentration from the crater.

It gives the possibility to measure the infiltration of due substances in the porous regions of filled tooth.

f. Resin Infiltration Method

The specimens are coated with nail polish to within 2.0 mm of the end of apex. The resin is prepared dissolving 1.4 gm of resorcinol in 2.0 ml of 40% formaldehyde solution and the pH adjusted to 8.2 with aqueous potassium hydroxide immediately before use. The teeth are immersed in resorcinol formaldehyde resin of 5 days at 4.0^0C and resin is allowed to polymerize completely for four days at room temperature. The nail polish is completely removed. They are then embedded in epoxy resin and sectioned horizontally. The cross-sections are transilluminated and viewed at magnification of 25 x with stereomicroscope. The photographs are taken for image analysis.

NANOLEAKAGE

Another type of leakage that is recently receiving a lot of special attention is the *'nanoleakage'*, This leakage occurs within the nanometrisized spaces around the collagen fibrils within the hybrid layer that have not been completely infiltrated by resin. It has been shown to occur both at the bottom of the hybrid layer and/or scattered along its entire width, depending upon the bonding system employed. It appears that bonding systems that etch deeper into dentin are likely to show higher degrees of nanoleakage. This could be the possible reason for reduced degree of leakage observed with self etching/self priming system than with systems that use an acidic conditioner as a separate step. The clinical significance of nanoleakage is not yet clear but it definitely indicates the inability of the adhesive resin to completely infiltrate the demineralized dentin thereby, leaving behind pores and spaces. Penetration pathways in nanoleakage are porosities in a range less than 50 μm. Poorly infiltrated hybrid layer contains voids that predispose to accumulation of water and oral fluids which may accelerate the degradation of the bond. When demineralized dentin is fully infiltrated with resin, its modulus of elasticity is much higher than the values of the original demineralized dentin. If the hybrid layer fails to be penetrated completely, its modulus of elasticity might fall in between that of adhesive resin and the un-infiltrated dentin collagen. Contact with water and oral fluids would provide a gradual decrease in the modulus of elasticity of the bonded interface reducing the stress concentration in this area and hence preserving its integrity for short period, but due to slow hydrolysis the long term effect is jeopardized. Therefore, dentin bonding agents though are an effective measure in reducing microleakage, their long term performance under stress and continued exposure to oral fluids is still questionable.

The techniques used to determine nanoleakage are:

1. Tracer using Non Acidic Solution of Ammonical Silver Nitrate with Microscopy

Several silver dyes have been used to test the sealing ability of dentin adhesives; such as, silver nitrate, silver methenamine and ammonical silver nitrate. It is shown that the hybrid layer is somewhat porous and is accessible to a silver dye even in the absence of marginal gap. 50% aqueous solution of silver nitrate has been as the silver ion is very small in size and once it has diffused into a region it gets reduced to metallic silver which cannot diffuse away from the site. Nanoleakage, is a significant problem even with the newest adhesives. A few authors have confirmed that the penetration of the tracer is occurring because of incomplete resin penetration within hybrid layers. Furthermore, they have observed that leakage may occur because the newer adhesives have increased porosities from their high hydrophilicity. Researchers used these tracer dyes along with microscopes to study the nanoleakage within the hybrid layer.

2. Scanning Electron Microscopy (SEM)

The scanning electron microscope (SEM) is an electron microscope capable of producing high-resolution images of a sample surface. SEM images have a characteristic three-dimensional appearance and are useful for judging the surface structure of the sample. Materials to be viewed under an electron microscope may require processing to produce a suitable sample. The technique varies depending on the specimen and the analysis required:

- Cryofixation
- Dehydration
- Embedding
- Staining
- Conductive Coating

The SEM provides a means of direct visual observation of the adaptation of restorative materials to cavity margins because of its high magnification and depth of focus. The defects at sub-micron level can be observed at required magnification such as x200 or x1000.

Drying of specimens, dehydration and embedding which is usually needed for SEM analysis may result in artefacts, affecting the outcome of the images. Also cutting or breaking the sample might influence the surface morphology and, therefore, influence artificially the results of this type of investigation.

3. Transmission Electron Microscopy (TEM)

Phase contrast techniques have been used for high resolution biological transmission electron microscopy. Transmission Electron Microscopy (TEM) is an imaging technique whereby a beam of electrons is transmitted through a specimen, then an image is formed, magnified and directed to appear either on a fluorescent screen or layer of photographic film, or to be detected by a sensor such as a CCD camera. The specimens must be prepared as a thin foil, or etched so some portion of the specimen is thin enough for the beam to penetrate. Preparation techniques to obtain an electron transparent region include ion beam milling and wedge polishing. Because of these techniques, it is possible to mill very thin membranes from a specific area of a sample. Materials that have dimensions small enough to be electron transparent, such as powders or nanotubes, can be quickly produced by the deposition of a dilute sample containing the specimen onto support grids. The suspension is normally a volatile solvent, such as ethanol, ensuring that the solvent rapidly evaporates allowing a sample that can be rapidly analyzed. TEM can resolve object details smaller than one nm and is used to expose fine details in unstained thin samples.

4. Field Emission Scanning Electron Microscopy (FESEM)

A field-emission cathode in the electron gun of a Scanning Electron Microscope provides narrower probing beams at low as well as high electron energy, resulting in both improved spatial resolution and minimized sample charging along with minimal damage. FESEM produces clearer, less electrostatically distorted images with spatial resolution down to 1.5 nm., i.e. 3 to 6 times better than conventional SEM. Smaller-area contamination spots can be examined at electron accelerating voltages compatible with Energy Dispersive X-ray Spectroscopy. High quality, low voltage images are obtained with negligible electrical charging of samples in FESEM. Need for placing conducting coatings on insulating materials is virtually eliminated.

5. Confocal Laser Scanning Electron Microscopy (CLSEM)

Confocal Laser Scanning Electron Microscopy (CLSEM) merges the capabilities of the scanning, transmission and x-ray microscopes, and achieves unprecedented resolutions in optically dense materials, by implementing the technology of confocal imaging into an electron microscope. Thus this is a technique for obtaining high-resolution optical image. The key feature of confocal microscopy is its ability to produce in-focus images of thick specimens, a process known as optical sectioning. Images are acquired point-by-point and reconstructed with a computer, allowing three-dimensional reconstructions of topologically-complex objects. CLSEM has also been used in combination with fluorescent dye (Rhodamin B) to determine nanoleakage. The advantages of CLSEM are that, it is a non-destructive examination and drying of the samples is not necessary.

6. Coherent Diffraction Imaging (CDI)

Coherent Diffraction Imaging (CDI) is a "lensless" technique for 2D/3D imaging of nanoscale structures such as nanotubes, nanocrystals, defects, etc. In CDI, a highly coherent beam of electrons is incident on a sample to generate a diffraction pattern. This pattern is recorded electronically and then used to reconstruct an image. Effectively, the objective lens in a typical microscope is replaced with software to convert from the reciprocal space diffraction pattern into a real space image. Due to radiation damage, resolution is limited (for continuous illumination set-ups) to about 10 nm for frozen-hydrated biological samples but resolutions of as high as 1.0 to 2.0 nm should be possible for inorganic materials less sensitive to damage (using modern synchrotron sources). It has been proposed that radiation damage may be avoided by using ultra short pulses of x-rays where the time scale of the destruction mechanism is longer than the pulse duration. This may enable higher energy and therefore higher resolution of organic materials, such as proteins, etc. The advantage in using no lens is that the final image is aberration free..

BIBLIOGRAPHY

1. Alani, A.H. and Toh, C.G.: Detection of microleakage around dental restorations: A review. Oper. Dent.: 22, 173, 1997.
2. Amarante, D.C.D.A., Sinhoretti, M.A., Correr, S.L. and Consani, S.: Influence of methodology and evaluation criteria on determining microleakage in dentin-restorative interfaces. Clin. Oral Invest.: Aug, 2006.
3. Ben-Amar, A.: Reduction of microleakage around new amalgam restorations. J.A.D.A.: 119, 725, 1989.
4. Browne, R.M. and Tobias, R.S.: Microbial microleakage and pulpal inflammation. A review. Endod. Dent. Traumatol.: 2, 177, 1986.
5. Bullard, R.H., Leinfelder, K.F. and Russell, C.M.: Effect of coefficient of thermal expansion on microleakage. J.A.D.A.; 116, 871, 1988.
6. Cheung, G.S.P.: Reducing marginal leakage of posterior composite resin restorations: a review of clinical techniques. J. Prosth. Dent.: 63, 286, 1990.
7. Costa, J.F., Siqueira, W.L., Logueruo, A.D., Resi, A., Oliveira, E.F., Alves, C.M.C., Bauer, J.R.D.O. and Grande, R.H.M.: Characterization of aqueous silver nitrate solution for leakage tests. J. Appl. Oral Sci.: 19, 254, 2011.
8. Edgren, B.N. and Denehy, G.E.: Microleakage of amalgam restorations using amalgam bond and copalite. Am. J. Dent.: 5, 296, 1992.

9. Ginguanju: Nanoleakage determination techniques – A literature review. B.L.A.: 8, 976, 2008.
10. Hasenreisoglu, U., Sonmey, H., Uctasli, S. and Wilson, H.J.: Microleakage of direct and indirect inlays/onlays system. J. Oral Rehab.: 23, 66, 1996.
11. Iwani, Y., Yamamoto, H. and Ebisu, S.: A new electrical method for detecting marginal leakage of in vitro resin restorations. J. Dent.: 28, 241, 2000.
12. Iwani, Y., Yamamoto, H., Hayashi, M., Takeshige, F. and Ebisu, S.: Validity of electrical conductance measurement in evaluating marginal leakage around resin composite restorations. Oper. Dent.: 27, 606, 2002.
13. Larson, T.D.: The clinical significance and management of microleakage. Part II. North West Dent.: 84, 15, 2005.
14. Retief, D.H.: Do adhesives prevent microleakage? I.D.J.: 44, 19, 1994.
15. Sano, H., Takatsu, T., Ciucchi, B. and Homer, J.A.: Nanoleakage: Leakage within the hybrid layer. Oper. Dent.: 20, 18, 1995.
16. Sinescu, C., Negrutiu, M., Draganescu, G., Todea, C., Dodenciu, D., Florita, Z. and Pop, D.: Microleakage in dentistry: new methods for investigation the gaps in biomaterials. Proc. Of SPIE: 6843, 68430P, 2008.
17. Taylor, M.J. and Lynch, E.: Microleakage. A Review. J. Dent.: 20, 3, 1992.
18. Triadan, H.: When is microleakage a real clinical problem? Oper. Dent.: 12, 153, 1998.
19. Yavuz, I. and Aydin, H.: New direction for measurement of microleakaeg in cariology research. J. Int. Dent. Med. Res.: 3, 19, 2010.

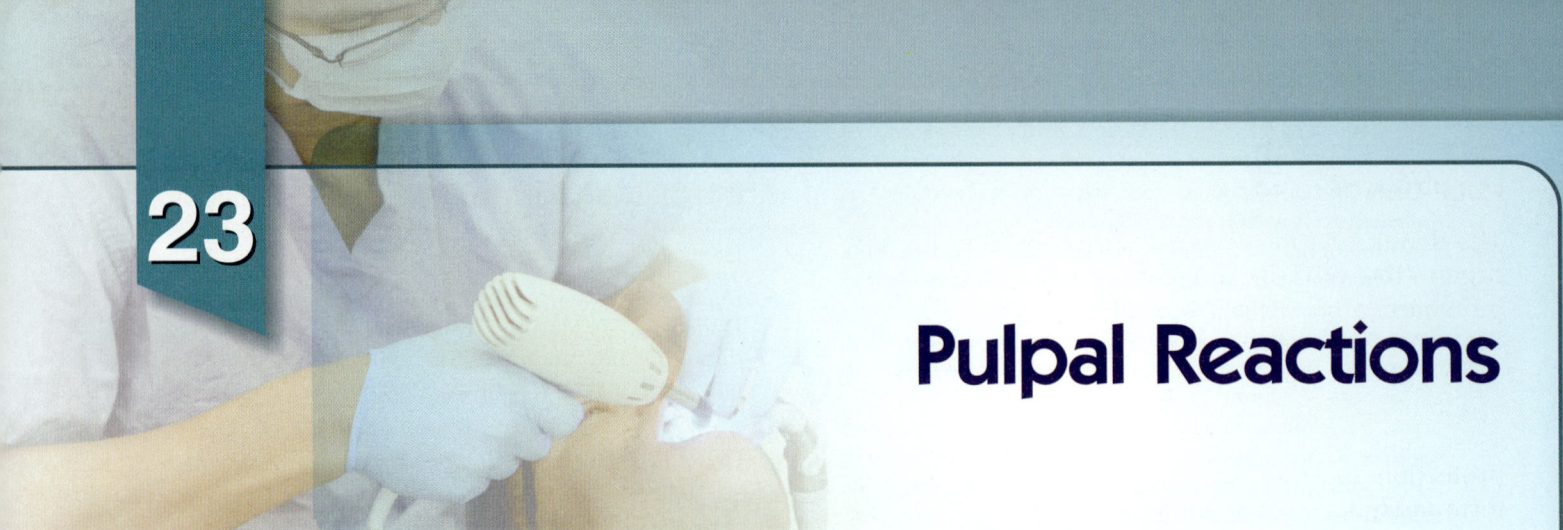

23
Pulpal Reactions

Pulp, a specialized connective tissue, is very sensitive to external stimuli. In addition to the dental procedures that threaten the integrity of the pulp, injury may also result from irritation by a noxious agent brought into contact with the exposed dentin or the pulpal tissue. Any stimulus over the exposed dentinal tubules affects the pulp. The reaction of the pulp, most of the times, is physiologic; however, depending upon the intensity of the stimulus pathological changes do occur in pulp.

It is biologically evident that the contact of a dental material with cytoplasmic cell process in dentin can induce odontoblastic alterations and transient inflammatory reactions. Over the past couple of years, there has been a gradual change of views on potential danger of the pulp from restorative materials. Earlier the acidic components from zinc phosphate & silicate cements and unreacted monomers from composite restorations were considered injurious to the pulp. Recently it is established that leakage of bacteria and their products from the oral environment along the gaps in the cavity/restoration interface are more toxic than the material itself.

Hence, with so many products already in the market and new ones continuously being introduced, it is necessary to know the comparative toxicity of all materials, such that materials that are kind to the pulp are chosen and measures undertaken to reduce the toxic effect of the materials. Further the effect of recently introduced cutting tools and other techniques utilized in restorative dentistry on the pulp should also be evaluated so as to guide the operator to use the same cautiously.

TERMINOLOGY

The commonly used terms in the context of safety of materials are:

i. Biocompatibility

The term 'biocompatible' is defined as being harmonious with life and not having toxic or injurious effects on biological functions. In general, biocompatibility is measured on the basis of localized cytotoxicity (such as pulp and mucosal response), systemic responses, allergenicity and carcinogenicity.

The dental materials or technique or any external stimulus should not be harmful to the pulp and soft tissues. It should not contain toxic diffusible substance that can be absorbed into the circulation to cause a systemic toxic response. Further it should have no carcinogenic potential and also should be free of potentially sensitizing agents that could cause an allergic response.

ii. Biomaterial

It can be defined as any substance, other than a drug, that can be used for any period as a part of a system that treats, augments or replaces any tissue, organ or function of a body. Dental materials are used in humans for short or long periods and collectively these must meet the requirements given in the definitions of a biomaterial and biocompatibility. The host environment for dental biomaterials is especially complicated because of the presence of bacteria and debris in the oral cavity and the corrosive properties of saliva and other fluids.

iii. Hazardous

A material is hazardous if placed in the body tissues has the potential to cause a problem. Hazardous materials are generally identified through screening tests, which place a material in direct contact with either cultured cells or animal tissues.

iv. Risk

Risk means the material is going to cause sufficient damage. A material which is hazardous may not pose a significant risk to the body, e.g. Zinc oxide eugenol may be hazardous but not risky. Risk may be reduced because of diffusion or dilution of the offending components, biological barriers, or a lack of sufficient time of contact between the offending components and susceptible tissues.

PULP-DENTIN ORGAN

The dentin and the pulp must be considered as one organ (the pulp-dentin complex) because of the intimate relationship between the cellular tissue within the dentin and the peripheral pulp tissue. Structure and response of dentin to injury are largely functions of the odontoblasts and other cells in the pulp, but these cells are dependent on the dentin for their protection and their state of differentiation. Normal form and function of one cannot be maintained without the other. The embryonic dental papilla is responsible for the formation of this coupled tissue. Hence it is obvious that the response of the pulp to any restorative material will be influenced by its surrounding dentin also. The dentinal tubules occupy 20–39% of dentin, and the dentinal fluid within them represents about 22% of the total volume of dentin. Dentinal fluid in the tubules, which is continuous with the extracellular fluid of the pulp serves as a medium for relaying injurious agents to the pulp to induce an inflammatory response. Thus anything that contacts the living dentin can be carried into the pulp. Also, either positive hydrostatic pressure or negative osmotic pressure may move the fluid in the dentinal tubules, which may displace the odontoblastic process or nerve endings resulting in pain.

Physiology of Pulp-Dentin Organ

As described earlier, the tissues of pulp and dentin are considered as one. The interstitial fluid of the pulp and the dentinal tubules are continuous and extend from dentino-enamel and dentino-cementum junction to the central part of the soft connective tissue of the pulp.

The pulp is vascularized as other organs of the body. A large arteriole passes through the root pulp to supply the coronal pulp. They branch as capillaries in the coronal sub-odontoblastic region. The blood capillaries have discontinuity in the endothelial walls. Such types of arrangements facilitate easy exchange of nutrients and the waste fluid. This exchange is important in case of pulp injury. The fluid flow from the pulp to exposed dentin is dependent on the hydraulic conductance of the dentinal fluid. Any reduction in this conductivity will reduce the dentin sensitivity.

Myelinated and un-myelinated nerves enter the pulp through apical foramen (Fig. 23.1). Usually the myelinated fibers and un-myelinated Aδ-fibers carry pain impulses. The sensory and the sympathetic nerve endings are activated at an early stage of the inflammatory process and are the initiators of vasodilatation. This is the start of the protective

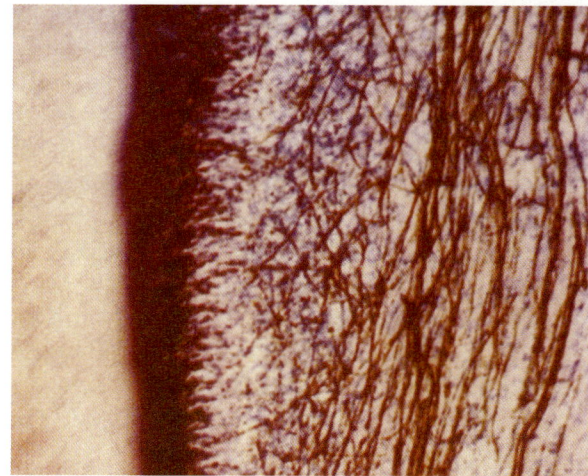

Fig. 23.1: Pulpal innervation

response to the injury by increasing blood volume and vascular permeability in the affected areas. Both the sympathetic and sensory nerve fibers have effect on the pulpal circulation. The number of nerve fibers decreases with age, which explains the reduced sensitivity in older adults.

Pulpal pain is characteristically pulsating, long lasting and of variable severity, very rarely excruciating. It is also affected by changes in blood pressure. The typical dentinal pain is short lasting, sharp and may be lancinating. The cold stimulus is considered more painful than the hot stimulus. In cold stimulus, there is outward fluid flow that results from shrinkage of the contents of the tubules. When heat is applied the contents of the tubules expand and an inward flow occurs, leading to comparatively less pain.

Composition of Dentin and Pulp

Dentin has an average of 45,000–90,000 tubules/mm^2 near the pulp, 30,000–35,000/mm^2 in the middle and 10,000–25,000/mm^2 at the periphery. At the pulp surface, the diameter of the tubules ranges from 2.5–3.0 µm and at the periphery to less than 1.0 µm. Each tubule is about 1.0 µm in diameter and 2.0–3.0 mm in length. The tubules have highly mineralized lining, the peritubular dentin which is not found in the pulpal part of the dentin of the newly erupted teeth. The highly mineralized peritubular dentin should be distinguished from the other mineralized component of dentin, the intertubular dentin that has much less collagen than the peritubular dentin. The growth of peritubular dentin, may be age related, or due to restorative procedures, leads to obliteration of the tubules. The occluded dentinal tubules referred to as dentin sclerosis, react differently to acid etching. The etching time here is to be modified to provide an adequate hybrid layer of collagen and resin.

The interface dentin with irregular, often atubular dentin, forms a barrier between the physiologic secondary and tertiary dentin. This barrier reduces the permeability of the affected dentin and may make it impermeable because the tubules from primary dentin do not cross the interface dentin. This phenomenon protects the pulp.

Branching of dentinal tubules differ as the number of tubules, depending upon the location within the tooth. In coronal dentin, the characteristic branching is found in peripheral 250 µm, where γ-shaped branches are evident. The fine branches are predominantly present in root dentin, but may be evident in other parts of the dentin such as cervical dentin.

The dentin in cervical area of cemento-enamel junction is usually covered by cementum. Sometimes cementum does not form, or the thin cementum wears out leading to exposure of dentin, which is always sensitive. This area is important as regards etching and the adhesive dentistry. The cementum and the dentin at the cemento-enamel junction and below may form inferior type of hybrid layer after etching because of low number of tubules and their branches. The thin hybrid layer may not provide good micromechanical attachment of the resin based restorative materials. Generally, dentin directly under the dentino-enamel junction is only 1% permeable, but permeability increases to 7.6% halfway to the pulp and upto 22.0% at the pulp surface. The dentinal tubules contain odontoblastic processes, which are direct extensions of the cell body of the odontoblasts underlying the predentin. It is these dentinal tubules and their contents that make operative dentistry so intimately related to the vitality of the pulp. The pulpal circulation maintains an intercellcular hydraulic pressure of about 24 mm of Hg, which causes the fluid flow in the tubules to be directed outwards from the pulp to the dentinoenamel junction. Chemical and bacterial products when introduced into unprotected dentinal tubules diffuse against the pressure gradient towards the pulp.

During cavity preparation by the operator, a layer is formed by the action of the cutting instrument on the calcified dentinal matrix called the 'smear layer'. This mat of organic and inorganic particles obliterates the tubules to some extent but can be removed by acid etching and other means.

The pulp is a connective tissue, which is derived from the mesenchyme, the dental papilla. The pulp is characterized by its specialized odontoblasts on the periphery beneath the predentin. Beneath the odontoblastic layer is the 'cell poor zone' or the 'Weil's layer' composed principally of young fibroblasts. The central portion of the pulp consists of many young fibroblasts and occasional lymphocytes. It is richly supplied by thin walled but wide capillaries. Bundles of myelinated nerve fibers accompany the blood vessels. Fibers predominantly present are collagenous and reticular types. Lying in close proximity to the blood vessels are many undifferentiated mesenchymal cells and histiocytes. These are believed to transform into secondary odontoblasts that form reparative dentin following the death of primary odontoblasts. When confronted with toxic bacterial or chemical products by way of dentinal tubules, the pulp usually responds first by transient pulpitis. The response resolves naturally if the injurious agent is removed or its concentration lowered. Differentiation of secondary odontoblasts may eventually lead to formation of reparative dentin. If pulpitis does not resolve, it may spread to involve the pulp in liquefaction necrosis or chronic inflammation.

FACTORS INFLUENCING PULPAL RESPONSE TO DENTAL RESTORATIVE MATERIAL

The risks of pulpal response associated with any dental material depend to a large extent on their ability to diffuse through dentin and accumulate in the pulp. It has been established that materials, which may not be toxic at low concentrations become toxic at high concentrations. Pulp reactions to the same irritant may vary not only between different persons but also between different teeth in the same mouth, and between opposing teeth of the similar anatomic form. Factors influencing pulpal responses are:

a. Dentin permeability

The rate of permeation of substances through dentin depends upon a number of factors like:

i. Location

Dentin permeability varies in different areas of the same tooth, e.g. it increases towards the pulpal side. This is because both the tubule diameter and the number increase towards the pulp chamber.

ii. Dentin Diffusional Surface Area

This is a product of tubule diameter and number, which directly influences the wetness and hence the hydrolytic dissolution of the restorative material.

iii. Smear Layer

The presence or absence of the 1.0–5.0 µm thick layer of microcrystalline debris on the cut dentin surface (smear layer) controls dentin permeability. Presence of smear layer reduces permeability.

iv. Intratubular Material

Such as mineral deposits, collagen fibrils, proteins, etc. may reduce permeability.

v. The Concentration and Solubility of the Diffusing Solutes

The substances with high molecular weight and size are less penetrating than the substances with low molecular size and weight. Solutes that are water soluble would show a rapid rate of penetration.

vi. Patency of the Dentinal Tubules

Sclerotic dentin is less permeable than the physiologic tubular dentin.

vii. Reparative Dentin

In cases where reparative dentin has been formed previously, the response of the pulp is less, probably because it reduces the penetration of the solute.

viii. Remaining Dentin Thickness

As the length of tubule increases the concentration of the solute reaching the pulp decreases. Whether this concentration would be injurious to the odontoblasts or pulpal cells will depend on the nature of the substance. It has been shown that a 0.5 mm thickness of dentin reduces the toxicity level of a material to 75% and an 1.0 mm thickness over 90%. Effective remaining dentin thickness of 2 mm provides an adequate insulating barrier against almost all the techniques and restorative materials.

b. Dentin Pretreatments

Preconditioning of dentin by acids (etchants and conditioners) might increase dentin permeability by removing smear layer and enlarging tubule orifices. The effect depends upon the concentration and the duration for which the etchant/conditioner is applied.

c. Age of the Patient

It is usually accepted that the inflammatory response of the older persons was slightly less extensive and the reparative dentin formation was also less than in the younger person. The older pulps are far less defensive in resolving a lesion and resisting infection. However, certain authors have shown that age differences do not affect the pulpal response of human teeth.

INTENSITY OF PULPAL RESPONSE

The response of pulp should be systematically established. There is need to record not only the location but also the severity of pulpal responses. The pulpal reactions are categorized into the following histopathological characteristics:

1. Cellular Displacement

It is characterized by movement of odontoblasts and leukocytes into the dentinal tubules. This occurs in the first few days and persists well over 30 days. It provides excellent evidence of the acuteness of initial response long after the leukocytes have degenerated and other characteristics of acute information have resolved.

2. Infilteration of Inflammatory Cells in the Superficial tissues (Odontoblastic Layer, Zone of Weil and Cell Rich Zone) and the Deeper Tissues

These specific features are usually arbitrarily graded for 0 to 3 degrees merely on the basis of the number of displaced cells or inflammatory cells present. When the response represents only one or two displaced cells or infilterating inflammatory cells, a graded value of one-half is given. Rarely, the intensity of the response is sufficiently great that grade-4 is utilized.

3. Predominantly Inflammatory Cells

The predominating type of infilterating inflammatory cells (Polymorphonucleated leukocyte, lymphocyte, eosinophil, monocyte and plasma cells) are usually recorded at the same time the intensity of the cellular inflammatory response is noted.

Eosinophils are grouped with the chronic cells because they usually appear at the same time in pulp lesions. As the lesion resolves, the acute inflammatory cells diminish in number and are replaced by smaller and deeper tissues. With extended post-operative intervals, the chronic inflammatory cells, gradually disappear in a resolving lesion with the formation of reparative dentin.

In some situations, the maximum response is reached in 1 to 2 days, in others it takes 3 to 6 days. With some restorative materials, post-operative period of 20 days or longer are required.

4. Special Histopathologic Characteristics

a. Abcess Formation

Occasionally, in a pre-operatively healthy pulp, there might occur beneath cavity preparation certain abscess like conditions (dense accumulations of leukocytes between the odontoblastic layer and the predentin), which will resolve, but any technique that produces either abscesses or abscess like conditions should be modified or eliminated. These characteristics are not necessarily localized, but sometimes they can be quite focal. Any lesion with an abscess is usually graded as having response of 4 degrees.

b. Foci of Necrosis

Initially, in burn areas and in lesions induced by toxic restorative materials or chemicals, a balancing out of all histologic features with loss of cellular detail, collapse of vascular channels and a paucity of inflammatory cells occurs. Subsequently, these lesions become heavily infiltrated by inflammatory cells and might either resolve with granulation tissue replacement or might undergo abscess formation.

c. Lesions of Delayed Healing

Such lesions usually present dense infilterations of chronic inflammatory cells and could possibly develop into abscess formation. These lesions are usually graded at 2 or 3 degrees in the longer time intervals, which is beyond 45 days.

d. Regeneration of Odontoblasts

With the resolution of a lesion, most or all of the inflammatory cells may disappear and leave behind an atrophic or degenerated odontoblastic layer, even exhibiting foci completely lacking in primary odontoblasts (Fig. 23.2). In some instances, only regenerated odontoblasts are found and a distinction needs to be made between these two types of layers.

e. Reparative (Tertiary) Dentin formation (Fig. 23.3)

The greater the degree of initial response due to irritation caused by cutting and placing of a restorative material, the greater the subsequent incidence of reparative dentin. With a very high-speed techniques used today, however, a very low incidence of reparative dentin results, leaving many primary dentinal tubules patent for the subsequent seepage of toxic products into the pulp.

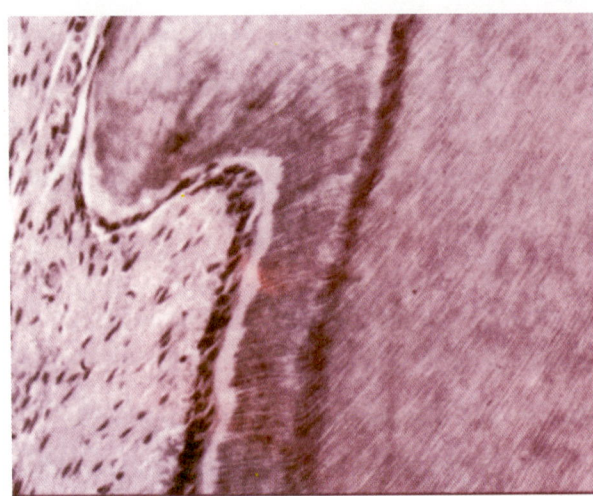

Fig. 23.3: Tertiary dentin formation

Reparative dentin seldom occurs in human pulp tissue sooner than 30 days. With some procedures, the lesions may so persist in intensity of inflammatory response that the differentiation of new odontoblasts is impossible and the incidence of reparative dentin is low, giving the false impression of a mild response.

f. Eosinophilic Staining

Another histologic characteristic usually seem is eosinophilic staining. The tissues involved remain histologically intact but are inundated by an amorphous material similar to that seen in capillaries. It is assumed that this is a plasma tranendate, which escapes through mildly injured capillaries.

This characteristic is found either in operative techniques capable of producing a low order of irritation or on the periphery of many larger pulpal lesions away from the center of greatest inflammation.

STAGES OF PULPAL INFLAMMATION

The reaction of the pulp to external stimuli is reflected in two broad processes: Inflammatory changes and secondary dentin formation. Various authors have graded these changes for evaluating pulpal response.

Whenever the pulp is subjected to external stimuli the immune system triggers inflammatory response to limit the tissue damage. The inflammation in pulp, the pulpitis, is similar to inflammation of any connective tissue in the body. The polymorphonuclear leucocytes are associated with acute reaction and also the mononuclear leucocytes, plasma cells and macrophages. Mast cells are only found in inflamed pulp, however, they are not there in normal pulp. The

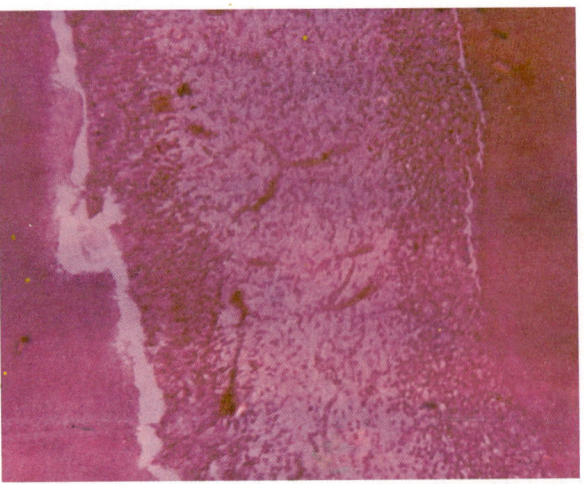

Fig. 23.2: Odontoblasts showing hydropic degeneration

inflammatory processes have been quantitatively divided into slight, moderate and severe.

Slight reaction recognizes the increased number of cells in the cell free zone and in the adjacent pulpal tissue. These cells are similar to fibroblasts and undifferentiated cells. However, few inflammatory cells are also observed. The increased number of capillaries means blood flow is also increased to the affected dentinal tubules. The irregularities in the odontoblastic layer are also observed (Fig. 23.4).

Moderate reaction is characterized by more cells around the injury site. The mononuclear leucocytes and the neutrophils invade the odontoblast-predentin area. Some odontoblastic nuclei can be seen in dentinal tubules. The number of capillaries increased along with the blood flow. The occasional haemorrhage in odontoblastic or subodontoblastic zone is also observed (Fig. 23.5).

Severe reaction is characterized by marked cellular infiltration, including abscess formation. The odontoblastic layer remains unidentified. This layer is either destroyed or greatly disrupted. The predentin is not formed. Numerous blood vessels are found in the tissues surrounding the cellular infiltration (Fig. 23.6).

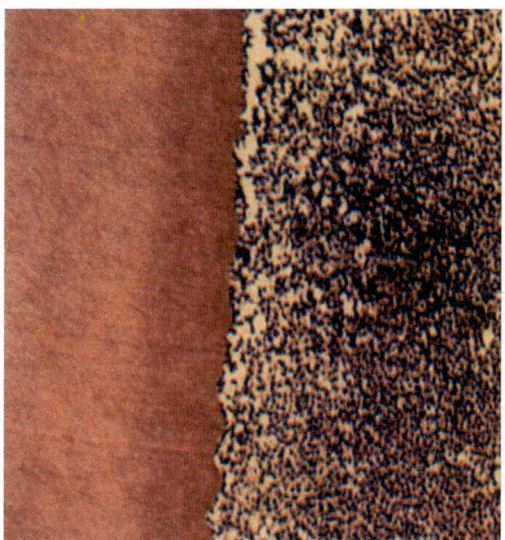

Fig. 23.6: Mononuclear cells predominates

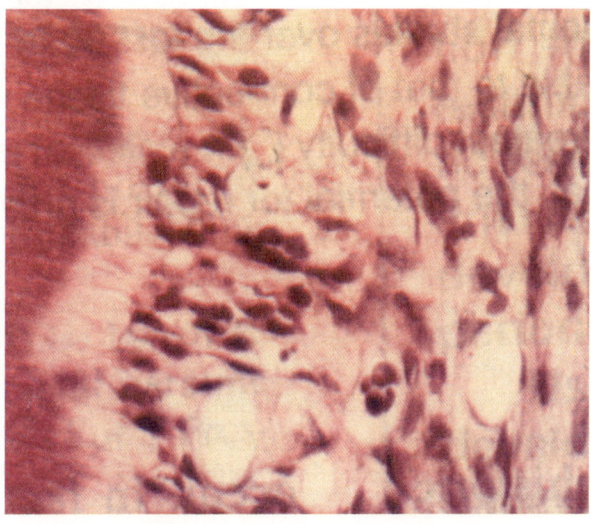

Fig. 23.4: Odontoblastic layer with more capillaries

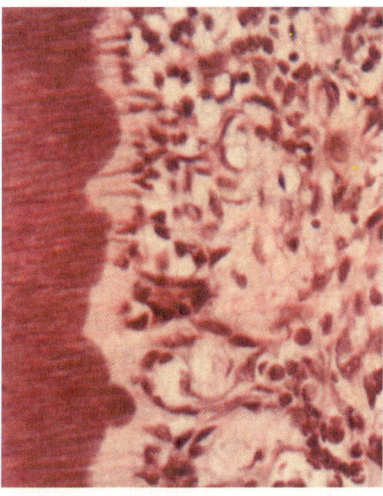

Fig. 23.5: Odontoblastic nuclei displaced

Another technique measuring the cytoplasm-nucleus ratio of the odontoblasts has also been used to quantify pulpal inflammation.

Earlier, plus sign was used to indicate the degree of infilteration of inflammatory cells in the odontoblastic layer and in the rest of the pulp. The plus sign was also used to indicate the different amounts of secondary dentin formation.

Later, the inflammation and secondary dentin formation was graded as I^0-I^3 and D^{-1}–D^3 respectively.

- I^0 Absence of inflammation and no disturbance of the odontoblastic layer.
- I^1 Involvement of the odontoblastic layer only, including aspiration of the nuclear debris.
- I^2 Extension of inflammation to the subodontoblastic layer.
- I^3 Involvement of the central pulp.
- D^{-1} Absence of secondary dentin formation and destruction of odontoblasts.
- D^0 A normal appearance of odontoblastic layer with a normal width of predentin (20–30 μms).
- D^1 A slight amount of secondary dentin formation (35–60 μms)
- D^2 A moderate amount of secondary dentin formation (60–90 μms)

- D³ A considerable amount of secondary dentin formation (> 90 μms)

TESTS FOR EVALUATION OF BIOCOMPATIBILITY

The aim of performing biocompatibility tests is to eliminate any product or a component of product than can damage the oral or maxillo-facial tissues. Earlier, toxicity was investigated by implanting the material in sub-dermal tissues. Later, improved version of these tests became available which were accepted worldwide as Pre-clinical evaluation of Biocompatibility of Medical devices used in Dentistry. The term 'irritation' and 'sensitization' must be understood and differentiated. *'Irritation'* is defined as an inflammation brought about without the intervention of an antibody or immune system where as *'sensitization'* is an inflammatory response requiring the participation of antibody system.

The material should pass all the three levels of biocompatibility testing before it is approved for final usage in the human oral cavity. The three levels are as follows:

Primary Tests

These are the most rapid and economical and include

a. Cytotoxicity tests
b. Genotoxicty tests

Secondary Tests

Only those materials that have passed the primary tests are subjected to secondary testing. These are slightly expensive and include:

a. Systemic toxicity testing
b. Inhalation toxicity testing
c. Skin irritation and sensitization tests
d. Implantation tests

Preclinical Usage Tests

These are the most expensive and include:

a. Pulp and dentin usage tests
b. Pulp capping and pulpotomy usage tests
c. Endodontic usage tests

Primary Tests

a. *Cytotoxicity tests:* Cytotoxicity tests include the placement of a dental material directly on to the tissue culture cells. The cells react metabolically depending upon the components that leach from these dental materials. The toxic response can be quantified by measurement of some biologic function such as DNA synthesis, protein synthesis, or the concentration of components that cause a decrease in cellular activity by 50% i.e. TC 50 concentration. TC 50 concentration is inversely proportional to the potency of the cytotoxic response i.e. lower the TC 50 concentration higher is the potency. These tests do not measure whether materials biodegrade over long periods of time as a result of the physical and chemical environment.

b. *Genotoxicity tests:* Mammalian or nonmammalian cells, bacteria, yeasts or fungi are used to determine specifically whether gene mutations, changes in chromosome structure, or other DNA or genetic changes are caused by the test materials, devices and extracts from materials, their extracts and other devices, if any.

Secondary Tests

a. *Systemic toxicity tests:* The test sample is administered daily to rats for 14 days either by oral lavage or by dietary inclusion. If 50% of the animals survive, the product is considered safe.

b. *Inhalation systemic toxicity tests:* These tests are performed on rats, rabbits, or guinea pigs in an exposure chamber with aerosol preparations. The spray material is released around the head and upper trunk of the animals for 30 seconds, each at 30 minutes intervals. After 10 consecutive exposures, the animals are observed for four days. If any animal dies within this period, the agent is considered toxic, otherwise safe.

c. *Skin irritation and sensitization tests:* The test material is held in contact with the shaved skin of albino rats for periods ranging from 24 (one exposure) to 90 days (with repeated exposures) for evaluating irritation effects.

However, for establishing allergic contact sensitization, the guinea pig is preferred animal. An allergen is defined as a substance that is not primarily irritating on the first exposure but produces reactions on subsequent exposures of similar concentrations. The stain reactions are evaluated after subsequent application of the test material.

d. *Implantation tests:* During the implantation techniques, the various physical properties of the product such as form, density, hardness and surface finish also influence the character of the tissue response. The animals are selected according to the duration of the test. The implant material is packed in plastic tubes and put into subcutaneous tissues or directly into bones in drilled holes. The reactions are evaluated.

Pre-clinical Usage Tests

a. *Pulp and dentin usage test:* The test is designed to assess the biocompatibility of dental materials placed in dentin adjacent to the dental pulp of non-rodent mammals like dogs, ferrets, etc. The material is placed in contact with open dentin 1.0 mm from the pulp and evaluated after given period of time. The specimens are examined regarding inflammatory response, reparative dentin formation and the number of microorganisms entrapped in the surrounding cavity walls and cut dentinal tubules. If an inflammatory response is produced, the time required for its disappearance is also measured.
b. *Pulp capping and pulpotomy usage tests:* The testing procedures are similar to the previous ones, except that the pulp is exposed. The animals are evaluated for dentin bridge formation, its quality and structure.
c. *Endodontic usage tests:* For this test, the pulp is completely removed from the pulp chamber and roots and replaced by the obturating test material and control material. The degree of inflammation is evaluated in the periapical tissues.

RESTORATIVE MATERIALS AND PULPAL REACTION

A. Zinc Oxide Eugenol

Zinc oxide eugenol is frequently used as a material in dentistry. It is generally considered bland or even therapeutic to the pulp and is routinely used as the non-toxic control in most invivo tooth tests of pulpal toxicity. It is highly cytotoxic in all tissue culture test systems that lack a dentin barrier. If it comes in direct contact with bone, the pain could be extremely severe so much so if extruded into the mandibular canal, it may damage the mandibular nerve.

Zinc oxide when mixed with eugenol leads to formation of zinc eugenolate matrix. The zinc eugenolate units are held together by van der Waal's forces and particle interlocking. When exposed to aqueous media such as saliva or dentinal fluid, hydrolysis of zinc eugenolate occurs yielding eugenol and zinc hydroxide. Eugenol liberated from zinc eugenolate can diffuse through dentin and into the saliva. It has been established that concentration of 10^{-2} mol/L of eugenol observed below the fillings in dentin and 10^{-4} mol/L in the pulp. These concentrations were maintained for more than one week. Calcium in the dentinal tubules chelates eugenol, limiting its ability to diffuse through dentin. Eugenol also binds with the organic matrix of dentin, especially collagen, which slows the diffusion rate. Modified ZOE cements have demonstrated less release of eugenol and fewer cytotoxic effects. It has been observed that acid etched dentin may facilitate diffusion of potentially toxic amounts of eugenol to the pulp.

Eugenol is bactericidal at relatively high concentration of 10^{-2} to 10^{-3} mol/L. Brief exposure to 10^{-2} mol/L and prolonged exposure to 10^{-3} mol/L of eugenol can kill mammalian cells. Even lower concentrations can inhibit cell respiration and cell division. Inhibitory eugenol concentrations are significantly higher than the one required for anti-inflammatory effects. The zinc oxide eugenol placed in direct contact with the pulp tissue result in chronic inflammation and necrosis. However, when placed against dentin, the cytotoxic effects are nil. Various mechanisms that explain the cytotoxicity of eugenol are:

- Eugenol can be oxidized by peroxidase enzymes, the product formed is toxic to hepatocytes.
- It has a high affinity to plasma membranes because of its lipid solubility, which can cause cell damage.
- Eugenol has shown to uncouple oxidative phosphorylation in mitochondria.

At concentration levels of 10^{-4} mol/L or just below it, eugenol has shown to inhibit prostaglandin synthesis and sensory nerve excitability. At low concentrations the intradental nerve activity is blocked reversibly just like a local anaesthetic, whereas at high concentrations of eugenol, nerve conduction is irreversibly blocked, indicating a neurotoxic effect. It exerts an antiinflammatory effect by the following mechanisms:

- Protects tissue from damage by inhibiting neutrophil function and chemotaxis.
- Inhibits prostaglandin and leukotriene synthesis, which are important mediators of inflammation by increasing blood flow and vascular permeability and lowering pain threshold.
- Eugenol causes vasodilation and decreases the response of these vessels to norepinephrine and histamine. Vasodilation would result in prevention of toxic accumulations and rapid removal of irritants.

Effects of Eugenol	
Toxic (High Dose)	*Beneficial (Low Dose)*
• Induces cell death	• Inhibits white cell chemotaxis
• Unknown vascular effect	• Inhibits prostaglandins synthesis
• Inhibits cell growth and respiration	• Inhibits nerve activity

Thus, it can be seen that the effect of eugenol is dose dependent.

The histologic response of a normal pulp to ZOE placed in standard cavity depths is a mild chronic inflammatory cell infiltration. At five interval weeks there is a persistence of inflammatory cells underlying the cavity floor and a little reparative dentin formation occurs. Since ZOE has a low compressive strength, different additives are added to reinforce the original formulation. These are having better physical properties, however more irritating to pulp.

B. Zinc Phosphate Cement

Zinc phosphate cement has been the most widely used dental cement. It is used as a luting agent for all indirect restorations and appliances. In deep cavities, it is used as a base as a substitute of lost dentin, because the thermal conductivity is approximately equal to that of enamel and considerably less than that of amalgam and gold.

When used as a thick base, it has a low toxicity level but when used as a luting agent in a thin state, it can be quite toxic. A young tooth or deep preparations with wide open tubules are more susceptible to intense inflammatory response to zinc phosphate cement, than in an older tooth, which has produced a considerable amount of sclerotic and reparative dentin that blocks the dentinal tubules and prevents acids from reaching the pulp. Zinc phosphate cement is irritating because of its low pH and the rapid penetration of its lower molecular weight phosphoric acid into the dentinal tubules and pulp tissues. The hydraulic forces, which are induced during the seating of the restoration or during functional movements phosphoric acid in large quantities is forced into the dentinal tubules. Since dentin can be penetrated by phosphoric acid to a depth of more than 1.0 mm, especially in luting procedures, insulating materials are indicated for deep preparations with narrow remaining dentin thickness. In deep preparations, a moderate to severe localized pulpal damage is produced within the first three days probably because the cement has an initially low pH on setting. The pH of the set cement approximates neutrality only at 48 hours. Resolution of inflammation occurs by 5 to 8 weeks.

The chemical toxicity of these materials may not completely explain the harmful effects on pulp, because it has been seen that in germ free rats no chronic inflammation or focal necrosis is induced but a dentin bridge is formed. These observations indicate that bacterial leakage would be an important factor for inducing pulpal damage around such restorations.

When zinc phosphate is used as a luting agent there occurs an intense diffuse infilterate of neutrophils throughout the pulp tissue. The initial pH of luting mixes ranged from 2.0–3.3, which changes to 3.0–4.2 after one hour. It has been established that such a low pH induced vascular thrombosis and necrosis in rodent pulp when the duration of exposure was prolonged over thin dentin. The pH for zinc phosphate, polycarboxylate and glass-ionomer cements rise during the first 15 minutes. The rise in pH was faster for the zinc phosphate and polycarboxylate cements but slower for the glass-ionomer cements. When the cement is used as a base with a remaining dentin as 1.0 mm, there occurs lifting of the odontoblastic layer and also the inflammatory cells become countable. In case the remaining dentin thickness is 1.5 mm, there occurs only moderate reaction with segmented odontoblastic layer and some reparative dentin formation.

C. Silicate Cements

Silicate cements, though widely used earlier, are rarely used these days. Slicates in set form consist of glass particles covered with a layer of alumino-silica gel and a matrix of amorphous insoluble phosphates and fluorides. The silicate cements are markedly cytotoxic and show severe pulpal reactions.

Its adverse effects are mainly because of the prolonged acidity due to phosphoric acid even 24 hours after the setting of the cement; and to some extent because of the release of fluoride. The pH of silicate cement at the time of insertion into the cavity is less than 3 and it remains below 7 even after 7 months. Fluoride ion concentrations of 15–25 μgm/ml are also known to reduce cell growth. Silicates implanted into subcutaneous tissue inhibit cell enzyme activity, elicit severe inflammatory responses and cause necrosis of tissue without fibrous capsule formation. In standard depth cavities, the initial response of the pulp to unlined silicates is a noticeable degree of acute inflammatory cell infiltration with disruption of the odontoblastic layer within one to three days after placement. After five to eight weeks the response shifts from moderate to severe, usually with abscess formation. The extent of remaining dentin is important. Cavities with 1.0 mm or more of remaining dentin reveal a moderate inflammatory response, whereas in deeper cavities dense concentrations of inflammatory cells border the cavity floor with loss of odontoblastic layer. It has been demonstrated that microleakage around the silicate may also be an important factor in inducing pulp response (Fig. 23.7).

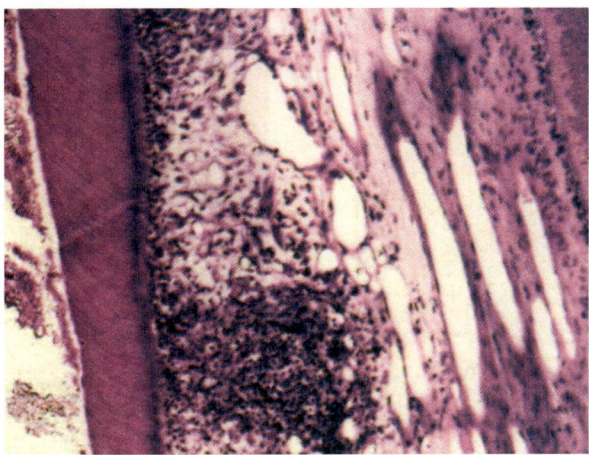

Fig. 23.7: Inflammation adjacent to silicate cement

D. Polycarboxylate Cements

Polycarboxylate cements are a combination of aqueous polyacrylic acid and zinc oxide. They have an excellent biocompatibility with the pulp and are almost equivalent to zinc oxide eugenol cements. Postoperative sensitivity effects are negligible with these cements. The pH of the cement liquid is approximately 1.7. The pH of the mix rises rapidly as the setting reaction proceeds. Despite the initial acidic nature of the polycarboxylate cements, these products produce minimal irritation to the pulp probably because the larger size of the polyacrylic acid molecule limits its diffusion through the dentinal tubules. At all times, the pH of the polycarboxylate cement is higher than the pH of the phosphate cements. Also, in the set cement the acrylic acid ions bind the metallic ions so tightly that they are not easily leached out from the set cement.

The pulpal response to polycarboxylate cements is slight to moderate inflammation at three days and only a mild chronic inflammation at five weeks. However, only minimal reparative dentin formation has been observed after five to eight weeks suggesting that they are not effective in stimulating dentin bridge formation. When these cements are placed directly on pulpal exposure varying degrees of inflammation have been noted. These reactions range from a mild chronic inflammation to the appearance of a localized liquefactive necrosis.

In short term tissue culture tests, a low degree of cytotoxicity in both freshly set and completely set cements has been found. On the other hand, subcutaneous and bone implant tests over one year period have not indicated long term toxicity of these cements. Thus, it appears that other mechanisms such as buffering and protein complexing of these materials neutralize the toxic effects in the long run. As a base material on dentin or as luting agent, almost all reports have mentioned mild pulpal reactions with polycarboxylate cements. However, pulp necrosis has also been reported.

E. Composites

The earlier resin bond materials, developed as a tooth colored materials, were detrimental to the pulp. The free monomer of the materials was injurious to the health of the pulp. Over the years, with the development of composites and also the tremendous improvements in the material aspect of these resins, the pulpal effects are minimum but not absent.

The bond strength of these materials is linked to the etching of the normal mineralized tissue. The effect of etching on pulp is minimum or negligible since the process is carried out for 10–15 seconds only (Fig. 23.8). To achieve optimal bonding to dentin, the adhesive material (bonding agents) must penetrate the demineralized dentin, enter the dentinal tubules and their branches (Figs 23.9A, B). The resin monomer enters the collagen fibers to completely infiltrate the deminearlized dentin forming the hybrid layer. Over this the composite is filled (Fig. 23.10).

The bonding materials have been tried as *'pulp capping'* with reasonably good results. It imparts healing process. However, the polymerization shrinkage of the composite creating vacuum in between the remaining dentin and the restoration might create problems for the pulp. It has been established that even after curing the monomer is leached from composites. This monomer is managed by the bonding agents and the remaining dentin thickness. In case the dentin thickness below the composites is less, the leaching monomer can affect the underlying pulp.

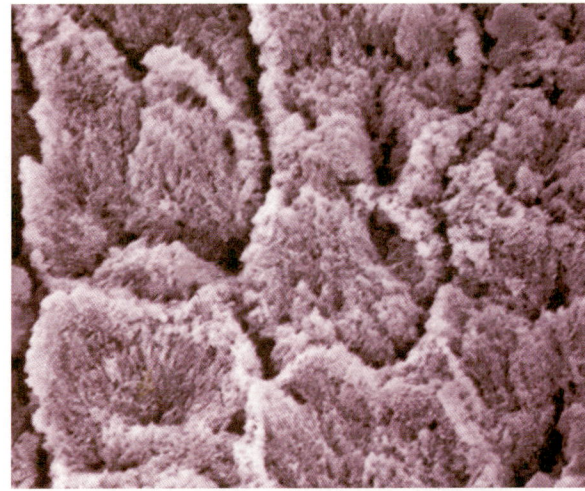

Fig. 23.8: Etched enamel surface. Demineralized rods and inter-rod tissues. X5000

F. Glass-Ionomer Cements

The glass-ionomer cement is a combination of fluoroalumino silicate and polyacrylic acid and water. The set material is composed of an inorganic-organic complex with high molecular weight. The material is considered biocompatible, since it is indicated in cavity bases and liners. The bonding of glass-ionomer material to dentin involves chemical and mechanical bonds. The chemical bond is based on exchange of ions between carboxyl group of substrate and calcium ions. The mechanical interlocking is based on the demineralization of exposed dentin by polyacrylic acid.

Various modified forms of glass-ionomers are also available. These are resin modified glass-ionomer cements or compomers. These materials achieve advantages of both the glass-ionomers and composites. After one week of placement of glass-ionomer cement the odontoblastic layer is disrupted and blood vessels seen in pulp area (Fig. 23.11). Bacterial penetration into tubules is also observed. After about a month the pulp tissue recovers and displays a normal appearance. The disruption of odontoblasts become normal.

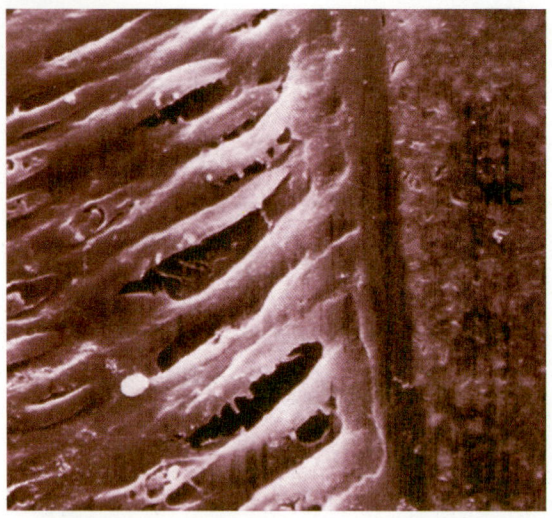

Fig. 23.9A: Dentin hybrid layer and resin tags. X1500

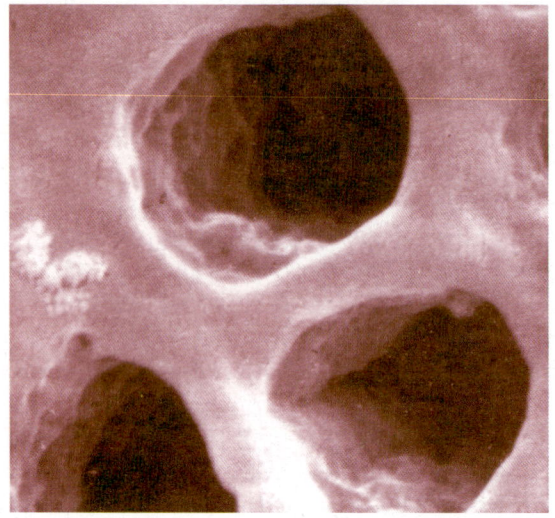

Fig. 23.9B: Dentin etching (open tubules). X10,000

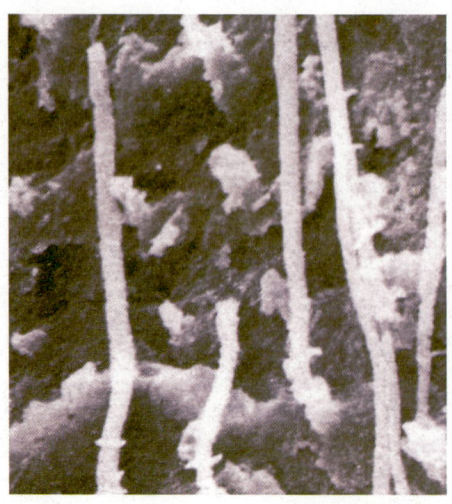

Fig. 23.10: Resin tags and modified smear layer

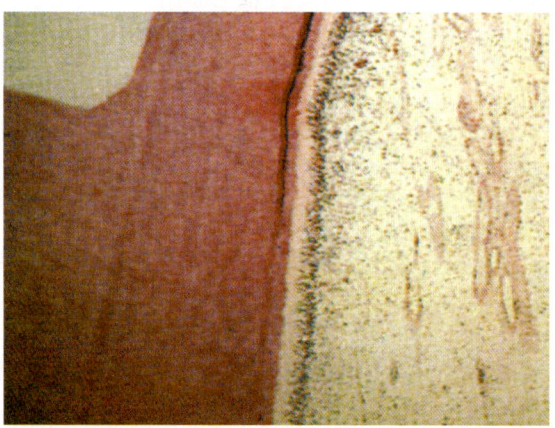

Fig. 23.11: Pulpal reaction with glass-ionomer cement

PULPAL REACTION TO TOOTH PREPARATION

In the recent past, high speed cutting instruments have largely been employed in cutting cavities and preparing tooth for crowns. Adequate cooling of the burs is essential to prevent injury to dentin and also to underlying odontoblastic region of the pulp. The water spray should reach at the site of cutting and bur. Light pressure with intermittent cooling can minimize temperature increase.

When the cooling is inadequate, the injury leads to displacement of odontoblastic nuclei into the dentinal tubules (Fig. 23.12). The odontoblasts appear disorganized. The cooling, if missing, or excessive pressure is utilized constantly, the burning of dentin becomes evident (Fig. 23.13). The cut section can

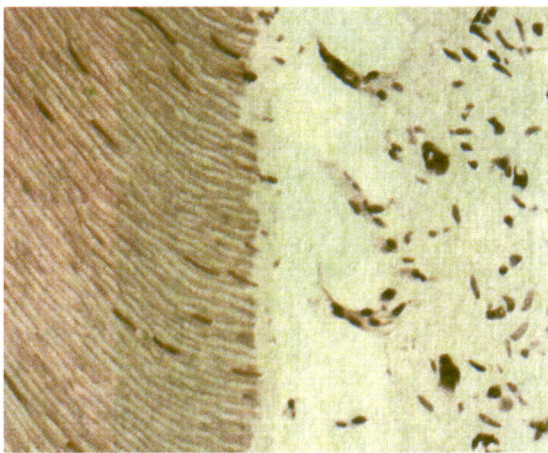

Fig. 23.12: Displacement of odontoblastic nuclei

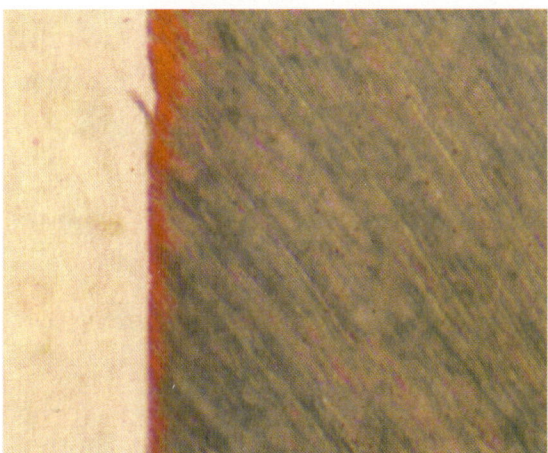

Fig. 23.13: Burning of dentin

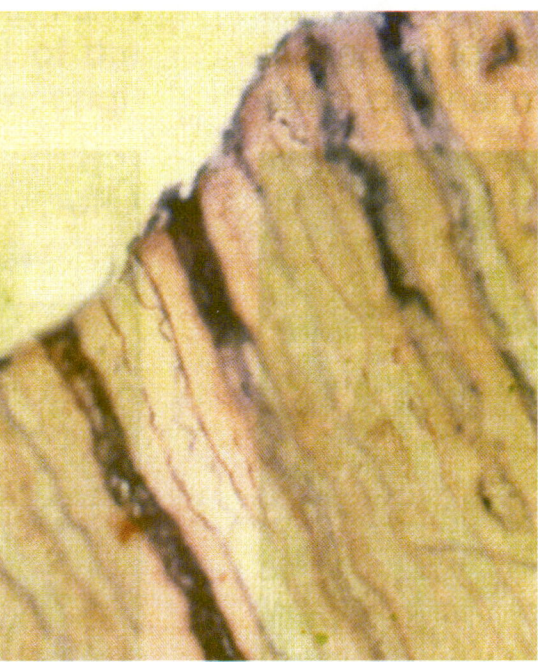

Fig. 23.14: Reaction of tubular contents

differentiate the color change at the margins. The most common feature in the reaction is the outward movement of the contents of the tubules (Fig. 23.14). This movement is also dependent on the tubules' openings, might be because of age or other developmental criteria. Many a times, the smear layer may obturate the opening of the tubules and reduce the extrusion of contents of dentinal fluids. It is established that such flow of fluid, later, is helpful in formation of peritubular dentin formation. The disturbance and redistribution of the cellular constituents, if continued, lead to degeneration of odontoblastic processes. This might form the basis for formation of 'dead tracts' and subsequently, formation of tertiary dentin.

Gentle grinding over the dentin leads to increased blood flow. Grinding halfway into the dentin causes much more increase in blood flow. However, grinding in the inner half leads to decrease in blood flow. The blood flow have been found to decrease after crown preparation, since the inner thickness of dentin might not be more than 1.0 mm.

In case the cavities are prepared deep and without coolant, vasoconstriction is noted. This vasoconstriction can be due to inhibition of sympathetic nerve stimulation. The flow of dentinal fluid plays an important role. The peripheral flow of fluid following cavity preparation allows plasma proteins to enter the tubules. This will lead to clotting of the tubules. Fibrinogen also causes obstruction of these tubules.

The displacement of odontoblastic nuclei into the dentinal tubules has been established. Earlier, 'aspiration of odontoblastic nuclei' was considered the phenomenon, but recently the accepted phenomenon is the 'displacement of odontoblasts'. The cavity depth or the remaining dentin thickness has always been the key factor in such reactions. A number of morphologic changes occur including intracellular disorganization of the odontoblasts. This can lead to disruption of odontoblastic layer. The exact mechanism of such movements might not be fully understood, however, mechanical distortion of the dentin can be the cause.

The alternative means of cavity preparation such as air abrasion and laser cavity preparation also affects the pulp. The generation of heat with the use of lasers is more detrimental. Laser is not a recommended procedure for cavity preparation, however, its effects on the other tissue is considerable.

PULPAL REACTION TO CARIES

The dental caries, may be in any form or at any site, affects the underlying pulp. The acidic environment of carious lesions cause both tissue dissolution and in aggressive lesions, cellular injury as well. The initiation of pulpal inflammation also stimulate the repair process. A balance usually occurs between repair and injury and deviation from the balance leads to changes in the dentin-pulp complex.

The cellular injury with caries arise from acidic environment created by diffusion of bacterial acids. The ability of the cells to withstand this acid environment depends upon hydrogen ion concentration. Local lymphatic drainage in the pulp may contribute to clearance of acid but the pulpal lymphatic system is not well developed. The odontoblasts are significantly reduced in size beneath the active enamel lesions whereas, at the site of arrested lesions such reduction is not exhibited. Before the caries lesion reaches dentino-enamel junction a significant reduction in cytoplasm to nucleus ratio of odontoblasts and also reduction in predentin thickness is observed. An increase in activity of phosphate enzyme is reported in odontoblasts and in predentin beneath the carious lesions.

Though the reaction in pulp varies according to intensity and progress of caries, the systematized classification of category of pulpal infection is not available. The terms *'slight'*, *'moderate'* and *'severe'* have the subjectivity and also, the varied interpretation of the histopathological results make it difficult to standardize the classification of pulpal reactions.

The onset of pulpal reactions to caries starts early, but its effect has not been documented properly. Pulpal reactions have been established even with the formation of white-spot lesions. There are marked changes in dentin with *'acute'* or rapidly progressing caries than with *'arrested'* or slow progressing caries. The odontoblasts in active lesions were significantly smaller than were, odontoblasts in other lesions. The cellular proliferation of the cell free zone is also observed in active lesions only. Changes in the subodontoblastic region also occur early and these changes might include early onset of neurogenic inflammatory reactions.

The active lesions do not show any marked changes in dentin mineralization. Slowly the demineralization of the affected dentin starts. Soon after the demineralization, the evidence of tertiary dentin can be noted at the pulp dentin border usually defined as *reactionary dentin*. The permeability of dentin plays an important role in these reactions. The initial entry to pulp for bacteria, bacterial antigens and toxic components is through the dentinal tubules.

The pulp adjacent to deep caries show the presence of chronic inflammatory exudates, including lymphocytes macrophages and plasma cells (Figs 23.15A, B). The localized increase in dentin thickness

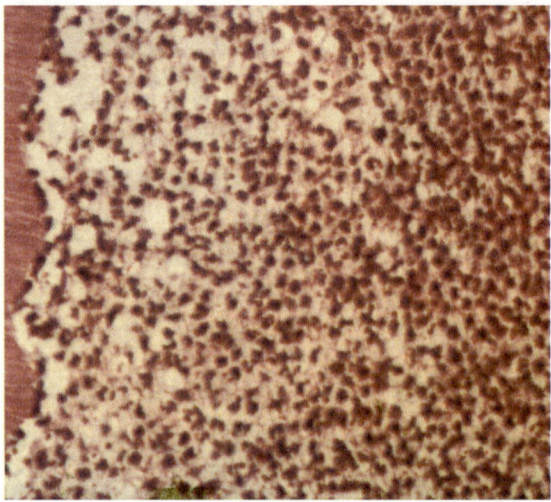

Fig. 23.15A: Polymorphonuclear leucocytes. X100

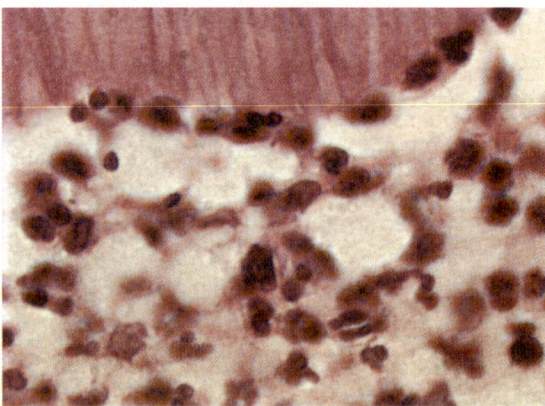

Fig. 23.15B: Leucocytes around dentinal tubules. X250

is often accompanied by reduced odonotoblastic layer in the affected area. The tertiary dentin can be seen at the affected site. The accumulation of inflammatory cells is particularly great whenever the bacteria associated with caries process reach the tertiary dentin. This stage corresponds to severe pulpal inflammation with minimum chances of healing. It may lead to pulp necrosis at a later stage. The flow chart illustrating the range of injury, defence and repair events associated with caries is depicted in Fig. 23.16 (Smith, 2002).

In case of rampant caries, the breakdown of affected enamel and dentin will occur within months. This leads to destruction of odontoblasts and lack of tertiary dentin formation. If the odontoblasts are destroyed slowly, there is formation of hard tissue, which is initially atubular with some cellular inclusions, defined as fibrodentin and interface dentin. The progress of caries, if halted, leads to formation of reparative dentin with differentiation of new secondary odontoblast like cells. If the lesion is allowed to progress, pulp necrosis may follow.

Pulpal Reactions

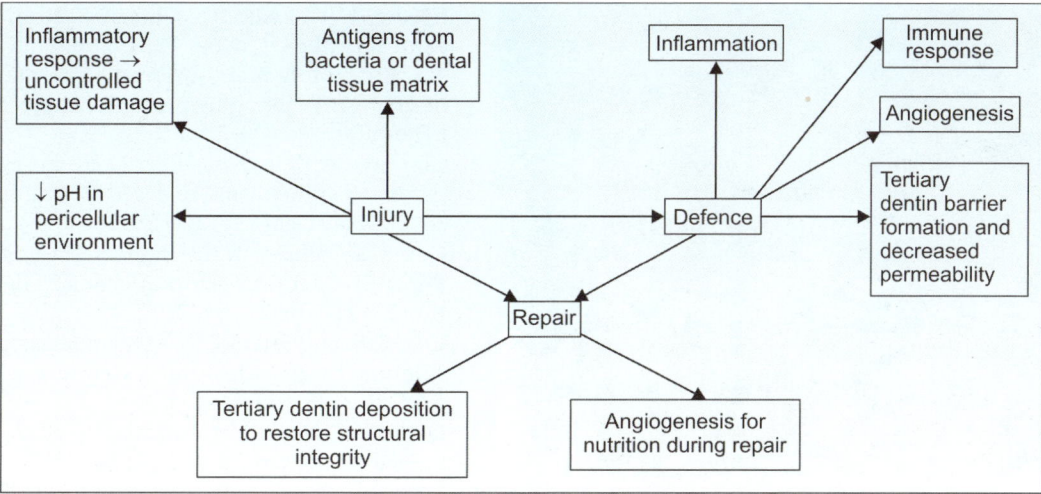

Fig. 23.16: Leucocytes around dentinal tubules. X250

The immune system helps in defence mechanism of pulp. In association with carious dentin, accumulation of immuno-competent cells has been demonstrated. During rapid lesion progression, accumulation of immuno-competent cells is observed in conjuction with reduced number of primary odontoblasts. In case the tertiary dentin develops, it is formed as an atubular dentin.

PULPAL REACTION TO TRAUMA

Physical trauma in the form of accidents is very common, especially during adolescent period. Trauma can be with wear, erosion, orthodontic movements and other occlusal traumas. Trauma may lead to future of enamel, dentin and exposure of pulp. Orthodontic tooth movements can be performed without any pulpal involvement but many a times, quick orthodontic movements cause changes in the pulp dentin complex.

The extensive trauma involves avulsion or displacement of the jaw bones. The pulp supply to the pulp is severed off. Either the pulp is necrosed with time or characterized by formation of hard tissues in the pulp chamber. These hard tissues have been labeled as ostodentin, because it has cellular infiltration similar to bone. In case of reimplantation, there occur degeneration of odontoblast and simultaneous loss of the adjacent cell free zone. This degeneration is accompanied by reduction of the width of predentin. In teeth with open apices, the odontoblasts can survive and produce reactionary dentin. A typical interface dentin is formed separating the primary dentin and reparative dentin.

The mechanism of cellular differentiation is similar to the analyzed and implanted teeth. The stimulation leads to differentiation of odontoblasts like cells or odontoblast like cells.

With the orthodontic movements of teeth putting pressure more than required there occurs increased blood flow in the pulp. Hyperaemia has been more marked in teeth adjacent to the one where force is applied (Figs 23.17A, B). Orthodontic treatment is becoming more common in adults these days with the root fully formed. These teeth are likely to have more pulpal changes than the teeth in young individuals.

The vacuolization of odontoblastic layer and the pulpal tissue are often the results in teeth subjected to heavy forces. These changes are suggestive of degeneration of pulp. The impaired predentin formation is also suggestive of degenerative changes. After the force is removed, the predentin formation starts.

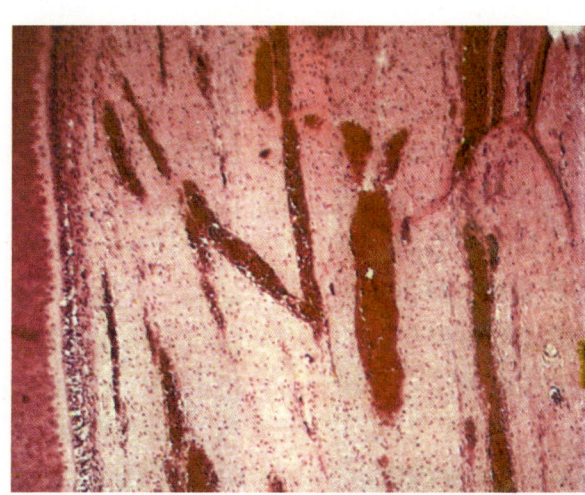

Fig. 23.17A: Severe hyperaemia

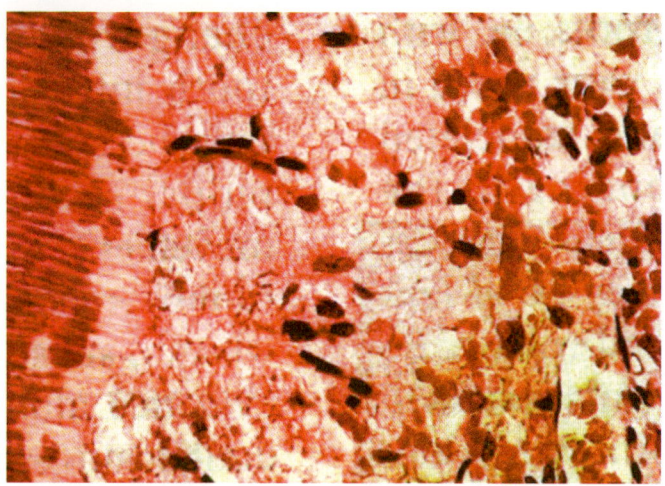

Fig. 23.17B: Haemorrhage in the odontoblastic layer

PULPAL REACTION TO VITAL BLEACHING

The vital tooth bleaching incorporates 10% carbamide solution in different modifications. Initial reaction of the pulp to bleaching includes less distinction of cell free zone. In areas on facial surface of these teeth, the cells migrate to these areas. Scattered leucocytes are observed along with irregularities in the pseudostratified odontoblastic layer. Only slight pulp reaction is observed. In any case even with high concentration, carbamide does not produce moderate or severe reactions. Few authors are of the view that using higher concentration of the hydrogen peroxide and heat is potentially harmful to pulp. The changes in pulp tissue are reversible after or within two weeks time. Therefore, two weeks of treatment with 10% carbamide peroxide used for nightguard vital bleaching is considered safe for the pulp.

BIBLIOGRAPHY

1. Bergenholtz, G.: Effect of bacterial products on inflammatory reaction in the dental pulp. Scand. J. Dent. Res.: 85, 122, 1977.
2. Bergenholtz, G.: Inflammatory response of the dental pulp to bacterial irritation. J. Endod.: 7, 100, 1981.
3. Bergenholtz, G.: Pathogenic mechanism in pulpal disease. J. Endo.: 16, 98, 1990.
4. Bjorndal, L.: Presence or absence of tertiary dentinogenesis in relation to caries progression. Adv. Dent. Res.: 15, 80, 2001.
5. Brannstrom, M. and Lind, P.O.: Pulpal response to early caries. J. Dent. Res.: 44, 1045, 1965.
6. Brannstrom, M. and Nyborg, H.: Pulpal reaction to composite resin restoration. J.P.D.: 27, 181, 1972.
7. Browne, R.M., Plant, C.G. and Tobias, R.S.: Quantification of the histologic features of pulpal damage. Int. Endod. J.: 13, 104, 1980.
8. Chogle, S.M.A., Goodis, H.E. and Kinaia, B.M.: pulpal and periradicular response to caries. Dent Clin North Am.: 6, 21, 2012.
9. Chung, H.Y., Lee, E.K., Choi, Y.J., Kim, J.M., Kim D.h., Kim, C.H., Lee, J., Kim, H.S., Kim, N.D., Jung, J.H. and Yu, B.P.: Molecular inflammation as an underlying mechanism of the aging process and age- related diseases. J Dent Res.: 90. 830, 2011.
10. Ciarlone, A.E. and Pashley, D.H.: Permeability of root dentin to epinephrine released from gingival retraction cord. Oper. Dent.: 17, 106, 1992.
11. Cox, C.F., Waite, K.C., Ramus, D.L. and Farmer, J.B.: Reparative dentin: Factors affecting its deposition. Quint. Int.: 23, 257, 1992.
12. Cox, C.F. and Suzuki, F.: Re-evaluating pulp protection: calcium hydroxide liner vs cohesive hybridization. J.A.D.A.: 125, 823, 1994.
13. Dahl, B.L.: Dentin pulp reaction to full crown preparation procedures. J. Oral Rehab.: 4, 247, 1977.
14. Dammascke, T., Stratmann, U. and Mokrigs, K.: Histocytological evaluation of the reaction of rat pulp-tissue to carisolv. J. Dent.: 29, 283, 2001.
15. Fugaro, J.O., Nordahl, I., Fugaro, O.J., Matis, B.A. and Six, N.: Pulp reaction to vital bleaching. Oper. Dent.: 29, 363, 2004.
16. Heyerass, K.: Blood flow and the vascular pressure in the dental pulp. Acta. Odont. Scand.: 38, 135, 1980.
17. Inokishi, S., Iwaku, M. and Fusayama, T.: Pulpal response to a new adhesive restorative resin. J.D.R.: 61, 1014, 1982.
18. Langeland, K.: Tissue response to dental caries. Endo. Dent. Traumat.: 3, 149, 1987.
19. Las fargues, J.J. and Goldberg, M.: In vivo study of the pulp reaction to Fuzi IX, a glass-ionomer cement. J. Dent.: 28, 413, 2000.
20. Leidal, T.I. and Eriksen, H.M.: Human pulp response to composite resin restoration. Endo. Dent. Traumat.: 1, 65, 1985.
21. Matthews, B. and Vogusavan, N.: Interaction between neural and hydrodynamic mechanism in dentine and pulp. Arch. Oral Biol.: 39, 875, 1994.
22. Mjor, I.A. and Tronstad, I.: The healing of experimentally induced pulpitis. O. Surg., O. Med., O. Path.: 38, 115, 1974.
23. Mjor, I.A.: The importance of methodology in the evaluation of pulp reactions. Int. Dent. J.: 30, 335, 1980.
24. Mjor, I.A., Nordahl, S. and Tronstad, L.: Glass ionomer cements and dental pulp. Endo. Dent. Traumat.: 7, 59, 1991.
25. Mjor, I.A. and Nordahl, I.: The dentistry and branches of dentinal tubules in human teeth. Arch. Oral Biol.: 41, 401, 1996.
26. Mjor, I.A., Sveen, S. and Ferrari, M.: Pulp dentin biology in restorative dentistry. Part 1–6. Quint. Int.: 427, 537 and 611, 2001, 74, 28, 39, 2002.
27. Murray, P.E, About, I., Lumlby, P.J. and Smith, G.: Postoperative pulpal and repair responses. J.A.D.A.: 131, 321, 2000.
28. Murray, P., About, I., Franquin, J.C. and Smith, A.J.: Restorative pulpal and repair responses. J.A.D.A.: 132, 482, 2001.
29. Pashley, D.H.: Dentin-Predentin complex and its permeability: physiologic overview. J. Dent. Res.: 64 (spl. Issue), 613, 1985.
30. Pashley, D.H.: The effect of acid etching on the pulpodentinal complex. Oper. Dent.: 17, 229, 1992.

31. Skogedal, O. and Mjor, I.A.: Pulp reaction to silicate cements in teeth with healing pulpitis. Scand. J. Dent. Res.: 85, 375, 1977.
32. Smith, A.J.: Pulpal responses to caries and dental repair. Caries Res.: 36, 223, 2002.
33. Sonoda, H., Sasafuchi, Y., Kitasako, Y., Arakawa, M., Otsuki, M. and Tagami, J.: Pulpal response to a fluoride releasing all-in one resin bonding systems. Oper. Dent.: 27, 271, 2002.
34. Stanley, H.R.: Design of human pulp. O. Surg., O. Med., O. Path.: 25, 633 and 756, 1968.
35. Stenvile, A. and Mjor, A.: Pulp and dentine reactions to experimentally tooth intrusion. A histologic study of the initial changes. Am. J. Orthod.: 57, 370, 1970.
36. Sulieman, M., Rees, J.S. and Addy, M.: Surface and pulp chamber temperature rise during tooth bleaching using a diode laser: a study in vitro. B.D.J.: 11, 631, 2006.
37. Suzuki, S., Cox, C.F. and White, K.C.: Pulpal responses after complete crown preparation, dentinal sealing and provisional restoration. Quint. Int.: 25, 477, 1994.
38. Trowbridge: Pathogenesis of pulpitis resulting from dental caries. J. Endod.: 7, 52, 1981.
39. Trowbridge, H., Edwall, L. and Panopoulas, P.: Effect of zinc oxide eugenol and calcium hydroxide on intradentinal nerve activity. J. Endod.: 8, 403, 1982.
40. Tziafus, D., Smith, A.J. and Lesot, H.: Designing new treatment strategies in vital pulp therapy. J. Dent.: 28, 77, 2000.
41. Van Hassel, H.J.: Physiology of the human dental pulp. O. Surg., O. Med., O. Path.: 32, 126, 1971.
42. Wedenberg, C. and Bornstein, R.: Pulpal reactions in rat incisors to caridex. Aust. Dent. J.: 35, 505, 1990.

24. Tooth Substance Loss

With the dramatic evolution of dental materials coupled with patient's awareness regarding preventive regimes, the individuals retaining their original dentition is increasing day by day. With the natural dentition and advancing age, the loss of tooth substance and its management is posing a challenge for the clinicians.

Apart from caries, non-carious processes such as attrition, abrasion and erosion may cause loss of tooth structure. The etiology, extent and clinical picture of this menace may vary among different individuals and may be associated with physiological or pathological processes.

Eccles suggested the term *'tooth substance loss'*, which can be used to encompass terms such as attrition, abrasion and erosion. Later, Smith and Knight (1984) proposed the term *'tooth wear'* so as to include all these conditions and their combination. They contended that the term tooth surface loss did not sufficiently reflect the severity of the condition and advocated the use of the term tooth wear. They also proposed a tooth wear index as depicted in Table 24.1. Later, Bardsley, et al (2004) simplified the tooth wear index for epidemiological studies (Table 24.2). The types of wear can be as follows.

ATTRITION

This term is derived from Latin word 'attitum', which describes the action of rubbing against something. Dental attrition is defined as *'the physiologic wearing of teeth resulting from tooth to tooth contact as in mastication. This is an age-related process that can occur at the incisal or occlusal surfaces and sometimes on proximal surfaces'*.

Clinically, the first manifestation is the appearance of a small polished facet on a cusp tip or ridge or an incisal edge. Severe attrition however can result in dentinal exposure, which may increase the rate of wear (Fig. 24.1).

Attrition may be hastened by a hard and abrasive diet; silica particles in tobacco or inorganic compounds in snuff can cause attrition. However, a few authors disagree with the concept where food is considered a major factor. Instead, they prefer to use the term

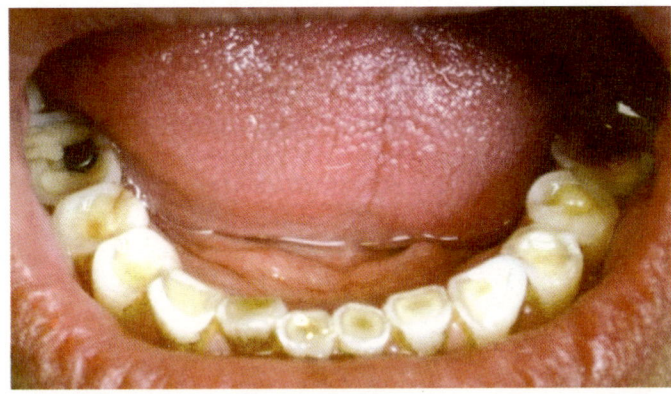

Fig. 24.1: Severe attrition involving dentin

	Table 24.1: Tooth wear index		
Score	Buccal/Lingual	Interproximal/occlusal	Cervical
0	No loss of enamel surface characteristics	No loss of enamel surface characteristics	No change in contour
1	Change in enamel surface characteristics	Change in enamel surface characteristics	Minimal loss of contour
2	Loss of 1/3rd of enamel surface	Loss of enamel fissure exposing dentin	Defect < 1.0 mm
3	Loss of more than 1/3rd of enamel surface	Exposure of dentin	1.0–2.0 mm deep defect
4	Complete loss of enamel surface; exposure of dentin	Substantial loss of dentin; no exposure of pulp	2.0–3.0 mm deep defect
5.	Pulp exposure	Pulp exposure	Pulp exposure

Tooth Substance Loss

Table 24.2: Simplified scoring criteria for tooth wear index

Score	Criteria
0	No wear into dentin
1	Dentin just visible (including cupping) or dentin exposed for less than 1/3 of surface
2	Dentin exposure greater than 1/3 of surface
3	Exposure of pulp or secondary dentin

demastication to describe the wearing away of tooth substance during mastication of food influenced by the abrasiveness of the individual food particles.

Some parafunctional habits like bruxism and clenching may also contribute to attrition. It has been reported that 5% to 96% of population may be affected by such habits. While a certain amount of attrition is physiologic, excessive destruction of tooth structure is pathologic. If occlusal wear occurs at a rate faster than the compensatory physiologic mechanisms, it is not considered as physiologic (Fig. 24.2).

At times, severe occlusal wear causes the amalgam or any other restoration to appear protruded while the surrounded occlusal surface is flattened (Fig. 24.3).

Caries can also superimpose at the attritional areas because of increased vulnerability of exposed dentinal surfaces (Fig. 24.4).

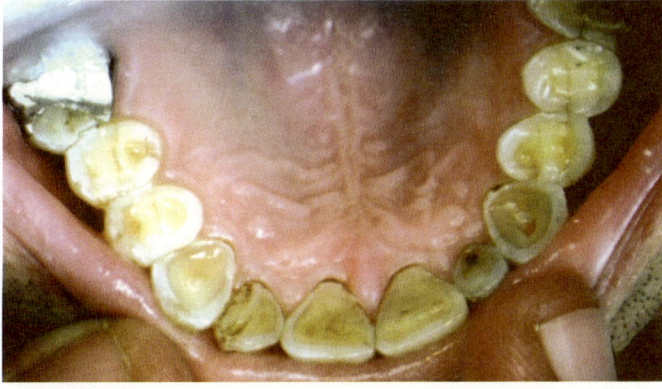

Fig. 24.2: Pathological attrition

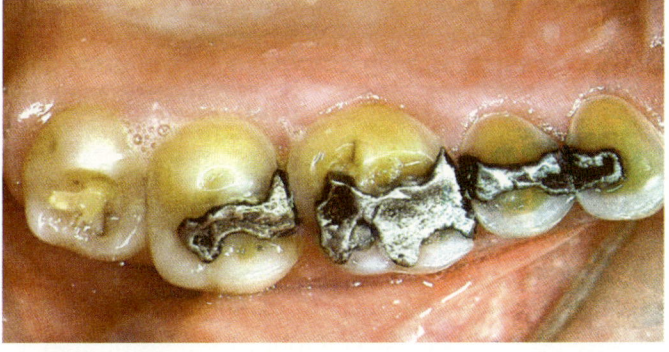

Fig. 24.3: Attrition of occlusal surfaces with protrusion of amalgam

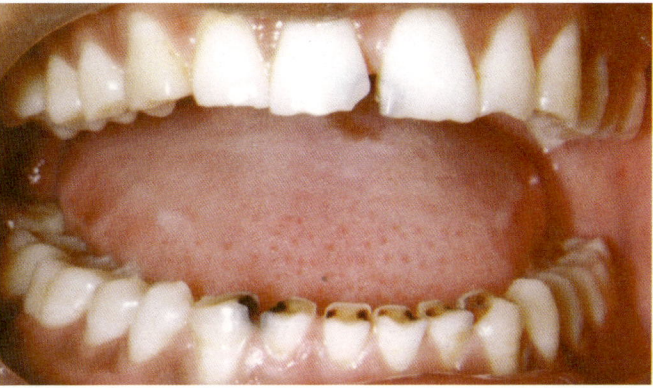

Fig. 24.4: Caries superimposing the attritioned incisors

An index for assessing attrition has been suggested

- 0 = No wear
- 1 = Minimal wear
- 2 = Noticeable flattening parallel to the occluding planes
- 3 = Flattening of cusps or grooves
- 4 = Total loss of contour and/or dentin exposure when identifiable

It should be borne in mind that the occurrence and pattern of tooth wear is related to educational, cultural, dietary, occupational and geographic factors. Other important factors are age and the function of occlusion.

Dental attrition has been used in archaeology and the forensic sciences to estimate human age. It is established that attrition has a multifactorial etiology along with age. The canine guided occlusion has significant influence in addition to crowding, occlusal slides, crossbites, chewing habits and diet (Figs 24.5, 24.6).

Experiments have shown that enamel wear is affected by changes in lubricating conditions (acidity) and loads. Enamel wear differs from dentin wear since dentin wear is associated with increasing load. It is also noted that attrition is a continuing process. It has been established that teeth continue to erupt in

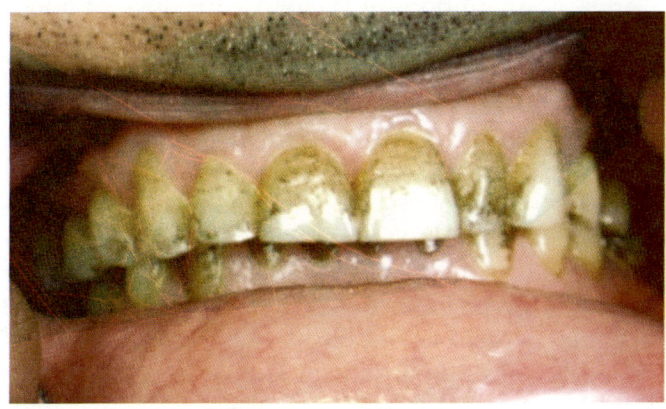

Fig. 24.5: Deep bite

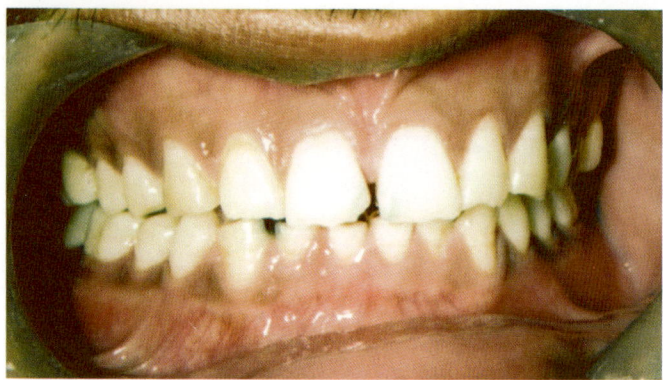

Fig. 24.6: Edge to edge bite

adulthood even in the absence of masticatory function and concomitant attrition.

CERVICAL LESIONS

Cervical lesions are the loss of hard tooth tissue at the cemento-enamel junction or in its adjoining one third portion of the tooth crown/root. It is a condition often encountered in the clinical practice. These can affect any surface of the tooth, i.e. facial, lingual or proximal. Defects arising on the cervical one third of the facial and lingual surfaces of any tooth are included in class V lesions. Those present on the cervical one third of the proximal surfaces of anterior and posterior teeth are included in class III and class II lesions respectively. The term '*cervical lesion*' should not be used to represent class V lesions. It is suggested that appropriate terminology be used whenever any reference is made to these lesions. Cervical lesions can be broadly classified into two categories:
   I. Carious cervical lesions
  II. Non-carious cervical lesions
     a. Abrasion lesions
     b. Erosion lesions
     c. Abfraction lesions

I. Carious Cervical Lesions

Caries is an important factor in the loss of tooth structure. Cervical carious lesions are smooth surface lesions, with their morphology and spread similar to carious smooth surface lesions in any other region of the tooth (Fig. 24.7). These begin over a broad surface area and converge towards the dentino-enamel junction. On reaching the junction, the lesion again spreads laterally. Depending upon the stage of progression, lesions may present with variable morphology. Incipient defects are seen as chalky white opacities, which become visible only when the enamel is dessicated, and partially or totally disappear when the surface is hydrated (wet). These have lost their translucency because of the extensive subsurface

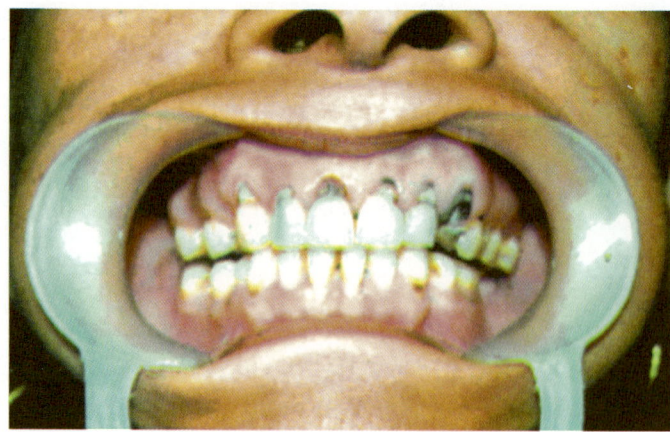

Fig. 24.7: Carious cervical lesions

porosity caused by demineralization. Their surface texture is unaltered and routinely cannot be detected by tactile examination with an explorer. At this stage, the lesion can generally be remineralized if adequate preventive measures are taken. A more advanced lesion is seen as a rough surface that is softer than the unaffected normal enamel. The lesion is then in an active stage. Further destruction of the tooth by caries results in frank cavitated lesions. Carious cervical lesions are often seen in regions of plaque accumulation. Both the incidence and severity of attack increases several fold in conditions of rampant caries or radiation induced xerostomia.

II. Non-carious Cervical Lesions

Tooth structure loss cannot be blamed entirely to caries. Many non-carious destructive processes that are an etiology to loss of tooth structure include attrition, abrasion, erosion, abfraction, demastication and resorption. Amongst these, abrasion, erosion and abfraction are the common ones, which are responsible for inducing cervical lesions. Miller was amongst the first to associate these etiologic factors to the presence of non-carious cervical lesions. Not necessarily, any one etiology can be isolated, but two or more may act together to initiate and promote the development of lesions. It is, therefore, emphasized to attain a detailed knowledge of the etiology of these defects for preventing further lesions and halting the progress of lesions already present. Also, treatment of lesions in the long run will be ineffective unless the etiologic factor(s) are eliminated.

Non-carious cervical lesions, depending upon their etiologic factors, present a variable morphology ranging from shallow grooves to broad dished out lesions to large notched or wedge shaped defects mostly on facial surfaces. Floor of the lesion may be flat, rounded or sharp angled. Rounded lesions are less frequently encountered than angular ones. The reported prevalence of non-carious cervical lesions, regardless of form and etiology, is shown to vary from 5% to 85%. Both prevalence and severity are known to increase with age. The older the patient population - larger is the percentage of individuals showing lesions, greater are the number of lesions in any one individual and deeper is the extent of lesions. The impact of these lesions on individual patients may also vary. Some patients present with no symptoms while others may complain of highly sensitive teeth. Severe lesions may affect the vitality of pulp and threaten the structural integrity of the tooth.

Why Non Carious Cervical Lesions are Usually on Facial Surface?

The relative thickness of bone on the lingual surfaces or palatal surfaces of teeth is consistently greater than the facial surface. The bone may deflect the load differently on the facial surfaces than on the lingual surfaces of teeth. This can be termed osteo-deflection (from "osteo" meaning bone and "deflection" being the displacement of a structural element under load). When a lateral force vector from a facial to a lingual direction begins to tip the tooth lingually, the tooth cannot move bodily due to the thickness of the bone, but rather must bend at the fulcrum (Fig. 24.8A). In doing so, this places the lingual cement-enamel junction (CEJ) area under compression and the facial CEJ area under tension. This tensile load is far more damaging than compressive load. Conversely, if the force vector comes from a lingual to a facial direction the tooth can more likely tip bodily because of lesser bone volume/thickness on the facial thus not concentrating as much tensile stress at the lingual CEJ (Fig. 24.8B). Recession is much more common on the facial and is generally accompanied by loss of vertical bone as well. This loss of bone on the facial allows the tooth to tip bodily in a facial direction even more, further reducing the tensile stress at the lingual CEJ. Conversely, forces that tend to move the tooth lingually are resisted by the lingual bone and the stresses at the facial CEJ can shift location. This change in the location of the fulcrum may cause the cervical notches to migrate incisally/occlusally or apically depending on the new site of the fulcrum.

ABRASION

Abrasion is defined as *'wearing away of the tooth substance because of grinding, rubbing or scraping caused by external mechanical means, like in repeated contact of the teeth with foreign objects or substances'*. Abrasion may affect one or more teeth, or the entire dentition. Any surface of the tooth may be affected but the most

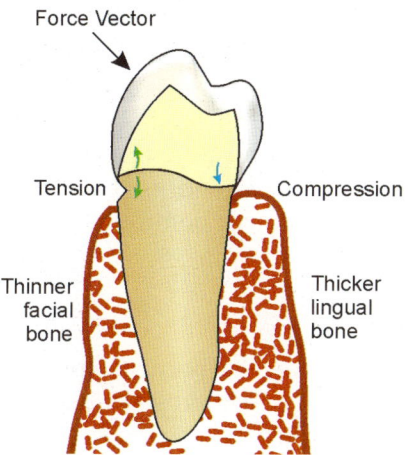

Fig. 24.8A: Direction of force from facial to lingual

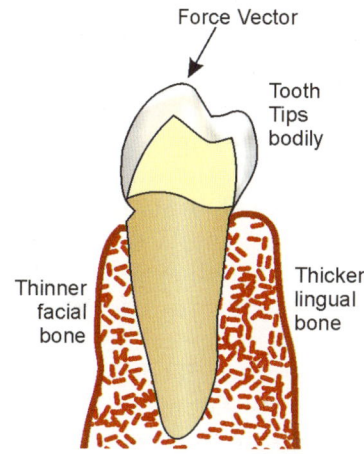

Fig. 24.8B: Direction of force from lingual to facial

frequently affected site is the cervical region. Causes for the cervical abrasion lesions may be as follows:

- Most common cause is faulty oral hygiene practice like horizontal brushing, excessive forces applied during brushing coupled with excessive time and frequency.
- Quality of tooth brush may be a contributing factor; for example, hardness and shape of tooth brush bristles, flexibility and length of the tooth brush handle affecting the grip of tooth brush and the grittiness. pH and amount of dentifrice used also affects the wear (Tooth powder is generally five times more abrasive).
- Ill-fitting clasps of partial dentures are also known to induce localized abrasion lesions.
- Cervical abrasive wear on the proximal surfaces of teeth is often caused by friction from objects such as toothpicks, inter-proximal brushes, etc.

Generally enamel is quite hard and not easily abraded; therefore, it serves as a protection for the underlying dentin, which is abraded 25 times faster.

Cementum is the softest of all tissues and shows an abrasion rate of 35 times higher than enamel. This explains for the higher prevalence and severity of cervical lesions in the older age. With increasing age, gingival recession exposes the cementum and as a result the tooth becomes highly susceptible to abrasion even under the previously non-damaging oral hygiene measures.

Effect of Tooth Brushing

Brushing technique has been considered to be an important factor in developing abrasion lesion. Using a horizontal or cross brushing technique significantly increases the frequency of cervical lesions compared to patients using a vertical or roll technique. Cross brushing produces more wear on dentin than vertical brushing as in the former technique, less force is applied yet the tooth brush bristles remain in contact with the tooth surface for a longer period and apply more consistent force. Horizontal brushing strokes usually produce V-shaped notches in dentin, independent of bristle stiffness and dentin abrasiveness. Vertical brushing strokes tend to produce U-shaped notches. Cervical lesions are also known to be associated with increased brushing frequency. Patients who brush quite often show more lesions irrespective of age group. The length of the time spent and forces applied during brushing may also influence the development of lesions, e.g. right handed individuals show a preponderance of lesions on the left side and vice versa. This may be because of easier access and more forces being applied on to the opposite side of the dental arch. The sequence in which teeth are brushed influences the location of lesions – more lesions are present in the quadrants brushed first. This finding reflects the greater force being applied in the earlier tooth brushing episodes. The amount of force used during brushing is determined by a number of factors like the age of the individual, brushing technique, hardness of bristles and individual habits.

A survey was conducted on 460 patients who visited Government Dental College and Hospital, Amritsar, (India). 11,040 teeth were examined for cervical abrasion lesions. 2760 teeth were found to be cervically abraded and the percentage of lesions increased with age: 9.34% (31–40 years), 30.43% (41–50 years), 42.02% (51–60 years) and 18.18% (61–70 years). Males were comparatively more affected than females. The frequency with which the lesions occurred was in the following decreasing order of the affected teeth – upper and lower first premolars, upper canines, upper and lower second premolars, lower canines and incisors, and molars. Premolars were more susceptible to abrasion probably because they were placed slightly protruded in the dental arch.

Effect of Dentifrices

The role of dentifrices has been established. A number of studies have confirmed the adverse effects of highly abrasive toothpastes and powders. The abrasive potential of a material varies among individuals. The amount of dentifrice applied, the degree of salivary dilution, technique and force applied during tooth brushing, all influence abrasion; thus not just a single factor but multiple factors work together to produce a lesion.

Morphology and location

Abrasion lesions are of varying morphology and may be classified as:

i. *Notch (N)/V-shaped defects*: Where oblique occlusal and cervical walls intersect at a certain depth with no definite axial wall in between them.
ii. *C-shaped defects (C)*: Where cross-section of the defect is C-shaped with rounded floors.
iii. *Undercut concave (UC)*: Where occlusal and cervical walls intersect with a definite axial wall in between them.
iv. *Divergent box (DB)*: Where a definite axial wall is present with the occlusal and cervical walls diverging toward the surface.

Cervical lesions thought to be because of abrasive forces generally have sharply defined margins, and hard smooth surfaces with burnished appearance. Occasionally, the surface may exhibit scratches. Hypersensitivity is intermittent in character, appearing or disappearing at intervals. In slowly progressive defects, reparative dentin formation occurs over a period of time making them asymptomatic. Lesions may show varying grades of depths like (i) Shallow (S): 0.1–0.5 mm in depth (ii) Deep (D): more than 0.5 mm but no pulp exposure and (iii) Exposure (E): Pulp is exposed.

Abrasion lesions are usually generalized and most commonly seen to damage facial surfaces of maxillary teeth, whereas lingual surfaces are rarely affected. The canines and the premolars exhibit the highest frequency. Occasionally, localized lesions may be present on teeth/tooth placed facial to the remaining dental arch.

EROSION

Erosion is defined as *'the defects arising because of dissolution of tooth structure subsequent to chemical attack of either endogenous or exogenous origin, or combined chemico-mechanical attack.'*

Eccles (1979) classified erosion lesions (Table 24.3) into three classes.

Bartlett, et al (2008) introduced Basic Erosive Wear Examination (BEWE) to be used for tooth scientific and clinical purposes.

The Basic Erosive Wear Examination (BEWE) was introduced to facilitate quantifying the risk of erosion. It can be used with the diagnostic criteria of most current indices and allows reanalysis and integration of results from existing studies. All teeth, except third molars, are examined in each case from the vestibular, occlusal, and palatal aspects for acid damage. The most severely affected surface in a sextant is recorded with a 4-level score (Table 24.4). The sum of the scores defines the severity of erosive wear and guides the further management of the condition (Table 24.5). The maximum score per subject is 18. Management includes identification and elimination of the main causative factor(s), prevention and monitoring, as well as symptomatic and operative intervention, where appropriate.

Recently, Vialati and Belser (2010) introduced anterior clinical erosive classification emphasizing on the maxillary anterior teeth. This classification system has been proposed to not only assess the severity of hard tissue loss but also to provide a guide to the treating clinician on how to appropriately restore the affected teeth. The classification, as shown by Table 24.6, establishes six levels of wear according to the level of dentin exposure in the palatal contact areas, the preservation of the incisal edges, the length of the remaining clinical crown, the preservation of enamel on the labial surfaces, and the vitality of the pulp. The 'sandwich approach' as listed in Table 24.6 refers to the application of a resin-based material to treat the palatal surface wear, followed by the application of a labial/facial ceramic veneer.

Table: 24.4: Criteria for grading erosive wear

Score	Criteria
0	No erosive tooth wear
1	Initial loss of surface texture
2[a]	Distinct defect, hard tissue loss <50% of the surface area
3[a]	Hard tissue loss >=50% of the surface area

[a] with scores 2 and 3, dentin is often involved.

Etiology

i. *Extrinsic (exogenous)*
   - Environmental/occupation – wine tasters, swimmers
   - Dietary – Soft drinks, Acidic food
   - Medication – Vitamin C, Mouth washes

ii. *Intrinsic (Endogenous)*
   - Gastric reflux – oesophagitis, hiatus hernia, increased gastric pressure, neuromuscular diseases
   - Vomiting – Psychosomatic, anorexia, bulimia, drug induced
   - Regurgitation

Table 24.3: Eccles index for dental erosion

Class	Surface	Criteria
Class I		Early stages of erosion, absence of development ridges, smooth, glazed surface occurring mainly on labial surfaces of maxillary incisors and canines
Class II	Facial	Dentin involved for less than one third surface: two types Type 1 (commonest): ovoid-crescentric in outline, concave in cross section at cervical region of surface. Must differentiate from wedge shaped abrasion lesions Type 2: irregular lesion entirely within crown. Punched out appearance, where enamel is absent from floor
Class IIIa	Facial	More extensive destruction of dentin, affecting anterior teeth particularly. Majority of lesions affect a large part of the surface, but some are localized and hollowed out
Class IIIb	Lingual or palatal	Dentin eroded for more than one third of the surface area. Gingival and proximal enamel margins have white, etched appearance. Incisal edges translucent due to loss of dentin. Dentin is smooth and anteriorly is flat or hollowed out, often extending into secondary dentin
Class IIIc	Incisal or occlusal	Surfaces involved into dentin, appearing flattened or with cupping. Incisal edges appear translucent due to undermined enamel; restorations are raised above surrounding tooth surface
Class IIId	All	Severely affected teeth, where both labial and lingual surfaces are extensively involved. Proximal surfaces may be affected; teeth are shortened

Table 24.5: Complexity levels as a guide to clinical management

Susceptibility Level	Cumulative Score of All Sextants	Management
	Less than or equal to 2	Routine maintenance and observation. Repeat at 3-year intervals
Low	3–8	Oral hygiene and dietary assessment and advice. Identify the main causative factor(s) and develop strategies to eliminate their effects, routine maintenance, and observation. Repeat at 1- to 2- year interval
Medium	9–13	As above plus Measures to increase the resistance of tooth surfaces Ideally, avoid the placement of restorations and monitor erosive wear with study casts, photographs, or silicone impressions. Repeat at 6- to 12- months.
High	More than or equal to 14	As above plus Especially in cases of severe progression consider special case, which may involve restorations. Repeat at 6- month intervals

Table 24.6: The ACE classification

Class	Palatal enamel	Palatal dentin	Incisal edge length	Facial enamel	Pulp vitality	Suggested therapy
Class I	Reduced	Not exposed	Preserved	Preserved	Preserved	No restorative treatment – prevention only
Class II	Lost in contact areas	Minimally exposed	Preserved	Preserved	Preserved	Palatal composites
Class III	Lost	Distinctly exposed	Lost less than 2.0 mm	Preserved	Preserved	Palatal onlays
Class IV	Lost	Extensively exposed	Lost greater than 2.0 mm	Preserved	Preserved	Sandwich approach
Class V	Lost	Extensively exposed	Lost greater than 2.0 mm	Distinctly reduced/lost	Preserved	Sandwich approach (experimental)
Class VI	Lost	Extensively exposed	Lost greater than 2.0 mm	Lost	Lost	Sandwich approach (highly experimental)

(Vialati and Belser-2010)

iii. *Idiopathic* (unknown)
   a. Clinical severity on tooth surface
     • Superficial lesion
     • Localized lesion
   b. Pathogenic activity of progression
     • Manifest or active
     • Latent or inactive

Depending upon the source of chemicals (usually acids), erosion may be intrinsic or extrinsic (Figs 24.9, 24.10, 24.11, 24.12). *Intrinsic erosion* is a result of endogenous acids and may be seen in situations like:

- Gastric acid contacting the teeth during recurrent vomiting, regurgitation or reflux. Such a condition is evidenced in psychosomatic disorders, e.g.

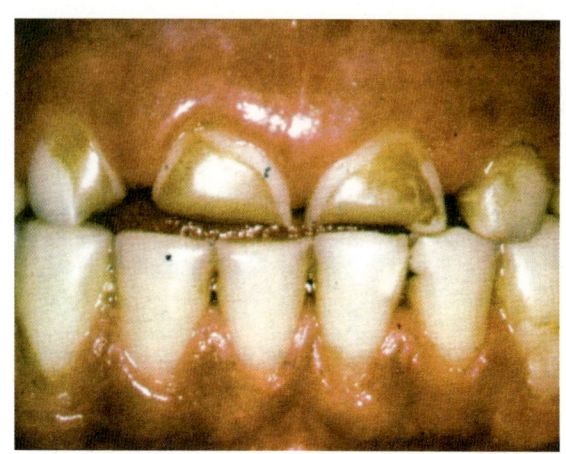

Fig. 24.9: Erosion involving labial surfaces of central incisors

Tooth Substance Loss

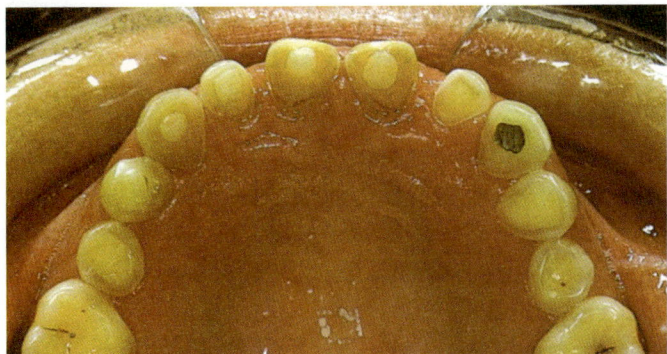

Fig. 24.10: Erosion involving palatal surfaces

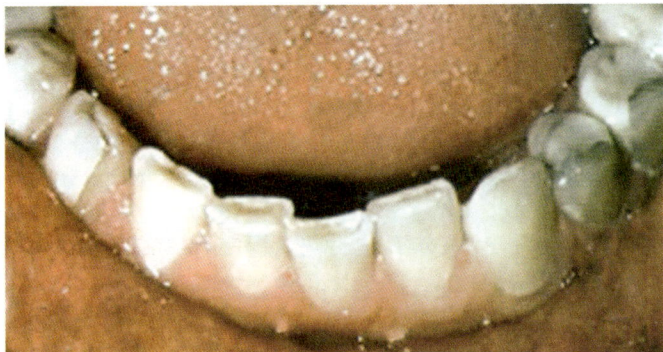

Fig. 24.11: Erosion involving incisal surfaces

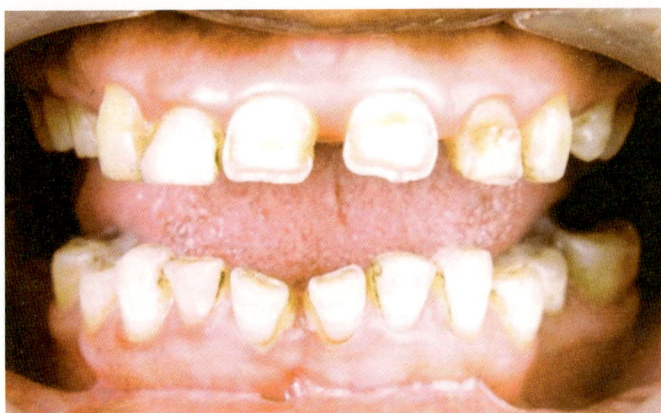

Fig. 24.12: Multisurface erosion

calcium phosphate from the labial/buccal mucous glands. This type of erosion usually is confined to the labial surfaces of anterior teeth though labial and buccal surfaces of entire dentition may be involved.
- Excess of acid salts present in the saliva from fermentation process.
- Acidity from a local acidosis in periodontal tissues as a result of traumatic occlusion.

Extrinsic erosion is a consequence of exogenous acids found as a contaminant in the work atmosphere (e.g. acid battery factories) or in chlorinated swimming pools, in low pH medications like iron tonics, aspirin, hydrochloric acid replacements, oral hygiene products and in the diet. The most commonly consumed, potentially damaging acidic diets are rich in fruits, fruit acids and phosphoric acids in fruit juices, lemons, vinegar and beverages (Tables 24.7 and 24.8). Ascorbic acid/citric acid added to a variety of drinks and candies have also been identified as a possible cause for erosion. The citrate ions are believed to bind with calcium in enamel and dentin forming soluble calcium citrate. Ironically, healthier diets, which include the consumption of more fruits and vegetables are an important factor in the etiology of dental erosion. Also, during fasting, the combination of acidic drinks and reduced salivary flow contribute to increased risk of erosion. Such lesions frequently present on the facial surfaces of anterior teeth. Fruits seem to affect anterior teeth while fruit juices may affect premolars

nervous vomiting, self induced anorexia nervosa, bulimia, etc; or in pregnancy, somatic disorders like, gastric dysfunction, chronic constipation, duodenal and peptic ulcers, etc. This type of intrinsic erosion is most likely seen on lingual surfaces of anterior teeth especially the maxillary teeth. Individuals having these disorders have also reported consuming diets rich in citrus fruits, juices and acidic carbonated beverages, which may be an additional contributing factor.
- Diseases because of lack of oxygen or faulty metabolism resulting in excessive formation and elimination of acid sodium phosphate and/or acid

Table 24.7: Acidity of common foods and beverages	
Pepsi/Coke	2.5–2.7
Fruit beer	3.0
Orange juice	2.8–3.8
Lemon juice	1.8–2.4
Pickles	2.5–3.0
Beer	4.0–5.0
Wine	2.2–3.5
Sauces	3.5–4.5

Table 24.8: Factors influencing erosive potential of foods and beverages	
Chemical	pH and buffering capacity Type of acid, adhesion to teeth, concentrations of acid
Behavioural	Drinking habits, excessive consumption of acid foods, oral hygiene measures
Biological	Salivary flow, buffering capacity, acquired pellicle dental anatomy, soft tissue movements

and molars. Cervical surfaces are most prone areas as they are close to the gingiva and less cleansable, and foods and beverages may harbour in their proximity for longer periods of time. Erosion because of air borne acids is comparatively very rare at the cervix. It is important to differentiate erosion lesions from carious lesions, the latter are characterized as a disease that occurs by the action of acids produced by plaque micro-organisms, while the former result from direct contact with acids of any origin excepting micro-organisms.

Erosion rarely is a factor that operates alone in causing tooth loss. Generally, such a lesion is multifactorial, i.e. once the surface of the tooth has been hypomineralized by erosion, wear resistance of dental hard tissues is lessened and they become more prone to damage by mechanical abrasion, demastication (abrasiveness of individual foods), friction from labial and buccal muscles and possibly abfraction. Because of the varied pathogenesis of cervical erosive lesions, it becomes increasingly difficult to differentiate between chemical and mechanical etiology. It is, therefore, critical to differentially diagnose the lesion before actual treatment is carried out. Fortunately, cervical erosive lesions are relatively rare.

Localization of Erosion
- Palatal and occlusal surface of maxillary teeth
- Buccal and occlusal surface of mandibular teeth

Intrinsic Factors Associated with Chronic Vomiting or Persistent Gastroesophageal Reflux (Table 24.9)
- Alimentary tract disorders (peptic ulcer, chronic gastritis, intestinal obstruction)
- Neurologic disorders (migraine, diabetic polyneuropathy)
- Metabolic and endocrine disorders (adrenal insufficiency)
- Drug side-effects (central emetic effects, gastric irritation)
- Psychosomatic disorders (stress-induced vomiting, eating disorders)

Table 24.9: Gastroesophageal reflux disease

Symptoms	
Adults	Children
Acid taste in mouth	Feeding problem
Vomiting	Laryngitis/bronchitis
Sore throat	Asthma
Excessive salivation	Recurrent pneumonia
Halitosis	Gastric pain

When teeth are exposed to an acid beverage of pH 2.8 for 15 minutes, 20 µm loss of enamel occurs.

A large number of studies have been carried out to determine the effect of beverages on erosion. The potential erosive effects of acidic juices when given for prolonged periods of time in some form of comforter or feeder have been documented.

The development of dental erosion is strongly influenced by:
- Determinant factors
    i. Biological
    ii. Behavioral
    iii. Chemical
- Modifying factors
    i. Knowledge
    ii. Systemic health
    iii. Socioeconomic status

i. Biological Factors

a. Saliva

Saliva plays an important role in modifying the erosive effects of dietary foods and beverages by the following mechanisms:
- Dilution and clearance of an erosive agent from the oral cavity
- Neutralization and buffering of dietary acids
- Formation of a pellicle layer on the surface of enamel which protects it from demineralization by dietary acids while enhancing remineralization by providing calcium, phosphate and fluoride to eroded enamel and dentin.

Both quantity and quality of saliva are known to control the extent of dental erosion. In mouths with decreased salivary flow and buffering capacity, erosion is expected to be higher. It has been suggested that saliva rich in mucin prevents precipitation of calcium phosphate that is beneficial in repairing minor acid injuries to enamel. Effect of compositional variation of saliva on erosion still needs to be explored fully.

b. Acquired Pellicle

Acquired pellicle is a protein-based layer that is rapidly formed on the tooth surface, shortly after its removal by tooth brushing, prophylaxis, or chemical dissolution. This pellicle protects teeth because it acts as a barrier, or a semipermeable membrane, which prevents the direct contact of erosive agents on the tooth surface and serves as reservoir of remineralizing electrolytes. It is important to instruct the patients, not to brush their teeth immediately before consuming acidic food or drink because it removes the acquired pellicle, thus leaving teeth less protected.

c. Tooth Structure

Susceptibility to dental erosion may vary according to each patient, as the developmental pattern of this disease may be influenced by the clinical history of each patient. This different developmental pattern is caused by different situations that can impair or modify the tooth, such as mechanical or chemical processes that include caries, erosion, abrasion, attrition, and abfraction. With regards to tooth composition, exposures to saliva and fluorides have demonstrated effectiveness on the remineralization of eroded enamel. Therefore, a structural difference, such as the formation of fluoroapatite, may influence and modulate the development of dental erosion.

d. Soft Tissues

Oral soft tissues and their movement influence the tooth sites that will contact acidic susbstances and affect clearance of acids in their proximity. Soft tissues may also promote tooth wear. Jarvinen (1992) observed severe erosion on palatal surfaces of teeth touched by tongue.

ii. Behavioral Factors

Behavioral patterns influence the biological response to erosive challenges because they are capable of modifying the oral environment by turning it more or less susceptible to the development of dental erosion. Behavioral aspects influence the intensity, localization and type of erosion lesions.

a. Unhealthy Lifestyles

Alcoholic individuals may be at risk of developing dental erosion due to the symptoms of alcoholism, such as recurrent vomiting and gastrointestinal reflux. The usage of drugs such as "ecstasy" (3,4–methylenedioxymethamphetamine) is known for causing tooth wear. Ecstasy users report symptoms such as dry mouth, hyperthermia, clenching, and grinding even hours after the mental effects of the drugs, indicating that the physical wear may continue for some time after the drug consumption.

b. Healthy Lifestyles

Although it seems to be contradictory that a healthy lifestyle may be linked to a disease, it is important to emphasize that people involved in sports and exercise may be at risk of developing dental erosion due to the consumption of sport drinks, replenishers, fruit juices, and other acidic beverages. Exercise increases the loss of body fluids and may lead to dehydration and a reduction of decreased salivary flow can create a proper condition for the development of dental erosion.

c. Nutritional Habits

The manner and frequency of acidic consumption is a factor of overriding importance. Prolonged contact of an acid with tooth surface increases its damaging potential. Certain agents are used only for short periods, yet an unusual or bizarre habit can modify their risk effects, e.g. a beverage may be swished or rinsed inside the oral cavity before final swallowing (Table 24.10). Habits such as lemon sucking and soft drink swishing expose enamel and dentin to an acidic environment for a longer period of time, which may cause greater demineralization. Phosphoric acid, usually found in soft drinks, is three times more erosive than organic acids. Citric, tartaric, maleic, and lactic acids are examples of organic acids. Citric and maleic acids are predominantly found in fruits and in their derivate products. Tartaric acid is present in grapes and wines. Dental erosion may occur when

Table: 24.10:	The erosion watch strategy for diet analysis and advice for patients with tooth wear (Young 2005)	
Water	Do you drink enough water?	Drink 2.5 litres pure water per day. 2 litres, 2 hours before a game or 1 litre, 1 hour before a game
Acids	Do you drink excess soft or sports drinks containinjg ascorbic, citric or phosphoric acid?	Avoid acid drinks when dehydrated in sports, work or when drugs shut off salivary protection
Taste	Do you eat enough fresh fruits daily?	Eat a piece of fruit with every breakfast to stimulate saliva
Calcium	Are you getting enough calcium in your diet?	Milk, cheese and yoghurt contain calcium and protect teeth against aicds
Health	Do you have a healthy lifestyle and diet?	Healthy lifestyles can be dehydrating. (Excess alcohol is dehydrating and causes gastric acid reflux)
	Do you have a health problem?	Drugs, given for asthma, depression, hypertension, etc. shut off saliva

any of these beverages or foods is abused. Roughness of foods also increases wear of the affected tooth surface. This can be particularly evidenced in lacto-vegetarian diets (healthy and rough foods), which show a greater incidence of erosive lesions. Prevalence rate of erosion lesions in lactovegetarians has shown to be 33.1%.

iii. Chemical Factors

The term "chemical factors" is used to describe parameters inherent to erosive beverages, food, and other products. In erosion, the amount of mineral dissolved from enamel depends upon the pH, buffering effect and the amount of calcium, phosphate and fluoride present in the drink. When there occurs a drop in pH, solubility of enamel apatite increases. At a pH of 3.0, solubility is 75 g/L, which rises sharply to 400 g/L at a pH of 2.5. When the pH is around 4.0, it is possible to counteract enamel dissolution by addition of calcium phosphate to the drink. Below this pH, since the solubility of enamel apatite increases steeply, not much benefit can be expected from calcium phosphate supplementation in counteracting enamel dissolution. Apart from these two factors, the ability of an acidic solution to dissolve enamel apatite depends upon its own capability of maintaining the pH at a lowered level and preventing it from being affected by dissolution of apatite and dilution with saliva. This property of the drink is known as its *buffering effect*. The higher the buffering effect, greater will be the apatite dissolved before neutral pH is reached and dissolution brought to an end. The buffering effect is directly proportional to the concentration of acid in the drink. Therefore, it seems likely that an acidic solution with a high buffering effect in the low phase pH range is more harmful than a solution with similar buffering effect but in the higher pH range.

Modifying Factors of Dental Erosion

i. Systemic Health

Some systemic diseases, such as Sjogren's syndrome; medicines, such as acetylsalicylic acid, diuretics and anti-depressive medicines and therapies that involve irradiation of salivary glands all adversely affect salivary production, thus interfering with the biological protection provided by saliva. Even without excessive exposure to erosive agents, hyposalivation may induce dental erosion.

ii. Knowledge

An awareness of the risks and activity of dental erosion, as well as an understanding of the erosive potential of drinks and foodstuff, is an important aspect in changing the initiation and progression of this disease. Patients who show signs and symptoms of dental erosion are often not aware of, and might be confused about, the erosive characteristics of items of their diet or about any modifying factors their dietary intake might have.

iii. Socioeconomic Status

Socioeconomic status might be linked to many of the previously mentioned factors, such as systemic health and knowledge, and thus indirectly influence development of dental erosion.

Clinical Consequences

Erosion lesions are most of the times observed as broad shallow saucer shaped excavations or depressions present in enamel and/or dentin, but with no sharp line angles and less well defined margins. At times, lesions may even be grooved, wedge shaped or irregular. As the progress of the lesion is very slow and because of the secondary mechanical factors mentioned earlier which act on the eroded areas, highly polished surfaces are produced with time. When the dentin is exposed, tubular calcification frequently occurs and discoloration often is seen. Hypersensitivity may be marked in rapid forms or in lesions where dentin is exposed with no underlying tubular calcification. In some instances caries may supervene and the characteristic features of erosion are lost.

Biological Consequences

i. Decrease in enamel microhardness: The result of constant exposure to erosive agents promotes changes in the physical properties of dental structures. The result of episodic exposure to acidic challenges decreases enamel microhardness, which upon exposure to mechanical forces, makes the dental surface more susceptible to disruption.
ii. Formation of reactionary dentin: The dentin-pulp complex responds to the attacks by producing reactionary dentin and occluding the dentinal tubules in order to compensate for the tissue loss. If the progression of dental erosion surpasses the dentin-pulp complex reparative capacity, there might be some complications, such as toothache, dental sensitivity, pulpal inflammation, pulp necrosis, and periapical lesion.

How Enamel and Dentin React to Attacks by Erosive Agents

Dental erosion is believed to be a result of demineralization of the inorganic matrix of the tooth.

Eroded enamel appears smooth and polished, perikymata on it are usually absent and the eroded area may or may not be discolored. Erosive demineralization of enamel is a centripetal process starting with the partial loss of surface mineral. On the enamel surface, the hydrogen ions or chelating agents start to dissolve the enamel crystal. First, the prism sheath area and then the prism core are dissolved, leaving a honeycomb appearance. Then, fresh and unionized acids will diffuse into the interprismatic areas of enamel and further dissolve the mineral content underneath the surface.

Usually, two erosive phases are seen on enamel. One is 'Manifest erosion' which is actively occurring and appears in micrographs as a hollowed out pitted surface resembling honeycomb. The pits characterize ends of enamel prisms that have been dissolved below the level of inter prismatic matrix. Second is 'Latent erosion' which is in an inactive stage and here the prisms are much less obvious. Manifest erosion is more common than latent erosion and is seen more frequently in females and young individuals.

The initial events in dentin demineralization are similar to those that occur in the enamel. However, because of the high organic content of dentin, diffusion of the demineralizing agents and mineral ions are partially stopped by the organic matrix, which acts as a barrier to acid diffusion and mineral release, thereby reducing the progression of the erosive process. This difference in erosive processes between enamel and dentin does not mean that the erosive process in dentin is slower; on the contrary, the dentin substrate is more susceptible to acid dissolution because its hydroxyapatite crystals are smaller than that of enamel. Thus, there is a large susceptible area for acid attack. Peritubular and intertubular dentin may also be demineralized in a lateral manner from the open tubules.

Recently, the term 'biocorrosion' is being used, which embraces the chemical, biochemical, and electrochemical degradation of tooth substance caused by endogenous/exogenous acids, proteolytic agents as well as the piezoelectric effects. The definition of erosion fails to recognize or account for proteolysis and piezoelectric effects, which respectively are also involved in the degradation of tooth substance which is better defined by the all encompassing term biocorrosion.

In addition, Biocorrosion is regarded as one of three major mechanisms for the development of non carious cervical lesions apart from stress and friction. It is the interplay of these mechanisms along with the modifying factors such as saliva, tongue action, and tooth form etc. that is responsible for the development of abfractions, abrasions and chemo-mechanical degradation of the tooth substance.

ABFRACTION

Abfraction is defined as *'wedge shaped defect in the cervical region of the tooth and is hypothesized to be a result of tensile stresses concentrated in this area consequent to occlusal forces in some remote area.'* The term *'abfraction'* for these lesions was first coined by *Grippo* (1991) to distinguish from abrasion and erosion. A few authors have also termed these lesions as *'idiopathic cervical erosions'*.

It is reported that the tensile stresses have definite role in developing cervical abfraction lesions.

Normally, during mastication, when moving from working side to centric occlusion, lingual slopes of the maxillary cusps contact buccal slopes of the mandibular cusps. This contact serves as an inclined plane and forces are generated perpendicular to the tangents drawn from the respective cusps. When these eccentrically placed lateral forces are resolved into their two components, the vertical component is directed along the long axis of the tooth and is well tolerated because it is compressive in nature, whereas horizontal component is perpendicular to the long axis. In a net result, the transverse force is responsible for creating deflection/flexure in the tooth structure, i.e. the tooth is compressed primarily on the side towards which it is being bent and is subjected to tensile stress on the side away from the direction of bending. For example, in lingually directed forces in a mandibular molar, lingual portion of the tooth is compressed while the buccal portion is stretched, with the fulcrum at the cemento-enamel junction. The region under greatest tensile stress is that closest to the fulcrum, while regions of greatest compressive stress are the occlusal contacts, fulcrum and the apex of the root.

Generally, these forces in ideal occlusion create deflection, which is within the tolerable limits of the tooth. However, the magnitude of transverse force (shown for buccal cusps only in the diagram) (Fig. 24.13) and the consequent bending movement increases with excessive cuspal slope and/or lingual inclination of the mandibular teeth. Also, masticatory forces in individuals with hyper or malocclusion and parafunctional forces in bruxism may expose one or more teeth to strong lateral forces beyond the capacity of the teeth to withstand, resulting in cervical lesions (Fig. 24.14). For example, in dentitions that lack canine disclusion, lateral forces are transmitted to the posterior teeth during excursive movements, thereby raising the chances of developing abfraction lesions. In bruxists, if canine disclusion is absent, the incidence

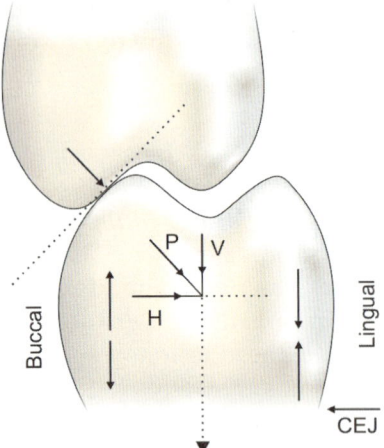

Fig. 24.13: Applied force on a cuspal incline (P) resolved into its vertical (V) and horizontal (H) components produces compression on the lingual side and tension on the buccal side

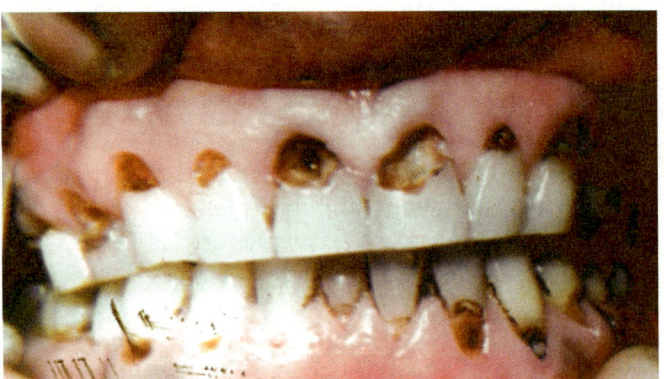

Fig. 24.14: Caries superimposed on abfraction lesions in bruxism

is further increased many fold. Abfraction lesions are mostly seen on the buccal surfaces of mandibular teeth as can be evidenced from the Fig. 24.13, in which the buccal surfaces of maxillary teeth will not be stressed to tension rather will be placed under compression.

How Abfraction Lesions Develop

The masticatory system during function exposes the teeth to three types of stresses: compressive, tensile and shear. As a general rule, both dentin and enamel have high compressive strengths but are relatively weak in tension. Enamel is 35 times stronger while dentin is 7 times stronger in compression than in tension. Even amongst the two, dentin is substantially stronger than enamel in counter-acting tensile stresses. The high resiliency and elasticity of the former enables it to withstand greater deformation without fracture. Comparatively, enamel moves as a rigid unit, is brittle and liable to fracture at small deformation loads. It is made up of three components: a mineral component

hydroxyapatite present in enamel rods, an organic matrix and water, either free or bound. The ability of enamel to withstand stresses depends significantly on the direction of forces in respect to orientation of enamel rods. Forces are best withstood when they are in line with the rods, whereas under tensile forces that tend to pull the rods away from each other, enamel generally surrenders. There occurs disruption of chemical bonds between hydroxyapatite crystals and as bonds are broken, small inter-cystalline spaces are created which allow penetration of water and other molecules. The disrupted crystalline structure is then much more susceptible to chemical dissolution and breakage from physical forces like brushing, compression, tension, mastication and bruxism (Fig. 24.15). It is a known fact that micro-cracks once initiated on the surface of a brittle material are easily propagated hence severely weakening its strength.

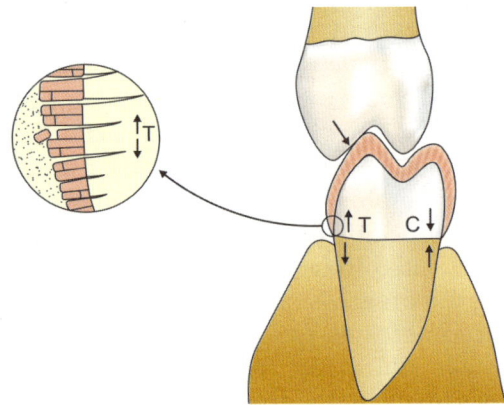

Fig. 24.15: Lateral forces create tension (T) and compression (C) at the cervix as indicated by arrows. In the enlarged section, disrupted bonds between enamel rods are shown

Two other possible mechanisms that contribute to loss of tooth tissue as a consequence of occlusal loading are (1) when a tooth is subject to tension or compression, electric potential gradient is generated between different regions of the tooth. The so called piezo-electric effect may promote loss of tooth substance. (2) The thickness of enamel and dentin varies over the cusps of posterior teeth, causing variation in the contour of dentino-enamel junction. A concavity on the dentino-enamel junction is usually found in the occlusal third of the facial cusps of mandibular premolar teeth and lingual cusps of maxillary premolar teeth. The location of this concavity corresponds to the most common functional location of premolar cervical lesions, i.e. below mandibular functional cusps and above maxillary nonfunctional cusps. When this concavity was eliminated in a finite element analysis of an artificial model, tensile stresses were also eliminated in the corresponding cervical area. This suggested that probably the cuspal contour of dentino-enamel junction had a role to play in determining the amount of stress produced at the cervix.

Characteristics of Abfraction Lesions

A lesion induced as a result of tooth flexure possesses certain characteristics. First, it is at or near the fulcrum. Second, its typical morphology is a wedge shaped lesion with sharp line angles and is the area of greatest tensile stress concentration. Local factors like abrasion, acid erosion, demastication, etc. may modify the shape of lesion but the overall pattern remains wedge shaped. Third, the direction of lateral forces determines the location of lesions, i.e. the number of lesions that can develop on the same tooth depend upon the number of directions of lateral forces, e.g. if there are two differently directed lateral forces acting on the same tooth, the final lesion would be a combination of two lesions generated by each of the two forces (Figs 24.16A and B). Fourth, the size of the lesion is determined by the magnitude and frequency of applied tensile force.

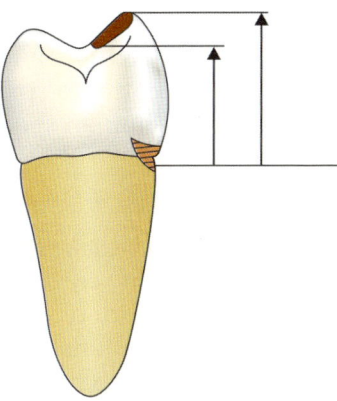

Fig. 24.17: Functioning along a contact plane: magnitude of tensile stress on tooth is a function of distance between applied force and fulcrum

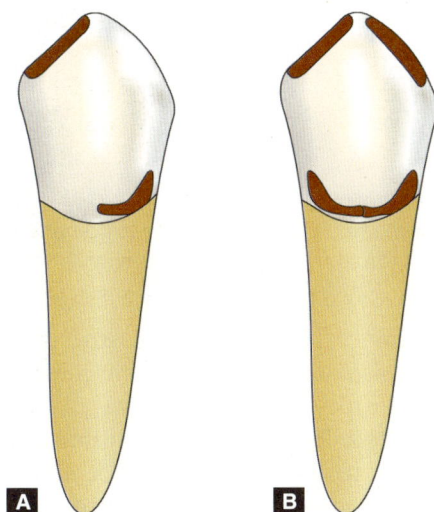

Figs 24.16A and B: (A) Morphology of lesion as dicated by the contact plane (B) Two differently directed lateral forces acting on the same tooth produces a combined lesion

The location of fulcrum determines the exact site of the lesion. For a given lateral force, magnitude of tensile stress is determined by the distance between the applied force and fulcrum. Greater this distance, larger is the tensile stress generated near the fulcrum and therefore larger the region of disruption in this region (Fig. 24.17). Also, it is well known that opposing teeth rarely contact at a single point, instead they usually contact over a surface area. As a consequence, the force is distributed along the contact plane, and the distance of any one point of force from the fulcrum is different from any other point in the plane. This exposes a large area of the tooth to tensile stresses and the lesion so formed is hence dictated by the area of contact.

Arguments Relating to Tooth Flexure Theory

1. Greater prevalence of cervical lesions in older individuals may be because of increased brittleness of enamel and dentin with increasing age which further exacerbates the effects of occlusal forces. Since damage to dental hard tissues is also a function of duration and magnitude of applied force, more lesions are likely to occur at older age.
2. More lesions are seen in bruxers compared to non-bruxers. Bruxism is a likely source of increased occlusal stress. It is reported that 80% of bruxers and 20% non-bruxers suffer from cervical lesions.
3. Increased loss of class V restorations is seen in patients with bruxism, malocclusion or some form of stressful occlusion. Debonding probably occurs because of tensile stresses generated by lateral deformation of teeth.
4. It is questionable as to how periodontal status affects the development of cervical lesions. Alveolar bone loss changes the fulcrum of bending moment causing the lesions to shift more apically. Conversely, loss of periodontal support leading to a high degree of tooth mobility may serve as a protective factor in that instead of flexing at the cemento-enamel junction, the entire tooth moves away from the occlusal force.
5. Likewise, it is not known how presence of restoration could relate to cervical lesions. Amalgam restorations on the occlusal surface are associated with increased cusp flexure and can weaken overall tooth structure. Any factor that decreases the resistance of tooth to withstand stresses probably helps in lesion formation.

6. The theory of tooth flexure in stress cervical lesions seems to explain the development of lesions on isolated or non-adjacent teeth, in subgingival regions, and also in non-human species.

BIOMECHANICS OF A CLASS V CAVITY

The early quotation '*The only known forces which tend to dislodge a well made class V filling are the pulling forces of sticky foods,*' reflected the widely held opinion of dentists that the class V restorations were not exposed to mechanical stresses. Similarly, the extrusion of a class V amalgam restoration was attributed to delayed expansion of amalgam due to water contamination. This hypothesis, however, could not explain all features and was considered incomplete as:

- Extrusion occurred even when rubber dam was used for placement of amalgam.
- Extrusion was commonly seen on the occlusal margin rather than on the wetter gingival margin.
- Extruded restorations were primarily confined to the buccal surfaces of lower premolars and molars.

Since the existing beliefs could not explain certain situations, the role of biomechanical interactions started gaining importance. Gabel was the first to consider the effect of mechanical forces disrupting class V restorations. According to him, when the slopes of the two opposing teeth meet each other in lateral excursive movements, the contact serves as an inclined plane and forces are produced perpendicular to this plane. On resolving this force into its two components: vertical component parallels long axis of the tooth while horizontal component is perpendicular to the long axis. The tooth being more or less firmly held in the alveolus, when subjected to a transverse force, behaves in a manner similar to a cantilever beam. This places one side, i.e. buccal or lingual in tension and the opposite side in compression.

Now, if a class V cavity is cut on the tooth surface, the width of the tooth being subjected to this horizontal force is reduced and as a result more deflection occurs under a given load than when the tooth is uncut. When subsequently a restoration is placed, it is also subjected to similar lateral deflecting forces. If the restoration is placed on the tooth side which is under tension, interface at the occlusal margin tends to open up and a wedge shaped defect is created between the tooth and the restoration (Fig. 24.18). Conversely, if it is placed on the side of the tooth being compressed, it would move out of the cavity because of pressure applied onto it (Fig. 24.19). Confirmation of this stressing effect has been obtained by placing pressure transducers in class V resin restorations in extracted teeth and simultaneously recording the occlusal loading and the response from pressure transducers. Authors have also observed changes in cervicoocclusal diameter of empty class V buccal cavities when occlusally loaded. It has been shown that there exists a minimum cavity size that does not alter the load deformation response of the tooth, but this size has not been quantified.

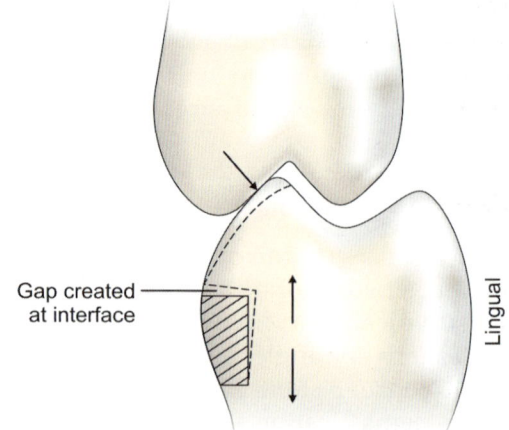

Fig. 24.18: Restoration being subjected to tensile forces and as a result, a gap is created at the interface

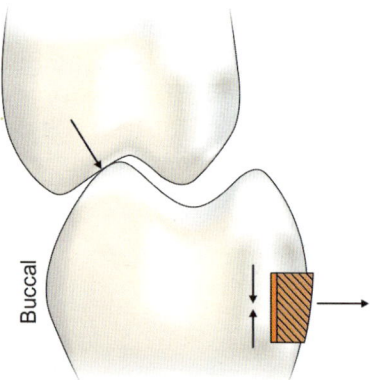

Fig. 24.19: Restoration being subjected to compressive forces and as a result could move out of the cavity

MEASURING TOOTH SUBSTANCE LOSS

The measurement of tooth substance loss has not been documented properly. Only macroscopic changes are quantified which might not be very accurate; however, it provides necessary information of the potential risk of the tooth wear. The methods and the instruments measuring tooth wear are as follows:

a. Measurement in-vitro

Since simulating an environment is difficult, most of the experiments have been carried out in-vitro. The in-vitro examination has the advantage such as variables like exposure time and nature of the agent can be controlled. And also more number of teeth can be involved.

The following are the methods for measuring the loss:

i. Polarized Light Microscopy

Direct viewing under polarized light has been tried as is being carried out for evaluation of caries. This method is useful in obtaining trends of tooth wear.

ii. Microhardness

The technique is employed to assess the hardness of the tooth before and after the erosion. This hardness data is qualitative and may not measure the full extent of the hard tissues loss by erosive attack.

iii. Surface Profilometry

The loss of the tooth material is measured by the surface profilometry by driving the spherical diamond tip onto the specimen. This method can measure the actual depth of the lesion and also the dissolution of the enamel.

iv. Microradiography

The subsurface demineralization of the area along with total mineral loss is being measured by microradiography, which is superior to surface profilometry.

v. Digital Image Analysis

The digital image analysis is useful in calculating the damage to the enamel. This technique is precise and sensitive and can be used both qualitatively and quantitatively. This technique measures the three dimensional loss of the tooth structure.

vi. Scanning Electron Microscope

The casts of the abraded or attritioned teeth are examined under the Scanning Electron Microscope. The impressions can also be examined by these methods. This method is precise, but only comparisons can be carried out at various intervals of time.

b. Measurement in-vivo

The in-vivo measurement of tooth substance loss is difficult since the wear is different at different location.

The examination is carried out inside the oral cavity. Certain indices are available which can give an idea of tooth wear qualitatively. The replicas of the tooth wear and the impressions can be studied under the electron microscope. With the development of Scanning Tunneling Microscope and also the Scanning Probe Microscope, the accurate measurements are becoming reality. The scanning probe microscope has the ability to probe the properties of the variety of materials. The new technology appears to facilitate improved accuracy of measurement, yet the goal of getting the accurate measurement has not been achieved.

TREATMENT OF TOOTH SUBSTANCE LOSS

Proper medical and dental history, which include history of bruxism, clenching, etc. is mandatory prior to treatment. This should be followed by thorough clinical examination both extra-orally and intra-orally.

A. Treatment of Carious Cervical Lesions

Smooth surface lesions in the cervical portion of the teeth are usually easy to detect visibly; but are often overlooked in a routine clinical examination unless the teeth are isolated with cotton rolls and dried with an air syringe and are free of debris. Radiographic diagnosis provides little benefit as the lesions extend bucco-lingually in a direction similar to that of the incident x-rays. The depth of the lesion cannot be ascertained on the radiograph, and also the radiolucency superimposes on the pulp giving the appearance of a pulpal exposure. Management of cervical caries involves institution of the same basic treatment procedures – prevention and restoration. However, depending upon the extent of lesion, i.e. if only superficial, restrict to preventive measures. Such measures may arrest further progress of lesions, at times reverting them to their original state.

Preventive Treatment

Generally, when an individual has caries in the cervical portions of the teeth, it is indicative of a high caries status. The local preventive measures need to be advocated and strictly followed or else the potential for the carious lesion to develop will continue.

Preventive measures include:
a. *Diet modification:* Advice patient to substantially reduce or eliminate sucrose from meals and consume more healthy foods. The sucrose consumed should be limited to meals and in-between snacks be avoided.
b. *Shift oral microbial flora from pathogenic to more of non-pathogenic* by using bactericidal mouth rinses like chlorhexidine, topical fluoride applications and rarely advising antibiotics like vancomycin, tetracyclin, etc.
c. *Periodontal treatment* is carried out to remove the already present deposits on the teeth and allow

for the gingiva to heal. Maintenance of attained oral hygiene standards is carried out by brushing, flossing and other interdental aids.

d. *Modification of the tooth surface*, i.e. increasing the resistance to demineralization and promoting remineralization is carried out by application of topical fluorides. Their continued usage prevents development of new lesions and allows remineralization of initial lesions on affected teeth, by precipitating fluorapatite which is much more resistant to acid attack in place of the highly soluble salts which contain manganese and carbonate.

e. *Stimulating salivary flow* increases its protective benefits; for example, clearing away of substrate and acids and promoting buffering, etc. It is carried out by consuming non-cariogenic food stuffs that require a lot of chewing, or chewing sugarless gum, etc.

Preventive treatment, as mentioned above, may prove beneficial for the lesions that are in their early stages. Incipient caries presenting as a chalky white lesion and where the probe cannot detect any roughness or break on the surface, may be treated by preventive measures. An affected enamel surface where the break or roughness extends only superficially can also be treated by smoothening with sandpaper discs, polishing and treating with a fluoride preparation.

Restorative Treatment

Once the caries has progressed sufficiently into enamel and beyond the dentino-enamel junction, preventive measures alone become ineffective. It becomes essential to clinically remove the infected area from the tooth and replace it with an adequate restoration. Combined preventive and restorative treatments are advised in such cases. In cases like rampant caries and radiation induced xerostomia, etc. where multiple acute caries lesions are rapidly progressing, treatment needs to be given on an emergency basis known as 'caries control'. This includes removing infected tooth structure, preferably at a single appointment, and restoring the defects with temporary restorations. Most of the infecting organisms are removed with this technique and further lesion formation is prevented. The caries control regime must be accompanied by previously discussed preventive measures, which further reduce and prevent micro-organism build up. Strict dietary counseling, intensive oral hygiene training and antibiotic cover is a must for such patients. Subsequently, the temporary restorations are replaced by permanent ones if adequate pulpal responses are obtained.

B. Treatment of Non-carious Cervical Lesions

The first and the foremost step in treatment of noncarious cervical lesions is a careful consideration of the etiology and progression of the condition. A correct diagnosis is prerequisite for management of these lesions. A detailed history should be taken comprising of the following aspects: dietary habits, gastric disturbances, acidic mouth taste, drugs, radiotherapy, salivary gland dysfunction, work related exposure to acidic environments, parafunctional habits, oral hygiene methods, etc. Dietary interviews are frequently insufficient as the patient himself may not be aware of the acidic consumption factors. To overcome this, the patients may be asked to maintain a diary noting the complete dietary intake for at least five consecutive days including a weekend and record the time, quality and quantity of all foods and beverages. Occlusion should be checked and a record of the study models made to monitor progression of lesions. After a thorough evaluation has been conducted, management is carried out in two phases, i.e. preventive and restorative. A brief overview of characteristics of different lesion is presented in Table 24.11.

Table 24.11: Characteristics of different cervical lesions

	Erosion	Abrasion	Abfraction
Location	Lingual or facial	Facial	Facial
Shape	U or dish shaped shallow	Wedged, notched or grooved	Single or overlapping wedge shape lesions
Margins	Smooth	Sharp	Sharp
Enamel surface	Smooth, may be polished	Smooth, may be scratched	Rough in initial stages, may have corrugated appearance

a. Preventive Aspects

The etiologic factors should first be removed. It cannot undo the damage already done but prevents development of fresh lesions and arrest the progress of old ones.

The preventive aspects include:

i. General Preventive Measures

Since constitutional disturbances are occasionally a factor in causing dental erosion, lesions because of these cannot be entirely prevented but definitely reduced by regulation of diet, exercise, fresh air, massage, administration of sodium bicarbonate (0.75–2.0 gms) thrice a day, etc. Plenty of plain water should be consumed.

ii. Local Preventive Measures

- Use soft tooth brushes along with low abrasive toothpastes and better techniques utilizing less force.
- Avoid ill fitting metal clasps.
- Manage parafunctional habits.
- Correct malocclusion.
- Regulate frequency of consumption of acid foods and beverages.
- Restrict acid foods to main meals.
- 'Drink only'; do not sip or swish acid beverages.
- Do not brush immediately following an acid intake.
- Use neutral pH fluoride mouth rinses daily.
- Relieve traumatic occlusion
- Enhance defense mechanism of the body by increasing salivary flow; for example, by chewing sugar free chewing gum.
- Enhance acid resistance and remineralization potential by topical fluoride agents.

The protective layer formed by the topical fluoride agents used in routine (sodium fluoride, strontium fluoride and acidulated phosphate fluoride) is not acid resistant and susceptible to acid attack. Recently, titaniumfluoride is being used to prevent erosive lesions and acts as a remineralizing agent.

Titanium tetrafluoride provides physical protection due to the formation of a glaze on the tooth surfaces, and chemical protection due to the reaction of fluoride with the tooth tissues. Different theories have been put forward for the chemistry of the glaze. Mundorff, et al (1972) suggested the involvement of organometallic complexes of titanium and organic material in enamel. Alternatively, the glaze could result from the formation of TiO_2 (Wei, et al., 1976). TiF_4 has been shown to reduce enamel solubility and enables high fluoride uptake. TiF_4 solutions of 1–4% (pH approx. 1) have been shown to reduce dental erosion.

Another, remineralizing agent casein is also recognized to prevent erosive lesions. Casein is the collective name for the caseinates, which comprises 70–80% of the total protein content. They consist of three subfractions, α-, β- and κ-casein, in the ratio of 8:6:1. The main physiological function of the caseins in milk is to stabilize calcium phosphate by forming micelles, proteins adhered to the enamel surface to form a protective layer which inhibits dissolution. There are a number of possible ways in which the protein layer could be protective against erosion. First, it could simply be physical, blocking access of H^+ ions to the enamel surface and preventing detachment of Ca^{2+} and PO_4^{3-} ions. If this is the case, the impact on dissolution may depend on the crystal face(s) to which the protein adsorbs. Second, it could act as a buffer. A number of the amino acid sequences found in the proteins (Phosphoserine, histidine, glutamate and aspartate) have H^+ accepting groups, and so when the proteins are bound to the enamel surface, they could act as a buffer, increasing the pH at the enamel surface. Any buffering effect is likely to diminish quickly, however, due to the small amount of adherent protein compared to the volume of acid. Thirdly, the adsorbed protein layer could act as an ion-retarding membrane, restricting the access of certain ions and allowing others to pass through, much like 'permselectivity' of the salivary pellicle. It is possible that a combination of buffering and 'permselectivity' is occurring here.

If a specific etiology can be ruled out, preventive measures pertaining to that particular cause are instituted. But generally, a multifactorial etiology is behind the lesion and a combination of measures are recommended.

Patients with non-carious cervical lesions also commonly complain of dentin sensitivity to both physical (cold, airblast, scratch) and hyper-osmotic (glucose solution) stimulation. This should be simultaneously treated by using desensitizing toothpastes, burnishing dentin with fluorides and applying bonding agents, etc.

Defects that may be left unrestored are superficial lesions whose sensitivity can be controlled with no evidence of soft tissue damage and there is affirmation that preventive treatment will prevent any further progress. The outcome of treatment should be monitored at regular intervals and in case the lesions increase in dimensions, it is most likely because of a missed or faulty diagnosis. Further attempts for arriving at a correct diagnosis are made. If unsuccessful, may be because of idiopathic factors or unable to eliminate the cause entirely, restoration should be considered.

b. Restorative Aspect

Prior to restoration the following factors should be considered:

i. *Structural integrity of the tooth*: If the notched/affected area is large/deep, strength of the root at the cervix is lessened. Bonded restoration is indicated in such cases.

ii. *Pulp Protection*: When the lesion is quite deep, endangering the vitality of pulp, pulp capping procedures should be carried out.

iii. *Sensitivity*: When sensitivity continues to exist despite use of desensitizing conservative treatments, lesions should be filled.

iv. *Esthetics*: Esthetics should be considered before planning restoration of these lesions.

- v. *Gingival health*: If the lesion seems to irritate the gingival tissue, the defect should be restored maintaining the gingival health.
- vi. *Caries*: If caries supervenes the lesion, it should be restored, unless it is incipient/superficial and can be treated by preventive measures alone.
- vii. *Presence of removable partial denture*: If the location of the lesion interferes with the design of removable partial denture, restoration is indicated.

Traditionally, non-carious cervical lesions were restored by preparing class V cavities and filling with amalgam, gold, porcelain and glass-ionomer, etc. All these materials have some disadvantages and generally require removal of moderate amounts of remaining tooth structure. With the advent of adhesive materials, the need for preparing a cavity has long been overcome and conservative treatments, which utilize bonding for retention are becoming popular. Materials having adhesion potential are composites, compomers, glass-ionomers, resin modified glass-ionomers and a combination of glass-ionomer and composite in sandwich technique. An important property desired of any restoration placed in non-carious cervical lesions is that it should be able to withstand degradation due to erosive attacks and toothbrush abrasion. Before the placement of any of these adhesive materials in the lesion, the principles of bonding dictate removal of contaminants from the surface such that a close union between the adhesive and the substrate is obtained. No smear layer will be present on un-instrumented lesions, but often adhesions in the form of bacterial plaque and food debris are present. These are removed with a slurry of pumice and water in a soft rubber cup. Pumice pastes shall not be used, as glycerin layer left on the surface could prevent proper etching of the cavity and wetting by the restorative material.

Restoration with composite resins offers the advantage of best esthetics and excellent mechanical attachment to etched enamel. Disadvantages include exacting and tedious placement, as well as doubtful long term bonding to dentin and cementum. Composites utilize the *'acid etch technique'* for mechanical bonding to enamel as a basis of their retention, eliminating the need for additional retentive aids. A layer of intervening enamel bonding agent may be employed to ensure good wetting and resin tag formation to etched enamel. For adhesion to dentin and cementum, dentin bonding agents are used. In a lesion that is surrounded by enamel on all sides, an adequate marginal seal is likely to be expected. But this is almost never the case and generally enamel is present only on the occlusal margins. The gingival margin either lacks enamel, being comprised of dentin and cementum, or the enamel is so thin that it serves no significant purpose in bonding. Since bonding to dentin or cementum is not as efficient as to enamel, microleakage and loss of retention is likely to occur at the gingival margin.

No instrumentation is desired in the non-carious cervical lesions when restoring with composite. It is demonstrated that V-shaped cavities are preferable over box shaped cavities as in the former the volume/area ratio is less and hence the amount of polymerization shrinkage of composite and subsequent gap formation is reduced. Since most of these cervical lesions are notched or V-shaped, the need for converting them into box shaped cavities is not required. A small amount of instrumentation may however be done on the incisal or occlusal margins with a tapering fissure bur to create a bevel on the enamel. This exposes enamel rod ends rather than lateral surfaces to the etching solution thereby improving retention. Placement of bevel is, however, controversial. Certain authors recommend placement of bevel while others have shown no differences between bevelled and non-bevelled interfaces. Improving retention at the non-enamel (gingival) margins of a class V cavity by placing slight undercut in dentin with a round bur can be considered. A groove additionally resists the effects of polymerization shrinkage and tooth flexure, hence increasing resistance to microleakage. This again is controversial as it is suggested that use of dentin bonding agents can provide sufficient retention, but their long term stability needs to be ascertained.

Prior to the restoration procedure, composite resin that best matches the tooth color is chosen. The tooth is isolated with a rubber dam or cotton rolls. Usually microfilled composite resins are selected as they provide the best surface smoothness and are more yielding compared to their counterparts. Increased flexibility allows the restoration to better counteract the effects of tooth flexure resulting from eccentric occlusal stresses. Matrix band is not used when restoring the class V cavity as the contour is controlled during insertion of material. After isolation has been attained, etching and conditioning/priming is done according to the manufacturer's instructions and a bonding agent applied and cured. Composite resin is then inserted with a hand instrument or a syringe. Incremental placement reduces the amount of polymerization shrinkage, with the first increment preferably being placed above the gingival margin. Subsequent increments are placed to fill the preparation and in the final increment, the contour of the tooth is established. Care should be taken to prevent material from overhanging the margins and should properly flush with the surrounding tooth. In deep cavities a suitable base of calcium hydroxide or glass-ionomer is given. The final restoration is finished and polished (Figs 24.20A, B).

Restoration with glass-ionomer offers the advantages of adhesion to enamel and dentin in wet environments and release of fluorides on a long term basis. Disadvantages include long time required to achieve maturity and less than adequate esthetics. Glass-ionomers adhere to the tooth surface through hydrogen and ionic bonding and hence mechanical retention is not required. Also, in the science of adhesion, union between two materials is best obtained in the presence of perfectly smooth surfaces with opposing polarity. Non-carious cervical lesions have surfaces that are usually very smooth and hence need not be instrumented. In addition, the dentinal tubules are closed to large extent by sclerosis thus minimizing the usual outward dentinal flow. The only instrumentation that has been suggested in non-carious cervical lesions is creating 0.5–1.0 mm deep finishing line on enamel margins to improve edge strength, and giving undercuts in dentin for retention. However, the role of both these features is controversial.

After the tooth surface has been cleaned off the adherent contaminants by pumice slurry in a rubber cup; conditioning with 10% polyacrylic acid may be carried out to enhance the wetting ability by forming hydrogen bonds with dentin and improving ionic exchange with the cement. Acid should not be applied for more than 10–15 seconds, as even low concentrations have an etching effect on enamel and could deprive it of calcium and phosphate ions. The surface is then washed thoroughly and dried. Since water is an important component in ionic exchange, the tooth should not be unduly dehydrated. Any traces of polyacrylic acid left on the surface are not harmful as the reaction liquid is polyacrylic acid itself.

Placement of cement under moderate pressure is desirable to ensure optimum adaptation of the cement to the underlying tooth structure. For this, a preformed soft tin matrix is recommended. Before mixing, a matrix of suitable size and shape is selected and curved slightly to confirm to the contour of the tooth. The material is inserted into the lesion either with a hand instrument or by a syringe and the matrix held in position until the cement shows an initial set. In certain cases the contour attained is such that no further adjustments are needed and the high gloss is retained. The restoration surface in its initial stages of setting is protected by applying cavity varnish or light cure resin bonding agents. Only gross excess at the margins should be removed at this appointment. The restoration is finally contoured and polished after at least one day and if possible after one week (Figs 24.21A, B and 24.22A, B).

Restorations with combined glass-ionomer and composite referred to as the '*sandwich or the laminate*

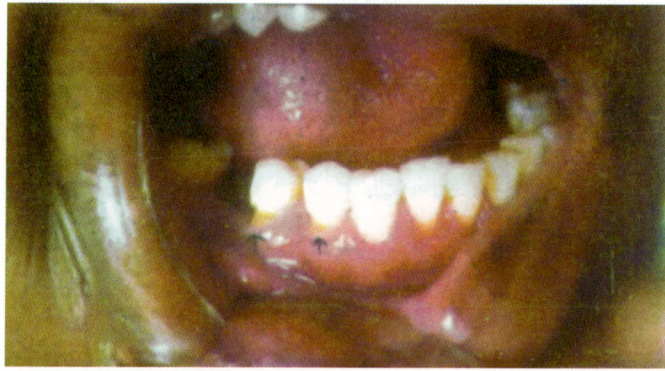

Fig. 24.20A: Abfraction lesions on right mandibular first and second premolars (pre-operative)

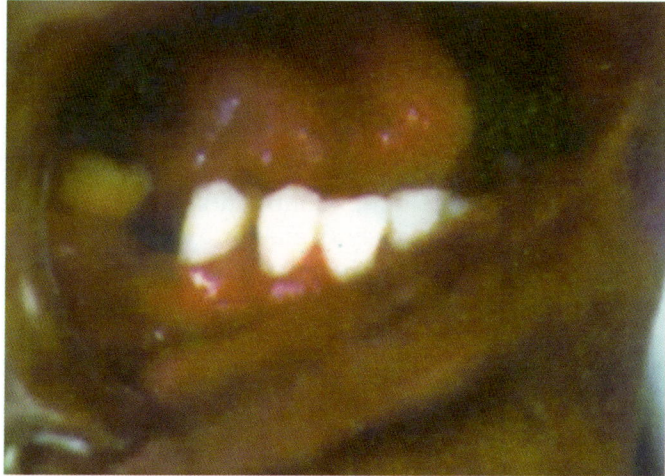

Fig. 24.20B: Restored abfraction lesions on right mandibular first and second premolars (post-operative)

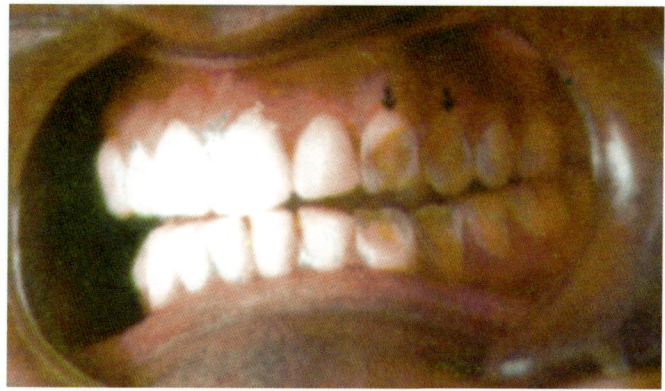

Fig. 24.21A: Erosion lesions on left maxillary canine and first premolar, and mandibular canine and premolars (pre-operative)

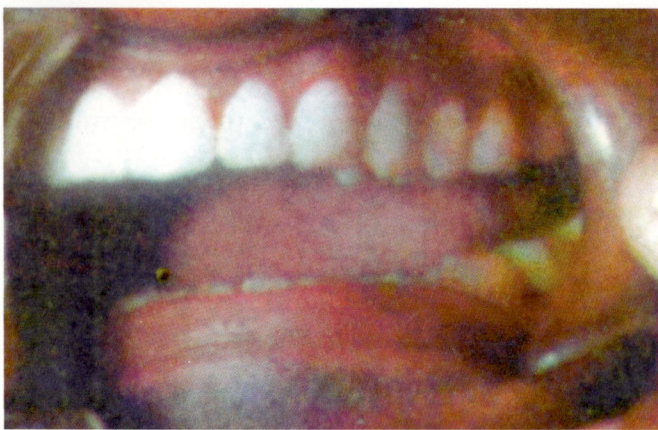

Fig. 24.21B: Restored erosion lesions on left maxillary canine and first premolar (post-operative)

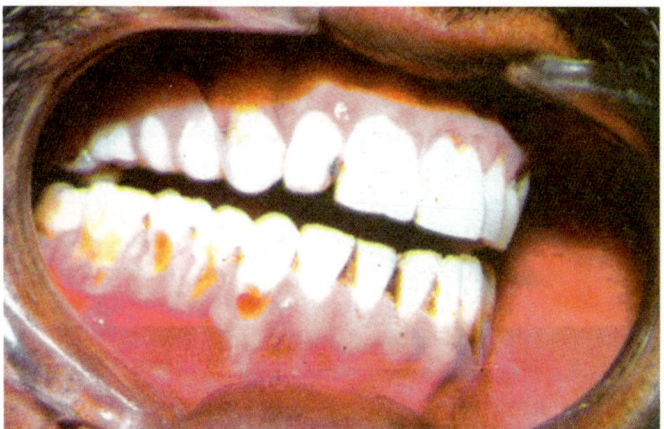

Fig. 24.22A: Abrasion lesions on mandibular right canine, first premolars and second premolars (pre-operative)

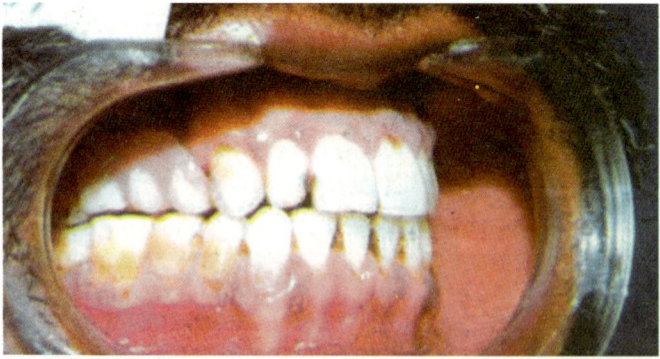

Fig. 24.22B: Restored abrasion lesions on mandibular right canine, first premolar and second premolar (post-operative)

technique' offer advantages of both the materials. Glass ionomer serves as a dentin replacement and provides chemical adhesion to the underlying tooth structure, where as composite provides control of contour and esthetics. The weak link in the dentin glass-ionomer-composite bond is usually the glass-ionomer cement itself, i.e. failure is generally cohesive in nature. This necessitates use of stronger glass-ionomer cements in adequate thickness. Type II restorative glass-ionomer cements fulfill the need for high strengths and also have a degree of translucency and color, thus minimizing the 'shine through' when veneered with a relatively translucent microfilled composite.

The lesion is modified by placing an undercut on non-enamel margins. Glass-ionomer cement is placed in the lesion using the above mentioned technique. If accurate color assessment is difficult, any further manipulation is delayed for at least a day to allow the cement to attain a high degree of maturity and final color characteristics. The tooth is then properly isolated with a rubber dam. Glass-ionomer cement is reduced using fine diamond burs under heavy air/water spray to expose the entire enamel margin and lightly bevel it. Cement should be reduced sufficiently enough to allow adequate room for composite resin. Do not expose the dentin, and leave about 1.0 mm of cement untouched at the gingival margin. This is followed by etching of the cement surface as well as the enamel margin with 37% orthophosphoric acid for 10–15 seconds. Wash thoroughly and dry lightly. Do not 'over-dry' as the glass-ionomer cement is still susceptible to dehydration and could result in crazing and cracking. Apply a thin layer of light activated low viscosity enamel bonding agent because of its superior qualities. Insert composite resin in bulk if lesion is small or in increments if lesion is large. The first increment is preferably placed at the enamel margin because this will be the strongest union. The restoration is then finally contoured and polished. Differences between the two materials on the surface should be recognized while finishing and polishing and care should be taken to avoid damaging the cement.

Light cured glass-ionomers are another possible alternative for restoration of non-carious cervical lesions. They overcome the disadvantages of conventional glass-ionomers in that they show a rapid initial set and hence are less sensitive to moisture contamination. Their properties are often between those of true glass-ionomers and compomers. Light cured glass-ionomers present with improved handling characteristics, but initial contraction towards light may be a disadvantage. Fortunately, expansion due to water uptake by the resin could compensate for the initial resin shrinkage to a little extent. Similar to the composite materials, the bond strength to dentin can be substantially improved by conditioning and priming. In sandwich restorations, resin modified glass-ionomers can be considered as these provide chemical attachment to the overlying composite resin compared to conventional glass-ionomers which provide only mechanical attachment.

Polyacid modified composites, i.e. compomers can also be used for restoration of non-carious cervical lesions. Their restoration process is similar to that for composite resins.

The management of generalized tooth wear, localized anterior tooth wear and localized posterior tooth wear is summarized in Figs 24.23, 24.24 and 24.25 respectively.

Cervical lesions continue to be a matter of great concern especially as more and more teeth are being retained in the older age and there is increased incidence and severity of lesions experienced. The multifactorial etiology has made the recognition of causal factors in individual patients quite problematic and thereby the prevention and treatment of these lesions has also remained haphazard. Adequate

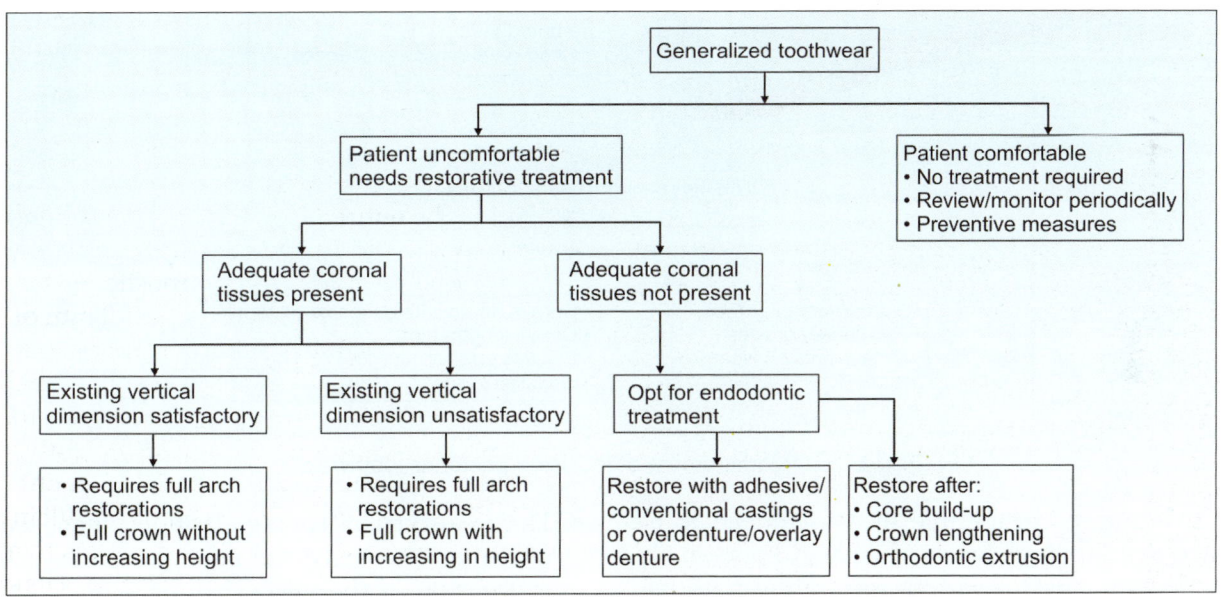

Fig. 24.23: Management of generalized toothwear

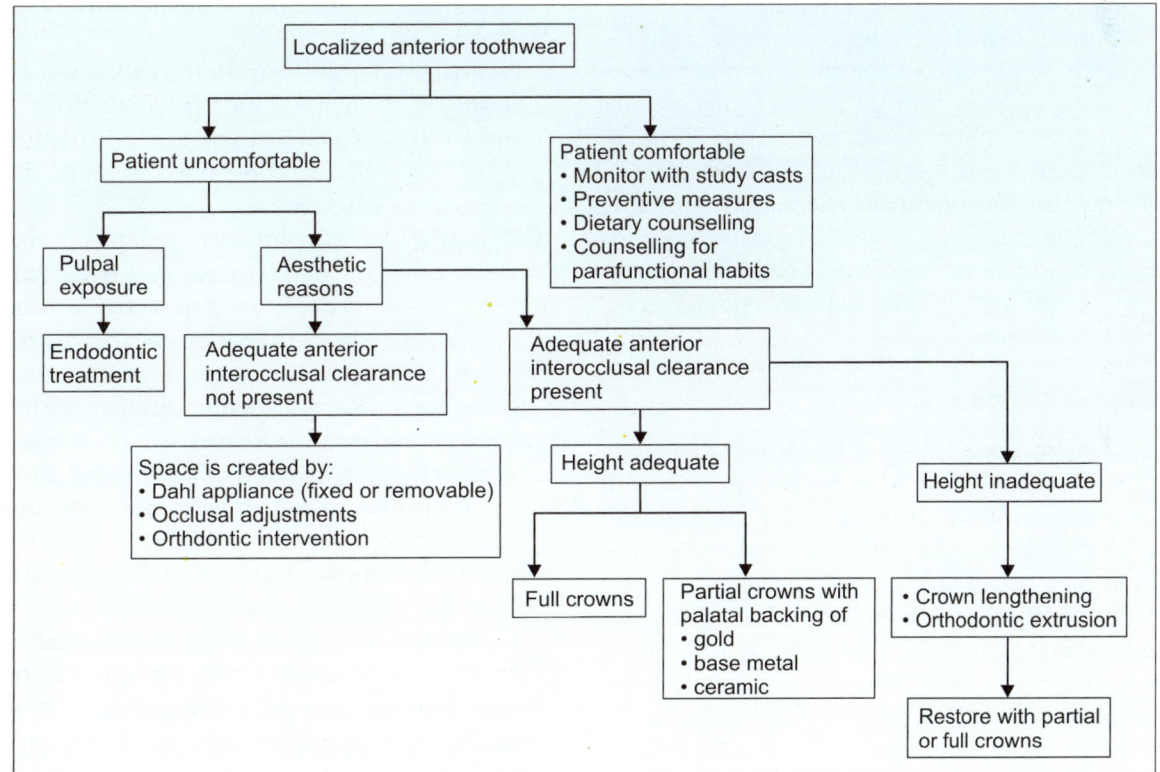

Fig. 24.24: Management of localized anterior toothwear

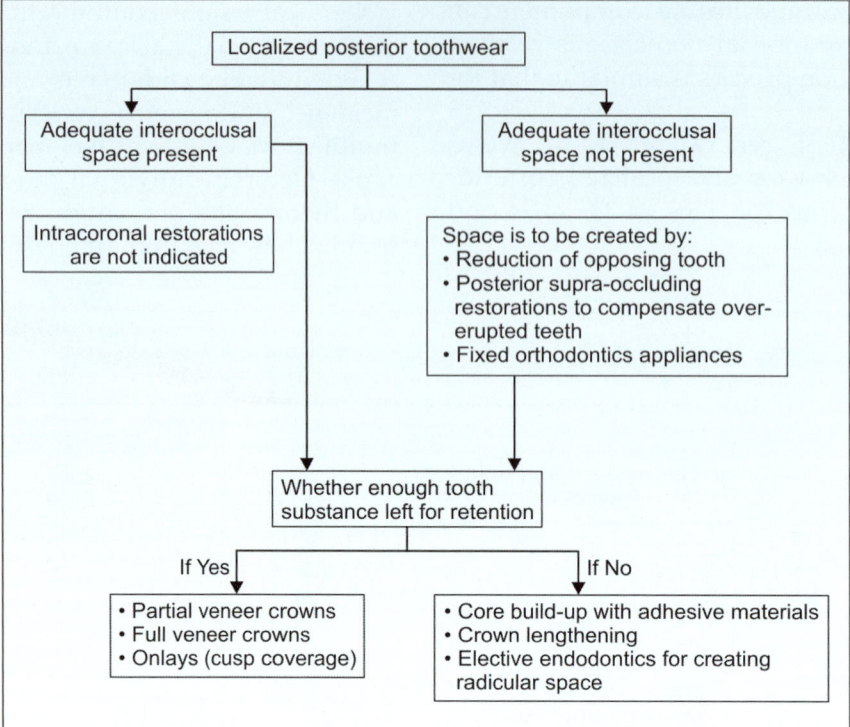

Fig. 24.25: Management of localized posterior toothwear

preventive and/or restorative measures need to be instituted to attain high levels of success. I personally believe that amongst the various restorative materials that have been discussed here, glass-ionomers are the best choice for restoration of cervical lesions. Resin modified glass-ionomers and polyacid modified composites still require extensive research to determine their long term durability as restorative materials. Also, in non-carious cervical lesions, a minimal amount of instrumentation in the form of bevels and retentive grooves should be carried out.

Though most of the retention is a function of the bonding between adhesive restorative material and tooth structure, additional undercuts or grooves will do no harm but definitely add to mechanical retention, yet being conservative.

C. Treatment of Attrition

- Normal attrition requires no treatment because formation of secondary dentin, tooth eruption and alveolar bone growth compensates for the occlusal attrition (physiologic) cementum may also be associated as a compensatory mechanism.
- When the attrition becomes pathologic, where it progresses fast, there can be loss of posterior support, malocclusion, bruxism, difficulty in mastication, pain in TMJ and/or total collapse of occlusion. In such instances occlusal adjustment and splint therapy may be indicated for the remaining dentition.
- The treatment of severe attrition where teeth are worn to the gingival margins, may require restoration of the vertical dimension to improve function and esthetics. Treatment options include extraction of affected teeth and replacement with conventional dentures, overdentures and overlay prosthesis, etc.

Treatment depends upon the following categories:

Category I: Appearance is satisfactory

Category II: Appearance is unsatisfactory and there is no need to raise the vertical height

Category III: Appearance is unsatisfactory but there is need to raise the vertical height, which in turn depends on the availability of space, whether it is present or needs to be created.

Category I (Appearance is satisfactory)
A. Counselling is required in patients with parafunctional habits. Habit breaking appliance should be given in patients with bruxism or clenching.
B. Conventional Restorative Treatment
  - Exposed pits are filled (Figs 24.26A, B)
  - Occlusal disharmony is corrected
  - Consideration to be given to crown lengthening procedure (Fig. 24.27)

Monitoring of such cases can be carried out by taking silicone rubber impressions every three months and evaluating the casts under microscope.

Category II (Appearance is unsatisfactory but there is no need to raise the vertical height).

- Teeth are restored, preferably with all ceramic crowns or laminates. The crowns can manage occlusal attrition as well as fractured cusps (Figs 24.28A, B)
- Occlusal guard for protection against nocdurnal clenching like bleaching trays, etc.

Category III (Appearance is unsatisfactory and there is a need to raise the vertical height) (Figs 24.29A, B).

- Generalized increase in vertical height is required.
- Orthodontic tooth movement can be used for over-eruption of posterior teeth creating space for the anterior teeth.
- Space has to be utilized in retruded cusp position (RCP) and intercuspal position (ICP).

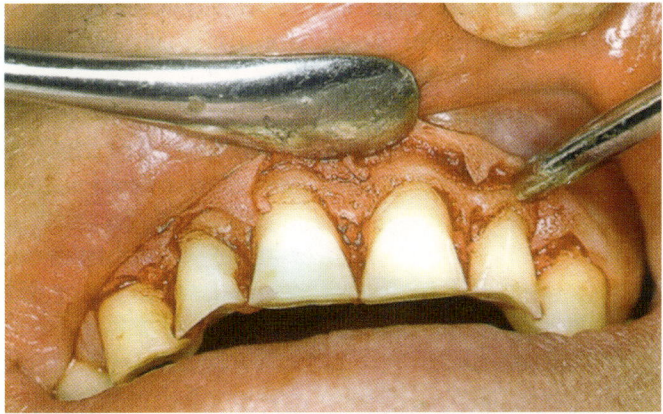

Fig. 24.27: Crown lengthening

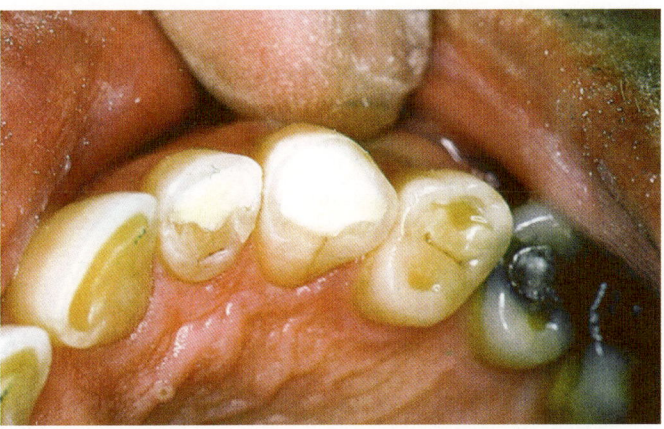

Fig. 24.26A: Incisal surface filled with glass-ionomer cement

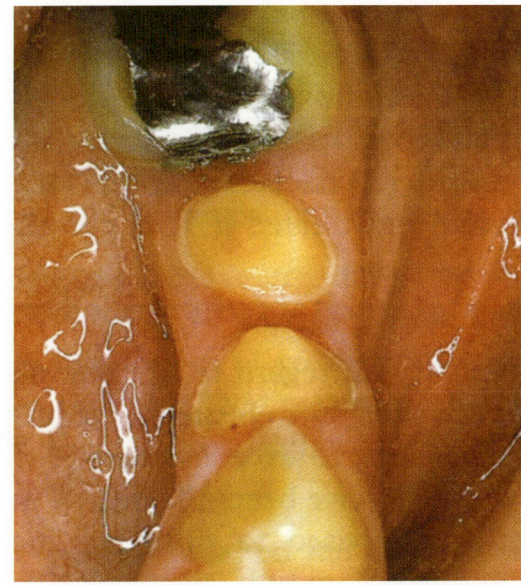

Fig. 24.28A: Tooth preparation for full crowns

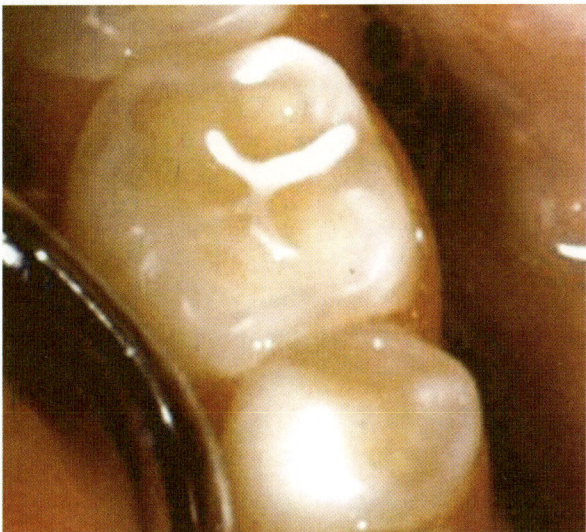

Fig. 24.26B: Occlusal pits filled with glass-ionomer cements

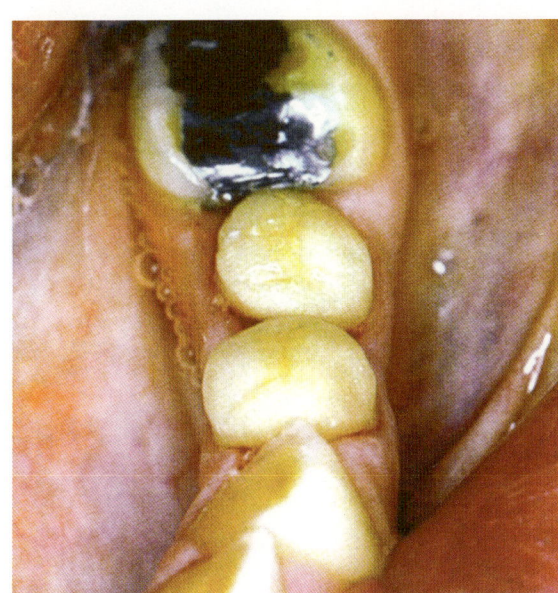

Fig. 24.28B: Crowns restored

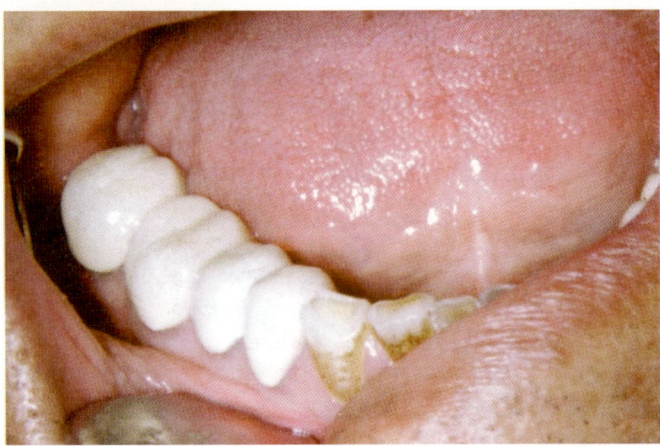

Fig. 24.29A: Raising vertical height, showing one side

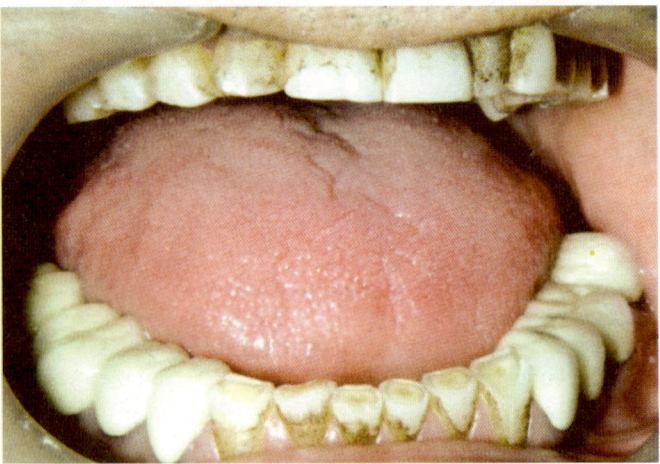

Fig. 24.29B: Raising vertical height, showing both sides

Dahl Concept

It is a method of gaining space in cases of localized tooth wear, where there is insufficient space available in either centric occlusion or centric relation. It refers to the relative axial movement that is observed to occur when a localized appliance or localized restoration is placed in supra-occlusion and occlusion re-establishes full arch contacts over a period of time. It was reported by Dahl and Krungstad that inter-occlusal space created occurs through a process of combined intrusion (40%) and extrusion (60%). Most of the cases re-establish occlusal contacts within 4–6 months but may take up to a period of 18–24 months in some cases.

Points to Remember

- No occlusal cutting; only spicules need to be removed or filled.
- No disturbance of inter-dental col area.
- Retention of the prosthesis is achieved by surface area.
- Buccal and lingual reduction takes care of periodontal health

BIBLIOGRAPHY

1. Abrahamsen, T.C.: The worn dentition – pathognomonic paterns of abrasion and erosion. Int. Dent. J.: 55, 268, 2005.
2. Bader, J.D., Levitch, L.C. and Shugars, D.A.: Dentist's classification and treatment of cervical lesions. J.A.D.A.: 124, 46, 1993.
3. Bardsley, P.F.: The evolution of tooth wear indices. Clin. Oral Invest.: 12, 15, 2008.
4. Bartlett, D., Gans, C. and Lussi, A.: Basic erosive wear examination (BEWE) L try a new scoring system for scientific and clinical needs. Clin. Oral Invest.: 12, 65, 2008.
5. Bartlett, D.W.: The role of erosion in tooth wear: aetiology, prevention and management. Int. Dent. J.: 55, 277, 2005.
6. Bartlett, D.: A proposed system for screening tooth wear. Br. Dent. J.: 208, 207, 2010.
7. Berry, D.C. and People, D.F.G.: Attrition: Possible mechanism of compensation. J. Oral Rehab.: 3, 201, 1976.
8. Blunck, U.: Improving cervical restorations: A review of material and technique. J. Adhes. Dent.: 3, 33, 2001.
9. Braem, M., Lambrechts, P. and Vanherle, G.: Stress induced cervical lesions. J. Prosth. Dent.: 67, 718, 1992.
10. Eccles, J.D.: Dental erosion of non-industrial origin: a clinical survey and classification. J. Prosthet. Dent.: 42, 649, 1979.
11. Gallien, G.S., Kaplan, I. and Owens, B.M.: A review of noncarious dental cervical lesions. Compend. Cont. Educ. Dent.: 16, 552, 1994.
12. Gallo, J.R. Burgess, J.O., Ripps, A.H., Walker, R.S., Ireland, E.J. and Mercantle, D.E.: Three year clinical evaluation of a compomer and a rest composite as class V filling materials. Oper. Dent.: 30, 275, 2005.
13. Gandara, B.K. and Truelove, E.L.: Diagnosis and Management of Dental erosion. J. Contemp. Dent. Practice: 1, 1, 1999.
14. Grippo, J.O.: Abfraction: a new classification of hard tissue lesions of teeth. J. Esth. Dent.: 3, 14, 1991.
15. Hattab, F.N. and Yassin, O.M.: Etiology and diagnosis of tooth wear: A literature review and presentation of selected cases. Int. J. Prosthod.: 13, 101, 2001.
16. Hemingway, C.A., White, A.J., Shelhi, R.P., Addy, M., Parker, D.M. and Barbour, M.E.: Enamel erosion in dietary acids: Inhibition by food proteins in vitro. Caries Res.: 44, 525, 2010.
17. Hong, F.L., Nu, Z.Y. and Xie, X.M.: Clinical classification and therapeutic design of dental cervical abrasion. Gerodontics: 4, 101, 1988.
18. Hood, J.A.A.: Biomechanics of the intact, prepared and restored teeth: some clinical implications. Int. Dent. J.: 41, 25, 1991.
19. Jaeggi, T., Gurninger, A. and Lussi, A.: Restorative therapy of erosion. Monog. Oral Sci.: 20, 200, 2006.
20. Jager D.H.J, Vissinik A., Timmer C.J., Bronkhorst E., Viera A.M. and Huysmans M.C.D.N.J.M: Reduction of erosion by protein-containing toothpastes. Caries Research 47, 135, 2013.

21. Johansson, A., Omar, R. and Carlsson, G.E.: Bruxism and prosthetic treatments: a critical review. J. Prosth. Rest.: 55, 127, 2011.
22. Knewitz, J.L. and Drisko, C.L.: Anorexia nervosa and bulimia: a review. Compend. Contin. Educ. Dent.: 9, 244, 1988.
23. Lussi, A., Jaeggi, T. and Zero, D.: The role of diet in the aetiology of dental erosion. Caries Res.: 38, 34, 2004.
24. Lussi, A., Schuleter, N., Rakhmatullina, E. and Ganss, C.: Dental erosion – an overview with emphasis on chemical and histopathological aspects. Caries Res.: 45, 2, 2011.
25. Mehta, S.B., Banerji, S., Millar, B.J. and Saweez-Feito, J.M.: Current concepts on the management of tooth wear: Part I. Assessment, treatment planning and strategies for the prevention and the passive management of tooth wear. Br. Dent. J.: 212, 17, 2012.
26. Mehta, S.B., Banerji, S., Millar, B.J. and Saweez-Feito, J.M.: Current concepts on the management of tooth wear: Part II. Active restorative care 1: the management of localized tooth wear. Br. Dent. J.: 212, 73, 2012.
27. Mehta, S.B., Banerji, S., Millar, B.J. and Saweez-Feito, J.M.: Current concepts on the management of tooth wear: Part III. Active restorative care 2. The management of generalized tooth wear. Br. Dent. J.: 212, 121, 2012.
28. Michael, J.A., Kaidonis, J.A. and Townsand, G.C.: Non carious cervical lesions on permanent anterior teeth: a new morphological classification. Aust. Dent. J.: 55, 134, 2010.
29. Milosevic, A.: Toothwear: Aetiology and presentation. Dent. Update: 25, 6, 1998.
30. Owen, B.M. and Gallien, G.S.: Non-carious dental 'abfraction' lesions in an aging population. Comped. Cont. Educ. Dent.: 16, 552, 1995.
31. Rees, J.S. and Jagger, D.C.: Abfraction lesion: Myth or Reality? J. Esthet. Dent.: 15, 263, 2003.
32. Sakoolnamarka, R., Burrow, M.F., Praver, S. and Tyas, M.J.: Raman spectroscopic study of non-carious cervical lesions. Odontology: 93, 35, 2005.
33. Schlueter, N., Gauss, C., De Sanctis, S. and Klimek, J.: Evaluation of a profilometric method for monitoring erosive tooth wear. Eur. J. Oral Sci.: 113, 505, 2005.
34. Shipley, S., Taylor, K. and Mitchell, W.: Identifying causes of dental erosion. Gen. Dent.: 53, 75, 2005.
35. Sikri, P. and Sikri, V.: Prevalence, classification and management of cervical abrasions. ISP Bulletin: 17, 1992.
36. Smith, B.G. and Knight, J.K.: An index for measuring the wear of teeth. B.D.J.: 156, 435, 1984.
37. Vailati, F. and Belser, U.C.: Classification and treatment of the anterior maxillary dentition affected by dental erosion: the ACE classification. Int. J. Periodontics and Restorative Dentistry: 30, 55, 2010.
38. VanDisken, J.W.: Durability of here simplified adhesive systems in class V non-carious cervical dentin lesions. Am. J. Dent.: 17, 27, 2004.
39. Wang, X. and Lussi, A.: Assessment and management of dental erosion. Dent. Cl. North Am.: 54, 565, 2010.
40. Wiegand, A. and Attin, J. Influence of fluoride on the prevention of erosive lesions: A review. Oral Health Prev. Dent.: 1, 245, 2003.
41. Young, W.G.: Tooth wear: Diet analysis and advice. Int. Dent. J.: 55, 68, 2005.
42. Zero, D.T. and Lussi, A.: Erosion – chemical and biological factors of importance to the dental practitioner. Int. Dent. J.: 55, 285, 2005.

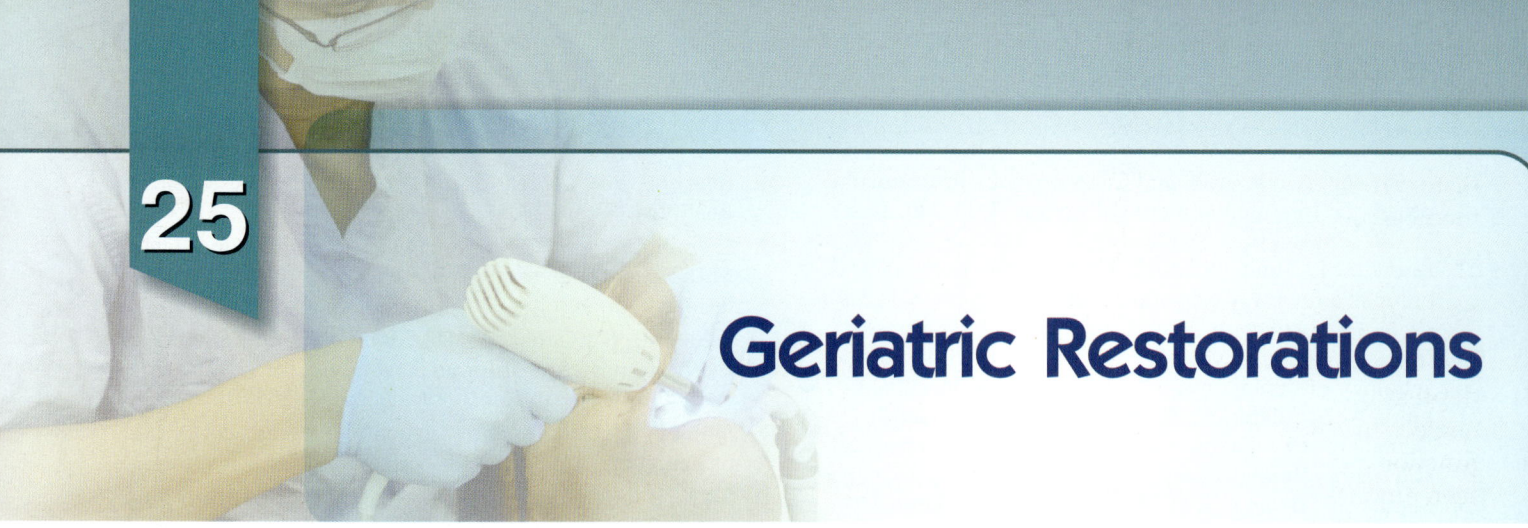

25. Geriatric Restorations

In the course of one's life, teeth are subjected to various physiological and pathological disease conditions leading to a compromised dentition. To lead a quality life in old age, one needs healthy dentition not only for the enjoyment of food but also for proper diet and nutrition. The relationship of the oral health/diseases with the systemic health; including cardiovascular, endocrine and pulmonary health, particularly in the elderly is well established. Therefore, retention of teeth can have an impressive value on the overall dental, physical and mental health of an individual. Moreover, the days are gone when elderly people cared less for their appearance. Now-a-days, an edentulous mouth with resultant sagging is one of the most often presenting complaints of the elderly.

The term geriatrics stems from a Greek word 'Geron' meaning 'old man' and 'Iatros' meaning 'healer'. Three groups of older subjects are identified on chronological age, i.e. Young old (65–74); Older old (75–84) and The Oldest old (greater than 85). *Geriatric dentistry* is 'the delivery of dental care to older adults involving diagnosis, prevention and treatment of problems associated with normal aging and age related diseases as part of an interdisciplinary team with other health care professionals'.

The World health organization documents that although the global population is growing at a rate of 17% annually, the aged population is galloping at a rate of 30%. These demographics suggest that there is an explosion in the population of the elderly. Life expectancy has doubled in the past century, more so in the last two decades. This improved life expectancy is a result of improved health awareness, accessibility, affordability and acceptability of improved medical care.

Old age is associated with several risk factors, both general as well as those specific to the oral cavity. Managing compromised dentition amidst multitude of risk factors is indeed a multi-faceted challenge. The general risk factors include various inter current medical problems, medication induced side effects and psychological problems. Those risk factors related specifically to oral cavity are gingival recession, presence of restorations, removable partial dentures and age related odontometric changes.

MEDICAL HISTORY

Most of the elderly people are on medication. The commonly seen medical conditions are diabetes, hypertension, cardiovascular diseases, arthritis and neuromuscular problems like Parkinson's disease and Alzheimer's disease. The health care providers should be familiar with the course and the complications associated with these disease conditions and the prophylactic guidelines provided for various medical conditions. For example, patients with some form of cardiovascular disease are vulnerable to physical or emotional stress, which may be encountered during dental treatment. Planning of dental treatment should include low stress protocols and shorter appointments. Some patients may not be able to tolerate reclining position on the chair. Since the elderly are more susceptible to orthostatic hypertension hence special attention has to be taken when they move from a reclining posture in the chair to a standing position. Vasoconstrictors should not be administered to patients with unstable angina, uncontrolled hypertension or people with recent myocardial infarction and coronary bypass graft surgery. Prophylactic antibiotics may be necessary for patients with history of high risk cardiac conditions while undertaking endodontic therapy. While restorations can be undertaken without discontinuing oral anti-coagulants, any surgical procedure should be carried out in consultation with a physician. Likewise all appointments for diabetic patients should be scheduled with consideration given to patients' normal meal and insulin schedule. Adverse drug reactions are more likely in this group of patients as many of them are under multiple drug therapy. Therefore careful evaluation of patients' medical/medication history, followed by consultation with the concerned medical professional is imperative to optimize patient care.

PSYCHOLOGICAL CONSIDERATIONS

The elderly individual may suffer from endogenous depression on account of loneliness or feeling of neglect. In addition there is a decline in their cognitive function. Senile dementia is a common phenomenon seen amongst the elderly. Senile dementia can cause memory loss, leading to confusion, difficulty in making decisions, comprehension and even alter the patient's ability to learn and concentrate on new tasks associated with the treatment modality.

AGE CHANGES IN DENTAL TISSUES

Aging of an individual is manifested at all levels of life. Age changes are considered to be the result of day-to-day biological activities. Age changes are slow or non-existent in tissues that do not exhibit biological reactivity. It is often difficult to differentiate between physiological age changes and the pathological age changes. Aging is the slowing down of natural function coupled with disintegration of the balanced control that characterizes the young individuals. Aging can be defined as the combination of process beyond development and maturation which results in a diminution of capacity of the tissues. The physical state of aging is referred to as *'senescence'* and the study of the aging process is known as *'gerontology.'*

General Effects of Aging

General features of aging are:
- Tissue desiccation
- Reduced elasticity
- Diminished reparative capacity
- Altered cell permeability
- Keratinization is diminished (Thin dermis and epidermis)
- Decreased blood supply
- Degeneration of nerve endings
- Capillaries appear to be more fragile, which may result in development of hematomas even after a minor trauma
- Bone undergoes osteoporosis; trabeculae are reduced in number, the cortical plates are thinned, vascularity is reduced, lacunae resorption is more prominent, and susceptibility to fracture is increased.

MECHANISM OF AGING

The mechanism of aging can be hypothesized into four types: (1) biologic clock type, (2) immunologic, (3) DNA damage-related and (4) aging related to damage of other cellular components (OCC).

These are enumerated as follows:

1. **Biologic clock**
   - *Genetic time table*
   - *Disposable soma*
   - *Immunologic theory*
   - *Watch-spring*
   - *Rate of living*
2. **Immunological**
   - *Immunologic theory*
3. **DNA damage related**
   - *DNA deterioration*
   - *Somatic mutation*
   - *Radiation theory*
   - *Wear-and-tear theory*
4. **Damage of other cellular components**
   - *Clinker theory*
   - *Falling domino theory*
   - *Thermal denaturation*
   - *Cellular loss theory*
   - *Enzyme/hormonal/glycoprotein theory*
   - *Disposable soma*
   - *Radiation theory*
   - *Immunologic theory*
   - *Nutritional theory*
   - *Macrophage theory*
   - *Wear-and-tear theory*
   - *Stress*

Cross-Linkage Theory

This theory purported to be the cause of aging of dental pulp, a major DNA- and OCC-damage theory. According to this theory, aging starts with the formation of cross-linkages in proteins and nucleic acids. Cross-linkages can also occur between molecules of collagen, which makes it tougher and more rigid. This theory also explains the aging phenomenon of skin, tendon, bone, blood vessels, lung tissue, and other body components. Cross-linked collagen is more readily infiltrated with calcium deposits. A previous aging theory known as the calcium theory linked aging to the gradual accumulation of calcium deposits throughout the body. Once a substance is cross-linked, it eventually loses its function. It is considered that cross-linkage prevents certain protein and nucleic acid molecules from being metabolized by the body's enzymes which then accumulate in the cells.

According to this theory, with aging an increased accumulation of cross-linkage agents occurs. These can be derived from foods, drugs, and pollutants. Purported cross-linkage agents include acetaldehyde, formaldehyde, glyceraldehyde, malonaldehyde, pyruvic acid, citric acid, succinic acid, ubiquinone, ortho-quinone, lipid peroxides and their derivatives, free radicals, silicon, lead, aluminum, copper, iron, man-ganese, cadmium, tin, titanium, calcium and zinc. Glucose can attach to proteins and nucleic acids to form cross-linkage products. The formed substances are known as advanced glycosylation end products. Tobacco smoke contains acrolein and glycerin, which are considered to be cross-linkage agents. Cross-linkages can induce somatic mutations and protein degeneration, and can change the immunologic behavior of proteins, which appears to be a prelude to autoimmunity.

Free-Radical Theory

This theory can relate to DNA damage, OCC damage, immunologic factors, and biologic clock mechanisms. The free-radical theory is steadily gaining acceptance as a plausible explanation of primary chemical reactions involved in aging. Free radicals can propagate through hundreds of thousands of molecules and wreak havoc before they finally encounter another free radical and become neutralized. Free radicals have been called the "great white sharks of the biochemical sea of life." If they are unchecked, free radicals can continue to create other free radicals from normal molecules, thereby disrupting vital functions. In this way free radicals can cause serious effects to cellular metabolism as a consequence of damage to DNA, RNA, enzymes, lipids, immune cells, and cell membranes. Free radicals are usually produced as unwarranted by-products of normal oxygen metabolism and lipid peroxidation of polyunsaturated fatty acids.

With respect to aging, this theory states that oxygen derived free radicals cause lipid peroxidation, which in turn damages cell membranes and other cellular structures. Mitochondria are the main source of free radicals. The body naturally contains antioxidant mechanisms (for example, superoxide dismutase, á-tocopherol, ascorbic acid, carotene, glutathione, glutathione peroxidase, etc.) that quench free radicals. With aging these mechanisms become less effective and more free radicals are generated. As a result of both occurrences, greater free radical damage occurs.

AGING AND DENTAL TISSUES

Different aspects of aging related to Dental tissues are discussed as follows:

I. Age Changes in Enamel

a. Wearing of the enamel (loss of vertical dimension and flattening of proximal contours)
b. The surfaces of recently erupted teeth are covered with pronounced rod ends and perikymata. As the age advances there is generalized loss of rod ends and flattening of the perikymata. Rate at which the structure is lost depends on the location of the surface of the tooth and on the location of the tooth in the oral cavity. Facial and lingual surfaces lose their structure much more rapidly than do proximal surfaces, and anterior teeth lose their structure more rapidly than posterior teeth.
c. Pronounced wear facets
d. Surface darkening (localized increase of nitrogen and fluoride and change in organic content lead to darkening of surface enamel)
e. Enamel becomes less permeable.

II. Age changes in Dentin

a. **Secondary dentin:** The major age changes in the dentin is the formation of secondary dentin. It occurs in as a part of response of the tooth to normal aging process. Secondary dentin is deposited only after completion of primary dentin.

A few authors describe secondary dentin as regular and irregular. The regular secondary dentin is considered physiological whereas irregular secondary dentin is considered as pathological. The irregular secondary dentin formed as result of abnormal irritation/stimulation has also been called as reactionary dentin or tertiary dentin. Reactionary dentin differs from reparative dentin as reactionary dentin is generalised deposition by the pre-existing odontoblasts and reparative dentin is localised deposition formed by newly differentiated odontoblasts in response to an aggressive local stimulus.

This process of secondary dentin formation results in gradual reduction in size of the pulp chamber and root canals. The number of dentinal tubules is also reduced since irregular secondary dentin, mainly deposited in the coronal regions, obliterates many tubule openings. Stimuli may not only induce additional formation of reparative dentin but also lead to protective changes in the existing dentin. The progress of caries, attrition, abrasion, erosion or cavity preparation generates sufficient stimuli causing deposition of collagen fibres and apatite crystals in the dentinal tubules. There is an evident decrease in tooth sensitivity when secondary dentin formation is extensive, as it is in elderly persons.

b. **Dentinal sclerosis:** The exact mechanism of dental sclerosis or the deposition of calcium salts in the tubules is not understood, although the most likely source of the calcium salts is the dental lymph within the tubules. The increased mineralization of the tooth decreases the conductivity of the odontoblastic processes. Apatite crystals are initially only sporadic in dentinal tubules but gradually the tubule becomes filled with a fine meshwork of crystals. Gradually the tubule lumen is obliterated with mineral which appear very much like peritubular dentin. Sclerosis reduces permeability of dentin and may help prolong pulp vitality. Sclerosis also slows an advancing carious process. Sclerotic dentin under a carious lesion is harder than adjacent normal dentin. Transparent or sclerotic dentin can be observed in teeth of elderly people, especially in roots. It appears transparent or light in transmitted light and dark in reflected light due to the equalization of the refractive indices of the sclerosed dentinal components.

c. **Dead Tracts:** When caries progresses rapidly, the odontoblasts degenerate. The dentinal tubules are no longer filled with living protoplasm, and dead tracts result. A similar occurrence is seen in:
   - Fracture of crowns
   - Severe operative injuries
   - Drug injuries

   The remaining vital odontoblasts or other pulp cells attempt to seal off the dead tracts by the elaboration of reparative dentin.

   Dead tracts are seen in ground sections of teeth and are manifested as a black zone by transmitted light and as a white zone in reflected light. This optical phenomenon is due to differences in the refractive indices of the affected tubules and normal tubules. The nature of the change in the affected tubules is not known, although these tubules are not calcified and are permeable to the penetration of dyes.

d. **Tertiary dentin:** Tertiary dentin develops when pulp irritants are more intense and secondary dentin forms in response to the slight aggressive effects of normal biological function. Tertiary dentin differs from secondary dentin in that it is localized exclusively adjacent to the irritated zone, its tubules being very irregular, tortuous, and reduced in number or absent.

III. Age Changes in Dental Pulp

a. **Reduction in size and volume of the pulp:**
   - The basic reduction in the coronal pulp areas is the result of a continual apposition of dentin occlusally as well at furcation area.
   - Deposition of dentin at furcation area is greater than that of occlusal dentin.
   - Secondary dentin formation occurs throughout life and may eventually result in almost complete pulpal obliteration (Figs 25.1A, B). In maxillary anterior teeth, the secondary dentin is formed on the lingual of the pulp chamber; in molar teeth the maximum deposition takes place on the floor of the chamber.

b. **Decrease in number of cells:**
   - Number of cells are reduced by 50% in aged pulps
   - Fibroblasts show degeneration with increasing age as characterized by small size and a decrease in number of organelles, including RER, mitochondria and Golgi complex
   - Odontoblasts exhibit degeneration with age
   - Increase in vacuole numbers and gradual degenerative changes leading to absence of cells over some or the entire pulpal surface.

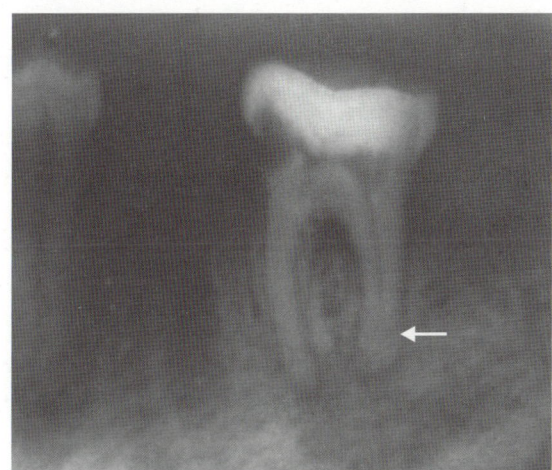

Fig. 25.1A: Pulpal obliteration in aged dental pulp (radiograph)

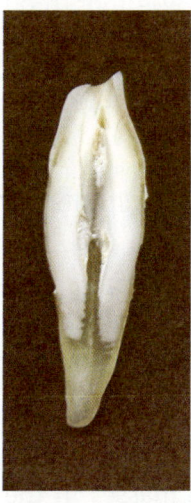

Fig. 25. 1B: Cut section of tooth showing reduced pulp space and sclerotic dentin

c. **Presence of calcifications:** as proposed by Kronfield, et al, there are two types of calcifications found in dental pulp:
  i. Discrete Calcification
  ii. Diffuse calcification

Discrete calcifications: Pulp stones or denticles are discrete calcifications found freely within the pulp tissue or attached to or embedded in dentin. Denticles are further classified as follows:
- *According to structure*
  a. True denticles: Denticles possessing a central cavity filled with epithelial remnants surrounded peripherally by odontoblasts
  b. False denticles: Pulp stones being compact degenerative masses of calcified tissues

The differences between the true and false denticles are summarized in Table 25.1

Table 25.1: Difference between true and false denticles

True denticles	False denticles
Attached to the wall of pulp chamber	Not attached to the wall of pulp chamber
Called as attached denticles	Called as free denticles
More common	Less common

- *According to location*
  a. Free denticle: freely lying in pulp chamber
  b. Attached denticle: attached to the dentinal walls
  c. Interstitial denticle: surrounded by secondary denticle

Etiology: The etiology of pulp stones is unknown. The incidence appears to increase with the age of the person but there is no definite association with pulpal irritation or inflammation such as that arising from caries or trauma. Few authors reported that an extreme high percentage of pulp stones yields a pure growth of streptococci upon culture. On that basis they suggested that microbes are responsible for the pulp stones. Various other authors hypothesized mechanism of thrombosis or vascular wall injury or both responsible for pulp stone formation.

Characteristic features:
- Common feature of old teeth from individuals over the age of 45 years
- Located in root pulp or coronal pulp or both.
- They are usually first seen in root pulp as an isolated calcified masses. Isolated masses coalesce to form large mass that fuse with dentin.
- The calcified masses in the coronal pulp may become larger in size and fuse together to obliterate the normal pulp architecture.
- There is a direct association of these masses with the collagen fibers. With increased cross linkage of collagen during advancing age there is an enhanced tendency for these fibers to become mineralized.

Diffuse calcification: Dystrophic or diffuse calcifications refers to the inappropriate biomineralization of the pulp in the absence of mineral imbalance. These are generally a pulpal response to trauma that is characterized by deposition of hard tissue within the root canal space and is commonly found in young adults in the anterior region of the mouth.

d. **Decreased vascular supply:**
  - Osteosclerotic changes are one of the first alterations to be observed to the small arteries in the root pulp in aging teeth. The intima of the vessel gets thickened resulting in smaller lumen. The old blood capillaries exhibited a widening of the basement membranes with strongly PAS-positive staining whereas the young vessels appeared to have thin lightly red stained membrane. In the process of diffuse calcification of the root pulp, the adventitia and media of the small arteries and veins as well as the walls of the capillaries become mineralized, eventually leading to loss of vessels in the old pulps.
  - Capillary permeability also decreases with age. Transfer of substances from blood to cells may be depleted during aging.

e. **Decreased nerve supply**

As with vascular system, the nerves within the root pulp also exhibit changes as a result of diffuse calcifications. The connective tissue sheath of the nerve bundles becomes mineralized. The cuspal nerves are decreased and their terminal branching is lost. Persistent nerve fibres show signs of degeneration such as reticulation, fragmentation and beading, etc.

IV. Age Changes in Cementum

Hypercementosis: It is an abnormal thickening of cementum. It may be diffuse or circumscribed. It may affect all the teeth of dentition, be confined to single tooth, or even effects only parts of one tooth. The thickness of the young apical cementum is 100 to 200µm and increases with age to two or three times of that thickness. Most common area involves the apical root area. Various causes of hypercementosis are:

- Accelerated elongation of tooth
- Inflammation around a tooth
- Tooth repair
- Paget's disease of bone

Accelerated elongation of tooth owing to loss of an antagonist accompanied by hyperplasia of cementum occurs apparently as a result of inherent tendency for the maintenance of the normal width of the periodontal ligament. Inflammation at the apex of the tooth root that usually occurs as a result of pulpal infection stimulates excessive deposition of cementum. In such cases cementum is laid down on the root surface at some distance above the apex. Moreover, tooth *repair does not, always, result in the deposition of remarkable amount of secondary cementum. On occasions, occlusal trauma results in mild root resorption. Such root resorption is repaired by deposition of cementum between the root fragments as well as on their periphery.*

V. Age Changes in Bone

- It is established that density of bone is decreased with advancing age; more so in women
- In addition to being less dense the bone is often more brittle
- Lamina dura is often lost and the cortical bone becomes thinner especially at the angle of the mandible
- Increased porosity, mainly due to increase in vascular spaces
- The volume occupied by each canaliculus remains constant or even decreased; however, the total canalicular volume is decreased
- Lacunar volume is increased despite a reduction in number of lacunae
- Walls of the blood capillaries get thickened with age
- Active cells of bone reduced in number.

VI. Age Changes in the Periodontium

a. In *gingiva* and other areas of the *oral mucosa*, following changes have been observed:
   - Diminished keratinization
   - Reduced or an unchanged amount of stippling
   - Increased width of attached gingiva
   - Decreased connective tissue cellularity
   - Increase in amount of intercellular substances
   - Reduced oxygen consumption
   - Increase or no change in mitotic index of gingival epithelium
   - Thinning of oral epithelium
   - Increased keratinization of lip and cheek mucosa
   - Atrophy of connective tissue with loss of elasticity
   - Decrease in number of protein bound hexoses and mucoproteins
   - Increase in number of mast cells.

b. In *Periodontal ligament*, the following changes are evident:
   - Increased number of elastic fibers
   - Decrease in vascularity, mitotic activity, fibroplasia, and the number of collagen fibers and mucopolysaccharides
   - Increase in arteriosclerotic changes
   - Reduction in width caused due to lower functional demand owing to the decrease in strength of the masticatory musculature
   - Increase in width caused due to availability of fewer teeth to support the entire functional load
   - Decreased width caused from encroachment on ligament by continuous deposition of cementum and bone.

CLINICAL IMPLICATIONS

The different clinical implications of the effects of aging are as follows:

I. Restorative Aspects

a. **Attrition:** With age, wearing of enamel surface takes place due to tooth to tooth contacts during various functional or parafunctional movements of the mandible. Attrition results in exposure of dentin and increased tooth sensitivity. Loss of vertical dimension of crown and flattening of proximal contour can occur. If abnormal attrition is present the patients' functional movements must be evaluated and inquiry should be made about his habits such as tooth grinding or bruxism. In order to preserve the attritioned teeth the best suitable treatment plan is to restore teeth with full coverage restorations.

b. **Cavity Design:** With age, transparent dentin formation occurs. Due to this dentin loses its resiliency power and chances of its fracture due to occlusal stresses or force are increased. Violating principles of cavity design combined with the loss of resiliency that results from reduced organic components of dentin can increase the susceptibility of tooth to cracks and cuspal fractures. Therefore, appropriate cavity preparation without any overhanging and unsupported enamel should be done.

c. **Bonding:** Partial or complete obliteration of the dentinal tubules with tube- or rod-like sclerotic casts is commonly observed. In the absence of undercut retention, cervical sclerotic dentin is more difficult to adhere to as compared to the normal dentin. Even after increasing the etching time, the sclerotic casts that obliterated the dentinal tubules cannot be completely removed after acid-conditioning of the sclerotic dentin, resulting in minimal or no resin tag formation. Furthermore, the zone of resin-impregnated sclerotic dentin was found to be thinner than those observed in normal dentin. Regional tensile bond strength to cervical sclerotic root dentin with some contemporary adhesives was found to be 20–45% lower than those bonded to artificial wedge-shaped lesions created in normal cervical root dentin. This was attributed to the presence of sclerotic casts within dentinal tubules that precluded optimal resin infiltration into the dentinal tubules and/or the presence of a surface hypermineralised layer that is more resistant to acid-etching

II. Pulp Testing

Slow and gentle testing should be done to determine pulp and periapical status. Vitality responses must correlate with clinical and radiographic findings and be interpreted as a supplement in developing clinical judgement. Vertically cracked teeth should always be considered when pulpal or periapical disease is observed. Cracks that are detected when the pulp is still vital can show better prognosis if restored with full coverage restorations. The reduced neural and vascular components of aged pulps, the overall reduced pulp volume and the change in character of the ground substance creates an environment that responds differently to both stimuli and irritants than that of younger pulps. Fewer nerve branches are present in older pulps due to retrogressive changes resulting from mineralization of the nerve and nerve sheath. The presence or absence of response is of limited value and must be correlated with other clinical tests, examination findings and radiographs. An alternative to electric pulp test is assessment of pulp vitality by applying thermal stimulus to the tooth surface. The electric pulp tester, CO_2 snow and dichlorodifluoromethane were found to be more reliable than ethyl chloride or ice in producing a positive response.

It is important to know that pulpal symptoms are usually chronic in older patients, and other sources of orofacial pain should be ruled out when pain is not soon localized. Diffuse pain of vague origin is uncommon in older pulps and limits the need for selective anaesthesia.

III. Radiographs

Indications for and techniques of taking radiographs do not differ much among adult age groups. However, several physiologic and anatomic changes can significantly affect their interpretation. The presence of tori, exostoses, and denser bone may require increased exposure times for proper diagnostic contrast. Digital radiography may be more useful than conventional in detecting early bone changes. Pulp recession is accelerated by reparative dentin so the depth of the pulp chamber should be measured from the occlusal surface and its mesiodistal position noted. Receding pulp horns that are apparent on a radiograph may remain microscopically much higher. Small canals are the rule in old patients. A mid-root disappearance of a detectable canal may indicate bifurcation rather than calcification. The narrowest point in the canal may be difficult to determine; it is positioned farther from the radiographic apex because of continued cementum deposition.

IV. Access Preparation and Working Length Determination

Adequate access and identification of canal orifices are probably the most difficult parts of providing root canal treatment for older patients. The decreased pulp chamber size makes the canal orifice location difficult. Also, the presence of pulp stone creates problems in the biomechanical preparation and cleaning and shaping of the root canals. Although the effects of aging and multiple restorations may reduce the volume and coronal extent of the chamber or canal orifice, its buccolingual and mesiodistal portions remain the same and can be predicted from radiographs and clinical examinations. In addition, the cemento-dentinal junction (CDJ) moves farther from the radiographic apex with continued cementum deposition leading to difficulty in accurate working length determination.

V. Tooth-periodontium Relationship

The most obvious change in the teeth with aging is a loss of tooth substance caused by attrition. Occlusal wear reduces cusp height and inclination with a resultant increase in food table area and loss of sluice ways. The degree of attrition is influenced by the:
  i. Musculature
  ii. Consistency of the food
  iii. The tooth hardness
  iv. Occupational factors
  v. Habits such as grinding (bruxism) and clenching.
- The rate of attrition may be coordinated with other aging related changes such as continuous tooth eruption and gingival recession. As the tooth erupts, cementum is usually deposited in the apical region of the root. The reduction in bone height that occurs with aging is not necessarily related to occlusal wear.

- If bone support is reduced the clinical crown tends to become disproportionately long and exerts excessive leverage on the bone. By reducing the clinical crown length, attrition appears to preserve the balance between tooth and its bony support.
- Wear of teeth also occurs on the proximal surfaces, accompanied by mesial migration of the teeth. Proximal wear reduces the antero-posterior length of the dental arch by approximately 0.5cm by the age of 40. Antero-posterior narrowing from proximal wear is greater in teeth that taper toward the cervical aspect, such as the incisors. Progressive attrition and proximal wear result in a reduced maxillary-mandibular overjet in the molar area and on edge-to-edge bite anteriorly.

VI. Masticatory Efficiency

- Slight atrophy of the buccal musculature has been described as a physiologic feature of aging.
- Reduced masticatory efficiency in aged individuals is due to:
   i. Unreplaced missing teeth.
   ii. Loose teeth.
   iii. Poorly fitting dentures.
   iv. Unwillingness to wear dentures.
- Reduced masticatory efficiency leads to poor chewing habits and the possibility of associated digestive disturbances.
- Avitaminosis is relatively common.
   i. An adequate intake of vitamin, calcium, iron and potassium is particularly important to geriatric patients and dietary supplementation may be advisable.
   ii. A diet high in fiber and vitamins and comparatively low in fat may also be beneficial.

VII. Root Caries

It is a continuum of changes ranging from needle point small, slightly softened and discolored spots on the root to extensive, brownish or very dark soft areas encircling the entire root surface also forming into cavity and even this cavity extends into pulp chamber. The lesions tend to spread laterally and often coalesce with neighbouring lesions. The lesions may eventually encircle the tooth in particular when they are located along cemento-enamel junction.

- Active root surface caries *(progressing lesions)*: It is well defined and shows yellowish, brownish or black discoloration. The lesion is mostly likely covered by visible plaque and presents a softened or leathery consistency on probing with medium pressure.
- Inactive root surface caries *(non-progressing lesions)*: Areas show a well-defined brownish or black discoloration. The surface of the lesion is smooth and shiny and appears hard on probing with moderate pressure.
- Risk factors
   i. Saliva: Aging per se has no significant clinical impact on salivary secretion. The most common cause of salivary hypo-function in the elderly is intake of medications and is most commonly associated with dental caries and fungal infections.
   ii. Gingival recession: Root surface caries cannot develop unless preceded by gingival recession. So it is common predominantly in age groups in which the loss of periodontal attachment is accompanied by gradual recession of gingival (Fig. 25.2).
   iii. Age and Sex: As gingival recession and age are associated so it is logical that root caries increases with the age. Men are generally more affected than women.

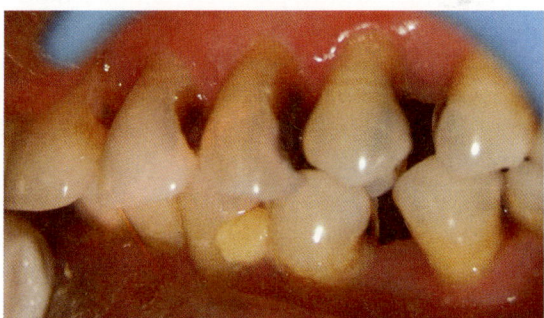

Fig. 25.2: Root caries with gingival recession

AGING AND CUMULATIVE EFFECTS OF DISEASES

Medical conditions are no more significant for endodontic procedures in the elderly (older) than for other types of treatment. It has been presumed that systemic conditions such as diabetes or immunosuppressant therapy would predispose an endodontic patient to infection or delayed healing. Osteoporosis is a common condition of older women. There is an evidence that osteoporosis is associated with a decrease in trabecular bone density in the jaws, particularly in the anterior maxilla and the posterior mandible. It is still not known whether patients with osteoporosis have delayed bony healing after root canal treatment or surgery. One important consideration is that older patients are more likely to be taking more and stronger medications. Caution is required, particularly while prescribing additional medications.

With time many chronic diseases can produce various oral changes such as gingival recession, tooth attrition, reduction in bone height, etc. In the elderly changes in the oral environment not only results from physiologic aging, but may result from disease and other factors in the oral cavity. Inflammation develops more rapidly in older individuals than in children. This may occur in part due to areas of recession which may favor plaque accumulation; it may also be due to a reduction in immune response with aging. Wound healing proceeds more slowly in old than in young with the same susceptibility to periodontal disease. Rapidly destructive forms of periodontal disease occur in young patients and are usually associated with deficient leukocyte function. In elderly it occurs as slowly progressive form of the disease and not due to impaired leukocyte function.

Dry mouth: Saliva plays a major role in oral homeostasis and is necessary to prevent oral diseases. There may be evidence of hypofunctioning due to aging; however, it is not a sequel to growing old. It is usually associated with use of medications such as anti-depressants, anti-hypertensive, anti-cholinergic and anti-asthmatics, etc. which are commonly taken by the elderly. Such conditions can significantly result in both local and systemic consequences leading to caries, periodontal disease, dysphagia, etc. In order to overcome this dryness they resort to sugar containing chewing lozenges which further worsens the situation.

Gingival recession: Periodontal disease with attachment loss is most commonly seen in the aged population. Gingival recession leads to food impaction and plaque accumulation on the rougher cemental surface rendering maintenance of oral hygiene difficult leading to dental caries and further progression of periodontal disease (Fig. 25.3).

Restorations: Old dentition generally has many restorations over a period of time. These old restorations with faulty margins coupled with poor oral hygiene and dry mouth increase the risk of secondary caries, especially with respect to the proximal gingival margins (Fig. 25.4).

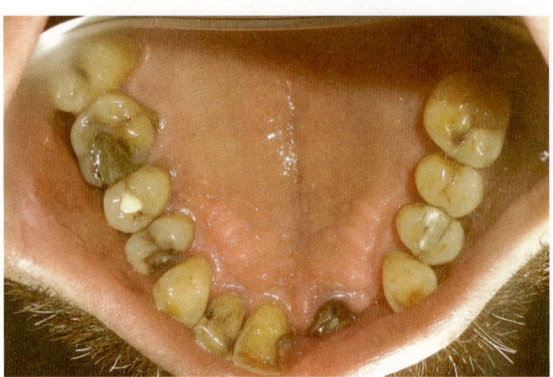

Fig. 25.4: Aged dentition with restorations and poor oral hygiene

Removable partial dentures: The retention clasps and junction of removable prosthesis and teeth can also act as retention sites for food and plaque.

Age related odontometric changes: As the age advances, tooth tissues and supporting structures undergo a number of changes. Many of these changes may not be age related but are as a result of incremental effects of wear, disease and habits. There is considerable reduction in density of odontoblasts and reparative capacity of the pulp following injury by tooth preparations, cytotoxic effects of dental materials, microleakage, etc. However the greater thickness of dentin in the elderly may compensate for the compromised response of the pulp by allowing the preparation to be deeper before an exposure or injury.

Compensatory changes occur as a result of aging or disease. These changes affect the tooth or periodontium that precedes the clinical condition. Attrition is a compensatory change that acts as a stabilizing factor between loss of bony support and the excessive leverage from occlusal forces. In addition, a reduction in the overjet of the teeth is seen manifesting as an edge to edge contact of anterior teeth.

All the above risk factors together with dry mouth and reduced physical ability of older individuals hinder the maintenance of oral hygiene, often encouraging the development of diseased conditions such as dental caries, periodontal disease, tooth wear, etc.

TREATMENT PLANNING FOR ELDERLY

Treatment planning in elderly involves both complexity and uncertainty. Patient's perceived needs and priorities as well as their expectations are to be

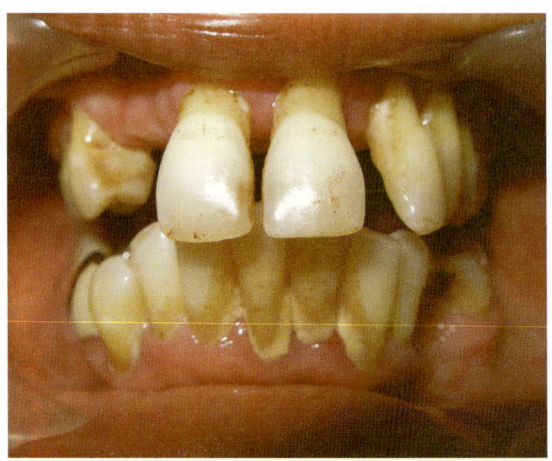

Fig. 25.3: Gingival recession

considered to ensure treatment success. The operator should concentrate on patient's quality of life within the four domains of need such as function, symptoms, pathology and esthetics.

Prior to any treatment planning, the following determinants need to be considered:

1. Desires and expectations
2. Types of patients' dental needs
3. Impact on patient's quality of life in terms of ability to eat, comfort level and esthetics.
4. Probability of positive treatment outcome (prognosis)
5. Availability of reasonable and less extensive alternatives
6. Ability to tolerate treatment stress
7. Ability to maintain oral health
8. Patients financial resources (whether individual has income or dependent on others)
9. Probable life span
10. Family support (living alone or with family members)

Kay has suggested four different types of needs for any dental treatment, viz. functional, psychological, perceived and normative. While treating the old, one should integrate these needs into a holistic approach to demonstrate the benefit, taking into account the impact of it on the patient's quality of life.

Geriatric patients can be grouped into three categories based on functional living disabilities while planning treatment strategies, viz. i) functionally independent, ii) frail and iii) functionally dependent.

The concept of staged treatment plan is preferred for geriatric patients.

Staged Treatment Plan

After collecting all data, the treatment is planned in following stages:

Stage I – Emergency car*e*:
Initially emergency treatment is carried out to relieve pain, if any.

Stage II – Maintenance and monitoring:
It includes management of chronic infection, root canal therapy, root planing and curettage, restoration of carious lesions, work related to dentures and patient education to improve oral health (such as changes in dietary habits, plaque control and fluorides). A further period of evaluation is required before one proceeds further.

Stage III – Rehabilitation phase:
It includes total mouth rehabilitation, reconstruction of occlusal plane and restoration of vertical dimension with fixed and removable prosthesis.

The stages provide the requisite care in increments that are appropriate to the resolution of the immediate problems. Once a critical dental problem is stabilized the dentist can consider undertaking the next appropriate step, which is providing more elaborate and comprehensive care.

Care of institutionalized or home bound patient: (Functionally dependent older adults)

These patients require assistance even for their normal day to day activities. Such patients should be given minimum treatment required to maintain physical and psychological comfort. Physician's presence may be necessary in patients who are severely diseased. If it involves too much of a medical risk it is better to hospitalize and do the necessary treatment. ART techniques may prove useful in these cases for restorative management.

RESTORATIVE MANAGEMENT OF COMMON ORAL DISEASES IN ELDERLY

I. Dental Caries

It is established that incidence of coronal caries in the old is more or less similar to the young, whereas the incidence of root caries is much higher (around 40–70%). It has been recognized that in the elderly, proportion of secondary caries predominates over primary caries. Mjor reported that 93% of recurrent caries associated with silver amalgam occurs at gingivo-proximal locations of class II restorations or crowns.

It is imperative to evaluate the risk factors involved in planning treatment of caries for the elderly. A thorough history of medical conditions and medication has to be analyzed. Salivary volume and buffering capacity tests can also be helpful. Treatment can be instituted in two phases.

a. **Restorative phase**
b. **Maintenance phase**

a. Restorative Phase

The following considerations should be kept in mind during restoration of teeth in elderly:

- *Restorative considerations for coronal caries:* In older adults, indirect restorations are generally not preferred. As far as possible direct restorative materials such as amalgam, composite, glass-ionomer, etc. should be used. These restorations can be readily modified, repaired or replaced as incidence of secondary caries is high in such patients. Owing to high incidence of caries, frequent maintenance of these restorations might be required, which is not possible in indirect restorations.

- *Restorative considerations for root caries:* Root carious lesions are predominantly seen on the proximal surfaces followed by the facial surface. It is imperative to act quickly because these lesions progress very rapidly and in a circumferential manner. The process of mineral loss can be twice as fast as that on enamel. The rapid progression coupled with the thinness of tooth structure on the root may lead to pulp exposure. Therefore, even a shallow lesion should be considered potentially deep. Billings, et al (1984) had categorized root caries into several grades and outlined the treatment plan that holds good even today (Table 25.2).

Glass-ionomer cement is the preferred restorative material since it possesses adhesive property, fluoride release, reasonable esthetics, biocompatibility and being less technique sensitive as compared to composites Figs 25.5 A,B depicts management of root caries with glass-ionomer cement. Alternative caries management strategies have been suggested. Ozone has successfully been used to inhibit root caries. Exposure of the lesion to ozone for 10–40 seconds is said to be anti-microbial. Use of Carisolv and Lasers for caries excavation has also been suggested especially for those who cannot tolerate local anesthetics; however, location of root caries may cause difficulties for the accomplishment of these procedures.

b. Maintenance Phase

Caries activity in elderly continues to remain high and unpredictable. So maintaining low caries activity amidst increasing risk factors for the rest of their life is challenging and many a times frustrating. It requires tremendous patience and effort from dentists, patients and family members. All possible preventive measures need to be undertaken in order to maintain both restored and unrestored teeth.

With the mechanism of caries being the same in the young and the old, preventive strategy also remains the same with minor modifications to suit the elderly. Daily use of fluoride dentifrices and fluoride rinses along with periodic topical fluoride application regime is advisable. Fluoride varnishes may be preferred over other forms. Chlorhexidine gel /mouth rinses / varnishes are advised. 10 % varnish is preferred over rinse/gel once a week for four weeks. New remineralisation products containing CPP-ACP, CPP-ACPF and BTCP, etc. may also be beneficial. Xylitol containing candies help not only in getting over the dryness but also prevent caries. All possible measures should be taken to prevent further loss of gingival tissue attachment which is most crucial to prevent root caries.

Preventive Regimen for Elderly with Dry Mouth

Most elderly suffer from some degree of xerostomia. If it is drug induced and is causing major discomfort, modifying the medication can be considered in consultation with the attending physician. For

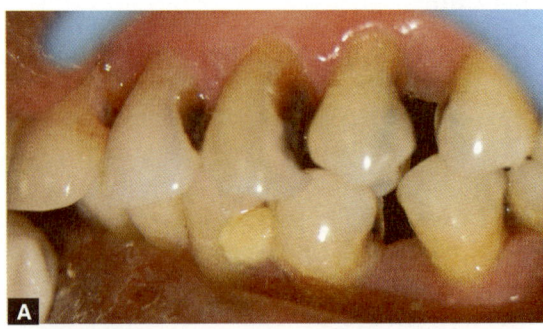

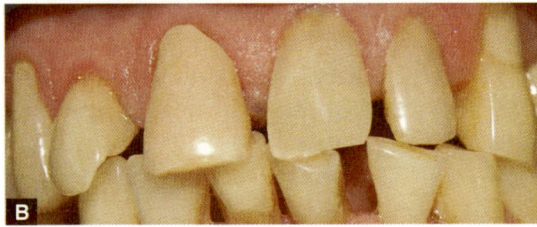

Fig. 25.5A and B: Management of root caries **(A)** Pre-operative view **(B)** Post-operative view

Table 25.2: Grade, description and management of root caries		
Grade	Description	Management
GRADE I	White or light brown, surface cannot be penetrated	Topical fluorides Re-mineralizing agents, frequent recall
GRADE II	Light brown, 0.5–1.0 mm penetration	Excavation of lesion, reshaping of margins, fluoride application
GRADE III	Dark brown Penetration>1.0 mm Not extending to pulp	Restoration with glass-ionomer cement
GRADE IV	Brown black Penetration into dental pulp	Root canal treatment or extraction

example, substituting the drug with one having lesser anti-cholinergic effect or altering the time of medication – (salivary flow is less in the night, therefore taking the medication in the morning may improve oral comfort. Clonazapine is an anti-psychotic that has marked reduced xerostomic side effect when compared to chlorpromazine). Symptomatic relief could be obtained by asking the patient to sip water frequently throughout the day and reduce caffeine containing beverages. The use of room humidifiers in dry weather may improve patient comfort. Instruct the patient not to use sugar containing lozenges and candies; instead replace them with xylitol containing gums and candies. In patients with severe salivary gland dysfunction artificial saliva can be prescribed for relief. Saliva substitutes are available in the form of gels, sprays and liquids for placement around dentures as well as on teeth and oral soft tissues.

II. Non Carious Tooth Tissue Loss

Tooth wear is one of the most common problems in the older adults. Attrition, abrasion and erosion may lead to tooth wear. These three elements are rarely seen isolated and one affects the other two and vice-versa. These teeth have been exposed to wear and tear of the oral environment for a relatively long period of time. Another important contributing factor is medication induced xerostomia which results in the loss of buffering action of saliva making the teeth more susceptible to acid erosion of teeth. With increasing age, gingival recession exposes the cementum, making it more susceptible to abrasion and erosion. Improper use of tooth brush and tooth pick, floss and partial denture clamps can also abrade the cemental surface. Caries can also superimpose in these worn out areas because of increased vulnerability of exposed dentinal surfaces. Lack of proper posterior support is another important factor in the elderly that gives rise to attrition in addition to normal physiological wear and tear.

Attrition can manifest as minimal wear to flattening of cusps and grooves and in severe cases total loss of contour, dentinal exposure, and reduction in clinical crown height. Abrasive lesions are of varying morphology and seen commonly on the cervical surfaces. Clinical characteristics of erosive lesions mostly depend on the cause. In general if source of acid is dietary, the labial surfaces of the upper anterior teeth will get affected and if the sources of acid are gastric in origin, the effects are generally seen on lingual, palatal and occlusal surfaces.

Consequences of tooth wear include unsightly appearance, possible development of caries in the exposed cemental / dentinal surfaces and sensitivity and reduction in clinical crown height. Reduction in the height of the crowns of teeth is usually accompanied by progressive eruption so that teeth continue to migrate incisally or occlusally together with the alveolar bone. This may result in long bulky alveolar processes that help to maintain the occlusal vertical dimension with the result that the height of clinical crowns may get reduced without concomitant reduction in vertical dimension. This effect may have some implications for restorative treatment.

The treatment for tooth wear is directed towards eliminating etiological factors and strengthening the modifying factors, that is implementation of preventive measures followed by restorative measures. The treatment may be either passive or active.

Passive treatment consists of monitoring and prevention. Monitoring helps one to know whether tooth surface loss is progressive or static. Periodic checkups, use of study casts, photographs, etc. made at different time periods helps in assessing the progress. Preventive treatment is to ensure that there is no further tooth tissue loss in future. The treatment plan varies for every patient. For example, if erosion is on account of excessive citrus fluid consumption, dietary modifications along with fluoride regimen can be suggested. Most patients can be successfully managed only by passive treatment.

Active treatment may be required in some patients for one or more of the following reasons such as sensitivity, aesthetics, functional difficulty & space loss in vertical dimension. Localized defects due to attrition, abrasion or erosion can be restored by using composite resin materials or glass-ionomers depending on the location, occlusal load and esthetic needs. Some occlusal adjustments may be necessary to prevent further tooth wear. Very few patients need advanced rehabilitative therapy (Figs 25.6A and B). An overenthusiastic attempt to restore teeth to their pre-diseased shape, contour and occlusion may end up with disastrous consequences. Careful selection of cases is essential after taking into consideration tolerability to stress and the time involved in the treatment process as well as the motivation and the financial status of the patient. Earlier severely worn out dentition were being rehabilitated with extensive crown and bridge work. Modern therapeutic concepts suggest that reconstructive restorative treatment should be adapted to the tooth and not vice-versa. With the advent of newer improved composite resin materials, small increase in vertical dimension (maximum 1.0–2.0 mm) can be achieved by reconstruction using direct composite build up. If it is more than that or if it involves more than one or two surfaces it is better to go for crown and bridge work.

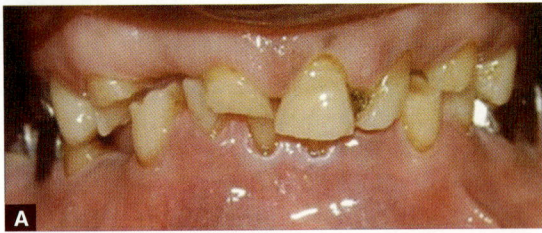
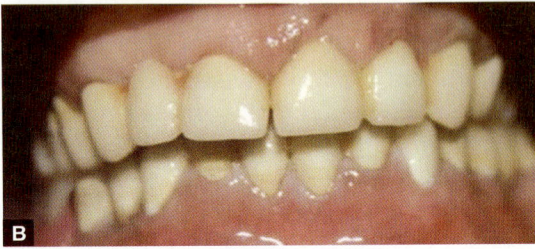

Figs 25.6A and B: Management of non-carious defects **(A)** Pre operative view **(B)** Post operative view

III. Treatment of Sensitivity

If there are symptoms of sensitivity, immediate active treatment may be warranted. Potassium containing desensitizing toothpastes are preferred for home use, while sodium and stannous fluorides have shown to be effective in office treatment (Fig. 25.7). Composites may be placed temporarily or semi-permanently over isolated exposed areas while the dentin bonding agents may be effective in reducing sensitivity and preventing further damage. Root canal treatment may be carried out as the last resort for extreme sensitivity that cannot be treated by conservative methods.

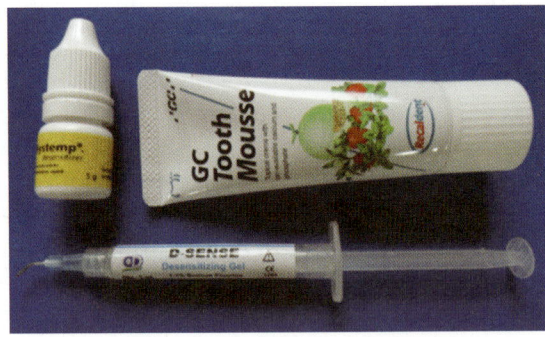

Fig 25.7: Desensitizing agents

IV. Esthetic Rehabilitation of the Elderly

Smile is one of the most important attributes of human beings and is carried throughout life. Even as people are aging most of them lead an independent social life and are therefore conscious about their appearance. If a patient wishes to improve his or her smile, the dental professionals have no right to deny or discourage as long as the patient can afford stress, time and the finances.

Teeth darken with age. This darkening can be caused by structural changes in the enamel, the addition of organic material to the enamel from the environment and due to the deepening of dentinal color seen through the progressive thinning of translucent enamel. Pigmented foods consumed over a period of many years may even darken teeth. The esthetic treatment for elderly could range from recontouring procedures to bleaching, laminates and crowns. Any major esthetic rehabilitation should be undertaken only after proper occlusal and esthetic analysis.

V. Chipping and Cracking of Tooth Structure

Chipping and cracking of tooth structure is a common phenomenon in the elderly. These areas take up stains easily and appear unsightly. Occlusal and incisal surfaces are worn out through enamel into dentin. The enamel may break along the lines of previous cracks leading to extension of cracks into dentin. The dentinal cracks are generally painful because of their access up to pulp. In such cases posterior teeth may require onlays and crowns to prevent further crack propagation and occasionally even endodontic therapy. In anterior teeth, bonded composites both direct and indirect are less invasive means of treating such cases.

CONSIDERATIONS FOR PRESCRIBING MEDICINES TO THE ELDERLY

Since the elderly are on several medications, drug interactions and adverse drug reactions are more likely in these groups of patients. Therefore the operator should take a careful history of their pharmacological status before prescribing any further medication. A simple policy is to ask the patient to bring all the drugs that is being taken, and then carefully prescribe minimum number of drugs with the simplest possible regime. The elderly are more sensitive to the depressant effects of drugs; hence the dosage of analgesics, anti-anxiety drugs, sedatives will need to be reduced. A decline in the renal function occurs in the elderly and requires that dosages of drugs whose principal route of elimination is the kidney be reduced. The operators should also be aware of the psychosocial considerations and be sensitive to such problems. There is possibility of forgetfulness and poor compliance in such patients. Special packaging, clear labeling and simplified dose regimens may improve compliance.

Increased life expectancy is causing an explosion of the aging population that will continue now and in the foreseeable future. Improved quality of life at old age will demand tooth retention and consequently the need for restorative care. Due diligence and interdisciplinary co-ordination among the dental and the medical professionals is crucial in providing safe, effective and appropriate care to the elderly.

The dental professionals should be conscious of the needs of the elderly dental patient, comprehend their psychological needs and offer them sympathetic behavior to ensure satisfaction, augment graceful dignity and inculcate a sense of well-being amongst them.

BIBLIOGRAPHY

1. Bernick S and Nedelman C.: Effect of aging on human pulp. J Endod., 1, 88, 1975.
2. Burgess JO.; Dental materials for the restoration of root surface caries. Am J Dent., 8, 342, 1995.
3. Burton P and Kay EJ.; Prevention of older dentate patients. British Dental J., 195, 237, 2003.
4. Chalmers JM. Minimal intervention dentistry: part 2.: Strategies for addressing restorative challenges in older patients. J Can Dent Assoc., 72, 430, 2006.
5. Chalmers JM.: Minimal interventions dentistry: part 1 Strategies for addressing the new caries challenge in older patient. J Can Dent Assoc.; 72, 427, 2006.
6. Chung, H.Y., Lee, E.K., Choi, Y.J., Kim, J.M., Kim D.h., Kim , C.H., Lee, J., Kim, H.S., Kim, N.D., Jung, J.H. and Yu, B.P.: Molecular inflammation as an underlying mechanism of the aging process and age- related diseases. J Dent Res.: 90. 830, 2011.
7. Douglass CW.: Future needs for dental restorative materials. Adv Dent Res.:, 6, 4, 1992.
8. Gilmour AG and Morgan CL.: Restorative management of the elderly patient. Prim Dent Care., 10, 45, 2003.
9. Heft MW and Mariotti AJ.: Geriatric pharmacology. Dent Clin N Am., 46,869, 2002.
10. Johnson G and Almqvist H.; Non invasive management of superficial carious lesion in disabled and infirm patients. J Oral Rehab., 35, 548, 2008.
11. Jones JA, Mash LK and Niessen LC.: Restorativeions considerations for special needs patients. Dent Clin North Am,: 37,483, 1993.
12. Lo EC, Luo Y and Tan HP.: ART and conventional root restorations in elders after 12 months. J Dent Res.: 85,929, 2006.
13. McComb D.: Operative dentistry consideration for the elderly. J Prosthet Dent.: 72, 517, 1994.
14. Nadig RR, Usha G, Kumar V, Rao R, and Bugalia A.: Geriatric restorative care-the need, the demand and the challenges. J Conser Dent., 14, 208, 2011.
15. Octavia A., Gonzalez M. and Novak J.: Effect of aging on apoptosis gene expression in oral mucosal tissues. Apoptosis 18, 3, 2013.
16. Patil M, Patil SB.: Psychological and emotional considerations during dental treatment. Gerodontology., 26, 72, 2009.
17. Preston, A.J.: Dental management of the elderly patient. Dent Update.: 3, 141, 2012.
18. Small BW.: Reparative dentistry or restorative dentistry? Gen Dent., 56, 126, 2008.
19. Vidal C., Pavan S., Brisso A. and Russo A.: Effects of three restorative techniques in the bond strength and nanoleakage at gingival wall of class II restorations subjected to simulated aging.: Clin Oral Invest, 17, 2, 2013.
20. Williams B, Kini J.: Medication use and prescribing considerations for elderly patients. Dent Clin N Am., 49, 411, 2005.
21. Yellowitz K.: Cognitive function, aging, and ethical decisions: recognizing change. Dent Clin N Am., 49, 389, 2005.

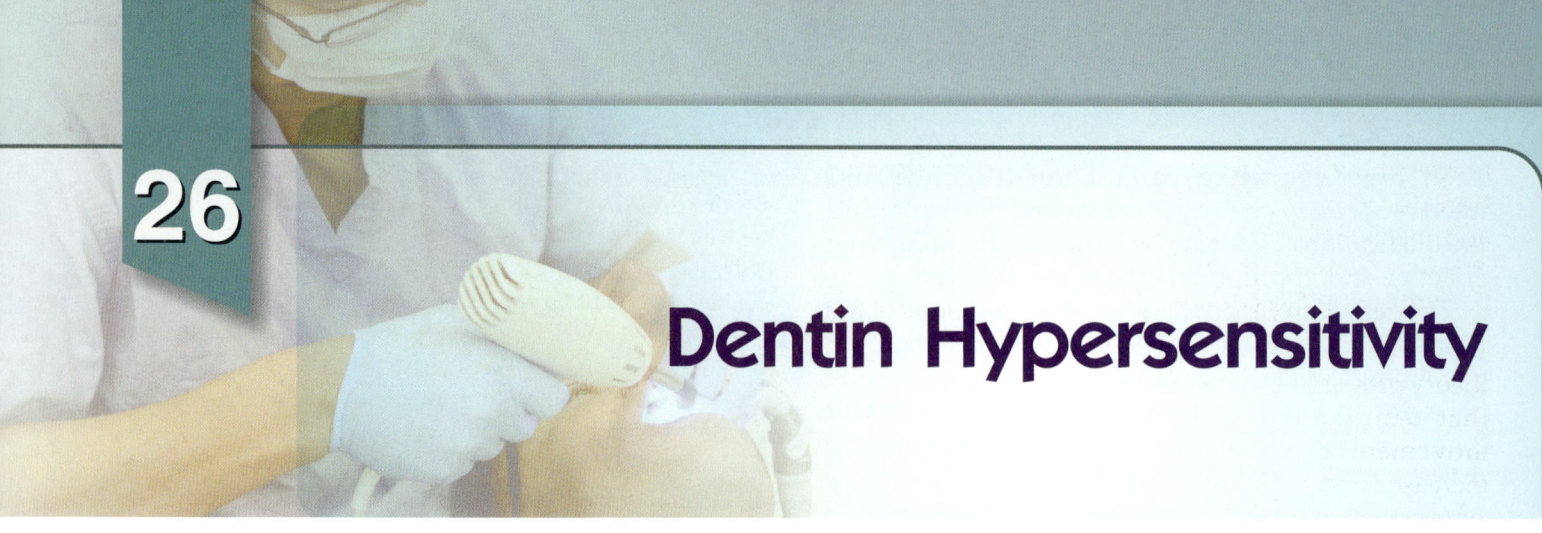

26. Dentin Hypersensitivity

With increase in life expectancy and increased retention of natural dentition, the incidence of dentin hypersensitivity is likely to become a frequent dental finding in future. Thus, the decline of tooth loss in the 20th century and the increasing longevity of the teeth with tooth wear in the 21st century will be far more demanding in the preventive and restorative skills of the dental professionals. One of the earliest citings of dentin hypersensitivity dates back to Blum in 1530. However, it was not until 1700 that this oral pain condition was more extensively investigated.

DEFINITION

Characteristic pain which arises from exposed dentin typically in response to a variety of stimuli, for example, thermal, evaporative, tactile, osmotic or chemical, which cannot be ascribed to any other form of dental defect or pathology is known as dentin hypersensitivity. Another term, root sensitivity, has been suggested for dentin hypersensitivity arising from gingival recession in periodontal disease and following periodontal treatment. This group of patients may have microorganisms invading the root dentinal tubules of periodontally involved teeth, with pain often occurring interdentally, coinciding with recession in these areas. Hence, this condition may be of different etiology but results in similar pain symptoms. Thus, recession linked to periodontal disease is often termed root sensitivity.

INCIDENCE AND PREVALENCE

Dentin hypersensitivity can be present from early to old age, with the majority of sufferers aged between 20 to 40 years with peak incidence between 30-39 years. Later in life, age-related changes in pulpal processes result in a reduction of sensitivity owing to reparative processes such as secondary dentin and tertiary dentin, fibrosis in the pulp and sclerosis of the tubules, which will decrease permeability and reduce the hydraulic conductance of dentin. Women are more frequently affected, which reflects oral hygiene and dietary practices and at a younger mean age. The reported prevalence of dentin hypersensitivity varies from 3 to 57%, however, the most consistent figure documented is 15%.

ETIOLOGY AND PREDISPOSING FACTORS

Typically, dentin hypersensitivity occurs when the external stimulus contacts exposed dentin, triggers a rapid outflow of dentinal fluid, and the resultant pressure change across the dentin activates interdental nerve fibers to cause immediate pain. Tactile, cold and osmotic stimuli all trigger rapid fluid outflow. Heat, on the other hand, triggers a slow retreat of dentin fluid and the resultant pressure change activates the nerve fibers in a less dramatic fashion, consistent with the observation that cold is generally more problematic to sufferers than is heat.

A number of theories have been proposed over the years to explain the pain mechanism of dentinal hypersensitivity.

1. Direct Neural Stimulation

An early hypothesis was the dentinal receptor mechanism theory, which suggests that dentin hypersensitivity is caused by the direct stimulation of sensory nerve endings in dentin. On the basis of microscopic and experimental data, it seems unlikely that neural cells exist in the sensory portion of the outer dentin. This theory is not well accepted.

2. Odontoblast Deformation Theory/Transducer Theory

The odontoblast transducer mechanism was proposed by Rapp et al. It suggested that odontoblasts act as receptor cells, mediating changes in the membrane potential of the odontoblasts via synaptic junctions with nerves. This could result in the sensation of pain from the nerve endings located in the pulpodentinal border; however, the evidence for the odontoblast transducer mechanism theory is generally lacking and inconclusive.

3. Hydrodynamic Theory

The current accepted hypothesis is the hydrodynamic theory proposed by Brannstrom. The hypothesis states that dentin hypersensitivity may be caused by movement of the dentinal tubule contents. An increased outward fluid flow causes a pressure change across the dentin, distorting the nerve fibres by a mechanoreceptor action, causing sharp, shooting pain (Figs 26.1A and B).

The width of the tubule is very important, as the rate of fluid flow is dependent on the fourth power of the radius. If the tubule diameter doubles, a 16-fold increase in fluid flow results. Sensitive teeth have many more (8 times) and wider (2 times) tubules at the buccal cervical area compared with non-sensitive teeth. A higher velocity of fluid flow also occurs in tubules of smaller diameter, possibly provoking pain sensations. Dentin will only be sensitive if the tubules are patent from the pulp to the oral environment, and this patency will change with production and removal of the smear layer, hence resulting in an episodic condition.

The trigeminal nerve supplies the pulp, with innervations from myelinated fibres (A-β and A-δ) and nonmyelinated C fibers. It is proposed that the larger myelinated fibres (A-β and A-δ) can respond to stimuli that displace the fluid in the dentinal tubule through a hydrodynamic mechanism, such as tactile, evaporative, osmotic or thermal challenges, to elicit short, sharp, stabbing pain that typically lasts for only a few seconds.

The classical pain experienced with dentin hypersensitivity can persist as a dull, throbbing ache for variable periods of time. Dentin hypersensitivity sufferers can readily be divided into two groups: those who have the sharp, shooting pain and those who have the subsequent dull, aching pain.

The poorly localized, dull, burning ache is thought to be caused by unmyelinated nerves, C-fibres and some of the slowest A-δ fibres.

The status of the pulp in dentin hypersensitivity is not known, although symptoms would suggest minor inflammation as a result of the length of time that symptoms persist without developing into a true pulpitis. It has been suggested that when the pain continues as a throbbing ache then a true pulpitis is present.

Dentin hypersensitivity results from dentin exposed from either coronal or radicular regions of the tooth.

Exposure of Dentin as a Result of Loss of Cementum

Gingival recession is a common finding both in populations with high standards of oral hygiene, as well as in populations with poor oral hygiene. The former type of recession can be attributed to overzealous toothbrushing and is predominantly found on the buccal surfaces of canines and premolars. Teeth and tooth surfaces that receive most brushing during the brushing cycle overall show the highest predilection for recession with a more common incidence on the left side where a high majority of subjects are right handed. Plaque scores derived from epidemiological and clinical studies also correlate with sites of gingival recession and dentin hypersensitivity, coinciding with the lowest plaque scores.

The latter type of recession is seen in periodontal patients both exhibiting the disease and following treatment. These lesions can be found anywhere around the root. Dentin hypersensitivity can be

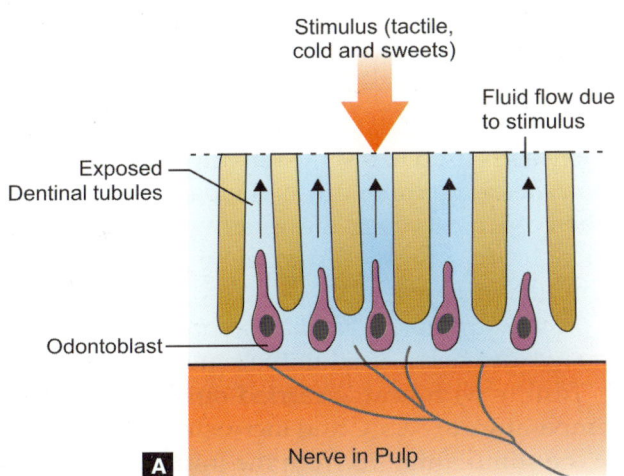
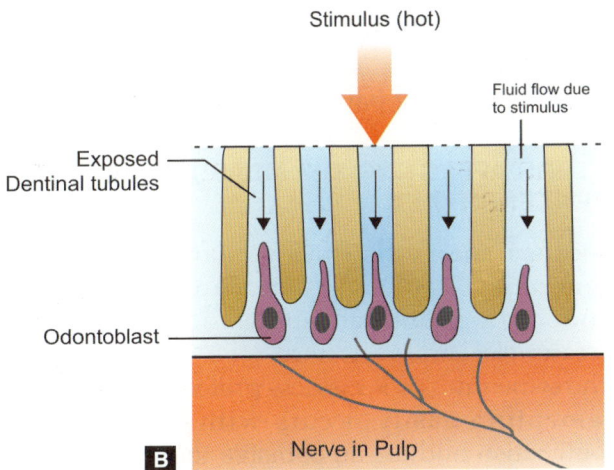

Figs 26.1A and B: Hydrodynamic theory: **(A)** outward flow of dentinal fluid; **(B)** inward flow of dentinal fluid

attributed to both types of recession but is most frequently associated with recession of the healthy gingiva. The two etiologies result in the same pain condition; however, they should be treated differently in terms of prevention, etiology and research.

Exposure of Dentin as a Result of Loss of Enamel

Tooth wear is usually multifactorial with one type of wear dominating over the other. Erosive tooth wear, in particular, is becoming increasingly significant to the longevity of the dentition. Lifestyles have dramatically changed the consumption characteristics of soft acidic drinks, and healthy (often acidic) diets are prominent. Emphasis of preventive dentistry has also increased, with the population spending more efforts on oral hygiene practices, which can result in the increased prevalence of tooth wear.

Enamel is highly susceptible to acid erosion, which is probably the most aggressive type of wear compared with abrasion and attrition. The acid may be derived from intrinsic, gastric, or more often, extrinsic sources that are dietary in origin. Individuals who consume 1 litre of soft drinks per day, which is not uncommon, can lose 1 mm of enamel over 2-20 years. When an acid comes into contact with the tooth, not only is there bulk loss of the hard tissues but also softening of the remaining surface. Surface softening can extend 3-5 microns and be susceptible to loss after a few brush strokes. So, if the erosive challenge is followed soon after with the abrasive challenge, the softened hard tissue will be easily removed and has no chance to reharden. This scenario is depicted well in individuals having a grapefruit for breakfast followed by brushing their teeth with brush and toothpaste. So, one should wait for at least half an hour for toothbrushing after having an acidic drink.

Toothbrushes alone have no measurable effects on enamel and dentin loss. But abrasive toothpastes accomplished with overzealous toothbrushing can lead to enamel loss. Attrition of tooth surfaces is usually the result of parafunctional acivity.

FACTORS AFFECTING THE MEASUREMENT OF HYPERSENSITIVITY

- Because enamel is thicker than cementum, it generally provides greater protection of the underlying dentinal tubules. It also provides greater electrical resistance.
- The cementum provides less protection. Loss of the cementum easily occurs with use of a hard toothbrush and/or an abrasive toothpaste, or by root scaling and planing during oral hygiene and periodontal therapy.
- Salivary calcium and phosphate ions facilitate obturation of the dentinal tubules. It affects the dentinal tubule permeability and, as a result, tooth sensitivity measurements, especially the electrical measurement.
- State of the pulp also affects the sensitivity. Inflamed pulpal tissue could result in a reading of greater sensitivity than normal, whereas necrotic pulp tissue generally results in readings of lower sensitivity or non-sensitivity.
- Longevity of the stimulus is also important feature. The time required for the tooth and pulp tissues to return to baseline values affects the tooth sensitivity.

METHODS USED TO MEASURE TOOTH HYPERSENSITIVITY

Various methods used to measure tooth hypersensitivity are:

Tactile

The tactile method implies lightly passing a sharp dental explorer over the sensitive area of a tooth (usually along the cemento-enamel junction). The patient's response is graded on a severity scale, generally 0 to 3 (a score of '0' is assigned if no pain is felt, '1' if there is slight pain or discomfort, '2' if there is severe pain, and '3' if there is severe pain that lasts for more than 10 seconds.

The force-sensitive electronic probe usually used to measure the depth of periodontal pockets at fixed pressures is also used to quantify the sensitivity. The operator can vary the force applied to the tip by regulating the amount of current and the tip position.

The probe force is controlled within ± 1 gram. The probe force can be increased in steps (say 5 gms) until the subject experiences discomfort. That point is taken as the pain threshold. If a maximum force of 70 grams is reached with no discomfort, the tooth is scored as non-sensitive. The probe emits a buzzing sound when a predetermined pressure is applied.

Thermal

Room air is used to test the sensitivity since it is cooler than the oral temperature. The patient will feel pain when cool air contacts the sensitive tooth. Blowing air on a tooth involves drying, which can also be stimulatory.

Tactile stimuli are applied before thermal stimuli if the two are being used in the same subject.

Testing with heat is carried out keeping the basic temperature at 37.5°C and increasing the temperature of the stimulating tip from the initial temperature of 37.5°C in increments of 1°C to the point at which pain is felt.

Osmotic

After isolation of the test tooth, a cotton applicator saturated with the sucrose solution is applied to the root surface of the tooth and allowed to remain in place for 10 seconds. The sensation as no pain (designed as '0') or pain (designated as '1') is recorded. The tooth surface is later rinsed with warm water.

Electrical

Electrical pulp testers are widely used to determine the vitality of tooth. The quantification of electric current can be used for measuring tooth sensitivity. Certain pulp testers may determine a condition known as pre-pain. The pre-pain sensation has been attributed to the larger, more rapidly conducting nerve fibers than the smaller diameter nerve fibers.

For safety reasons, any electrical current that is applied should be limited to less than 1 milliampere, preferably 0.5 milliampere (the approximate range of the human body's threshold of current perception). The voltage pulses with a width of 0.05 to 0.20 millisecond each and spaced at 5 to 10 millisecond intervals will provide a stimulus of pre-pain instead of pain.

Air Indexing Method

The air indexing method was designed to quantify dentin hypersensitivity. A restricted air stream was directed toward the cementoenamel junction at approximately 45° angle for 0.5 to 1.0 second. The tip is kept at a distance of 0.5 cm from the tooth cervix. The duration of the air exposure is for shorter possible duration to avoid neurogenic inflammation or evaporative phenomenon. The air is applied for fluid control block hole (Different holes have different pressures, viz. No.1: 2-3 psi, No.2: 4-6 psi, No.3: 11-17 psi, No.4: 25-20 psi and No.5: 35-40 psi). Usually number one hole is used to initiate the response. If no response is elicited, then the next number is used. The least air pressure necessary for detection of sensitive tooth is termed as 'threshold patient response.' These threshold response values were determined by the patient and recorded as none (0), slight (1), moderate (2) or severe (3).

The same method is then used for lingual surfaces. Resultant threshold response can be noted. The changes in response over time is evaluated before planning treatment for dentinal sensitivity.

DIAGNOSIS

In 1982, dentin hypersensitivity was described as an enigma, because it was frequently encountered and poorly understood. For the diagnosis and management of dentin hypersensitivity, the dental professional is advised to follow six steps with their patients:

- Correct diagnosis of dentin hypersensitivity based upon history and clinical examination;
- Differential diagnosis, to exclude other conditions giving rise to similar pain symptoms;
- Treatment of all secondary conditions with symptoms similar to dentin hypersensitivity;
- Identification of etiologic and predisposing factors, particularly dietary and oral hygiene habits, pertinent to erosion and abrasion;
- Removal or minimization of etiologic and predisposing factors through dietary advice and oral hygiene instructions;
- Recommendation or provision of treatment based upon individual needs.

Differential Diagnosis

Prior to advocating treatment regimens it is important to consider confirmation of the correct diagnosis and exclude the differential diagnosis. A number of other dental conditions can give rise to pain symptoms similar to those of dentin hypersensitivity. Indeed, a definitive diagnosis of dentin hypersensitivity is reached through exclusion of the following conditions, which need a variety of treatment options for resolution.

- Cracked tooth syndrome, often in heavily restored teeth.
- Incorrect placement of dentin adhesives in restorative dentistry, leading to nanoleakage.
- Fractured restorations and incorrectly placed dentin pins.
- Pulpal response to caries and to restorative treatment.
- Inappropriate application of various medicaments during cavity preparation.
- Lack of care while contouring restorations so the tooth is left in traumatic occlusion.
- Palatogingival groove and other enamel invaginations.
- Chipped teeth causing exposed dentin.
- Vital bleaching.

MANAGEMENT OF HYPERSENSITIVITY

Management of hypersensitive dentin involves the following steps along with specific treatment modalities.

1. Dietary Counselling

Dietary acids are capable of causing erosive loss of tooth structure, subsequently opening the dentinal tubules. Dietary counseling should focus on the quantity and frequency of acid intake. It is established that wine, citrus fruit juices, apple juice, and yogurt were capable of dissolving the smear layer; however, tannic acids, low-pH carbonated drinks and Coca-Cola had no effect on smear layer. Loss of dentin is greatly increased when brushing is performed immediately after exposure of the tooth to dietary acids.

2. Tooth Brushing Techniques

Incorrect tooth brushing, especially using hard bristles, may lead to abrasion and the hypersensitivity. Instruction of proper brushing techniques can prevent loss of dentin and the resulting hypersensitivity.

3. Plaque Control

Saliva contains calcium and phosphate ions and is therefore able to contribute to the formation of mineral deposits within exposed dentinal tubules. The presence of plaque may interfere with this process, as plaque bacteria, produce acid and dissolve any mineral precipitates, thus opening dentinal tubules.

TREATMENT MODALITIES FOR DENTINAL HYPERSENSITIVITY

Various desensitizing agents (Fig. 26.2) have been used and are currently being used to treat dentin sensitivity. Dentin fluid flow rate is proportional to the fourth power of the tubule radius, so the difference in tubule diameter between 'sensitive' and 'non-sensitive' teeth is certainly of clinical relevance to the treatment of dentin hypersensitivity.

The requisites of desensitizing agents are:
- Provides immediate and lasting relief of pain
- Easy to apply
- Well tolerated by patients
- Not injurious to the pulp
- Not discolor the tooth
- Relatively inexpensive

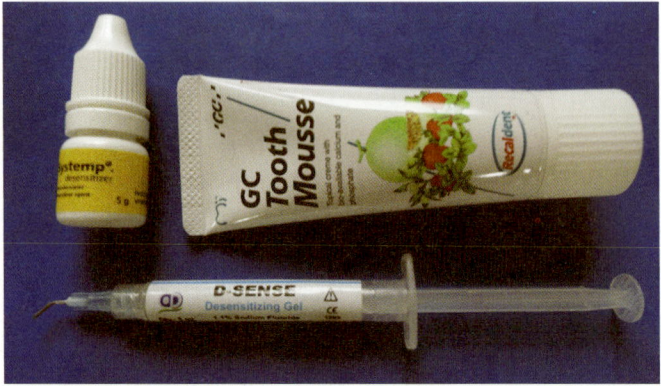

Fig. 26.2: Desensitizing agents

The treatment procedures are differentiated as over the counter dentifrices and in-office treatment procedures.

a. Over the Counter Dentifrices

A dentifrice is defined as an agent, usually incorporated in toothpastes, helps in cleaning the accessible surfaces of the teeth. The agent containing desensitizing formulation in a dentifrice can be used for alleviating symptoms of tooth sensitivity.

Dentifrice usually have abrasive, surfactant and thickener, etc. Therapeutic dentifrices contain drug agents in addition to the other items.

Abrasives are solid particles that clean or polish the tooth surface, for example calcium phosphate, pyrophosphate, sodium metaphosphate and alumina. Recently silicas are being preferred because of their compatibility with fluoride. Dentifrice abrasives are essential to prevent tooth staining.

The taste of a dentifrice is one of the most important factors related to the continuous use of a particular dentifrice.

There are two mechanisms of action of desensitizing agents.

a. blocking dentinal fluid movement by occluding dentinal tubules
b. blocking pulpal nerves activity by altering the excitability of sensory nerves.

Various agents used as desensitizing agents are:

1. Strontium Chloride

Strontium chloride (10%) was the first tubule blocking ingredient to be introduced into toothpaste, being commercialized as Sensodyne, approximately 50 years ago. The literature suggests three potential mechanisms of action for strontium salts. First, nerve depolarization is possible. Second, because of its chemical similarity to calcium, strontium could, in principle, replace lost calcium in the hydroxyapatite lattice to strengthen demineralized enamel and/or dentin. Third, strontium salts may deposit a layer of fine particles to occlude tubules. The third has been proposed to be the most likely of the three mechanisms. It has, however, been concluded that strontium salts appear to have only a minimal effect in reducing the symptoms of dentin hypersensitivity.

2. Potassium Salts

Potassium salts are now the most commonly used agents in pastes. The mechanism of action of potassium salts is that they can dramatically reduce the excitability of intra-dental nerves. Specifically, raising the concentration of potassium ion significantly above the physiological level in the extracellular fluid induces depolarization of the nerve cells, a brief excitatory burst, following which the nerves become unresponsive to excitatory stimuli. Some divalent cations, such as calcium and strontium, are also able to suppress nerve activity in vitro, but they do so to a much lesser extent than potassium. The potassium ion has to diffuse from the oral cavity into the dentin tubules, then through the dentin tubules against the flow of dentin fluid to the site of action at the interface of the inner dentin surface and the pulp chamber, i.e., the nerve endings. Further, to induce depolarization of the nerves and achieve significant pain relief, the concentration of potassium must build up in the fluid surrounding the nerve ending, which typically takes a period of 4 to 8 weeks, and be maintained at that level on an ongoing basis. If and when treatment with potassium-based products is ceased, elevated levels of potassium the site of action are diffused, and sensitivity relief is lost.

3. Oxalates

The mode of action of oxalates has been proposed as tubule occlusion by oxalate ions reacting with calcium ions in the dentinal fluid to form insoluble calcium oxalate crystals. However, these are acid labile and can be easily washed from the surface of dentin.

4. Silica Abrasives

Silica abrasives can also occlude dentin tubules and can reduce sensitivity.

5. Fluoride Salts

It has been suggested that fluoride may mechanically block the tubules, or that labile fluoride in the organic matrix of the dentin could block the transmission of stimuli. Sodium fluoride is superior to sodium monofluorophosphate in fluoride deposition on the teeth.

b. In-office Treatment Procedures

Treatment of hypersensitive teeth should be directed toward reducing the functional diameter of the tubules so as to limit fluid movement. In order to accomplish this objective the possible approaches are:

- Formation of a smear layer by brushing the exposed root surface.
- Topical application of agents that form insoluble precipitates within the tubules.
- Impregnation of tubules with plastic resins.
- Application of dental bonding agents to seal off the tubules.

Although most agents that are effective in reducing dentinal hypersensitivity are also effective in partially occluding the dentinal tubules (Potassium nitrate is an exception) (Table 26.1).

In-office treatment procedures include:

  i. Cavity varnishes
 ii. Corticosteroids
iii. Procedures/Chemical agents that can obturate dentinal tubules
   - Burnishing of dentin
   - Silver nitrate/Zinc chloride/strontium chloride/potassium oxalate
   - Calcium hydroxide/Dibasic calcium phosphate
   - Sodium fluoride/Sodium silicofluoride/Stannous fluoride
 iv. Primers/Bonding agents
  v. Iontophoresis
 vi. Lasers
vii. Restorative methods

Prior to treating sensitive root surfaces, hard or soft deposits should be removed from the teeth. Root planing may cause considerable discomfort, in that case teeth should be anesthetized prior to treatment. The teeth should be isolated and dried with warm air. When using desensitizing agents that have a caustic effect on soft tissue, care must be exercised to prevent them from contacting the alveolar mucosa.

i. Cavity Varnishes

Dentin often becomes insensitive when open tubules are covered with a thin film of varnish. This may be an effective means of providing temporary relief.

A fluoride-containing varnish (Duraflor) can be used for sustained relief.

ii. Corticosteroids

Steroids have been widely used to treat dentinal hypersensitivity. It is reported that steroids cause complete obliteration of tubules thus decreasing dentin permeability.

iii. Procedures/Chemical Agents that can Obturate Dentinal Tubules

Burnishing of dentin results in the formation of a smear layer that partially occludes the dentinal tubules. Usually wooden sticks are used to burnish dentin. It is observed that burnishing creates a partial smear layer that reduce fluid movement across dentin by 50 to 80 per cent.

Silver nitrate/zinc chloride: Certain salts react with tooth structure to form crystals on the surface of the dentin. Such crystallization should occur within 1 to

Table 26.1: Dentin desensitizers and mode of action

Chemical used	Brand name	Mode of action	Evaluation
Oxalate products	Sensodyne sealant, MS-coat	Tubule occlusion	Air blast, tactile
Calcium phosphate products	Quell desensitizer	Tubule occlusion	Quantitative permeability reduction
HEMA + Glutaraidehyde and others	Gluma desensitizer, hema desensitizer HemaSeal G Gluma, Fuji VII	Protein precipitation tubule occlusion	Tactile, air blast quantitative permeability reduction
Fluorides of sodium and stannous	Dentin bloc	Tubule occlusion	Air blast, tactile
Fluoride varnish (5% NaF)	Durphant, cavity shield, all solutions fluoride varnish	Tubule occlusion	Tactile, cold, air blast ice
Light-cure adhesives	Gluma, single bond prime and bond 2.1	Tubule occlusion	Air blast, tactile, cold, quantitative permeability
Glass-ionomer cements	Vitrabond, gluma Fuji VII	Tubule occlusion	Tactile, cold, air blast
Potassium-containing products (potassium nitrate alone and in combination with other salts)	Radent, relief	Lower nerve sensitivity	Air blast, cold, tactile

2 minutes and the crystals should be able to enter the tubules.

Silver nitrate has long been used as desensitizing agent. Silver nitrate precipitates protein constituents of odontoblast processes, thereby partially blocking the tubules.

Zinc chloride alone or zinc chloride – potassium ferrocyanide combination has also been used. 40% solution of aqueous zinc chloride followed by 20% solution of aqueous potassium ferrocyanide has been successfully used as desensitizing agent.

Calcium hydroxide/Calcium phosphate: Calcium hydroxide is being routinely used for the treatment of dentin hypersensitivity. The exact mechanism of action is unknown, however, it is hypothetized that it may block dentinal tubules or promote peritubular dentin formation.

Increasing the concentration of calcium ions around nerve fibers may results in decreased nerve excitability; therefore, calcium hydroxide might be capable of suppressing nerve activity.

Calcium phosphate has also been successfully tried as a desensitizing agent.

Sodium fluoride/Stannous fluoride: 2.0% sodium fluoride has been routinely used as a desensitizing agent.

The dentinal fluid is saturated with calcium and phosphate ions and the application of sodium fluoride to dentin leads to precipitation of calcium fluoride crystals, thus reducing the functional radius of the dentinal tubules. The crystal size of calcium fluoride is very small (approximately 0.5 μm), and therefore less effective as compared to potassium oxalate that give rise to larger crystals. Furthermore, it has been shown that fluoride is lost fairly rapidly following application of sodium fluoride to dentin.

Sodium silicofluoride was more effective than sodium fluoride.

10 per cent solution of stannous fluoride has also been successfully used.

iv. Primers/bonding Agents

The primers/bonding agents are used to seal the dentinal tubules.

The area of sensitive dentin is cleansed and etched with an acid conditioner for 5 seconds. The dentin is then dehydrated with a continuous blast of air for at least 15 to 20 seconds in order to dry the outer part of the dentinal tubules. A drop of a bonding agent is then applied to the dentin and cured.

Glass-ionomer luting cement has been successfully used to desensitize the dentin because it is hydrophilic, adheres well and it is esthetically pleasing.

v. Iontophoresis

Iontophoresis is a term applied to the use of an electrical potential to transfer ions into the body for therapeutic purposes.

When a direct current passes through an electrolyte, positive ions travel toward the negative electrode (cathode) and negative ions towards the positive electrode (anode).

Iontophoresis involves the placement of a negative electrode to dentin and a positive electrode to the patient's face or arm. If the negative electrode makes contact with saliva, gingival tissue or a metallic restoration, the flow of current will follow the path of least resistance and stream around the dentin rather than through. It is recommended that teeth be isolated with plastic strips or cotton rolls, rather than with rubber dam. The moisture that accumulate between the tooth and the rubber dam, may provide a low resistance pathway for the current.

The chemical is applied to the tooth surface after proper isolation and the current passed through negative electrode using a 0.5 mA current.

Potassium oxalate (30%) and ferric oxalate (6%) solutions make available oxalate ions that react with calcium ions in the dentinal fluid to form insoluble calcium oxalate crystals. These crystals blade the dentinal tubules.

It is hypothetized that the larger crystals are only effective in obturating wide open tubules, whereas the smaller crystals are capable of obturating open as well as partially close tubules. Application of potassium oxalate to the etched dentin reduced sensory nerve excitability to the level of unetched dentin.

vi. Lasers

The advent of Lasers has provided another possible treatment option for dentin hypersensitivity.

The various types of Lasers used are

- CO_2 Laser
- Nd:YAG Laser
- Er:YAG Laser
- He:Ne Laser

Lasers occlude the dentinal tubules by producing local changes around the exposed dentin and also produce changes in the central pulp neuron.

Disadvantage

- Expensive
- Not available for routine use

vii. Restorative methods

The exposed dentin is restored with glass-ionomer cement/composite resins, especially in case of recession. A routine conservative cavity is prepared and restored with any of these cements.

PREVENTION

Suggestions for Patients

- Avoid gingival recession by practicing good oral hygiene measures.
- Avoid using large amounts of dentifrices
- Avoid toothbrushes with hard bristles
- Avoid brushing teeth immediately following ingestion of acidic food or beverages
- Avoid over brushing with excessive pressure for prolonged periods of time
- Avoid excessive flossing or incorrect use of other interproximal cleaning devices
- Avoid frequent use of toothpicks

Suggestions for Professionals

- Avoid over instrumenting the root surfaces during calculus removal and scaling and root planning
- Avoid over polishing the exposed roots during stain removal
- Avoid violating the biologic width when placing crown margins causing subsequent recession
- Avoid 'burning' the gingival tissue during in-office tooth whitening or bleaching procedures

NEWER TECHNIQUES

1. Pro-Argin Technology

It is established that saliva transports calcium and phosphate into dentin tubules inducing tubule plugging. A new "saliva-based composition" containing arginine (an amino acid which is positively charged at physiological pH), bicarbonate (a pH buffer) and calcium carbonate (a source of calcium) is developed to massage sensitivity. A product (ProClude[c]) based upon this composition has recently been marketed. Clinical studies have shown that this desensitizing paste is effective in providing instant sensitivity relief and that this sensitivity relief lasts for at least 28 days.

Colgate has further improved this technology by combining arginine and calcium carbonate, with fluoride to provide a significant advance in treatment of dentin hypersensitivity. A new dentifrice containing 8.0% arginine, calcium carbonate, and 1450 ppm fluoride, as MFP, has been clinically proven to provide lasting relief to sensitivity.

Confocal laser scanning microscopy (CLSM) has confirmed that the Pro-Argin technology effectively plugs and seals dentin tubules and that the occlusion achieved is resistant to acid challenge. CLSM studies have also shown that the arginine is delivered to the inner surfaces of dentin tubules within the occluded dentin plug. Hydraulic conductance has shown that the occlusion achieved with the arginine-containing toothpaste results in reduced dentin fluid flow and inhibition of the hydrodynamic mechanism.

A new variant of this desensitizing toothpaste, containing the Pro-Argin technology, fluoride and calcium carbonate has been developed.

The Pro-Argin technology is clinically proven to provide instant sensitivity relief prior to and after dental procedures, such as scaling and root planning.

2. NovaMin

NovaMin is bioactive glass ceramic material that provides calcium and phosphate. The active ingredient is calcium sodium phosphosilicate that reacts when exposed to aqueous medium and provide calcium and phosphate ions that form hydroxy-carbonate apatite with time.

NovaMin is successfully used to treat dentinal hypersensitivity. The calcium and phosphate ions block the dentinal tubules, thereby reducing the flow of dentinal fluid. NovaMin has been used with and without fluoride (Oravive). NovaMin in combination with 5% sodium fluoride (Renew: 5 wt% NovaMin and 5000 ppm fluoride) is also marketed. The manufacturers also claim its ability to whiten and remineralize the affected dentin.

3. Casein Derivatives

Casein is the predominant phosphoprotein in bovine milk and accounts for almost 80% of its total protein. Under alkaline conditions the calcium phosphate is present as an alkaline amorphous phase along with calcium phosphate, referred to as casein phosphopeptide-amorphous calcium phosphate (CPP-ACP). They have the ability to stabilize high concentrations of calcium and phosphate in metastable solutions. CPP-ACP is a useful cariostatic agent for the control of dental caries as it contains calcium and phosphate in a bio-available form. CPP-ACP can be used as an:

- Adjunct preventive therapy to reduce caries in high risk patients
- Reduce dental erosion in patients with gastric reflux
- To repair enamel involving white spot lesions
- Orthodontic decalcification
- Desensitizing agent

CONCLUSION

- Preventive measures should be followed as indicated.
- Clinically there are many treatment modalities for dentin hypersensitivity that the clinician finds successful in alleviating the pain of dentin hypersensitivity.
- The first line of treatment should be the least invasive, such as a low abrasive strontium-based or potassium-based toothpaste.
- High fluoride products can be utilized.
- If these treatment modalities fail, varnishes/resins can be used followed by conventional restorative procedures.
- Unfortunately, no single treatment seems to suit all. The least invasive treatments are usually advocated first followed by the professionally led treatment.

BIBLIOGRAPHY

1. Addy, M.: Dentin hypersensitivity: new perspectives on an old problem. Int. Dent. J.: 52, 367, 2002.
2. Addy, M.: Oral hygiene products: Potential for harm to oral and systemic health. Periodontology 2000: 48, 54, 2008.
3. Addy, M.: Tooth brushing, tooth wear and dentin hypersensitivity – are they associated ? Int. Dent. J.: 55, 261, 2005.
4. Amarasena, N., Spencer, J., Du, Y. and Brennan, D.: Dentin hypersensitivity in a private practice patient population in Australia. J. Oral Rehab.: 38, 52, 2011.
5. Arrais, C.A., Micheloni, C.D., Giannini, M. and Chan, D.C.: Occluding effect of dentifrices on dentinal tubules. J. Dent.: 31, 577, 2003.
6. Banfield, N. and Addy, M.: Dentin hypersensitivity: Development and evaluation of a model in situ to study tubule patency. J. Clin. Periodontol.: 31, 325, 2004.
7. Bartold, P.M.: Dentinal hypersensitivity: a review. Aust. Dent. J.: 51, 212, 2006.
8. Coleman TA, Kinderknecht KE. Cervical dentin hypersensitivity. Part I: The air indexing method. Quintessence Int 31, 461, 2000.
9. Cruz, J.C., Stout, J.R., Heaton, L.J. and Wataha, J.C.: Dentin hypersensitivity and oxalates : a systematic review. J Dent Res.: 90, 304, 2011
10. Cummins, D.: Dentin hypersensitivity: From diagnosis to a breakthrough therapy for everyday sensitivity relief. J. Clin. Dent.: 20, 1, 2009.
11. Cummins, D.: Recent advances in dentin hypersensitivity. Clinically proven treatments for intact and lasting sensitivity relief. Am. J. Dent.: 23, sp. Issue 3A, 2010.
12. Cummins, D.: The efficacy of a new dentifrice containing 8.0% arginine, calcium carbonate, and 1450 ppm fluoride in delivering instant and lasting relief of dentin hypersensitivity. J. Clin. Dent.; 20, 109, 2009.
13. Cummins, D.: Recent advances in dentin hypersensitivity: clinically proven treatments for instant and lasting sensitivity relief. Am J Dent.: 23, 3A, 2010

14. Cunha-Cruz, J., Stout, J.R., Heaton, L.J. and Wataha, J.C.: Dentin hypersensitivity and oxalate: a systematic review. J. Dent. Res.: 90, 304, 2011.
15. Dababneh, R.H., Khouri, A.T. and Addy, M.: Dentin hypersensitivity. An enigma? A review of terminology, epidemiology, mechanisms, aetiology and management. Br. Dent. J.: 187, 606, 1999.
16. Drisko, C.H.: Dentin hypersensitivity – Dental hygiene and periodontal considerations. Int. Dent. J.: 52, 385, 2002.
17. Duran I. and Sengun, A.: The long-term effectiveness of five current desensitizing products on cervical dentin sensitivity. J. Oral Rehabil.: 31, 351, 2004.
18. Gandolfi, M.G., Farascioni, S., Pashley, D.H., Giorgio, G. and Prati, C.: Calcium silicate coating derived from Portland cement as treatment for hypersensitive dentin. J. Dent.: 36, 565, 2008.
19. Gillam, D.G. and Orchardson, R.: Advances in the treatment of root dentin sensitivity: mechanisms and treatment principles. Endod. Topics: 13, 13, 2006.
20. Hu, D., Zhang, Y.P., Chaknis, P., Petrone, M.E., Volpe, A.R. and DeVizio, W.: Comparative investigation of the desensitizing efficacy of a new dentifrice containing potassium citrate: An eight-week clinical study. J. Clin. Dent.: 15, 6, 2004.
21. Kimura, Y., Wilder-Smith, P., Yonaga, K. and Matsumoto, K.: Treatment of dentin hypersensitivity by lasers: a review. J. Clin. Periodontol.: 27, 715, 2000.
22. Lavender, S., Petrou, I., Heu, R., Stranick, M., Cummins, D., Kilpatrick-Liverman, L., Sullivan, R.J., Santarpia III P.: Mode of action studies on a new desensitizing dentifrice, containing the Pro-Argin technology, with a gentle whitening benefit. Am. J. Dent.: 23, 14A, 2010.
23. Markowitz, K. and Pashley, D.H.: Discovering new treatments for sensitive teeth: The long path from biology to therapy. J. Oral Rehabil.: 35, 300, 2007.
24. Markowitz, K.: The original desensitizers: Strontium and potassium salts. J. Clin. Dent.: 20, 145, 2009.
25. Orchardson, R. and Gillam, D.G.: The efficacy of potassium salts as agents for treating dentin hypersensitivity J. Orofac Pain: 14, 9, 2000.
26. Orchardson, R. and Gillam, D.G.: Managing dentin hypersensitivity. J Am Dent Assoc.: 137, 990, 2006.
27. Pashley, D.H.: Mechanisms of dentin sensitivity. Dent. Clin. North Am.: 34, 449, 1990.
28. Porto, I.C.M., Andrade, A.K.M. and Monets, A.J.R.: Diagnosis and treatment of dentinal sensitivity. J. Oral Sciences: 51, 323, 2009.
29. Suge, T., Kawasaki, A., Ishikawa, K., Matsuo, T. and Ebisu, S.: Ammonium hexafluorosilicate elicits calcium phosphate precipitation and shows continuous dentin tubule occlusion. Dent. Mater.: 24, 192, 2008.
30. Umberto R , Claudia R, Gaspare P, Gianluca T and Alessandro DV.: Treatment of dentin hypersensitivity by diode laser : A clinical study. : Int J Dent. 85, 8950, 2012
31. von Troil, B., Needleman, I. and Sanz, M.: A systematic review of the prevalence of root sensitivity following periodontal therapy. J. Clin. Periodontol.: 29, 173, 2002.
32. Walters, P.A.: Dentin hypersensitivity: A review. J. Contemp. Dent. Pract.: 6, 1, 2005.
33. Wang, S.H.Y., Hu, D. and Li, X.: Effectiveness of Laser therapy and topical desensitizing agents in treating dentin hypersensitivity: a systematic review. J. Oral Rehab.: 38, 348, 2011.
34. Wefel, J.S.: Novamin: Likely clinical success. Adv. Dent. Res.: 21, 40, 2009.

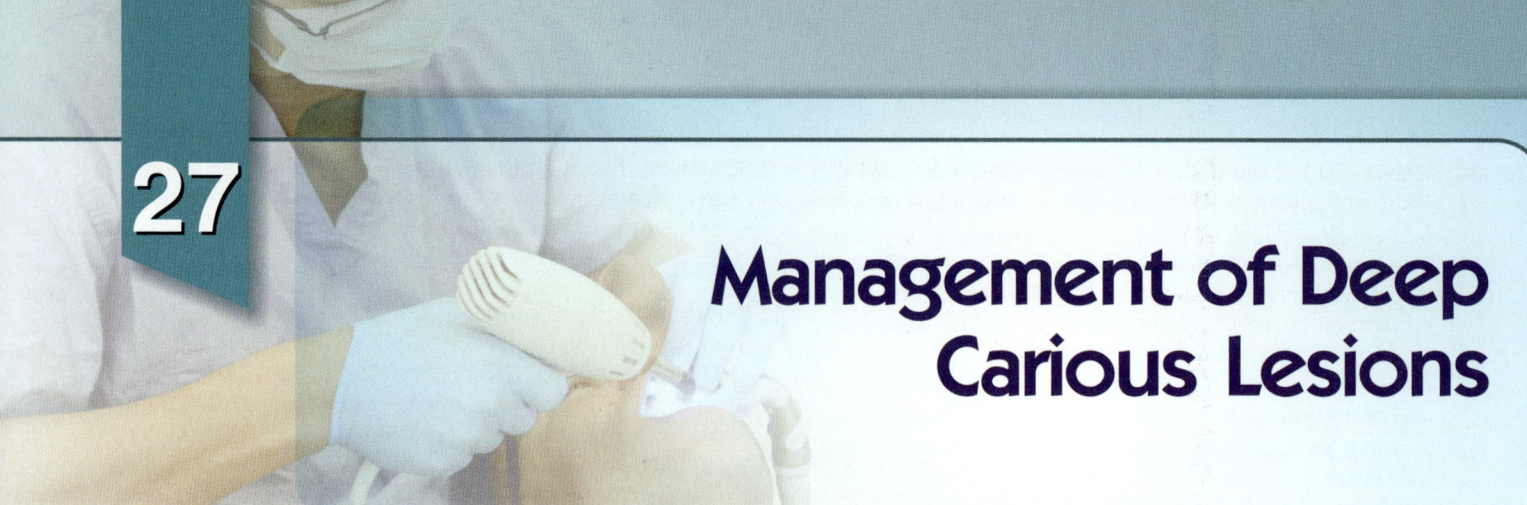

27. Management of Deep Carious Lesions

An important issue prior to restorative or endodontic treatment of carious teeth is the assessment of static and anatomical considerations of the location of the caries lesion, as well as the dynamic activity and extent of caries process. Presently major focus has been on improving the technical aspects of cavity design and choice of restorative materials, however, very less attention has been paid to the pathology of caries in relation to restorative treatment offered.

RESPONSE OF PULPO-DENTINAL COMPLEX IN DIFFERENT STAGES OF LESION PROGRESSION

The changes in pulpo-dentinal complex start appearing subjacent to lesions in enamel only, even before alterations in dentin have occurred.

a. Carious lesion advancing in enamel
- A reduction of the odontoblast predentin region can be observed as the very first cellular changes subjacent to active progressing enamel lesions.
- Size of odontoblasts decrease, as compared to unaffected odontoblasts.
- Pulpal cells proliferate into the cell free zone.
- Dentin tubular hypermineralization occurs, as the demineralization in enamel is reaching the dentino-enamel junction.

b. Carious lesion advancing in dentin
- Demineralization of dentin is initiated, as the enamel lesion comes in contact with the dentino-enamel junction. It presents as a brownish discoloration of dentin. This appearance is not lateral spread of the lesion. It has been shown never to extend beyond the limits of the enamel lesion contact area with the dentino-enamel junction. This dentin demineralization is a reaction of bacterial byproducts passing through enamel prisms.
- The advancing front of dentinal caries follows the direction of dentinal tubules, this being the primary route for dissolution of the hard dentinal tissue. Consequently the zone of dentin demineralization subjacent to non-cavitated lesions narrows as it progresses toward the pulp.
- The initial dentin demineralization takes place without the presence of bacteria in the dentin. As bacteria are still far too large to penetrate the demineralized rod and inter-rod enamel. However, when the enamel crumbles, bacterial invasion of the demineralized enamel occurs.

On the basis of oral hygiene status of the patient, persistence of the plaque biofilm and other related factors, caries may progress as an active lesion, or slow progressing lesion or may attain quiescence as arrested caries. The differences between active and slow progressing carious lesion are given in Table 27.1

ARRESTED CARIES

The conditions under which the arrest of an active lesion occur are still very not clear and being studied. An arrested dentinal lesion differs from an active lesion by its darker pigmentation, absence of visible bacteria within the tubule and impermeability to dyes and isotopes.

Following layers are identified:
1. A narrow surface layer, brown in color and leathery in consistency.
2. The widest zone, dark brown in color and hard in consistency.
3. Sclerotic layer, white in color and often harder than normal dentin.

One of the major characteristics of an arrested caries is its high degree of mineralization. The possible ways by which the accumulation of minerals occur can be:

a. Remineralization of the surface layer – source can be saliva from where calcium and phosphate are absorbed.

b. Reprecipitation of dissolved apatite – the minerals dissolved by bacterial acids in the upper demineralized layer reprecipitate to form large crystals in the area just below.

Management of Deep Carious Lesions

Table 27.1: Differences between acute and chronic carious lesions

Acute Caries/Active lesion	Chronic caries/slow progressing lesion
Dentin – yellowish, light brown in color	It has a darker brown color
The hardness of carious dentin decreases considerably	Relatively less softening of dentin occurs
Proliferation of cells takes place from the sub-odontoblastic cell rich zone into cell free zone.	It is not so evident in slow progressing lesions
Odontolbasts necrosis occurs at a faster rate followed by atubular dentin or fibrodentin deposition by newly formed odontoblasts	Tertiary dentin formed is tubular dentin at the pulpal site. It appears as a result of reactionary dentinogenesis and dentin produced by new odontoblast like cells
Rapid demineralization and tissue destruction occurs	Organic tissue is more resistance. Defensive process predominates

c. Sclerosis of intratubular calcification and obliteration of tubules of deeper layers underneath the lesion. Probably minerals are mediated by odontoblastic processes through blood supply.

In arrested lesions, the bacterial bodies are coalesced into homogenous masses, degenerated and disintegrated. Another characteristic is the presence of deep pigmentation. The degenerated bacteria or the degradation products of their proteins and nucleic acids are the possible sources of pigmentation.

HISTOPATHOLOGY OF DENTINAL CARIES

The pathological changes occurring in dentin, have been divided into various zones, starting from surface. These are:

A. Zone of decomposed dentin
B. Zone of bacterial invasion
C. Zone of demineralization
D. Zone of dentinal sclerosis or hypermineralization
E. Zone of fatty degeneration of Tome's fibers

A. Zone of Decomposed Dentin

- Completely devoid of minerals; more so in acute caries than in chronic caries
- Organic matrix decomposed completely
- High concentration of micro-organisms in the destructed dentin mass with substantial amounts of residual plaque deposits.
- Chronic lesions may be more odiferous, due to extensive lysis and darker in color due to longer duration of the decay process.
- Soft consistency

B. Zone of Bacterial Invasion

- Highest concentration of micro-organisms
- Dentinal tubules are extremely widened and cavitated
- This layer may have a slightly greater dimension in chronic than in acute decay
- Soft consistency, more soft in acute lesion

C. Zone of Demineralization

- Dentin is only demineralized, with the dentinal matrix intact
- Dentinal tubules may have normal dimensions
- Dimension of this zone is greater in acute lesion (1750 µm) than a chronic lesion (50 µm)
- Remineralization process is seen to accompany the demineralization activity in this zone, less so pronounced in acute decay
- Color in acute decay is straw color, and for chronic decay, the color is always yellow-brown or dark brown depending upon the time it has been subjected to microbial and environmental staining.
- Consistency and hardness in acute decay is much less than in chronic decay.

D. Zone of Dentinal Sclerosis or Hypermineralization

- Appears transparent in ground section and opaque in radiograph.
- Area of undisturbed mineralization repair
- Zone of dentinal sclerosis and calcific barrier, the two most impermeable types of dentin
- More pronounced in chronic decay
- Extremely hard when compared with normal dentin (15 times harder) and more so in chronic lesions.

E. Zone of fatty degeneration

- Intratubular fatty degeneration with lipid deposits being precipitated from fatty degeneration of the peripheral odontoblastic processes
- This degeneration predisposes to the sclerosis of the dentinal tubules
- More pronounced in acute lesions and will appear radiolucent in radiograph

The chronic or acute status of a lesion can be changed if there is a change in the environment (presence of bacterial substrates) encouraging one condition over the other.

EFFECTIVE DEPTH (REMAINING DENTIN) AND PULPAL RESPONSE

The effective depth is the area of minimum thickness of sound dentin separating the pulpal tissue from the carious lesion.

If remaining dentin thickness is more than 1.0mm, no significant disturbance in the pulp is seen. 0.25 to 0.5 mm remaining dentin leads to maximal reparative dentin formation and remineralization of demineralized dentin, whereas 0.25 mm or less remaining dentin provokes bacterial growth in pulp. Reparative dentin formation and remineralization is greatly decreased.

PROGNOSIS OF DEEP CARIOUS LESIONS

The outcome of the treatment of a deep carious lesion depends on various factors:
- Reparative capacity of pulpo-dentinal complex
- Soundness of the dentin in the preparation floors and walls
- Reparative capacity of unsound affected dentin
- Type and extent of any degeneration in the pulpo-dentinal complex
- Sealability of the restorative materials to be used
- Potential further irritation to the pulpo-dentinal complex resulting from preparation instrumentation, restorative materials and procedures

REPARABILITY OF PULPO-DENTINAL COMPLEX

The reparative capacity of pulpo-dentinal complex is the main agent determining the fate of a carious lesion advancing into dentin. It is further dependent on various factors:

I. Status of Pulp

a. Pain: Pain could serve as a tool to assess the pulpal status. The absence of toothache cannot be used as a deciding criterion for the pulpal health. The presence or absence of pain varies with different pathological conditions of pulp.
  - Spontaneous pain not initiated by thermal/chemical stimulation – indicative of pulpo-dentinal degeneration.
  - Pain initiated by thermal/chemical stimulation of pulpo-dentinal organ that disappears immediately after the removal of the stimulation is a possible indication of much lesser degree of degenerative changes.

2. Radiographs: A radiograph can indicate:
   a. Proximity of the carious lesion to the pulp chamber and root canal system.
   b. The effective depth or the thickness of the dentin bridge can be evaluated.
   c. Any pulpal changes in the form of intrapulpal and peripulpal calcification (it denotes the consumption of and reduction of the reparative capacity of the pulp; as it reduces/prevents the flow of fluids into or out of the pulp/root canal system).
   d. Periradicular status- the thickening of the periodontal ligament with an intact lamina-dura, especially periapically will indicate increased vascularity and consequently increased reparative capacity. Discontinuity in lamina dura indicates degeneration.
   e. Size of pulp chamber compared to size of tooth– the higher the pulp size/tooth ratio, the better will be the reparative capabilities of the pulpo-dentinal organ (It must be mentioned that unusually high ratio in comparison to other teeth may indicate complete cessation of reparative capacity).
   f. Size of pulp exposure – Size of pulp exposure in relation to pulp chamber/root canal system is a major factor determining the reparability via dentinal bridging.
   g. Permeability of dentin or evaluation of mineralization – Sclerotic dentin and calcific barrier can be identified radiologically as radio-opaque regions. Tertiary dentin, appears as a localized thickening of the dentinal bridge, pulpal to lesion creating irregularities in the pulp chamber.
3. Pulp testing
   a. Thermal pulp testing
      Application of heat or cold stimulates the nerves present in the pulp to elicit the symptoms of pain. The character of this pain, helps in arriving at a primitive diagnosis regarding the condition of the pulp.
   b. Electric pulp testing
      The objective of electric pulp testing is to stimulate a response by electric excitation of the neural elements within the pulp by subjecting the tooth to an increase degree of electric current.
      Positive response   - indicates vitality of pulp
      No response   - pulp necrosis

II. Extent of Pulpal Exposure

1. Pin point exposure; sound dentin at periphery, no haemorrhage, vital pulp, no pulpal inflammation

or mild inflammation restricted to exposure site – successful repair possible.
2. Exposure having infected dentin at periphery – reparability doubtful.
3. Exposure with profuse haemorrhage – beyond repair
4. Exposure with inflammatory fluid/pus – beyond repair
5. Exposure near to the anatomical constrictions in root canals – lesser will be the reparability locally because of the diminished availability of nutrients

III. Type of Dentin

The type of dentin is assessed visually and also using tactile methods. Presence of a calcific barrier/sclerotic dentin indicates formation of reparative dentin. Generalized discolored dentin ranging from grayish to grayish-brown may indicate necrosis of underlying pulp.

Caries Indicator Dyes

Various types of dyes are used to indicate the extent of progress of caries. 0.5% basic fuschin in propylene glycol applied to dentin for 10 seconds and washing it off with water may guide an operator as to where to stop in excavating dentin from cavity walls and floors.

It is the nature of collagen fibers that differ in infected and affected dentin that accounts for the different stainability of the two. The affected dentin will have intact collagen fibers oriented for remineralization and will not stain with dye. The infected dentin or the irreparable damaged collagen, stains red. 1% acid solution in propylene glycol can also be used.

TREATMENT MODALITIES OF DEEP CARIES LESIONS

Various treatment modalities are:
1. Indirect pulp capping/indirect rule treatment
2. Indirect pulp capping using stepwise excavation
3. Direct pulp capping
4. Atraumatic restorative treatment (ART)
5. Pulp curettage
6. Partial pulpotomy
7. Partial pulpotomy after carious exopsure

1. Indirect Pulp Capping/Indirect Pulp Treatment

Indirect pulp capping implies treating pulps, which are near exposure; whereas indirect pulp treatment is a technique in which an effort is made to avoid exposure during the treatment of teeth with deep carious lesions without any evidence of pulpal degeneration or periapical pathology. Indirect pulp capping is a two appointment procedure, whereas indirect pulp treatment is a single appointment procedure.

Indications

- Deep carious lesion with minimal pulpal inflammation.
- Where complete removal of caries may lead to pulp exposure.

Contraindications

- A tooth with existing pulp inflammation
- A tooth with periapical pathosis

Objectives

- Minimize pulp injury
- Promote dentin sclerosis
- Minimize post operative sensitivity
- Arrest carious lesion
- Stimulation of reparative dentin formation
- Remineralize affected dentin

Rationale

In a carious lesion, dentin decalcification precedes bacterial invasion within dentin. In an active carious lesion, two distinct layers are seen (Fig. 27.1):
  i. *Infected dentin:* It is necrotic, soft dentin, not painful to stimulation and grossly infected with bacteria. Collagen is irreversibly denatured.
  ii. *Affected dentin:* It is demineralized, discolored but hard dentin, painful to stimulation containing very few bacteria. It is reversibly denatured and capable of being remineralized.

When outer layer is removed, most of the bacteria are removed and the substrate on which they thrive is also removed. When cavity is sealed with a suitable material, any remaining bacteria are either killed or lie in a stage of dormancy. However affected dentin can be left on pulpal and axial walls and never on dentinoenamel junction and cavity margins. The two

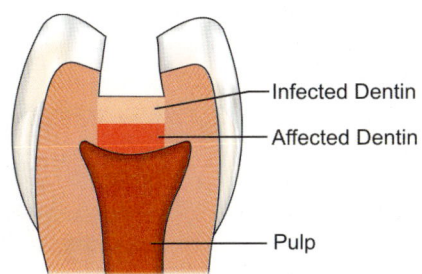

Fig. 27.1: Infected and affected dentin

layers can be differentiated with either 0.5% basic fuschin or 1.0% acid red dyes. Acid red is preferred since basic fuschin has carcinogenic potential.

Technique

The technique involves the following steps:

Removal of Caries

1. Mechanical Method

- Soft caries can be removed with a spoon excavator by removing flakes of carious dentin in layers.
- The discolored dentin can be removed with large round steel bur revolving at slow speed. Pulp damage may result from reaction of frictional heat with the use of bur while excessive pressure with a spoon excavator may force the micro organisms into the dentinal tubules or expose the pulp. Removal of infected dentin should continue until the remaining dentin feels as hard as normal dentin.

2. Chemomechanical Methods

It is the chemical softening of carious dentin followed by gentle excavation. It is especially indicated in deciduous teeth, dental phobics and medically compromised patients. Carisolv and Caridex are the two agents available which soften the carious dentin.

Two-appointment Technique

Ist Sitting

Local anaesthesia is administered and the tooth is isolated with a rubber dam. Cavity outline is established with a high-speed handpiece. Peripheral carious dentin/infected dentin should be removed with sharp spoon excavators; however, Cohen recommends the use of a large round bur for better results (Fig. 27.2A). Cavity should be irrigated and dried with cotton followed by placement of hard setting calcium hydroxide over the remaining affected dentin. The remainder of the cavity is filled with reinforced zinc oxide eugenol cement or a glass-ionomer cement to achieve a good seal (Fig. 27.2B). This seal should not be disturbed for 6–8 weeks, as the carious process in the deeper layer gets arrested.

IInd Sitting, (6–8 weeks later)

In the second sitting, carefully all temporary filling material, especially the Calcium hydroxide dressing over the deep portions of the cavity floor is removed. The color changes from deep red rose to light gray/light brown. The texture would change from spongy to hard and caries appear to be dehydrated. Thus, the remaining affected carious dentin appearing dehydrated and "flaky" should be removed. Do not disturb predentin, which is the area around the potential exposure appearing whitish and may be soft. The cavity preparation should be restored in the similar way as 1st sitting (Fig. 27.2C).

Re-enter or Not?

The re-entry restorative procedure is still questionable. It is recommended only if the tooth is asymptomatic, surrounding soft tissues are free from swelling, temporary filling is intact, bitewing radiographs of the treated tooth showing the presence of reparative dentin. Research has shown that carious dentin will remineralize within the restoration. If patient is asymptomatic on recall, the restoration should be redone.

With re-entry there should be a risk of creating pulp exposure and further insult to the pulp. If a pulp exposure occurs during re-entry, a more invasive vital pulp therapy techniques such as direct pulp capping or pulpotomy would be indicated.

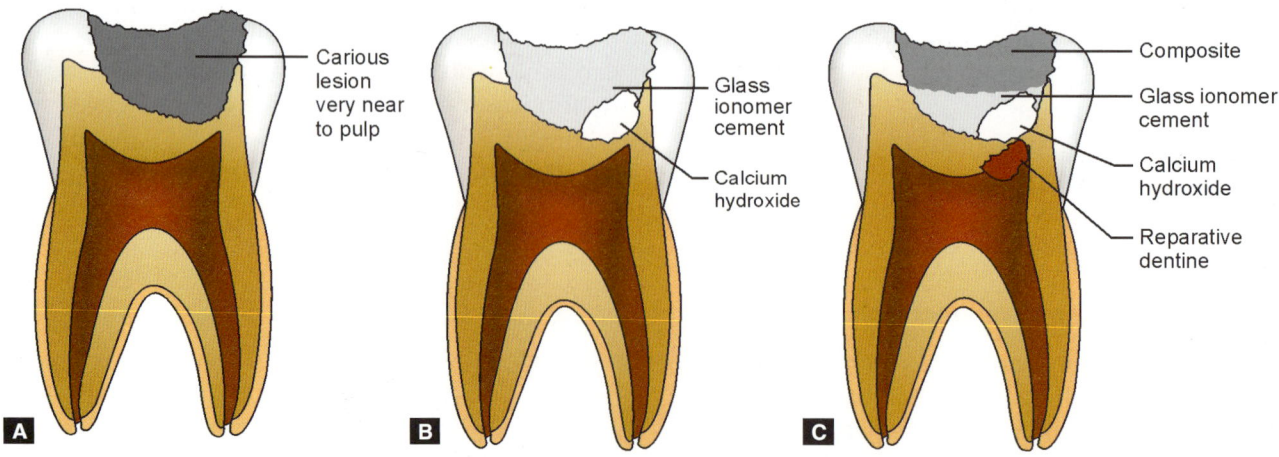

Figs 27.2A, B and C: Indirect pulp capping

One Appointment Technique

Indirect pulp capping is now termed as indirect pulp treatment. The selection for one-appointment indirect pulp treatment must be based on clinical judgement and experience with many cases. In recent years, rather than complete caries removal in two appointments, the focus has been to excavate caries as close as possible to the pulp, i.e. some caries be left in the tooth to avoid an exposure, placement of a protective liner, and restoring the tooth without a subsequent re-entry to remove any remaining caries.

2. Indirect Pulp Capping Using Step-wise Excavation

More recently, the step-wise excavation of deep caries has been revisited and shown to be successfully in managing reversible pulpitis without pulpal perforation and/or endodontic therapy. This approach involves a 2-step process.

a. The first step is the removal of carious dentin along the dentino-enamel junction (DEJ) and excavation of only the outermost infected dentin, leaving a carious mass over the pulp. The objective is to change the cariogenic environment in order to decrease the number of bacteria, close the remaining caries from the biofilm of the oral cavity, and slow or arrest the caries development. This allows time for pulp-dentin complex reactions to take place so that at the second excavation visit, there is less likelyhood of pulpal exposure. It is also suggested that changing the cavity environment from an active lesion into the condition of a slowly progressing lesion, a more regular and tubular tertiary dentin formation occurs.

b. The second step is the removal of the remaining caries and placement of a final restoration. The most common recommendation for the interval between steps is 3–6 months, allowing sufficient time for the formation of tertiary dentin and a definitive pulpal diagnosis. Critical to both steps of excavation is the placement of a well-sealed restoration. Since the research available is inconclusive on which approach is the most successful over time. The decision to use a one-appointment caries excavation or a step-wise technique should be based on the individual patient circumstances.

3. Direct Pulp Capping

Direct pulp capping implies treating exposed pulps. Exposure caused by trauma or by operators' fault during tooth preparation can be successfully treated; whereas, exposure caused by caries usually need root canal treatment. The younger the patient, the better are the chances of healing and repair.

Indications

- Size of exposure should be less than 0.5 mm
- No profuse haemorrhage or serous/purulent exudates
- In case of trauma, it is not more than few hours old
- Non tender to percussion (a recently traumatized tooth may be reversibly tender to percussion).

Contraindications

- Instrument has not penetrated the pulp, since infected dentin chips may settle in the pulp
- Tooth should not be periodontally involved
- Symptoms of irreversible pulpitis

Ideal Requirements of Pulp Capping Material

- Stimulate reparative dentin formation
- Maintain pulp vitality
- Bactericidal/Bacteriostatic
- Release fluoride to prevent secondary caries
- Adhere to dentin/restorative material
- Resist forces during restoration placement
- Provide appropriate seal
- Radiopaque

Technique

Tooth is isolated with rubber dam. Caries, if present, are removed from side walls using spoon excavators (Fig. 27.3A). The exposed pulp is not allowed to dry. The exposed site is washed with weak disinfectant and covered with a moist cotton pellet dipped in disinfectant solution. Bleeding is controlled with 5% sodium hypochlorite. After controlling bleeding, pulp capping material is placed (Fig. 27.3B). (It is placed with little pressure because displacement of capping material/dentin chips into the pulp may lead to further pulpal damage). It is followed by a restoration that seals the tooth from microleakage (Fig. 27.3C). It is established that bacterial leakage is responsible for pulpal response rather than toxicity of materials which results in only mild and transitory pulpal response. Hypersensitivity to temperature change may persist for a day or so. Tooth is tested periodically for pulp vitality. Symptoms usually subside in 4–6 weeks. If tooth remains vital, a permanent restoration may be placed. If tooth becomes painful, or exhibits decreased reading on vitality testing or becomes non vital, root canal treatment becomes mandatory.

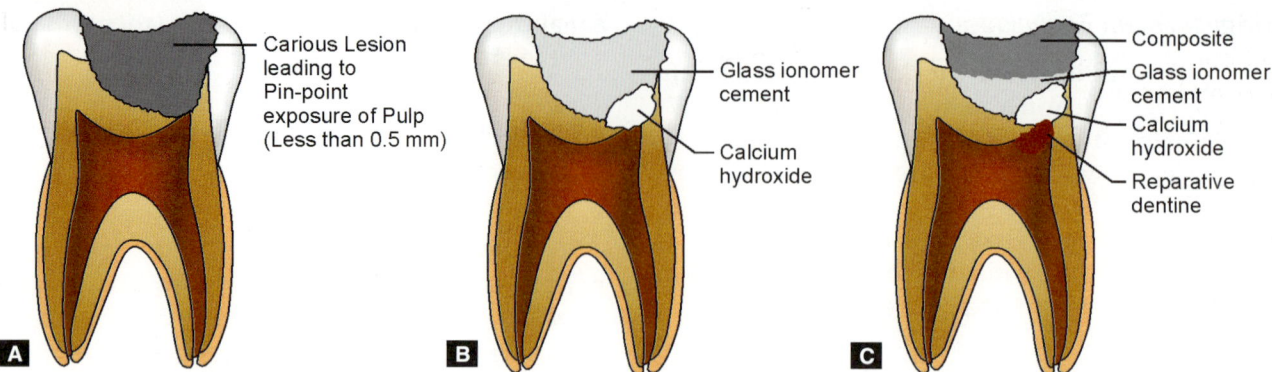

Figs 27.3A, B and C: Direct pulp capping **(A)** Pin point carious exposure, **(B)** Placement of pulp capping material, **(C)** Formation of reparative dentin

Materials used

a. Calcium hydroxide
b. Mineral trioxide aggregate (MTA)
c. Bonding agents
d. Resin-resorcinol

a. Calcium Hydroxide

Herman (1930) demonstrated that when vital pulps were covered with calcium hydroxide, it led to the formation of secondary dentin. When calcium hydroxide is applied directly to pulp tissue, coagulation necrosis of adjacent tissues occur. Beneath the region of coagulation necorsis, cells of underlying pulp differentiate into odontoblasts and other cells, which help forming dentin matrix. However a blood clot should not be left between calcium hydroxide and pulp. In these cases, hydroxyl ions trapped in the clot do not allow differentiation of odontoblasts. Calcium hydroxide maintains a local state of alkalinity necessary for bone/dentin formation. Earlier, it was postulated that calcium (Ca) from calcium hydroxide would diffuse into pulp and participate in the formation of reparative dentin. Later, it was established that calcium ions from calcium hydroxide do not enter into the formation of new dentin; however, it may come from blood. Commercially available pastes of calcium hydroxide are less alkaline and less caustic, therefore, tissue created by the action of these pastes is resorbed first and bridge is formed in contact with capping material. The altered tissue degenerates and disappears having a void between the capping material and the dentin bridge. Calcium hydroxide induced dentinal bridge contains multiple tunnel defects facilitating bacterial microleakage. Also calcium hydroxide becomes softened and allows leakage resulting in pulpal inflammation and necrosis after one to two years. Such teeth may show evidence of calcification or internal resorption; subsequently root canal treatment may be initiated.

b. Mineral Trioxide Aggregate (MTA)

It is modified Portland cement. It is of following three types:
- Gray
- White
- Modified

Properties

- Setting time: sets within 24 hours
- Compressive strength: 70 MPa after one day
- pH of the set MTA: 11–13 after setting
- Biocompatible and non-mutagenic
- Antibacterial effect is similar to calcium hydroxide

Manipulation

MTA powder is mixed with sterile water at a ratio of 3:1 on a glass slab or paper pad a plastic/metal spatula. It is placed over exposure site using plastic/metal spatula. The chamber is filled with flowable composite and other interim restorative materials. MTA is a difficult material to handle. Once it starts to dry it looses its cohesiveness and becomes hard to handle. When compared with calcium hydroxide, MTA produces more dentinal bridging in a short period of time with significantly less inflammation. It resists microleakage better than calcium hydroxide. Presence of blood has little impact on leakage of MTA.

C. Bonding Agents

It is established that healing is directly related to capacity of pulp capping agent to provide a biological seal against immediate and long term micorleakage. Adhesive bonding agents have been tried as pulp capping agent. They provide immediate seal. However, when adhesive agents were compared with calcium hydroxide, they showed more pulp necrosis. Histological studies have shown persistent inflammatory reactions and hyaline alteration of extracellulr matix inhibiting complete pulpal repair or bridge formation when bonding agents were used. Direct bonding agents are not preferred as these can lead to inflammatory reaction, delay in pulpal healing and failure of dentin bridge formation.

d. Resin-resorcinol

Resin-resorcinol has also been successfully tried as pulp capping material. The exposure site is washed immediately with normal saline solution and isolated with sterilized cotton rolls. The exposure site and the rest of the cavity is wiped with cresophene. Two drops of freshly prepared resinifying solution is poured over the exposure site and allowed to set. The rest of the cavity is filled with Kalzinol, zinc phosphate cement or any other restorative material.

The effectiveness of resinifying agent as pulp capping material has been histologically proved. Histological sections revealed areas of fibrosis and hyalinization in the pulp in the coronal area; however, in the middle and apical third of the sections, normal pulpal tissue was evident. The fibroblastic activities present at the coronal sites are suggestive of the healing process. The normal pulp tissue, without any sign of necrosis, present in the middle and apical part of the root confirms that the resinifying agent can successfully be sued in direct pulp capping.

4. Atraumatic Restorative Treatment (ART)

This is considered as one form of indirect pulp treatment. The procedure is based on excavating and removing caries using hand instruments only and then restoring the tooth with an adhesive filling material.

Pulp Protection

Because the ingress of bacteria is most commonly associated with various pulp responses, more emphasis should be given to complete sealing of prepared dentinal tubules.

The materials used for pulp protection are:
- Calcium hydroxide
- Zinc oxide eugenol
- Glass-ionomer cement
- Cyanoacrylates
- Thymol
- Polycarboxylate cements
- Tricalcium phosphate
- Resin resorcinol

All these materials lead to the formation of reparative dentin and decrease the dentin permeability. Zinc oxide eugenol has a sedative, palliative and obtundant effect; however, pulp beneath zinc oxide eugenol has been observed to show chronic inflammation with less likelyhood of bridge formation. Calcium hydroxide has been shown to increase pH of residual dentin, decrease permeability of dentinal tubules and increase remineralization. Wider and earlier formation of reparative dentin has been seen as compared to other materials. Other materials are also useful in forming reparative dentin. Dentin bonding agents also have been used for direct and indirect pulp treatment. New strategies using bioactive molecules such as enamel matrix protein or TGF beta have been used experimentally to stimulate tertiary dentin permeability but are not in use clinically. Dentin can also be used as pulp capping agent because bioactive molecules released from dentin can promote dentinogenesis. When EDTA demineralized dentin was used as pulp capping material, odontoblasts like cells and reparative dentin formed.

5. Pulp Curettage

It is well documented that pulp exposure due to caries usually lead to pulp necrosis with passage of time. During caries removal, carious dentin chips may be inadvertently pushed into pulp tissue resulting in inflammation, resorption and encapsulation of dentin chips which after capping may show foreign body reaction. It is suggested to remove superficial layer of pulp tissue by enlargement of the exposure site. This procedure is known as 'Pulp curettage'. It is followed by control of haemorrhage, placement of a pulp capping material and sealing of the cavity as in direct pulp capping.

Advantages
- It preserves cell zone due to minimal excision, hence chances of better healing.
- Physiologic apposition of dentin is maintained.
- Natural color/translucency of tooth is maintained.
- Less chance of root canal obliteration.

6. Partial Pulpotomy

It is the removal of only outer layer of damaged hyperemic tissues in exposed pulps. If 2.0 – 3.0 mm of pulp is removed it is called partial pulpotomy.

Rationale

Based on the rationale that following surgical amputation of the affected or infected pulp tissue at the exposure site, the remaining tissue is capable of healing.

Indications

- A small and recent pulpal exposure of upto approximately 14 days in a non-carious primary incisor

- Highly indicated in a very young tooth with a wide-open apex and very thin root dentin walls
- Only if sufficient tooth structure is present to allow proper restoration and full coverage of the crown with a bonded resin-composite strip crown

Contraindications

If the exposure is very large or when more than two weeks have passed between injury and treatment time allowing oral contaminants to cause extension infection or inflammation beyond 2.0 to 3.0 mm of the exposure.

Advantages
• This procedure is quick and easy to perform • It maintains the natural tooth color and preserves the tooth structure for better retention of restoration. • It is advantageous over complete pulpotomy in the preservation of cell-rich coronal pulp tissue. • Its successful outcome will allow the continuation of normal development of the tooth, including further root development and maturation.

7. Partial Pulpotomy After Carious Exposures

Indications

In a young permanent tooth for a carious pulp exposure (Fig. 27.4A) in which the pulpal bleeding can be controlled within several minutes. The tooth must be vital, with a diagnosis of normal pulp or reversible pulpitis.

Procedure

In this procedure, the inflamed pulp beneath an exposure is removed to a depth of 1.0 to 3.0 mm or deeper to reach healthy pulp tissue (Fig. 27.4B). Pulpal bleeding is controlled by irrigation with a bactericidal agent such as sodium hypochlorite or chlorhexidine. Later, the site is covered with calcium hydroxide or MTA.

Calcium Hydroxide

A dressing of calcium hydroxide paste should be placed followed by a base-liner of glass-ionomer (Fig. 27.4C). The tooth is restored using a bonded resin-composite strip crown. Scheduled follow-ups should be made after 1 month, 3 months, and then every 6 months. A dentin bridge will begin to form, separating the exposure site from the rest of the pulp. The bridge may be evidenced radiographically after 6 to 8 weeks.

MTA

After haemorrhage control, MTA is paced over the pulp stump. A thin layer of flowable composite is placed over it and light cured. The tooth is then sealed

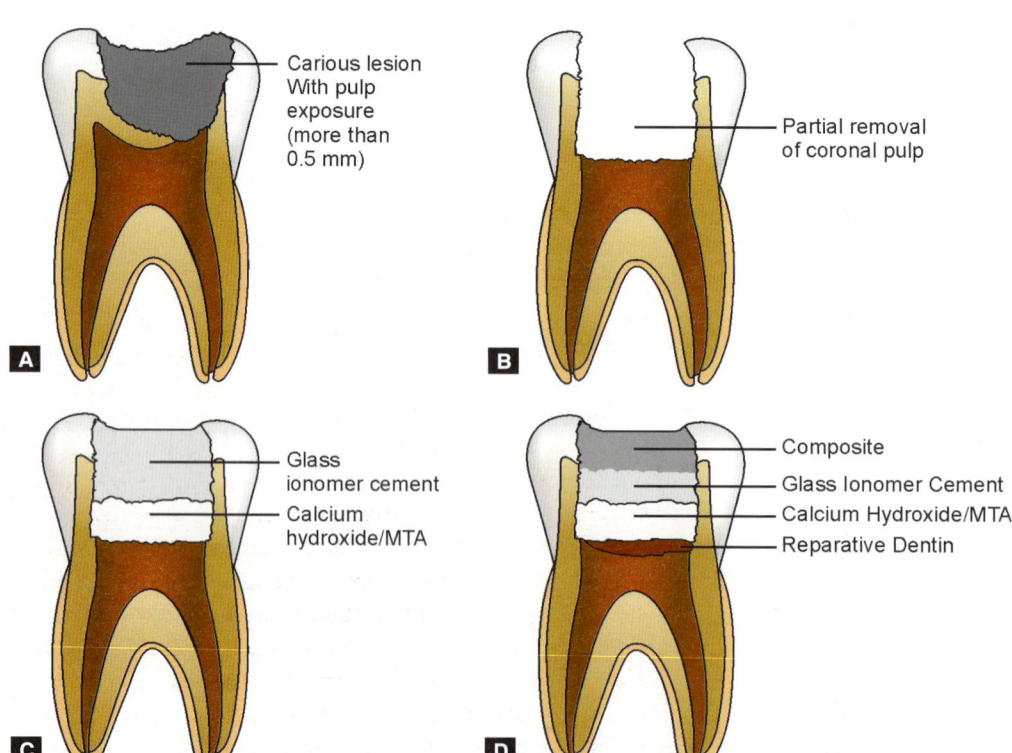

Figs 27.4A to D: Partial pulpotomy after carious exposure **(A)** Pulp exposure, **(B)** Partial removal of coronal pulp, **(C)** Placement of Calcium hydroxide/ MTA, **(D)** formation of reparative dentin

with etched bonded composite restoration. While calcium hydroxide has been demonstrated to have long-term success, MTA has shown more predictable dentin bridging and pulp health.

BIBLIOGRAPHY

1. Bjorndal, L.: Dentin and pulp reactions to caries and operative treatment: biological variables affecting treatment outcome. Endodontic Topics: 2, 10, 2002.
2. Bjorndal, L.: Dental caries: Progression and clinical management. Oper. Dent.: 27, 211, 2002.
3. Bjorndal, L.: The caries process and its effect on the pulp: The science is changing and so is our understanding. J. Endod.: 34, 52, 2008.
4. Bjorndal, l.: Indirect pulp therapy and stepwise excavation. J. Endodo.: 34, S29, 2008.
5. Borges, B.C., Borges, J.S., Araujo, L., Machado, C.T., Santos, A.J. and Pinhiero, I.V.A.: Update on non-surgical ultraconservative approaches to treat effective non-cavitated lesions in permanent teeth. Eur. J. Dent.: 5, 229, 2011.
6. Carounanidy, U. and Sathyanarayanan, R.: Dental caries: a complete changeover (Part II) – Changeover in the diagnosis and prognosis. J. Conserv. Dent.: 12, 87, 2009.
7. Cate, J.M.: Remineralization of deep caries enamel dentine caries lesions. Aust. Dent. J.: 53, 281, 2008.
8. Derksen E.K., Chen C.F., Majewski R., Tootla R.G.H. and Boynton J.R.: Reinforced Zinc Oxide Eugenol pulptomy: A retrospective study. Pediatric Dent.: 35, 43, 2013
9. Fachin, E.V.F., Filho, E.O. and Cavarlho, T.P.: Caries removal based on pulp biology. Electronic Journal of Endodontics Rosario: 1, 1, 2007.
10. Featherstone, J.D.B.: The continuum of dental caries – evidence for a dynamic dislase process. Jr. Dent. Res.: 83, C39, 2004.
11. Hayashi, M., Fujitani, M., Yamaki, C. and Moncoi, Y.: Ways of enhancing pulp preservation by stepwise excavation – a systematic review. J. Dent.: 39, 95, 2011.
12. Hilton, T.J.: Keys to clinical success with pulp capping: A review of literature. Oper. Dent.: 34, 615, 2009.
13. Hojo, S., Komatsu, M., Okuda, R., Takahashi, N. and Yamada, T.: Acid profiles and pH of carious dentin in active and arrested lesions. J. Dent. Res.: 73, 1853, 1994.
14. Javaheri, M., Kambakhsh, S., Elemad-Moghadam, S.: Efficacy of two caries detector dyese in the diagnosis of dental caries. J. Dent.: 7, 71, 2010.
15. Kamal, M., Okiji, T., Kawashima, N. and Suda, H.: Defense response of dentin/pulp complex to experimentally induced caries in rat molars: An immunohistochemical study on kinetics of pulpal 1a Antigen-expressing cells and macrophages. J. Endod.: 23, 115, 1997.
16. Kidd, E.A.M. and Fyirskov, O.: What constitutes dental caries ? Histopathology of carious enamel and dentin related to the action of cariogenic biofilms. J. Dent. Res.: 83, C35, 2004.
17. Maltz, M., Oliveira, E.F., Fontenella, V. and Corminatti, G.: Deep caries lesions after incomplete dentine caries removal: 40 month follow-up study. Caries Res.: 41, 493–96, 2007.
18. Medeiros, E. and Rosemblatt, A.: Differential diagnosis between active and arrested decayed lesion in dentin. Odontolgia: 5, 27, 2006.
19. Murray, P. and Godoy, F.: The incidence of pulp healing defects with direct capping materials. Am. J. Dent.: 19, 171, 2006.
20. Oliviera, E.F., Carminati, G., Fontanella, V. and Maltz, M.: The monitoring of deep caries lesions after incomplete dentine caries removal: results after 14–18 months. Clin. Oral Invest.: 10, 134, 2006.
21. Orhan, A.I., Oz T Eirdevs, Ozcelik, B. and Orhan, K.: A clinical and microbiological comparative study of deep carious lesion treatment in deciduous and young permanent molars. Clin. Oral Invest.: 12, 369, 2008.
22. Ricketts, D.: Management of the deep carious lesion and the vital pulp dentin complex. Br. Dent. J.: 191, 606, 2001.
23. Ritter , A.V., Browning, W.D., : Partial Caries Excavation. J Esthet Restor Dent.: 24, 148, 2012.
24. Thompson, V., Craig, R., Cuaro, F., Green, W. and Ship, J.: Treatment of deep carious lesions by complete excavation or partial removal: A critical review. J. Am. Dent. Assoc.: 139, 705, 2008.
25. Tran X.V., Gorin C., Willig C., Baroukh B., Pellat B., Decup F., Vital S.O., Chaussain C and Boukpessi T.: Effect of a calcium silicate based restorative cement on pulp repair. J Dent Res.: 91, 1166, 2012

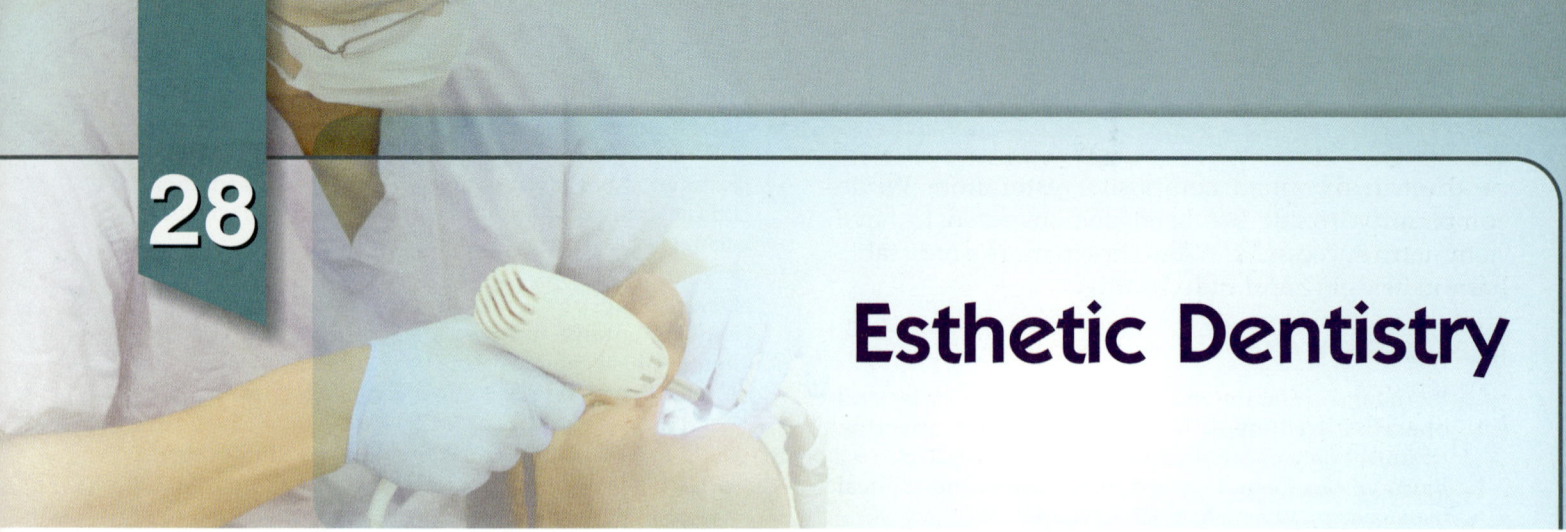

28

Esthetic Dentistry

The clinical practice of dentistry no longer revolves only around prevention and treatment of dental diseases. It also emphasizes on the esthetic components too. Dental treatment plans involve morphological, functional and esthetical components. Esthetics is an intellectual phenomenon, which deals with scientific knowledge, principles and perception of essential and natural beauty in nature and art. *Esthetic dentistry is the 'art and science of dentistry applied to create or enhance the beauty of an individual within functional and physiological limits'*. It involves the skills and techniques used to improve the art and symmetry of the teeth and face to enhance the appearance as well as the function of the teeth, oral cavity and face.

The history of initiation of esthetic concepts dates back to more than 4000 years. Philosophers like Plato and Aristotle introduced esthetics as the study of beauty and philosophy of attraction. Later, as the dentistry advanced and emerged as a specialty, researchers got interested in esthetic materials and restorations. In early nineteenth century, fixed crown and other ceramic restorations were being popularized. With the advent of composites and glass-ionomer cements the restorations could be made esthetically pleasing.

ESTHETIC PRINCIPLES

The basic principles of esthetics are:
    I. Composition
    II. Proportion
    III. Illusion
    IV. Color and translucency

I. Composition

It means the act of combining elements to form a whole. In dental esthetics, it can be defined as the relation that exists between the teeth, when illuminated, due to attributes of contrasts in color, lines and texture. Any dental composition can be esthetic or non-esthetic depending on how these elements are combined.

The various attributes of the elements of composition that impart the esthetic value are-

a. **Unity or oneness:** It gives different parts of the composition the effect of a whole. A dentition appears pleasing when teeth are arranged in repetitions of their shape(outline form), line(axial inclination and position) and color. This repetitive fashion in right and left sides of the mouth gives unity to the composition.

b. **Subtle variation:** The unity of the composition when viewed from the frontal view is not static but dynamic, such that nature never achieves absolute bilateral symmetry. There exist subtle variations in right and left halves of the dentitions such that we perceive dynamic unity without monotony.

c. **Dominance:** It is the means by which we achieve unity. Dominance implies when a strong structure in the centre is surrounded by well demarcated structures. The centrally placed structure dominates the visual perception.

    For example, when numerous anterior natural dentitions are viewed, then one feature that will be dominant in all is maxillary central incisor. *(Color, shape and size are the factors that control the dominance).*

d. **Contrast:** It is the element factor that makes the various elements of a composition visible. The eye can differentiate the parts of an object due to contrast of colors, lines, patterns etc.

e. **Symmetry:** It is the regularity of arrangement of objects either in horizontal/vertical direction, or from a central point to either side like a mirror image (radiating symmetry). In a dento-facial composition radiating symmetry of the teeth is esthetically more appealing.

II. Proportion

The term proportion is used to give a certain mathematical representation to express the relationship of the various units that combine to make a combination.

In natural dentition though each individual tooth has a different shape and size, they are related to one another and the entire dental composition relates to face in a certain proportion, that must be pleasing and harmonious. The proportion in esthetics is the key tool in shaping the dental and facial components.

The routinely used ratios applied in dentistry are:
a. Golden proportion
b. Golden percentage or mean
c. Red proportion

a. Golden Proportion

The golden proportion was described by the Pythagoreans in the sixth century BC. It represents the most agreeable proportion of two measurements. This ratio is approximately 1.61803:1; that is, the smaller section is about 62% the size of the larger. The uniqueness of this ratio is that the ratio of the smaller part to the larger part is the same as the ratio of the larger part to the whole. It is rounded to a mathematical figure- 1.618. Phidias, a greek sculptor has labeled this number as phi, using greek symbol φ.

- It is a natural law, describes how our eyes evaluate a pleasing proportion.
- Pacioli gave its name 'divine proportion'
- It is applied in arts, architecture and anatomy.
- The parts organized in this proportion seem to display maximum beauty and ultimate efficiency in function
- Derived from Fibonacci series.

It was not until the 13th century, when the Westernworld adopted Arabic numbers, that this divine relationship was translated into mathematical terms by Filius Bonaccio. This mathematical phenomenon is also called the 'magic numbers.' To create the series, begin with the simple addition equation of 0+1=1. The second number to be added in that equation, 1, and the sum of that equation, also 1, are added together, in that order, to create the next line (1+1=2). The sums of each line—1, 2, 3, 5, 8, 13, etc., are the Fibonacci series.

$$0 + 1 = 1$$
$$1 + 1 = 2$$
$$1 + 2 = 3$$
$$2 + 3 = 5$$
$$3 + 5 = 8$$
$$5 + 8 = 13 \text{ etc}$$

This pattern is not a simple arithmetic progression; it follows an exponential law that can be applied to esthetic dentistry. This progression is most pleasing to the senses and provides a unique relationship. The Fibonacci numbers, after the thirteenth in the series, increase in an unchanging proportion of 1.0 to 1.61803. Therefore, in that part of the series, the Fibonacci numbers are golden to their neighbors.

Divide:
0 / 1 = 0	34 / 21 = 1.61904
1 / 1 = 1	55 / 34 = 1.6176
2 / 1 = 2	89 / 55 = 1.61818
3 / 2 = 1.5	144 / 89 = 1.61797
5 / 3 = 1.666	233 / 144 = 1.61805
8 / 5 = 1.6	377 / 233 = 1.61802
13 / 8 = 1.625	610 / 377 = 1.61803
21 / 13 = 1.615	987 / 610 = 1.61803

How the proportion works clinically
- The upper central incisor has a golden ratio to the lower central incisor, if the lower central incisor is taken as a starting reference.
- The total width of both lower centrals is golden to that of the upper incisors.
- Similar series of proportions lies with the widths of all four upper incisors to lower four incisors.
- Width of lower incisor segment to the upper canine width appears in golden ratio.
- Similar relationship is present from the distal of the lower canines to the buccal groove on the upper molar.
- Width of the maxillary lateral incisor, as viewed from the front, should be in golden proportion to the width of maxillary central incisor. The maxillary lateral incisor should be 62% of the width of the maxillary central incisor. Similarly, the width of maxillary canine, as viewed from front should be 62% of the width of resulting lateral incisor (Fig. 28.1).

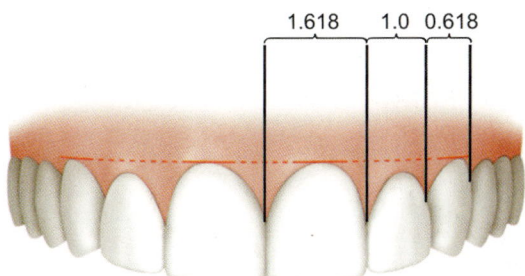

Fig. 28.1: Golden proportion

b. Golden Percentage or Golden Mean

This theory states that the width of the maxillary central incisor should be 25% of the total width from the distal of the maxillary canine on one side to the distal of canine on the contralateral side. Each maxillary lateral incisor should be 15% and each maxillary canine 10% of the inter-canine distance as viewed from the front (Fig. 28.2).

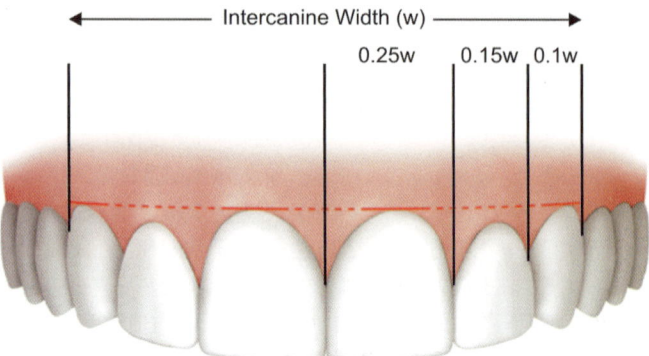

Fig. 28.2: Golden mean

c. Red proportion (Recurring Esthetic Dental Proportion)

The red proportion states that the proportion of the successive widths of the maxillary teeth as viewed from the front should remain constant, progressing distally. The width of the lateral incisor is reduced by a selected percentage from the width of the central incisor, and the width of each tooth distally is reduced by this same percentage from its mesial tooth. The 70% Red proportion has been recommended for normal length teeth with a 78% width/ height ratio of the maxillary central incisors. When using the 70% Red proportion, the width of the maxillary lateral incisor is 70% of the frontal view width of the maxillary central incisor, and the maxillary canine is 70% of the width of the resulting lateral incisor (Fig. 28.3)

- 70% red proportion is recommended for normal length
- 62% red proportion is recommended for very small teeth
- 80% red proportion is recommended for small teeth

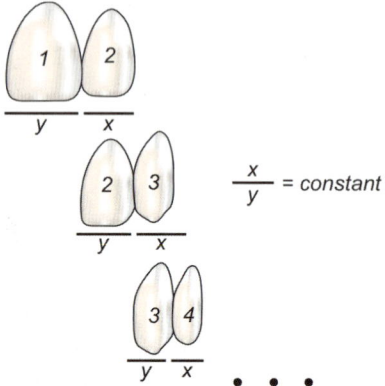

Fig. 28.3: Red Proportion

III. Illusion

It is a figment of imagination where a perception of an object is created. The art of creating illusion consists of changing perception, to cause an object to appear different from what it actually is. Teeth can be made to appear smaller, larger, wider, narrower, shorter, longer, younger, older, masculine or feminine.

For example:

a. *Illusion achieved from the principle of gradation of size:* The central incisor closest to the viewer appears the largest, whereas the premolar appears smaller because they are farther away from the viewer, even though both teeth may have the same occluso-gingival length.

Any discrepancy in this arrangement leads to destruction of illusion of front to back gradation and creates visual tension.

b. *Illusion achieved from light/Illusion of transillumination:* An object exhibits two dimensions, that is, length and width when subjected to light. True natural light is multi-directional and on striking the surface of the object, also reveals texture and shadows, this adds third life like dimension of depth.
- The horizontal lines illuminated under light make the object wider and vertical lines make the object appear longer (principle of line).
- Shadows created as light strikes the facial surface of the tooth begin at the transitional line angles; these shadows delineate the boundaries of the facial form. Thus the apparent face is that portion of the face that is visible to the observer from any single view. When maxillary anterior teeth are viewed from the front only the mesial half of canine is visible however the entire incisor is visible.

IV. Color and Translucency

*Color-*Color is the most complex and least understood artistic element. Teeth are typically composed of multitude of colors. A gradation of color usually occurs from gingival to incisal, with the gingival region being typically darker because of thinner enamel. The use of several different shades of restorative material may be required to esthetically restore a tooth.

Translucency- The degree of translucency is related to how deeply light penetrates into the tooth before it gets reflected outward. Normally light penetrates through the enamel into dentin before it gets reflected outward. This affords the life like vitality characteristic of normal, unrestored tooth. Shallow penetration often results in loss of esthetic vitality. *Illusion of translucency*

Esthetic Dentistry

can also be created to enhance the realism of restoration (addition of tints or opacifiers).

ANALYSIS OF ESTHETIC SMILE

A. Facial Analysis

a. *Facial height*: The face height is divided into three equal thirds:
   - from forehead to brow line
   - from brow line to the base of the nose
   - from base of the nose to base of the chin (Fig. 28.4).
b. *Facial width*: The width of the face is typically the width of five "eyes" (Fig. 28.4).
c. *Lateral facial profiles*: It can be straight, convex, or concave. A cephalometric analysis of the head in frontal and lateral views is useful in determining bony relationships of the face and the mandible, and their relationship to the teeth in the alveolar bone.
d. The facial features related to *gender and age* involves the soft tissues and includes the texture, complexion, and tissue integrity of the epithelial tissues.
e. Facial features that have a particularly important impact on the dental–facial composition are those that relate the interpupillary plane with the commissure line and the occlusal plane.

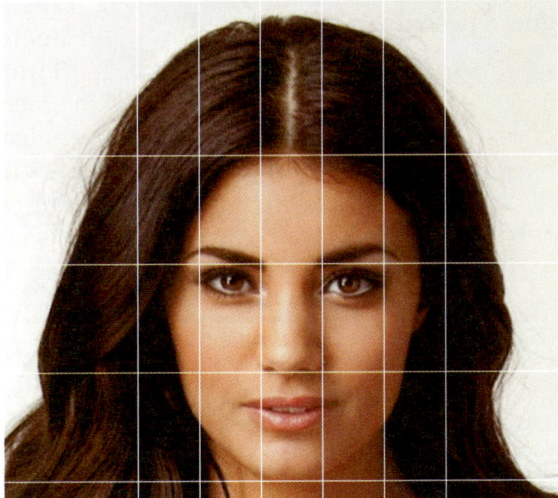

Fig. 28.4: Facial Analysis

B. Lip Analysis

a. *Lip morphology*: Width, fullness and symmetry.
b. *Lip line*: The inferior border of the lip as it relates to the teeth and gingival tissues is called the lip line
   - *Average lip line* exposes the maxillary teeth and only the interdental papillae.
   - A *high lip line* exposes the teeth in full display as well as gingival tissues above the gingival margins. (gummy smile)
   - A *low lip line* displays no gingival tissues when smiling.

   In most cases, the lip line is acceptable if it is within a range of 2.0 mm apical to the height of the gingival on the maxillary centrals
c. *Incisal display*: The incisal display refers to the amount of visible tooth displayed when the lips and lower jaw are in the rest position. The average incisal display of the maxillary centrals for males is 1.91 mm and the average for females is 3.40 mm. With age, the amount of incisal display of the maxillary centrals diminishes and the amount of incisal display of the mandibular centrals increases. Therefore, the amount of incisal display is an important factor in a youthful smile.

C. Gingival Tissue Analysis

a. *Gingival Contour*: The gingival contours should be symmetric and the marginal gingival tissues of the maxillary anterior teeth should be located along a horizontal line extending from canine to canine. Ideally, the laterals reach slightly short of that line. It is also acceptable, although not ideal, to have the gingival height of all six anteriors equal in gingival height on the same plane (Fig. 28.5).

   Ideally the papillary contour should be pointed and should fill the interdental spaces to the contact point. An unfilled interdental space creates an unwanted black interdental triangle in the gingival embrasure and makes a smile less attractive.
b. *Zenith point*: The gingival zenith point is the most apical point of the gingival tissues along the long axis of the tooth (Fig. 28.6). Zenith point can enhance:

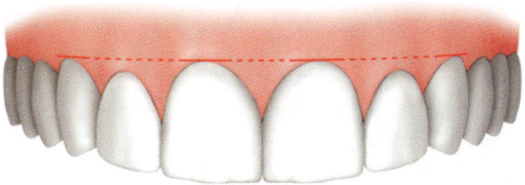

Fig. 28.5: Gingival contour

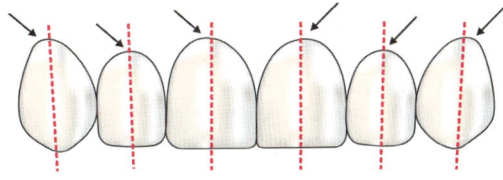

Fig. 28.6: Zenith point

- Preparation of tooth axis
- Length of the tooth
- Gingival shapes

Importance of zenith point

  i. When closing diastemas or changing the mesial or distal tilt position of the tooth(these are examples of moving zenith points horizontally)
  ii. In case where tooth needs to be shown longer or more taper at the gingival 1/3rd, zenith point can move apically.

c. *Biological width*: *Biological width* is defined as the combination of junctional epithelium and connective tissue elements of dento-gingival unit that occupy the space between the base of the gingival crevice and the alveolar crest; the total dimension would be 2.04 mm. It was better termed as biologic zone by Kois (3.0 mm in healthy normal gingiva).

  i. Epithelial compartment
     - Gingival epithelium
     - Sulcular epithelium
     - Sulcus depth- 0.69 mm
     - Functional epithelium- 0.97 mm
  ii. Connective tissue compartment
     It represents fibrous attachment of the gingiva to the hard tissue wall and support to the epithelium of the dento-gingival junction (Fig. 28.7).

D. Smile Line

The smile line can be defined as an imaginary line drawn along the incisal edges of the maxillary anterior teeth (Fig. 28.8).

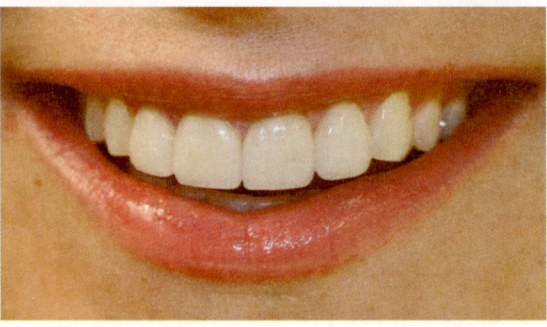

Fig. 28.8: Smile line and Buccal Corridor

- In an ideal tooth arrangement, that line should coincide or follow the curvature of the lower lip while smiling
- Another frame of reference suggests that the centrals are slightly longer than the cuspids
- In a reverse smile line, the centrals appear shorter than the cuspids along the incisal plane and create an aged or worn appearance

E. Midline

The midline refers to a vertical line formed by the contact of the maxillary central incisors. The midline should be perpendicular to the incisal plane and parallel or coincident to the midline of the face (Fig. 28.9).

Several anatomical landmarks can be useful guides to assess the midline of the face as it relates to dental midline. These include:

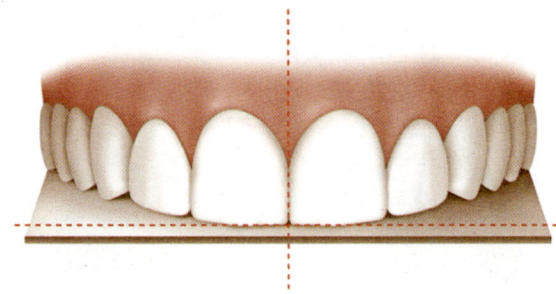

Fig. 28.9: Midline

- Midline of the nose, forehead
- Inter-pupillary plane
- Philtrum
- Chin

The *philtrum of the lip* is considered to be one of the most accurate anatomical guide as it is always in the center of the face.

F. Axial Inclination

- The axial inclination of the anterior teeth tends to incline mesially toward the midline and become

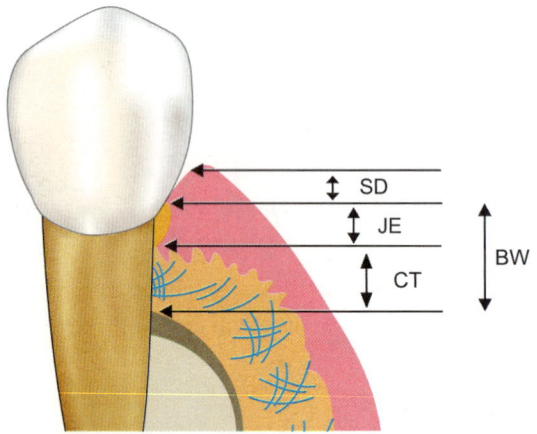

SD : Sulcular Depth
JE : Junctional Epithelium
CT : Connective Tissue
BW : Biological Width

Fig. 28.7: Biological width

more pronounced from the central incisors to the canines
- The axial inclination of the posterior teeth from the frontal view exhibits the same mesial inclination toward the midline as the cuspid
- This creates a natural visual gradation, making the teeth appear to diminish in size as they progress posteriorly

G. Buccal Corridor

The area between the corners of the mouth during smile formation and the buccal surfaces of the maxillary teeth (particularly the bicuspids and molars) form a space known as the buccal corridor. The greater and more pronounced this negative space becomes, the more these posterior teeth are concealed, restricting the full breadth of the smile. A full and symmetric buccal corridor is an important element of an esthetic smile. In these posterior segments, the artistic perception of esthetics can be used to alter the typical inclinations to produce an enhanced esthetic effect (Fig. 28.8).

H. Anatomy of Anterior Teeth

a. *Labial contour:* The labial contour of these teeth should exhibit three planes when viewed from a lateral profile (with differing reflections of light, giving a natural appearance) (Fig. 28.10). The anterior teeth could be flat or convex, square shaped or fan-shaped when viewed from front.

b. *Incisal embrasure:* With ideal anatomy and alignment of these six teeth, an open space is formed between the proximal surfaces of incisal edges from the contact points. This area is called an incisal embrasure. The incisal embrasure spaces of the anterior teeth display a natural and progressive increase in depth from the central incisor to the canine.

c. *Texture:* The characterization of the tooth surface is a function of various anatomical grooves, facets, prominences along with Perikymata, stippling and rippling that may affect the enamel surfaces.

d. *Mesio-distal width:* This dimension is much more critical dimension than inciso-gingival length for anterior tooth placement.

e. *Inciso-gingival height:* The incisal edge of the maxillary central incisor is an important determinant in creation of a smile. It serves to determine the proper tooth proportion and gingival level. Position of the incisal edge acts as the parameter upon which rest of the treatment is built. Average anatomic crown length for maxillary central incisors 10.4–11.2 mm. The ideal ratio of inciso-gingival height and mesio-distal width of central incisors is shown in Fig. 28.11. Ideally the mesio-distal width of the tooth must be 80% of the inciso-gingival height of the tooth.

   i. Elongation of the incisal edge indicated in:
   - Incisal wear
   - Inadequate tooth display
   - Displeasing tooth or crown proportion

   ii. Shortening of the incisal edge may be required:
   - To correct excessive tooth display
   - Displeasing tooth or crown portion
   - To compensate for unaesthetic elongation created by periodontal recession.

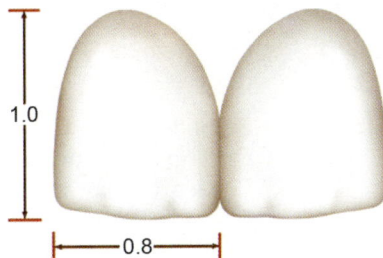

Fig. 28.11: Ratio of mesiodistal width to incisogingival height of maxillary central incisor

EXAMINING THE DENTOFACIAL COMPOSITION

To achieve a successful, healthy, and functional result requires an understanding of the interrelationship among all the supporting oral structures, including the muscles, bones, joints, gingival tissues, and occlusion. Gaining this understanding requires collecting all the data necessary to properly evaluate all the structures of the oral complex.

Aids for examining dento-facial composition
- Radiographs
- Diagnostic and Mock-up casts

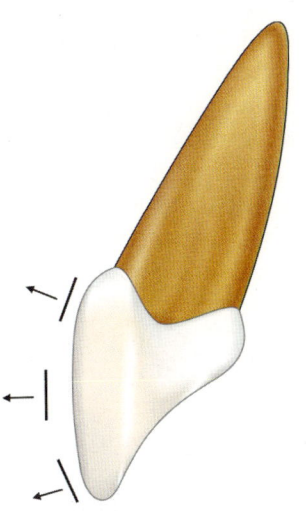

Fig. 28.10: Labial contour reflects light in three planes

- Photographic records
- Computer aided analysis

TREATMENT PLANNING IN ESTHETIC DENTISTRY

Before planning the esthetic aspect, the following features should be analyzed:

- Thorough knowledge about esthetic principles
- Patients' needs and expectations
- Esthetic perception of the patient
- Morpho-psychology of the patient
- Components of dento-facial complex
- Physiology of occlusion and mastication
- Affordability

Treatment planning starts with evaluation of entire stomatognathic system; however, following three components are mandatory for planning esthetics.

- Evaluation of the teeth and arch
- Evaluation of the periodontal status
- Analysis of facial structure

Various esthetic problems and the indicated treatment modalities are given in Table 28.1

Table 28.1: Treatment options for various esthetic problems

Esthetic problems	Treatment modalities
Problems with tooth morphology and alignment	Bleaching, microabrasion etc. Esthetic recontouring Composite resin restorations Composite/ceramic veneers Esthetic inlays, onlays and crowns
Stomatognathic problems	Orthodontic treatment Orthognathic surgery Post-core restorations
Color problems	Bleaching Veneers Crowns
Traumatic injuries	Splinting Surgical corrections Periodontal therapy Veneers/ Crowns
Gingival/ periodontal esthetic problems	Gingival recontouring, electro-surgery Gingival grafting Periodontal therapy Frenectomy
Missing teeth	Dentures Implants
Dermatological problems	Cosmetic skin resurfacing Plastic surgery

COSMETIC CONTOURING

Cosmetic contouring is the reshaping of the natural teeth for esthetic purposes. Such reshaping does not merely consist of filing and leveling the incisal edges, but it involves shaping the mesial, distal, labial and lingual surfaces as well. Cosmetic reshaping provides an excellent compromise in many situations when other procedures are prohibitively expensive. It is perhaps the most inexpensive cosmetic treatment. It is a rapid procedure that gives immediate and long lasting results and it is nearly painless and therefore requires no anaesthesia.

Indications
- Alteration of tooth structure
- Correction of Developmental Anomalies
- Substitute for crowning
- Minor orthodontic problems
- Removal of stains and other discolorations
- Periodontal problems
- Bruxism
- Attrited incisal edges
- Minor facture of tooth structure

Contraindications
- Hypersensitive teeth
- Large pulp canals
- Thin enamel
- Deeply pigmented stains
- Large anterior restorations
- Susceptibility to caries
- Excessive anterior crowding or occlusal disharmony

Treatment Procedure

- Photographs, study models, computer aided esthetic designing, mock up casts, line drawings serve helpful in treatment planning and estimating outcome.
- Feminine characteristics of esthetically pleasing anterior teeth include narrow teeth, rounded incisal angles, prominent or open incisal embrasure
- Masculine characteristics include wider incisors, sharp incisal angles or minimally open incisal embrasures.
- Reshaping is restricted to enamel only.
- Diamond burs and abrasive disks are used to bring about the necessary changes in the contour or embrasure of tooth.
- Marking the outline on the teeth in the mouth enables the patient and clinician to envision the potential improvement.
- Protrusive occlusion should be evaluated prior to initiation of treatment.
- Finishing and polishing to highest degree must be carried out to ensure long term results.

DIASTEMA CLOSURE

The presence of a space, or diastema, between anterior teeth is a common feature of adult dentitions. The spaces usually distort a pleasing smile by concentrating the observer's attention not on the overall dental composition, but on the diastema.

Etiology

The etiological factors can be summarized as follows:
- *Developmental*: microdontia, missing laterals, mesiodens, macroglossia, macro-hypertrophic fibrous frenum;
- *Pathological*: midline cysts, tumours and periodontitis;
- *Neuromuscular*: oral habits, such as tongue thrusting during speech, swallowing or abnormal pressure during rest.

Treatment

The specific goals of treating a diastema are creating a tooth form that is in harmony with adjacent teeth, arch, and facial form, maintaining gingival health with a stable and functional occlusion. Many forms of therapy can be used for diastema closure such as porcelain laminate or veneers, composite veneers, direct bonding, and crowns, both with and without orthodontics. A comparison between Composite veneer and Porcelain veneer is enlisted in Table 28.2.

Table 28.2: Comparison between direct composite veneers and ceramic veneers for diastema closure

Direct Composite Veneers	Ceramic veneers
Advantages	**Advantages**
• Conservative treatment modality • Satisfactory esthetic • No or minimal tooth preparation required results • Ease of intraoral repair • Economical • Single visit treatment	• Excellent esthetics • Maximum control over shade, contours and proportions
Disadvantages	**Disadvantages**
• Needs multiple replacements in lifetime due to color instability • Given in patients with excellent oral hygiene status only	• High cost • Two appointments needed

Diastema Closure with Direct Bonding Composite Application

Step by step diastema closure procedure:
1. Clean teeth to be treated and adjacent teeth. Select shade by using shade tabs under appropriate light conditions or by using trial restorations before placement of ruber dam and retraction clamps.
2. Verify desired mesial-distal width of teeth after restoration by measuring with a vernier caliper and record dimension.
3. Etch first tooth to be treated while protecting the adjacent tooth with a mylar strip. Apply bonding material, air dry and cure.
4. Build up contour of first tooth using previous selected shade and verify mesial-distal dimension by measuring.
5. Remove facial, lingual, incisal and gingival excess. Sof-Lex disc can be used to remove facial, incisal and interproximal excesses. To remove lingual excess, a football shaped bur can be used. Blade no. 12 is used to carve out gingival contour.
6. Polish interproximal contact area with finishing strips and fine and extra-fine Sof-Lex discs.
7. Repeat the similar steps for the adjacent tooth.
8. To maintain the separation between the adjacent teeth keep the mylar strip in place during placement of increments in the proximal area.
9. Contour transitional angles of teeth with disc and blade. Evaluate for contour from incisal, facial and lingual aspect.
10. Finish and polish the final restoration. Verify smoothness of contact area and gingival margin with floss.
11. Remove rubber dam. Check and adjust centric and excursive contacts with articulating material.
    - Care must be taken to prevent mesio-distal enlargement of teeth, or tooth on either side of the gap.
    - To maintain proper length to width ratios, teeth need to be lengthened in a diastema closure, it is possible to lengthen the anterior teeth either apically, with periodontal procedures, or incisally with a restorative addition.
    - If the incisal edge position is correct and to be maintained, and there is no periodontal intervention, closing the diastema results in short appearing clinical crowns with disproportional, unattractive teeth. Frequently these patients benefit from a more aggressive restorative approach. It may be necessary to include 4, 6, or more teeth in the restorative plan. The distal surface of the teeth in these cases is reduced with addition to the mesial surface. This approach keeps individual tooth

proportion appropriate, while at the same time moves the dental midline to the right position. Gingival zenith point location must be a part of the treatment planning for these cases. If the zenith points are left unchanged from their pretreatment position, they appear to be too far distal. The result is teeth that appear to be mesially tilted. To avoid this outcome, the zenith points have to be relocated with either a periodontal procedure or by recontouring the gingival trough in the provisional restorations.

The procedural steps for composite veneers and ceramic veneer techniques are given in Chapters 17 and 20 respectively.

GUIDELINES FOR ADHESIVE ANTERIOR RESTORATION

For composite restorations to mimic natural tooth structure, the clinician must have a comprehensive understanding of the material science and techniques involved in direct bonding procedures. Material science can be broken down to include various types of composites, tints, opaquers, adhesive systems, and armamentarium. The necessary techniques involve an understanding of color, adhesive principles, layering to create polychromicity, incisal effects, perfect imperfections and finishing and polishing.

The indications of various types of tints and opaquers and composites are given in Tables 28.3 and 28.4 respectively.

LAYERING TECHNIQUES

Composite mirroring is the natural replacement of teeth with minimal or no additional removal of the intact, health dentition to normal form and function with tooth-colored material. With this approach, the restorative dentist must indulge the optical, anatomic, and functional characteristics of natural teeth. In a layering technique, the dentist chooses an enamel and dentin replacement material that emulates the missing tooth structure in optical properties and strength (Fig. 28.12 A).

This simplified form of layering technique can be modified in following ways, according to esthetic requirements and affordability of patient:

Modification 1

Two shaded materials, one for enamel and one for dentin are used with an additional layer of incisal shaded material (Fig. 28.12 B).

Modification 2

Two shaded materials with different chromas are used to replace dentin, with an enamel layer for enamel effects. Another layer of incisal shaded material is also placed (Fig. 28.12 C).

Modification 3

Two shaded materials with different chromas are used to replace dentin with two shaded materials with different chromas for the enamel layer for enamel effects, and another layer uses incisal shaded material.

Table 28.3: Indications of tints and opaquers

Tints	Opaquers
• Match natural tooth structure in polychromicity and maverick colors	• Block dark tooth color in thin layer
• Help mask out tooth-restorative interface	• Help mask out tooth-restorative interface
• Lower the value	• Block excessive translucency in Class III and IV restorations
	• Raise the value

Table 28.4: Indications, advantages and disadvantages of the three major categories of composite resins

Classification	Indications	Advantages	Disadvantages
MICROHYBRID	Layer the desired shade deep within the restoration to mimic dentin and enamel morphology. Provide strength in any functional area	Strength: less likely to chip off in high-strength area Refractory properties: opacity similar to enamel and dentin	Polishability: does not sustain for long time
MICROFILLED	Replace enamel in color and translucency; Polishability; Wear resistance and surface texture	Polishability: high shine for the long-term Wear resistance better than microhybrids Refractory properties: translucency similar to enamel	Lacks strength for some functional areas Can be too translucent
NANOFILLER	All anterior and posterior restorative applications	Potential advantages of MicroHybrid and MicroFill	No in vivo long-term studies

A characterization layer is placed between the two enamel layers. Tints are placed internally to mirror the unique characterizations of the natural tooth, such as subsurface staining or demarcations of any color, shape, or size (Fig. 28.12 D).

DIRECT COMPOSITE PREFABRICATED VENEERS (COMPONEER)

Componeer are pre-poylmerized, prefabricated nano-hybrid composite enamel shells that combine the advantages of direct composite restoration with the advantages of prefabricated veneers. The pre-shaped componeer veneers are available in different sizes and are easy to use for single-tooth reconstruction as well as complete reconstruction in the anterior region. Time-consuming forming of the anatomical shape and surface and elaborate trimming are no longer required. Componeer can be customized to individual requirements with composite at any time. The extremely thin veneers (as thin as 0.3 mm) allow a high level of conservation of hard tooth substance during preparation.

Advantages
• Easy and efficient to use
• Only one session required
• Quality dental restoration with better esthetic results
• No laboratory work
• Optimum customization (choice of color, highlighting shape and structure)
• Economical

LUMINEERS

Lumineers are made from special patented cerinate porcelain that is very strong but much thinner than traditional laboratory-fabricated veneers. Their thickness is comparable to contact lenses, and so they are often called contact lenses for teeth. The main advantage of these ultra-thin veneers is that minimal tooth preparation is required. This technique is best used with patients who have spacing in their smile and only minor tooth rotations. Often Lumineers do not require any grinding, cutting or filing down any tooth structure for proper placement. The veneers are adhesively bonded to the "facial (front) surface" of the teeth, making the process as much of a minimally invasive procedure as possible.

Advantages
• Minimal or no preparation required
• Reversible procedure as no cutting is often made
• Can be used over bridges and crowns without their removal
• Excellent esthetics
• A painless procedure
• Sensitivity-free results

Indications
- Chipped or cracked teeth
- Stained or discolored teeth
- Spaced teeth
- Mis-shapen teeth
- Slightly crowded teeth
- Worn teeth
- Small teeth

LASERS IN ESTHETIC DENTISTRY

Dental lasers have evolved considerably as an adjunctive and alternative treatment to safely, conservatively, and reliably decrease bacterial levels and improve the hard and soft tissue contours. Minimally invasive laser procedures, with precise restorative planning and technique, can satisfy esthetic and functional parameters. The advantages and disadvantages of lasers are summarized in Table 28.5.

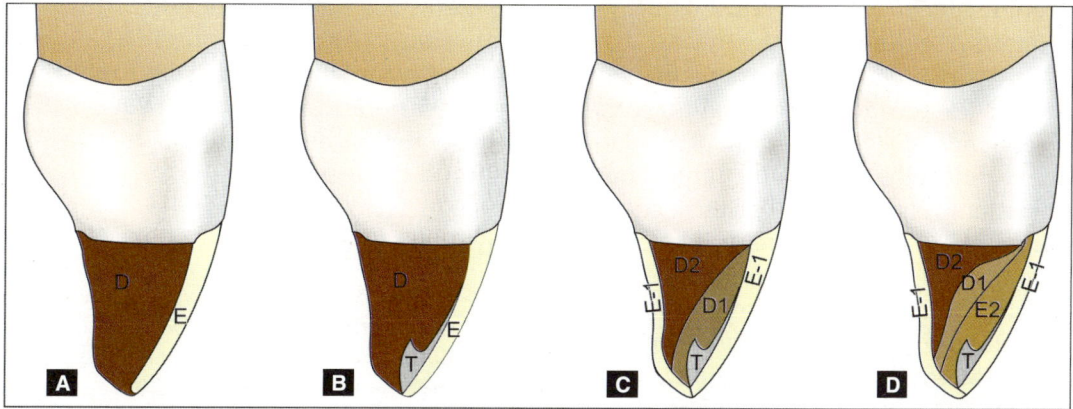

Figs 28.12A to D: Layering techniques: **(A)** Simple; **(B)** Modification 1; **(C)** Modification 2, **(D)** Modification 3. (E- Enamel; D-Dentin; T- Translucent)

Table 28.5: Advantages and disadvantages of lasers

	Advantages	Disadvantages
Soft tissue laser	• No suturing • Little/no bleeding • Painless • Quicker • Atraumatic	• Technique sensitive
Hard tissue laser	• Quicker • More accurate • More comfortable • Better results	• Crack formation • Carbonization of dentin • Damage to dental pulp • Technique sensitive

There are essentially five types of lasers currently in the armamentarium for the aesthetic dental practice. This list includes argon, CO_2, diode, erbium, and pulsed Nd:YAG lasers.

1. **Argon lasers**: They are used for curing of composite restorations and bonding cements; transillumination of teeth for the purpose of detecting tooth fractures and carious lesions
2. **Carbon dioxide lasers**: They are used for cutting, and coagulation of soft tissue, which includes gross tissue debulking, frenectomy, gingivoplasty, gingivectomy, etc.
3. **Diode laser**: They are used for rapid cutting, vaporizing, and bacterial reduction of tissue adjacent to tooth structure.
4. **Erbium: YAG laser**: They are used to cut soft tissue, tooth structure, and bone, bleaching of teeth, etching and for treatment of dentin hypersensitivity.
5. **Nd:YAG laser**: They are used as a hard and soft tissue laser and for selective removal of initial caries with little interaction to the surrounding healthy enamel.

ETHICS AND ESTHETIC DENTISTRY

Ethics is a generic term used for various ways of understanding and examining the moral life. In healthcare ethical considerations centre on the values that are intrinsic to the act of caring for others. Obligations like beneficence, promotion of autonomy and truthfulness reflect the underlying ethical nature of the dentist-patient relationship. The term cosmetic procedure refers to essentially elective procedures performed on normal tissue in order to enhance appearance while maintaining functional integrity.

Prior to undertaking any elective, 'cosmetic' dental procedures, it is vital for the treating dentist to discuss the merits and drawbacks of all viable options. It is important that the patient understands what the consequences and limitations of treatment are likely to be, and what the potential failures could entail later in his/her life. Informed consent should be obtained (preferably in writing) and the clinical notes and records should be clearly documented, with accurate and concise details provided of all the investigations carried out, and their findings, as well as including details of the various discussions that have taken place. Dentists need to be aware of the existence of heightened expectations in this group of patients and be cautious about accepting patients who have unrealistic 'cosmetic' expectations. Where possible, cosmetic or aesthetic dental treatment should be provided which is minimally destructive and, in the longterm, be in the 'best interests' of the patient. Important matters such as the gaining of informed consent and maintaining meticulous, contemporaneous dental records will also be emphasized.

Ethical Issues Associated with Esthetic Procedures

- The use of false or non-recognized credentials promoted by non-accredited institutions
- Reliance on unproved science to promote treatments
- Exaggeration of clinical skills and education
- Unnecessary treatment and services
- Lack of full informed consent
- Harmful practices, such as the unnecessary removal of tooth structure and the replacement of highly clinically successful materials with inferior, untested restorative materials
- Exposing patients to the unknown risks of overtreatment
- Excessive fee
- Failure to refer to specialist

When considering elective cosmetic enhancement, patient health always should come first in the mind of practitioners and always should trump patients' cosmetic desires, even at the expense of patient autonomy. As a professional, a dentist has an ethical duty to weigh the benefits and the risks of any procedure, and if the potential harm or risks outweigh the benefits, even patients' requests for treatment should be declined.

BIBLIOGRAPHY

1. Albino JE and Tedsco LA: Patient perception of dental-facial esthetics. J Prosth Dent 9, 52, 1984.
2. Berland G: Dentistry is challenging; Aesthetic dentistry even more. Dent Today, 4, 2011.
3. Bhuvaneshwan M: Principles of smile design. J Cons Dent 13,225,2010.
4. Davis NC: Smile design. Dent Clin N Am 51,299, 2007.

5. Denry I L: Recent advances in ceramics in dentistry. Crit Rev Oral Biol Med 7,134, 1996.
6. Edward A M: What are the indications of feldspthic veneers. Compend 32, 44, 2011.
7. Flax H: Smile enhancement with laser- a case report. J Cosmetic Dent. 23, 94, 2007.
8. Gerrad P: All ceramic crowns and adjacent veneers. Int J Cosmetic Dent. 1, 18, 2010.
9. Gutnetch N: A Novel Er:YAG Laser-Assisted Tooth Whitening Method. J Laser Health Acad. 1, 1, 2011.
10. Kelleher M: Ethical issues, dilemmas and controversies in cosmetic or aesthetic dentistry. A personal opinion. Br. Dent J. 212 ,365, 2012.
11. Kelleher M: Ethical marketing in aesthetic or cosmetic dentistry part 2. Dental Update. 313, 2012.
12. LeSage B and Milnar A: Achieving the epitome of composite art: creating natural tooth texture, color and anatomy using appropriate preparation and layering technique. J Cosmetic Dent 24, 132, 2008.
13. Lesage B: Minimally invasive dentistry: a paradigm shift in dentistry. Prac Proced Aesthet Dent 21, 97, 2009.
14. LeSage B: Revisiting the design of minimal and no-preparation veneers- A step by step technique. CDA J 38, 561, 2010.
15. Levin EI: Dental esthetics and the golden proportion. J Prosth Dent. 40,244, 1978.
16. Lombardi R: Visual perception and dental esthetics. J Prosth Dent. 29, 352, 1973.
17. Peyton JH: Direct restoration of anterior teeth: review of the clinical technique and case presentation. Pract Proced Aesthet Dent. 14, 203, 2002.
18. Pini N.B., De Marchi L.M., Gribel B.F., Ubaldini A.L.M, Pascotto R.B.: Analysis of the Golden Proportion and width/ height of Maxillary anterior dentition in patients with lateral incisor agenesis. J Esthet and Restor Dent 24, 402, 2012.
19. Ritter AV: Masters of Esthetic Dentistry: posterior composites revisited. Journal Comp 20, 57, 2008.
20. Seymour, D.W., Patel, E. and Chan, F.W.y: Aesthetic Preview: A novel approach. Dent Update.: 4,423, 2012.
21. Simonsen K: Commerce versus care: troubling trends in the ethics of esthetic dentistry. Dent Clin North Am 51, 281, 2007.
22. Spear M and Kokich VG: A multidisciplinary approach to esthetic dentistry. Dent Clin N Am 51, 487, 2007.
23. Stephan J: Clinical Steps to Predictable Color Management in Aesthetic Restorative Dentistry. Dent Clin North Am 51, 473, 2007.
24. Turgut S, Bagis B, Turkaslan S, Bagis Y.: Effect of Ultraviolet Aging on Translucency of Resin-Cemented Ceramic Veneers: An In Vitro Study. J. of prosthodontics 22, 4, 2013.
25. Wells D and LeSage B: Myths vs reality: prep-less veneers and veneers. J Cosmetic Dent, 27, 66, 2011
26. White J: Lasers for use in dentistry. J Esthet Rest Dent. 17, 61, 2005.

29

Color and Its Application

Restorative dentistry is a blend of science and art. The success of restorative dentistry is determined on the basis of functional and esthetic results. To achieve esthetics, four basic determinants are required in sequence; viz. position, contour, texture and color. Color makes an object more appealing, attractive and gives the pleasure of observing. Since aesthetic dentistry imposes several demands on the artistic abilities of the dentist and the technician, knowledge of underlying scientific principles of color is essential. Color combination not only improves esthetics, but also makes the restoration appear natural and attractive. Continued research on the human visual system has given us greater insight into how color discrimination is affected by environment and other features like disease, drugs and aging. The basic fundamentals of color and light, the radiation spectrum and the optical characteristics of the object is to be understood before evaluating and selecting proper color shade for the restoration.

Rarely has color been taught as a separate subject and no clinical courses on color have ever been conducted as a part of dental curriculum. Research work and publications have also not focused much on this subject. The result is that most dentists, even the post-graduates and well experienced clinicians fear color matching and are apprehensive before placement of the final restorations. Color and its clinical application is mainly explained in reference to dental porcelain and/or composites.

SOURCE OF LIGHT

Light is mandatory for any color to exist. Light is a form of electromagnetic energy which is a small part of the large and continuous radiation spectrum (Fig. 29.1). Sunlight or the light of a glowing body is not single type of wavelength but a combination of different wavelengths (measured in nanometers, i.e. millionths of a millimeter). Light in the wavelength range of 380 nm to 760 nm is referred to as the *visible*

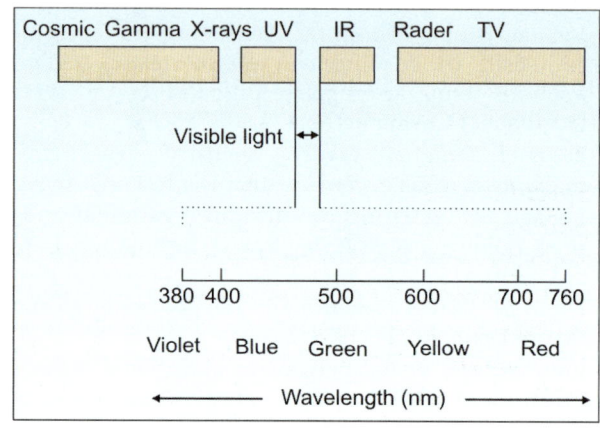

Fig. 29.1: Radiation spectrum

light. Wavelengths less than 380 nm are in the *ultraviolet* range (cosmic rays, gamma rays and x-rays). Wavelengths above 760 nm are in the *infrared* range (radar waves, TV waves and radio waves).

A beam of light when passed through a glass prism gets broken down into its component parts depending upon the wavelength. On projecting these on a screen, they are viewed as a series of glowing spectral colors ranging from violet, blue, green, yellow, orange and red without any clear demarcation between them. White light is produced when all these colors are combined together without the preponderance of any. The wavelength range of different colors is shown in Table 29.1.

OPTICAL CHARACTERISTICS

What happens when light falls on an object? It is either reflected, transmitted or absorbed. If all the light is reflected, the object appears white. On the contrary, if the light is entirely absorbed, the object appears black. Greater the intensity of the direct light source, or greater the amount of light reflected, higher is the brightness of the object being viewed. The final effect is however greatly determined by the transparent, translucent or opaque characteristics of the object.

Table 29.1: Wavelength range of different colors	
Color	Wavelength range
Violet	380 nm–450 nm
Blue	450 nm–480 nm
Blue-green	480 nm–510 nm
Green	510 nm–550 nm
Yellow-green	550 nm–570 nm
Yellow	570 nm–590 nm
Orange	590 nm–630 nm
Red	630 nm–750 nm

Reflection

Reflected light rays are those rays which bounce back from the surface of the object being hit instead of being transmitted or absorbed. Reflection can be of two types:

i. *Specular reflection*: The light is reflected from the point of incidence in a single direction (Fig. 29.2). Such type of reflection is seen on perfectly smooth surfaces. Mirror reflection is an example of specular reflection.

ii. *Diffuse reflection*: The light is reflected from the point of incidence in various directions at angles different from the angle of incidence (Fig. 29.3). Diffuse reflection is seen on rough surfaces. These reflections carry information about the color of an object whereas specular reflections are devoid of any information about color.

Transmission

When light emerges through an object, the process is called 'transmission' (Fig. 29.4).

Refraction

When light travels from one medium into another medium, the velocity changes and the light ray is bent. This process is known as refraction and the ratio between velocities as the index of refraction (Fig. 29.5).

Transparency

A medium is said to be transparent when it allows maximum transmission of light without any distortion, i.e. regular transmission (Fig. 29.6). A clear window glass through which the object can be viewed distinctly is said to be transparent. When regular transmission occurs, it indicates that the density and index of refraction are uniform throughout the body of the material.

Translucency

A medium is said to be translucent when it allows transmission of light in a diffused manner (Fig. 29.7). A frosted glass through which an object is viewed

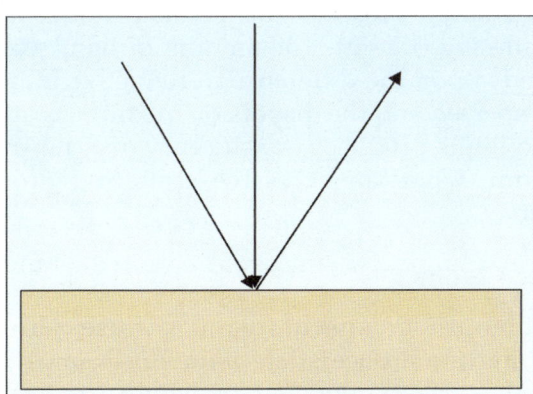

Fig. 29.2: Specular reflection

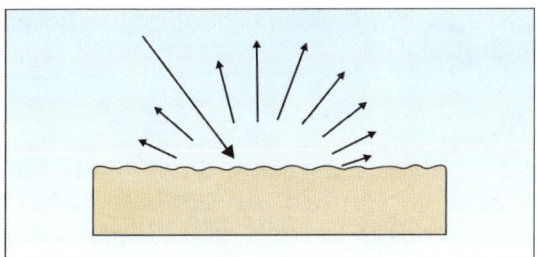

Fig. 29.3: Diffuse reflection

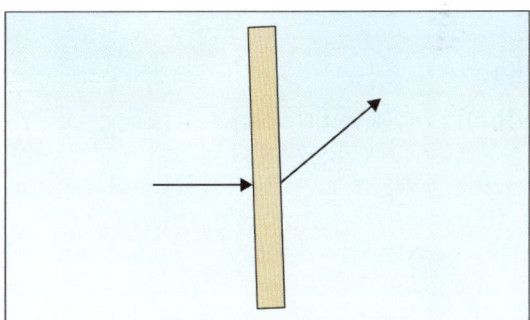

Fig. 29.4: Transmission

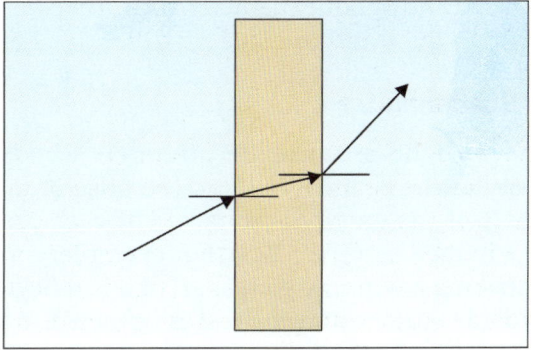

Fig. 29.5: Refraction

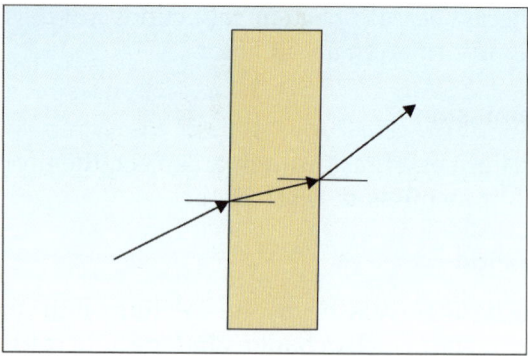

Fig. 29.6: Transparent

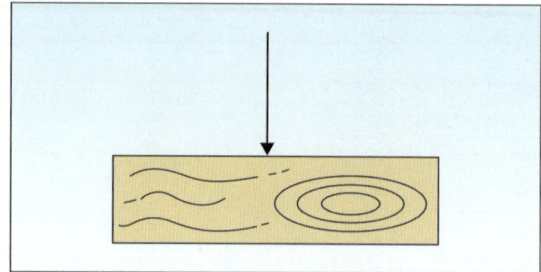

Fig. 29.8: Opaque

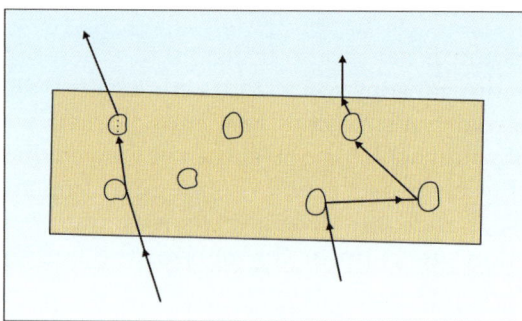

Fig. 29.7: Translucent

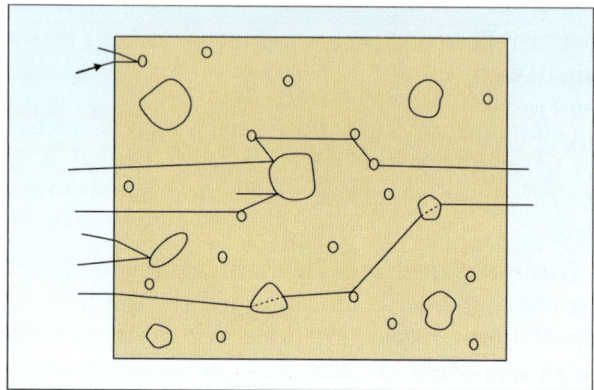

Fig. 29.9: Diagram showing scattering of light due to several internal reflections and refractions

indistinctly is said to be translucent. Diffuse transmission of light is because of the enormous number of internal reflections, external reflections as well as refractions that occur in an object.

Opacity

A medium is said to be opaque when it transmits no light, whatsoever (Fig. 29.8), for example a brick wall. The incident light is either refracted or absorbed depending upon the nature of the medium. The degree of translucency can be defined more accurately by the measurement of the degree of opacity. A body that transmits no light is said to be 100% opaque, whereas one which transmits, say 30% light is said to be 70% opaque. In dentistry, we are more concerned with the translucent and opaque characteristics of a restoration rather than the transparency.

Light Scattering

Whenever light is transmitted through a body, the intensity of the beam is reduced, because of the fact that part of the energy is refracted at each point of change in medium (Fig. 29.9). For example, consider light striking a window glass. Part of it is reflected on the outside surface and the rest is refracted towards the glass pane. As the light leaves the pane to enter air, another portion is reflected and the remainder is refracted in the air. When the medium is heterogeneous, the number of reflections and refractions occurring inside the medium are considerably increased. This phenomenon is known as scattering of light. The amount of light scattered depends upon the difference in refractive indices of the dispersed and the dispersion medium. Scattering within limits produces translucency in a transparent medium, while an excessive scattering produces opacity.

Surface Gloss

The amount of specular and diffuse reflection occurring on a surface is determined by its smoothness. Ceramic surfaces always have slight irregularities, hence the reflection at the surface is usually a combination of specular and diffuse types. On a glazed surface, specular reflection predominates whereas on a rough surface diffuse reflection predominates (Figs 29.10A & B).

COLOR

Color is the property of a surface or substance due to the absorption of certain light rays and reflection of others within the range of wavelengths (380 nm to 760 nm) adequate to excite the retinal receptors. Briefly, it can be said that color is a result of selective absorption and

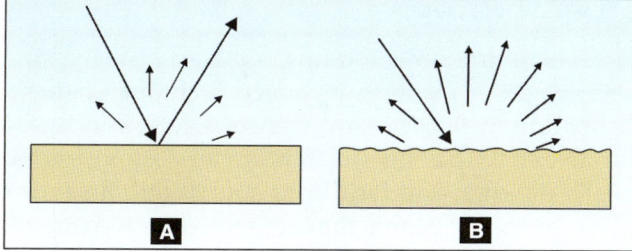

Figs 29.10A and B: Diagram showing **(A)** predominance of specular reflection on smooth glazed surface and **(B)** predominance of diffuse reflection on rough surface

selective reflection. For example an object appears red when it absorbs all constituent lights of the spectrum except red which is reflected back and reaches the eye. Color perception is psychophysical process – *'a psychological response to a physical stimulus, i.e. it involves both objective and subjective phenomenon'*. Objective is the falling of light rays on the retina and subjective is its interpretation by the brain. Since color determination involves a psychological response, it is quite evident that an object may appear to be differently colored when viewed by different observers.

STRUCTURE AND FUNCTION OF EYE

The main features of human eye are shown in Fig. 29.11. Light enters the eye through the cornea. Immediately behind the cornea is the iris. It is a fibrous membrane with central circular aperture which contracts or expands to control the amount of light entering the eye. This compensating property of the eye is known as *chromic adaptation*. Eye lens is situated behind the iris and has sufficient refracting power to focus the image of the object on the retina. Ciliary muscles control the focal length of the eye lens. Various layers of the retina are shown in Fig. 29.12. From inside to outside, these consist of pigment cells, photosensitive receptors, i.e. rods (rod shaped) and cones (cone shaped), bipolar cells, ganglion cells and optic nerve. Cones are responsible for perceiving the

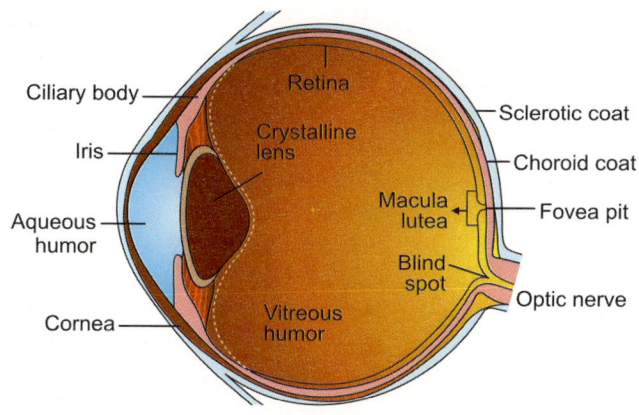

Fig. 29.11: The human eye

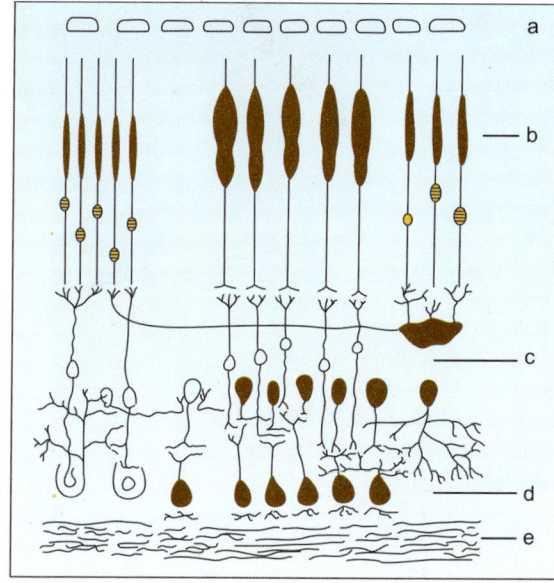

Fig. 29.12: Structure of retina. **(a)** Pigment layer; **(b)** rods and cones; **(c)** bipolar cells; **(d)** ganglion cells and **(e)** optic nerve

chromatic aspects of an object, i.e. its color. Present in the retina are 7 million cones, most of which are packed in the fovea. There are three types of cone receptors: blue sensitive cones, green sensitive cones and red sensitive cones. The ultimate color depends upon the relative amount of stimulation of these three color receptors.

Cones are the only receptors in the fovea, each cell having an individual nerve fiber. In the region immediately surrounding the fovea, both rods and cones are present. Moving more towards the periphery, the ratio of rods to cones increases and multiple receptor cells are supplied by a single fiber. Consequently, color of the image is most distinct when light rays fall in the centre and becomes progressively less distinct when they fall at the periphery.

Irrespective of the nature of light source, color results only from a reflected or transmitted beam of white light or a portion of it. There should be enough light to elicit a color. No object appears colored at low levels of illumination. This is because at low lights, the more sensitive rods get functional which are unable to differentiate color.

PERCEPTION OF COLOR

Color perception involves series of following events (i) the light source (ii) surface viewed (iii) individual observer (eye and brain) and (iv) conditions under which the object is being viewed (Fig. 29.13). All these factors are interrelated and a variation in any one of them can affect the color perception.

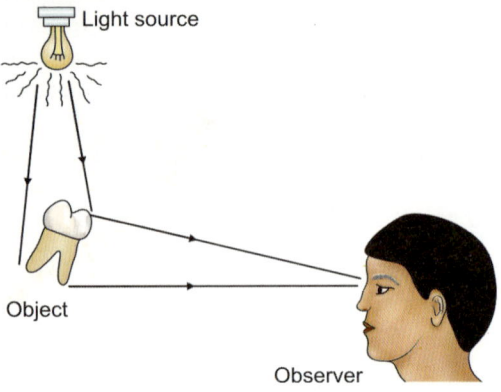

Fig. 29.13: Perception of color

i. The Light Source

The clinician should use a source of light that contains full spectrum of rays without the dominance of any wavelength; because when an object is viewed under lights dominating in particular wavelengths (color bands), that specific color becomes dominant to the observer. Different types of lights and their designation by CIE (Commission International de'Eclairage) are given in Table 29.2.

Table 29.2: Different types of lights and their designation as given by CIE (Commission International de'Eclairage)

Light type	Color temperature K	Light source
A	2856	Incandescent bulb
B	4860	Midday sunlight
C	6770	Average northern sunlight
D	6500	Average daylight (overcast)
E	5455	Equal energy radiator
F	3000	Fluorescent tube "warm-white"

Sunlight is the most preferred light for shade selection. However it may vary in its spectral distribution throughout the day depending upon the time and weather. Average northern daylight with a slightly overcast sky having an intensity of 1500 Lx is considered ideal for shade determination. Light at dawn and dusk is rich in the red-yellow spectrum. Fluorescent lamps are gas discharge lamps and their specturm includes narrow band widths of wavelengths that are elicited by the atoms of the respective gas within the tube. Incandescent (tungsten) bulbs show a spectrum of wavelengths that are dominant in the orange red energy. It is observed that an object when viewed under tungsten lights would possess a greater orange red color, compared to a more neutral greyish blue color when viewed under average daylight.

ii. Surface Viewed

Surface of an object being viewed affects color determination through its spectral characteristics of absorption, reflection and transmission. The surface is analyzed with a spectrophotometer – a device which breaks down a standard light source into a series of monochromatic beams that are then directed onto the surface. The percentage of reflectance compared with the total amount of light incident on the surface at any given wavelength across the visible spectrum is recorded. The location of a peak in spectral reflectance curve so obtained determines the hue of the object. Achromatic objects with white, grey and black do not exhibit any peak in their spectral reflectance curves. In case where the spectral curves are different; a change in the light source or observer or angle of viewing can cause a seemingly accurate color match to disappear. Such a phenomenon is referred to as 'spectral metamerism'.

iii. Individual Observer

Eye is most sensitive to brightness in wavelength regions between 540–570 nm (yellow-green) and thereon the brightness diminishes in both directions. Interpretation of color by the brain differs for different observers. The color perceived is also affected by the eye fatigue. Prolonged viewing of a color for 15–30 seconds strains the cones and causes depletion of photopigments. Fatigue to a particular color sensitizes the eye to its complimentary color. Therefore the cones can be made resensitive to the desired color by gazing at the complementary color until the eye gets fatigued to the latter.

iv. Surrounding Conditions

The surrounding conditions also influence the interpretation of the color. These include: the oral background, wet or dry conditions, angle and intensity of illumination, etc.

METAMERISM

Metamerism is defined as 'the phenomenon when color of two objects appear to match under one set of viewing conditions but differ under different set of conditions like a change in light source or the observer'. Metamerism should not be confused with color changes that occur when a single object is viewed under different types of lights or by different observers. In metamerism, there should always be present two objects whose spectrophotometric curves are different. An exact match is almost impossible when two different materials are used (e.g. natural tooth enamel and porcelain) but the more closer the curves are matched, the fewer are the metameric problems. A consideration should be given to all those possible means that can help prevent metamerism like surface characteristics, individual observer and the light source.

Various forms of metamerism are:
- Illuminant metamerism (due to different lightening conditions)
- Observer metamerism (due to difference in interpretation by different observers)
- Geometric metamerism (due to change in angle of view)
- Field size metamerism (due to change in area of view)

FLUORESCENCE

Fluorescence is the absorption of radiation of a particular wavelength and its re-emission as a radiation of longer wavelength.

Natural tooth has fluorescing qualities believed to be because of its organic content. It absorbs wavelengths between 300 to 400 nm (ultraviolet range). Sunlight, photoflash lamps, UV lights and certain types of vapor lamps are sources of ultraviolet radiations. The energy absorbed by the tooth is then released as radiations of longer wavelengths, generally in the range of 400–500 nm (yellow white fluorescence). Because of fluorescence, the human tooth has the much appreciable brightness and life like appearance. Any restoration that is to replace natural tooth structure should therefore contain fluorescing agents. It also emphasizes the importance of matching the shade under two or more lighting conditions, out of which one should have adequate UV component (incandescent lights).

In porcelains, the fluorescing effects can be reasonably simulated by addition of small amounts of sodium diuranate, of which uranium content is usually 0.15% or less. Uranium produces a brilliant carnary yellow fluorescence. Addition of cerium salts results in blue fluorescence damping the yellowness to a certain extent.

OPALESCENCE

Opalescence is the phenomenon in which a material appears to be of one color when light is reflected from it and of another color when light is transmitted through it. Opals act like prisms and refract different wavelengths to varying degrees. The shorter wavelengths refract more and require a higher critical angle to escape an optically dense material than the longer wavelength. The hydroxyapatite crystals of enamel also act as prisms. Wavelengths of light have different degrees of translucency through teeth and dental materials. When illuminated, opals and enamel will transilluminate the reds and scatter the blues within its body; thus, enamel appears bluish even though it is colorless. The opalescent effects of enamel brighten the tooth and give it optical depth and vitality.

BASIC COLOR SCHEMES

The **color wheel** or **color circle** (Fig. 29.14) is the basic tool for combining colors. The first circular color diagram was designed by Sir Isaac Newton in 1666. Over the years, many variations of the basic design have been made, but the most common version is a wheel of 12 colors, the **primary colors** being red, yellow and blue. Three **secondary colors** (green, orange and purple) are created by mixing two primary colors. Six **tertiary colors** are created by mixing primary and secondary colors.

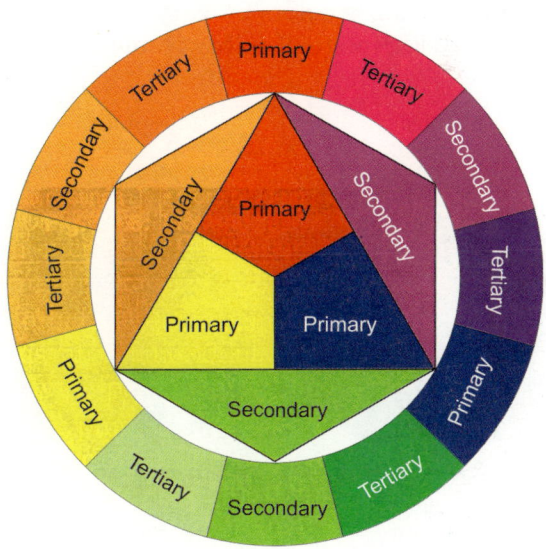

Fig. 29.14: The color wheel

COLOR HARMONIES

The color combinations that are considered pleasing are called **color harmonies** or **color chords**. They consist of two or more colors having fixed relation in the color wheel.

These are:
- Complementary color scheme (Colors that are opposite to each other on the color wheel are considered to be complementary colors; for example, red and green).
- Analogous color scheme (colors that are next to each other on the color wheel).
- Triadic color scheme (three colors that are evenly spaced around the color wheel).
- Tetradic or rectangular color scheme (four colors arranged into two complementary pairs).

- Split complementary color scheme (In addition to the base color, it uses two colors adjacent to its complement).
- Square color scheme (similar to rectangle, but all four colors spaced evenly around the color circle).

Additive Color Theory

The additive primary colors are **red, green and blue** (RGB). Combining one of these additive primary colors with equal amounts of another one results in the **additive secondary colors of cyan, magenta and yellow** (Fig. 29.15). Combining all three additive primary colors in equal amounts will produce the color white. Remember combining additive colors creates lighter colors; so adding all three primary colors results in a color so "light", it's actually seen as white (Table 29.3). By changing the brightness of each of the three primary colors by varying degrees, you can make a wide range of colors (Table 29.4).

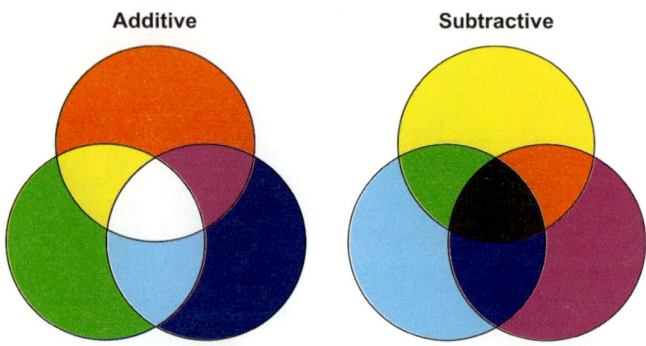

Fig. 29.15: Additive and subtractive color mixing

Table 29.3: Additive colors combined in equal parts

Blue + Green	=	Cyan
Red + Blue	=	Magenta
Green + Red	=	Yellow
Red + Green + Blue	=	White

Table 29.4: Additive colors combined in unequal parts

1 Green + 2 Red	=	Orange
1 Red + 2 Green	=	Lime
1 Green + 1 Blue + 4 Red	=	Brown

Subtractive Color Theory

The subtractive primary colors are **cyan, magenta and yellow** (Fig. 29.15). Subtractive color mixing occurs when light is reflected off a surface or is filtered through a translucent object. For example, a red surface only appears red because it **absorbs (subtracts)** all of the light that is not red and only **reflects or allows** the red light.

Mixing of two subtractive primary colors result in a color, which is complimentary to the remaining primary. For example, if cyan and magenta is mixed it will form blue which is complimentary to the yellow (third subtractive primary color) Table 29.5.

Table 29.5: Subtractive colors mixing

Combine	Absorbs	Leaves
Cyan + Magenta	Red + Green	Blue
Cyan + Yellow	Red + Blue	Green
Magenta + Yellow	Green + Blue	Red
Cyan + Magenta + Yellow	Red + Green + Blue	Black

COLOR SYSTEMS

A system for representing color is required for tooth color. A tooth color atlas can then be produced as colored samples organized according to this specified arrangement.

Color, perceived when light reflected from an object enters the eye, consists of quantity and quality. Quantity is the variable lightness (value) and is the total amount of light reflected from an object. It is indicated by the relative nearness of a color to white or black on an achromatic grey scale such as a black and white photograph. Quality is the chromatic component of color consisting of two variables which can be represented in two dimensions.

1. Munsell Color System

A color order system describing colors by hue, saturation and lightness was proposed by *Albert H. Munsell* (1961), which came to be known as the Munsell color system. This is presently the most widely used visual color order system. The method arranges the three dimensions of the color in orderly scales of equal visual steps.

The Munsell color solid can be likened to a sphere or a cylinder as it is an irregular three dimensional figure with characteristics of both. To simplify its understanding, it is considered as a cylinder in this chapter (Fig. 29.16). The Munsell cylinder may be formed by a series of wheels stacked one upon the other. The hub of each wheel represents the value axis. When placed on top of each other, a colorless or achromatic axis extends through the centre of the cylinder, pure white at the top (assigned a value of 10) and pure black at the bottom (assigned a value of 0).

Color and Its Application

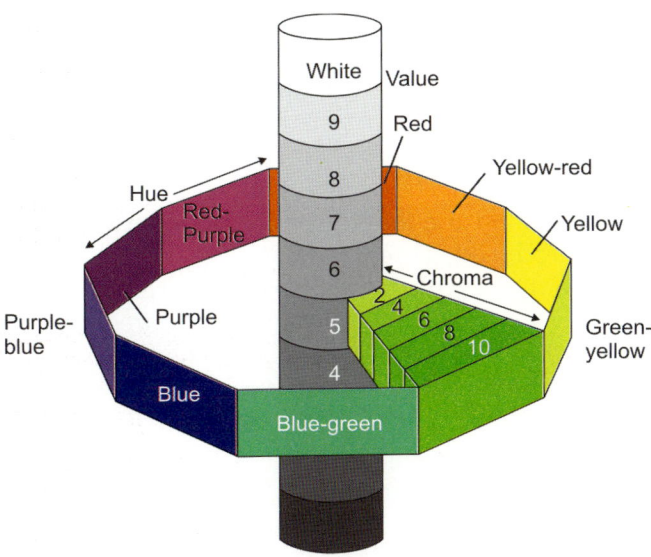

Fig. 29.16: Munsell color system

A series of greys progressing from black to white in equal visual steps connects these extremities. 5 represents middle grey. Hues are arranged sequentially around the rim of the wheel. There are 100 hues in this scale: 10 major hues - (5 principal and 5 intermediate hues) positioned 10 steps apart: Red (R), Yellow (Y), Green (G), Blue (B) and Purple (P) are the principal hues where as Yellow-red (YR), Green-yellow (GY), Blue-green (BG), Purple-blue (PB) and Red-purple (RP) are the intermediate hues. Within each hue, the colors are arranged in scales according to their lightness/darkness (value) and their purity (saturation). Colors with lower value numbers are known as dark colors and are arranged towards the bottom. Conversely, colors with higher value numbers are known as light colors and are arranged towards the top.

The spokes of the wheel represent the saturation (chroma) of a color. Purest colors are arranged towards the periphery. Any newer purer color that is created can be added at the periphery easily and this is responsible for the different projections beyond the surface of the solid. The chroma scale starts from zero and till today extends to a maximum of fourteen.

The designation of any particular color located in the Munsell color solid is given by the notation HV/C, where H stands for hue, V for value and C for chroma, e.g. 8R3/7 would mean hue is 8 red, value is 3 and chroma is 7. The scale of value extends from 0/, 1/, 2/ …. 10/ and chroma from /0, /1, /2 ….../14 or farther. A color differing only in value and being darker would be placed directly below the previous one. Most of the dental shade guides are based on a section of the Munsell color system that includes color range of the natural teeth.

Dimensions of Color

Color is usually described according to Munsell color space in three dimensions – *Hue, Chroma and Value.* When color is determined using Munsell system value is determined first, followed by chroma. Hue is described last by matching with shade tabs of value and chroma already determined.

Hue

Hue is that quality by which we distinguish one color family from another, e.g. red, yellow, blue, etc. In simple words, hue is the type of color. It is specified as the dominant range of wavelengths in the visible spectrum that yield the perceived color. Hue is represented by A, B, C and D on the commercial vita shade guide (Fig. 29.17A).

Chroma

Chroma is that quality by which we distinguish a strong color from a weak one. In simple words, it is the saturation or intensity of a hue (Fig. 29.17B). This dimension can be more easily explained by employing the concept of painting a box. Suppose one side of the box is painted in pure red. Now before painting the second side, a little amount of grey is added to the previous red, the color then perceived is weak red. Similarly, while painting the third side, the same gray is added more, the color now becomes more weak, i.e. greyer. Adding grey reduces the chroma while the hue remains same.

Value

Value is the amount of light returned from an object. It is that quality by which we distinguish whiteness from blackness, i.e. achromatic aspects of a color. A color of high value is transmitted as light grey and that of a low value as dark grey (Fig. 29.17C). It is considered the most important dimension while making a color match. If a series of colors have the same values, all of them would be composed of the same greys. A younger tooth is generally whiter and brighter than its older counterpart. This demands use of more whitening agents like zirconium oxide in porcelain while replacing younger teeth. Increase in the thickness of opaque or core porcelain raises the value whereas an increase in enamel (translucent) porcelain reduces the value. Lowering value means less light returns from the illuminated object and the rest is being absorbed or scattered elsewhere.

The value of a specific color is the value levels of grey added to the original color. If the grey of same value is added each time, no change in value occurs,

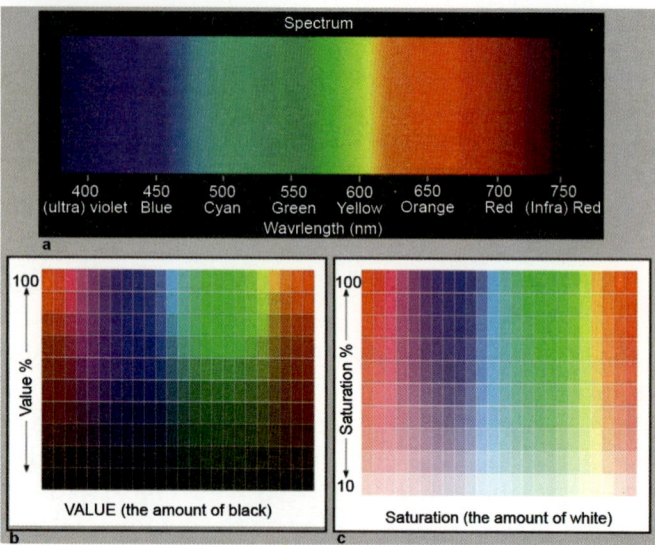

Figs 29.17A, B and C: Dimensions of color: **(A)** Hue, **(B)** Value, **(C)** Chroma

only the chroma reduces. On adding a value higher than the original value of the color, the resulting color has the same hue, reduced chroma and higher value. On adding a value lower than the original value, the resulting color has the same hue, reduced chroma and reduced value.

Judd and Wyszecki (1975) opined that polar coordinate systems, such as Munsell should be avoided due to the inherent chromatic distortions where the distance between colors of the same hue increase as the chroma increases. Spacing the samples requires a non-distorting color space such as the more recently developed internationally accepted colorimetric for reflective materials, CIELAB (CIE 1978). It was designed for small color differences as a cartesian coordinate system of opponent colors.

2. CIE 1931 System

In 1931, the CIE introduced a system of instrumental color measurement for describing colors. It is based on the fundamental property of trichromacy. The rationale involved is that a color sensation can be matched by the mixing of three colored lights or three primary wavelengths. If the three primaries, red, green and blue, are represented by [R], [G] and [B] then when these are used to match a given color [C], the amount of the primaries needed to imitate the color will be R, G and B. Thus, C units of color [C] can be matched by R units of the red primary [R] additively mixed with G units of the green primary [G] and B units of the blue primary [B]. This is represented as

C[C] = R[R] + G[G] + B[B]

The amount of the three primaries used (i.e. R, G and B) are known as the tristimulus values of the color [C]. In the 1931 CIE system, a series of (human) observers were employed, using a 2° viewing angle (so that light illuminated only the fovea). The observers determined the amount of the three primaries that were needed to match all spectral colors within the visible spectrum. The results obtained for the observers were collected and the concept of a standard observer was introduced. Three curves were obtained which represent the color vision characteristics of the observers because the amount of the three primary lights needed to match the spectral colors was related to the response character of the cone receptors. These curves are known as the color matching functions of the observer. The 1931 CIE system uses the following terminology.

Primaries: Three imaginary primaries are used, specified as [X], [Y] and [Z].

Color matching functions: These characterize the response of the cone receptors in the observer and are denoted $\bar{x}$, $\bar{y}$, and $\bar{z}$.

Standard observer: Although a 2° viewing angle was initially used, in 1964, the CIE introduced a 10° standard observer which has been adopted in most countries.

Tristimulus values: These are denoted as X, Y and Z. It was earlier mentioned that the perception of the color of an object depends on three elements, namely the light source, the object and the observer. The color of an object depends on:

- The spectral energy distribution of the light that illuminates the sample (S)
- The reflectance characteristics of the sample (R)
- The sensitivity of the observer (color matching functions).

As mentioned, in the CIE system, the tristimulus value is the amount of a primary that will match the color of a given object. The given color is matched by:

X[X] + Y[Y] + Z[Z]

As the color of that object also depends on the characteristics of the illuminant, object and observer, it follows that the tristimulus values are related to S, R and $\bar{x}$, $\bar{y}$, and $\bar{z}$. For a given wavelength, λ, then:

$X = S_\lambda R \bar{x}_\lambda$
$Y = S_\lambda R \bar{y}_\lambda$
$Z = S_\lambda R \bar{z}_\lambda$

Thus, if a given colored sample is illuminated with a known light [a CIE standard illuminant of defined SED (S)] and the reflected light (R) is viewed by a known observer (a CIE standard observer of defined $\bar{x}$, $\bar{y}$ and $\bar{z}$); the tristimulus values can be calculated.

Chromaticity

As mentioned, color is three-dimensional, with the three attributes of color being hue, value and chroma. This means that the CIE system must be three-dimensional which gives rise to the concept of color space. In the CIE system, the Y tristimulus value represents the luminance of the object and is normalized to 100. To represent the other two dimensions of color, the concept of chromaticity is used. To represent hue and chroma, chromaticity coordinates are calculated and displayed on a chromaticity diagram. The chromaticity coordinates are defined as x, y and z where

x + y + z = 1:

$$x = \frac{X}{X + Y + Z}$$

$$x = \frac{Y}{X + Y + Z}$$

$$x = \frac{Z}{X + Y + Z}$$

In practice a plot of x versus y is constructed that exhibits a horse shoe shaped area and which contains all real colors. Neutral colors occupy a central position and moving from this region to the spectral locus the colors increase in chroma. Achromatic colors are represented by a neutral point. While the chromaticity diagram represents the hue and chroma of a color, the third dimension of color (value) is imagined as the Y tristimulus value perpendicular to the plane of the chromaticity diagram. This is of great significance with regards to the description of color difference. Clearly, what is required is for distances in color space (i.e. differences between x, y or Y values) to correspond to the same visually perceived differences. Various attempts have been made to improve the 1931 CIE system and in 1976, the CIE proposed the use of the CIE L*a*b* color space.

3. CIE L*a*b* Color Space

In this system, which is now far more widely used than the 1931CIE system, the tristimulus values of the sample are transformed into L*, a* and b* coordinates as mutually perpendicular axes. In this three-dimensional color space, lightness is represented by L* on a scale of 0 for black to 100 for white. The hue and chroma of a sample are represented on an a* versus b* plot. a* is the red/green coordinate with +a* indicating red and -a* indicating green. b* is the yellow/blue coordinate, with +b* indicating yellow and -b* indicating blue (Fig. 29.18). The CIE L*a*b* color space can be used to specify color differences via the equation:

$$\Delta E^{*ab} = [(\Delta L^*)^2 + (\Delta a^*)^2 + (\Delta b^*)^2]^{0.5}$$

where ΔL*, Δa* and Δb* represent the differences between the corresponding coordinates of two samples. According to this system, a color difference of one ΔE^{*ab} unit or greater is just perceivable.

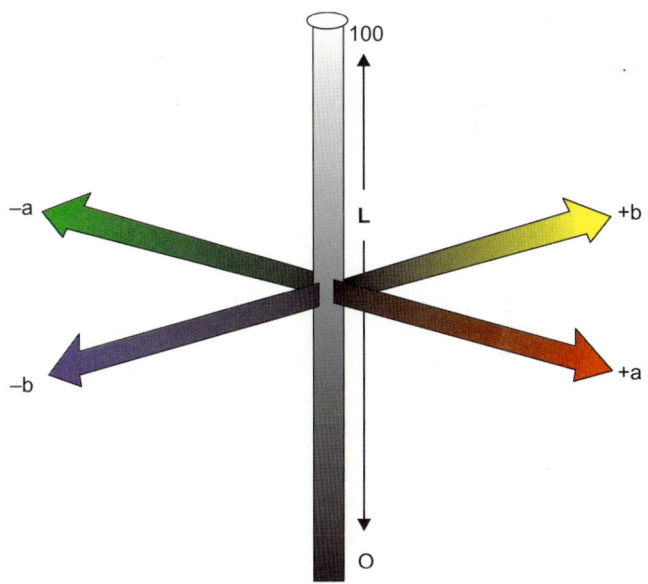

Fig. 29.18: CIE L*a*b* color space

4. CIE L*C*h° Color Difference

The cartesian coordinates, L*, a* and b*, can be transformed into the cylindrical coordinates L*, C* and h°. The lightness (L*) coordinate is the same as in L*, a*, b* space, with the chroma (C*) coordinate being perpendicular to the lightness axis and the hue angle (h°) expressed in degrees (0° at the +a* axis, 90° at the +b* axis, 180° at the –a* axis, 270° for –b* and back to 360° = 0°).

Color difference is expressed in this system by:

$$\Delta E^{*ab} = [(\Delta L^*)^2 + (\Delta C^*)^2 + (\Delta H^*)^2]^{0.5}$$

where ΔH* is the metric hue difference as opposed to the angular difference, Δh°. Color differences (ΔE^{*ab}) are the same for any pair of samples whether CIE L*a*b* or CIE L*C*h° are used. However, CIE L*a*b* color space (and thus CIE L*C*h° color space) is visually non-uniform with the result that differences between colors at the edges of the color space may not agree with visually judged color differences. Consequently, several alternative color spaces have been devised though none has, as yet, been recommended by the CIE to replace CIEL*a*b* color space. In essence, the alternative color space systems seek to improve the accuracy of color difference description and modify the ΔL*, ΔC* and ΔH* coordinates obtained using the CIE L*a*b* equations.

OPTICS OF NATURAL TEETH

Enamel is translucent compared to dentin and may be optically considered as a veneer formed by a bundle of translucent rods, with the outer ends of the rods on the tooth surface and inner ends adjacent to less translucent dentin. Histologically, enamel is constituted of approximately 97 percent by weight of inorganic matter mostly present as hydroxyapatite $[Ca_{10}(PO_4)_6(OH)_2]$ crystals. Other mineral forms like fluorapatite, calcium carbonate, calcium fluoride may also be present in minor amounts. These inorganic crystallites are quite small and are 3000–5000Å in length by 50–1200Å in width. The extremely small size results in high surface area to volume ratio. Enamel crystallites are grouped together into rods which are held together by organic matrix (i.e. collagen), the latter constituting about one percent of the total enamel. The remaining 2–3 percent is water. Because of the different constituents in enamel that have different refractive indices, it is likely that reflection and refraction occur within the medium but are limited to an extent of 30% in 1.0 mm specimen. The rest of the light about 70% is transmitted and the enamel thus exhibits a translucent quality.

On the contrary, dentin has less inorganic content (about 70 wt%) of hydroxyapatite and the apatite crystallites are much smaller than those in enamel: 200–300 Å in length and 40–70 Å in width which results in an even higher surface area: volume ratio compared to enamel. The organic matrix is collagen and constitutes about 20 wt% and the water about 10 wt% of the total tissue. Because the area over which the difference in refractive indices has increased, light transmitted is only about 30% through 1.0 mm thick specimens and dentin hence tends to be less translucent. It is also quite possible that the smaller size of apatite crystals in dentin render the particle size close to the wavelength of the incident light, thereby increasing the opacity values.

The color space of natural tooth has been described by Clark as a hue range of 6YR to 9.3Y, a value range of 4/ to 8/ and a chroma range of /10 to / 7. Color of natural tooth is a result of light reflected directly from the tooth surface combined with light reflected from the dentin and a minor contribution from the oral background. Dentin is the primary source of color and the rays reflected from it transmitted via enamel are modified by the thickness and degree of enamel translucency. The effect of enamel thickness and translucency on tooth color is evident in the incisal, middle and cervical thirds of the tooth, which needs to be duplicated in porcelain restorations (Fig. 29.19A) using translucent, opaque, enamel and dentin porcelain (Fig. 29.19B).

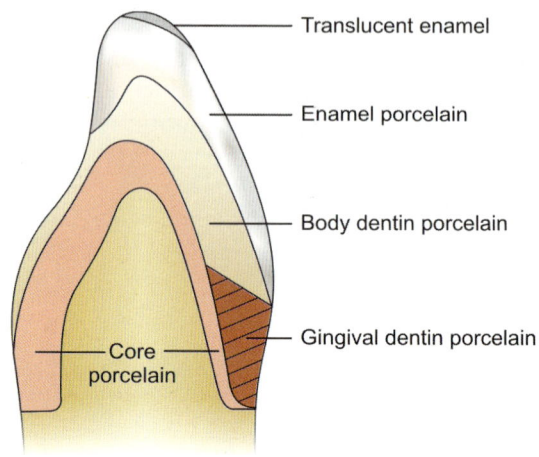

Fig. 29.19A: Diagram showing the gingival, dentin and enamel colors along with the tracing of enamel outline

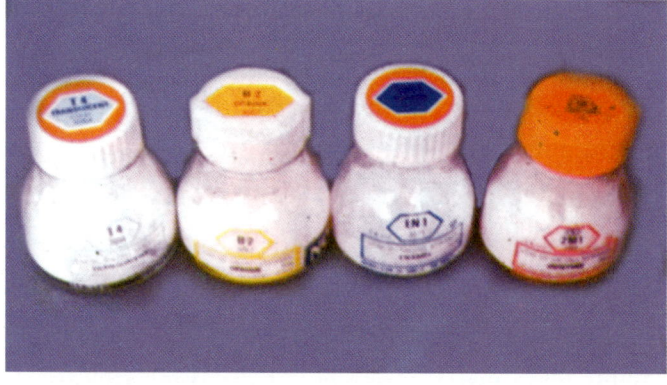

Fig. 29.19B: Translucent, opaque, enamel and dentin porcelain powders

Incisal third of tooth: This is primarily composed of translucent enamel and the shade may hence vary from light to dark gray to bluish. The translucency and consequently the greyness is seen to extend into approximal areas. At times the underlying extension of dentin may also be visible through the overlying enamel. The color of incisal third is referred to as the *enamel color.*

Middle third of tooth: This area is primarily composed of dentin. The final color of the middle third region is hence determined by the dentin hue having been modified by the overlying translucent blue grey enamel. It generally falls in the range of orange red, blue yellow or gray yellow. The color of middle third is referred to as the *body dentin color*.

Cervical third of tooth: In this area, the enamel thins out extremely and the underlying dentin color is hence quite marked. The color of the cervical half region is referred to as the *gingival dentin color* and is in the range of orange yellow to brown, depending upon the amount of calcification that has taken place.

DENTAL SHADE GUIDES

Dental shade guides are a collection of various color combinations available from the manufacturers of denture teeth, restorative resins and porcelain; which aid the dentist in selecting the most acceptable color match with the tooth or teeth in question. Their reliable use is closely associated with the adequacy of the shade guide plus the familiarity of the dentist with the basic color matching procedures. Shades guides are best based on the Munsell color order system. Prime requirements for any shade guide as given by Sproull which include (1) a logical arrangement of colors in the color space and (2) an adequate distribution of colors in color space. An ideal color space is one in which each color is the centre of a sphere of colors, and the next closest matches in color surrounding it. A guide that does not meet the above mentioned requirements results in problems like:

- It takes too long to decide where to begin.
- It is impossible to rapidly or logically check the chosen match for accuracy.
- The volume of color space occupied by the materials to be matched may be impossible to reach within the guide.

Most shade guides in the market usually do not extend through the volume of color space required; an orderly or systematic arrangement between tabs is usually lacking and there is clustering or duplication of colors in certain areas of color space and deficiencies in other regions. Most manufacturers provide shade guides for their material and it is advisable that these should not be used for shade matching of materials from other manufacturers. Variations may be evident in different batches of the same material also. Many shade guide systems use hue as the basis to define color. Within each hue there are various levels of chroma (or saturation) to select from with no consideration for the ΔE difference between tabs. The third and most critical component for color selection (value) typically has no accountability and is not addressed in most shade guides. The VITA Classical Shade Guide is the most commonly used shade guide, but it's flawed because it does not address value. It was not until 1997 that value was added to a shade guide and used as the primary source of shade selection, with chroma and hue having less impact on the selection process. The VITA 3D Master Shade Guide revolutionized shade selection, making the process easier by basing color selection on value. With the 3D-MasterGuide, as each color component is selected, it is held constant while the next color component is found. There's no other system available that allows this to be done. However, simply knowing the correct color will not provide a perfectly matching restoration. It's easier to understand where to place ceramic when fabricating a restoration if there is some visual input. This is why a photograph issued to help determine where color changes occur. This information is invaluable for the technician to see color shifts, regardless of whether or not a photograph is color accurate. The traditional VITA Classical Shade Guide has 16 shade tabs with ΔE's close together, and can be difficult for proper shade selection. It's also unable to produce all of the colors necessary in dentistry. The total VITA Classical Shade Guide range has a coverage rated at 17 ΔE* divergence. The 34 ΔE coverage of the VITA Bleachedguide 3D-Master allows for considerably more interpretation. VITA has also introduced the VITA Linear - guide, which simplifies the arrangement of the original VITA 3D-Master by separating the value tabs into their own holders. The chroma and hue tabs are arranged separately within each value group. This allows quick determination of the value of the restoration before moving on to chroma and hue, and removes any potential confusion caused by the nonlinear arrangement of shade tabs in the current 3D-Master system (Fig. 29.20).

Shofu offered the Natural Color Concept (NCC). *Egger* conducted a worldwide clinical study in which

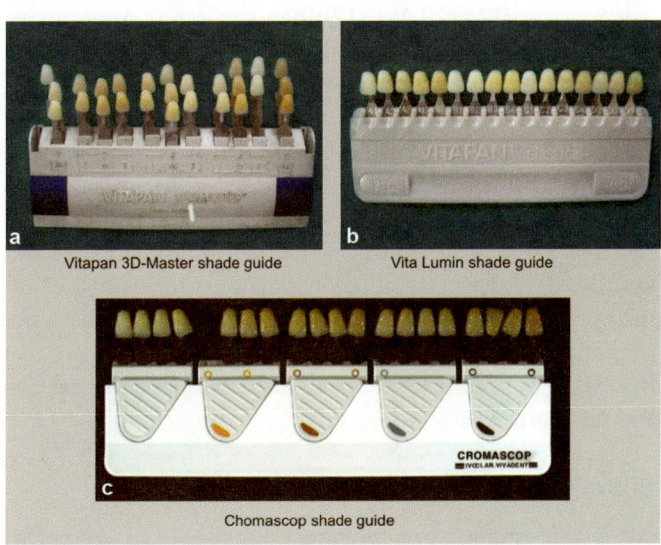

Fig. 29.20: Various shade guides

the tooth shades of more than 3500 patients were recorded and analyzed spectrophotometrically. The NCC color indicator was derived from these data, which served as the basis for the dental color space. The NCC system consists of 208 color blends based on 38 basic shades. The manufacturer purports that these blends are logically arranged in L*a*b* color space according to Munsell Hue, Chroma, and Value.

A shade guide meant for porcelain should not be used for metal ceramic restorations. Shade guides can be of two types: key ring guides and metal slotted type fixed in plastic holders. The latter are preferred. Though a reasonable color match can be obtained, the use of shade guides have numerous inherent flaws like:

1. Because of reflectance, refractiveness, opacity, translucency and transparency, a given shade button will probably never match a tooth exactly.
2. The thickness of the porcelain tab may be different from that of the prosthesis to be made.
3. Porcelain of a given shade from the same manufacturer may vary from batch to batch.
4. The size and surface texture of a tooth and shade button may not be in harmony.
5. Most shade buttons have a shape of maxillary central incisor thereby introducing another variable in shade matching.
6. Difficulty in conveying the information to the laboratory technician.
7. The necks of the shade tabs are usually darker in shade and hence need to be ground off.

SHADE-TAKING DEVICES

These devices have been designed to aid clinicians and technicians in the specification and control of tooth color (Fig. 29.21). The earliest color-measuring device designed specifically for clinical dental use was a filter colorimeter. The Chromascan (Sterngold, Stamford, Connecticut) was introduced in the early 1980s but enjoyed limited success due to its inadequate design and accuracy. Further development was hindered primarily by lack of resources and commitment on industry's side—the market was too small. Now, with esthetics as a major focus of dental marketing and with the availability of improved color-measuring optics, companies are willing to make the investment required to apply advanced technology to the challenge of shade control.

Basic Design

All color-measuring devices consist of a detector, signal conditioner, and software that process the signal

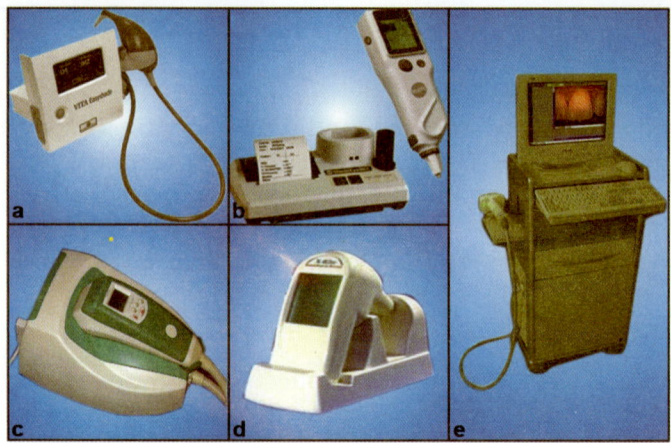

a. Vita easyshade   b. Shade eye NCC   c. Shadescan
d. Shaderie dental vision system   e. Spactroshade

Fig. 29.21: Shade - taking devices

in a manner that makes the data usable in the dental operatory or laboratory. Because of the complex relationship between these elements, accurate colorimetric analysis is difficult at best.

Colorimeters

Filter colorimeters generally use three or four silicon photodiodes that have spectral correction filters that closely simulate the standard observer functions. These filters act as analog function generators that limit the spectral characteristics of the light that strikes the detector surface. The inability to exactly match the standard observer functions with filters while retaining adequate sensitivity for low light levels is the reason that the absolute accuracy of filter colorimeters is considered inferior to scanning devices such as spectrophotometers and spectroradiometers. However, because of their consistent and rapid sensing nature, these devices can be precise with differential measurements. This is why they often are used for quality control.

Digital Cameras as Filter Colorimeters

The newest devices used for dental shade matching are based on digital camera technology. Instead of focusing light upon film to create a chemical reaction, digital cameras capture images using CCDs, which contain many thousands or even millions of microscopically small light-sensitive elements (photosites). Like the photodiodes, each photosite responds only to the total light intensity that strikes its surface. To get a full color image, most sensors use filtering to look at the light in its three primary colors in a manner analogous to the filtered colorimeter described previously. There are several ways of recording the three colors in a digital camera. The highest-quality cameras use three separate sensors, each with a different filter over it. Light is directed to the different filter/sensor combinations by placing a beam splitter in the camera. The beam splitter allows each detector to see the image simultaneously. The advantage of this method is that the camera records each of the three colors at each pixel location.

Spectrophotometers and Spectroradiometers

Spectrophotometers and spectroradiometers are instruments designed to produce the most accurate color measurements. Spectrophotometers differ from spectroradiometers primarily because they include a stable light source. There are two types of basic designs commonly used for these instruments. The traditional scanning instrument consists of a single photodiode detector that records the amount of light at each wavelength. The light is divided into small wavelength intervals by passing through a monochromator. A more recent design uses a diode array with a dedicated element for each wavelength. This design allows for the simultaneous integration of all wavelengths. Both designs are considerably slower than filter colorimeters but remain the tools that are required to examine and develop accurate color-measuring devices.

The difference between Colorimeter and Spectrophotometer is tabulated in Table 29.6.

GUIDELINES FOR CLINICAL SHADE SELECTION

A precise color match between artificial color samples and a natural tooth can best be approximated only if strict guidelines are followed, such as:

1. Lighting of the operatory

The traditional light source considered optimal for color matching is – Northern exposure sunlight in the middle of the day with a slight overcast sky (intensity-1500). This exposure contains an almost equal blend of all wavelengths of light compared to morning and evening exposures which are rich in blue wavelength and reddish yellow wavelengths respectively.

Since, the intensity of day light varies, artificial systems that have the same spectrum as natural daylight have been proposed. The capacity of an artificial light to reproduce natural light is measured by using color temperature and color rendering index (CRI).

White light, which is considered the best source for color comparison, is assigned a Color Rendering Index (CRI) of 100. Any artificial sources with an index over 90 are considered adequate.

Several *color corrected fluorescent lamps* with a CRI of over 90 are available that provide an environment conducive to optimal color matching. Chair light is not recommended for color matching procedures.

Before proceeding for color selection, it should be ascertained as to which lights are critical to the patient, e.g. whether the person works indoors under fluorescent lamps? Whether the patient is an actor and works on stage? Whether he/she is exposed more to sunlight? Whether he/she is a night club performer? Those lights should be selected which closely simulate his working conditions, e.g. a night club performer should be viewed under incandescent and fluorescent light sources to achieve harmony of shade. The patient

Table: 29.6 Difference between Colorimeter and Spectrophotometer	
Colorimeter	*Spectrophotometer*
An instrument for psychophysical analysis – provides measurements that correlate with human eye-brain perception. Colorimetric data is directly read and provided as tristimulus values	An instrument for physical analysis – provides wavelength by wavelength spectral analysis of the reflecting and/or transmitting properties of objects without interpretation by human
Consists of sensor and simple data processor	Consists of sensor plus data processor or computer with software
Has a set illuminant and observer combination usually 2°	Has many available illuminant/observer combinations
Isolates a broad band of wavelength using a tristimulus absorption filter	Isolates a narrow band of wavelength using a prism or interference filter
Less complex instrument	More complex instrument
Works well for routine comparisons of similar colors and for adjustment of small color differences under constant conditions. Optimal for quality inspection	Works well for color formulation, measurement of metamerism and variable illuminant/observer conditions. Optimal for both quality inspection and research and development.

should be informed that the particular color match was done to provide the most satisfactory appearance in the most critical light and that a slight mismatch might be expected under other light sources.

Intensity of light is also important. The ratio of intra-oral to extra-oral illumination should be 3 to 5:1 with extra oral light intensity of 200–300 foot candles. This amount of lighting also reduces eye fatigue by decreasing the difference in brightness levels of the light needed for execution of intra oral procedures and the immediate surroundings.

The location of light can be from ceiling or surface mounted installation away from ceiling.

All luminous ceiling is achieved by having the entire ceiling of the room illuminated by fluorescent lighting. *Open perimeter surface mounted installation* involves using fluorescent fixtures only at the perimeter of the ceiling and not in the centre. *Open perimeter recessed installation* restricts lateral and upward loss of light by providing a proper reflective surface to project the light downwards.

2. Surrounding Environment

Bright colored surroundings greatly influence the colors in the reflected light and hence interfere with proper color matching. The bright colored curtains, walls, etc. should be avoided in the dental operatory. The dentist and the patient are advised not to wear bright clothes. A drape can be used to mask an undesirable color in the patient's clothing, provided the drape itself does not introduce an undesirable reflecting color. Lipstick should be removed so that it does not affect the perceived color. A portable color corrected light source can be employed to provide oral lightning. *Light grey* is an ideal background for color matching. Surfaces with high gloss produce disturbing glares and should be avoided.

3. Tooth Condition

The concerned tooth and a few adjoining teeth on both sides should be free of plaque and surface stains prior to color matching. The tooth should be moist while selecting the shade as dehydration results in a whiter appearance. Dehydration also results in loss of loosely bound water from enamel which increases the internal scattering of light and consequently the amount of reflected light reaching the operator. Dehydration becomes a specific problem when considerably long time is spent in arriving at a final color match. Under such situations the patient is suggested to close the mouth between comparisons so that the teeth are moistened by running the tongue over them.

Shade matching should be carried out before the application of rubber dam. It prevents any light reflected from the dam to interfere with shade selection and provides a more natural environment. Also, an isolated tooth under rubber dam tends to dehydrate in 15 to 20 minutes and takes approximately 30 minutes to regain its original appearance after the isolation has been removed.

4. Selection Distance

The shade selection is carried out at 3 to 6 feet distance, which is considered as the distance from which the patients teeth are usually observed.

5. Patient Position

The patient should be seated upright with his mouth at the observer's eye level. The dentist should stand directly in front of the patient when selecting a shade.

6. Time of Selection

The color selection process should be performed by the dentist when he is able to devote sufficient time. The shade matching should be given equal importance and performed at the beginning of the day when eye fatigue has not set in.

PROCEDURE FOR SHADE MATCHING IN PORCELAIN RESTORATIONS

Before initiating shade matching, patient's position, tooth condition and lightning requirements should be proper. Any bleaching procedures, if necessary, should be performed prior to shade selection. The color selection in this section is explained using Vita shade guides, Vita VMK shade indicator chart and ring tabs. Vita shade guide system is currently a universally adopted system. Its shade indicator chart and ring tabs consist of individually fired buttons of opaque, dentin and incisal porcelains, which are about 1.0–2.0 mm in thickness. The shade guide is arranged according to four basic hues: A, B, C and D (Table 29.7). Further in each hue, there are divisions like A1, A2, A3, A3.5 and A4 which represent different chroma, and similarly so in B, C and D. Another less common arrangement in the shade guide is according to the value: B1, A1, B2, D2, C1, C2, D4, A3, D3, A3.5, B4, C3, A4 and C4.

Table 29.7: Four basic hues in the VITA shads guide

Groups	Hue
A	Brownish tones
B	Yellowish tones
C	Grey tones
D	Reddish tones

The first step is to select the hue. Since there is not much difference amongst the different hues, and to simplify the procedure, *'the four hues technique'* is used. In this, the maximum chromas of each hue, i.e. A4, B4, C4 and D4 are selected and placed at equal distances. This permits one to effectively visualise the differences in hue because chromas of maximum intensity are placed besides each other. The shade is selected in no more than five seconds to avoid fatigue of cones in the retina. Gaze at a blue card or napkin between each shade evaluation. Fatigue to blue color accentuates its complimentary color, i.e. yellow orange sensitivity, which is the dominant hue of teeth.

After the basic hue has been determined, a color that closely matches the tooth, i.e. chroma is chosen. For this, all the different chromas of the selected tab, say B, i.e. B1, B2, B3, B3.5 and B4 are placed one by one alongside the tooth to be restored. For simulating natural conditions more closely, the shade tab is covered with the patient's lips or operator's thumb to create a shadow effect. A general guideline that may assist the clinician while selecting a chroma is:

- Maxillary incisors and premolars are similar in chroma, with the central incisors being the lightest.
- Mandibualar incisors are generally one chroma lighter than the maxillary incisors.
- Maxillary Canines are at least two chroma darker than the maxillary incisors. This applies particularly to the dentin shade.

The second shade guide (arranged according to value) is used to select the value. Avoid considering the hue and chroma when choosing for a value. Squinting aids in selection as it sensitizes the more sensitive black and white rods. The value is selected and the results again evaluated by matching against the corresponding opaque shade.

At times when one experiences difficulty in chosing a hue, shades that are fractionally darker in hue are selected, since lighter hues are readily discernible in the oral cavity. After a hue has been properly selected, difficulty may also arise in matching the chroma and value. In such cases, a shade is chosen that is of a lower chroma and a higher value.

Surface Texture

The surface texture of the restoration should be so designed that it simulates the reflectance pattern of adjacent teeth. This not only creates a natural appearance but also hides slight color differences. A smooth surface reflects most of the incident light back to the observer whereas a roughened surface scatters light in many directions.

Newly erupted teeth have a rough surface texture. The vertical ridges are formed by the fusion of developmental lobes traversed by fine horizontal lines (perikymata). As the age increases, these surface features are gradually worn down by tooth brushing or occlusal wear. The tooth appears smooth with a highly reflective glossy surface. The surface characteristics should be simulated for a particular age group so as to achieve a life like restoration.

Esthetics Prescription form

The esthetics prescription form contains detailed directions from the dentist. A grid is provided below the teeth for recording the basic shade and selected shade numbers of opaque, body and incisal porcelains (Fig. 29.22). An elaborate diagram describes the location and pattern of the different characteristics like incisal translucency patterns, areas of high chroma, hypocalcified areas, craze lines and stains. If additional depth of translucency is required, it is better to mark in an overlay of transparent porcelain over the enamel. An increase in the thickness of enamel porcelain may alter the shade considerably, whereas a thin layer of overlying clear glassy porcelain will increase the depth of translucency with little alteration in the shade. The translucency of the incisal tip can be accentuated by placing translucent porcelain behind the incisal edge. 'Stain colors' can now be marked to represent areas of craze lines, hypocalcified areas, etc.

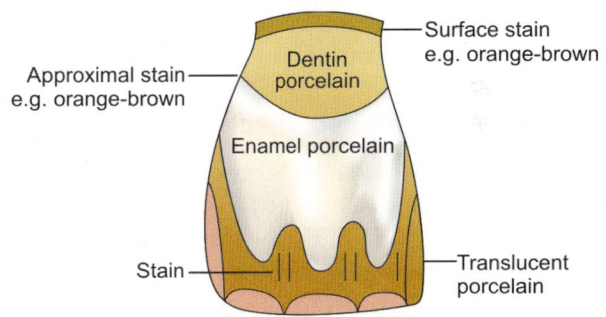

Fig. 29.22: Diagram describing the location and pattern of different characteristics like incisal translucency, craze lines and stains

Identification Tab

The identification tab is a simple method for visualising the end results. Discrepancies in the shade or patient's desires can be noted before the final try-in and hence the appropriate shade alterations made.

A tab mold using maxillary incisor is fabricated. To make the tab, a thin layer of porcelain is coated on the mold. The selected opaque, dentin and incisal porcelains are then layered in prescribed thickness. Characterizations such as deep translucency created with transparent porcelains, mamelons, craze lines and hypocalcification patterns can be incorporated into the identification tab for evaluation.

Characterization Map

When hypocalcification or translucency patterns need to be duplicated in a ceramic restoration, a means of recording their exact location is needed. The hypocalcification or translucency patterns are drawn on the contralateral tooth of the working side using Boley gauge. An alternative procedure is to paste transparent tape on the contralateral tooth and draw the desired pattern on the tape.

Staining of Porcelain

Ceramic stains used for surface modifications are usually colored metallic oxide pigments. These are similar in composition to the colorants used in opaque and body porcelains. Ceramic stains belong to the partitive system, which is a process of separating colors into very small particles and then mixing the particles.

Stains can be applied on the natural glazed porcelain or on to a surface where the glaze has been removed. When applied to an unglazed surface, the stain penetrates to a much greater depth creating a more diffused appearance. Therefore for more intense changes, glaze should be removed. For subdued changes, the stain may be applied directly over the glaze. An airbrush containing aluminium oxide powder can be used for removing the glaze. No matter to what surface the stain is applied, it should be absolutely clean and devoid of any contaminants.

Modification of Selected Shades

The shade modifications are carried out by the application of stains. Different stain kits are available with wide variations in the number and intensity of stains. First, these stain powders are mixed with just enough liquid medium to produce a heavy creamy consistency. A brush cleaned thoroughly with the medium is used to wet the surface of the restoration. Subsequently, a small increment of stain is picked up with the brush tip and applied. Any excess is removed with the brush itself. Again clean the brush off the stain and wet it with medium. Wipe the surface with the wetted brush. If too much liquid remains on the surface, the stain will puddle; and if too little then the color will not appear accurately.

The foremost rule for shade modification with stain is *moderation*. Only minor changes should be attempted. The dentist should avoid changing the basic hue as he may lose control over the selected color. Complementary hue when added reduces both the chroma and value with a minimal loss in translucency. An over addition of complement also change the basic hue.

BIBLIOGRAPHY

1. Bayindir F., Gozalo-Diaz, D., Kim-Pusateri, S and Wee, AG.: Incisal translucency of vital natural unrestored teeth : A clinical study. J Esthet Restor Dent.: 24, 335, 2012
2. Bona, A.D., Barrett, A.A., Rosa, V. and Pinzetta, C.: Visual and instrumental agreement in dental shade selection: Three distinct observer populations and shade matching protocols. Dental Materials: 25, 276, 2009.
3. Brewer, J.D. and Wee, A.S.: Advances in color matching. Dent. Clin. North Am.: 48, 341, 2004.
4. Burkinshaw, S.M.: Color in relation to dentistry. Fundamentals of color science. British Dent. J.: 33, 196, 2004.
5. Cal, E., Guneri, P. and Kose, T.: Comparison of digital and spectrophotometric measurements of color shade guides. J. Oral Rehabil.: 33, 221, 29006.
6. Cal, E., Sonugelen, M., Guneri, P., Kesercioglu, A. and Kose, T.: Application of a digital technique in evaluating the reliability of shade guides. J. Oral Rehabil.: 31, 483, 2004.
7. Denissen, H. and Dozie, A.: Photometric assessment of tooth color using commonly available software. Eur. J. Esthet. Dent.: 5, 204, 2010.
8. Dozic, A.: Relation in color of three regions of vital human incisors. Dent. Mater.: 10, 1016, 2004.
9. Dozic, A., Kleverlaan, J., Aartman, I.H.A. and Feilzer, A.J.: Relation in color among maxillary incisors and canines. Dent. Mater.: 21, 187, 2005.
10. Egger, B.: Natural color concept: A systematic approach to visual shade selection. QDT: 26, 161, 2003.
11. Fondriest, J.: Shade matching in restorative dentistry: The science and strategies. Int. J. Periodont. Restorative Dent.: 23, 467, 2003.
12. Hindle, J.P. and Harrison, A.: Tooth color analysis by a new opto-electronic system. Eur. J. Prosth. Rest. Dent.: 8, 57, 2000.
13. Joiner, A.: Tooth color: a review of the literature. J. Dent.: 32, 3, 2004.
14. Lee, Y.K., Lu, Huan, Powers, J.M.: Measurement of opalescence of resin composites. Dent. Mater.: 21, 1068, 2005.
15. Mayekar, S.: Shades of a color: illusion or reality ? D.C.N.A.: 45, 155, 2001.
16. Mc Cullock, A.J. and Mc Cullock, R.M.: Communicating shades: A clinical and technical perspective. Dent. Update: 26, 247, 1999.
17. McLaren, E.A.: Provisionalization and the 3D communication of shade and shape. Contemp. Esthet. Restorative Pract.: 5, 48, 2000.
18. Moser, J.B., Wozniak, T.P. and Moore, B.K.: Use of Munsell system to complete color differences in composite resins. J. Dent. Res.: 57, 958, 1978.
19. Odiara, C., Itoh, S. and Ishibashi, K.: Clinical evaluation of a dental color analysis system: The Crystaleye Spectrophotometer. J Prosth Research.: 55, 199, 2011
20. Park, J.H., Lee, Y.K. and Lim, B.S.: Influence of illuminants on the color distribution of shade guide. J. Prosthet Dent.: 96, 402, 2006.

21. Pensler, A.V.: Shade selection: Problems and solutions. Compend. Contin. Educ. Dent.: 19, 387, 1998.
22. Pizzamiglio, E.: A color selection technique. J.P.D.: 66, 592, 1991.
23. Reno, E.A., Sunberg, R.J., Black, R.P. and Bush, R.D.: The influence of lip/gum color on subject perception of tooth color. J.D.R.: 79, 381, 2000.
24. Russell, M.D., Gulfraz, M. and Moss, B.W.: In vivo measurement of color changes in natural teeth. J. Oral Rehab.: 27, 786, 2000.
25. Sproull, R.C.: Color matching in dentistry-Part I. The three dimensional nature of color. J.P.D.: 86, 453, 2001.
26. Stephen J.: Precision shade technology; contemporary strategies in shade selection. Prac Proced Aesthet. Dent.: 14, 79, 2002.
27. Yuan, J.C.C., Brewer, J.D., Monaco, E.D. and Davis, E.L.: Defining a natural tooth color space based on a 3-dimensional shade system. J. Prosthet. Dent.: 98, 110, 2007.

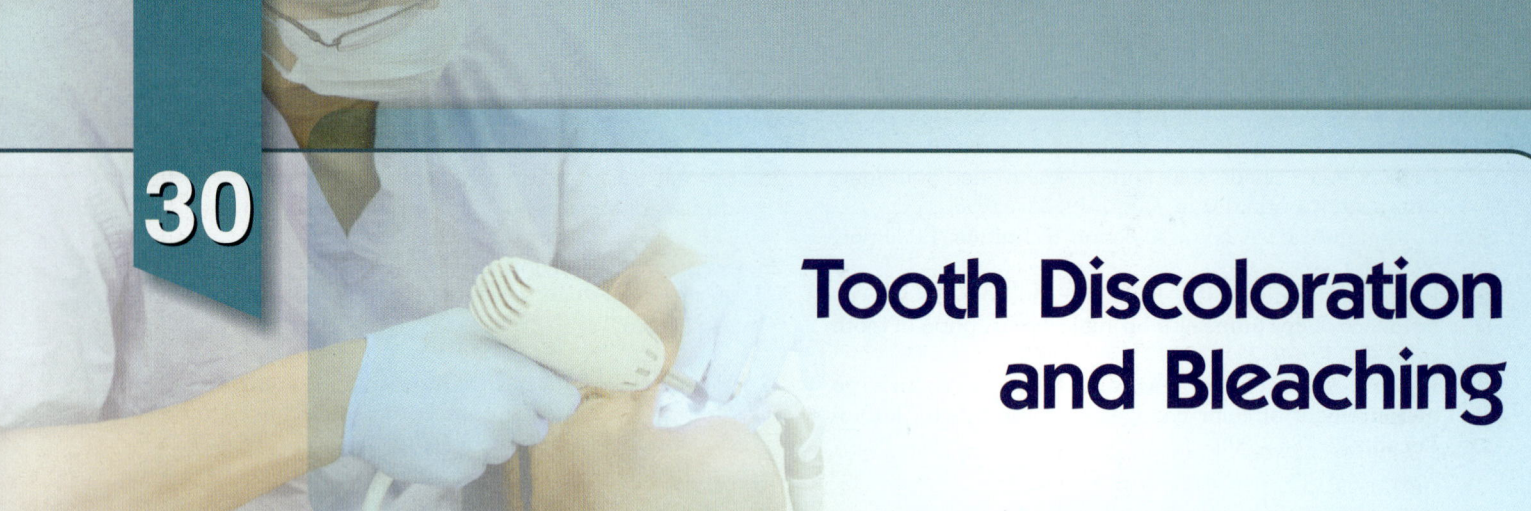

30

Tooth Discoloration and Bleaching

Esthetics is the science of beauty. Esthetic dentistry not only relates to disfigured teeth but also involves the needs of a normal appearing individual who wishes to look younger, healthier and confident. The perception and description of color in a given object, coupled with need and desire of the people forms the basis of esthetics. One of the most frequent reasons warranting dental care is discolored anterior teeth. The increasing public interest coupled with better technical ability of the dentists, has paved the way for improving the esthetics by lightening the stained teeth. The lightening of stained teeth without disturbing the biological tissues and the periodontal environment is the goal, which is being achieved successfully.

The lightening of the color of a tooth through the application of a chemical agent to oxidize the organic pigmentation in the tooth is referred to as 'Bleaching'. American Dental Association defined bleaching as 'the treatment, usually involving an oxidative chemical that alters the light absorbing and/or light reflecting nature of the material structure, thereby increasing its value (whiteness)'.

Bleaching or tooth whitening dates back to 18th century when chloride of lime was used as bleaching agent. Different authors, over the years, tried various materials and techniques to aid in bleaching. In early nineteenth century, hydrogen peroxide alone and in combination with other materials, was used as bleaching agent. Recently, LASERS have also been tried.

TOOTH DISCOLORATION AND STAINING

Various factors are responsible for tooth discoloration and staining. A thorough knowledge of the etiology of tooth staining is essential in order to make a correct diagnosis. The factors and extent of discoloration influence the treatment options and also determine the prognosis. The vital and non-vital aspects of the tooth also affect the treatment options.

Classification of Tooth Discoloration

The tooth discoloration is broadly divided into intrinsic and extrinsic stains.

A. Intrinsic Discoloration

a. Enamel hypoplasia: Enamel hypoplasia may occur because of local and/or general factors:

Local factors
  i. Trauma
  ii. Infection

General factors
  i. Hereditary and idiopathic hypoplasia, Amelogenesis imperfecta
  ii. General diseases of genetic or idiopathic origin–Epidermolysis bullosa, Cleidocranial dysostosis, Osteogenesis imperfecta, Osteopetrosis, Morquio's disease, etc.
  iii. Prenatal or congenital syphilis
  iv. Trophic disturbances like infantile tetany, rickets, vitamin C deficiency, etc.
  v. Endemic fluorosis

b. *Fluorosis:* It has been established that high concentration of fluorides (more than 4 ppm) causes moderate to severe discoloration. The incisors are more prevalent followed by premolars and molars. Fluorosis is further categorized as mild, moderate and severe. Mild fluorosis exhibits brown pigmentation on a smooth surface, moderate shows flecks on the enamel surface along with staining whereas severe shows pigmentation with pitted enamel surfaces. The severe form of fluorosis does not respond to bleaching.

c. *Tetracycline staining*: Tetracyclines are widely used for the treatment of various infections. Discoloration due to tetracycline ingestion was reported in early 50's and later confirmed by various authors. It was also established that the dose of tetracycline was more important than the duration. The different varieties of tetracyclines produce yellow to yellowish brown stains, which fluoresce under ultraviolet light. However doxycyclines do not produce any stain.

d. **Pulpal haemorrhagic products:** Pulpal haemorrhage and disintegration products like iron sulphide enter dentinal tubules and cause discoloration.
e. **Ageing:** As age increases, changes take place in enamel and dentin which lead to eventual discoloration of the teeth.
f. **Trauma:** Trauma leads to pulpal hameorrhage which causes greyish discoloration of the teeth. It may cause obliteration of the pulp canal which leads to dark yellow discoloration of the teeth.
g. **Amelogenesis imperfecta:** It presents with abnormal formation of enamel. It is of three types.
   i. Hypoplastic Type
   ii. Hypomineralization
   iii. Hypomaturation Type
h. **Dentinogenesis Imperfecta:** Colour of teeth varies from grey to brownish violet to yellowish brown with a characteristic usual translucent or opalescent hue. It is an autosomal dominant developmental disturbance of the dentin.
i. **Dentin dysplasia:** It is a rare disturbance of dentin formation characterized by atypical dentin formation. It may lead to slight amber translucency of teeth.
j. **Congenital Hyperbilirubinemia:** It is a condition where there is a high level of bilirubin in the blood. It causes yellow green discoloration of the teeth.
k. **Congenital erythropoietic porphyria:** It is a rare inborn error of porphyrin-heme synthesis, inherited as an autosomal recessive trait. It leads to red brown/purplish red discoloration of the teeth.
l. **Alkaptonuria:** It is a rare, inherited genetic disorder of phenylalanine and tyrosine metabolism. It gives brown discoloration to the teeth.

B. Extrinsic Discoloration

Various authors have classified extrinsic discoloration depending upon different criteria:

a. *Classification according to the cause*
   - Direct staining mainly with chromogenic microorganisms derived from dietary sources, though other factors are also responsible.
   - Indirect staining is associated with cationic antiseptics and metal salts.

b. *Classification given by Nathoo*
   - Type 1 (N1): Chromogens bind to tooth surface and cause discoloration. The color of the chromogen is similar to that of dental stains caused by tea, coffee, wine and other chromogenic bacteria.
   - Type 2 (N2): Chromogen changes color after binding up to teeth. The stain darkens with time.
   - Type 3 (N3): Prechromogen (colorless material) binds to tooth and undergoes chemical reaction to cause the staining.

c. *Non-metallic Stains*
   - Tea, coffee, blackcurrant juice, cola drinks, etc.
   - Due to chemicals like chlorhexidine.

d. *Metallic Stains*
   - Black staining seen in people using iron supplement and in iron foundry workers.
   - Copper causes green stain in mouth after rinsing with copper salts.
   - Potassium permanganate produces violet to black color.
   - Silver nitrate salt causes grey discoloration.
   - Stannous fluoride causes golden brown discoloration.

C. Internalized Discoloration

It occurs due to incorporation of extrinsic stains within the tooth substance following some dental pathology. It occurs in enamel defects and in the porous surface of exposed dentin such as developmental defects like fluorosis, hypoplasia, enamel hypocalcification. These types of defects can also be seen in tooth wear, gingival recession and caries, etc.

BLEACHING OF TEETH

Bleaching is believed to be linked to the degradation of high molecular weight and complex organic molecules that reflect a specific wavelength of light, which is responsible for the color of the stain. The resulting degradation products are of lower molecular weight that reflect less light, resulting in reduction or elimination of discoloration.

Average life of a bleaching regimen ranges from 1–3 years. The bleaching modalities are further divided into vital and non-vital tooth bleaching.

I. Vital Tooth Bleaching

a. In-office bleaching
   i. Thermocatalytic vital tooth bleaching
   ii. Power bleaching
   iii. Non-thermocatalytic vital tooth bleaching
   iv. Microabrasion assisted bleaching

b. Dentist prescribed home bleaching (Night guard vital bleaching)

II. Non-vital Tooth Bleaching

a. Thermocatalytic in office technique
b. Walking bleach technique
c. Modified walking bleach technique
d. Combination technique

III. Laser Assisted Bleaching

IV. Over the counter products

I. VITAL TOOTH BLEACHING

Vital bleaching technique requires use of materials that do not endanger the tooth structure and the soft tissue.

Bleaching Agents for Vital Bleaching

1. Hydrogen Peroxide (30–35%): It is a strong oxidizing agent. Ionization of H_2O_2 produces different type of free radicals, such as Hydroxyl ions (OH^-) and Perhydroxyl ions (OOH^-)
2. Hydrochloric acid (18%–36%): The hydrochloric acid causes decalcification of tooth substance along with removal of stain.
3. Other bleaching agents: for example, Fuji Hilite dual cure material (it is green-blue in color and on activation loses oxygen and color of particle changes to white). It can be used in office or at home.

Methods of Vital Bleaching

The two basic methods of vital bleaching are:
a. In office bleaching
   i. Thermocatalytic
   ii. Power bleaching
   iii. Non-Thermocatalytic
   iv. Microabrasion assisted
b. Dentist prescribed bleaching (Night guard bleaching)

a. In-office Bleaching

Indications

i. Superficial extrinsic color discrepancies
ii. Extrinsic and Intrinsic stains of moderately darkened and moderate intense color characteristics
iii. General yellow to brown discoloration

Contraindications

i. Severe discoloration from amalgam corrosion
ii. Tetracycline stains
iii. Extensive restorations or caries
iv. Inherent sensitivity of the patient to bleaching agents

Advantages

i. Treatment is totally under dentist's control.
ii. Potential for early results.
iii. Soft tissue is generally protected from the process.

Disadvantages

i. Cost factor.
ii. Unknown duration of the treatment.
iii. Discomfort of rubber dam.
iv. Potential for soft tissue damage to patient and operator.
v. Adverse effects of thermocatalytic temperature rise on the pulp.
vi. Resultant post treatment sensitivity.
vii. If etching is performed with bleaching, polishing is required after each visit resulting in small amount of enamel loss.

Preparation of the Patient for Bleaching

- Shade of the patient's existing dentition is recorded with a standardized shade guide tab and a photograph of patient's teeth is taken for records.
- Thorough Prophylaxis is performed.
- The patient is draped with a protective cape and is made to wear protective eye glasses.
- No local anaesthesia is administered.
- Teeth are isolated with heavy gauge rubber dam.
- Before rubber dam application, oraseal (a light cured resin) or orabase paste is applied to protect the labial and lingual tissue.
- Oraseal can also be applied to amalgam restorations reducing the risk of build up of heat from the light source.
- Vaseline is applied to the patient's lips before mounting the rubber dam frame.
- Wet gauze is placed over the patient's lips to prevent thermal trauma.

i. Thermocatalytic Bleaching

The thermocatalytic bleaching involves the use of heat alone or heat and light both. The units are;

1. *Heat light unit:* The bleaching light provides high intensity light and heat, needed to activate bleaching agents. A narrow beam of light is concentrated in one section of the mouth at a distance of approximately 13–15 inches. Calibrated rheostat controls the amount of light and heat.
2. *Heat unit:* Heat unit with accurate temperature control and continuous read out is used to activate the bleaching agent. Two tips are available – one

to fit the contour of labial surface of a non-vital tooth and one is inserted in the coronal access opening. Temperature recommended is:
  i. Non-vital teeth – 60°C to 70°C
  ii. Vital teeth – 46°C to 60°C

Do not exceed 30 minutes of treatment in each appointment. After removing the heat source, tooth is allowed to cool to avoid sudden temperature change that can be deleterious to the pulp. After five minutes tooth is washed with warm water for one minute. Bleaching appointments are scheduled 2–4 weeks apart. A minimum of three treatments is required. However, not more than ten treatments are recommended. Color is checked one week after the third treatment.

The source of heat can be:
  i. Photoflood lamp
  ii. Polymerization light
  iii. Spirit lamp
  iv. Commercial bleaching units
  v. Light-heat lamp
  vi. Lasers (Argon and Diode)

Some of the commercial preparation systems utilizing different activating light sources are:

1. *Quartz tungsten halogen curing light:* The standard curing light provides heat to simulate the chemical reaction by activating light sensitive chemicals in the bleaching agent. Each application is used for 40–60 seconds.
2. *Plasma arc:* It provides intensity of light similar to or slightly higher than halogen curing temperature. An application of four seconds leads to an intrapulpal temperature rise of 2.2°C. Maximum allowable time of application is 30 seconds per tooth.
3. *Rembrandt tooth whitening system:* This system includes the use of a plasma arc light (named **Rembrandt Sapphire**). This bleaching can be fitted with a **Rembrandt Whitening Crystal** so as to enable the dentist to treat both the arches simultaneously. The wavelength of light emitted from this source is in the range of 400–525 nm (blue green coloration).
4. *Beyond whitening accelerator:* This system uses high intensity blue light at a wavelength of 480–520 nm. The light is filtered to remove infrared and ultraviolet light. It is used with special whitening formula, the half hour procedure rapidly oxidizes 16 or more teeth. It leads to substantial improvement.
5. *The Zoom! Teeth whitening system:* This system includes the use of mercury metal halide light with a wavelength of 300–450 nm (violet coloration). The Zoom! Light unit has an infrared filter, which filters these radiations, thereby minimizing the amount of heat generated at the surface of tooth during the whitening treatment.

Technique (Figs 30.1A, B and C)

- Using an eye dropper, a small amount of the bleaching solution (30–35% H_2O_2) is placed into a dappen dish.
- The teeth are properly isolated preferably with rubber dam.

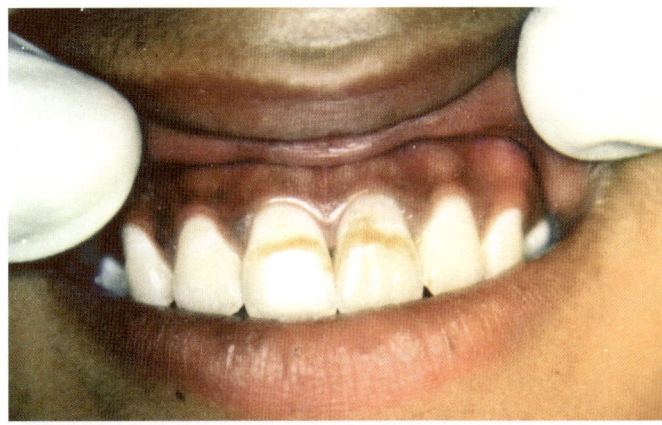

(A) Pre-operative

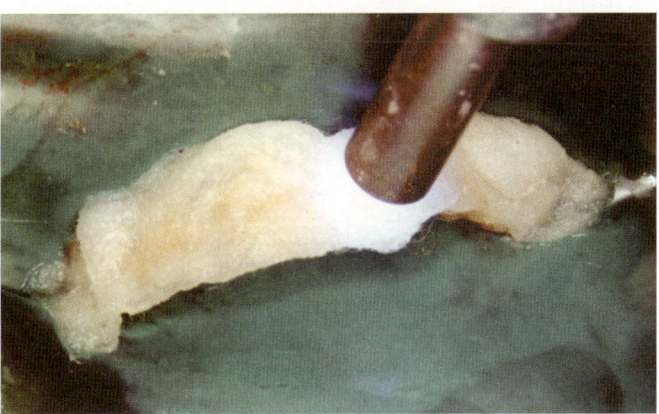

(B) Application of bleaching agent

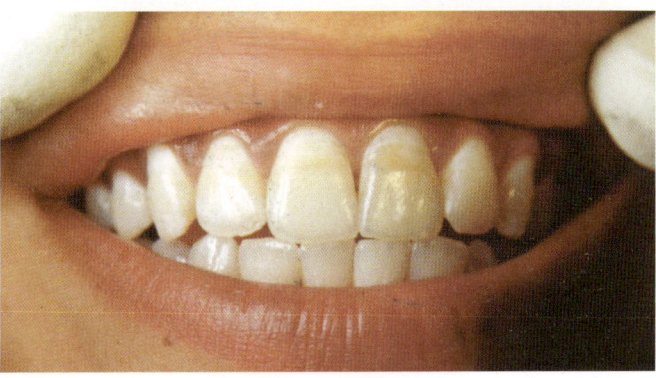

(C) Post-operative

Figs 30.1A, B and C: Vital bleaching (Thermocatalytic bleaching technique)

- The cotton or gauze piece, held in cotton pliers is dipped into the dish and the saturated bleaching solution is carried and placed onto the tooth surface.
- With a small plastic instrument, the cotton or gauze is pressed and shaped to cover the entire surface.
- The selected heating unit is positioned.
- When the photo lamp is used, the solution is applied every 4 to 5 minutes.
- When the heat unit is used, the solution is applied after every heating cycle.
- After removing the gauze/cotton, the teeth and the entire rubber dam are washed with warm water and a high volume vacuum aspirator.
- The floss is removed either by slipping the explorer under each knot or can be cut with scalpel and removed slowly with cotton pliers.
- The rubber dam is stretched apically and labially to gain access to the inter-proximal areas. The clamps are removed and the rubber dam sheet is gently teased off from the teeth.
- Wet, warm gauze squares are used to remove the excess orabase/oraseal.
- The solution residues on teeth are neutralized with a mild warm solution of ½ teaspoon salt, ½ cup warm water and ½ teaspoon sodium bicarbonate.
- Instruct the patient to avoid coffee, tea and cola drinks for two weeks.

ii. Power Bleaching

In this technique, high intensity light, which was used as a heat source, is replaced with conventional halogen units, plasma arc lamps, LED lights, Xe-halogen lights and Lasers. There are specific situations, such as single tooth bleaching within an arch, or even small areas on teeth that need to be lightened.

Advantages
- The time factor; produces immediate results.
- Avoiding problems with home bleaching procedures such as:
  a. Wearing trays that cause patients to gag.
  b. Distaste for home bleaching gel.

Disadvantages
- The caustic nature of the 30–35% H_2O_2 makes isolation and protection mandatory.
- Expensive
- Dehydration of teeth may occur, thereby, giving a falsely lighter shade immediately post-treatment.

iii. Non-Thermocatalytic Bleaching

The non-thermocatalytic technique does not utilize heat sources.

The different solutions used are:
i. Superoxol (5 parts of H_2O_2 + 1 part of ether)
ii. McInnes Solution: 5 parts of 36% HCl (increases the penetration of solution) + 5 parts 30% H_2O_2 (bleaches the enamel by process of oxidation) + 1 part of 0.2% anaesthetic ether (removes the surface debris)).
iii. Modified McInnes bleaching solution consisting of 30% H_2O_2 and 20% NaOH in 1:1 ratio along with 0.2% ether has been introduced to overcome the deleterious effects of hydrochloric acid.
iv. Self activating bleaching agent for vital teeth

The bleaching agent as prepared by Matsuba (1996) contains 35% H_2O_2 0.4 ml, CaO 0.12 gms, Aerosil 0.32, 0.48 or 0.64 gm (to alter/control the viscosity)

Technique (Figs 30.2A to E)

After rubber dam application, paste is applied on the teeth for five minutes and reapplication is done as required followed by copious irrigation of warm water and polishing.

iv. Microabrasion Assisted Bleaching

Microabrasion is a procedure involving the surface dissolution of the stains of enamel by an acid (preferably 18% HCl) along with abrasives (preferably pumice powder). Microabrasion is indicated for improvement of particular tooth color. This is also used in cases where routine bleaching is not effective.

Advantages
- It helps to remove superficial stains and discoloration.
- The result is achieved with minimal patient discomfort and operator difficulty.
- The treated teeth display a smooth texture and shine.

Disadvantages
- Microabrasion removes enamel layer.
- Only effective on those stains confined to outer layer of enamel, i.e. not effective for deeper stains
- Since it removes enamel layer, teeth sometimes appear more yellow after treatment.

b. Dentist Prescribed Bleaching (Night Guard Vital Bleaching)

Night guard bleaching was introduced in the late 60's. The earlier authors used 10% carbamide peroxide, delivered in a custom fitting mouth tray. The patient is asked to keep the tray along with the medicament over the teeth during night time (Fig. 30.3).

Tooth Discoloration and Bleaching

Indications

- Persons dissatisfied with the original color of their otherwise sound teeth.
- For brown fluorosis stains.
- For discolored teeth that have darkened from trauma but are still vital or have a poor endodontic prognosis.
- As retreatment of walking bleach after reversal of the treatment.
- For discolored teeth even though considered for the placement of porcelain or other esthetic veneer.
- For teeth affected with dentinogenesis imperfecta.
- To lighten natural teeth to match existing ceramic crowns, fixed partial dentures, etc.

Advantages

- Patience convenience
- Cost effective

Disadvantages

- Patient compliance is mandatory
- Difficult for dentist to monitor the amount of time the trays are used as well as the color change.

Bleaching agent used is carbamide peroxide in different concentrations. As the solution is flown onto the tooth surface, carbamide peroxide being unstable dissociates into water, urea and/or oxygen. The carbamide peroxide dissociates into H_2O_2 and urea, in different concentrations depending upon the concentration of the carbamide peroxide. The H_2O_2 further dissociates into water and oxygen. The oxygen

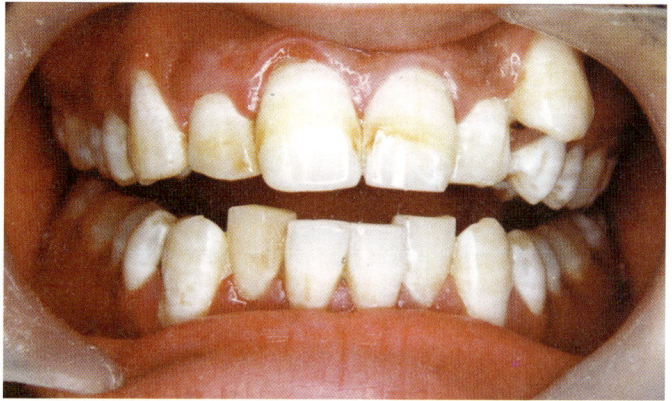

(A) Pre-operative

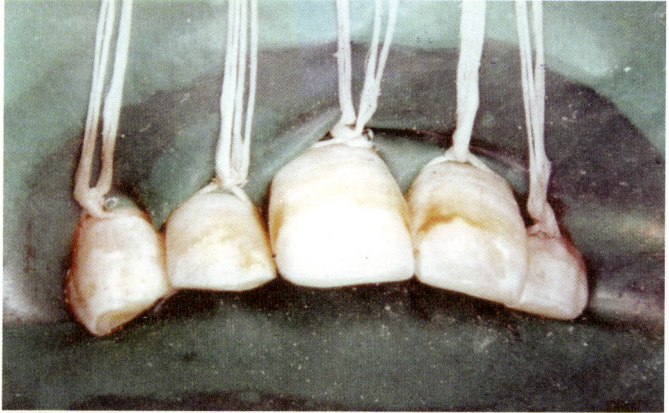

(B) Rubber dam application

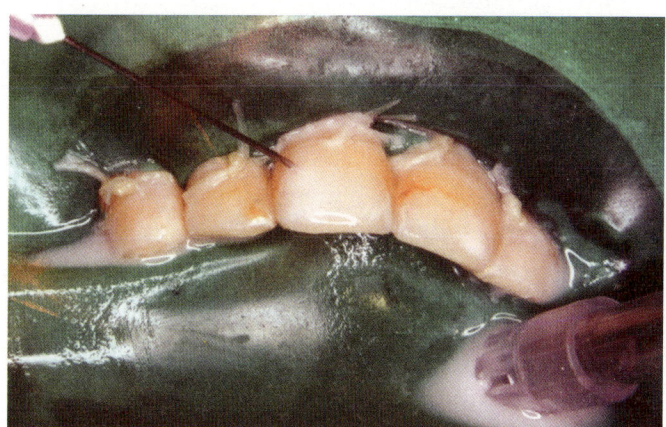

(D) Irrigation

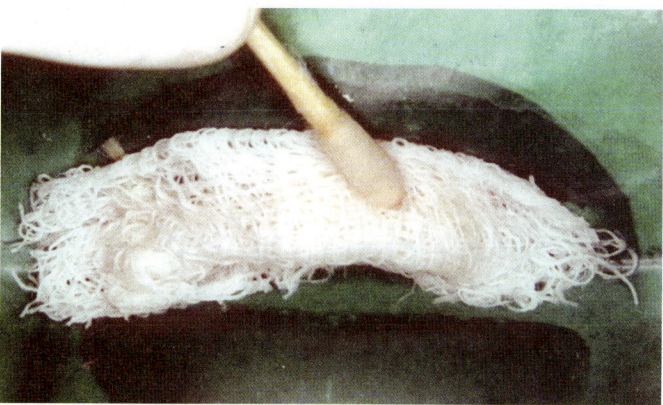

(C) Application of bleaching agent

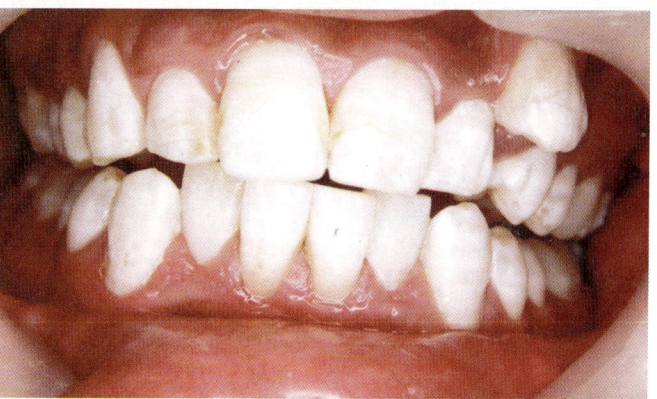

(E) Post-operative

Figs 30.2A to E: Vital bleaching (Non-thermocatalytic bleaching technique)

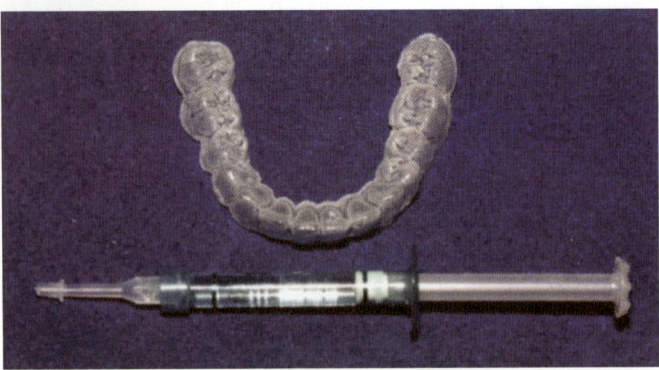

Fig. 30.3: Tray and syringe

radicals cause oxidation of pigmentation in the tooth. The urea degrades into ammonia and carbon dioxide. An agent, carbopol is added to prolong the release of oxygen, counter carbon dioxide released by urea and improve tissue adherence.

Commercial Preparations

- 10% carbamide peroxide with carbopol (Proxigel, ultralite, etc.)
- 10% carbamide peroxide without carbopol (fast oxygen releasing, e.g. Glyoxide, Dentalite, etc.)
- 15% carbamide peroxide, e.g. Nu smile.
- 1.0%–10% H_2O_2 (Peroxyl, Brite smile, etc.)

Technique

There are three basic regimens for the application of the whitening solutions.

i. Sleeping with the night guard tray filled with the bleaching solution and the solution is changed each night.
ii. Wearing the loaded night guard tray during the day while changing the solution every 1.5–2 hours.
iii. Polyethylene strips impregnated with 5.25% of H_2O_2 is also used without tray.

The night guard vital bleaching procedures usually require three appointments.

First Appointment

The initial shade examination and evaluation of the adjacent structures is carried out before the treatment. Then the cast is formed after taking impressions with suitable materials and the tray material is selected. Usually 0.040 inch or 0.035 inch ethyl vinyl acetate is used for fabricating the tray, however 0.020 inch polypropylene has also been used.

After selection of the tray material, the cast is placed on the suction grid. The tray material is placed in the retainer frame on the vacuum forming unit. When the tray material (53" × 53" sheet) is sufficiently softened by heating it and sags approximately one inch, the heated sheet is pulled down and adapted slowly and gently.

The tray material is allowed to cool on the casts. The night guard is trimmed by scalloping the tray in a smooth curve until only about 2.0 mm of tissue apical to gingival crest is covered facially and lingually.

Variations in Tray Fabrication

i. Round bur no. ½ is used to cut groove along the gingival tooth margin on the cast.
ii. A gel trench is built into the tray by stretching a rectangular rubber band (2 mm × 2 mm) around the crest, centered on the clinical crowns of the teeth. This trench functions as blocked out reservoir.
iii. Night guard is also prepared using reservoir space
   - The reservoirs are created using a viscous light cure composite gel.
   - The viscous composite spacer gel is applied to the selected teeth on the cast.
   - Only the facial surface of the teeth is painted 1.0 mm from the gingival margin with a thickness of 0.5 mm.
   - The spacer gel is not allowed to flow onto the incisal edge or occlusal surface.
   - A light curing oven or the clinical light curing wand can be used for curing the spacer.
   - The surface is washed or the oxygen inhibited resin layer is wiped away from the spacer.
   - Tray material is selected and night guard constructed in a vacuum forming machine.
   - The space of spacer gel in the bleaching trays forms the reservoir.

Advantages of reservoir
- Provides space for the bleaching agent. - Allows seating of tray when more viscous solution is used. - Minimizes tooth sensitivity by avoiding the pinching effect of a light tray. - Allows the transfer of bleaching gel in area of higher concentration.

Disadvantages
- Increased cost of fabrication and time. - Decreased tray retention. - Gel leakage and irritation of gingiva.

The tray also is formed using foam liners, which are placed on the selected area of the cast. The trays are then prepared in a vacuum forming machine.

Advantages of foam liner
• Soft on patients' gingival tissues • 50% reduction in bleaching time

Disadvantages
• Aesthetically less pleasing • Occlusal discrepancies are common • Does not help in retention

Second Appointment

The second appointment involves inserting and fitting the night guard. The bleaching material is applied into the night guard as follows:

- Two to three drops of bleaching material is placed into the area of each tooth to be bleached.
- After inserting the night guard, the excess material is wiped out.
- Patient is instructed not to drink or rinse during treatment.
- The bleaching solution is replaced every one and half to two hours during daytime regimen.
- A single application of bleaching material at bedtime is indicated, if worn at night.
- The daytime regimen requires one to three weeks and four to six weeks are required for night time bleaching.

Third Appointment

This appointment includes postoperative photographs, patient's satisfaction and consent, a decision whether future bleaching or restorative treatment is required (Figs 30.4A, B).

Side Effects of Vital Bleaching

a. *Sensitivity*: The most common side effect associated with vital bleaching is a transient or prolonged sensitivity. It has been established that the bleaching procedure increases intrapulpal temperature, which is detrimental to pulp. The heat when applied to H_2O_2 can lead to diffusion of H_2O_2 into the pulp. However inflammatory changes get recovered within one month.

In-office bleaching procedures with high concentrations of hydrogen peroxide were associated with high sensitivity; however, night guard bleaching with lower concentration of hydrogen peroxide (3.0%) or carbamide peroxide (10%) has resulted in decreased sensitivity.

The pH of the solution and dessication of the tooth surface are the factors aiding in sensitivity. Introduction of potassium nitrate and sodium fluoride added to 10% carbamide peroxide have been found to considerably reduce sensitivity without any significant change in bleaching results.

b. Hydrogen peroxide and hydrochloric acid can result in removal of the surface enamel. Alterations in the enamel structure can affect adhesion of composites and glass-ionomer cement to the tooth surface. This problem is prevalent immediately after bleaching.
c. Caries progression
d. Minor ulceration of the gingival tissues. It may lead to pharyngitis, etc.

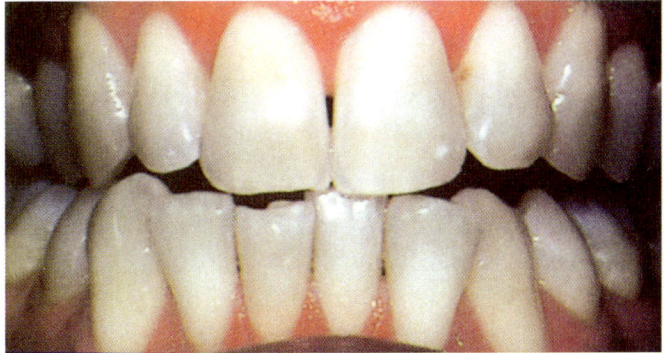

(A) Pre-operative

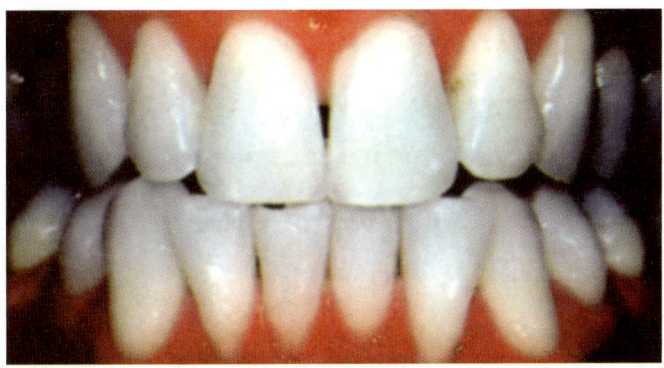

(B) Post-operative

Figs 30.4A and B: Night guard vital bleaching

II. NON-VITAL TOOTH BLEACHING

The non-vital bleaching involves bleaching of nonvital teeth, which are discolored because of pulpal necrosis and related complications. Many a times, to achieve better results in deeply stained teeth (tetracycline stains), intentional root canal treatment is done so as to bleach the tooth from both inside and outside. Calcified root canals without any root canal treatment are also candidates for non-vital bleaching. However, this modality is contraindicated in teeth, which are discolored due to corrosion products and/or large restorations. The commonly used solutions are:

- Hydrogen peroxide
  - Superoxol (30% H_2O_2)
  - Pyrozone (25% H_2O_2 and ether)

- Sodium perborate
- Sodium percarbonate

Preparation of the Tooth

- The restoration, if any, is removed from the coronal opening and from within the pulp chamber.
- Approximately 2.0–3.0 mm of root canal restorative material is also removed in an apical direction beyond cemento-enamel junction.
- The tooth is washed with 3% H_2O_2 solution, rinsed with water and dried.
- 0.5–1.0 mm thick calcium hydroxide plug is sealed in direct contact with the root obturation material.
- The rest of the root canal is filled with dual cure glass-ionomer cement.
- The pulp chamber is then cleaned and superficial dentin, if present, is removed.

a. Thermocatalytic Technique (Figs 30.5A to D)

- Cotton pellet is placed against labial aspect of the tooth.
- The bleaching agent, either superoxol and sodium perborate separately or a combination of both is introduced.
- The solution is heated with a bleaching wand at low to medium setting. A dry endodontic spreader or heated spatula can also be used. Light heating units are also employed.
- The process is repeated as required with the total treatment time per appointment ranging from not more than 20–30 minutes along with remoistening of the cotton pellets at regular intervals.
- The tooth is rinsed with water. A fresh, dry cotton pellet is placed in the pulp chamber and sealed with temporary sealing agent.
- The patient is recalled after one to three weeks.
- The final restoration of the cavity is carried out preferably with composite resin of the shade esthetically compatible with the tooth. It is recommended that acetone based adhesive systems be used because these have been shown to reverse the adverse effects of bleaching on enamel bond strengths.

Variations of the Thermocatalytic Technique

i. A mixture of one part 95% ethyl alcohol and two parts chloroform is used to desiccate all the exposed enamel and dentin for two minutes. This is followed by placement of cotton pellet saturated with pyrozone in the access cavity and on the labial and lingual surfaces of the teeth. A thermocatalytic source, (a photoflood lamp) is used for about 20 minutes. After this a dressing of 30% H_2O_2 is placed

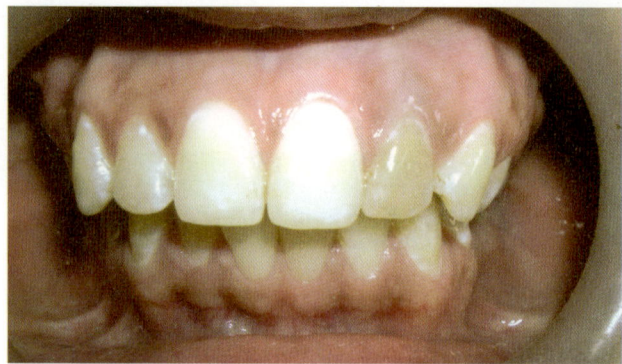

(A) Pre-operative

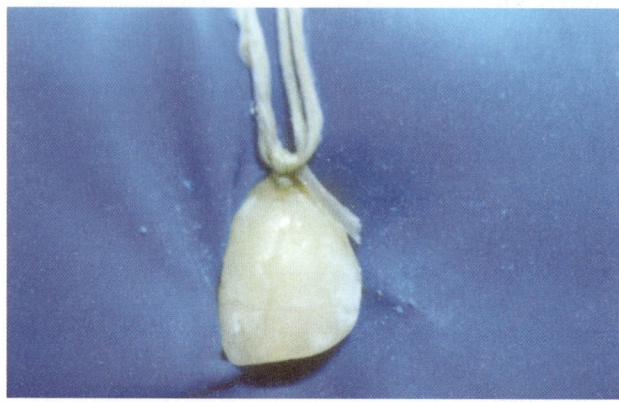

(B) Rubber dam application

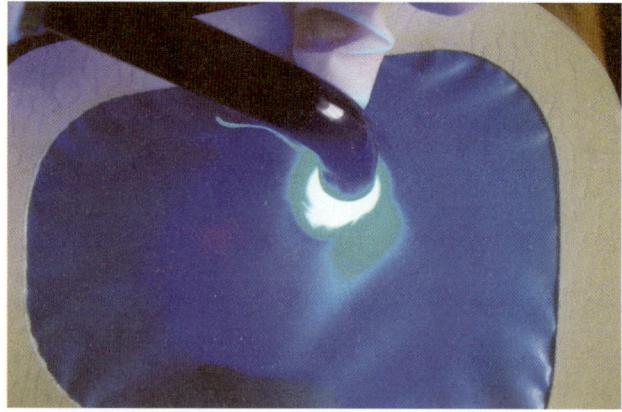

(C) Application of heat

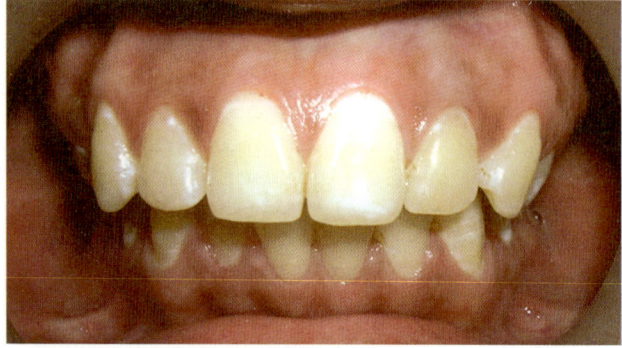

(D) Post-operative

Figs 30.5A to D: Non-vital bleaching (Thermocatalytic bleaching technique) in pulp chamber and sealed with zinc phosphate cement. This technique of thermo-catalytic bleaching was modified by different authors using different combination of materials.

ii. A soldering iron coupled to a rheostat, encased in a metal case whose temperature can be regulated by adjusting the voltage has also been used. The bleaching solution used is four part 30% H_2O_2 and one part ethyl ether.

iii. The dentinal tubules are dehydrated with 90% ethyl alcohol. After this a vulcanite rubber cone is pressed for 1–2 minutes over the cotton saturated with superoxol or pyrozone into the pulp chamber. The bleaching agent is activated with a light source (lamp) for a period of 30–40 minutes.

iv. A mixture of 95% ethyl alcohol and chloroform (3:1) is used for dehydrating the dentin and enamel. A 30% H_2O_2 saturated cotton pellet is placed into the access cavity. This bleaching agent is activated with ultraviolet light for two minutes. After the desirable results, the cavity is filled with guttapercha within 1.5 mm of its margins followed by composite resin.

v. A combination of 35% H_2O_2, manganese sulphate as photo activator, and iron sulphate as the chemical activator has also been used.

b. Walking Bleach technique

It employs a bleaching regimen, which involves placement of the bleaching agents in the pulp chamber over an extended period of time ranging from 24–48 hours to 7–10 days. The pulp chamber is sealed with temporary materials. The commonly employed agents are superoxol, sodium perborate and their combinations.

Technique

- A thick paste of sodium perborate and 35% H_2O_2 is applied into the pulp chamber.
- The lingual access is sealed with a material capable of providing a good marginal seal. It should also create pressure as pressure in the pulp chamber is required for bleaching. The commonly used sealing agents are fast setting zinc oxide eugenol, zinc phosphate cement, glass-ionomer cement, etc.

c. Modified Walking Bleach Technique

i. Aldecoa and Mayordomo (1992) described a modified technique for severe tetracycline discoloration. After a desired result is obtained by walking bleach technique, a mixture of 10% carbamide peroxide and sodium perborate is placed in the pulp chamber for 4 to 6 weeks.

ii. Liebenberg (1997) introduced a modified technique that relies on patient's cooperation. He administered intracoronal 10% carbamide peroxide gel in a splint constructed from 0.0203" poly-propylene coping material. The splint is used to retain the bleaching agent and to prevent ingress of debris into the access cavity.

d. Combination Bleaching Technique

This technique involves the combined use of thermocatalytic in office non-vital bleaching technique followed by walking bleach regimen using a mixture of sodium perborate and superoxol. It provides synergistic effect and is effective in 90% of cases (Figs 30.6A to G).

Side Effects of Non-vital Bleaching

The non-vital bleaching procedure adversely affects the marginal seal leading to marginal leakage.

Another commonly seen complication of such type of bleaching is cervical resorption. The incidence of cervical root resorption after non-vital bleaching ranges from 0 to 7%. This is more commonly seen in teeth which become pulpless at a young age and when no barrier is placed between endodontic filling material and pulp chamber during bleaching. In such cases, the dentinal tubules remain patent and communicate with periodontal space through the defects of cemento-enamel junction. This allows the bleach solution to reach the periodontal ligament from root canal system and an inflammatory reaction can be initiated, resulting in external cervical root resorption.

The features affecting the root resorption are:

- 10% of anterior teeth have cervical areas in which enamel and cementum do not meet.
- Cervical resorption is observed coronal to the endodontic seal.

The critical region is the proximal area where the cemento-enamel junction dips and cervical root resorption begins. Location, shape and material of a bleach barrier between endodontic filling material and the pulp chamber can effectively curtail this problem.

The barrier transfer technique involves three areas of periodontal probing, i.e. *labial*, *mesial* and distal aspects. The probing is carried out from the epithelial attachment of the tooth with a periodontal probe customized to conform to the labial contour of the tooth. The internal level of barrier is placed one millimeter incisal to the corresponding external probings of the epithelial attachment. Facial outline of the barrier resembles a tunnel and proximally the

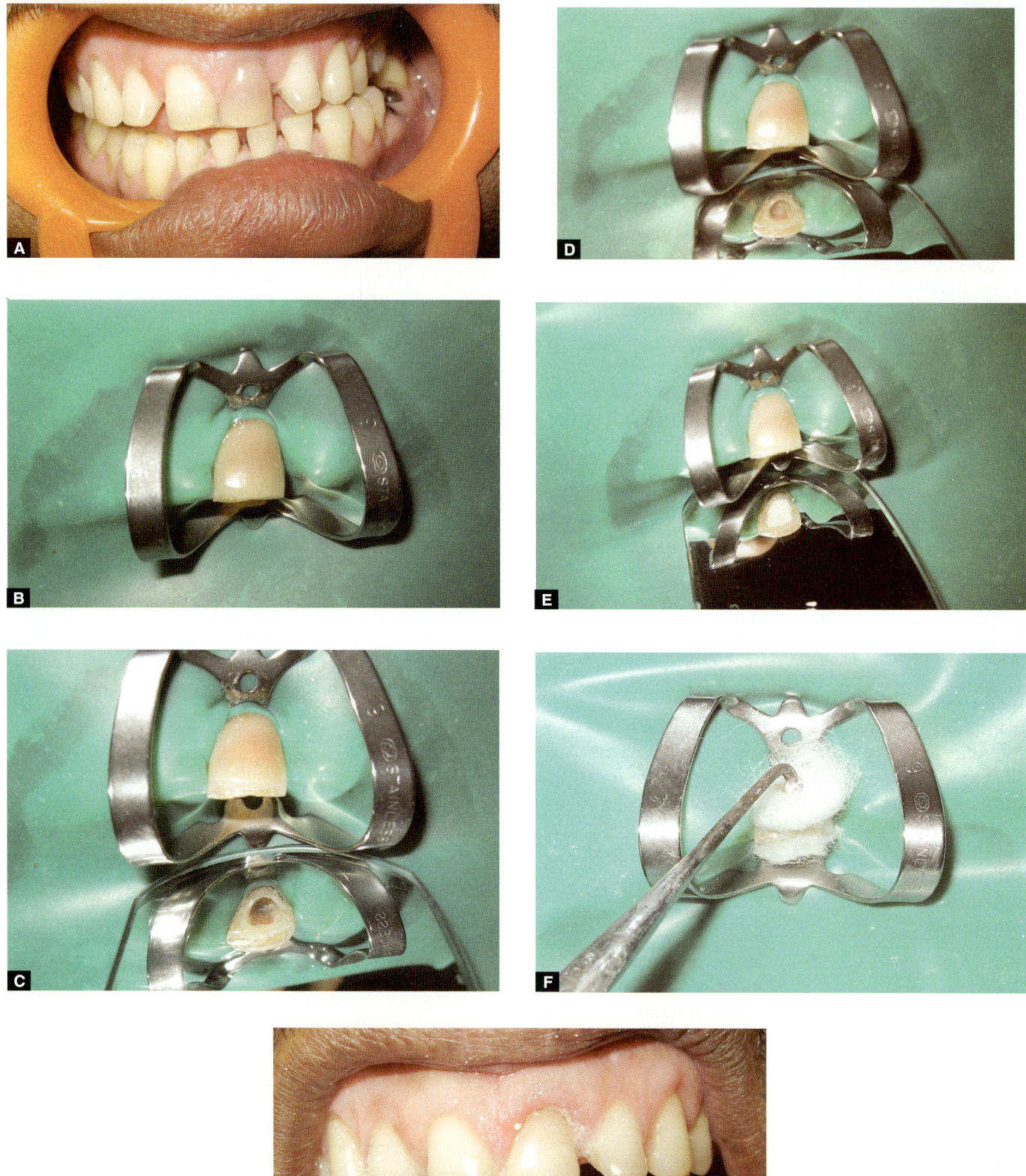

Figs 30.6A to G: **(A)** Pre-operative; **(B)** Isolation with rubber dam **(C)** Removal of coronal restoration **(D)** Sealing of cervical part with GIC **(E)** Placement of bleaching agent **(F)** Application of heat **(G)** Post-operative

outline appears as a slope. This can be verified radiographically.

The intention of barrier transfer is to cover dentinal tubules apical to the epithelial attachment so that the bleaching agents are contained within the pulp chamber.

Cavit and light cured glass-ionomer cements are the most promising barrier materials currently under research.

III. LASER ASSISTED TOOTH WHITENING

The objective of laser bleaching is to achieve the ultimate power bleaching process utilizing efficient energy source and also avoiding any adverse effects. Laser tooth whitening is not a very new phenomenon. It started in the past one decade. The procedure utilizes 30–35% H_2O_2 which is usually applicable in routine bleaching. Laser whitening Gel has a unique mix of Thermal Absorption Crystals integrated into gel of highly processed fumed silica and 35% H_2O_2.

Bleaching gel is applied and is activated by high intensity light source or plasma arc light. Crystals in gel absorb thermal energy from light, allowing better dissociation of oxygen and easy penetration into the enamel matrix thus increasing the lighting effect on teeth.

Three dental laser wavelengths have been cleared by the Food and Drug Administration (FDA) for tooth whitening.
  i. Argon Laser – 488 nm
 ii. CO_2 – 10,600 nm
iii. GaAlAs diode laser – 980 nm
    (Gallium-Aluminium-Arsenide)
 iv. Photochemical laser whitening – smart bleach

i. Argon Laser

Argon lasers are in the form of a blue light with the wavelength of 480 nm in the visible part of the spectrum. Such a spectrum is absorbed by dark color. The affinity to dark stains ensures that the yellow brown color can be easily removed.

The Argon laser rapidly excites the already unstable and reactive H_2O_2 molecule; the energy then is absorbed into all intramolecular bonds. The H_2O_2 molecules fall apart into extremely reactive ionic fragments that swiftly combine with the chromophilic structure of the organic molecules, altering them and producing simpler chemical chains. The result is a visually whitened tooth surface.

Advantages
Argon lasers emit fairly short wavelengths (480 nm) with higher energy photons; conversely plasma arc lamps, halogen lamps and other heat lamps emit short wavelengths as well as longer invisible infrared thermal wavelength (750 nm – 1.0 μm) with longer energy photons and predictable high thermal character. This high energy can create unfavourable pulpal responses which does not happen in case of Argon Laser.

ii. CO_2 Laser

The CO_2 lasers having wavelength of 10,600 nm are basically used for enhancing the effect of Argon lasers. It is unrelated to the color of the tooth and the energy is emitted in the form of the heat. The laser penetrates only 0.1 mm into water and H_2O_2, where it gets absorbed. This energy can enhance the effect of the whitening agent after the initial Argon laser process. The Argon laser, which emits a visible blue light is used first to activate the bleaching gel. This blue light will be absorbed by the dark stains and becomes less effective as the tooth whitens because the blue light will be reflected rather than absorbed by the whiter tooth surface. Then the CO_2 laser, which emits invisible infrared energy is used to achieve deeper penetration of the energized oxygen resulting in a deeper, more efficient tooth whitening.

It was previously approved by FDA for bleaching, however, its use has been discontinued because of its thermal effect on the pulp.

iii. Diode Laser

These are semiconductor lasers with varying wavelengths, 980 nm wave length is usually used for bleaching procedure. Different forms of diode lasers are available.

- Infrared diode has wavelength of 790 nm.
- Laser with blue light emission diode has wavelength of 467 nm. The bleaching agent used is 38% hydrogen peroxide.
- GaAlAs diode: The diode works at different watts. The surface temperature can be raised from 36°C at 1W to 86°C with 3W. Pulpal temperature increased from 4.3°C to 16°C. The bleaching agent utilizes 38% H_2O_2.

iv. Photochemical Laser Whitening

The routinely used lasers provide a greater shade improvement than in-office or home bleaching with trays.

- The commercial hydrogen peroxide system has the potential to affect dental enamel because of the acidic pH of the solution in its native form, which ranges from 5.0 to 6.0.

- The concentrated solutions of hydrogen peroxide (30%) can transiently reduce the microhardness of enamel and dentin.
- The lasers also result in post-treatment sensitivity.

With the new Smart bleach technique (KTP Smart bleach) these problems do not occur as the pH of the bleaching gel is alkaline (approximately 9.5). The primary action of Smart bleaching is photochemical and not photothermal. The perhydroxyl radical is produced compared to superoxide, which is more reactive than the superoxide and other radicals. Also under alkaline conditions, etching of the tooth surface does not occur and the results obtained with KTP and argon lasers are equal to photobleaching.

Smart bleach is particularly useful in bleaching tetracycline stained teeth. The chelate formed between tetracyclines and hydroxyapatite is a red quinone product dimethylamino tetracycline. This colored product is relatively resistant to oxidation from peroxide, but can be broken down (photo-oxidised) by green light in a particular narrow spectral range (512 to 540 nm). Because this energy aligns particularly well with the wavelength of KTP laser (532 nm), energy from this laser can cause terminal photo-oxidation of the quinone molecule, which renders it colorless. The use of the KTP laser in combination with a hydrogen peroxide based gel ensures that complete and irreversible bleaching of red quinone occurs.

In addition to driving photo-oxidation reactions within the tooth, some of the visible green laser energy applied to the site is absorbed in Rhodamine B red dye, which is present within the bleaching gel (0.5% w/w). This is a photochemical process resulting in the production of free oxygen radicals. A portion of the KTP laser energy absorbed into the Rhodamine B dye is also transferred from the excited molecule into the bleaching gel in the form of thermal energy. This transfer results in controlled heating of the gel and not the tooth, minimizing the possibility of thermal insult to the dental pulp. This superficial heating of the gel accelerates the breakdown of H_2O_2, which further boosts the overall yield or free oxygen radicals over a given time.

Examples of currently marketed whitening system are:

i. Laser Smile Whitening System (Biolase)

- A purple gel is applied to one to several teeth at a time, then the dental dam gel is applied, which will protect the gums.
- After these applications are complete, laser light is then applied to the teeth for as little as two minutes collectively for average whitening cases.

ii. Pearlinbrite Laser Whitening System

- This system utilizes Energy Transfer Crystals, or ETCs. ETCs actually absorb the laser's energy and transfers the energy to the hydrogen peroxide molecules of the gel.
- This whitens the stains in the teeth with oxygen on a much higher level than carbamide peroxide gels.
- Usually several applications, lasting up to 30s per tooth is needed per session.

Temperature Changes during Bleaching

1. *Plasma arc light:* The temperature was increased to 39.3°C above baseline, when colorant was used and was 37.1°C when no colorant was used.
2. *QTH light:* The temperature rise was 24.8°C above baseline when colorant was used and 11.5°C when no colorant was used.
3. *Conventional QTH light:* It increased fresh bleach temperature by 17.7°C above baseline when colorant was used and 11.1°C when no colorant was used.
4. *Argon laser:* It increased the temperature by 9.4°C irrespective of the use of colorant.
5. *Diode laser:* The increase in temperature recorded was 37°C at 1W and 28.6°C at 3W. The presence of bleaching gel, however, reduces the increased temperature.

IV. OVER THE COUNTER PRODUCTS

A variety of tooth whitening products, mainly tooth polish, toothpastes and bleaching kits are available in the market. Mostly the tooth polish and tooth pastes, contain ingredients that remove extrinsic stains on teeth rather than bleaching them, although a few products do contain bleaching agents. Extrinsic stain removal from teeth by toothpastes (Close-up whitening, Amway whitener, Shine and smile, etc.) is mainly achieved by physical means, though some commercial products claim removal of stains from teeth by chemical means through organic solvents. The readymade bleaching kits supply preformed trays with the bleaching agent dispensed in tubes (Colgate Platinum). The instructions on these kits recommend the use of kit for a particular span of time period.

Recently wearable bleaching device and tooth whitening pen have been introduced.

Wearable bleaching device: The iPower is the first wearable and portable thermal diffusion bleaching device. It is safe, powerful, cost effective, painfree and easy to use. It uses thermal diffusion technology to deliver optimum results. An accurate amount of thermal energy is delivered onto the bleaching gel is painted on the patient's teeth. A thermal gradient thus

Tooth Discoloration and Bleaching

created in the gel increased the diffusion rate of bleaching agent into the enamel structure, speeding up the entire process.

Tooth whitening pen: It is an easy and convenient way for fast and effective whitening of the teeth. The whitening gel comes in a pen like applicator which is easy to use and carry.

The whitening gel usually contain carbamide peroxide bur hydrogen peroxide based pens are also available.

The gel can be selectively applied to individual teeth or just top or bottom of a tooth as needed, e.g. Listerine whitening pen, White ice whitner stick.

ADDITIONAL MATERIALS USED DURING BLEACHING PROCEDURE

1. Orabase Protective Paste

Orabase is composed of gelatin, pectin and sodium carboxymethylcellulose in Plastibase (plasticized hydrocarbon gel).

By virtue of its superior adhesive properties ORABASE paste adheres tenaciously and remains in intimate contact with mucous membranes of the mouth and gums, protecting the affected area in the mouth against further irritation from chewing, swallowing and other normal mouth activity. It acts like an invisible bandage.

Indications

To protect gingiva and oral mucosa during bleaching.

Directions for use

A small dab of ORABASE paste is taken and the area is coated. It is held in position until it becomes sticky. It is not rubbed. It should not be applied too thickly in the mouth as the excess simply peels off leaving a thin film in contact with the sore spot.

2. Gingival Dam

The polymerizable isolation barriers are useful for many types of dental procedures. The polymerizable isolation barrier compositions comprise:

a. Monomers
b. Curing agents (0.01–2%)
c. Polymerization strength reducers (1–30%)
d. Tissue adherence accentuators (0.01–9%)
e. Reflective materials (1–50%)

a. Monomers

The monomer can be single or a selection of monomers depending upon the specific applications. Examples of monomers include alkylmethacrylates, alkylhydroxymethacrylates, and triethylene glycol dimethacrylate.

b. Curing Agents

A curing agent is provided to include the monomer to cross link upon exposure to adequate light radiant energy. Curing agents include photoinitiators and amine additives as needed.

Examples of photoinitiators include camphorquinone, benzoin methyl ether, 2-hydroxy-2-methyl-1-phenyl-1-propanone, diphenyl trimethylbenzoyl phosphine oxide, benzoin ethyl ether, benzophenone and equivalents.

Optional activities such as amine additives are preferred in formulating curing agents to assist the curing agents. Examples of amine additives include dimethyl amino ethyl methacrylate, triethylamine, 2-dimethylamino ethanol, diethyl amino ethyl methacrylate, trihexyl amine, N,N-dimethyl-ptoluidine, N-methylethanolamines and equivalents.

c. Polymerization Strength Reducers

A weakened isolation barrier has the advantage of easy removal after completion of the dental procedure. The clinician can take hold of the polymerized isolation barrier by hand or with an instrument like tweezers and remove it in discrete segments or as integral unit. The size of the discrete segments is generally about one-half the area that the isolation barrier is isolating. For example, when the whole arch is being isolated, it is preferable that the discrete segments are at least about one-fourth the length of the arch, more preferable at least about one-half the length of the arch, and most preferably the isolation barrier will be removed as an integral unit. When a hydrophobic isolation barrier is used, removal after the procedure takes only one or a few removal steps and any small portions that may crumble are easily rinsed away after being dislodged. Examples of suitable polymerization strength reducers include oils such as mineral oils, alcohols, its derivatives and equivalents. Yet other suitable examples include polyols such as polyethylene glycols, polypropylene glycols, propylene glycol, derivatives thereof, and equivalents. Of the polymerization strength reducers, the preferred includes acetyl alcohol.

d. Tissue Adherence Accentuators

With preferred tissue adherence accentuators, the isolation barrier composition continues to gently adhere to wetted tissue even when the monomer becomes substantially polymerized. An advantage of this feature is that a substantially conformal isolation barrier can be laid up against the tooth to isolate it and it will adhere adequately to tissues during a time period for standard isolation treatment procedures.

Examples of tissue adherence accentuators include gums such as xanthan gum, guar gum, tragacanth gum and their derivatives, cellulose materials such as ethyl cellulose, hydroxypropyl methyl cellulose and their derivatives. Yet other examples include polymers such as carboxy poly methylene, polysiloxanes, watersoluble polyethylene oxide polymers, derivatives and equivalents. The water-soluble polyethylene oxides preferably have molecular weights of around 100,000 or more even up to several million. The preferred water-soluble polyethylene oxide polymer is marketed as Polyox R by Union Carbide. Additionally, high molecular weight polyols can function as tissue adherence accentuators such as polypropylene glycols and polyethylene glycols. The preferred tissue adherence accentuator is xanthan gum.

e. Reflective Materials

Another method of lowering harmful amounts of heat released during polymerization is to reflect some of the light radiant energy of the dental light away from the isolation barrier composition. Dental curing lights and laser treatment lights typically come with only intense light radiation settings, which is desirable in certain applications such as peroxide teeth bleaching. It was found that the addition of reflective materials causes a portion of the dental light to be reflected, thereby reducing heating of the isolation barrier during polymerization. Thus, the composition absorbs less light radiant energy, the isolation barrier is less energized than would be otherwise, the underlying gum tissue is not subjected to undue heating during a dental procedure that uses a curing or laser light and light is even reflected away from the underlying gums or other protected tissue.

Examples of reflective materials include metals such as gold flake, aluminium flake, titanium flake, and equivalents. Other examples include metal oxides such as aluminium oxide, titanium dioxide, precipitated silica, ceria, thoria and equivalents. Yet other examples include micas and equivalents. The preferred reflective material comprises micas.

Composition of Barriers

The polymerizable isolation barrier consists of at least one monomer; providing at least one curing agent for curing one monomer; and by providing at least one of three preferred additives that include the organic polymerization strength reducer, the tissue adherence accentuator, or the reflective material. The ingredients are blended in a container until homogeneous, and the homogeneous mixture is placed in a container that is resistant to light energy. The polymerizable isolation barrier material is preferably stored at or below room temperature. The polymerizable isolation barrier material is stable enough to be stored under normal conditions at the operatory until activated by suitable light radiant energy.

Methods of use of Isolation Barrier

The polymerizable isolation barrier material is made in a paste or gel form that is rheologically able to be expressed from a dental syringe. The components of the isolation barrier material depends upon selection of a preferred application. The inventive polymerizable isolation barrier material is also preferably made in a roll or tape form of a curable putty that is rolled onto the gums, pressed into place, for example with finger pressure, carved to isolate hard tissue, and then cured with light radiant energy. The components of this isolation barrier material form either an emulsion, dispersion or suspension solution depending upon selection of a preferred application.

3. Diamond Polishing Paste

The diamond polishing paste contains:

- Fiber points: It incorporates a blend of very fine abrasive particles in each starch of fibre thus forming a three dimensional open weave design. This provides finishing and polishing in one step.
- Diamond paste contains supercharged diamond particles.

4. First Aid Kit

It contains antioxidants such as vitamin E in liquid or capsule form and aloe-vera gel. A single spill of a droplet of H_2O_2 blanches and burns the gingival tissue. Vitamin E oil quickly relieves the symptoms within one minute.

SAFETY ISSUES IN BLEACHING

The intensity of light used for bleaching must be blocked out with glasses with proper optimal density for specific wavelengths. Everyone in the operatory must wear these glasses.

Adverse Effects of Bleaching

Contemporary tooth whitening (tooth bleaching) systems are based primarily on hydrogen peroxide (H_2O_2) or one of its precursors, carbamide peroxide. These bleach the chromogens within the dentin, thereby reducing the body color of the tooth and are often used in combination with an activating agent such as heat and/or light. Such agents can be applied externally to the teeth (vital bleaching) or internally within the pulp chamber (non-vital bleaching).

The predictable tooth whitening can be achieved using a 10% carbamide peroxide gel in a bleaching tray at night (the night guard vital bleaching technique), H_2O_2 strips and 'power bleaching' using 35% H_2O_2 with or without light and/or heat activation. The 'walking bleach' technique involves sealing a mixture of sodium perborate and water into the pulp chamber between patients' visits. The method was later modified; the water was replaced by 30–35% H_2O_2 to improve the whitening effect. Concerns have been expressed over the potential adverse effects of the use of H_2O_2 tooth whitening agents. The adverse effects that have been reported in cellular, animal and human studies include:

- Cervical root resorption associated with nonvital bleaching
- Increased tooth sensitivity associated with vital bleaching
- Alteration in the surface topography of enamel
- Reduction in bond strength of resin based materials
- The possibility that H_2O_2 may have carcinogenic or tumor promoting capabilities.

a. Hydrogen Peroxide Toxicity

i. 30% H_2O_2 can cause severe irritation or burns on contact with skin or eyes. Following application of 30% H_2O_2 at 15 minute intervals (Four applications) to the tip of rat tongue, oedema was followed by intraepithelial and some subepithelial vesiculation, changes preventable by prior administration of catalase.

ii. Following inadvertent irritation of H_2O_2 into the periodontal ligament during root canal treatment, contact of the H_2O_2 with blood and tissue proteins produces effervescence, liberating oxygen and causing tissue emphysema.

iii. Hydrogen peroxide mouth rinses can be responsible for objective and subjective adverse effects including mouth irritation and discomfort, dryness, loss of taste, elongation of filiform papillae and diffuse mucosal whitening.

iv. There are also changes in epithelial proliferation rate and morphological changes with epithelial thickening but fewer epithelial ridges. The PCNA (Proliferating cell nuclear antigen) index, an indication of cell proliferation, increases in basal and parabasal layers of epithelium. At baseline, although smokers had a significantly higher PCNA index than non-smokers, this difference disappeared following bleaching, indicating simulation of cell division activity by peroxide similar to that produced by smoke. In view of this, it was concluded that 10% carbamide peroxide would act as a tumor promoter in the presence of mutated cells.

v. Dental pulp is reported to have a low peroxidase enzyme activity due to a sparse cell population of fibroblasts. Studies have reported the inhibition as well as inactivation of pulpal enzymes by H_2O_2. The quantity of peroxides penetrating the pulp chamber of extracted teeth is sufficient to produce toxic effects on cultured fibroblasts. Though there have been few reports of untoward pulpal responses, this suggests caution is warranted.

b. Cervical Root Resorption after Internal (Non-Vital) Tooth Bleaching

An adverse affect that has been reported following internal tooth bleaching is cervical root resorption (as inflammatory-mediated external resorption of the root).

c. Increased Sensitivity after External (Vital) Tooth Bleaching

Vital tooth bleaching can be performed by dentist administered bleaching – the use of a high concentration of hydrogen peroxide (35–50%) or carbamide peroxide (35–40%), often supplemented with a heat source; dentist-supervised home bleaching – using a bleaching tray containing a high concentration of carbamide peroxide (10%–10.22%). Tooth sensitivity is a common adverse effect of external tooth bleaching. Data from various studies of 10% carbamide peroxide indicate that from 15–65% of patients reported increased tooth sensitivity. Higher incidences of tooth sensitivity (from 67–78%) were reported after bleaching with H_2O_2 in combination with heat.

The mechanisms that could account for the tooth sensitivity after external tooth bleaching have not yet been fully established, but an in vitro experiment has shown that peroxide can penetrate enamel and dentine and enter the pulp chamber.

d. Effect of Bleaching on the Structure of Enamel

Significant surface alterations in enamel topography follow vital bleaching using carbamide peroxide or H_2O_2. High concentrations of carbamide peroxide damage enamel surface integrity, but lesser than phosphoric acid etch. As a result of this increased surface roughness it is possible that teeth may be more susceptible to extrinsic discoloration after bleaching.

e. Effect of Bleaching on Dentin

1. Tooth color: It is primarily determined by dentin and can be changed by bleaching treatments. In a study by McCaslin, et al, 1999 using 10% carbamide peroxide placed directly on enamel to validate the color change in dentin and to assess whether color changed uniformly, it was noted that a color change occurred throughout the dentin and the color change was uniform.
2. Surface texture: The majority of studies investigated that surface morphology of dentin using SEM found no significant changes. However, Zalkind, et al (1996) found that $CaPO_4$ ratio of dentin was modified following 7 days of continuous treatment with 30% H_2O_2 or 10% carbamide peroxide solutions compared to saline control.
3. Surface microhardness: A transient decrease in surface microhardness has been observed in some studies but recovered following remineralization period or 0.05% fluoride solution treatment

f. Effect of Bleaching on Pulp

A 3% solution of H_2O_2 is capable of causing transient reduction in pulpal blood circulation and occlusion of pulpal blood vessels. The most common side effect experienced by patients using home bleaching technique is mild, transient temperature sensitivity. The sensitivity appears to be dose related rather than pH related.

g. Effect of Bleaching of the Gingiva and Mucosa

Gingival irritation from custom made trays has been reported in 21–40% of patients during treatment. Bleaching trays which are ill-fitting, overextended, or not properly trimmed, can irritiate soft tissue directly or through bleaching agents leaking on to gingival soft tissues. Effective protection of gingiva and mucosa, with good isolation will minimize the risk of irritation.

h. Effects of Tooth Bleaching on Tooth Restorations

Bleaching causes surface roughening and etching on composites.

IRM on exposure to H_2O_2 become cracked or swollen

Microstructural changes in amalgam is also seen with bleaching

Bleaching may increase the solubility of glass-ionomer and other cements. It may reduce the bond strength between enamel and resin-based fillings in the first 24 hours, but not later. Following bleaching, H_2O_2 residues in the enamel may inhibit the polymerization of resin-based materials and reduce bond strength. Thus tooth-bleaching agents should not be used (for 24 hours) prior to treatment with resin-based materials.

ADVANCEMENTS IN BLEACHING

i. Tooth Bleaching with Non-thermal Atmospheric Plasma

Plasma is considered as the fourth state of matter and it is the most abundant state in the universe. The term was introduced into physics by Irving-Langmuir in 1928, because it resembles the ionic liquids in biology and medicine. Plasma can be divided into two main categories: hot plasma (near-equilibrium plasma) and cold plasma (non-equilibrium plasma). Hot plasma consists of very high temperature particles and they are close to the maximal degree of ionization. Cold plasma is composed of low temperature particles and relatively high temperature electrons and they have low degree of ionization (Tendero, et al, 2006). Lee, et al (2009) demonstrated that room temperature plasma could be used for tooth bleaching. The authors concluded that the tooth bleaching method with plasma can be complementary to conventional method because it provides effective bleaching without thermal damage.

ii. Bleching Technique Modified by Casein Phosphopeptide Amorphous Calcium Phosphate (CPP-ACP)

Side effects such as hypersensitivity and dental remineralization remain a problem in bleaching therapy. Remineralization techniques in association with vital tooth bleaching regimens such as using CPP-ACP based substances during and after bleaching have been advocated to overcome these problems.

Majority of these products do not reveal the ingredients of the product for the sake of professional secrecy.

The major disadvantage is that the abrasive constituents not only remove the stains but also abrade the tooth structure. This makes the teeth more susceptible to further permeability to extrinsic stains and internalized stains. Excess and vigorous use of pastes may also cause hypersensitive dentin because of loss of enamel.

Regarding the bleaching kits, apart from few instructions, there is no thorough knowledge provided to the patient in relation to the whitening process and exact manner of use. The prefabricated trays may not fit accurately in the patients' mouth and this causes occlusal discrepancies, Temporomandibular joint dysfunction, leaching out of the bleaching agent causing soft tissue injury.

Since, over the counter products are not monitored by the dentists, so their potential, efficacy, results and side effects are not thoroughly known. The academic research is needed before finally accepting these professionally.

iii. Enzymatic Bleaching Dentifrice

Enzymatic activation is a new method to improve the bleaching procedure. Enzymes can be used as bleaching catalyst by decreasing the activation energy of bleaching reactions or by generating hydrogen peroxide in situ, thereby enabling a reduction in peroxide concentrations and the risk of possible toxic effects from treatments.

BIBLIOGRAPHY

1. Alkmin, Y.T., Sartoralli, R. and Florio, F.M.: Comparative study of the effects of two bleaching agents on oral microbiota. Oper. Dent.: 30, 417, 2005.
2. Almas, K. and Al-Harbi, M.: The effect of 10% carbamide peroxide home bleaching system on the gingival health. J. Contemp. Dent. Pract.: 1, 32, 2003.
3. Alonsodela, V. and Balboa, C.O.: Comparison of the clinical efficacy and safety of carbamide peroxide and hydrogen peroxide in at-home bleaching gels. Quint. Int.: 37, 551, 2006.
4. Al-Qunaian, T.: The effects of whitening agents on caries susceptibility of human enamel. Oper. Dent.: 30, 265, 2005.
5. Attin, T., Paque, F., Ajan, F. and Lemon, A.M.: Review of the current status of tooth whitening with the walking bleach technique. Int. Endod. J.: 36, 313, 2003.
6. Attin, T., Hanning, C. and Wiegand, A.: Effect of bleaching on restorative materials and restoration – a systematic review. Dent. Mater.: 20, 852, 2004.
7. Auschill, T.M., Hellwig, E., Schmidale, S., Sculean, A. and Arweiler, N.B.: Efficacy, side effects and patients acceptance of different bleaching techniques (OTC, in office, at home). Oper. Dent.: 30, 156, 2005.
8. Bartlett, J.D., Dwyer, S.E., Beniash, E., Skobe, Z. and Ferreira, T.L.: Fluorosis: A new model and new insights. J.D.R.: 84, 832, 2005.
9. Borges, B.C., devasconselos, A.A., Cunha, A.G., Pinheiro, F.H., Machado, C.T. and Santos, A.J.: Preliminary clinical reports of a novel night-guard tooth blaeching technique modified by Casein phosphopeptide-amorphous calcium phosphate (CPP-ACP). Eur. J. Esthet. Dent.: 6, 446, 2011.
10. Browning W.D., Cho S.D. and Descepper E.J.: Effect of a nano-hydroxyapatite paste on bleaching related tooth sensitivity. J Esthet Restor Dent.: 24, 268, 2012.
11. Deliperi, S., Bardwell, D.N. and Papathanasiou, A.: Clinical evaluation of a combined in-office and take home bleaching system. J.A.D.A.: 135, 628, 2004.
12. Dietschi, D., Rossier, S. and Krejci, I.: In vitro calorimetric evaluation of the efficacy of various bleaching methods and products. Quint. Int.: 37, 515, 2006.
13. Forner, L., Amengual, J., Llena, C. and Riutord, P.: Therapeutic effectiveness of a new enzymatic bleaching dentifrice. Eur. J. Esthet. Dent.: 7, 63, 2012.
14. Gianluca, G., Luca, T. and Giovanni, D.: Clinical evaluation of a novel liquid tooth whitening gel. Am. J. Dent.: 16, 147, 2003.
15. Joiner, A.: Review of effects of peroxide on enamel and dentin properties. J. Dent.: 35, 889, 2007.
16. Kathernine, A.K., Ingvar, M., Matthew, L.B. and Robert, W.G.: Placebo controlled clinical trial of a 19% sodium percarbonate whitening film: Initial and sustained whitening. Am. J. Dent.: 16, 12B, 2003.
17. Lee, H.W., Kim, G.J., Kim, J.M., Park, J.K., Lee, J.K. and Kim, G.C.: Tooth bleaching with non-thermal atmospheric pressure plasma. J. Endod.: 351, 587, 2009.
18. Matis, B.A., Cochran, M.A., Wang, G., Franco, M. and Eckert, G.J.: A clinical evaluation of bleaching using whitening wraps and strips. Oper. Dent.: 30, 588, 2005.
19. Mokhlio, G.R., Matis, B.A., Cochrm, M.A. and Eckert, G.J.: A clinical evaluation of carbamide peroxide and hydrogen peroxide whitening agents during day time. J.A.D.A.: 131, 1269, 2000.
20. Muydeci, A. and Gokay, O.: Effect of bleaching agents on the mircohardness of tooth colored restorative materials. J.P.D.: 95, 286, 2006.
21. Naik, S., Tredwin, C.J. and Scully, C.: H_2O_2 tooth-whitening (bleaching): Review of study in relation to possible carciongenesis. Oral Oncology: 42, 668, 2006.
22. Pleffken P.R., Borges A.B., Goncalves S.E.D.P. and Torres C.R.G.: The effectiveness of low intensity red laser for activating a bleaching gel and its effect in temperature of the bleaching gel and the dental pulp. J Esthet Restor Dent.: 24, 126, 2012.
23. Polydorou O, Wirsching M, Wokewitz M and Hahn P.: Three-Month Evaluation of Vital Tooth Bleaching Using Light Units—A Randomized Clinical Study. Oper Dent 38, 1, 2013.
24. Pretty, I.A., Ellwood, R.P., Brunton, P.A. and Aminian, A.: Vital tooth bleaching in dental practice: 1. Professional bleaching. Dent. Update: 33, 293, 2006.
25. Qunaian TA: The effect of Whitening agents on caries susceptibility of human enamel. Oper. Dent. 30, 265, 2005.
26. Rosentritt, M., Lang, R., Plein, T. and Michael, B.: Discoloration of restorative materials after bleaching application. Quint. Int.: pg. 26, 2005.
27. Silva, G.M.S., Brackett, M.G. and Haywood, V.B.: Number of in-office light activated bleaching treatment needed to achieve patient satisfaction. Quint. Int.: 37, 115, 2006.
28. Sulieman, M.: An overview of two bleaching techniques: Night guard vital bleaching and non-vital bleaching. Dent. Update: 32, 37, 2005.
29. Sulieman, M.: An overview of tooth discoloration: Extrinsic, intrinsic and internalized stains. Dent. Update: 32, 463, 2005.
30. Timpawaqt, S., Nipattamanon, C., Kijsamanmith, K. and Messer, h.H.: Effect of bleaching agents on bonding to pulp chamber dentin. Int. Endod. J.: 38, 211, 2005.
31. Tredwin, C.J., Naik, S., Lewis, N.J. and Scully, C.: Hydrogen peroxide tooth whitening (bleaching) products: review of adverse effects and safety issues. B.D.J.: 200, 371, 2006.
32. Villalta, P., Lu, H., Okte, Z., Garcia-Godoy, F. and Powers, J.M.: Effects of staining and bleaching on color changes of dental composite resins. J.P.D.: 95, 137, 2006.
33. Walsh, L.J., Liu, J.Y. and Verhejen, P.: Tooth discoloration and its treatment using KTP laser assisted tooth whitening. J. Oral Laser Appl.: 4, 7, 2004.
34. Watts, A. and Addy, M.: Tooth discoloration and staining: A review of the literature. B.D.J.: 190, 309, 2001.
35. Yarborough, D.K.: The safety and efficacy of tooth bleaching. A review of literature. Compend.: 12, 191, 1991.

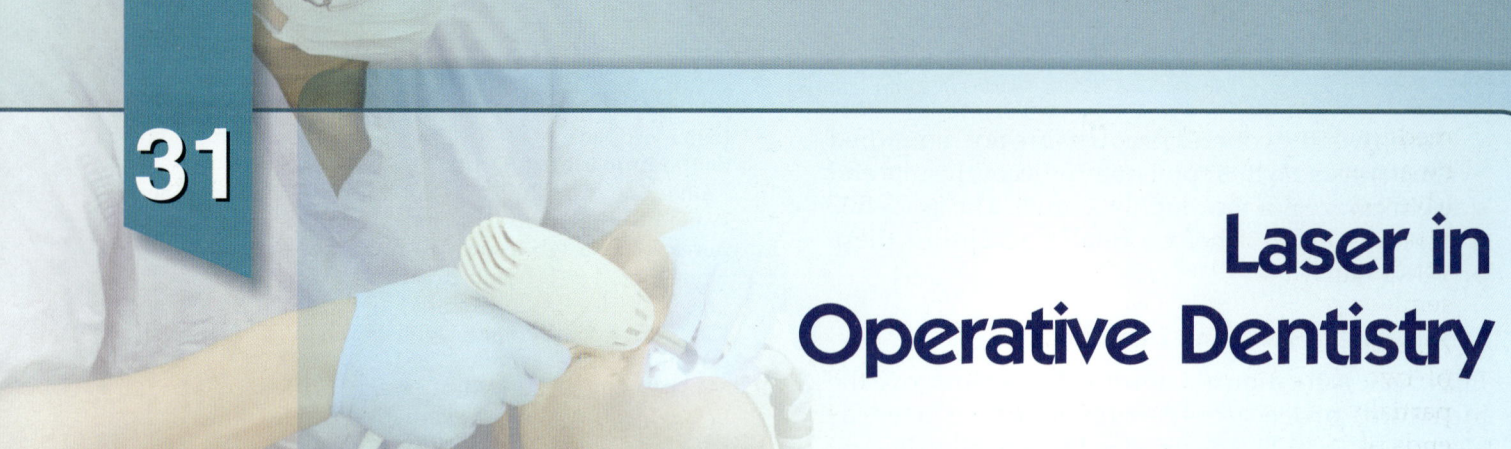

31

Laser in Operative Dentistry

Laser is being widely used in dentistry. The investigators have been studying their effects on oral hard and soft tissues. Food and drug administration has approved the use of Laser on soft and hard tissues.

Laser is a device that transforms light of various frequencies into a chromatic radiation in the visible, infrared and ultraviolet regions with all the waves in a phase capable of mobilizing immense heat and power when focused at a close range.

LASER is acronym for 'Light amplification by stimulated emission of radiation'. The first Laser was fabricated by Theodore Harold Maiman in 1960 using synthetic Ruby (Aluminium oxide doped with chromium oxide). The light emitted was 107 times stronger than the solar light. The first Lasers marketed for intraoral use were CO_2 lasers.

PRINCIPLE OF LASER

If a microwave beam containing photons passes through a cloud of ammonia gas, the gas molecules will be raised to a higher energy state as energy is absorbed. Earlier, Einstein predicted that if a photon of correct size struck a molecule already in an excited state, that molecule would fall back to lower energy level and would emit a photon of exactly the same size and moving in the same direction as the entering photon. Thus, in case of ammonia gas, the molecules can undergo two possible changes, i.e. either moving to a higher state or being pushed back to a lower one. Normally, the first process would predominate but if the majority of molecules are already in a higher energy state (termed as population inversion) then the released photon will speed on with the original photon. These two photons will strike two further molecules causing production of another two photons and a cascade reaction starts. This effect is known as Maser (Microwave Amplification by Stimulated Emission of Radiation). This principle was applied to the electromagnetic waves of wavelength of light and the process was called as Laser.

LASER DEVICE

The Laser device (Fig. 31.1) consists of the following:
a. *A Laser medium:* This is what determines the wavelength of the light emitted from Laser. The names of dental Lasers are based on the active

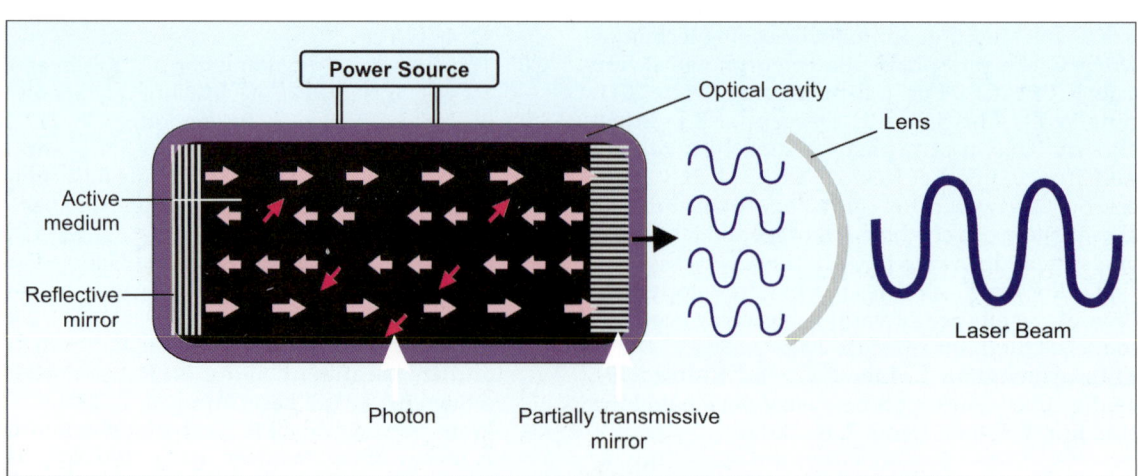

Fig. 31.1: The Laser device

medium that is stimulated. The active medium can be a gas [(e.g. Argon, Carbon dioxide), a liquid (dyes) or a solid state crystal rod [e.g. Neodymium yttrium aluminium garnet (Nd:YAG), Erbium yttrium aluminium garnet (Er: YAG) or a semiconductor (diode lasers)].

b. *An optical cavity/Laser tube/optical screen:* It consists of two mirrors: one fully reflective and other partially transmissive, that are located on the either ends of the optical cavity.

c. *Power Source:* The power source excites or pumps the atoms of Laser medium to their higher energy levels.

A population inversion happens when there are more atoms in the excited state rather than non-excited state. Atoms in excited state spontaneously emit photons of light which bounce back and forth between the two mirrors in laser tube. As they bounce, they strike other atoms, stimulating more photons emissions. Photons as energy, wavelength and frequency escape through transmissive mirror as a laser beam. The beam is directed via a flexible fiber optic light pipe or mirror train to the point of application where it is focused by a lens to focal area near the tip. Energy impact that produces population inversion is called pumping. Gas lasers are pumped by electrode discharge between electrodes. Laser is a beam of very high intensity light. It is monochromatic, coherent and collimated (Directional).

- Monochromatic: Radiation in which the waves have same wavelength.
- Coherent: The waves are in a certain phase relationship to each other, both in space and time.
- Collimated (Directional): The emitted waves have low divergence (nearly parallel).

LASER DELIVERY SYSTEM

There are three delivery systems:

a. *Articulated arms (with mirror at joints):* For UV, visible and infrared Lasers.

b. *Flexible hollow waveguide:* A flexible hollow waveguide or tube has an interior mirror finish. The Laser energy is reflected along this tube and it exits through the handpiece at the surgical end with the beam striking the tissue in a non-contact fashion.

c. *Glass fiberoptic cable:* The third delivery system is a glass fiber optic cable. This cable can be more pliant than the waveguide as it has a corresponding decrease in weight and resistance to movement, and is usually smaller in diameter (the delivery system of choice).

LASER EMISSION MODES

The dental Laser device can emit the light energy in three modalities as a function of time:

a. *'Constant on' Emission:* It is the continuous wave in which the beam is emitted at only one power level for as long as the operator depresses the foot switch.

b. *'Pushed on and off' Emission:* This is a gated pulse mode having periodic alterations of the Laser energy, much like a blinking light. This mode is achieved by the opening and closing of a mechanical shutter in front of the beam pathway of a continuous wave emission.

c. *Free running pulse mode:* In this mode a very large Laser energy is emitted for an extremely short span, in microseconds followed by a relatively long time in which the Laser is off.

MECHANISM OF ACTION

The possible mechanisms of action of Laser can be:

- *Photo-thermal ablation:* This occurs with high powered Lasers, when used to vaporize or coagulate tissue through absorption in a major tissue component.
- *Photo-mechanical ablation:* It causes the disruption of tissues due to a range of phenomena, such as Shock wave formation, Cavitations, etc.
- *Photo-chemical effects:* Use light sensitive substances to treat conditions such as cancer.

LASER-TISSUE INTERACTION

This is the interaction of photons with the atoms or molecules of the target. Lasers have four different interactions with the target tissue. These interactions depend on the optical properties of the tissue.

a. *Photobiological interactions:* The photobiological interactions of Lasers on tissues are further of four types:
   i. Reflection: During reflection, the incident laser beam redirects itself without affecting the target tissues.
   ii. Absorption: The second interaction is the absorption of laser energy by the intended target tissue. This effect is desirable and the amount of energy that is absorbed by the tissue depends on the tissue characteristics, such as pigmentation and water content; and on the laser wavelength and emission mode. Argon has a high affinity for melanin and haemoglobin in soft tissue.
   iii. Transmission: The third interaction is the transmission of laser energy directly through the tissue without affecting it.

iv. *Scattering:* The fourth interaction is scattering. Scattering of the reflected light weakens the intended energy and possibly produces no useful biologic effect.
b. *Photochemical interactions:* The basic principle of photochemical process is that specific wavelength of laser light is absorbed by naturally occurring chromophores, which are able to induce certain biochemical reactions. Photosensitive compounds when exposed to laser energy can produce a single oxygen radical for disinfection of the endodontic canals.
c. *Photothermal interactions:* The radiant energy absorbed by tissue substances are transformed into heat energy, which then produces the tissue effects (Table 31.1).
d. *Photomechanical and photoelectrical interactions:* These include photodisruption, photoplasmolysis and photoacoustic interactions. In photoacoustic effects, the pulse of laser energy on the dental tissues can produce a shock wave. When this shock wave explodes or pulverizes the tissue, it creates an abraded crater. Photoplasmolysis describes the removal of tissues is through the formation of electrically charged ions.

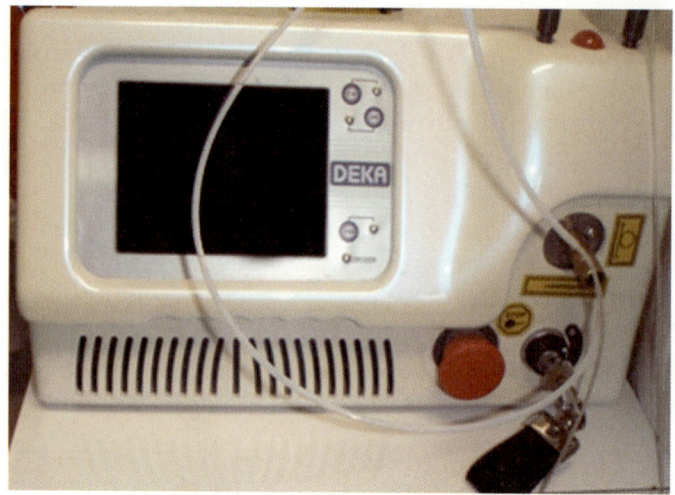

Fig. 31.2: Soft Laser unit

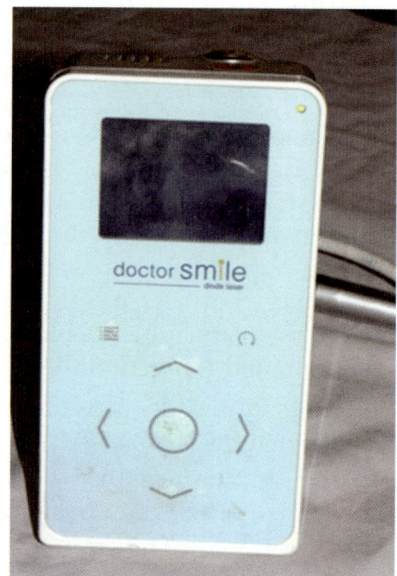

Fig. 31.3: Soft Laser unit

Table 31.1: Tissue effects with rise in temperature

Tissue temperature (°C)	Observed effect
<100°C	Water in soft and hard tissue boils producing explosive expansion
>100°C	Protein denaturation, hemolysis, coagulation, shrinkage
>400°C	Carbonization of organic material occurs
400–1400°C	Inorganic constituents may melt and/or recrystallize and may vaporize

TYPES OF LASERS

Lasers are generally of two types:
I. Soft Laser
II. Hard Laser

I. Soft Lasers

These are athermic, low energy Lasers that generally utilize the semi-conductor Laser diodes (Figs 31.2 and 31.3). They are of the wavelength, which stimulates cellular activity. They aid in tissue regeneration and wound healing by increasing collagen production by fibroblast stimulation.

The soft Lasers are:
- Helium – Neon (He-Ne) Laser
- Gallium – Arsenide (Ga-Ar) Laser
- Gallium – Aluminium – Arsenide (Ga-Al-Ar) Laser

II. Hard Lasers

The Hard Lasers are thermic and of high energy, that are utilized in surgery as precise energy source, i.e. cut, coagulate and vaporize (Fig. 31.4).

The Hard Lasers are:
- Argon Laser
- CO_2 Laser
- Nd-YAG Laser

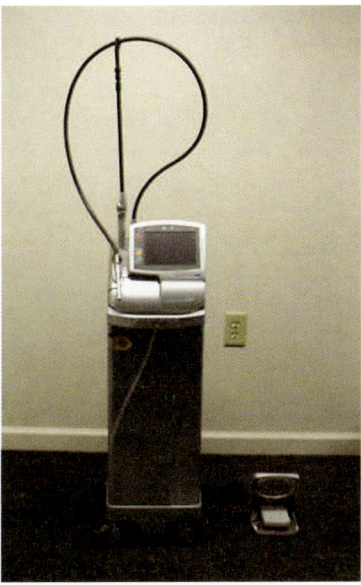

Fig. 31.4: Hard Laser unit

ROUTINELY USED LASERS

CO_2 Laser

CO_2 Laser was thought to be suitable for selected surface applications on teeth such as sealing of pit and fissures, welding of ceramic materials to enamel and prevention of dental caries since it is well absorbed by enamel because of its wavelength (10.6 µm) (Fig. 31.5). Later, these applications were found to be unsuccessful due to the generation of extremely high surface temperatures and their inability to be transmitted via a fiber optic cable to a handpiece approaching the size of a traditional dental instrument. As principally absorbed by water molecules, it can cut many hard and soft tissues. The wavelength has the highest absorption in hydroxyapatite out of any dental laser. Therefore, structures adjacent to surgical site must be shielded from laser beam. CO_2 Laser has been used successfully in soft tissue surgeries.

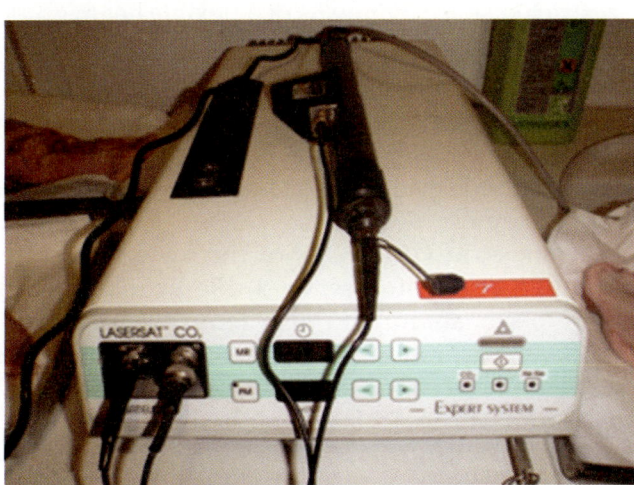

Fig. 31.5: CO_2 Laser unit

Nd:YAG Laser

Nd:YAG Laser systems are usually large and bulky. This system emits its pulsed energy at 1064 nm and this energy is directed through a 320µ silica fiber, using the high peak powers of a free running pulse emission. Its common clinical applications are for cutting and coagulation of the dental soft tissues. It has an affinity for pigmented tissues. It minimizes the heat build-up in tissues.

Argon Laser

The Argon Laser uses argon gas as the active medium. Energy passing through the gas laser head and reflective mirrors generate coherent visible light with primary wavelengths of 488 and 514.55 nm. These visible blue green laser light wavelengths have peak absorption in red pigment such as Heamoglobin; thus, laser light is well absorbed in pigmented tissues with abundance of Haemoglobin, Haemosiderin and Melanin. Argon laser light is not well absorbed by enamel and dentin or other non-pigmented tissues. These characteristics make argon laser energy very useful for cutting, vaporizing, coagulating and providing haemostasis on gingival and oral mucosa. The argon laser is primarily used for root planning and curettage, gingival retraction, gingivectomy/gingivoplasty, frenectomy, treatment of oral lesions and tissue welding.

Er: YAG Laser

It is a promising laser system because of its emission wavelength of 2.94 µ which coincides with main absorption peak of water, resulting in good absorption in all biologic tissues including enamel and dentin. Previous studies with infrared laser systems like continuous wave CO_2 or Nd:YAG laser have reported the presence of zones of carbonization and necrosis due to high temperatures. In contrast, Er:YAG laser treatment do not induce any thermal changes. Water has a very high absorption for Er:YAG laser light. The incident laser radiation is absorbed in a thin surface layer causing sudden heating and vaporization of water. A high steam pressure then leads to micro-explosions with erupting particles. Because the tissue is not vaporized completely but only disintegrated into fragments, radiant energy is converted into ablation that alters the morphological structure of tissue. Er:YAG laser can be used for the removal of healthy hard tissue as well as carious decay without causing any thermal injury to adjacent tissues. Restorative materials like composites and cements can be ablated without using mechanical bur. Gold crowns and cast fillings cannot be removed because the laser beam is reflected by metals. No ablation effect is observed on ceramics. This Laser is recommended for osteotomy, cyst removal and apicoectomy because of bone healing properties.

The thermal side effects are greatly reduced with Er:YAG laser. However, this laser beam is not easily transmitted through optical fibers and therefore is usually applied via mirror and arm delivery systems. A root canal preparation is not possible due to lack of suitable delivery system (Figs 31.6A, B).

The preparation of dental hard tissue with laser has been tried with Excimer lasers emitted in UV spectral range. They work by the process of ablative photodecomposition which describes the bond breaking of molecules with minimal thermal side effects, caused by high energy photon application emitted by UV Excimer lasers. Residual energy is converted into kinetic energy by expansion of residual gaseous phase.

Laser type, wavelength and their clinical potential are summarized in Table 31.2

USES OF LASER IN OPERATIVE (CONSERVATIVE) DENTISTRY

a. Preventive effects
   (CO_2, Nd:YAG, Excimers)
b. Caries treatment
   (CO_2, Nd:YAG, Excimers, Er:YAG)
c. Composite Resin Light Curing
   (Argon, Dye)
d. Tooth surface Conditioning
   (Excimers, CO_2, Nd:YAG, Er:YAG)

a. Preventive Effects

Dental caries is characterized by subsurface enamel demineralization. Laser energy has the potential to alter the enamel to make it less susceptible to this subsurface demineralization.

Commonly used Lasers for this purpose are CO_2, Nd:YAG and Excimers.

CO_2 laser is thought to be ideally suitable since its long wavelength can easily be absorbed by enamel. Only the shallow depth is affected thereby minimizing possible harmful effects on the pulp. The most effective wavelength for inhibiting artificial caries was found to be 9.3 μm to 10.6 μm.

Nd:YAG Laser is used as pit and fissure sealant. It removes inorganic and organic debris in pit and fissure without injuring the surrounding healthy enamel. The laser effect would weld hydroxyl apatite crystals blocking the pits/fissures.

Following two features are important for Lasers to help in caries prevention:

- Minimum energy density is required to avoid damaging the soft tissues especially dental pulp.
- The ability to direct the Laser beam within the restricted space by means of a flexible beam guide.

Various hypothesis were put forward explaining how Lasers prevent caries.

Earlier authors opined that Nd:YAG Laser may increase the acid resistance of tooth enamel. This effect is caused by melting of a thin glaze like surface layer of enamel.

Nelson, et al (1978) was of the view that caries preventive effect of Laser was due to reduction of enamel permeability and also reduction of enamel solubility. Formation of pyrophosphate on lased enamel reducing enamel solubility was also suggested.

Oho and Morio Ka (1990) observed that the lased enamel was found to have a high positive birefringence, which might be due to presence of micropores. The loss of water, carbonate and organic

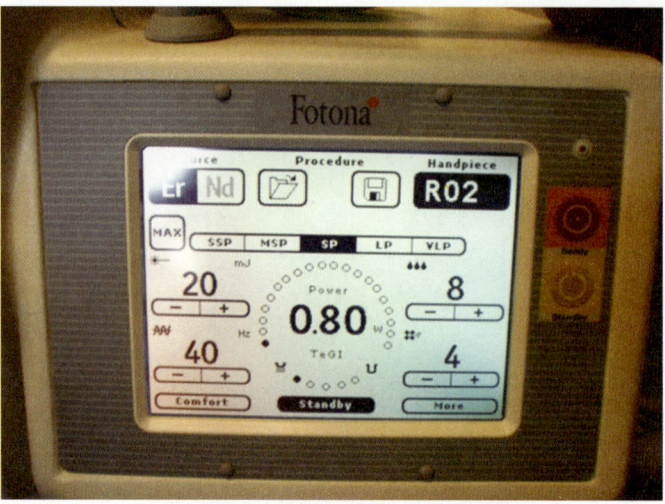

Fig. 31.6B: Er: YAG Laser unit (screen)

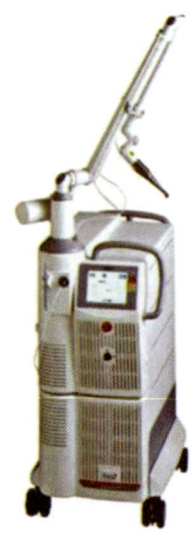

Fig. 31.6A: Er: YAG Laser unit

Laser in Operative Dentistry

Table 31.2: Laser type, wavelength and their clinical potential

Medium	Wavelength (nm)	Enamel characteristics	Clinical Potential
CO_2	10,600	• Surface fusion • Roughness • Partially fused crystallizes • Charring • Cracking	• Resin bonding • Enamel etching • Caries reduction
Er:YAG	2,900	• Etched, scaly or flacky, rough surface	• Cavitation • Enamel etching
Nd:YAG	1,064	• Reflection of beam is seen, until photoabsorptive is placed	• Decay removal • Etching
Ruby	693	• Cratering • Irregular cavitated surface, charring	• Resin polymerization
Argon	514	• Reflection of beam produces minimal effect on surface	
ArF	193	• Slight etching, smooth, lacking in charring, planed enamel prisms	• Cavitation • Enamel etching

substances from enamel might have caused formation of micropores.

The micropores were thought to act as sites for deposition of ions released by an acid attack. During the treatment with lactate buffer, acid solution penetrates the enamel and Ca^{2+} ions are released by acid decalcification. In unlased enamel, released ions diffuse to the surrounding surface.

On the other hand in lased enamel, some of released ions would be trapped in microspaces which lead to remineralization which is responsible for changes of birefringence.

It is now established that Laser act in the following ways:

- The enamel surface gets sealed and becomes less permeable to diffusion by ions into and out of enamel during demineralization.
- The composition of enamel is altered (reduced carbonate content of apatite crystals), which reduces its solubility and permeability.

The application of Laser is most effective when the emitted Laser light is matched to the absorption of target tissue. The degree of difference between these two wavelengths determine the amount of Laser energy, i.e. reflected or absorbed into the target tissue; for example, when applied to enamel and dentin, treatment of tooth is different. Enamel and dentin have different peak absorption values of 9.6 µm and 2.9 µm respectively. As a result, no single Laser has proven fully versatile when applied to oral tissues.

Unfortunately, commercial available Lasers operate at one predetermined wavelength that cannot be changed to accommodate the absorption values of treated teeth. The transmission wavelength of Er:YAG Laser is equal to absorption of water (2.94 µm). The new generation laser (Mark III Free Electron Laser (FEL) can be adjusted in the range of 1.4–10 µm which enhances its application in medical treatment.

Cavity Preparation

CO_2 Laser has been successfully used to remove carious dentin without damage to pulp.

Nd:YAG Laser is being used to remove caries. A small amount of Laser initiatior was applied to enamel to facilitate absorption of laser energy. The patient feels slightly warm sensation.

Usually Lasers when used for operative cavity preparations produced too much heat, melted the enamel and damaged the pulp.

When dentition is vaporized by Laser, its surface becomes darkened by carbonization. This can be easily removed by applying a steady stream of water while simultaneously lasing the area.

Advantages

- Laser induced analgesia (No need for local anaesthesia).
- Less post-operative sensitivity because dentin may be fused.
- Access to subgingival caries is greatly improved since Lasers vaporize gingival tissues.

Due to alteration of surface structure, the lased tooth becomes resistant to decay. In case of root caries, the placement of restorative material may not be necessary after Laser application.

The Er:YAG laser has shown more promising results. It is absorbed by water and hydroxyapatite, which partially accounts for its efficiency in cutting enamel and dentin.

It has also been suggested that laser is pulsed at intervals that are shorter than the stimulation period required to trigger nerve pulse transmission. When cutting the vital tooth, it can be lased for about 10 seconds and after that cutting or cavity preparation can be carried out without discomfort (Figs 31.7A, B, and C).

Cozean, et al (1997) reported that Er:YAG laser was equivalent to high speed drill in its ability to make cavity preparations in enamel and dentin. The procedure can be carried out without anaesthesia.

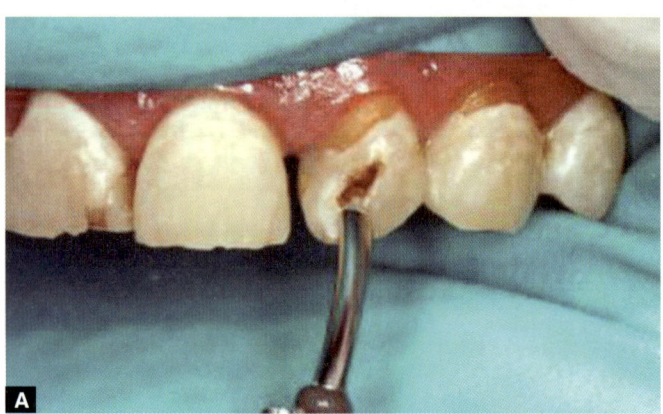
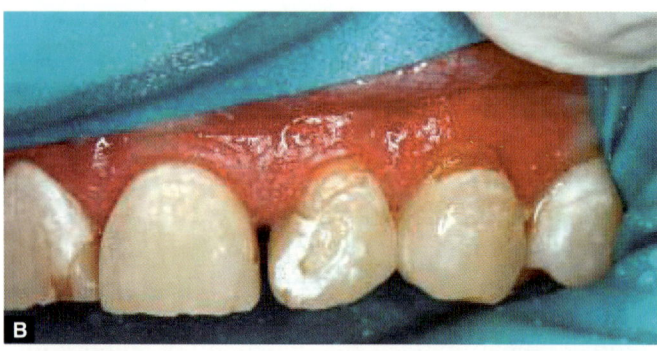
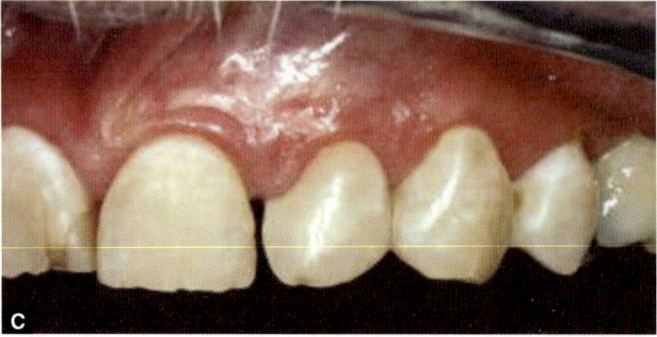

Figs 31.7A, B, and C: Cavity preparation with Laser: (A) Cavity preparation on maxillary lateral incisor using Er:Yag Laser; (B) Prepared cavity; (C) Restored cavity

Caries Detection

It is established that intact enamel is luminous when exposed to Argon Laser at a wavelength of 488 nm. The carious lesions appear as dark areas. Proximate lesions between contacting teeth may be visualized using Laser before demineralization could be evident on radiographs.

Diagnodent is a low pulsed caries detector. It exhibits 90% accuracy in diagnosing caries as compared with conventional diagnostic modalities. This device also has limitations because depth of penetration of light is limited to about 2.0 mm. Another drawback is that it only detects occlusal lesion and cannot identify interproximal lesions.

Etching/Conditioning

CO_2 and Nd:YAG Laser are being used for etching of enamel. CO_2 laser is preferred because of its favourable absorption characteristics in dental hard tissue (Fig. 31.8).

In addition, CO_2 laser can be placed at localized area when used with appropriate delivery system. This results in etching to a specific area of enamel, whereas acid gels usually overextend the area.

A black dye is placed on enamel surface to increase absorption of Laser beam. Total clinical time is reduced (seven seconds for conditioning and fifteen seconds for acid etching) as there is no need of washing or drying.

Curing of Composites

Lasers have been used to cure composites. The Laser used is Argon with a wavelength of 488 nm. This is near the wavelength of initiator used (comphoroquinone) in composite resins.

Advantages
• Shorter curing time
• Better physical properties
• Increased depth of cure
• Better polymerization
• Reduced polymerization shrinkage

Dentin Bonding

It is established that dentinal bonding is substantially increased (upto 300%) if the dentin is pretreated with a pulsed CO_2 laser prior to bonding. Improved dentin-bonding with Argon or Nd:YAG Lasers has also been reported. The enamel surface to receive composite can first be Laser etched to provide enamel the desired roughness. After restoration, the restoration-tooth

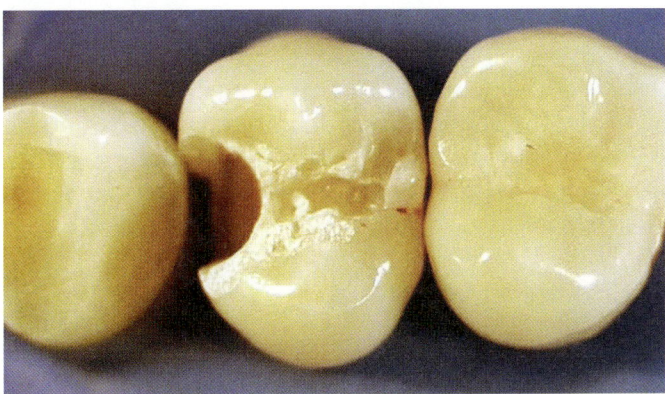

Fig. 31.8: Etching with Laser

interface is Laser treated to reduce the marginal gap, subsequently the recurrent caries.

Bleaching

Two types of Lasers are usually used:

The Argon Laser that emits a visible blue light and CO_2 Laser that emits invisible infrared light.

The Laser energy rapidly decompose H_2O_2 to O_2 and H_2O. Argon laser is best for removal of initial dark stains than CO_2 laser.

Dentin Hypersensitivity

The advent of Lasers has provided another possible treatment option for dentin hypersensitivity (Fig. 31.9).

The various types of Lasers used are

- CO_2 Laser
- Nd:YAG Laser
- Er:YAG Laser
- He:Ne Laser

Lasers occlude the dentinal tubules by producing local changes around the exposed dentin and also produce changes in the central pulp neuron

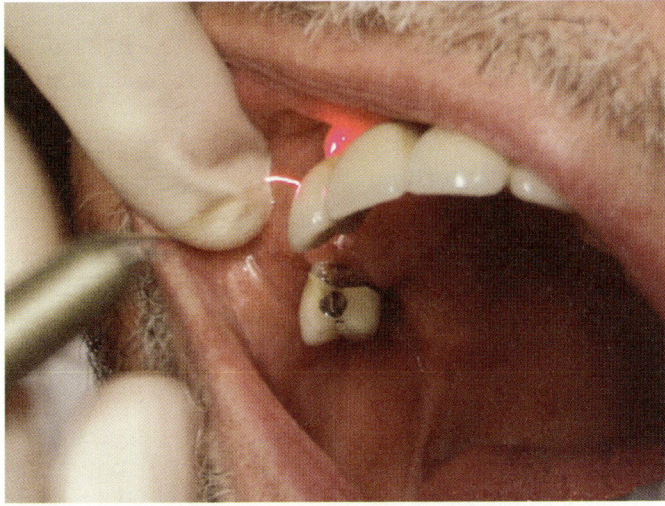

Fig. 31.9: Densensitization using Laser

Miscellaneous

Laser can be used in variety of other fields such as:

i. Nd:YAG Laser is widely used for welding
ii. CO_2, Nd:YAG, Argon Laser can be used to sterilize dental instruments and to kill bacteria on culture media, glass slides, etc.
iii. Exposure of dentin to Laser leads to activation of dentinogenesis.
iv. Laser can produce 3-D images of objects. These images are called holograms. The study casts, etc. can be saved as holograms. The three dimensional co-ordinates of a crown can be relayed to a computer, which controls a milling machine designed to produce the final restoration.
v. The cavity treated with laser offers better adaptation of glass-ionomer cements.
vi. Laser produces effective analgesia and has replaced the need for local anaesthesia.
vii. Laser is effective in soft tissue management during cavity and crown preparations.
viii. Effective in detecting vertical root fractures.

EXCIMER LASER

The following limitation of CO_2 and Nd:YAG Laser led to the development of Excimer laser.

- Vaporization and carbonization of dental tissue.
- Thermal side effect, which may damage pulp and periodontal tissue (Temperature may rise up to 65°C).
- Caries removal leads to structural changes such as cracks, zones of necrosis, etc.

Excimers work by the process of ablative photo decomposition, which implies bond breaking of molecules with minimal thermal side effects (Temperature increase is approximately 12°C). Residual energy is converted into kinetic energy by expansion of residual gaseous phase. Excimers are emitted in UV spectral range.

The available Excimers are:

ArF	-	193 nm
KrF	-	248 nm
XeCl	-	308 nm
XeF	-	351 nm

Argon-fluorine Excimer laser has the following advantages:

- Thermal effects are minimal (The temperature rise of pulp was 5°C).
- Prepare cavities in dental hard tissue without side effects.
- It has bacteriological effect on prepared surface.

- The possibility of tissue identification during the treatment process in selective removal of affected tissues.
- The zone of necrosis is small so there is no residual debris.
- The experiments have observed no carcinogenic effect.

Disadvantage
- Expensive

LASER HAZARDS

The beneficial effects of Lasers have been accepted in day-to-day practice; however, continuous use may have certain hazards. The hazards can be:

a. Effect on eyes
b. Effect on skin and other tissues
c. Environmental hazards
d. Electrical hazards

a. Effect on Eyes

Potential injury to the eye can occur either by direct emission from Laser or by reflection from a specular surface. The primary ocular injury that may result from a Laser accident is a retinal or corneal damage. Retinal injury is possible with emissions in the visible (400–780 nm) and near infrared (780–1400 nm) wavelengths. It may cause 'scotoma' (loss of vision in the path of visual field; blind spot).

b. Effect on Skin and other Tissues

Laser may damage skin and other tissues as a result from thermal interaction of radiant energy with tissue proteins. Temperature elevation of 21°C above normal body temperature can produce cell destruction by denaturation of cellular enzyme and structural proteins, which interrupts basic metabolic processes.

Factors affecting laser-tissue interaction are:
- The relative absorption and transmission of particular wavelength.
- The pulse duration and pulse repetition rate.
- The level of radiation exposure.
- The relative degree of vascularity of tissue.

The deleterious effects of Lasers on enamel and dentin are:
- Enamel exhibits gross cratering from 0.1–1.1 mm deep depending on amount of energy delivered to target area. In deeper penetration, dark speckling of exposed dentin can be seen. Examination under polarized light may show crystallographic changes.
- Dentin shows shallow, irregular craters 0.1 mm deep. Three distinct zones of dentinal destruction are: central zone of complete dentinal destruction; an immediate surrounding area of partial dentinal destruction and a scattered zone of dark speckling beyond first two zones.

c. Environmental Hazards

Inhaled air borne contaminants can be emitted in the form of smoke or fume generated through thermal interaction of Laser with tissue or through accidental escape of toxic chemical and gases from Laser itself. These damage the functioning of respiratory system.

d. Electrical Hazards

Because Laser use high currents and high voltage power supplies, these are potentially hazardous. Electrical hazards of Lasers can be grouped as electrical shock hazards, electrical fire hazards or explosion hazards.

Laser Safety

American National Standard Institute (ANSI) has classified Lasers on their safety parameters.

- Class I denotes Laser system, which under normal conditions do not pose hazard.
- Class II denotes low power visible Laser system, they usually do not present hazard; but may have potential for hazard, if viewed directly or extended period of time.
- Class III (a) denotes Laser system having 'caution' label that normally would not injure the eye if viewed momentarily; but present hazard if viewed using collecting optics.
- Class III(b) denotes Laser system that is hazardous, if viewed directly.
- Class IV denotes Laser system that is hazardous not only from direct reflection, but also produce significant skin hazards, etc.

ANSI has specified 'Maximum Permissible Exposure', i.e. the level of radiation to which a person may be exposed without hazardous effects on adverse biologic changes. In some applications open beams are required making it necessary to define an area of potentially hazardous laser radiation. This is Normal Hazard Zone (NHZ) which is defined as a space within which the level of direct, scattered or reflected laser exceeds the MPE.

The safety requirements include:
- A Laser warning signal outside the clinic.
- Use of barriers within the operatory.

- Use of eyewear to protect against reflected Laser light or accidental direct exposure.
- The residue left after tissue ablation should be evacuated using high volume suction.
- Equipment should be serviced and checked regularly.
- The operator should take adequate precautions to prevent injury or damage to adjacent soft and hard tissue or to the pulp and periodontal apparatus.

BIBLIOGRAPHY

1. Attrill, D.C., Davies, R.M. and King, T.A.: Thermal effects of Er:YAG laser on simulated dental pulp: a quantitative evaluation of effects of water spray. J. Dent.: 32, 35, 2004.
2. Cankat Kara and Recep Orbak: Comparative evaluation of Nd:YAG laser and fluoride varnish for treatment of dentin hypersensitivity. J. Endod.: 35, 971, 2009.
3. Corona, S.A., Borsatto, M. and Dibb, R.G., et al: Microleakage of class V resin composite restoration after bur, air-abrasion or Er:YAG Laser preparation. Oper. Dent.: 26, 491, 2001.
4. Evans, D.J., Matthews, S. and Pitts, N.B., et al: A clinical evaluation of an Er: YAG Laser for dental cavity preparation. Br. Dent. J.: 188, 677, 2000.
5. Hibst, R.: Lasers for caries removal and cavity preparation: state of art and future directions. J. Oral Laser Applications: 2, 203, 2002.
6. Hibst, R., Paulus, R. and Lussi, A.: Detection of occlusal caries by Laser fluorescence. Basic and clinical investigations. Med. Las. App.: 16, 205, 2001.
7. Kimura, Y., Tanabe, M., Amano, Y., Kinoshita, J., Yamada, Y. and Masuda, Y.: Basic study of the use of Laser on detection of vertical root fracture. J. Dent.: 37, 909, 2009.
8. Linc, C.H., Chou, T.M. and Chen, J.H.: Evaluation of effect of laser tooth whitening. Int. J. Prosthodont.: 21, 415, 2008.
9. Lussi, A., Imwinkelried,S., Pitts, N.B., Longbottom, C. and Reich, E.: Performance and reproducibility of a Laser fluorescence system for detection of occlusal caries in vitro. Caries Research: 33, 261, 1999.
10. Marcelo Thorne Schein, Bocangel, J.S. and Nogueria, G.E.C.: SEM evaluation of interaction pattern between dentin and resin after cavity preparation using Er:YAG laser. J. Dent.: 31, 127, 2003.
11. Marchesan, M.A., et al: Effects of 980-nanometer diode laser on root canal permeability after dentin treatment with different chemical solutions. J. Endod.: 34, 721, 2008.
12. Mat, S.: Expanding Laser application – faster technological evolution. Photonics Spectra: 1, 102, 1991.
13. Powell, G.L. and Blankenau, R.J.: Laser curing of dental materials. J. Oral Laser Appliactions: 1, 7, 2001.
14. Rodriguesa, L.K.A., Santos, M.N., Pereira, D., Assaf, A.V. and Pardi, V.: Carbon dioxide Laser in dental caries prevention. J. Dent.: 32, 531, 2004.
15. Roy George: Lasers in dentistry – Review. Int. J. Dent. Clinics.: 1, 13, 2009.
16. Schwartz, F., Arweiler, N. and Georg, T., et al: Desensitizing effect of an Er:YAG Laser on hypersensitive dentine. J. Clin. Periodontology: 29, 211, 2002.
17. Schwass D, Leichter W.: Evaluating the efficiency of caries removal using an Er:YAG laser driven by fluorescence feedback control. Archives of oral biology 58, 6, 2013.
18. Walsh, L.J.: The current status of low level laser therapy in dentistry Part I. Soft tissue applications. Aust. Dent. J.: 42, 247, 1997.
19. Walsh, L.J.: The current status of low level laser therapy in dentistry Part 2. Soft tissue applications. Aust. Dent. J.: 42, 302, 1997.
20. Wang Hong Lan, Bor Shiunn Lee, Hsin Cheng Liu: Morphological study of Nd:YAG laser usage in treatment of dentinal hypersensitivity. J. Endod.: 30, 131, 2004.

Appendix

Table of Weights and Measure

Length

1 milimeter (mm)	=	0.001 meter
1 centimeter (cm)	=	0.01 meter
1 yard (yd)	=	0.9144 meter
1 inch (in)	=	2.54 centimeters
1 micrometer (mm)	=	0.001 milimeter
1 micrometer (mm)	=	10,000 Angstrom units
1 Angstrom unit (Å)	=	0.1 nanometer

Weight

1 miligram (mg)	=	0.001 gram
1 gram (gm)	=	0.0022 pound
1 gram (gm)	=	0.035 ounce
1 kilogram (kg)	=	1000 grams
1 ounce (oz)	=	28.35 grams
1 pound (ib)	=	453.59 grams
1 grain	=	0.0645 gram
1 Newton	=	0.2248 pound = 0.102 kg
1 dyne	=	0.00102 gram

Capacity (liquid)

1 mililiter	=	1 cubic centimeter
1 liter (I)	=	1000 cubic centimeters
1 quart (qt)	=	0.946 liter
1 ounce (oz)	=	29.6 milimeters
1 cubic foot (cu ft)	=	28.32 liters

Conversion factors (linear)

	Mm	cm
1 Angstrom unit (Å)	0.0000001	0.00000001
1 nanometer (nm)	0.000001	0.0000001
1 micrometer (mm)	0.001	0.0001

Conversion factor (force per area)

- To change kilograms per square centimeter (kg/cm^2) to pounds per square inch (ib/in^2), multiply by 14.223 (1 kg/cm^2 = 14.223 ib/in^2).
- To change pounds kilograms per square centimeter (kg/cm^2) to megapascals (Mpa), multiply by 0.0981 (1 kg/cm$_2$ = 0.0981 Mpa). Note 1 MN/m^2 = 1 Mpa.
- To chage pounds per suqre inch (ib/in^2) to kilograms per centimeter (kg/cm^2), multiply by 0.070307 (1 ib/in = 0.0703 kg/cm^2).
- To chage meganewtons per squre meter (MN/m^2) to giganewtons per squre meter (GN/m^2), divide by 1000, = 1.273 kg/cm^2 = 18.22 ib/in ^{2}.

From	To	Multiply by
psi	Mpa (MN/m^2)	0.006895
psi	kg/cm^2	0.0703
kg/cm^2	Mpa (MN/m^2)	0.09807
kg/cm^2	psi	14.2233
MN/m^2	psi	145.0
MN/m^2	kg/cm^2	10.1968

Conversion of thermometer scales

- Temperature Fahrenheit (°F) = 9/5 Temperature Celsius + 32°
- Temperature Celsius (°C) = 5/9 Temperature Fahrenheit − 32° or (°C × 1.8) + 32 = °F

$$\frac{°F - 32°}{1.8} = °C$$

Index

A
Abfraction 12, 541
Abrasion 12, 533
Abrasive cutting 125
Abrasive efficiency 124
Abrasive instruments 123, 124
Abrasive materials 481
Absorbent pads/wafers 163, 170
Accelerator 365
Acetone 346
Acetylene 277
Acid conditioners 341, 355, 365
Acid etching 380
Acid-base reaction 406
Acidogenic theory 65
Acute caries 12
Acute trauma from occlusion 90
Addition silicones 259
Additive colour theory 608
Add-on porcelain 442
Adherend 335
Adhesion 335, 496
Admixed/Blended alloy 212
Advanced/cavitated caries 12
Affected and infected dentin 12
Air abrasion 428
Air driven handpieces 116
Air firing procedure 441
Air indexing method 573
Air pressure casting machine 274
Air pressure 509
Alban test 88
Alcohol flame 318
All ceramic systems 447
Alloy mercury reaction 213
Aluminium chloride 175
Aluminium or copper collars 158
Aluminium oxide 365
Aluminosilicates 364
Aluminous porcelain (Hi Ceram) 443
Amalgam blues 251
Amalgam bonding agents 500
Amalgam dies 265
Amalgam knives 114
Amalgam pledge 3
Amalgapins 290
Amelogenesis imperfecta 12
Amide resins 422
Ammonium bifluoride 506
Analogous systems 463
Anatomic matrix 157
Anatomic tooth root 10
Anatomical tooth crown 10
Angle former 111
Annealing 315, 317
Anorexia nervosa 537
Anti sialogogues 163
Antibacterial composites 367
Anti-cariogenicity 408
Argon 641
Arkansas stones 115
Army system (nomenclature) 89
Arrested caries 64, 75
ART (Atraumatic Restorative Treatment) 404, 426
Art glass 394
Articulating papers 39
Articulator 31, 33
Asbestos 272
ASPA 417
Astringents and styptics 174
Attrition 12, 561, 530
Autoclave 135
Autoglazing 438, 509
Automatrix 160
Auto-mix technique 260
Auxiliary slice 255
Axial line angle 17

B
Back pressure porosity 280
Balanced occlusion 23
Bandlish theory 69
Base metal 244
Bases 186
Basic fuschin 175
Beaver tail burnisher 325, 328
Beilby layer 476
Belleglass HP 394
Belt driven handpieces 116
Bennett shift 29
Benzoin methyl ether 365
Benzoyl peroxide 365
Beta propiolactone 140
Beta quartz glass inserts 503
Bevels 17, 254, 375, 377, 390, 400

Bilateral balanced occlusion 30
Bilayered/sandwich restorations 421
Bio corrosion 541
Biocompatibility 514
Biological width 53
Biomaterial 514
BisGMA 360, 374
Bisque 447
Bite-fork 47
Bite-wing radiography 94
Black's classification 19
Blade angle 109, 121
Blade/Nib 109
Bladed cutting 125
Bleaching 620
Blebs 439
Body dentin colour 613
Body of the lesion 22
Bonded amalgam restorations 226, 235
Bonding 335
Boric oxide 436, 443
Boron carbide 481, 527
Borosilicates 364
Bosworth system (nomenclature) 8, 9
Box preparation 255
Box's classification of occlusion 90
Brilliant blue 103
Broken arm principle 275
Bruxism 531, 541
Buccal corridor 595
Buffing 476
Bulimia 535
Bulk annealing 318
Bur sizes, shape and design 119, 120
Burlew's wheel 491
Burnishing 230, 477
Burnout procedure 277

C
CAD-CAM technology 463, 493
Calcifications 560
Calcium hydroxide 5, 87, 208
Canine and incisor guidance 29
Canine guidance 32
Canine protected occlusion 30
Carbon dioxide snow 82
Carbon steel 108

Carbonized gold foil 316
Carborundum disc 290
Caries activity tests 86
Caries control 546
Caries of cementum 75
Caries of dentin 75
Caries of enamel 74
Caries risk assessment and susceptibility 84
Casein derivatives 425
Casein deviation 578
Cast gold pins 289
Castable apatite ceramic (Cera Pearl) 462
Castable glass ceramic (Dicor) 453, 468
Casting defects 280
Casting machines 268
Casting procedures 244
Casting techniques 277
Cavit 202
Cavitated caries 10
Cavities on the incisal and cusp tips 22
Cavity preparation 13, 214
Cavity varnish 188
Cavosurface angle 17
Celay 456, 472, 493, 543
Celluloid or plastic wedges 153, 154
Cellulose liners 272
Cellulose wafers 169
Cemented pins 287
Cemento-enamel junction 54
Centric holding cusps 31
Centric occlusion 26
Centric relation 25
Centric stop 38
Centrix syringe 415
Ceramic fibers 366
Ceramic liners 276
Ceramming 447
Cerec vitablocs Mark 449
Cerec vitablocs Mark II 449
Cerec 493
Ceromatic II 463
Cervical lesions 532
Cervicoincisal location of contact areas 55
Chameleon effect 448
Chamfer 252
Chamois wheel 490
Cheek and lip retractors 173
Chelators 342
Chemical adhesion 335
Chemical conditioning 342
Chemical tracers 508
Chemical/Parasitic theory 65
Chip spaces 120
Chisels 111
Chlorhexidine 367
Cholesteric liquid crystals 84
Chroma 609
Chromic adaptation 605
Chronic caries 142, 581
Chronic trauma from occlusion 58

Circumferential tie 253
Circumferentially bevelled instruments 111
Citric acid 340
Class V cavity preparation (composite) 378
Classification of caries 9
Clearance angle and face 121
Cleoid discoid 111
Clinical tooth crown 10
Clinical tooth root 10
CO_2 laser 103, 641
Coagulation 175
Coated abrasives 476
Coated discs and strips 480
Coherent diffraction imaging 512
Cohesive gold 316, 318
Cold welding 315
Collagen smear layer 340
Color 604
Coloring agents 365
Coloring tints 391
Colour harmonies 607
Colour rendering index 615
Coltene brilliant system 394
Compaction technique for gold foil 332
Complex cavities 13
Compomers 368
Componeer 599
Composite inlay 393, 504
Composite laminates and veneers 390
Composition of alloy 211
Compound cavities 13
Computer image analysis 90, 96
Concentricity 122
Concrescence 81
Condensable composites 366
Condensation 233
Conditioners 341
Conditioning agents (GIC) 414
Condylar guidance 28
Cone-socket instrument 109
Configuration factor 373
Confocal laser SEM 512
Contact angle 336
Contacts 54
Contours 53
Contra-angling 111
Contributory factors in dental caries 71
Controlled water technique 278
Convenience form 185
Conventional cavity preparation 377
Conventional cured inlays 394
Conventional radiography 94
Copper bands 155
Copper plating 264
Copy milling 433, 463
Cords 174, 171
Corrugated foil 315, 316
Cosmetic contouring 596
Cotton pellets 164, 175
Cotton rolls and holder 163, 169, 173
Coupling agents 364
Cove 294
Cracked tooth syndrome 84

Crevicular epithelium 53
Critical pH 72
Cross linkage theory 557
Crosscuts 120
Crucible former 271
Crystalline gold 327
C-shaped defect 505, 534
Curve of Spee 29
Curve of Wilson 30
Cusher clamp 165
Cusp angle 40
Cusp capping 255
Custom trays 25
Cutting edge angle 109
Cutting effectiveness 121
Cutting operation 476
Cuttle fish bone 481
Cuttlefish finishing strip 484

D

Dahl concept 554
Dead tracts 559
Debonding 357
Deflective occlusal contacts 37, 38
Degassing 317
Delayed expansion 233
Demineralization 581
Dens in dente 81
Dental caries 63, 11
Dental cements 197, 199
Dental floss 165
Dental shade guides 613
Denticles 560
Dentin bonding 340
Dentin permeability 337, 341
Dentin substitute 404
Dentinal cracks 305
Dentinal sclerosis 558
Dentino-enamel junction 14
Dentinogenesis imperfecta 12
Dento-gingival unit 52
Desiccation 136, 175
Determinants of cusp heights and fossa depths 41
Determinants of intercuspation 41
Determinants of ridge and groove directions 42
Diagnosis 80
Diamond abrasive instruments 486
Diamond hone 141
Diastema 597
Diazoresorcinol 87
Dicalcium phosphate dihydrate 351
Dichloro-difluoro methane 562
Dicor MGC 449
Die spacer 264
Die 263
Diffuse reflection 603
Diffusible gas firing 442
Digital imaging 100
Digital subtraction radiography 90
Digital systems 463
Dimethyl-p-toluidine 365
Direct filling gold 324
Direct neural stimulation 570

Index

Direct pins 287
Discoid 137
Discoloration 620
Dispensing of alloy and mercury 227
Dispensing of powder and liquid (GIC) 415
Dispersion strengthening 43
Disposable diamond abrasives 124
Ditching 458
Divergent box 534
Double-planed instruments 110
Dovetail 250
Dowel pin system 262
Drill breakage 304
Dry brush technique 440
Dual cure composite 395
Duceram LFC 443
Dye enhanced laser fluorescence 100
Dye penetration method 103, 507
Dyes 103, 507

E

Edge enhancement 96
EDTA 356
Effect of dentifrices 534
Elastic bonding 358
Elastic compression 183
Electralloy 317
Electric annealers 318
Electric malleting 320
Electric pulp testing 83
Electrical resistance 97
Electroformed dies 264
Electrolytic precipitated gold 315, 317
Electron clouds 335
Electronic caries monitor 8
Elliot separator 156
Embrasures/Spillways 55
Enamel colour 612
Enamel hatchet 112, 113
Enamel hypoplasia 12
Enameloplasty 180
Endoscope/Videoscope 102
Endoscopy 102
Epoxy resin dies 266
Epoxy resins 365, 368, 369
Er.YAG 641
Erosion method 464
Erosion 12, 532
Esthetics 590
Etchants 337
Etching 176
Ethanol 346
Ethics 600
Ethyl chloride 62
Etiology of dental caries 65
Evacuation systems 170
Excavators 111
Excimer laser 645
Expanding matrix resins 368
Extension for prevention 177, 179
External outline form 177
Extracoronal cavity preparation 13
Extra retentive devices 285

F

Fabrication of tray 259
Failures in composite restorations 387
Failures of dental amalgam 230
Faulty cavity preparation 230
Faulty contacts 44
FDI System 9
Feldspar 435
Feldspathic porcelains 435
Ferrier double-bow 153
Ferrier's design 326, 329
Fiberoptic transillumination 100
Field emission SEM 512
Fillers 364
Final cavity preparation 188
Finishing and carving 230
Finishing and polishing 476
Finishing burs 479
Finishing knives 114
Firing procedure 441
Flowable composites 365
Fluorescence 607
Fluorescent microscopy 509
Fluoridated cements 206
Fluoride in glass ionomer 408
Fluorosis 82
Flute 120
Flux 276
FNP system 346
Foci of necrosis 518
Foil 330
Food impaction 54, 61
Forces acting on the tooth 190
Fracture lines 246
Free gingival margin 53
Free radicals 365
Friction locked pins 289
Frozen slab method 196
Fulgration 175
Full veneer crown 245
Functional occlusion 23, 24

G

Gait 80
Gallium alloys 500
Galvanic deterioration of amalgam 247
Galvanism 233
Gamma-2 free amalgams 234
Gap grading system 445
Garnet 480
Gas inclusion porosity 283
Gastro-eosophageal reflux disease 538
Gear driven handpiece 142
Gel etchant 352
Geometry of the tooth preparation 250
Geriatric caries 11
Geriatric dentistry 556
Gerontology 557
Gingival bevels 253
Gingival crevice 82
Gingival enlargement 91
Gingival margin trimmer 137
Gingival recession 91, 564

Glass cermets 422
Glass formers 439
Glass ionomer bonding agents 559
Glass modifiers 440
Glazes 442
Glenoid fossa 50, 29
Gold alloy 244
Gold beating 315
Gold calcium alloy 317
Gold foil 330
Gold knife 330
Golden mean 590
Golden percentage 591
Golden proportion 591
Goldent 325, 328
Grinder's disease 526
Grooves 184, 285
Grooving 62
Group function guidance 30
Group function occlusion 30
Guards 115
Guidance of occlusion 23
Guiding cusps 25
Guiding inclines 23
Gutta percha 196, 197
Gypsum 263

H

Haderup's system 8
Hall technique 427
Hand condensation 320, 229
Hand cutting instruments 108
Hand lasers 640
Hand malleting 320
Hand trituration 227
Handle or shaft 109
Hatchets 111
Heat generation 305
Heat tests 61
Heat treatment of steel 108
Height of epithelial attachment 154
HEMA 356, 360
High fusing porcelains 440
Hoe chisel 111
Hollenback carver 112
Homogenization heat treatment 206
Horizontal relations 42
Host defense factors 553
Hotsalt sterilizer 133
Hot air oven 133
Hot spot 286
Hue 490
Hybrid layer 354, 357, 362
Hybridoid regions 367
Hydrochloric acid 259
hydrodynamic theory 571
Hydrofluoric acid 467
Hydrogen bonds 356, 385
Hydrothermal low fusing ceramic 450
Hygroscopic expansion technique 281
Hyper cementosis 560
Hyper occlusion 231
Hyper sensitivity 534, 570
Hypocalcification 12

I

Ideal occlusion 24
Illumination 391
Illusion 391
Impression tray 261
Incipient caries 10, 117, 118
Incisal guidance 39
Inclined planes 177
Increment placement for composites 382, 387
Indirect acrylic restorations 201
Indirect pins 289
Indirect pulp capping 175
Indirect veneers 392
Infilterable ceramic/High alumina ceramic (in ceram) 443, 446
Ingraham design 329
Initiator 365
Injection moulded glass ceramic 446
Inlay taper 249
Inlay 245
In-office bleaching 622
Instrument design 111
Instrument formula 110
Instrument grasps 114
Instrument nomenclature 110
Interceptive contacts 94
Inter-condylar distance 39
Intercuspal contact position (ICP) 37
Intermediate oxides 441
Internal outline form 167, 248
Interpin distance 299
Inter-proximal finishing strips 484
Interruption of crack propagation 444
Intracoronal cavity preparation 121
Intra-oral periapical radiography 70
Intratubular penetration 357
Intrinsic discoloration 620
Inverted bevel 125, 254
Inverted pen grasp 140
Iodine penetration method 78
Ion leachable glass 418
Irreversible pulpitis 63
Isolation from moisture 163
Isolation from the soft tissues 173
Itaconic acid 405
Ivory matrix holder 159

J

Junctional epithelium 53

K

Kaolin 435
Kieselguhr 481
Knives 111
Kulzer inlay system 394

L

Lab system 611
Lack of maintaining contact 388
Lactobacillus count test 87
Lamina dura 61
Lamina propria 52
Laminate technique 420
Laminated foil 315
Laminated gold foil 316
Land 121
Lanthanum fluoride 394
Laser auto fluorescence 100
Laser curing 372
Laser emission modes 639
Laser etching 340
Laser hazards 646
Laser microspectral analysis 510
Lasers 340
Latent erosion 541
Lateral cutting instruments 135
Lateral functional occlusion 24
Lateral non-functional occlusion 25
Layering techniques 598
Leucite reinforced hot pressed glass ceramic 435
Leucite reinforced porcelain (Optec HSP) 445
Leucite 435
Levine's theory 69
Light cure calcium hydroxide 208
Light cure glass ionomers 410
Light curing units 370
Light scattering 604
Lighting of the operatory 615
Line angle 17
Liner 198
Lingual dove tail 223
Liquefying bath 261
Localized shrinkage porosity 280
Location of lightening 495
Locks or partial vertical grooves 283
Loma linda design 329
Long bevel 249
Long centric 26
Loose pins 304
Lubricant 166
Lumineer 599

M

Machinable ceramic 449
Machined ceramic inlays 463
Macro abrasion 477
Macrotags 338
Macula lutea 605
Maleic acid 405
Manifest erosion 541
Manufacturing of alloy 213
Marginal discolouration 496
Marginal fracture 230
Marginal ridge 55
Margins 56
Mat foil 317
Mat gold 315
Matrices 154
Matrix retainers 158
Mechanical adhesion 348
Mechanical condensation 236
Mechanical retainers 159
Mechanism of dentin bonding 340
Mega fillers 503
Mercury allergy 241
Mercury alloy ratio 232
Mercury concentration in urine and blood 241
Mercury exposure 241
Mercury management 240
Mercury sniffer 241
Mercury toxicity 241
Mercury vapour 483
Metamerism 606
Mica trays 318
Micro abrasion 477
Micro abrasion assisted bleaching 624
Micro etching 466
Micro porosity 280
Microbial plaque 52
Microleakage coefficient 510
Microleakage 495
Microradiography 545
Microtags 340
Microwave sterilization 134
Minibox preparation 428
Minikin pins 289
Minim pins 289
Minimal intervention dentistry 226, 423
Minuta pins 289
Miracle mix 409
Modelling compound 259
Modification of the cervical cavities 388
Modified flare preparation 255
Modified zinc oxide eugenol cement 198
Monel metal 109
Monitoring mercury levels 241
Morphologic occlusion 23
Mount classification 2
MTA 587
Mulling 225
Munsell colour system 608

N

Nanoleakage 511
Natural gas 277
Navy system (nomenclature) 115
Nd:YAG 641
Neutron activation analysis 508
Nib 109
Nichrome 109
Night guard vital bleaching 624
Nitrocellulose 424
Non critical items 130
Non functional occlusion 25
Non parallel pins 287
Non physiologic occlusion 25
Non-cohesive form of gold 317
Non-interfering true separator 153
Non-supporting cusps 26
Non-thermocatalytic bleaching 624
Non-vital bleaching 627
Notched defects 534
Notched effect 448
NovaMin 425, 578
NPG-GMA 359
NTG-GMA 363

Index

Nygaard ostby frame 165
Nystrom's retainer 159

O

Occlusal adjustment 59
Occlusal disharmony 59
Occlusal radiographs 70
Occlusal records 50
Occlusal reduction 46
Occlusal schemes 37
Occlusal table 44
Occlusal wear 49
Odontoblast deformation theory 570
Oligodynamic action 367, 392
Onlay 245, 255
Opacity 604
Opaquer 390
Optics of natural teeth 612
Optidam 167
Optradam 166
Organic silanes 365
Ormocer 368
Outer barrier 76
Outer lesion 78, 566
Outline form 177, 221, 247
Overbite 26
Overglazing 492
Overjet 26
Over-wetting phenomenon 354

P

Packable composites 366
Packaging 131
Pain perception 510
Palm and thumb grasp 115
Palmer's notation 7
Panoramic radiographs 81, 94
Parafunctional forces 541
Parallel pins 287
Parallelogram condensers 320, 325
Parasite theory 65
Pasteurization 134
Pellets 315
Pellicle 337
Pen grasp 114
Peracetic acid 139
Perception of colour 605
Perforation 287, 292
Performic acid 140
Pericementitis 59
Periodontal abscess 59
Personal barrier tech 195
Phenols 139
Phosphate bonding systems 344
Phosphoric acid 337
Phosphorous oxychloride 346
Physical adhesion 335
Physiological occlusion 90
Physiological xerostomia 19
Pickling 279
Piece method 318
Pilot holes 295
Pin amalgam foundation 299
Pin bending 296
Pin breakage 304

Pin channels 285
Pin diameter 294
Pin fractures 307
Pin ledge casting 308
Pin length 295
Pin number 292
Pin orientation 303
Pin placement 297
Pin removal 296
Pin restoration surface 304
Pin site 292
Pin trimming 296
Pin 185
Pinhole porosity 280
Pinholes 295
Pioneer bacteria 75
Pit and fissure caries 10, 63
Pit and fissure cavities 13
Plane of occlusion 29
Planning the cavity preparation 180
Plasma ster 140
Platinized foil 315
Platinum matrix adaptation 464
Plexus of Rashkow 63
Plunger cusps 32
Pneumatic malleting 320
Poded contacts 26
Point angle 17
Polarized light microscopy 545
Polyacid modified composite resins 410
Polyacrylic acid co-polymer 405
Polyacrylic acid 199
Polyacrylic gel 489
Polyalkenoate cement 206
Polycarbonate crowns 209
Polycarboxylate cement 404
Polyether material 261
Polymerization shrinkage 496
Polysulfide 260
Polytetra-fluoroethylene 336
Polyvinyl siloxane 260
Porcelain inlays 451
Porcelain laminates/veneers 466
Porosity 283, 446
Post carve burnishing 230, 524
Postholes 250
Powdered gold 317, 322
Pre-carve burnishing 230, 524
Prefabricated aluminium crowns 209
Prefabricated crowns 209
Prefabricated plastic matrices 157
Premature contacts 37, 93
Prepolymerised composite ball 503
Presoaking 130
Pressable ceramic 443
Pressed glass ceramic (IPS empress) 446
Preventive resin restoration 366
Prima 496
Primary caries 10
Primary flare 254
Primary resistance and retention form 181
Primers 342
Priming 342
PRIMM 366

Principle of laser 638
Proargin technology 577
Procion 77
Production of aerosol 483
Prophylactic odontotomy 127
Proportioning of alloy and mercury 227
Proteolysis chelation theory 66
Proteolytic theory 66
Protrusive functional occlusion 24
Protrusive non-functional occlusion 25
Proximal contact areas 54
Proximal contours 54
Pulp protection 186
Pulp vitality tests 84
Pulpal inflammation 518
Pulpal line angle 17
Pulpal pathology 496
Pulpal reaction 514
Pulpdentin organ 515
Pumice 481
Pure gold 314
Putty silicon technique 260
Pyroplastic flow 436

Q

Quartz 375, 440, 528
Quaternary alloys 212

R

Radial clearance 121
Radiation caries 64
Radioactive isotopes 508
Radiographic method 93
Radio-visio-graphy (RVG) 96
Rake angle 120, 121
Rake face 120, 121
Rampant caries 10, 19
Rapid or immediate separation 153
Rarefaction of bone 59
Recurrent caries 388
Red proportion 592
Reducing flux 276
Reference image 97
Reflection 603
Refractory dies 459
Removing carious dentin 177
Repair of defective restoration 223
Reparative dentin 582
Reservoir 260, 270
Residual caries 11
Residual compressive stresses 444
Resin interdiffusion zone 357
Resin matrix 374
Resin modified glass ionomer cements 500
Resin reinforced layer 343
Resin resorcinol 587
Resin tags 343
Resistance and retention form 181
Rests 149
Retina 605
Reverse bevel 249
Reverse curve 218
Reverse diffusion method 510
Reverse step 217

Reversible caries 11
Reversible hydrocolloid 261
Reversible pulpitis 63
Rods 605
Role of contact areas 54
Rolled cotton twills 163
Rolling 315
Root caries 9, 19, 71, 118
Ropes 315
Rotary instruments 115
Rouge 490
Rubber dam 163
Rubber dam application 167
Rubber dam armamentarium 163
Rubber dam clamps 164
Rubber dam holder 165
Rubber dam punch 165
Rubber dam retainer forcep 165
Rubber dam sheets 163
Rubber dam template/stamp 165
Run-out 122

S

Safe-T-frame 165
Saliva ejector 171
Salivary reductase test 87
Sandwich technique 421
Saucerized preparation 394
Scanning electron microscopy 509
Scanning probe microscope 545
Scanning tunneling microscope 545
Secondary caries/recurrent caries 11, 76
Secondary cured inlays 408
Secondary dentin 570
Secondary flare 248
Secondary reaction stage 406
Secondary retentive devices 183
Sectional matrix system 155
Selective interfacial amalgamation liner 235
Self etching/self priming agents 342
Self glazing 438
Self rewetting effect 353
Self sealing restoration 498
Semicohesive gold form 327
Semicritical items 130
Senescence 557
Senile caries 72
Shade indicator chart 616
Shade selection 606, 615
Shank 109, 117
Sharpening of instruments 115
Shear cusps 28
Sheets 315
Short bevel 187
Shoulder 41
Silica 435
Silicon carbide - Carborundum 481, 482
Silicophosphate cement dies 266
Silicosis 434
Silver amalgam 211
Silver cermet 405
Silver cyanide bath 265
Silver plating 265
Simple cavities 13
Single bevelled instruments 111
Single composition/All in one alloy 212
Single planed instrument 110
Sintering 440
Sjogren's syndrome 18
Skirt extensions 183
Slice preparation 255
Slide in centric 24
Slimming of a drill 295
Slip 439
Slots or horizontal grooves 183
Slow separation 152
Slump test 415
Smear layer 497
Smear plugs 497
Smear unit 337
Smile line 594
Smooth surface caries 11
Smooth surface cavities 121
Smudges 62
Snyder Test 87
Sodium diuranate 607
Sof-lex discs 488
Soft lasers 640
Soft start polymerization 503
Soft steel 108
Soft tin matrix 517
Sonotrodes 473
Spatulation method 440
Specificity 80
Spectrophotometer 615
Specular reflection 603
Speed ranges 117
Spherical eutectic 212
Spheroiding 62
Spinel 446
Spiral angle 122
Spiro orthocarbonates 368
Spoon excavator 111
Spratley blade carver 489
Spratley burnisher 477, 489
Sprue former attachment 271
Sprue former diameter 270
Sprue former length 270
Sprue former location 270
Sprue former material 269
Sprue former number 271
Sprue former 268
SR Isosit system 394
Stabilizing cord 163
Staining of porcelain 500
Stainless steel 108
Stains and colour modifiers 442
Stamp cusps 28
Starter gold 334
Static relationship 23
Steam cleaner 490
Steel squiveland self-adjusting matrix 159
Stein's knife 114
Stellite 109
Stepping 319, 321
Stereographic tracing 48
Sterilization of cavity walls 188
Sterilization 130
Sticky wax 268
Stillman's clefts 92
Stippling 92
Stock impression trays 259
Stomatognathic system 23
Stopping stick 61
Storage bath 261
Strain hardening 324
Strengthening dental porcelain 444
Streptococcus mutans 72
Stress concentration areas 444
Stress concentration 251
Strip technique 262
Stroboscopic light 394
Structure and function of eye 605
Study model 259
Subclass 110
Subgingival lesions 246
Suborder 110
Subsurface demineralisation 68
Subsurface porosity 280
Subtraction radiography 90
Subtractive colour theory 608
Sulphuric acid 339
Superdioxide water 140
Superficial inlays 394
Sunlight 136
Supporting cusps 26, 28
Surface energy 336, 340
Surface finish and texture 57
Surface irregularities 476
Surface layer 22
Surface profilometry 545
Surface protection 416
Surface temperature of a tooth 84
Surface wetting agent 260
Surfacine 139
Surgical means 176
Synthetic smear layer 498
Systemic theory 70

T

T Scan system 42
Tactile evidence of caries 69, 84
Tannic acid 175
Taper 249
Tarno 109
Tartaric acid 605
Teflon 366, 382
TEGDMA 374
Tempering bath 261
Temporizations 470
Terminal arc of closure 26
Terminal hinge axis 26
Ternary alloys 212
Tertiary amines 365
Tertiary dentin 558
Thermal conditioning 342
Thermal conductivity 314, 333
Thermal expansion technique 277
Thermal sensitivity 84
Thermal tests 84

Index

Thermodynamic equilibrium 213
Thielemann's formula 29
Threaded pins 289
Three increment design 382
Throat screens 170
Tiger clamp 164
Time temperature graph 65
Tin 211
Tissue coagulants 175
Titanium alloys 245
Titanium dioxide 365
TMS system 290
Tofflemire universal retainer 159
Toilet of the cavity 176
Tongue depressors 173
Tongue guards 173
Tooth flexure 543
Tooth fracture 60
Tooth guidance 25
Tooth separators 153
Topical application of fluoride 21
Torque 44
Traction principle 153
Transducer theory 570
Transferable records 46
Transillumination 103
Translation 29
Translucent zone 74
Transluncency 603
Transmission 603
Transparency 603
Transparent crown form matrices 157
Trauma from occlusion 57
Tray adhesives 260
Tri carballylic acid 405
Trial impression 252
Triple angle chisel 111
Triangular fossae 27
Tricalcium phosphate 425
Triclosan 367
Triple-bevelled instruments 111
Tripoli 481
Trituration 227
Tuckers technique 256
Tunnel restorations 427
Twin table technique 50

Twist drills 305
Two digit system 9

U

UDMA 374
Ultra short/partial bevel 17, 253
Ultrasonic cleaner 130
Ultrasonic condensation 228
Ultrasonic detection 90
Ultrasonic imaging 90
Ultraviolet illumination 100
Undercontoured restorations 54
Undercut concave (UC) 534
Unfilled resin 345
Universal system 8
Use of cavity liners and bases 504
UV light 365

V

Vacuum casting machine 275
Vacuum firing 441
Vacuum investing 274
Vacuum mixer 274
Value 609
Vander Waals forces 336
Vasoconstrictors 174
Venting 271
Vertical relations 41
Vertical/angular bone loss 92
Vibration method 441
Videoscope 102
Vimal Sikri classification 21, 22
Visio Gem 394
Vision 391
Visual examination 81
VITA shade guide 609
Vital tooth bleaching 622
Vitality 84
Vitrification 439
V-shaped defect 534

W

Wall lesion 78
Washer disinfector 131
Water bath technique 278
Water driven handpiece 116
Water tree 350

Water treeing phenomenon 359
Wax impressions 269
Wax pattern 267
Wedelstaedt chisel 111
Wedge principle 153
Wedges 159, 174, 201
Wedget 166
Wedging 194
Wet bonding 336, 356
Wet field technique 261
Wetting 351
Whipping method 440
White light endoscopy 102
Wide centric 26
Wilson's knife 114
Winged retainers 164
Wingless retainers 164
Woodbury design 329
Wooden wedges 161
Woodward's screw matrix 154
Work hardening 314
Working tooth guidance 29
Worm theory 65
Wrought precious metal pins 288

X

Xenon lamps 372
Xero radiography 95
Xerostomia 566

Y

Yitterbium trifluoride 364
Yttrium trifluoride 364
Young's frame 165

Z

Zenith point 593
Zinc chloride 131
Zinc oxide eugenol cement 197
Zinc phosphate cement 203
Zinc silico phosphate cements 206
Zirconium dioxide 364
Zirconium silicate 481
Zone of decomposed dentin 75
Zsigmondy–Palmer notation system 7

Reader's Note

Reader's Note

Reader's Note